Core Curriculum
for Oncology
Nursing

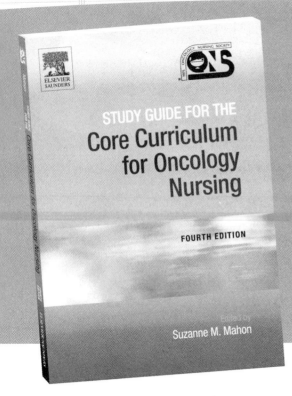

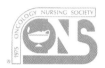

Core Curriculum for Oncology Nursing

FOURTH EDITION

Edited by

JOANNE K. ITANO, RN, PhD, OCN®
Associate Professor of Nursing and
Director, Academic Support Services
University of Hawaii
Honolulu, Hawaii

KAREN N. TAOKA, RN, MN, AOCN®
Nursing Clinical Team Lead, HIS Project
The Queen's Medical Center
Honolulu, Hawaii

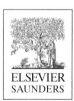

ELSEVIER
SAUNDERS

ELSEVIER
SAUNDERS

11830 Westline Industrial Drive
St. Louis, Missouri 63146

NOTICE

Previous editions copyrighted 1998, 1992, 1987 by Oncology Nursing Society.

Library of Congress Cataloging-in-Publication Data

Itano, Joanne.
Core curriculum for oncology nursing/Joanne K. Itano, Karen N. Taoka. –4th ed.
   p.   cm.
     Includes bibliographical references and index.
     ISBN 0-7216-0357-2
   1. Cancer–Nursing. 2. Cancer. I. Taoka, Karen N. II. Title.

RC266.I87 2005
616.99'40231–dc22   2004062948

Executive Publisher: Barbara Nelson Cullen
Acquisitions Editor: Sandra Clark Brown
Senior Developmental Editor: Cindi Anderson
Publishing Services Manager: Catherine Jackson
Senior Project Manager: Anne Konopka
Designer: Teresa McBryan

Printed in the United States of America.

Last digit is the print number: 9 8 7 6 5 4 3 2 1

Working together to grow
libraries in developing countries

www.elsevier.com | www.bookaid.org | www.sabre.org

ELSEVIER   BOOK AID International   Sabre Foundation

Contributors

PATRICIA AGRE, RN, EdD
Director of Patient/Family Education
Memorial Sloan-Kettering Cancer Center
New York, New York
The Education Process

MARILYNN BERENDT, RN, BSN, EdM
Administrator
Department of Home Health
Children's Memorial Hospital
Chicago, Illinois
Alterations in Nutrition

MARJORIE BERNICE, RN-C, MSN, APRN
Women's Health Care Nurse Practitioner
The Queen Emma Clinics
The Queen's Medical Center
Honolulu, Hawaii
Nursing Care of the Client with Breast Cancer

JEANNINE M. BRANT, RN, MS, AOCN®
Oncology Clinical Nurse Specialist
Pain Consultant
St. Vincent Healthcare
Billings, Montana
Comfort

KATHLEEN A. CALZONE, RN, MSN, APNG
Senior Nurse Specialist (Research)
Center for Cancer Research, Genetics Branch
National Cancer Institute
Bethesda, Maryland
Genetics

DAWN CAMP-SORRELL, MSN, FNP, AOCN®
Oncology Nurse Practitioner
Central Alabama Oncology, LLC
Alabaster, Alabama
Myelosuppression

ELLEN CARR, RN, MSN, AOCN®
Case Manager
Head/Neck Oncology
Rebecca and John Moores Cancer Center
University of California, San Diego
San Diego, California
*Nursing Care of the Client with Head and
    Neck Cancer*
*Nursing Care of the Client with Bone and Soft
    Tissue Cancers*

MARGARET J. CROWLEY, MSEd, RN, OCN®
Clinical Nurse Specialist
Department of Education
Pennsylvania Hospital
Philadelphia, Pennsylvania
Supportive Care: Dying and Death

SHERRI D'AGOSTINO, RN, MSN, CPON
Clinical Manager
Department of Home Health
Children's Memorial Hospital
Chicago, Illinois
Alterations in Nutrition

DENISE MURRAY EDWARDS, CS, ARNP, MA, MEd, MTS
Mental Health Nurse Practitioner
The Center for Health and Well-Being
Iowa Health Systems
West Des Moines, Iowa
*Supportive Care: Nonpharmacologic
    Interventions*

JEAN M. ELLSWORTH-WOLK, RN, MS, AOCN®
Oncology Clinical Nurse Specialist
Lakewood Hospital
Lakewood, Ohio
*Principles of Preparation, Administration, and
    Disposal of Hazardous Drugs*

SUSAN EZZONE, MS, RN, CNP
Nurse Practitioner
Bone & Marrow Transplant Program
Arthur G. James Cancer Hospital and
    Richard Solove Institute
The Ohio State University Medical Center
Columbus, Ohio
Nursing Care of the Client with Leukemia

MARIE FLANNERY, RN, PhD, AOCN®
Senior Nurse Practitioner
James P. Wilmot Cancer Center
Assistant Professor
University of Rochester School of Nursing
Rochester, New York
Nursing Care of the Client with Lung Cancer

BETH A. FREITAS, RN, MN, OCN®
Clinical Nurse Specialist
Pain and Palliative Care Department
The Queen's Medical Center
Honolulu, Hawaii
Coping: Altered Body Image and Alopecia

SUE L. FRYMARK, RN, BS
Executive Director
Cancer Care Resources/Northwest Cancer
 Specialists Foundation
Portland, Oregon
Supportive Care: Rehabilitation and Resources

DANIELLE M. GALE, RN, ND, FNP-CS
Manager—Oncology Clinical Coordinator
 Program
Department of BioOncology
Genentech, Inc.
South San Francisco, California
*Nursing Implications of Biotherapy and
 Molecular Targeted Therapy*

JACQUELINE J. GLOVER, PhD
Associate Professor
Department of Pediatrics
Center for Bioethics and Humanities
School of Medicine
University of Colorado Health Sciences
 Center
Denver, Colorado
Selected Ethical Issues in Cancer Care

BARBARA HOLMES GOBEL, RN, MS, AOCN®
Oncology Clinical Nurse Specialist
Northwestern Memorial Hospital
Chicago, Illinois
Metabolic Emergencies

PATRICIA M. GRIMM, PhD, RN, APRN, BC
Clinical Staff
HopeWELL Cancer Support
Baltimore, Maryland
Coping: Psychosocial Issues

MARY MAGEE GULLATTE, RN, MN, AOCN®, ANP, FAAMA
Director of Nursing
Inpatient Oncology and Transplant Services
Emory University Hospital and
 Crawford Long Hospital
Director, Oncology Data Center
Winship Cancer Institute of Emory University
Adjunct Clinical Faculty
Nell Hodgson Woodruff School of Nursing
Emory University
Atlanta, Georgia
Legal Issues Influencing Cancer Care

JANE C. HUNTER, RN, MN, ANP
Adult Nurse Practitioner
Head and Neck Cancer Program
Carolinas HealthCare System
Charlotte, North Carolina
Structural Emergencies

ROBERT J. IGNOFFO, PharmD, FASHP, FCSHP
Clinical Professor
Department of Clinical Pharmacy
University of California, San Francisco
San Francisco, California
Supportive Care: Pharmacologic Interventions

DIANNE N. ISHIDA, PhD, APRN, CMC
Associate Professor
School of Nursing
University of Hawaii at Manoa
Manoa, Hawaii
Professional Issues in Cancer Care

JOANNE K. ITANO, RN, PhD, OCN®
Associate Professor of Nursing and
 Director, Academic Support Services
University of Hawaii
Honolulu, Hawaii
Coping: Cultural Issues

RYAN R. IWAMOTO, ARNP, MN, AOCN®
Oncology Clinical Coordinator
Genentech BioOncology
Seattle, Washington
*Nursing Care of the Client with Lymphoma or
 Multiple Myeloma*

SHIRLEY J. KERN, RN, MSN, AOCN®, APRN-BC
Oncology Clinical Nurse Specialist
Lung Cancer Program
North Memorial Medical Center
Minneapolis, Minnesota
*Nursing Care of the Client with Cancers of the
 Neurologic System*

LINDA U. KREBS, RN, PhD, AOCN®
Associate Professor
School of Nursing
University of Colorado at Denver and
 Health Sciences Center
Denver, Colorado
Application of the Statement on the Scope
 and Standards of Oncology Nursing
 Practice *and Evidence-Based Practice*

ANNETTE W. KUCK, RN, MS, CS, AOCN®
Nurse Practitioner
Georgia Cancer Specialists
Atlanta, Georgia
Alterations in Elimination

SUSAN LEIGH, BSN, RN
Cancer Survivorship Consultant
Tucson, Arizona
*Coping: Survivorship Issues and Financial
Concerns*

MOLLY LONEY, RN, MSN, AOCN®
Clinical Nurse Specialist
Hillcrest Hospital
The Cleveland Clinic Health System
Cleveland, Ohio
Cancer Economics and Health Care Reform

ALICE J. LONGMAN, RN, EdD, FAAN
Professor Emeritus
The University of Arizona College of Nursing
Tucson, Arizona
Nursing Care of the Client with Skin Cancer

LESLIE V. MATTHEWS, RN, MS, ANP, AOCN®
Nurse Practitioner
Winthrop Oncology/Hematology
Mineola, New York
Alterations in Ventilation

JAN HAWTHORNE MAXSON, RN, MSN, AOCN®
Nurse Practitioner
Division of Gynecologic Oncology
University Hospitals of Cleveland
Cleveland, Ohio
*Principles of Preparation, Administration, and
Disposal of Hazardous Drugs*

MOLLY J. MORAN, MS, APRN, BC
Clinical Nurse Specialist
Department of Oncology Nursing
James Cancer Hospital and Solove Research
Institute
Columbus, Ohio
Nursing Care of the Client with Leukemia

THERESA A. MORAN, RN, MN, FNP
Nurse Practitioner III
Department of Hematology/Oncology
University of California, San Francisco
San Francisco, California
*Nursing Care of the Client with HIV-Related
Cancers*

CANDIS MORRISON, PhD, CRNP
Associate Professor
School of Nursing/Oncology
Johns Hopkins University
Baltimore, Maryland
Early Detection of Cancer

PAULA NELSON-MARTEN, RN, PhD, AOCN®
Associate Professor
School of Nursing
University of Colorado Health Sciences Center
Denver, Colorado
Selected Ethical Issues in Cancer Care

ZOE NGO, PharmD
Oncology Pharmacist
Assistant Clinical Professor
Department of Clinical Pharmacy
UCSF Comprehensive Cancer Center
San Francisco, California
Supportive Care: Pharmacologic Interventions

PATRICIA W. NISHIMOTO, BSN, MPH, DNS
Adult Oncology Clinical Nurse Specialist
Department of Medicine
Tripler Army Medical Center
Honolulu, Hawaii
Sexuality

SHARON J. OLSEN, MS, CS, NP, AOCN®
Assistant Professor
School of Nursing
Johns Hopkins University
Baltimore, Maryland
Doctoral Student
The Catholic University of America
Washington, DC
Epidemiology and Prevention of Cancer

MAUREEN E. O'ROURKE, RN, PhD
Associate Clinical Professor of Nursing
University of North Carolina
Greensboro, North Carolina
Adjunct Assistant Professor of Medicine
Hematology Oncology
Wake Forest University Medical School
Winston-Salem, North Carolina
*Nursing Care of the Client with Cancers of the
Urinary System*

JENNIFER DOUGLAS PEARCE, RN, MSN, CNS
Associate Professor
Department of Nursing
University of Cincinnati
Raymond Walters College
Cincinnati, Ohio
*Alterations in Mobility, Skin Integrity, and
Neurologic Status*

JANIS M. PETREE, RN, MS, FNP
Oncology Nurse Practitioner
Department of Medical Oncology
Stanford University Hospital and Clinics
Stanford, California
*Supportive Care: Support Therapies and
Procedures*

BARBARA C. PONIATOWSKI, MS, RN,C, AOCN®
Senior Clinical Nurse Educator
Oncology Division
GlaxoSmithKline
Philadelphia, Pennsylvania
*Nursing Implications of Antineoplastic
Therapy*

ELISA RICCIARDI, BA, MS
Patient Care Manager
Wound, Ostomy, Continence Nurse
Department of Hematology/Oncology,
Inpatient Unit
Childrens Hospitals and Clinics
Minneapolis, Minnesota
Alterations in Elimination

PAUL JAY ROSS, APRN, MA, MSN, ANP-CS, OCN®
Director, Oncology Services
St. Francis Medical Center
Adjunct Instructor
Department of Anthropology
University of Hawaii
Honolulu, Hawaii
Complementary and Alternative Medicines

KRISTI V. SCHMIDT, MN, RN, AOCN®
Clinical Trainer
Commercial Excellence, Leadership, and
Learning
Genentech
South San Francisco, California
Immunology

TERRY WIKLE SHAPIRO, MSN, CRNP
Nurse Practitioner
Bone Marrow Transplant Program
University of Arizona
Tucson, Arizona
*Nursing Implications of Hematopoietic Stem
Cell Transplantation*

KRISTINE TURNER STORY, RN, MSN, APRN
Nurse Practitioner
Department of Internal Medicine
Physicians Clinic, Internal Medicine Health
West
Omaha, Nebraska
Alterations in Circulation

ROBERTA ANNE STROHL, RN, MN, AOCN®
Senior Training Manager, Oncology
Schering-Plough
Baltimore, Maryland
*Nursing Care of the Client with Cancers of the
Gastrointestinal Tract*

THOMAS J. SZOPA, RN, MS, WOCN
Clinical Nurse Specialist
Oncology and Ostomy/Wound
Management
Elliot Hospital
Manchester, New Hampshire
Nursing Implications of Surgical Treatment

SUSAN VOGT TEMPLE, RN, MSN, ETN, AOCN®
Senior Clinical Educator
GlaxoSmithKline Oncology
Seale, Alabama
*Nursing Care of the Client with Cancers of the
Reproductive System*
*Nursing Implications of Antineoplastic
Therapy*

CYNTHIA H. UMSTEAD, RN, MSN, OCN®
Senior Clinical Educator
GlaxoSmithKline Pharmaceuticals
Philadelphia, Pennsylvania
*Nursing Care of the Client with Cancers of the
Reproductive System*

CAROL S. VIELE, RN, MS
Clinical Nurse Specialist
Department of Hematology-Oncology-Bone
Marrow Transplant
Assistant Clinical Professor
Department of Physiological Nursing
School of Nursing
University of California, San Francisco
San Francisco, California
Supportive Care: Pharmacologic Interventions

DEBORAH L. VOLKER, RN, PhD, AOCN®
Assistant Professor
School of Nursing
The University of Texas at Austin
Austin, Texas
Biology of Cancer and Carcinogenesis

MARY ELLYN WITT, RN, MS, AOCN®
Clinical Research Nurse
Department of Radiation Oncology
University of Chicago Hospital
Chicago, Illinois
Nursing Implications of Radiation Therapy

Reviewers

PATRICIA C. BUCHSEL, RN, MSN, FAAN
Clinical Faculty
University of Washington, School of Nursing
Seattle, Washington

ELAINE S. DEMEYER RN, MSN, AOCN®
Independent Oncology Nurse Consultant
President and CEO, Creative Cancer
    Concepts, Inc.
Rockwall, Texas

PAT GILLETT, RN, MSN, ACNP
Clinical Instructor
College of Nursing
The University of New Mexico
Albuquerque, New Mexico

**JEANNE HELD-WARMKESSEL, MSN, RN, AOCN®,
    APRN, BC**
Clinical Nurse Specialist
Fox Chase Cancer Center
Philadelphia, Pennsylvania

**BERNADETTE M. LOMBARDI, RN, MSN, MA,
    MS, PhD(c)**
Assistant Director
Northeast Health Albany and Samaritan
    Hospitals School of Nursing
Albany, New York

JULIE D. PAINTER, RNC, MSN, OCN®
Clinical Nurse Specialist
Community Health Network
Indianapolis, Indiana

PHYLLIS G. PETERSON, RN, MN, AOCN®
Assistant Professor
Division of Nursing
Our Lady of Holy Cross College
New Orleans, Louisiana

CARMENCITA M. POE, RN, EdD, CD, OCN®, CHPN
Clinical Nurse Manager
Department of Oncology/Medical-Surgical
    Nursing
Bon Secours DePaul Medical Center
Norfolk, Virginia

CHERYL REGGIO, RN, OCN®
Clinical Staff Nurse
Department of Hematology/Oncology
Children's National Medical Center
Silver Spring, Maryland

NOEMI SALCIDO, RN, BSN
El Paso Cancer Treatment Center
El Paso, Texas

PATTI C. SIMMONS, RN, MN
Assistant Professor of Nursing
Department of Nursing
North Georgia College and State University
Dahlonega, Georgia

MIRIAM E. SLEVEN, RN, MS, OCN®
Oncology Nurse Consultant
Clovis, California

SUSAN K. STEELE, DNS, RN, AOCN®
Assistant Professor of Nursing
School of Nursing
Louisiana State University Health Sciences
    Center
New Orleans, Louisiana

SCOTT CARTER THIGPEN, RN, MSN, CCRN, CEN
Assistant Professor of Nursing
Division of Nursing
South Georgia College
Douglas, Georgia

CONSTANCE VISOVSKY PhD, RN, ACNP
Assistant Professor of Nursing
Case Western Reserve University
Cleveland, Ohio

M. LINDA WORKMAN, RN, PhD, FAAN
The Gertrude Perkins Olivia Professor of
    Oncology Nursing
Case Western Reserve University
Cleveland, Ohio

Preface

The fourth edition of the *Core Curriculum for Oncology Nursing* is completely revised, updated, and expanded to reflect the current state of oncology nursing practice. It describes the essential content for the generalist in cancer nursing. It establishes the knowledge base from which nurses at the generalist level support their practice.

This edition is based on the revised OCN® Test Blueprint, making it a powerful study tool for the OCN® certification examination, which is offered by the Oncology Nursing Certification Corporation (ONCC). It presents a comprehensive coverage of the entire scope of the specialty plus new and expanded information on nonpharmacologic interventions and alternative therapies.

The test blueprint directed the organization of the book. As in the third edition, most chapters begin with a theory section that outlines the knowledge necessary to understand a content area and provides the foundation from which the practice of cancer nursing is based. Subsequent sections on assessment, nursing diagnoses, outcome identification, planning and implementation, and evaluation reflect the nursing process and the standards for oncology nursing practice. The outcome identification section provides the benchmarks that may be used to determine the degree of outcome achievement.

The book is a valuable resource for generalist and advanced practice cancer nurses. With its outline format, it is an easy-to-use reference tool when nurses are faced with questions in practice. Many nurses will use this text to prepare education materials. A reference list is provided at the end of each chapter, and many chapters include websites for additional sources of information.

We are excited about the currency and relevancy of the chapters. Contributors brought their expertise to the text, representing the best in cancer nursing from throughout the United States. Reviewers assisted by critically critiquing the chapters. We feel the final product reflects the most current information for the generalist in cancer nursing.

Our mahalo (thank you) to the Oncology Nursing Society (ONS) for providing us with the opportunity to edit this book. It has been our privilege to work with the contributors and reviewers. We have increased our knowledge and have had an enjoyable experience collaborating with our cancer nursing colleagues. Our special thanks to Barbara Sigler of the ONS; Cindi Anderson and Anne Konopka of Elsevier; and our good friend and colleague, Ryan Iwamoto. They all played significant roles in helping us complete this book.

Aloha,
Joanne K. Itano
Karen N. Taoka

Contents

13 Myelosuppression, 259

DAWN CAMP-SORRELL

PART THREE
GASTROINTESTINAL AND URINARY FUNCTION

14 Alterations in Nutrition, 277

MARILYNN BERENDT AND SHERRI D'AGOSTINO

15 Alterations in Elimination, 318

ANNETTE W. KUCK AND ELISA RICCIARDI

PART FOUR
CARDIOPULMONARY FUNCTION

16 Alterations in Ventilation, 347

LESLIE V. MATTHEWS

PART ONE

QUALITY OF LIFE

1 Comfort

JEANNINE M. BRANT

PAIN

Theory

I. Overview.
   A. Definition.
      1. Unpleasant sensory and emotional experience associated with actual or potential tissue damage (Merskey, 1986).
      2. Pain is whatever the person says it is, existing whenever he/she says it does (McCaffery, 1968).
   B. Characteristics of pain.
      1. Acute pain—usually lasts less than 6 months; etiology of the pain is often known; objective pain behaviors are more frequently exhibited.
      2. Chronic nonmalignant pain—usually lasts longer than 3 months; etiology of the pain is often unknown; fatigue and depression are common.
      3. Cancer pain—includes acute cancer-related pain caused by the cancer or cancer therapy and chronic cancer-related pain from tumor progression or cancer therapy; increased pain may precipitate fear of cancer progression; increased pain worsens anxiety, hopelessness, and depression.
   C. Types of pain (McCaffery & Pasero, 1999).
      1. Nociceptive pain—result of activation of nociceptors (pain fibers) in deep and cutaneous tissues.
         a. Somatic pain—arises from the bone, joint, or connective tissue, usually well localized, characterized by an aching or gnawing sensation.
         b. Visceral pain—result of nociceptor activation in thoracic or abdominal tissue; arises from the viscera such as the pancreas, liver, and gastrointestinal (GI) tract; usually poorly localized; characterized by a cramping or aching sensation.
      2. Neuropathic pain—result of compression or injury to peripheral, sympathetic, and/or central nervous system (CNS) (Dworkin, 2002).
         a. Peripheral neuropathic pain—caused by injury and pain along the peripheral nerves, often characterized by a numbness and tingling sensation.
         b. Centrally mediated pain—characterized by radiating and shooting sensations with a background of burning and aching.
         c. Sympathetically maintained pain—centrally generated, caused by autonomic dysregulation, referred to as complex regional pain syndrome (CRPS).
II. Physiology (McCaffery & Pasero, 1999) (Figure 1-1).
   A. Transduction.
      1. Initiated by a mechanical, thermal, or chemical noxious stimulus at the periphery that sensitizes nociceptors (receptors sensitive to noxious stimuli).

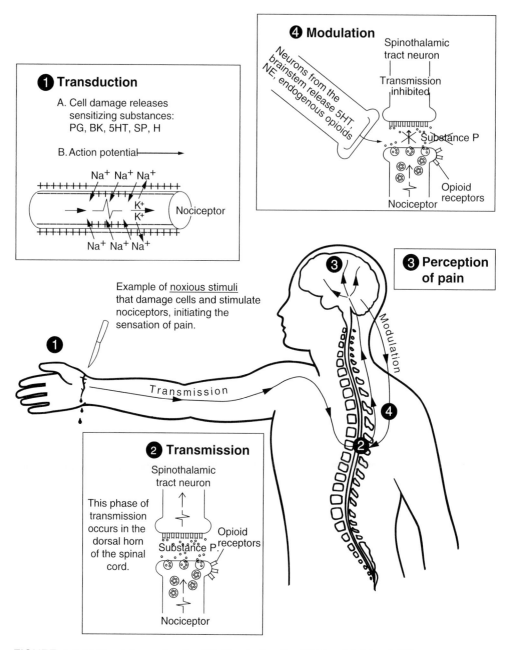

FIGURE 1-1 ■ Physiology of pain. *PG,* Prostaglandin; *BK,* bradykinin; *5-HT,* serotonin; *SP,* substance P; *H,* histamine; *NE,* norepinephrine (From McCaffery M, Pasero C: *Pain: clinical manual,* ed 2, St Louis, 1999, Mosby.)

2. Neurotransmitters are released at the time of injury: prostaglandins (PG), bradykinin (BK), serotonin (5-HT), substance P (SP), histamine (H).
3. An action potential is generated along the neuron when sodium moves into the cell and potassium out of the cell, and the pain message begins its way to the CNS.

B. Transmission.
  1. Action potential continues to the dorsal horn, where nociceptors terminate.
  2. Some neurons continue the message to the thalamus, and others carry the message to various centers in the brain.
  3. The thalamus transmits the message to the cerebral cortex.
C. Perception—the cerebral cortex processes the experience of pain.
D. Modulation.
  1. Descending neurons originating in the brainstem travel to the dorsal horn and release neuromediators—endogenous opioids, norepinephrine, serotonin.
  2. The neuromediators inhibit nociception at the dorsal horn.
III. Risk factors.
  A. Disease-related factors.
    1. Bone metastases are the most common source of cancer pain.
      a. Breast, prostate, and lung cancer and multiple myeloma have the greatest incidence of bone metastases.
      b. Bone destruction or compression of the bone on nerves and soft tissue.
    2. Abdominal visceral pain—may be caused by tumor obstruction of the bowel, liver metastasis, blood flow occlusion to visceral organs, and other causes.
    3. Nerve compression or injury to peripheral, sympathetic, and/or central nerves.
      a. Spinal cord compression.
      b. Plexopathies—pain is often a first sign followed by extremity weakness and sensory loss.
      c. Peripheral neuropathies—characterized by painful numbness, tingling, weakness, sensory loss.
  B. Treatment-related factors.
    1. Chemotherapy-related pain.
      a. Mucositis.
      b. Peripheral neuropathies.
        (1) Vinca alkaloids, cisplatin, taxanes, and thalidomide have the highest incidence (Brown et al., 2001; Nielsen & Brant, 2002).
        (2) Characterized by burning and numbness on the hands and feet.
      c. Herpetic neuralgia—often occurs from the immunosuppression of chemotherapy; characterized by burning, aching, and shocklike pain in the area of the lesions.
    2. Radiation therapy–related pain (Shih et al, 2002).
      a. Mucositis often occurs with radiation therapy to the head and neck.
      b. Radiation may induce peripheral nerve tumors characterized by a painful, enlarging mass in a previously irradiated area.
      c. Radiation skin changes—radiation enhancement and radiation recall.
    3. Chronic pain related to cancer surgery (Jacox, 1994).
      a. Postmastectomy—characterized by tightness in the axilla, medial upper arm, and/or chest; often exacerbated with movement, extending, reaching, lifting, pulling, and pushing.
      b. Postthoracotomy—characterized by aching, sensory loss characterized by numbness and/or burning in the incisional area.
      c. Postradical neck dissection—characterized by tightness, burning, shocklike pain.

      d. Postnephrectomy—characterized by flank, groin, or abdominal heaviness or numbness.

      e. Postlimb amputation—characterized by phantom or stump pain; may be neuropathic in nature.

C. Personal and psychosocial factors.

    1. Client-related fears.

      a. Reluctance to take opioid drugs for fear and misunderstanding of "analgesic tolerance" and "addiction."

      b. Fear that pain may be a sign of progressive disease; denial prevents client from taking adequate analgesia.

      c. Do not want to burden the health care provider—desire to be a "good patient."

    2. Provider-related factors.

      a. Misunderstanding of "addiction" (psychologic dependence), "analgesic tolerance," "physical dependence."

      b. Reluctance to prescribe—fear of discrimination by opioid regulatory agencies.

      c. Inadequate pain management curricula in nursing and medical schools.

    3. Age—elderly are at higher risk for chronic pain and inadequate pain management (O'Leary, 2002).

    4. Culture—influences the perceptions and expression of pain.

Assessment (American Pain Society, 2003; Jacox, 1994)

I. Special populations.

  A. Elderly population.

    1. Obtain a comprehensive medication history because many elderly clients are taking numerous medications.

    2. Start with lower doses, and titrate up slowly because advanced age results in a prolonged half-life and metabolism of the drug.

    3. Consider presence of confusion and poor vision, availability of home supervision, and cost when planning analgesics for the elderly; FLACC (face, legs, activity, cry, consolability) scale may be used for clients who cannot communicate.

  B. Pediatric population.

    1. Developmental age provides the basis for pain assessment.

    2. Pain scales

      a. Pain faces are usually used in children ages 7 years and younger.

      b. The "0 to 10" scale is sometimes used for school-aged and older children.

      c. The FLACC behavioral pain assessment scale for children who cannot verbalize pain is also used.

    3. Starting dosage should be calculated according to weight; infants less than 6 months old are at risk for apnea when taking opioids.

II. Clinical pain assessment (Figure 1-2).

  A. Location, intensity, quality, temporality (Table 1-1).

  B. Affective or emotional dimension—how pain affects the client's affect (i.e., depression, anxiety, hopelessness, fear).

  C. Behavioral dimension—how pain prevents specific behaviors (i.e., mobility); how the client uses self-care behaviors to relieve pain.

Pain Assessment Tool

Date _____

Patient's Name _____ Age _____ Room _____

Diagnosis _____ Physician _____

                                              Nurse _____

1. LOCATION: Patient or nurse marks drawing.

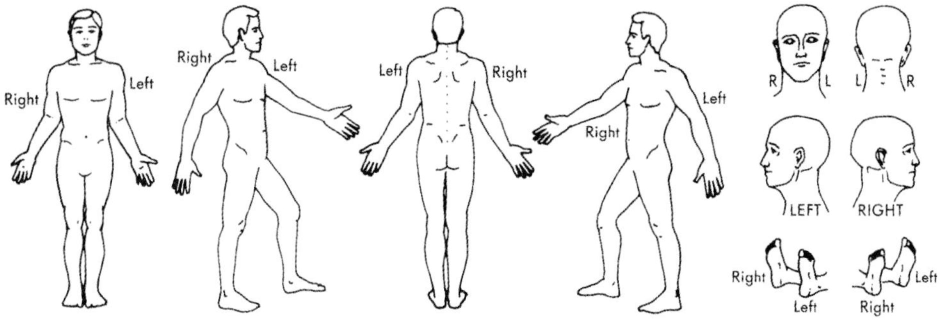

2. INTENSITY: Patient rates the pain. Scale used _____

   Present: _____
   Worst pain gets: _____
   Best pain gets: _____
   Acceptable level of pain: _____

3. QUALITY: (Use patient's own words, e.g., prick, ache, burn, throb, pull, sharp) _____
   _____

4. ONSET, DURATION, VARIATIONS, RHYTHMS: _____
   _____

5. MANNER OF EXPRESSING PAIN: _____
   _____

6. WHAT RELIEVES THE PAIN? _____
   _____

7. WHAT CAUSES OR INCREASES THE PAIN? _____
   _____

8. EFFECTS OF PAIN: (Note decreased function, decreased quality of life.)
   Accompanying symptoms (e.g., nausea) _____
   Sleep _____
   Appetite _____
   Physical activity _____
   Relationship with others (e.g., irritability) _____
   Emotions (e.g., anger, suicidal, crying) _____
   Concentration _____
   Other _____

9. OTHER COMMENTS: _____
   _____

10. PLAN: _____
    _____

FIGURE 1-2 ■ Initial pain assessment tool. (From McCaffery M, Pasero C: *Pain: clinical manual,* ed 2, St Louis, 1999, Mosby.)

TABLE 1-1
Pain Assessment Parameters

Pain Assessment Component	Description	Clinical Usefulness
Location	Client points to the exact location of pain or draws pain location on a body diagram	Useful to assess multiple pain syndromes, exact locations of pain, and focal vs. referred patterns
Intensity	Client rates individual pain intensity using a 0-10 scale with 0 being no pain and 10 being the worst possible pain; mild— moderate—severe or other simple descriptive scale may be used if the patient cannot conceptualize the 0-10 scale	Allows caregivers the ability to objectively determine the amount of pain and to assess effectiveness of the current medication regimen
Quality	Client describes how the pain feels (i.e., constant, dull, aching, burning, radiating)	Provides the clinician with information to diagnose and manage specific pain syndromes
Temporality	Client describes how the pain changes over time, including the onset, duration, exacerbating and relieving factors	Provides data on the nature of the pain that can be used in the pain management plan of care (i.e., patients with constant pain should receive long-acting analgesics)

Modified from Brant J, Brumit J, Forseth J: *Pain and symptom management in the terminally ill*, Billings, Mont, 1996, Big Sky Hospice.

   D. Cognitive and mental dimension—what pain means to the client, how medications affect cognitive functioning (i.e., inability to concentrate, disorientation).
   E. Social evaluation—how pain affects finances, roles, family dynamics.
III. History and physical examination.
   A. Evaluation of computerized transaxial tomography (CT), magnetic resonance imaging (MRI), tumor markers.
   B. Physical and neurologic examination—assess pain behaviors, changes in muscle tone, vital signs.
   C. Assess for alterations in the following systems:
      1. Respiratory status—decreased rate and ventilatory volume, increased CO_2 levels.
      2. CNS changes—sedation, euphoria, coordination, mood.
      3. Cardiovascular system—hypotension.
      4. GI system—constipation, inability to evacuate stool, nausea.
      5. Genitourinary system—urinary retention, difficult urination.
      6. Dermatologic system—cutaneous reactions, diaphoresis, facial flushing, pruritus.
IV. Evaluation and reassessment of pain (Jacox , 1994).
   A. Pain should be assessed in each client with cancer on admission to the hospital or during each home or outpatient clinic visit.

B. Pain should be assessed with each new report or increase in pain.
C. Pain should be reassessed after appropriate intervals following pain interventions (e.g., evaluation of an oral medication should be approximately 1 hour after administration).
D. Consider assessing pain as the fifth vital sign.

Nursing Diagnoses

I. Acute or chronic pain.
II. Deficient knowledge of effective pain management strategies.
III. Impaired physical mobility.
IV. Disturbed sleep pattern or sleep deprivation.

Outcome Identification

I. Client states that the pain is reduced or relieved to his/her satisfaction.
   A. Client recognizes importance of preventing and controlling pain.
   B. Client communicates pain intensity and temporality using standardized measures.
II. Client uses appropriate pharmacologic and complementary interventions to control pain.
III. Client participates in the usual daily lifestyle with appropriate modifications, as needed.
IV. Client reports adequate amounts of sleep and feeling rested.

Planning and Implementation

I. Pharmacologic and nonpharmacologic management.
   A. Treat underlying cause of pain.
   B. Plan the pain management care according to the client's individualized pain assessment (Brant, 2002; Lucas & Lipman, 2002; Mercadante, 2001).
      1. Administer long-acting analgesics around the clock for pain that is constant.
      2. Distinguish and manage breakthrough pain (McMillan, 2001).
         a. Breakthrough pain—a flare in the pain pattern that occurs in conjunction with persistent pain.
            (1) Oral opioids: administer 5% to 20% of the 24-hour dose as needed.
            (2) Parenteral opioids: administer 25% to 50% of the hourly infusion rate; may be higher for incident pain that is predominant.
         b. Incident pain—transient pain precipitated by any movement or activity.
            (1) Administer analgesics at appropriate intervals to allow analgesics to work before anticipated pain-inducing activities (incident pain).
            (2) Use breakthrough analgesics with a fast onset; consider transmucosal fentanyl, immediate-release opioids, or subcutaneous/intravenous (IV) patient-controlled analgesia.
         c. End-of-dose pain—pain that increases before the next scheduled dose.
      3. Use equianalgesic conversion tables as a guide to convert one opioid to another.
      4. Begin with least invasive route of administration (oral preferred, transdermal, rectal); change routes if intolerable side effects or intractable pain occurs despite escalating doses.

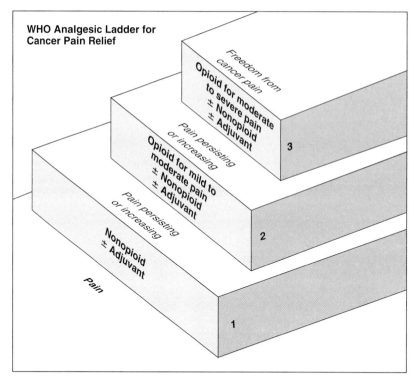

WHO Analgesic Ladder for Cancer Pain Relief

Freedom from cancer pain

Opioid for moderate to severe pain
± Nonopioid
± Adjuvant

3

Pain persisting or increasing

Opioid for mild to moderate pain
± Nonopioid
± Adjuvant

2

Pain persisting or increasing

Nonopioid
± Adjuvant

1

Pain

FIGURE 1-3 ■ The WHO three-step analgesic ladder. (Reproduced by permission of WHO. From *Cancer pain relief,* ed 2, Geneva, 1996, World Health Organization.)

     5. Implement strategies to minimize side effects of analgesic therapy: stool softener with bowel stimulant, antiemetics, H_2 antagonists, CNS stimulants.
  C. Pharmacologic pain management—use the World Health Organization (WHO) analgesic ladder to manage pain (Figure 1-3) (American Pain Society, 2003; Jacox, 1994).
    1. Step 1—nonopioid analgesics.
      a. Use for mild pain or as adjuvants with opioid medications.
      b. Examples: acetaminophen (Tylenol), acetylsalicylic acid (aspirin and ASA), nonsteroidal antiinflammatory drugs (NSAIDs).
    2. Step 2—opioid analgesics.
      a. Use opioids for mild to moderate pain or if pain persists or increases from step 1 of the WHO ladder.
      b. Examples: hydrocodone and oxycodone in fixed combinations with acetaminophen or aspirin.
      c. Opioids with acetaminophen combinations have a ceiling dose; acetaminophen should not exceed 4000 mg in 24 hours.
      d. Avoid propoxyphene (Darvon); the metabolite norpropoxyphene may accumulate and cause CNS toxicity.
      e. Agonist-antagonists (pentazocine [Talwin], nalbuphine [Nubain], butorphanol [Stadol]) are not recommended for cancer pain management.
    3. Step 3—opioid analgesics.
      a. For severe pain or if pain persists or increases from step 2 of the ladder.

    b. Examples: morphine, oxycodone (OxyContin), hydromorphone (Dilaudid), fentanyl (Duragesic), levorphanol (Levo-Dromoran).

    c. Used most commonly for cancer pain management.

    d. Avoid meperidine (Demerol) for cancer pain management; the metabolite normeperidine may accumulate and cause CNS toxicity.

  4. Analgesic adjuvant: use on each step of the WHO ladder to enhance analgesia, relieve concurrent symptoms that exacerbate pain, and/or relieve side effects associated with opioid drugs (Table 1-2).

TABLE 1-2
Analgesic Adjuvants

Drug Classifications	Indications	Side Effects
Acetaminophen (Tylenol)	Mild to moderate pain, fever	Hepatotoxicity, increased risk with alcohol consumption. Maximum recommended dose is 4000 mg/day
α_2-Agonist: clonidine hydrochloride (Catapres)	Epidural analgesia for neuropathic pain, postsurgical pain	Hypotension, bradycardia, central nervous system depression, dry mouth
Antiarrhythmic: mexiletine (Mexitil)	Neuropathic pain	Hypotension, bradycardia, ataxia, tremors, arrhythmias
CNS STIMULANTS Dextroamphetamine (Dexedrine) Methylphenidate (Ritalin)	Counteract psychomotor retardation, reduce sedation side effects of opioids	Nervousness, sleep disorder, hypertension, palpitations, anxiety
ANTICONVULSANTS Gabapentin (Neurontin) Phenytoin (Dilantin) Carbamazepine (Tegretol) Lamotrigine (Lamictal) Topiramate (Topamax) Divalproex sodium (Depakote)	Neuropathic pain, trigeminal neuralgia, postherpetic neuralgia, brachial and lumbosacral plexopathies, chemoimmunotherapy-related neuropathies	Sedation, bone marrow depression, nausea, rash, confusion, drowsiness, ataxia
ANTIDEPRESSANTS Amitriptyline (Elavil) Desipramine (Norpramin) Nortriptyline (Pamelor) Venlafaxine (Effexor)	Neuropathic pain, postherpetic neuralgia, postsurgical neuropathies, chemoimmunotherapy-related neuropathies	Dry mouth, sedation, constipation, agitation, delirium, tachycardia, orthostatic hypotension, worsening of cardiac conduction abnormalities
ANTIHISTAMINES Hydroxyzine (Vistaril, Atarax) Diphenhydramine (Benadryl) Orphenadrine (Norflex)	Uses include pruritic pain, musculoskeletal pain, anxiety, nausea associated with pain Hydroxyzine: use oral route	Dry mouth, sedation, dizziness, blurred vision, tachycardia

(Continued)

TABLE 1-2
Analgesic Adjuvants—cont'd

Drug Classifications	Indications	Side Effects
ANTISPASMODICS Belladonna and opium supprettes Scopolamine (Transderm-Scop, Isopto-Hyoscine) Dicyclomine (Bentyl)	GI spasm, bladder spasm	Dry mouth, sedation, constipation, tachycardia, urinary retention
ANTISPASTIC AGENT Baclofen (Lioresal)	Spastic pain, centrally mediated pain from spinal lesions	Drowsiness, slurred speech, hypotension, constipation, urinary retention
BENZODIAZEPINES Alprazolam (Xanax) Clonazepam (Klonopin) Diazepam (Valium) Lorazepam (Ativan) Midazolam hydrochloride (Versed)	Anxiety associated with pain, panic attack, muscle spasm, procedure-related pain	Sedation, dementia, delirium, motor incoordination, hypotension, dizziness, respiratory depression
CORTICOSTEROIDS Betamethasone (Celestone) Dexamethasone (Decadron) Prednisone (Deltasone, Orasone) Methylprednisolone (Solu-Medrol)	Nerve compression (brachial and lumbosacral plexopathies), lymphedema and visceral distention, increased intracranial pressure	Gastritis, fluid retention, insomnia, hypertension, hyperglycemia, psychosis, euphoria, increased appetite, candidiasis
LOCAL ANESTHETICS Lidocaine intravenous infusion, hydrochloride jelly (Anestacon), or patch 5% (Lidoderm) EMLA cream	Lidocaine for postherpetic neuralgia, peripheral neuropathy, postsurgical neuropathies EMLA cream for topical dermal anesthesia	Lidocaine patch may cause a mild rash at the application site
MUSCLE RELAXANTS Methocarbamol (Robaxin) Carisoprodol (Soma) Tizanidine (Zanaflex)	Should be used short term for musculoskeletal pain, tetanus Tizanidine may be used for longer periods of time	Sedation, light-headedness, blurred vision, hypotension, akathisia
***N*-METHYL-D-ASPARTATE (NMDA) ANTAGONISTS** Dextromethorphan with morphine (Morphidex) Ketamine	Neuropathic pain, synergistic with opioids, may be helpful in preventing tolerance to opioids Note: methadone also has NMDA activity	Psychotomimetic side effects, hallucinations, drowsiness, dizziness

TABLE 1-2
Analgesic Adjuvants—cont'd

Drug Classifications	Indications	Side Effects
NSAIDs COX-2 INHIBITORS Celecoxib (Celebrex) Rofecoxib (Vioxx) Valdecoxib (Bextra) COX-1 INHIBITORS Ibuprofen (Advil, Motrin, Nuprin) Indomethacin (Indocin) Ketorolac (Toradol) Flurbiprofen (Ansaid) Diflunisal (Dolobid) Naproxen (Naprosyn, Aleve, Anaprox) Choline magnesium trisalicylate (Trilisate) Sulindac (Clinoril)	Bone metastases, soft tissue infiltration, tumor, fever, inflammation	COX-1 inhibitors may cause inhibition of platelet aggregation, gastric ulceration, renal toxicity. COX-2 NSAIDs are more selective and cause fewer side effects

Data from American Pain Society: *Principles of analgesic use in the treatment of acute pain and cancer pain*, ed 5, Glenview, Ill, 2003, American Pain Society; Goldstein F: Adjuncts to opioid therapy, *J Am Osteopath Assoc* 102: S15-S21, 2002; Lucas L, Lipman AG: Recent advances in pharmacotherapy for cancer pain management, *Cancer Pract* 10:S14-S20, 2002.
CNS, Central nervous system; *GI*, gastrointestinal; *NSAIDs*, nonsteroidal antiinflammatory drugs.

5. Miscellaneous interventions.
   a. Pharmaceuticals for bone metastases.
      (1) Strontium 89 for pain relief in disseminated metastatic bone cancer.
      (2) Bisphosphonates (e.g., pamidronate [Aredia], zoledronic acid [Zometa]) for relief of pain in osteolytic bone metastases (Body & Mancini, 2002).
6. Intraspinal analgesia (Bennet et al., 2000a, 2000b).
   a. Epidural—percutaneous catheters.
   b. Intrathecal—percutaneous catheters, implantable pumps, or Ommaya reservoir.
7. Radiation therapy may alleviate painful bone metastases and large bulky tumors (Saarto et al., 2002).
8. Surgical interventions (Cullinane & Chu, 2002).
   a. Peripheral nervous system blocks—destruction of peripheral nerves; example: chest wall pain.
   b. Autonomic celiac plexus block—for pain with pancreatic cancer; relief reported at greater than 80%.
   c. Dorsal rhizotomy—ablation of sensory nerve root fibers; examples: lung, head and neck cancer pain; visceral pain.
   d. Anterolateral cordotomy—ablation of pain-conductive tracts involving sensory and thermal fibers; examples: visceral, somatic, unilateral pain.

        e. Commissural myelotomy—ablation of a polysynaptic pain pathway involving sensory and thermal fibers; examples: midline pelvic and perineal pain.

        f. Sympathectomy—interruption or partial removal of the sympathetic nervous system; example: visceral pain.

   D. Nonpharmacologic interventions.

      1. Transcutaneous electrical nerve stimulation (TENS).

      2. Occupational and physical therapy, cancer rehabilitation, acupuncture.

      3. Complementary therapies—distraction, music, guided imagery, hypnosis, massage.

II. Measures to increase comfort and client and family knowledge.

   A. Educate clients and families about strategies to prevent and manage of pain (Sutton et al., 2002).

      1. Discuss a positive philosophy of pain management with the client and family and the importance of good pain management in attaining optimal quality of life.

      2. Educate clients and families regarding the use of standardized pain rating scales to communicate pain and the responsiveness to interventions (see Figure 1-2).

      3. Encourage the client to take analgesics early in the pain experience to avoid severe pain.

      4. Begin a bowel regimen on initiation of opioid analgesics; include a stool softener and bowel stimulant.

      5. Educate the client and family about state-of-the-art technology available to control pain: nonopioids, opioids, adjuvant analgesics, other modalities.

      6. Collaborate with family leaders, minister, spiritual leader, or healer as appropriate.

   B. Differentiate among analgesic tolerance, physical dependence, addiction, and other pain terms (Federation of State Medical Boards, 1998; McCaffery & Pasero, 1999).

      1. Analgesic tolerance—a physiologic phenomenon, the need to increase the dose of opioid to achieve the same level of analgesia.

      2. Physical dependence—a physiologic state of neuroadaptation that is characterized by the emergence of a withdrawal syndrome if drug use is stopped or decreased abruptly or if an antagonist is administered.

      3. Addiction—a neurobehavioral syndrome with genetic and environmental influences that results in psychologic dependence on the use of substances for their psychic effects and is characterized by compulsive use despite harm.

   C. Monitor the client for safety.

      1. Monitor for side effects of opioid therapy including respiratory depression.

      2. Educate clients who are at high risk for spinal cord compression to notify the health care team if signs of impending compression occur.

III. Measures to facilitate coping.

   A. Manage psychologic distress that can exacerbate pain (Sutton et al., 2002).

   B. Use complementary therapies to augment optimal pain management.

      1. Use adjunct therapies such as bubbles, pop-up books, magic gloves, and puppets to decrease pain perception in the pediatric population.

      2. Provide information about additional complementary therapies including relaxation, massage, hypnosis, guided imagery, and deep breathing as appropriate (Smith et al., 2002).

    C. Incorporate self-care behaviors and cultural and spiritual preferences into the plan of care.

Evaluation

The oncology nurse systematically and regularly evaluates the client's and/or family's responses to interventions to determine progress toward the achievement of expected outcomes. Relevant data are collected, and actual findings are compared with expected findings. Nursing diagnoses, outcomes, and plans of care are reviewed and revised as necessary.

FATIGUE

Theory

  I. Definition—"self-recognized state in which an individual experiences an overwhelming sustained sense of exhaustion and decreased capacity for physical and mental work that is not relieved by rest" (Carpenito, 1995, p. 379).
  II. Physiology
    A. The physiology of cancer-related fatigue is unclear—may result from endogenous cytokines that act on tumor growth factors and cause fatigue-related conditions: cachexia, anemia, infection, depression (Barnes & Bruera, 2002).
    B. Anemia-related fatigue—caused by a decrease in the hemoglobin and hematocrit level that causes fatigue and shortness of breath (see Chapter 17).
    C. Anemia and fatigue may impact cognitive functioning; erythropoietin crosses the blood-brain barrier and serves as a neuroprotector; lack of erythropoietin may contribute to cognitive impairment; erythropoietic agents may provide positive cognitive effects (Brines et al., 2000; O'Shaughnessy et al., 2002).
  III. Risk factors (Sobrero et al., 2001).
    A. Disease-related factors.
      1. Most frequently experienced symptom of cancer.
      2. Precede and accompany most malignancies; dependent on stage and duration of illness.
      3. Electrolyte imbalance, dehydration, pain, and other deleterious symptoms.
    B. Treatment-related factors.
      1. Chemotherapy (Brown et al., 2001).
        a. Fatigue is most common side effect of chemotherapy.
        b. Fatigue generally peaks 3 to 4 days following the nadir and can occur with each cycle.
      2. Immunotherapy.
        a. Common side effect of interferon, interleukin-2, thalidomide (Thalomid), monoclonal antibodies.
        b. Rare reports of fatigue with hematopoietic growth factors, such as granulocyte-macrophage colony-stimulating factor.
      3. Radiation therapy—fatigue affects almost 100% of clients and is cumulative over the course of treatment; onset at approximately 2 weeks and peaks at 6 weeks.
      4. Surgery.
        a. Altered cardiovascular function, nutritional status, and neuromuscular function contribute to postoperative fatigue.

       b. Fear, anticipation of surgery, and surgical outcomes contribute to pre-operative and postoperative fatigue.

    5. Medications—opioids, hypnotics, anxiolytics, antihistamines, antiemetics.

  C. Lifestyle related.

    1. Stress, anxiety, depression, insomnia (Redeker et al., 2000).

    2. Employment and financial difficulty, often related to the cancer diagnosis.

    3. Inactivity and sedentary lifestyle.

Assessment

  I. Clinical fatigue assessment (Lee, 2001).

    A. Temporal assessment—assess for various patterns of fatigue, including circadian pattern, timing, onset, duration.

    B. Perception of fatigue.

      1. Assess the client's individual symptoms and the impact on activities of daily living (ADLs)—bathing, hygiene, shopping, cooking.

      2. Degree of unpleasantness—impact on mood, depression, social isolation, motivation.

      3. Impact of fatigue on quality of life (QOL)—management of fatigue and anemia symptoms found to markedly enhance QOL (Demetri, 2001; Demetri et al., 1998).

    C. Cognitive and mental dimension assessment—assess impact on concentration, memory, alertness.

    D. Methods of assessment.

      1. Client's self-report.

      2. Symptom distress scales with descriptors—mild, moderate, severe; use of "0 to 10" scale; encourage fatigue as the sixth vital sign.

      3. Depression scales.

      4. Performance scales, ADL and functional scales.

      5. Neurocognitive screening—recall of words, orientation (name, date, place, time), attention (count backward by threes), memory (repeat words given in recall).

    E. Fatigue assessment tools available.

      1. Functional Assessment of Cancer Therapy Fatigue (Cella, 1997).

      2. Piper Fatigue Scale (Piper et al., 1998).

      3. Schwartz Cancer Fatigue Scale (Schwartz, 1998).

 II. History and physical examination.

    A. Potential physical examination findings.

      1. General appearance is overall tiredness.

      2. Review radiology scan data for progressive disease.

      3. Surface electromyogram (EMG) results may be abnormal.

      4. Increased melatonin, a sign of insomnia.

    B. Potential laboratory findings (Holzner et al., 2002).

      1. Decreased red blood cell (RBC), hemoglobin, hematocrit levels.

      2. Decreased O_2 or increased CO_2 on the arterial blood gas report.

      3. Hypoglycemia, hyponatremia, hypercalcemia, hypothyroidism.

Nursing Diagnoses

  I. Activity intolerance.

 II. Fatigue.

III. Deficient knowledge of effective fatigue management strategies.

Outcome Identification

I. Client performs ADLs and participates in desired activities at his/her level of ability or adapts to decreased energy levels.

II. Client recognizes fatigue as a manifestation of cancer and a side effect of cancer treatment.

    A. Client copes with fatigue using individual and community support resources.

III. Client describes self-care measures for the management of fatigue.

Planning and Implementation

I. Pharmacologic and nonpharmacologic management.

    A. Treatment of the malignancy or the underlying cause.

    B. RBC growth factors to manage anemia.

        1. Recombinant human erythropoietin (rHuEPO) (Epogen, Procrit).

            a. Stimulates the production of RBCs in the bone marrow.

            b. Starting dose 150 units/kg subcutaneously three times per week or 40,000 units/wk; may be titrated to 60,000 units/wk (Gabrilove et al., 2001).

        2. Darbepoetin alfa (Aranesp).

            a. Prolonged serum half-life, approximately 40 hours, allows less frequent dosing.

            b. Dosing is variable; 200 mcg often used every 2 weeks and titrated to 300 mcg if response is a rise in hemoglobin (Hgb) of less than 1 g (Glaspy et al., 2002).

    C. Psychostimulants (caffeine, pemoline [Cylert], methylphenidate [Ritalin], modafinil (Provigil), dextroamphetamine [Dexedrine]) being tested to determine their effectiveness in the management of fatigue (Nail, 2002).

    D. Vitamins and herbs commonly used for fatigue include iron, folate, B-complex vitamins, ginseng, vitamin C, flaxseed oil, magnesium, amino acid complex, others.

    E. RBC transfusions.

    F. Nonpharmacologic management (Nail, 2002).

        1. Oxygen therapy.

        2. Adequate nutrition and rest.

        3. Exercise balanced with energy conservation.

        4. Psychosocial support.

II. Measures to increase knowledge of client and family.

    A. Discuss the potential for fatigue at the time of diagnosis and at treatment initiation.

    B. Inform the client and family of therapies known to cause fatigue.

    C. Provide information about medical interventions used to treat fatigue-related anemia that interferes with ventilation, including erythropoietin, RBC administration, and oxygen therapy.

    D. Educate the client and family about the management of fatigue.

        1. Energy conservation—assist the client in prioritizing needs, planning, using proper body mechanics, pacing the daily schedule, and modifying plans if needed.

        2. Exercise—maintain adequate activity to increase energy stores.

        3. Nutrition—maintain adequate nutrition to promote ideal weight and body energy.

       4. Restoration of attention—reduce environmental demands (information, stimuli, distractions) to conserve attention for priority needs.

       5. Sleep and rest—maintain adequate sleep and rest.

III. Measures to facilitate client and family coping.

    A. Encourage the client and family to discuss fatigue and its impact on ADLs.

    B. Consult with psychosocial services when fatigue may be related to psychologic and social factors, such as depression, stress, or difficulty coping with the disease.

    C. Administer medical interventions in a timely and appropriate manner.

    D. Acknowledge the potential for fatigue to interfere with sexuality.

Evaluation

The oncology nurse systematically and regularly evaluates the client's and/or family's responses to interventions to determine progress toward the achievement of expected outcomes. Relevant data are collected, and actual findings are compared with expected findings. Nursing diagnoses, outcomes, and plans of care are reviewed and revised as necessary.

PRURITUS

Theory

  I. Definition—itching.

 II. Physiology (Krajnik & Zylicz, 2001; Lidstone & Thorns, 2001).

    A. Mediators.

       1. Histamine is released from mast cells and acts on H_1 receptors on C-fibers.

       2. Prostaglandins E_2 and H_2 potentiate pruritus.

       3. Substance P is synthesized in C-fibers and mediates pruritus.

       4. Opioids mediate pruritus along the afferent pathway.

    B. Neural pathways.

       1. The physiology of pruritus is closely linked to the physiology of pain.

       2. Polymodal C-nociceptors are the neurons responsible for itch; they include 20% of the C-fiber population.

       3. C-fibers are sensitive to histamine.

       4. Impulse travels from the C-fibers to the ipsilateral dorsal root ganglia to the opposite anterolateral spinothalamic tract to the posterolateral ventral thalamic nucleus and ends at the cortex.

       5. The stimuli can originate anywhere along the afferent pathway.

III. Risk factors (Table 1-3).

Assessment

  I. Clinical assessment (Lidstone & Thorns, 2001).

    A. Review medication history and potential allergies.

    B. Presence of underlying disease.

    C. Temporal patterns.

       1. Patterns of pruritus including circadian occurrence (pruritus typically increases at night), timing, onset, duration.

TABLE 1-3
Risk Factors of Pruritus

Client- or Disease-Related Factors	Treatment-Related Factors	Lifestyle-Related Factors
CANCER RELATED	**CHEMOTHERAPY**	**PSYCHOLOGIC**
Hematologic malignancies: Hodgkin's lymphoma (30%), non-Hodgkin's lymphoma, leukemia, multiple myeloma	L-asparaginase, cisplatin, cytarabine	Stress, anxiety, depression, boredom, psychoses
Solid tumors: lung, colon, breast, stomach	Allergic reaction and related pruritus may occur with any agent	**ENVIRONMENTAL**
Melanoma		Dry atmospheric conditions
Anal and vulvar tumors (local itch)	**RADIATION THERAPY**	Dehydration
Prostate cancer (perineal and scrotal itch)	Skin reactions and pruritus are most common when the radiation dosage is >20 Gy	Clothing and laundering practices (chemical allergy)
Gliomas (face or nostril itch)		Overheating
Age: itch is experienced by 50%-70% of patients over 70 yr	**IMMUNOTHERAPY**	
Infection	**SURGERY**	
	Postsurgical wound healing	
OTHER DISEASES	**MEDICATIONS**	
Iron deficiency	Opioids, aspirin, erythromycin, hormonal therapy, phenothiazines	
Cholestasis		
Polycythemia vera (30%-50%)		
Renal and hepatic disease		
Mycosis fungoides		
Thyroid dysfunction (Graves' disease or hypothyroidism)		
Diabetes (peripheral neuropathy)		

Data from Krajnik M, Zylicz Z: Pruritus in advanced internal diseases: pathogenesis and treatment, *Neth J Med* 58:27-40, 2001; Lidstone V, Thorns A: Pruritus in cancer patients, *Cancer Treat Rev* 27:305-312, 2001.

   2. Aggravating and alleviating factors.
   3. Impact of pruritus on daily activities.
   4. Methods of assessment.
      a. Client's self-report.
      b. Adjective lists describing pruritus: constant, intermittent, transient, burning, numbness.
II. History and physical examination (Bleiker & Graham-Brown, 2000; Krajnik & Zylicz, 2001).
   A. Potential laboratory findings.
      1. Complete blood count—elevated white blood cell (WBC) count, anemia, eosinophilia, polycythemia.
      2. Blood chemistries—hyperglycemia, hyperuricemia, elevated blood urea nitrogen (BUN) or creatinine levels, abnormal liver function test results.

3. Thyroid function tests—hypoactive or hyperactive thyroid.
4. Other—low ferritin level, increased sedimentation rate.
5. Urinalysis—glucosuria.
B. Physical and psychosocial findings.
   1. New diagnosis of a malignancy—pruritus may be the presenting symptom.
   2. Skin assessment—scratch marks, erythema, excoriation, thickening, dryness.
   3. Vaginal discharge and erythema.
   4. Presence of urea or bilirubin on the skin.
   5. Presence of stress and anxiety.

Nursing Diagnoses

I. Impaired skin integrity.
II. Ineffective coping.
III. Deficient knowledge of effective management strategies for pruritus.
IV. Disturbed sleep pattern.

Outcome Identification

I. Client's skin remains intact.
   A. Client reports alleviation of pruritus and increased comfort.
II. Client and the family contact an appropriate health care team member when pruritus interrupts protective mechanisms and psychologic well-being.
III. Client states the potential for pruritus with specific cancers, cancer therapies, and other related disease entities.
   A. Client and the family describe interventions to manage pruritus and maximize comfort.
IV. Client reports adequate amount of sleep.

Planning and Implementation

I. Pharmacologic and nonpharmacologic management (Table 1-4).
   A. Treat or remove the underlying cause.
   B. Pharmacologic management.
      1. Use pharmacologic agents to manage the underlying reaction and enhance comfort.
      2. Drug or allergic reaction: antihistamines, corticosteroids.
      3. Comfort—antihistamines, corticosteroids, tranquilizers.
   C. Nonpharmacologic management.
      1. Take medicated baths with antipruritics.
      2. Apply creams and emollient lotions for comfort.
II. Measures to increase the client and family knowledge base.
   A. Educate about therapies that may cause pruritus.
   B. Inform about the signs and symptoms of infection related to pruritus: fever, erythema, edema, pain, purulent drainage.
   C. Educate about self-care interventions to decrease the severity of pruritus.
III. Measures to maximize comfort.
   A. Modify the environment to prevent and minimize pruritus.
      1. Keep the room humidity at 30% to 40%.

TABLE 1-4
Phamacologic and Nonpharmacologic Management of Pruritus

PHARMACOLOGIC AGENTS	COMMENTS
SYSTEMIC AGENTS	
Diphenhydramine (Benadryl)	H_1-receptor antagonists are the first drugs of choice for pruritus
Cimetidine (Tagamet), ranitidine (Zantac)	H_2-receptor antagonists may be helpful; use for itch related to lymphoma
Doxepin (Prudoxin, Sinequan, Zonalon)	Tricyclic antidepressant and potent antihistamine; use for atopic dermatitis and other generalized pruritus
Opioid antagonists (naltrexone [ReVia]) or agonist/antagonists (e.g., nalbuphine [Nubain])	For opioid-induced pruritus; especially helpful for itching with intraspinal analgesia
Serotonin antagonists (ondansetron [Zofran])	Helpful for opioid-induced pruritus and cholestasis
Intraspinal droperidol (Inapsine)	For opioid-induced pruritus
Cholestyramine (Questran)	Used with pruritus related to biliary obstruction and cholestasis
Thalidomide (Thalomid)	For pruritus related to uremia
TOPICAL AGENTS	
Corticosteroid creams	For inflammation associated with pruritus
Capsaicin (Zostrix) (0.025%)	For uremia, branchioradial pruritus and counterirritants
Menthol (0.25%-2%)	For uremia, branchioradial pruritus and counterirritants
NONPHARMACOLOGIC MODALITIES	
Ultraviolet B light	For cholestatic and uremic pruritus
Hypnotherapy	To ease anxiety, psychologic issues associated with pruritus
Transcutaneous electrical nerve stimulation (TENS), acupuncture	Case studies report positive results

Data from Bleiker TO, Graham-Brown RAC: Diagnosing skin disease in the elderly, *Practitioner* 244:974-981, 2000; Friedman JD, Dello Buono FA: Opioid antagonists in the treatment of opioid-induced constipation and pruritus, *Ann Pharmacother* 35:85-91, 2001; Krajnik M, Zylicz Z: Pruritus in advanced internal diseases: pathogenesis and treatment, *Neth J Med* 58:27-40, 2001; Lidstone V, Thorns A: Pruritus in cancer patients, *Cancer Treat Rev* 27:305-312, 2001.

2. Keep the room temperature cool to prevent vasodilation and limit sweating that may exacerbate itch; use fans to circulate the air.
3. Use cotton clothing and sheets.
4. Use hypoallergenic soaps.
5. Avoid alcohol and spicy foods that may exacerbate itch.
B. Minimize vasodilation.
   1. Encourage cool baths, showers, and environmental conditions.
   2. Avoid alcohol and caffeine intake.
   3. Reduce stress and anxiety.
C. Promote skin integrity.
   1. Encourage fluid intake of 3000 ml/day.
   2. Encourage a diet high in iron, zinc, and protein.
   3. Wear loose-fitting clothing.
   4. Avoid scratching; wear cotton gloves at night to avoid skin trauma.
IV. Measures to protect client from potential sequelae.
   A. Use massage, pressure, and rubbing as alternatives to scratching.

    B. Cut the fingernails short and file smooth.

    C. Instruct others about the importance of good hand washing.

    D. Assess the pruritic areas for signs of infection.

  V. Measures to facilitate client and family coping.

    A. Teach behavioral interventions that may distract from the pruritus: imagery, television, reading, crafts.

    B. Encourage relaxation, stress reduction; refer to psychosocial services if needed.

Evaluation

The oncology nurse systematically and regularly evaluates the client's and/or family's responses to interventions to determine progress toward the achievement of expected outcomes. Relevant data are collected, and actual findings are compared with expected findings. Nursing diagnoses, outcomes, and plans of care are reviewed and revised as necessary.

SLEEP DISORDERS

Theory

  I. Definition (Savard & Morin, 2001).

    A. Sleep—natural suspension of consciousness in which processes of the body are restored.

    B. Sleep disorder—interruption in the amount or quality of sleep: inability to go to sleep, stay asleep, sleep long enough, and feel restored and relaxed on awakening.

  II. Physiology.

    A. Stages of sleep (Savard & Morin, 2001).

      1. Non–rapid-eye movement (NREM)—also called quiet sleep, the first sleep phase.

        a. Stage 1—transition between wakefulness and sleep.

        b. Stage 2—nonequivocal physiologic sleep.

        c. Stages 3 and 4—also called delta or slow-wave pattern; sequence moves from stage 2 to 3 to 4 and then back to stage 3 and stage 2, which leads to the first rapid eye movement (REM) cycle.

      2. REM sleep—also called paradoxical sleep.

        a. Biologic activity—electroencephalographic activation, muscle atony, dreams.

        b. Cycle length is approximately 90 minutes, repeated four or five times per night with the latter REM episodes increasing in duration.

    B. Other regulatory processes.

      1. Melatonin—hormone released by the pineal gland and mediator of night and day rhythms, sensitive to external light (Rohr & Herold, 2002).

        a. Low levels are frequently associated with depression, insomnia.

        b. Levels decrease with age.

        c. Some studies suggest that low levels are associated with an increased incidence of cancer and high levels may be protective against cancer.

      2. Environmental factors—light regulates the sleep cycle with decreased levels of melatonin during daylight.

III. Risk factors.
  A. Disease-related factors.
     1. Approximately 30% to 50% of clients who are newly diagnosed or recently treated for cancer experience sleep disorder (Davidson et al., 2002; Savard & Morin, 2001).
     2. Presence of concurrent symptoms such as pain, pruritus, fever, nausea, night sweats, shortness of breath, leg restlessness, and fatigue (Davidson et al., 2002; Lee, 2001).
     3. Paraneoplastic syndromes with an increase in corticosteroid production.
     4. Electrolyte disturbances.
     5. Delirium, confusion, altered mental status.
     6. Clients with lung cancer, brain tumors, and head and neck cancer (Davidson et al., 2002; Desuter et al., 2002; Friedman et al., 2001; Ioos, 2001).
  B. Treatment-related factors (Savard & Morin, 2001).
     1. Chemotherapy, hormonal therapy, radiation therapy, surgery.
     2. Medications—antimetabolites, steroids, tamoxifen (Nolvadex) (hot flashes), analeptics used as adjuvants in pain management, dopamine antagonists (associated with extrapyramidal side effects), sedatives.
     3. Perimenopause and menopause—may be treatment related; sleep disorder is caused by a decreased estrogen and melatonin level (Rohr & Herold, 2002).
     4. Hospitalization—interruption of normal routine, increased IV or oral fluids, increased frequency of voiding.
  C. Lifestyle-related and personal factors.
     1. Medical illness with a succession of severe stressors such as cancer (thoughts about cancer and the future, physical effects, finances) (Davidson et al., 2002).
     2. Increased age (Naeim & Reuben, 2001), female gender, family history.
     3. Depression, stress, anxiety, psychiatric disorder (Redeker et al., 2000).
     4. Physical inactivity, irregular sleep-wake schedule, naps, excessive time in bed.
     5. Alcohol intake.

Assessment

I. Clinical assessment.
  A. Usual pattern of sleep.
     1. Time when retiring to bed.
     2. Amount of time needed to fall asleep, duration of sleep.
     3. Time(s) of awakening—include reason for awakening, ability to return to sleep.
     4. Quantity and quality of daytime naps, time spent in bed.
     5. Exacerbating and relieving factors.
     6. Exercise patterns.
  B. Sleeping environment—light and noise factors, room temperature, other potential disturbances.
  C. Bedtime routine.
     1. Exercise versus relaxation within 2 hours of retiring.
     2. Caffeine and alcohol intake in afternoon or evening.
     3. Food and fluid intake before retiring.
     4. Use of sleeping aids: medications, warm milk.

    D. Impact of insomnia on daily living: self-care, concentration, cognitive functioning, fatigue, mood, depression, restlessness, irritability, anxiety.
    E. Family perception and involvement with the sleep disorder.
    F. Caregiver sleep problems (Carter, 2002; Carter & Chang, 2000).
    G. Relationships with others, role performance alterations, perceived reasons for inability to sleep.
II. History and physical examination.
    A. Client observation—dark circles under the eyes, expressionless face, nystagmus, ptosis of the eyelids, frequent yawning, slurred speech, incorrect word usage.
    B. Sleep studies—polysomnography.

Nursing Diagnosis

I. Disturbed sleep pattern.

Outcome Identification

I. Client reports adequate sleep patterns.
    A. Client states the risk factors of disease and treatment that may alter sleep patterns.
    B. Client identifies pharmacologic strategies to facilitate sleep.
    C. Client describes specific behavioral and cognitive interventions to promote sleep.

Planning and Implementation

I. Pharmacologic interventions.
    A. Medications to induce and maintain sleep.
        1. Hypnotics.
            a. Generalized side effects—tolerance and dependence.
            b. Recommended use is for situational insomnia.
            c. Benzodiazepines—flurazepam, temazepam, triazolam.
                (1) Short-term use recommended because of side effects—residual drowsiness and light-headedness, cognitive impairments, delirium, liver toxicity.
                (2) Higher side effect profile in the elderly.
            d. Nonbenzodiazepine hypnotics—zolpidem (Ambien), zopiclone (Imovane), zaleplon (Sonata).
                (1) More selective hypnotic mechanism, fewer residual side effects the next day.
        2. Sedating antidepressants—trazodone (Desyrel), amitriptyline (Elavil), doxepin (Prudoxin, Sinequan, Zonalon).
    B. Medications for symptom management: analgesics, antihistamines, anxiolytics.
II. Nonpharmacologic interventions (Table 1-5).
    A. Teach the client and family stimulus control techniques (Davidson et al., 2001).
        1. Go to bed when sleepy, not before the scheduled time.
        2. Do not use the bed for activities other than sleep (sexual activity is the exception).
        3. If the client cannot fall asleep or go back to sleep within 10 to 20 minutes, leave the bed for a while and return when sleepy.
        4. Arise at the same time each morning.
        5. Client may take a short nap (<1 hour) if excessively sleepy in the afternoon.

TABLE 1-5
Nonpharmacologic Sleep Interventions

Intervention	Goal	Procedure
Stimulus control therapy	■ Reassociate temporal (bedtime) and environmental (bed and bedroom) stimuli with rapid sleep onsets ■ Establish a regular circadian sleep-wake rhythm	Keep at least 1 hr before going to bed to relax; develop a ritual to do before going to bed; go to bed only when sleepy; when unable to fall asleep or go back to sleep within 15-20 min, get out of bed and leave the bedroom, and return to bed only when sleepy; maintain a regular arising time in the morning; use the bed/bedroom for sleep and sex only (do not watch television, listen to the radio, eat, or read in the bed); do not nap during the day
Sleep restriction procedures	■ Curtail time in bed to the actual sleep time, thereby creating mild sleep deprivation, which results in more consolidated and more efficient sleep	Restrict the amount of time spent in bed to the actual amount of time asleep; time in bed is progressively increased as sleep efficiency improves
Relaxation training	■ Reduce somatic and cognitive arousal interfering with sleep	Progressive muscle relaxation, autogenic training, biofeedback, imagery training, hypnosis, thought stopping
Cognitive therapy	■ Change dysfunctional beliefs and attitudes about sleep and insomnia that exacerbate emotional arousal, performance anxiety, and learned helplessness related to sleep (unrealistic sleep requirement expectations, faulty appraisals of sleep difficulties, misattributions of daytime impairments, misconceptions about the causes of insomnia)	Identify sleep cognitive distortions (mainly by self-monitoring); challenge the validity of sleep cognitions (by using probing questions such as "What is the evidence that supports this idea?" or "Is there an alternative explanation?"); reframe dysfunctional cognitions into more adaptive thoughts by using cognitive restructuring techniques (e.g., decatastrophizing, reattribution, reappraisal, attention shifting)
Sleep hygiene education	■ Change health practices and environmental factors that interfere with sleep	Avoid stimulants (e.g., caffeine, nicotine) and alcohol around bedtime; do not eat heavy or spicy meals too close to bedtime; exercise regularly but not too late in the evening; maintain a dark, quiet, comfortable sleep environment

From Savard J, Morin CM: Insomnia in the context of cancer: a review of a neglected problem, *J Clin Oncol* 19:895-908, 2001.

B. Provide the client with behavioral and cognitive strategies to sleep—counting and word games, loading Noah's Ark with animals, prayer and meditation.

C. Educate the client about relaxation techniques, such as progressive muscle relaxation and imagery.

D. Encourage regular exercise during the day, avoid 2 hours before bedtime (Lee, 2001).

III. Measures to increase the knowledge base of the client and family.
   A. Inform the client about the need to report sleep disorders.
   B. Inform the client about strategies for stimulus control and improved sleep.
IV. Measures to maximize client comfort (Davidson et al., 2001; Savard & Morin, 2001).
   A. Plan nursing interventions succinctly to prevent unnecessary interruption of sleep.
   B. Implement pain and symptom management interventions in a timely and appropriate manner to control pain and concurrent symptoms.
   C. Administer sleeping medications in a timely and appropriate manner.
   D. Provide a restful environment.
      1. Decrease light and noise factors.
      2. Maintain the client's room temperature.
      3. Straighten and provide clean bed linens.
      4. Encourage the practice of a normal bedtime routine when the client is hospitalized: sleepwear, reading before bedtime, warm milk, medications.
   E. Provide or promote relaxation before bedtime.
      1. Bathing, relaxation techniques, reading, television, small snack, warm milk.
      2. Avoid eating large amounts of food, caffeine, stimulants, excessive fluids.

Evaluation

The oncology nurse systematically and regularly evaluates the client's and/or family's responses to interventions to determine progress toward the achievement of expected outcomes. Relevant data are collected, and actual findings are compared with expected findings. Nursing diagnoses, outcomes, and plans of care are reviewed and revised as necessary.

See Chapter 13 for information on fever and chills and Chapter 16 for information on dyspnea.

REFERENCES

American Pain Society. (2003). *Principles of analgesic use in the treatment of acute pain and cancer pain* (5th ed.). Glenview, IL: American Pain Society.

Barnes, E.A., & Bruera, E. (2002). Fatigue in patients with advanced cancer: A review. *International Journal of Gynecologic Cancer 12*(5), 424-428.

Bennet, G., Burchiel, K., Buchser, E., et al. (2000a). Clinical guidelines for intraspinal infusion: Report of an expert panel. *Journal of Pain and Symptom Management 20*, S37-S43.

Bennet, G., Deer, T., Dupen, S., et al. (2000b). Future directions in the management of pain by intraspinal drug delivery. *Journal of Pain and Symptom Management 20*, S44-S50.

Bleiker, T.O., & Graham-Brown, R.A.C. (2000). Diagnosing skin disease in the elderly. *The Practitioner 244*, 974-981.

Body, J.J., & Mancini, I. (2002). Bisphosphonates for cancer patients: Why, how, and when? *Supportive Care in Cancer 10*, 399-407.

Brant, J. (2002). Pain management at the end of life. In M. O'Connor & S. Aranda (Eds.). *Palliative care nursing: A guide to practice*. Melbourne, Australia: Ausmed Publications.

Brines, M.L., Ghezzi, P., Keenan, S., et al. (2000). Erythropoietin crosses the blood-brain barrier to protect against experimental brain injury. *Proceedings of the National Academy of Science USA 97*, 10526-10531.

Brown, K., Espar, P., Kelleher, L., et al. (2001). *Chemotherapy and biotherapy guidelines and recommendations for practice*. Pittsburgh: Oncology Nursing Press.

Carpenito, L.J. (1995). *Nursing diagnosis: Application to clinical practice*. Philadelphia: Lippincott.

Carter, P.A. (2002). Caregivers' descriptions of sleep changes and depressive symptoms. *Oncology Nursing Forum 29,* 1277-1283.

Carter, P.A., & Chang, B.L. (2000). Sleep and depression in cancer caregivers. *Cancer Nursing 23,* 410-415.

Cella D. (1997). The Functional Assessment of Cancer Therapy-Anemia (FACT-An) Scale: A new tool for the assessment of outcomes in cancer anemia and fatigue. *Seminars in Hematology 34*(3, Suppl. 2), 13-19.

Cullinane, C., & Chu, D.Z.J. (2002). Current surgical options in the control of cancer pain. *Cancer Practice 10,* S21-S26.

Davidson, J.R., MacLean, A.W., Brundage, M.D., & Schulze, K. (2002). Sleep disturbance in cancer patients. *Social Science and Medicine 54,* 1309-1321.

Davidson, J.R., Waisberg, J.L., Brundage, M.D., & MacLean, W. (2001). Nonpharmacologic group treatment of insomnia: A preliminary study with cancer survivors. *Psycho-Oncology 10,* 389-397.

Demetri, G.D. (2001). Anemia and its functional consequences in cancer patients: Current challenges in management and prospects for improving therapy. *British Journal of Cancer 84*(Suppl. 1), 31-37.

Demetri, G., Kris, M., Wade, J., et al. (1998). Quality-of-life benefit in chemotherapy patients treated with epoetin alfa is independent of disease response or tumor type: Results from a prospective community oncology study. *Journal of Clinical Oncology 16,* 3412-3425.

Desuter, G., Castelein, S., de Toeuf, C., et al. (2002). Parapharyngeal causes of sleep apnea syndrome: Two case reports and review of the literature. *Acta Oto-Rhino-Laryngologica Belgica 56,* 189-194.

Dworkin, R.H. (2002). An overview of neuropathic pain: Syndromes, symptoms, signs, and several mechanisms. *The Clinical Journal of Pain 18,* 343-349.

Federation of State Medical Boards. (1998). *Model guidelines for the use of controlled substances for the treatment of pain.* Euless, TX: Federation of State Medical Boards of the United States.

Friedman, M., Landsberg, R., Pryor, S., et al. (2001). The occurrence of sleep-disordered breathing among patients with head and neck cancer. *Laryngoscope 111,* 1917-1919.

Gabrilove, J.L., Cleeland, C., Livingston, R.B., et al. (2001). Clinical evaluation of once weekly dosing of epoetin alfa in chemotherapy patients: Improvements in hemoglobin and quality of life are similar in three times weekly dosing. *Journal of Clinical Oncology 19,* 2875-2882.

Glaspy, J., Jadeja, J., & Justice, G. (2002). Randomized, active-controlled, phase I/II, dose-escalation study of darbepoetin alpha every 2 weeks in patients with solid tumors. *European Journal of Cancer 37*(Suppl. 6), 353-358.

Holzner, B., Kemmler, G., Greil, R., et al. (2002). The impact of hemoglobin levels on fatigue and quality of life in cancer patients. *Annals of Oncology 13,* 965-973.

Ioos, C. (2001). Sleep disorders caused by brainstem tumor: Case report. *Journal of Child Neurology 16,* 767-770.

Jacox, A, Carr, D.B., Payne, R., et al. (1994). *Management of cancer pain, clinical practice guideline number 9 AHCPR Publication No. 94-0592,* Rockville, MD: U.S. Department of Health and Human Services.

Krajnik, M., & Zylicz, Z. (2001). Pruritus in advanced internal diseases: Pathogenesis and treatment. *The Netherlands Journal of Medicine 58,* 27-40.

Lee, K.A. (2001). Sleep and fatigue. In J.J. Fitzpatrick, D. Taylor, & N.F. Woods (Eds.). *Annual Review of Nursing Research.* New York: Springer Publishing Co.

Lidstone, V., & Thorns, A. (2001). Pruritus in cancer patients. *Cancer Treatment Reviews 27,* 305-312.

Lucas, L., & Lipman, A.G. (2002). Recent advances in pharmacotherapy for cancer pain management. *Cancer Practice 10,* S14-S20.

McCaffery, M. (1968). *Nursing practice theories related to cognition, bodily pain, and man-environment interactions.* Los Angeles: Student Store.

McCaffery, M., & Pasero, C. (1999). *Pain: Clinical manual* (2nd ed.). St. Louis: Mosby.

McMillan, C. (2001). Breakthrough pain: Assessment and management in cancer patients. *British Journal of Nursing 10,* 860-866.

Mercadante, S. (2001). Recent progress in the pharmacotherapy of cancer pain. *Expert Reviews in Anticancer Therapy 1*, 487-494.

Merskey, H. (Ed.). (1986). Classification of chronic pain: Description of chronic pain syndromes and definitions of pain terms. *Pain Suppl. 3*, S217.

Naeim, A., & Reuben, D. (2001). Geriatric syndromes and assessment in older cancer patients. *Oncology 15*, 1567-1591.

Nail, L. (2002). Fatigue in patients with cancer. *Oncology Nursing Forum 29*, 537-546.

Nielsen, E., & Brant, J. (2002). Chemotherapy-induced neurotoxicity. *American Journal of Nursing* April Suppl., 16-19.

O'Leary, U. (2002). Psychosocial influences on pain perceptions in cancer. *Nursing Times 98*, 36-38.

O'Shaughnessy, J., Vukelja, S., Savin, M., et al. (2002). Effects of epoetin alfa (Procrit) on cognitive function, mood, asthenia and quality of life. *Proceedings of the American Society of Clinical Oncology 21*(Abstract No. 1449), 363a.

Piper B.F., Dibble S.L., Dodd M.J., et al. (1998). The revised Piper Fatigue Scale: Psychometric evaluation in women with breast cancer. *Oncology Nursing Forum 25*, 677-684.

Redeker, N.S., Lev, E.L., & Ruggiero, J. (2000). Insomnia, fatigue, anxiety, depression, and quality of life of cancer patients undergoing chemotherapy. *Scholarly Inquiry for Nursing Practice: An International Journal 14*, 275-290.

Rohr, U.D., & Herold, J. (2002). Melatonin deficiencies in women. *Maturitas, 41*, S85-S104.

Savard, J., & Morin, C.M. (2001). Insomnia in the context of cancer: A review of a neglected problem. *Journal of Clinical Oncology 19*, 895-908.

Saarto, T., Janes, R., Tenhunen, M., & Kouri, M. (2002). Palliative radiotherapy in the treatment of skeletal metastases. *European Journal of Pain 6*, 323-330.

Schwartz, A.L. (1998). The Schwartz Cancer Fatigue Scale: Testing reliability and validity. *Oncology Nursing Forum 25*, 711-717.

Shih, A., Miaskowski, C., Dodd, M.J., et al. (2002). A research review of the current treatments for radiation-induced oral mucositis in patients with head and neck cancer. *Oncology Nursing Forum 29*, 1063-1080.

Smith, M.C., Kemp, J., Hemphill, L., & Vojir, C.P. (2002). Outcomes of therapeutic massage for hospitalized cancer patients. *Image: The Journal of Nursing Scholarship 34*, 257-262.

Sobrero. A., Puglisi, F, & Gulielmi, A. (2001). Fatigue: A main component of anemia symptomlogy. *Seminars in Oncology 28*(Suppl. 8), 15-18.

Sutton, L.M., Porter, L.S., & Keefe, F.J. (2002). Cancer pain at the end of life: A biopsychosocial perspective. *Pain 99*, 5-10.

2 Coping: Psychosocial Issues

PATRICIA M. GRIMM

EMOTIONAL DISTRESS

Theory

I. Definition—a pattern of expected changes in thinking, feelings, and behaviors that occur in response to the diagnosis, prognosis, treatment, and events that occur in the clinical course of cancer.
   A. Changes are related to a specific stressor or stressors and to diagnosis and treatment of cancer.
   B. Duration of feelings is not as long and intensity of feelings is not as severe as with clinical anxiety or depression.
II. Risk factors (Bush, 1998b, Holland, 1998).
   A. Disease related and treatment related.
      1. Site, stage, clinical course.
      2. Nature of dysfunction and symptoms produced.
      3. Treatment required (i.e., surgery, chemotherapy, radiotherapy, combined modalities, bone marrow transplant [BMT], biotherapy).
      4. Rehabilitative options.
      5. Psychologic management by the health care team.
   B. Situational.
      1. Social attitudes about cancer, its stigma, and the meaning attached.
      2. Nature and availability of social supports: family, friends, affiliated groups.
      3. Changes in family communication, roles, functional responsibilities.
   C. Developmental.
      1. Age-specific developmental life tasks threatened or disrupted by cancer.
      2. Personality, prior coping ability in response to major life stresses.
III. General treatment approaches (Bush, 1998b).
   A. Psychologic support.
   B. Individual or family psychotherapy.
   C. Spiritual counseling.
   D. Cognitive and behavioral interventions, such as support groups, relaxation training, guided imagery.
   E. Occupational or recreational therapy.
   F. Pharmacologic management of symptoms with sedatives, anxiolytics, and/or antidepressants (see Chapter 10).
IV. Potential sequelae of emotional distress.
   A. Chronic emotional distress.
   B. Development of major psychiatric disorders: anxiety or depression, with risk for suicide.

C. Somatic symptoms, such as gastrointestinal (GI) disturbances, headaches, dizziness, chest pain, insomnia.
D. Interference with performance at home, school, or work.
E. Decreased compliance with the recommended treatment regimen.

Assessment

I. History.
  A. Presence of risk factors.
  B. Presence of discomforting thoughts, feelings, and behaviors—nervousness, worry, jitteriness, tearfulness, hopelessness, difficulty concentrating, social withdrawal, difficulties with school and work.
II. Pattern of emotional distress.
  A. Onset; frequency; intensity; associated symptoms; precipitating, aggravating, and alleviating factors.
  B. Duration—not considered major psychiatric disorder if it is assessed as a normally expected response to current stressors and it is episodic in nature.
III. Perceived effect on client and family functioning—physical, lifestyle, interpersonal, work, or school.

Nursing Diagnoses

I. Deficient knowledge of diagnosis, treatment approaches, community resources.
II. Ineffective coping.
III. Fear.
IV. Situational low self-esteem.

Outcome Identification

I. Client and family identify expected symptoms and side effects of the disease and its treatment.
  A. Client and family identify community resources that meet their needs.
II. Client manages emotional distress.
  A. Verbalizes emotional responses to cancer diagnosis and treatment.
  B. Makes decisions and follows through with appropriate interventions to manage emotional distress.
III. Client verbalizes a reduction or absence of fear.
IV. Client identifies personal strengths and support systems available for managing emotional distress.

Planning and Implementation

I. Interventions to minimize risk and severity of emotional distress (Carpenito, 2002; NCCN, 1999).
  A. Discuss concerns that may be precipitating emotional distress.
  B. Discuss the meaning of disease and treatment to client.
  C. Provide teaching regarding cancer diagnosis, treatment, and expected outcomes to reduce fear of the unknown.
  D. Explore past coping responses to stressful events, and support use of those responses that have been successful in the past.

E. Inform of appropriate resources for emotional distress management—psychotherapy, support groups, relaxation training.

F. Encourage use of support groups, relaxation, psychotherapy.

II. Interventions to maximize comfort during emotional distress (Carpenito, 2002; NCCN, 1999).

A. Provide a safe, comfortable, supportive environment.

B. Allow the client to discuss thoughts, feelings, fears.

C. Listen attentively, conveying genuineness and empathy.

D. Encourage use of self-help interventions, such as relaxation, distraction, or exercise.

III. Interventions to monitor for complications related to emotional distress (Carpenito, 2002; NCCN, 1999).

A. Observe for somatic symptoms, and discuss treatment with the health care team.

B. Observe for indications of major psychiatric disorders: anxiety, depression, risk for suicide.

C. Observe for untoward effects of pharmacologic management of symptoms—sedatives, anxiolytics, and/or antidepressants (see Chapter 10).

D. Report indications of psychiatric disorders and untoward effects of medications to the appropriate member of the health team.

E. Monitor compliance with the recommended treatment regimen.

IV. Interventions to enhance adaptation and rehabilitation (Carpenito, 2002; NCCN, 1999).

A. Provide ongoing teaching regarding the client's treatment plan and expected responses.

B. Promote ongoing discussion of the client's thoughts, feelings, and fears regarding diagnosis and treatment.

C. Provide positive feedback for use of alternative coping approaches that lessen emotional distress, such as relaxation, distraction, exercise.

D. Implement strategies to manage symptoms and side effects of cancer and treatment, and psychotropic medications.

V. Interventions to increase client and family involvement with care (Carpenito, 2002; NCCN, 1999).

A. Assist family members to identify experiences and thoughts that result in emotional distress.

B. Provide teaching regarding the client's and family's role in the client's care—encourage a sense of control over these aspects of the treatment plan.

C. Instruct the client and family in recreational and diversional outlets for emotional energy.

D. Provide information on educational materials and community resources available through the American Cancer Society, National Cancer Institute, other hospital programs and community agencies, and Internet websites (see Box 2-1 and Chapter 8).

Evaluation

The oncology nurse systematically and regularly evaluates the client's and/or family's responses to interventions to determine progress toward the achievement of expected outcomes. Relevant data are collected, and actual findings are compared with expected findings. Nursing diagnoses, outcomes, and plans of care are reviewed and revised as necessary.

BOX 2-1
CANCER RESOURCES: SELECTED WEBSITES

American Cancer Society	www.cancer.org
Cancer Care, Inc.	www.cancercare.org
Leukemia and Lymphoma Society	www.leukemia-lymphoma.org
National Alliance of Breast Cancer Organizations	www.nabco.org
National Cancer Institute	www.cancer.gov
National Coalition for Cancer Survivorship	www.cansearch.org
National Comprehensive Cancer Network	www.nccn.org
National Hospice Organization	www.nho.org

ANXIETY

Theory

I. Definition—a state of feeling uneasy and apprehensive in response to a vague, nonspecific, or unidentifiable threat.

II. Risk factors (Bush, 1998a).
   A. Disease related.
      1. Uncertainty of prognosis and/or social stigma of diagnosis.
      2. Inadequate symptom control—pain, insomnia, nausea and/or vomiting.
      3. Abnormal metabolic states—hypoxia, pulmonary embolus, sepsis, delirium, hypoglycemia, bleeding, heart failure, and so on.
      4. Hormone-secreting tumors.
      5. Recurrence of disease.
      6. Progression of disease—paraneoplastic syndrome, cachexia.
      7. Brain metastases—in area that affects physical comfort, breathing, or circulation.
   B. Treatment related.
      1. Prolonged treatment regimen and hospitalization.
      2. Intensive therapy—mutilating surgery, combination therapy, bone marrow transplantation.
      3. Anxiety-producing drugs—corticosteroids, neuroleptics used as antiemetics, thyroxine, bronchodilators, antihistamines/decongestants, β-adrenergic stimulants, opiate pain medications.
      4. Untoward effects or side effects—alopecia, immunosuppression.
      5. Failure or termination of therapy.
   C. Lifestyle and situational.
      1. Disease-related losses—health, status, finances, family relationships and roles, social interaction.
      2. Exposure to the new situations and relationships of cancer treatment.
      3. Excessive intake of caffeine and nicotine.
      4. Withdrawal from alcohol and narcotic or sedative/hypnotic drugs.
   D. Developmental.
      1. Preexisting anxiety disorder—generalized anxiety, phobias, panic attacks, posttraumatic stress.
      2. Low self-esteem or intense fears in childhood.
      3. Blocked age-specific expectations, needs, or goals.

III. General treatment approaches (ACS, 2000; APA, 2000; Bush, 1998a).
   A. Individual or family psychotherapy.
   B. Pharmacologic management with anxiolytics such as benzodiazepines, anti-depressants (see Chapter 10).
   C. Complementary and alternative therapies—aromatherapy, herbal remedies, massage, breathing exercises, music (see Chapters 11 and 41).
   D. Cognitive and behavioral interventions—biofeedback, relaxation training, guided imagery, support groups.
   E. Occupational or recreational therapy—diversional activities, exercises.
IV. Potential sequelae of anxiety (APA, 2000).
   A. Somatic symptoms—nausea, vomiting, headaches, GI distress.
   B. Behavioral—substance use, eating disturbances, self-destructive activities.
   C. Cognitive changes—problems with concentration and decision making, memory difficulties, disorientation.
   D. Chronic anxiety disorders—generalized anxiety, panic attacks, phobias, obsessive-compulsive disorder.
   E. Psychosomatic illnesses—gastric ulcers, colitis, migraine headaches.
   F. Interference with performance at home, school, or work.

Assessment

I. History.
   A. Presence of risk factors.
   B. History of defining characteristics of anxiety (APA, 2000).
      1. Physical—flushing, sweating, tenseness, tremors, pacing, overactivity or immobility, changes in weight (loss or gain), changes in sleep patterns (insomnia, hypersomnia), shortness of breath, vomiting, diarrhea, muscle aches, feelings of heaviness, headaches, dry mouth, palpitations, decreased hearing or visual acuity.
      2. Emotional—irritability, feeling "keyed up," cries easily, self-doubting and blaming.
      3. Cognitive and behavioral—changes in perceptual field (hypervigilant or narrowly focused), difficulty with problem solving and decision making, compulsiveness, anger, withdrawal.
   C. Patterns of anxiety—past experiences; onset; frequency; severity; associated symptoms; precipitating, aggravating, and alleviating factors.
   D. Previous responses to anxiety, perceived effectiveness of these responses (constructive, destructive).
   E. Anxiety management strategies used—medication, relaxation, biofeedback, psychotherapy.
   F. Perceived effect of anxiety on client and family functioning—physical, lifestyle, interpersonal, work or school.
II. Symptoms and signs (APA, 2000; Bush, 1998a; NCCN, 1999).
   A. Appearance and behavior—flushed face, tense or worried expression, restlessness, signs of nail biting, sweating.
   B. Neurologic—poor concentration and memory, decreased interest in usual activities, irritability, dizziness, weakness, exhaustion, fine tremors, insomnia, nightmares, headaches, drowsiness.
   C. Other physical symptoms and signs—palpitations, elevated blood pressure, hyperventilation, dyspnea, anorexia, heartburn.

III. Laboratory findings.
    A. Increased blood sugar level.
    B. Increased epinephrine level.

Nursing Diagnoses

  I. Anxiety (including Death anxiety).
 II. Ineffective coping.
III. Disturbed sleep pattern.

Outcome Identification

  I. Client identifies anxiety-provoking situations and responses.
    A. Identifies sources of anxiety.
    B. Ventilates feelings of anxiety to others.
    C. Identifies effective and ineffective coping responses.
    D. Discusses the disease and treatment accurately.
 II. Client participates in anxiety-reducing interventions.
    A. Describes methods to decrease feelings of anxiety.
    B. Omits or limits alcohol, caffeine, and nicotine intake.
    C. Complies with pharmacologic and/or behavioral interventions.
    D. Utilizes complementary therapies as discussed with health care practitioner.
    E. Identifies support systems within the family and community.
III. Client participates in sleep-promoting interventions.
    A. Describes methods to promote sleep.
    B. Complies with pharmacologic and/or behavioral interventions.
    C. Utilizes complementary therapies as discussed with health care practitioner.

Planning and Implementation (Bush, 1998a; Carpenito, 2002; NCCN, 1999; Noyes et al., 1998)

 I. Interventions to minimize risk and severity of anxiety.
    A. Use of interpersonal skills related to management of anxiety.
      1. Use calm, reassuring approach.
      2. Listen attentively.
      3. Help the client identify situations that precipitate anxiety.
      4. Seek to understand the client's perspective of a stressful situation.
      5. Encourage verbalization of feelings, perceptions, fears.
      6. Explore similarities between the present situation and successful resolution of problems in the past.
    B. Institute measures to enhance management of anxiety.
      1. Provide factual information concerning diagnosis, treatment, prognosis.
      2. Explain all procedures, including sensations likely to be experienced during the procedure.
      3. Use diversional activities or relaxation techniques as appropriate.
      4. Administer prescribed medications to reduce anxiety.
 II. Interventions to maximize client safety with anxiety.
    A. Assess the level of the client's anxiety.
    B. Provide a safe, supportive, predictable environment.
    C. During periods of high anxiety, stay with the client to promote safety and reduce fear.
    D. Assist with self-care as needed.

     E. Refrain from asking the client to make decisions during high anxiety states.
     F. Set limits to minimize risks to the client.
     G. Report critical changes in the results of client assessment to the appropriate health team member.
        1. Panic attacks.
        2. Withdrawal, noncompliance with cancer therapeutic regimen.
        3. Untoward effects of anxiolytic drug therapy.
        4. Abrupt discontinuance of anxiolytics.
        5. Suicidal attempts or ideation.

III. Interventions to monitor for complications related to anxiety and its treatment.
     A. Observe for severe anxiety reactions—panic attacks, decreased level of orientation, concentration, hallucinations, fight-or-flight responses of anger, hyperactivity.
     B. Observe for untoward effects of anxiolytic medications—dry mouth, drowsiness, dizziness, memory losses.
     C. Observe for symptoms of withdrawal if use of anxiolytics is abruptly discontinued.

IV. Interventions to enhance adaptation and rehabilitation.
     A. Discuss possible secondary gains of anxious behavior.
     B. Discuss interference with daily functioning regarding use or ineffective coping responses—overeating, overactivity.
     C. Limit or discontinue intake of alcohol, caffeine, nicotine.
     D. Promote sleep with comfort measures and/or medications, balanced diet, regular physical exercise.
     E. Implement strategies to manage side effects of anxiolytic and/or antidepressant medications.
        1. Dry mouth—fluid intake increase, frequent mouth care, use of sugarless gum or hard candies.
        2. Constipation—fluid intake increase, high-fiber diet, exercise.
        3. Blurred vision—will improve over time; new glasses should not be needed.
        4. Drowsiness—take medication at bedtime; symptom usually improves with time; caution about operating a motor vehicle or other machinery.
        5. Dizziness—avoid rapid movements of the head and change positions slowly.

  V. Interventions to incorporate the client and family in care.
     A. Assist the client and family to identify feelings of anxiety, to discuss these feelings, and to seek support in their management.
     B. Instruct the client and family in the importance of recreational and leisure activity outlets for emotional energy.
     C. Provide information on resources for support in managing anxiety—individual and/or family therapy, crisis intervention hotlines, emergency rooms, support groups and programs, such as *I Can Cope*.

Evaluation

The oncology nurse systematically and regularly evaluates the client's and/or family's responses to interventions to determine progress toward the achievement of expected outcomes. Relevant data are collected, and actual findings are compared with expected findings. Nursing diagnoses, outcomes, and plans of care are reviewed and revised as necessary.

DEPRESSION

Theory (APA, 2000)

I. Definition—a state of feeling sad, discouraged, hopeless, and worthless, which may vary from transient emotional distress to a major psychiatric illness with possible suicidal ideation.
  A. Primary symptoms are depressed mood and loss of interest or pleasure.
  B. Symptoms have persisted over the same 2-week period.
  C. Symptoms represent a change from the previous level of functioning.
  D. Important to differentiate from delirium, which has an acute onset, induces impaired cognitive function, and typically waxes and wanes.

II. Risk factors (Massie, 1998).
  A. Disease related.
    1. Type of cancer—lung, pancreas, central nervous system (CNS).
    2. Differences in prognosis with different types of cancer—lung and pancreas versus skin and cervical.
    3. Status of cancer—stage, recurrence, progression.
    4. Inadequate symptom control, particularly pain.
  B. Treatment related.
    1. Prolonged or difficult treatment.
    2. Chemotherapeutic or biotherapeutic agents—vincristine (Oncovin), vinblastine (Velban), procarbazine (Matulane), asparaginase (Elspar), ifosfamide (Ifex), and interferon alpha.
    3. Medications—corticosteroids, antihypertensives, benzodiazepines, β-blockers (propranolol), opiates, estrogens.
  C. Other medical conditions—anemia, dehydration, sleep deprivation, alcoholism, hypertension, thyroid dysfunction, electrolyte abnormalities, neurologic disorders, infectious diseases.
  D. Situational and developmental.
    1. History of depression (client or family).
    2. History of suicide attempts (client or family).
    3. History of, or concurrent, substance abuse.
    4. Perceived or actual loss of personal control.
    5. Cumulative crises in family or crises related to illness.
    6. Perceived, or actual, lack of social support.
    7. Changes in family and social roles and relationships.

III. General treatment approaches (ACS, 2000; Massie, 1998; Moore & Schmais, 2001; NCCN, 1999).
  A. Treatment of underlying medical conditions.
  B. Modification of pharmacologic influences.
  C. Individual or family psychotherapy.
  D. Pharmacologic management of depression with antidepressants, stimulants; management of other symptoms (insomnia, restlessness) with anxiolytics, sedatives.
  E. Complementary therapies—aromatherapy, herbal remedies, meditation, massage, breathing exercises, nutritional supplements (see Chapters 11 and 41).
  F. Cognitive and behavioral interventions, such as support groups, relaxation, cognitive restructuring.
  G. Occupational or recreational therapy: diversional activities, exercise.

IV. Potential sequelae of depression (Massie, 1998).
  A. Somatic problems related to changes in appetite and sleep patterns.
  B. Severe psychologic regression, loss of function, somatic delusions.

C. Suicidal ideation and/or attempts.
D. Interference with the role of the client functioning at home, work, or school.
E. Decreased compliance with the recommended medical regimen.

Assessment

I. History (APA, 2000; Massie, 1998).
  A. Presence of risk factors for depression.
  B. Presence of five or more of the defining symptoms of depression for a period of 2 consecutive weeks or more.
    1. Depressed mood (feeling sad or tearful).
    2. Decreased interest or pleasure in activities.
    3. Weight loss or gain, increased or decreased appetite.
    4. Insomnia or hypersomnia.
    5. Psychomotor agitation or retardation.
    6. Fatigue, loss of energy.
    7. Sense of worthlessness or excessive guilt.
    8. Decreased concentration, indecisiveness.
    9. Recurrent thoughts of death.
  C. Presence of delirium as the etiology of depression-like symptoms.
  D. Patterns of symptoms of depression—previous history, onset, frequency, severity, associated symptoms, and precipitating, aggravating, and alleviating factors.
  E. Presence of suicidal ideation, suicide plan, means to accomplish the plan.
  F. Perceived effectiveness of strategies to relieve symptoms.
  G. Perceived meaning of depression for the client and family.
  H. Perceived effect of depression on client and family functioning—physical, lifestyle, interpersonal, work, or school.
II. Symptoms and signs (APA, 2000; Massie, 1998).
  A. Appearance and behavior—flat affect, lack of spontaneity, changes in eye contact (consider cultural differences), slowed speech or minimal verbalizations, inactivity or agitation.
  B. Emotional and cognitive—crying, labile emotions; verbalization of self-reproach, pessimism, guilt, hopelessness; problems with concentration and decision making.
III. Laboratory or measurement findings (APA, 2000).
  A. Changes in cortisol levels.
  B. Mental status examination changes may be indicative of delirium, not depression.

Nursing Diagnoses

I. Deficient knowledge related to depression and its management.
II. Situational low self-esteem.
III. Ineffective role performance.
IV. Social isolation.
V. Risk for suicide

Outcome Identification

I. Client identifies signs and symptoms of depression.
  A. Client describes personal risk factors for depression.

    B. Client lists strategies to decrease risks or complications of depression.

    C. Client participates in recommended treatment interventions for depression.

  II. Client identifies realistic ways to exert control and influence outcomes in current life situation.

 III. Client and family discuss the impact of depression on client and family functioning—physical, emotional, social; at home, work, or school.

 IV. Client develops plan to become more involved with others.

    A. Client and family identify personal, family, community, and professional resources to assist in increasing social interaction.

  V. Client and family identify situations that require professional interventions.

    A. Acute changes in ability to control physical and psychologic responses.

    B. Rapid deterioration of physical status.

    C. Indications of suicidal ideation or attempts.

Planning and Implementation (Carpenito, 2002; Massie, 1998; Moore & Schmais, 2001)

  I. Interventions to minimize risk of symptom occurrence and severity of depression.

    A. Enhance client and family sense of control by informing them of the diagnosis and treatment or of changes in diagnosis and treatment and by offering choices in treatment and self-care when possible.

    B. Spend time with the client—listen and communicate acceptance.

    C. Validate thoughts, feelings, and self-perceptions as needed.

    D. Encourage the client to express feelings and ask for help when needed.

    E. Foster communications among client, family, and health team by formulating a list of concerns, facilitating care conferences, or other strategies.

    F. Initiate appropriate symptom management—pain (see Chapter 1), sleep disturbances (see Chapter 1), nausea and vomiting (see Chapter 14).

    G. Assist the client and family to redefine their goals and self-beliefs in terms of the reality of the disease, treatment, and resources.

    H. Initiate referrals to spiritual, occupational, and psychologic resources, when appropriate.

  II. Interventions to maximize client safety and comfort.

    A. Assess the client's mental status to rule out delirium as the causative factor for symptoms.

    B. Attend to dietary needs and activities of daily living (ADLs) if the client is extremely withdrawn or apathetic.

    C. Consider all discussions of suicide as serious, and report them to appropriate members of the health team.

    D. Review medications for any contribution to depressive symptoms—corticosteroids, chemotherapeutic agents, antihypertensives, benzodiazepines, β-blockers, opiates, estrogens.

    E. Monitor and report reactions to antidepressants, sedatives, anxiolytics.

    F. Caution the client against abrupt discontinuance of antidepressants and use of alcohol while taking these drugs.

    G. Report critical changes in client behaviors to appropriate health care members.

      1. Marked changes in mood or interactions, either withdrawal or agitation.

      2. Weight changes—loss or gain of 10% or more of body weight.

      3. Cognitive and physiologic changes related to insomnia that impede functioning or progress.

III. Interventions to monitor responses to depression and its treatment.
  A. Monitor physiologic changes that may explain somatic complaints.
  B. Monitor for side effects or adverse reactions to antidepressants.
  C. Observe for symptoms of withdrawal of antidepressants.
  D. Monitor behavioral changes that indicate improvement or persistence of depression.
IV. Interventions to enhance adaptation and rehabilitation.
  A. Assist with problem solving and information gathering.
  B. Provide positive reinforcement for behaviors that approximate goal achievement.
  C. Accept verbalized anger or negative feelings; try to avoid personalizing.
  D. Teach and assist the client to manage side effects of antidepressants.
      1. Dry mouth—fluid intake increase, frequent mouth care, use of sugarless gum or hard candies.
      2. Constipation—increased fluid intake, high-fiber diet, exercise.
      3. Blurred vision—will improve over time; new glasses should not be needed.
      4. Drowsiness—take medication at bedtime, symptom usually improves with time; caution about operating a motor vehicle or other machinery.
      5. Dizziness—avoid rapid movements of the head, and change positions slowly.
V. Interventions to increase client and family involvement with care.
  A. Teach the client and family to recognize the signs and symptoms of depression.
  B. Initiate referral to self-help and support groups as appropriate.
  C. Inform the client and family of telephone hotlines for crisis intervention.
  D. Teach alternative coping strategies, such as relaxation, music, or recreational activities.
  E. Assist the client to focus energy constructively by participating in health care, verbalizing feelings, and instituting health promotion activities—sleep, diet, exercise.

Evaluation

The oncology nurse systematically and regularly evaluates the client's and/or family's responses to interventions to determine progress toward the achievement of expected outcomes. Relevant data are collected, and actual findings are compared with expected findings. Nursing diagnoses, outcomes, and plans of care are reviewed and revised as necessary.

SPIRITUAL DISTRESS

Theory (Carson, 1989)

  I. Definition—state of experiencing a disturbance in one's belief or value system that provides strength, hope, and meaning in life.
  A. Presence of a spiritual self allows transcendence of immediate circumstances, such as cancer and treatment.
  B. Cultural or ethnic background influences client and family perceptions of spiritual distress.
  C. May be misdiagnosed as psychologic distress when it more correctly stems from a spiritual crisis of loss of faith or meaning.

II. Risk factors.
   A. Disease related and treatment related.
      1. Site, stage, clinical course.
      2. Nature of dysfunction and symptoms produced.
      3. Treatment required (i.e., surgery, blood transfusions, dietary restrictions, isolation).
   B. Situational.
      1. Conflict between client and family spiritual beliefs and prescribed treatment regimen.
      2. Hospital and treatment barriers to practicing spiritual rituals.
         a. Restrictions of setting (e.g., isolation, intensive care).
         b. Confinement to the bed or room, lack of privacy.
         c. Lack of availability of special foods and usual diet.
         d. Lack of understanding of, or opposition to, beliefs by family, peers, health care providers.
      3. Embarrassment at practicing spiritual rituals.
      4. Availability of spiritual resources.
III. General treatment approaches.
   A. Spiritual counseling.
   B. Performance of spiritual rites or services by an appropriate spiritual leader.
   C. Maintenance of dietary restrictions.
IV. Potential sequelae of spiritual distress.
   A. Decreased compliance with the recommended medical regimen.
   B. Loneliness and social isolation.
   C. Development of major psychiatric disorders: anxiety or depression, with a risk for suicide.

Assessment

I. History (Carpenito, 2002; Carson, 1989).
   A. Presence of risk factors.
   B. Presence of defining characteristics.
      1. Expresses concern with the meaning of life and death, suffering, or a belief system.
      2. Verbalizes inner conflict about beliefs and the relationship with a deity.
      3. Questions meaning of his/her own existence.
      4. Expresses anger toward religious representatives, God.
      5. Questions moral or ethical implications of the treatment regimen.
      6. Alterations of behavior or mood: anger, crying, withdrawal, preoccupation, anxiety, apathy.
   C. Pattern of spiritual distress: onset; frequency; intensity; precipitating, aggravating, and alleviating factors.
   D. Perceived effect of spiritual distress on client and family functioning—lifestyle, interpersonal, work, or school.

Nursing Diagnoses

I. Spiritual distress.
II. Readiness for enhancement of spiritual well-being.

Outcome Identification

I. Client expresses satisfaction with his/her own belief system and inner resources.
II. Client experiences positive meaning of his/her existence within the present circumstances and continues spiritual practices supportive to health.

Planning and Implementation (Carpenito, 2002; Carson, 1989)

I. Interventions to minimize risk and severity of spiritual distress.
  A. Eliminate or reduce barriers to spiritual practice.
    1. Provide privacy and quiet for daily prayers or other rituals.
    2. Contact the client's spiritual leader to clarify practices.
  B. Encourage spiritual practices not detrimental to health.
    1. Facilitate contacts with spiritual leaders and folk healers.
    2. Maintain the diet within spiritual restrictions when not contraindicated.
    3. Encourage spiritual practices and rituals.
    4. Contact the spiritual leader to meet with client.
  C. Be open to expressions of loneliness and powerlessness.
    1. Be available to listen and express empathy.
    2. Use values clarification to help the client identify beliefs and values.
    3. Assure the client that the nurse and others will be available to support the client in time of suffering.
    4. Be open to the client's discussion of illness and/or death.
II. Interventions to maximize safety and comfort.
  A. Provide privacy and quiet for daily prayers and rituals and visits with spiritual leaders.
  B. Provide spiritual articles according to client preferences.
  C. Facilitate the client's use of meditation, prayer, and other religious traditions and rituals.
III. Interventions to monitor complications of spiritual distress.
  A. Encourage verbalization of thoughts and feelings regarding spiritual comfort.
  B. Assess the client for lessening or continuation of feelings of fear, guilt, or anxiety.
  C. Evaluate the client for development of major psychiatric disorders—anxiety, depression, suicidal ideation.
  D. Report critical changes in emotional state to appropriate health team members—make appropriate referrals.
IV. Interventions to increase client and family involvement with care.
  A. Seek opinions and suggestions about spiritual needs from the client and family.
  B. Encourage the client and family to participate in spiritual practices together.
  C. Encourage the family to continue usual spiritual practices in the health care setting as much as possible.
  D. Discuss the treatment regimen with the client and family to identify potential areas of difficulty resulting from conflicts with spiritual beliefs.
  E. Encourage the family to participate in care of client in keeping with spiritual beliefs and practices.
  F. Discuss with the client and family the spiritual meaning illness has for them.

Evaluation

The oncology nurse systematically and regularly evaluates the client's and/or family's responses to interventions to determine progress toward the achievement of expected outcomes. Relevant data are collected, and actual findings are compared with expected findings. Nursing diagnoses, outcomes, and plans of care are reviewed and revised as necessary.

LOSS OF PERSONAL CONTROL

Theory

I. Definition—perception that one's own actions will not significantly affect an outcome; a perceived lack of control over certain events or situations that affect outlook, goals, and lifestyle (Carpenito, 2002).
   A. Each individual has a desire for control.
   B. Response to loss of personal control depends on the meaning of loss, the individual patterns of coping, personal characteristics, and the response of others.

II. Risk factors (Raines, 1998).
   A. Disease related.
      1. Lack of knowledge about the disease process or health status.
      2. Physiologic and psychologic demands of disease.
      3. Perceived loss of part of the self.
      4. Progressive, debilitating disease.
   B. Treatment related.
      1. Lack of knowledge about the treatment course, demands, and expected outcomes.
         a. Physiologic and psychologic demands of treatment.
      2. Uncontrolled symptoms and side effects of treatment (i.e., pain, nausea and vomiting, fatigue).
      3. Loss of ability to perform daily activities and roles.
   C. Situational.
      1. Loss of ability to manage one's own health care.
      2. Loss of control in decision-making matters.
      3. Hospital or institutional limitations—control relinquished to others, no privacy, altered personal space, relocation for treatment.
      4. Ineffective interpersonal interactions.
   D. Developmental.
      1. Control highly valued as part of personality.
      2. Lifestyle of dependency.
      3. Age-specific considerations.
         a. Adolescent—dependence on peers, independence from family.
         b. Young adult—marriage, parenthood.
         c. Adult—adolescent children, signs of aging, career pressures.
         d. Elderly—retirement, sensory and motor deficits, losses.

III. General treatment approaches (Raines, 1998).
   A. Inclusion of the client and family in decision making about medical treatment and care.
   B. Individual or family psychotherapy.

IV. Potential sequelae of prolonged loss of personal control.
   A. Lowered self-esteem.

    B. Helplessness.
    C. Hopelessness.
    D. Development of depression.

Assessment

  I. History (Carpenito, 2002; Raines, 1998).
    A. Presence of risk factors.
    B. Presence of subjective characteristics of loss of personal control.
      1. Expression of dissatisfaction over inability to control a situation—work, illness, prognosis, care, recovery.
      2. Expression of dissatisfaction or frustration with the negative impact of the inability to have control on outlook, goals, and lifestyle.
    C. Presence of objective characteristics of loss of personal control.
      1. Refusal or reluctance to participate in decision making.
      2. Refusal or reluctance to participate in ADLs.
      3. Refusal or reluctance to express emotions.
      4. Emotional responses may include apathy, resignation, withdrawal, uneasiness, anxiety, aggression.
      5. Responses to limitations on personal control may include attempts to circumvent limits, increased attempts to exercise control, ignoring of limits.
      6. Noncompliance with the medical treatment regimen.
    D. Perceived impact of loss of personal control on client and family ADLs, lifestyle, relationships, role responsibilities, work, or school.

Nursing Diagnoses

  I. Situational low self-esteem.
 II. Powerlessness.
III. Ineffective coping.

Outcome Identification

  I. Client begins to recognize, accept, and verbalize positive aspects of self and his/her own capabilities.
    A. Client participates in measures to minimize the risk, occurrence, severity, and complications of loss of personal control.
 II. Client expresses sense of control and participates in decisions regarding own care.
    A. Client identifies factors that can be controlled by self.
III. Client describes and initiates alternative coping strategies.

Planning and Implementation (Carpenito, 2002; Raines, 1998)

  I. Interventions to minimize the risk of occurrence, severity, or complications of a loss of personal control.
    A. Provide the client with information regarding disease, treatment, responses, and hospital or clinic routines.
    B. Provide the client and family with opportunities to participate in decision making about care.
    C. Identify factors that contribute to loss of personal control for the client.

    D. Provide consistent communications about changes in health status and the treatment regimen.

    E. Encourage client and family to express feelings related to living with cancer.

    F. Maintain personal articles, a call light, and a telephone within reach of client.

    G. Provide successful management of symptoms—pain, nausea and vomiting, sleep disturbances.

    H. Encourage the client to identify areas over which control can be maintained and to exercise decision-making skills in these areas.

  II. Interventions to monitor for complications related to loss of personal control.

    A. Elicit subjective responses of the client and family about satisfaction with amount of information received, interpersonal communications, and opportunities to participate in decision making.

    B. Assess the client's level of participation in decision-making and information-seeking activities.

    C. Assess for outcomes of loss of personal control—hopelessness, depression, suicidal intentions.

    D. Report critical changes in assessment data to appropriate health team members—inability to participate in decision making and health care, verbal expressions of despair, or suicidal intentions.

 III. Interventions to incorporate the client and family in care.

    A. Seek opinions and suggestions about care from the client and family members.

    B. Reinforce participation in decision making by the client and family members.

    C. Encourage the client and family to be responsible for portions of care, as appropriate for condition.

Evaluation

The oncology nurse systematically and regularly evaluates the client's and/or family's responses to interventions to determine progress toward the achievement of expected outcomes. Relevant data are collected, and actual findings are compared with expected findings. Nursing diagnoses, outcomes, and plans of care are reviewed and revised as necessary.

LOSS AND GRIEF

Theory

  I. Definitions (Brown-Saltzman, 1998).

    A. Loss—an experience in which an individual relinquishes a connection to a valued person, object, relationship, or situation.

      1. Loss can occur without death.

      2. Any loss can result in grief and mourning.

    B. Grief is the emotional response to loss; grief work is the adaptive process of mourning. Grief work is a process.

      1. Expressed as changes in thoughts, feelings, and behaviors experienced as a natural human response to an actual or perceived loss of a loved person, relationship, object, function, status, or identity.

      2. Affected by many factors—personality, loss history, intimacy of the lost relationship, personal resources.

  II. Risk factors (Brown-Saltzman, 1998; Carpenito, 2002).

    A. Disease related and treatment related.

1. Diagnosis of cancer, poor prognosis, uncertain outcome, likelihood of recurrence.
        2. Perceived or actual changes in body structure and function—amputation, mastectomy, colostomy, alopecia, cachexia, cognition.
        3. Chronic pain.
    B. Situational and social.
        1. Loss of persons through death, divorce, or separation.
        2. Loss of objects such as pets, home, or possessions.
        3. Nature of the relationship with the lost person or object.
        4. Multiple losses or crises and unanticipated losses.
        5. Perceived or actual loss of, or inadequate, support system.
        6. Employment losses—demotion, firing, retirement, or bankruptcy.
    C. Developmental.
        1. Aging—loss of friends, occupation, function, home.
        2. Symbolic losses—hope, dreams, autonomy or independence, loss of normalcy owing to illness.
        3. History of psychiatric illness.
III. General treatment approaches (Brown-Saltzman, 1998; Moore & Schmais, 2001).
    A. Individual or family psychotherapy.
    B. Spiritual counseling.
    C. Pharmacologic management of symptoms—anxiolytics, antidepressants, sedatives (see Chapter 10).
    D. Complementary therapies—homeopathy.
    E. Behavioral and cognitive interventions—support groups, relaxation training.
    F. Occupational or recreational therapy.
IV. Potential sequelae of loss and grief.
    A. Anticipatory grief—the experiencing of grief in response to an anticipated loss.
    B. Dysfunctional grief responses.
        1. Failure to resolve grief, resulting in detrimental activities.
            a. Prolonged denial of loss, preoccupation with images of the lost person or object, refusal to mourn.
            b. Lasting loss of normal patterns of behavior.
            c. Somatic symptoms—GI disorders, shortness of breath, muscle tension.
        2. Behavioral—abuse of substances; obsessive-compulsive behavior; phobias; difficulties with concentration, attention, and decision making.
    C. Development of psychiatric disorder—depression, suicidal ideation or attempts.

Assessment (Brown-Saltzman, 1998)

I. History.
    A. Presence of risk factors.
    B. Presence of defining physical and emotional characteristics of loss and grief.
        1. Shock and disbelief—emotional and physical immobility and denial of loss.
        2. Developing awareness—crying, angry outbursts, shortness of breath, choked feelings, sighing, flashes of anguish, retelling the story, painful dejection, and changes in eating, sleeping, and sexual interest.
        3. Bargaining and restitution—idealizing the loss and contracting for reprieval or deliverance.

   4. Accepting the loss—reliving past experiences, preoccupation with thoughts of loss, painful void in life, crying, somatic symptoms, dreams or nightmares.
   5. Resolving the loss—establishing new relationships, planning for the future, recalling rich memories or past experiences, affirming oneself, resuming previous roles.
 II. Patterns of loss and grief response.
   A. Duration.
   B. Previous losses and patterns of resolution.
   C. Presence or potential for cumulative losses.
   D. Sociocultural factors that influence the grief response—ethnicity, spiritual beliefs, religion.
   E. Potential strengths and weaknesses that may facilitate or impede the grief process, such as coping patterns, family patterns of interaction, social support system, availability of community resources.
 III. Client and family knowledge and understanding of expected thoughts, feelings, and behaviors involved with loss and grief.
 IV. Perceived meaning of the losses for the client and family.
  V. Perceived effect of losses and grief on client and family functioning—roles, relationships, ADLs, work, or school.

Nursing Diagnoses

   I. Anticipatory or dysfunctional grieving.
  II. Interrupted family processes.

Outcome Identification

   I. Client and family identify perceived losses, significance of losses, and adaptive coping strategies.
   A. Client and family discuss stages of the normal grief response.
   B. Client and family describe personal strengths and resources for dealing with loss and grief.
   C. Client and family identify institutional and community resources to deal with loss and grief.
  II. Family maintains a functional system of support for each member of the family.
   A. Family verbalizes thoughts and feelings to health care team and each other regarding the illness of the family member and its effects on the family.
   B. Family uses appropriate health agency, community, and other resources as needed.

Planning and Implementation (Brown-Saltzman, 1998; Carpenito, 2002)

   I. Interventions to minimize risk of occurrence and severity of dysfunctional grief.
   A. Use interpersonal relationship skills appropriate to the stage of the grief process.
     1. Encourage talking about perceived or actual losses.
     2. Actively listen to subjective responses to losses.
     3. Provide a supportive, nonjudgmental atmosphere to facilitate expression of negative emotions and minimize feelings of guilt.

4. Validate perceptions of responses.
5. Give the client permission to grieve and to resolve the loss.
   B. Institute measures to facilitate coping.
1. Assist the client to identify effective personal coping strategies.
2. Teach relaxation techniques.
3. Encourage participation in support groups.
4. Refer for counseling as indicated.
5. Give the client permission to resume past roles and establish new relationships.
   C. Identify a means to channel energy constructively.
II. Interventions to maximize client safety and comfort.
   A. Encourage the client to implement cultural, religious, and social customs and rituals associated with loss and grief.
   B. Advocate avoidance of conditions that block resolution of the grief process: oversedation, closed communications, social isolation.
   C. Report critical changes in behavior to appropriate members of the health care team.
1. Oversedation.
2. Withdrawal or social isolation.
3. Extreme emotional reactions—guilt, anger, hostility, depression.
4. Substance abuse—alcohol or other drugs.
5. Expression of suicidal ideations.
III. Interventions to monitor for complications related to loss and grief.
   A. Monitor for weight changes—gain or loss.
   B. Monitor changes in sleep, rest, eating patterns.
   C. Assess for a decline in physical and psychosocial functioning.
   D. Observe for withdrawal from social relationships.
IV. Interventions to enhance adaptation and rehabilitation.
   A. Encourage expression of anticipatory grief.
   B. Allow the client and family to experience the discomforts of the loss within a supportive environment.
   C. Assist in identifying modifications that will be needed in lifestyle.
   D. Provide bereavement care to assist in resolving secondary losses, attend to unfinished business, and incorporate loss into life.
   E. Support progression through the personal grieving stages.
   F. Encourage referral for support groups or psychotherapy as indicated.
V. Interventions to incorporate the client and family in care.
   A. Use teaching aids on loss and grief.
   B. Encourage the client and family to discuss their thoughts and feelings with each other.
   C. Include the family in discussion and decisions as appropriate.
   D. Provide or refer the client and family to family counseling and bereavement care.

Evaluation

The oncology nurse systematically and regularly evaluates the client's and/or family's responses to interventions to determine progress toward the achievement of expected outcomes. Relevant data are collected, and actual findings are compared with expected findings. Nursing diagnoses, outcomes, and plans of care are reviewed and revised as necessary.

SOCIAL DYSFUNCTION (CLIENT AND FAMILY)

Theory

I. Definition—a state of being unable to interact effectively with one's social environment—family, work or school, and community (Carpenito, 2002).
   A. Effective reality testing, ability to solve problems, and various coping skills are necessary for the client and family to be socially functional.
   B. The client, or family, and the environment may contribute to social dysfunction. One may be able to function in one environment or situation but not in others.
   C. Family members interact in a variety of roles that result from individual and group needs: spouse, parent, sibling, teacher, friend. Illness of one member may cause significant changes, putting the family at risk for social dysfunction.

II. Risk factors (Carpenito, 2002).
   A. Disease related and treatment related.
      1. Perceived or actual change in body structure or function.
      2. Untoward effects and side effects of treatment.
      3. Inadequate symptom control of pain, nausea and vomiting, fatigue.
      4. Chronicity of cancer.
   B. Situational.
      1. Social isolation, living alone.
      2. Language and/or cultural differences from the community and the health care environment.
      3. Prolonged treatment and hospitalization.
      4. History of substance abuse, violence, legal difficulties.
   C. Developmental.
      1. Poorly developed social and interpersonal skills.
      2. Age-related issues.
         a. Child and adolescent—altered appearance, separation from family.
         b. Adult—loss of ability to be employed.
         c. Elderly—retirement, death of spouse, friends.
      3. History of psychiatric disorder—anxiety, depression, antisocial personality, psychotic disorders, prior difficulties within the family or other interpersonal relationships.
   D. Family.
      1. Dysfunctional responses to the changing health status of family member.
      2. Dysfunctional responses to the role changes resulting from illness.
      3. Limited social support; a pattern of isolation from community, extended family, friends.
      4. Disruption of family routines because of illness.
      5. Changes in income—loss of a job, inadequate income.
      6. History of psychiatric illness or family dysfunction—depression, psychosis, violence, substance abuse, conflicting relationships, inadequate decision making and problem solving, legal difficulties.

III. General treatment approaches (Carpenito, 2002).
   A. Management of disease and treatment symptoms and their side effects.
   B. Individual, family, and group psychotherapy.
   C. Spiritual counseling.
   D. Social and financial counseling.

    E. Cognitive and behavioral interventions—behavior modification, relaxation training, support groups.

    F. Occupational and recreational therapy.

IV. Potential sequelae of social dysfunction (Carpenito, 2002).

    A. Caregiver burden—inability of family member to care for the client, changes in health of the caregiver.

    B. Social and emotional isolation of the client and family.

    C. Noncompliance with the medical treatment regimen.

    D. Interference with the client and family role while functioning at home, work, or school.

    E. Development of social deviant behavior—substance abuse, violence.

    F. Development of psychiatric disorders—anxiety, depression, suicidal ideation and/or attempts.

    G. Disruption of family relationships—separation, divorce.

Assessment (Carpenito, 2002)

I. History.

    A. Presence of client risk factors.

    B. Presence of family risk factors.

II. Presence of client behaviors or characteristics indicative of social dysfunction.

    A. Interpersonal patterns and skills.

        1. Egocentricity.

        2. Lack of self-care.

        3. Superficial relationships, blames others for interpersonal difficulties.

        4. Social isolation.

        5. Employment difficulties.

    B. Response to cancer diagnosis and treatment—anxiety, dependency, hopelessness.

    C. Support system.

        1. Living alone, alienation from family and friends.

        2. Lack of compliance with the treatment regimen.

    D. Coping skills

        1. Poor problem-solving and decision-making skills.

        2. Aggression, violence, substance abuse, legal difficulties.

        3. Psychiatric history—depression, suicidal ideation and/or attempts, antisocial personality, psychoses.

III. Presence of family characteristics or behaviors indicative of social dysfunction.

    A. Identification of family—developmental level, health status of members, caregiving abilities, current roles and relationships.

    B. Understanding of the cancer experience.

        1. Perceived threat of pain, disability, or death.

        2. Understanding of treatment and side effects.

        3. Beliefs regarding prognosis and the client's potential for regaining health.

    C. Meaning of the cancer experience.

        1. Perceived impact of cancer on family roles and relationships—role conflict, role strain, conflict, family violence.

        2. Perceived emotional impact of cancer—frustration, helplessness, guilt, grieving.

        3. Perceived impact on family decision making and problem solving—evaluation of effectiveness.

    D. Family resources.
      1. Limited or threatened financial resources—unemployment, social service agency involvement, insurance limitations.
      2. Limited social and emotional resources.
        a. Socially isolated.
        b. Estranged or troubled relationships with extended family.
        c. Minimal connection with community support systems (i.e., churches, social service agencies, neighborhood activities).
      3. Ineffective family coping.
        a. Family conflict and/or violence, substance abuse.
      4. Legal difficulties, involvement of social service agencies.

Nursing Diagnoses

  I. Impaired social interaction.
 II. Ineffective role performance.
III. Interrupted family processes.

Outcome Identification

 I. Client describes the impact of disease and its treatment on the ability to function socially.
    A. Client discusses strategies to promote more effective social functioning.
II. Family maintains a functional system of support for each member of the family.
    A. Family verbalizes thoughts and feelings to health care team and each other regarding the illness of the family member and its effects on the family.
    B. Family uses appropriate health agency, community, and other resources as needed.

Planning and Implementation

I. Interventions to minimize risk and severity of social dysfunction (Carpenito, 2002).
    A. Client-centered interventions.
      1. Instruct regarding disease, treatment regimen and expected responses, symptoms and side effects.
      2. Discuss effects of disease and treatment on the ability to function socially.
        a. Assist the client in managing disease-related and treatment-related stresses, including symptom management.
      3. Help the client identify how stress precipitates problems with social functioning.
      4. Encourage an increase in awareness of strengths and limitations in communicating to others, analyzing which approaches work best.
      5. Support appropriate interpersonal communication.
      6. Encourage respect for the rights of others—family members, friends, health team members.
      7. Encourage involvement in already established relationships.
      8. Encourage involvement in social and community activities.
      9. Refer to appropriate agencies and services for support of optimal social functioning—financial counseling, social services, community activities, support groups, psychiatric services, substance abuse programs.
    B. Family-focused interventions.
      1. Instruct regarding the disease, treatment regimen, and expected client responses—symptoms and side effects.

2. Discuss the effect of the client's illness and treatment on family functioning—physical; emotional; role; activities at home, work, or school.
3. Assist the family in managing stresses stemming from the client's illness.
4. Encourage family members to discuss thoughts and feelings regarding the illness and its effects with each other and with the client.
5. Encourage the family to continue relationships with others, including those who are extended family and friends, and to continue community activities.
6. Support the family in maintaining functional family routines as much as possible.
7. Refer the family to appropriate resources—support groups, financial counseling, social services, individual or family psychiatric services, substance abuse programs.

II. Interventions to maximize safety and comfort related to social function or dysfunction (Carpenito, 2002).
   A. Communicate empathy and understanding regarding the impact of diagnosis and treatment on social functioning.
   B. Establish limits on problematic client and family behaviors that interfere with social functioning.
      1. Social isolation, withdrawal.
      2. Lack of self-care, lack of compliance with treatment regimen.
      3. Inappropriate expressions of anger and violence.
      4. Substance abuse.
      5. Suicidal attempts and/or ideation.
   C. Provide positive feedback for compliance with limits on socially dysfunctional behavior.
   D. Report changes in behavior that threaten client and family social functioning to the appropriate health team members.

III. Interventions to enhance adaptation and rehabilitation (Carpenito, 2002).
   A. Create a private and supportive care environment for the client and family.
   B. Assist the client and family in identifying their strengths in managing the demands of illness and its treatment.
   C. Discuss with the client and family the family's limitations in providing care for the client—risk of caregiver burden, available resources to assist with care.
   D. Identify, with the client and family, cultural and spiritual beliefs and practices that may be judged by others as interfering with social functioning.
   E. Educate the health care team as to cultural and spiritual beliefs and practices.
   F. Support family cohesiveness.
   G. Make appropriate referrals to needed agency and community resources.

IV. Interventions to incorporate the client and family in care (Carpenito, 2002).
   A. Provide the client and family with knowledge and skills required for provision of day-to-day care.
   B. Facilitate family strengths related to care of the client.
      1. Acknowledge the family's ability to care for the client.
      2. Involve the family in care of the client as desired.
      3. Involve the family in the decision-making process with health team members regarding care.
   C. Encourage the client to participate in self-care within limits of the physical condition.
   D. Assess outcomes of caregiving activities—effects on caregiver, effects on social functioning of client and family members.

Evaluation

The oncology nurse systematically and regularly evaluates the client's and/or family's responses to interventions to determine progress toward the achievement of expected outcomes. Relevant data are collected, and actual findings are compared with expected findings. Nursing diagnoses, outcomes, and plans of care are reviewed and revised as necessary.

REFERENCES

American Cancer Society (ACS). (2000). *Complementary and alternative cancer methods.* Atlanta: Author.

American Psychiatric Association (APA). (2000). *Diagnostic and statistical manual of mental disorders* (4th ed., text revision). Washington, DC: Author.

Brown-Saltzman, K. (1998). Transforming the grief experience. In Carroll-Johnson, Gorman, & Bush (Eds.). *Psychosocial nursing care: Along the cancer continuum.* Pittsburgh: Oncology Nursing Press, pp. 192-214.

Bush, N. (1998a). Anxiety and the cancer experience. In Carroll-Johnson, Gorman, & Bush (Eds.). *Psychosocial nursing care: Along the cancer continuum.* Pittsburgh: Oncology Nursing Press, pp. 125-138.

Bush, N. (1998b). Coping and adaptation. In Carroll-Johnson, Gorman, & Bush (Eds.). *Psychosocial nursing care: Along the cancer continuum.* Pittsburgh: Oncology Nursing Press, pp. 35-52.

Carpenito, L.J. (Ed.). (2002). *Nursing diagnosis: Application to clinical practice* (9th ed.). Philadelphia: Lippincott, Williams & Wilkins.

Carson, V. (1989). *Spiritual dimensions of nursing practice.* Philadelphia: W.B. Saunders.

Holland, J. (Ed.). (1998). Clinical course of cancer. In J. Holland (Ed.). *Psycho-Oncology.* New York: Oxford University Press.

Massie, M.J. (1998). Depression. In J. Holland (Ed.). *Psycho-Oncology.* New York: Oxford University Press.

Moore, K., & Schmais, L. (2001). *Living well with cancer.* New York: G.P. Putnam's Sons.

National Comprehensive Cancer Network (NCCN). (1999). NCCN practice guidelines for management of psychosocial distress (NCCN Proceedings). *Oncology 13*(5A), 113-147.

Noyes, R., Holt, C., & Massie, M.J. (1998). Anxiety disorders. In J. Holland (Ed.). *Psycho-Oncology.* New York: Oxford University Press.

Raines, M. (1998). Powerlessness. In Carroll-Johnson, Gorman, & Bush (Eds.). *Psychosocial nursing care: Along the cancer continuum.* Pittsburgh: Oncology Nursing Press, pp. 253-263.

3 Coping: Altered Body Image and Alopecia

BETH A. FREITAS

BODY IMAGE

Theory

I. Body image is the dynamic perception and feelings related to one's appearance, body function, and sensations (Dropkin, 1999).

II. Risk factors.
   A. Actual or perceived changes in body reality (Weber et al., 2001).
      1. Altered physiology: cachexia, cognitive dysfunction, sterility.
      2. Treatment and side effects, such as surgical scars/amputation, weight loss or gain.
      3. Symptoms: pain, discomfort, fatigue, nausea and vomiting.
      4. Normal development: growth spurts, dependency with aging, or maturation of client.
      5. Body function changes, that is, sexual dysfunction.
   B. Actual or perceived changes in social network (Price, 2000).
   C. Lack of decision making in amount of disfigurement.
   D. Limited positive compensatory behaviors.

III. Principles of medical management.
   A. Preventive and reconstructive procedures to minimize disease or treatment effects.
   B. Prosthetic devices.
   C. Medications, such as antianxiety or antidepressant agents.
   D. Behavioral interventions, such as self-help groups or relaxation therapy.
   E. Psychotherapy either as an individual or in a group (Price, 2000).

IV. Potential sequelae of disturbed body image.
   A. Role abandonment or ineffectiveness.
   B. Social isolation and loneliness.
   C. Sexual dysfunction.
   D. Emotional distress—anxiety.
   E. Depression.

Assessment

I. Presence of risk factors.

II. Perception of specific client before body image change regarding overall attractiveness, self-confidence, self-concept, and sexuality; assumption that women with breast conservation therapy have a better body image than mastectomy clients is not always accurate (Kraus, 1999).

III. Responses of significant others, work and social contacts regarding body image changes (Price, 2000).
IV. Defining characteristics of body image changes.
  A. Physical changes.
    1. Neglect or compulsive attention to self-care or grooming; ask how feeling versus assumption based on appearance (Cohen et al., 1998).
    2. Weight gain or loss.
    3. Insomnia or hypersomnia.
  B. Cognitive changes.
    1. Decreased attention span, problems with concentration, or forgetfulness.
    2. Difficulty with problem solving, decision making, or memory loss.
  C. Psychosocial changes.
    1. Dysfunctional grieving.
    2. Expressions of self-doubt, self-negation, or fear of rejection.
    3. Hesitancy or discomfort in social interactions—avoidance of social contact.
    4. Self-destructive behaviors, such as self-neglect, alcoholism, or other drug misuse.
    5. Sexual dysfunction, such as impotence or frigidity.
    6. Refusal to look at or touch the changed body part (Newell, 2002).
    7. Refusal to assume responsibility for the changed body function (e.g., to care for a stoma).

Nursing Diagnoses

  I. Disturbed body image.
  II. Situational low self-esteem.
  III. Ineffective sexuality patterns.
  IV. Impaired social interaction.

Outcome Identification

  I. Client identifies body image changes, significance of changes, and adaptive coping strategies.
    A. Client utilizes community resources to deal with changes and achieve maximal functioning.
  II. Client recognizes, accepts, and verbalizes positive aspects of self and his/her own capabilities.
    A. Client discusses plans for reintegration of roles and social interactions.
  III. Client or couple expresses satisfaction with the way they express intimacy.
  IV. Client begins to become actively involved with others.

Planning and Implementation

  I. Interventions to minimize risk of severity of body image disturbance.
    A. Provide an opportunity to discuss losses and meaning to self and significant others (Cohen et al., 1998; Newell, 2002).
    B. Give permission to grieve and to resolve losses.
    C. Allow the client to ventilate negative emotions, such as anger and guilt.
    D. Monitor responses of others that imply rejection of the client or negative reactions to body changes.

E. Educate the client about potential body image changes and reactions before treatment.
F. Educate the client and significant others as to concerns related to body image changes that may be priorities to each at different times.
G. Stress the temporary nature of some side effects and limit in function.
H. Allow children time to play with dolls to work out feelings.
I. Discuss with teenagers the impact of their body change on their peer group and ways to reintegrate.
II. Interventions to enhance adaptation and rehabilitation—prepare the client and family for changes in structure or function.
  A. Ensure participation in the informed consent and treatment decision-making processes.
  B. Initiate referral to client and family services, such as United Ostomy Association, Reach to Recovery, or International Association of Laryngectomees. Patient's focus may be survival and not body image or function until after surgery and initial recovery.
  C. Determine readiness to view changes and assume responsibility for self-care. Head and neck patients have identified the following as important: facial expression of emotions, ability to communicate, identity preservation, and the ability to continue to articulate their intellect (Dropkin, 1999).
  D. Support the client and family during the initial viewing of changes.
    1. Provide literature, videos, audiotapes, resource referrals (e.g., *I Can Cope*, National Cancer Institute Information Line, American Cancer Society [ACS], Look Good Feel Better Program), community peer support resources.
    2. Initiate discharge planning that facilitates reintegration to work, the school system, or social settings (Price, 2000).
    3. Provide resources for product and prosthesis sources.
III. Interventions to incorporate the client and family in care.
  A. Teach use of restorative devices and rehabilitation procedures.
  B. Observe client and family return demonstrations of self-care.
  C. Teach the client and family strategies to identify destructive behaviors and resources to assist in management.
  D. Use active listening and nonjudgmental acceptance to facilitate discussion of concerns such as intimacy, resumption of sexual activity, and explanations to significant others (Cohen et al., 1998).
  E. Encourage positive family coping behaviors: open communication, distraction, humor.

Evaluation

The oncology nurse systematically and regularly evaluates the client's and/or family's responses to interventions to determine progress toward the achievement of expected outcomes. Relevant data are collected, and actual findings are compared with expected findings. Nursing diagnoses, outcomes, and plans of care are reviewed and revised as necessary.

ALOPECIA

Theory

I. Alopecia is loss of hair (scalp, facial, axillary, pubic, eyebrow, eyelash, nasal, body).

II. Risk factors.
  A. Treatments that impact rapidly dividing cells damage hair follicles, causing temporary/permanent hair loss (Pickard-Holley, 1995).
  B. Radiation therapy dosage greater than 30 to 35 gray (Gy) may cause temporary hair loss, and dosage greater than 40 Gy may cause permanent hair loss in the area being treated (Alley et al., 2002).
  C. Hair loss associated with chemotherapy generally is temporary and agent/dose dependent (Pickard-Holley, 1995).
  D. Chemotherapeutic agents that often or commonly cause alopecia are bleomycin (Blenoxane), cyclophosphamide (Cytoxan), daunorubicin (Cerubidine, DaunoXome), docetaxel (Taxotere), doxorubicin (Adriamycin), etoposide (VP-16), idarubicin (Idamycin), ifosfamide (Ifex), mechlorethamine (Mustargen), methotrexate (Mexate, Folex), mitoxantrone (Novantrone), and paclitaxel (Paxene, Taxol) (Alley et al., 2002).
  E. Administration of multiple chemotherapy agents increases the chances of total alopecia.
III. Principles of medical management.
  A. No significant data exist that scalp hypothermia or scalp tourniquet decreases hair loss; however, scalp hypothermia or scalp tourniquet may increase the risk of scalp metastases (Batchelor, 2001).
IV. Potential sequelae of alopecia.
  A. Increased heat loss through scalp.
  B. Loss of eyelashes and nasal hair decreases the body's natural resistors.
  C. Impaired self-concept.
  D. Decreased sexual and social interaction.

Assessment

  I. History.
  A. Current hair growth, style, color.
 II. Physical examination.
  A. Thinning of hair or complete hair loss.
  B. Location of hair loss.
III. Psychosocial examination.
  A. Perceptions of client before and after hair loss about self-concept, body image, perceived sexuality and responses of significant others including social and work acquaintances to hair loss.
    1. Reactions of teenagers and children also need to be assessed.
  B. Impact on social interaction.

Nursing Diagnoses

  I. Disturbed body image.
 II. Risk for situational low self-esteem.

Outcome Identification

  I. Client discusses potential effects of alopecia on body image, sexuality, social interaction, and body function.
  A. Client identifies community resources, such as the ACS's Toppers program, insurance benefits available, and peers who also have dealt with hair loss issues.
  B. Client identifies measures to adapt to alopecia.

II. Client identifies impact of alopecia on self and implements strategies to avoid low self-esteem.

Planning and Implementation

I. Interventions to maximize coping with alopecia.
  A. Provide anticipatory guidance related to hair loss (Batchelor, 2001).
   1. Provide information related to hair loss and regrowth.
     a. Hair loss occurs 2 to 3 weeks after treatment begins.
     b. Loss occurs over a period of days to weeks or may occur in 1 day.
     c. Regrowth usually starts 6 to 8 weeks after completion of therapy.
     d. Color and texture of regrown hair may differ from hair growth before loss.
   2. Encourage clients to obtain scarves, turbans, caps, hats, and/or wigs before hair loss. Cotton products let scalp breathe.
   3. Encourage clients to experiment with new hairstyles/colors before hair loss. Some salons have computerized systems to "visualize" a new look (McGarvey et al., 2001).
   4. No physical or pharmacologic interventions prevent alopecia (Pickard-Holley, 1995).
  B. Other measures to decrease side effects of hair loss (Batchelor, 2001).
   1. Ski cap or other head cover to prevent heat loss in cold climates.
   2. A large-brimmed hat or sunscreen (SPF 30) on the scalp to protect from the sun.
   3. Glasses, sunglasses, and eye drops to protect eyes.
II. Implement strategies to enhance adaptation and rehabilitation.
  A. Identify community and personal resources for financial assistance with head coverings.
  B. Refer to programs that provide tools for the client to improve physical appearance.
  C. Encourage discussion of responses to alopecia among clients and significant others and with the health care team (Pickard-Holley, 1995).
  D. Inform client that products that supposedly promote hair regrowth, such as vitamin E or gelatin, have not been proven helpful. Encourage a healthy diet.

Evaluation

The oncology nurse systematically and regularly evaluates the client's and/or family's responses to interventions to determine progress toward the achievement of expected outcomes. Relevant data are collected, and actual findings are compared with expected findings. Nursing diagnoses, outcomes, and plans of care are reviewed and revised as necessary.

REFERENCES

Alley, E., Green, R., & Schuchter, L. (2002). Cutaneous toxicities of cancer therapy. *Current Opinions in Oncology 14*(2), 212-216.

Batchelor, D. (2001). Hair and cancer chemotherapy: Consequences and nursing care—a literature study. *European Journal of Cancer Care 10*, 147-163.

Cohen, M.Z., Kahn, D.L., & Steeves, R.H. (1998). Beyond body image: The experience of breast cancer. *Oncology Nursing Forum 25*(5), 835-841.

Dropkin, M.J. (1999). Body image and quality of life after head and neck cancer surgery. *Cancer Practice 7*(6), 309-313.

Kraus, P.L. (1999). Body image, decision making, and breast cancer treatment. *Cancer Nursing* 22(6), 421-427.

McGarvey, E.L., Baum, L.D., Pinkerton, R.C., & Rogers, L.M. (2001). Psychological sequela and alopecia among women with cancer. *Cancer Practice* 9(6), 283-289.

Newell, R. (2002). Terminal illness and body image. *Nursing Times* 98(14), 36-37.

Pickard-Holley, S. (1995). The symptom experience of alopecia. *Seminars in Oncology Nursing* 11(4), 235-238, 298.

Price, B. (2000). Altered body image: Managing social encounters. *International Journal of Palliative Nursing* 6(4), 179-185.

Weber, C., Bronner, E., Their, P., et al. (2001). Body experience and mental representation of body image in patients with haematological malignancies and cancer as assessed with the body grid. *British Journal of Medical Psychology 74,* 507-521.

4 Coping: Cultural Issues

JOANNE K. ITANO

Theory

I. Demographics of the United States (U.S.) population have shifted dramatically with marked increases in the number of ethnic minorities (Simmonds, 2003; White, 2001).

  A. Until recently, the cultural diversity of the United States was largely limited to Caucasian immigrants from Europe who made up the majority of the population.

  B. In the 1950s, nine out of ten Americans were of European descent.

  C. According to the U.S. Census Bureau, by the year 2050, it is estimated that Hispanics will account for almost 25% of the population; African Americans, Asian and Pacific Islanders, and American Indians/Alaskan Natives will combine to total another 25% of the population.

  D. Nurses are providing care to an increasingly culturally diverse client population and must develop an understanding about culture and its relevance to competent nursing practice.

II. Definitions.

  A. Culture is the values, beliefs, norms, and practices of a particular group that are learned and shared. It guides thinking, decisions, and actions in a patterned way (Leininger, 1991).

    1. The cancer experience cannot be understood as an objective event separated from its cultural context. Culture affects the following (Kagawa-Singer, 1996):

      a. The client's and family's beliefs about the cause and meaning of the cancer.

      b. How the client and family respond to the diagnosis and the likely changes to their lifestyle and to treatments and their side effects.

      c. Concepts of body image and sexuality, public and private behavior, interactions with authority figures.

      d. Who constitutes the family and the dynamics that occur within the family unit.

  B. Ethnicity is a cultural group's perception of itself or a group identity (Potter & Perry, 2001; White, 2001).

    1. Refers to groups whose members share a common social and cultural heritage that is passed on to successive generations.

    2. The group feels a sense of identity.

III. Poverty is a major social barrier that affects entry into the health care system (ACS, 1989a, 1989b; Freeman, 2004).

  A. Poverty, not ethnicity, accounts for a 10% to 15% lower survival rate from cancer in many cultural groups.

  B. Impact of poverty on cancer is felt in ethnic minority groups because a disproportionate number of ethnic minority groups comprise the poor of America.

C. "Culture of poverty" includes unemployment; unskilled occupations; no savings; no health insurance; frequent daily food purchases in small amounts; crowded living quarters; women as single parents; low education level; critical attitudes toward the dominant class; feelings of helplessness, inferiority, fatalism, and dependency; or a present time orientation with inability to defer gratification.

D. Poverty contributes to increased cancer incidence and mortality through risk factors of chronic malnutrition, occupational exposure through unskilled jobs, early initiation into sex and multiple partners, smoking, and alcoholism.

E. Secondary prevention may be absent because of a present orientation in which survival needs take precedence over screening and early detection practices.

F. Critical attitudes toward middle class and sense of fatalism may decrease participation in screening programs.

G. Tertiary prevention (treatment) may be delayed because of lack of insurance, inability to pay fee-for-service, or limited health care access.

H. Emergency rooms used inappropriately and referral to clinics may result in fragmented care, impersonal service, long waiting hours, transportation and child care problems.

IV. Oncology nursing practice reflects respect for the unique cultural background of the client and family by providing culturally competent care (ONS, 1999).

  A. Culturally competent care (Purnell & Paulanka, 2003).

    1. Consists of the following:

      a. Developing an awareness of one's own existence, sensations, thoughts, and environment without letting it have an undue influence on those from other backgrounds.

      b. Demonstrating knowledge and understanding of the client's culture, health-related needs, and meanings of health and illness.

      c. Accepting and respecting cultural differences.

      d. Not assuming that the health care provider's beliefs and values are the same as the client's.

      e. Resisting judgmental attitudes such as "different is not as good."

      f. Being open to cultural encounters.

      g. Adapting care to be congruent with the client's culture.

    2. Is a conscious process that is ongoing.

  B. Barriers to developing cultural competence.

    1. Ethnocentrism is the tendency to view people unconsciously by using one's group and one's own customs as the standard for all judgments. May include the following (Kozier et al., 2000; White, 2001):

      a. The belief that the only valid and legitimate health care beliefs are those held by the traditional health care culture.

        (1) These beliefs and values reflect the dominant culture in the United States, that of Caucasian, middle-class Protestants of European ancestry. Common values include the following:

          (a) Achievement and success.

          (b) Individualism, independence, self-reliance.

          (c) Activity, work, ownership.

          (d) Efficiency, practicality, reliance on technology.

          (e) Material comfort.

          (f) Competition, achievement.

          (g) Youth, beauty.

    b. The health provider's own cultural background may be used as the standard for all judgments.

  2. Stereotyping is assuming that all members of the cultural group are alike.

    a. Ignores that wide variation exists within cultural groups.

V. Differences among cultural groups.

  A. African Americans (ACS, 2003a; Jemal et al., 2003; U.S. Census Bureau, 2001a, 2001b).

    1. Include immigrants from African countries, the West Indies, the Dominican Republic, Haiti, Jamaica.

    2. According to the 2000 census, there are an estimated 36.6 million African Americans in the United States, about 12.9% of the total U.S. population.

      a. About 6% are foreign born.

      b. Increased by about 6.7 million between 1990 and 2000.

      c. Poverty rate in 2001 was 22.7% for African Americans compared with 7.8% for Caucasians.

      d. 19% of African Americans have no health insurance coverage compared with 10% in Caucasians.

    3. Incidence.

      a. About 132,700 new cancer cases expected to be diagnosed in African Americans in 2003.

        (1) Most commonly diagnosed cancers among African American men are prostate (39%), lung (16%), and colon and rectum (9%).

        (2) In women, breast cancer is highest (31%), followed by lung (13%) and colon and rectum (13%) cancers.

      b. Highest cancer incidence rate of all sites in comparison to other ethnic groups (Table 4-1).

        (1) About 10% higher than Caucasians, 50% to 60% higher than in Hispanics and Asian and Pacific Islanders, and more than twice as high as the rate for American Indians/Alaskan Natives.

        (2) African American men have a 20% higher incidence rate and a 40% higher death rate from all cancers combined compared with Caucasian men.

      c. Proportion of African Americans who are diagnosed with more advanced stages of cancer is higher than Caucasians.

        (1) Other factors include unequal access to health care, a higher prevalence of coexisting conditions, and differences in tumor biology.

      d. From 1992 through 1999, cancer incidence rates decreased by 1.3%/year for African Americans compared with a decline of 0.9%/year for Caucasians.

    4. Mortality.

      a. About 63,100 African Americans are expected to die from cancer in 2003.

      b. Lung cancer accounts for the largest number of deaths for both African American men (29%) and African American women (21%), followed by prostate cancer (16%) in men and breast cancer in women (19%); then colon and rectum cancer and pancreatic cancer are third and fourth.

      c. Death rates among African Americans for all cancer sites declined by 1.2%/year between 1992 and 1999.

      d. Highest death rate from all cancers combined compared with other ethnic groups (see Table 4-1).

        (1) 30% higher when compared with Caucasians.

        (2) More than twice as high as Asian and Pacific Islanders, American Indians/Alaskan Natives and Hispanics.

TABLE 4-1

Age-Standardized Incidence and Mortality Rates* for Selected Cancer Sites by Ethnicity, U.S., 1996 to 2000

	White	African American	Asian/Pacific Islander	American Indian/Alaskan Native	Hispanic-Latino[†]
INCIDENCE					
All Sites					
Males	555.9	696.8	392.0	259.0	419.3
Females	431.8	406.3	306.9	229.2	312.2
Breast (female)	140.8	121.7	97.2	58.0	89.8
Colon and rectum					
Males	64.1	72.4	57.2	37.5	49.8
Females	46.2	56.2	38.8	32.6	32.9
Lung and bronchus					
Males	79.4	120.4	62.1	45.6	46.1
Females	51.9	54.8	28.4	23.4	24.4
Prostate	164.3	272.1	100.0	53.6	137.2
Stomach					
Males	11.2	19.9	23.0	14.4	18.1
Females	5.1	9.9	12.8	8.3	10.0
Liver					
Males	7.3	11.0	21.1	6.1	13.8
Females	2.8	3.9	7.7	5.5	5.6
Uterine cervix	9.2	12.4	10.2	6.9	16.8
MORTALITY					
All Sites					
Males	249.5	356.2	154.8	172.3	176.7
Females	166.9	198.6	102.0	115.8	112.4
Breast (female)	27.2	35.9	12.5	14.9	17.9
Colon and rectum					
Males	25.3	34.6	15.8	18.5	18.4
Females	17.5	24.6	11.0	12.1	11.4
Lung and bronchus					
Males	78.1	107.0	40.9	52.9	40.7
Females	41.5	40.0	19.1	26.2	15.1
Prostate	30.2	73.0	13.9	21.9	24.1
Stomach					
Males	6.1	14.0	12.5	7.0	9.9
Females	2.9	6.5	7.4	4.2	5.3
Liver					
Males	6.0	9.3	16.1	7.6	10.5
Females	2.7	3.7	6.7	4.3	5.0
Uterine cervix	2.7	5.9	2.9	2.9	3.7

Ries LA et al: *SEER cancer statistics review,* 1975-2000. Bethesda, MD, 2003, National Cancer Institute.
*Rates are per 100,000 and age-adjusted to the 2000 U.S. standard population.
[†]Hispanics-Latinos are not mutually exclusive from Whites, African Americans, Asian/Pacific Islanders, and American Indians/Alaskan Natives.

  e. Except for female breast cancer incidence and lung cancer death rates, where rates are highest in Caucasian females, ethnic- and gender-specific incidence and death rates for the most common cancer types are higher for African Americans than for any other ethnic minority groups.

  f. Annual mortality rates declined 1.2% in African Americans compared with a decrease of 0.9% among Caucasians.

 5. Lower 5-year relative survival rates than Caucasians for all cancer sites and at all stages of diagnosis.

  a. Believed to be caused by poverty, disparities in treatment, reduced access to health care, or diagnosis at a later stage (Bach et al., 2002; Bradley, et al., 2001; Shavers & Brown, 2002; Smedley et al., 2002).

B. Hispanics or Latinos (ACS, 2003b; Jemal et al., 2003; O'Brien et al., 2003).

 1. Are a heterogeneous group who trace their ancestry to Mexico (66%), Puerto Rico (9%), Cuba (4%), and other counties in Central and South America (15%) or other Spanish cultures (6%).

 2. Approximately 35.3 million Hispanics comprised about 12.5% of the total U.S. population according to the 2000 census.

  a. Increased from 9% of population in 1990; thus it is the nation's fastest growing minority group.

 3. Cancer occurrence and risk factors vary among Hispanics based on whether they are U.S. or foreign born, country of origin or heritage, degree of acculturation, and socioeconomic status.

 4. Incidence.

  a. In 2003 estimated 67,400 new cases of cancer.

  b. Lower incidence from all cancers combined and from the four most common cancers (breast, prostate, lung and bronchus, colon and rectum) than non-Hispanic Caucasians (see Table 4-1).

   (1) For men, prostate cancer (27%) is the most common cancer, followed by colon and rectum cancer (12%) and lung and bronchus cancer (7%).

   (2) For women, breast cancer (30%) is the highest, followed by cancers of the colon and rectum (9%) and lung and bronchus (6%).

   (3) Have higher incidence and mortality rates from cancers of the stomach, liver, uterine cervix and gallbladder.

    (a) Cancers of stomach, liver, and uterine cervix are more common in developing countries in Central and South America where Hispanics may migrate from.

    (b) Cancers of stomach, liver, and uterine cervix are particularly high among first-generation Hispanic migrants to United States.

    (c) May reflect greater exposure to specific infectious agents and lower rates of screening for cervical cancer as well as dietary patterns and possible genetic factors.

    (d) Lower utilization of Pap screening among Hispanic women may contribute to higher rates of cervical cancer; and women in the United States who were born in Mexico have a higher prevalence of human papillomavirus (HPV) (Giuliano et al., 1999).

    (e) Variations in incidence of stomach cancer may be related to prevalence of *Helicobacter pylori* infection and to diets rich in smoked foods, salted meat or fish, and pickled vegetables and low in fresh vegetables.

(i) Higher prevalence of *H. pylori* infection documented among Hispanics in the United States.

(f) Obesity and high number of pregnancies are associated with higher risk of gallbladder cancer.

(i) Hispanic women are more likely to be overweight and have a higher fertility rate than other racial/ethnic groups.

c. Mortality.

(1) In 2003, 22,100 cancer deaths estimated.

(2) Lower mortality from all cancers combined and from the four most common cancers (breast, prostate, lung and bronchus, colon and rectum) than non-Hispanic Caucasians (see Table 4-1).

(3) Lung cancer is leading cause of death among Hispanic men (22%) followed by colon and rectum and prostate cancers (10% each).

(4) For women, mortality is highest from breast cancer (16%), followed by lung (13%) and colon and rectum cancers (11%).

d. Trends.

(1) Between 1992 and 1999.

(a) Incidence rates decreased by 1.6 %/year compared with 0.8% for Caucasians.

(b) Mortality rates declined by 1.2%/year compared with 0.7% among Caucasians.

C. Asian and Pacific Islanders (U.S. Census Bureau, 2003; U.S. Department of Commerce, May 2001, February 2002).

1. Asian and Pacific Islanders have been combined as one group until the 2000 census designated the Native Hawaiians and other Pacific Islanders as a separate group.

2. Asian refers to people having origins in any of the original peoples of the Far East, Southeast Asia, or the Indian subcontinent.

a. The category includes Asian Indian, Chinese, Cambodian, Filipino, Korean, Japanese, Vietnamese, Hmong, Laotian, Thai, and other Asian (Bangladeshi, Burmese, Indonesian, Pakistani, Sri Lankan).

b. Of the U.S. population 3.6%, or 10.2 million, are Asians according to the 2000 census.

c. More than 30 different languages are spoken.

d. More than half of all people who reported being Asian live in three states: Hawaii, California, Washington.

(1) The percentage of Hawaii's population that is Asian is the highest in the nation (42%); California follows with 11%.

3. The term *Native Hawaiians and other Pacific Islanders* refers to people having origins in any of the original peoples of Hawaii, Guam, Samoa, and other Pacific Islanders (Tahitian, Northern Mariana Islander, Palauan, Fujian, or cultural groups such as Melanesian, Micronesian, or Polynesian) (U.S. Department of Commerce, May 2001, December 2001).

a. There are approximately 874,400 Native Hawaiians and other Pacific Islanders alone or in combination with one or more other races, or 0.3% of total U.S. population

b. More than half of this group lives in Hawaii and California.

4. Data (1996 to 2000) from the Surveillance Research Program of the National Cancer Institute (SEER, 2003) (see Table 4-1) indicate that as a group:

a. Asian and Pacific Islanders are fourth in cancer incidence behind African Americans, Whites, and Hispanics.

    b. Asian and Pacific Islanders have the lowest mortality rate compared with African Americans, Caucasians, Hispanics, and American Indians/Alaskan Natives.

    c. However, given the diversity of the group, there are differences in incidence and mortality rates among the different subgroups of the diverse group of Asian and Pacific Islanders. For example,

        (1) There are variations in the age-adjusted incidence rate in the top five cancers for Asian groups compared with Caucasians (Miller et al., 1996).

            (a) Stomach cancer is included for the Chinese, Japanese, Korean, Vietnamese men, and liver cancer appears in the Chinese, Filipino, Korean, Vietnamese men.

            (b) Thyroid and cervical cancers are in the top five for Filipino women.

            (c) Uterine cancer is first in incidence for Vietnamese women.

        (2) There are variations in the age-adjusted mortality rates in the top five cancers for Asian groups compared with Caucasians (Miller et al., 1996).

            (a) In Chinese men, esophageal cancer is in the top five.

            (b) For Filipino men, liver cancer is in the top five.

            (c) For Japanese men and women and Chinese women, stomach cancer is in the top five.

        (3) The state of Hawaii has a high concentration of Asians and Native Hawaiians. Data from the Hawaii Tumor Registry indicate variations among Caucasians, Hawaiian/part Hawaiian, Japanese, Chinese, and Filipinos (Hernandez, 2003).

            (a) Cancer incidence (1995 to 2000) in men is highest for Caucasians, followed by Filipinos, Hawaiians, Japanese, Chinese.

                (i) For women, cancer incidence is highest for Hawaiian women, followed by Caucasians, Japanese, Chinese, Filipinos.

            (b) Overall mortality rate (1995 to 2000) is highest for the Hawaiians, followed by the Filipinos, Caucasians, Japanese, Chinese.

            (c) Mortality trends from 1975 to 2000 show a reduction in mortality rates for all groups except the Hawaiians, which increased from a rate of 119.9 (1975 to 1979) per 100,000 population, age adjusted to the 2000 U.S. population to 220.09 (1995 to 2000).

            (d) Japanese men have the highest rates of stomach cancer and rectal cancers in Hawaii.

            (e) A substantial increase in colon cancer is noted in Filipino men.

            (f) Hawaiian women have the highest rate of lung and breast cancers.

            (g) Filipino women continue to have the highest incidence of thyroid cancer compared with both men and women of all ethnic groups.

D. American Indians/Alaskan Natives (Eberhardt et al., 2001; Keppel, et al., 2002; U.S. Census Bureau, 2001a, 2001b; U.S. Department of Commerce, May 2001).

    1. Include person having origins in any of the original peoples of North and South America including Central America and who maintain tribal affiliation or community attachment.

2. Total 2.5 million, or 0.9% of U.S. population, according to the 2000 census.
3. Lowest cancer incidence rates and third lowest cancer mortality rates among African Americans, Caucasians, Asian and Pacific Islanders, Hispanics (see Table 4-1).
   a. Percentage of deaths from lung cancer increased 28.1% between 1990 and 1998.
      (1) Higher percentage of adults who smoke cigarettes.
         (a) Men—38.8% compared with 26.1% for all races.
         (b) Women—31.7% compared with 21.9% for all races.
   b. Other major health issues affecting this group.
      (1) Age-adjusted death rates (1992 to 1994) for the following causes were much higher compared with the U.S. population (Spector, 2004).
         (a) Alcoholism—579%.
         (b) Tuberculosis—475%.
         (c) Diabetes—231%.
         (d) Accidents—212%.
         (e) Suicide—70%.
         (f) Pneumonia and influenza—61%.
         (g) Homicide—41%.
   c. Other factors influencing health.
      (1) Poverty rate in 2001 was 24.5%; higher than non-Hispanic Caucasians (7.8%), Asian and Pacific Islanders (10.2%), Hispanics of any race (21.4%), African Americans (22.7%).
      (2) Less likely to have health insurance than other racial groups based on 3-year average (1999 to 2001): 72.9% compared with 66.8% for Hispanics, 80.8% for African Americans, 81.5% for Asian and Pacific Islanders, 90.2% for non-Hispanic Caucasians.

VI. Six cultural phenomena that may vary among cultural groups and affect health care and are present in all cultural groups (Giger & Davidhizar, 2004).
   A. Communication (Giger & Davidhizar, 2004; Spector, 2004).
      1. Means by which culture is transmitted and preserved.
      2. Consists of verbal, nonverbal, and written words.
      3. Most obvious cultural difference is language.
         a. Most important factor in culturally competent care because it affects the nurse-client relationship and all phases of the nursing process.
         b. If the nurse does not speak the client's language, a translator may be needed.
      4. Common nurse responses to inability to communicate verbally with client.
         a. Avoid clients.
         b. Shout the same words louder.
         c. Focus on tasks rather than the clients.
         d. Stop talking with clients.
            (1) Start doing things for them instead of with them.
            (2) May be interpreted as implying client inferiority.
         e. Result is isolation of clients who do not speak the dominant language with possible reactions of withdrawal, hostility or belligerence, or uncooperativeness.
      5. Nonverbal communication includes use of touch, facial expressions, eye movement, body language, silence.
         a. Need to know the meaning of nonspecific nonverbal behaviors in the client's culture.

B. Space (Giger & Davidhizar, 2004; Potter & Perry, 2001).
  1. Includes the individual's body, space around the body as well as the surrounding environment, objects within that environment.
  2. In the United States, three categories of personal space.
    a. Intimate zone is within 18 inches of the body.
      (1) Used for comforting, protecting, or counseling and usually reserved for someone with whom there is great trust.
    b. Personal zone is 18 inches to 3 feet from the body.
      (1) Used for friends and some counseling.
    c. Social zone is 3 to 6 feet from the body.
      (1) Used for impersonal business being conducted.
  3. Individuals are by nature territorial.
    a. For territoriality needs to be met, the individual must be in control of some space, must establish some rules for the space, and must be able to defend it against invasion or misuse by others.
    b. The nurse often invades this personal space.
  4. Cultures vary in their use of personal space and often are not conscious of their requirements regarding personal space.
    a. May react unconsciously negatively when personal space is entered.
C. Social organization (Giger & Davidhizar, 2004; Potter & Perry, 2001).
  1. Social environment where people grow up, live, and play.
    a. Children learn their cultural responses to life events from the family in the social environment.
    b. How cultural group organizes itself around units such as families, ethnic groups, religious groups, and community or social groups.
  2. Family may be nuclear, single parent, extended or include others beyond normal bloodlines.
    a. Includes family roles and functioning.
  3. Next to family, religion is second most important social organization.
    a. Religion and religious practices may be integrated within social activity; the church may serve as a social as well as a religious organization for some groups.
    b. Religious beliefs and practices also dictate culturally accepted roles of different members of the group and rules of behavior.
  4. Behaviors are prescribed for significant life events, such as birth, death, childbearing, child rearing, role and care of the elderly, illness.
D. Time (Giger & Davidhizar, 2004; Harkreader & Hogan, 2000).
  1. Meaning and influence of time from a cultural perspective.
    a. Developed early in life as a result of experiences linked to the individual's culture.
    b. Results from learning and becomes a part of human nature.
  2. May be present, past, or future.
    a. In present orientation, time is flexible and events begin when the client arrives, which may result in client arriving late for appointments.
      (1) May have little concern for long-term preventive health practices and may respond better to short-term goals.
    b. Past orientation emphasizes influence of past events and ancestors on present events.
      (1) If traditions conflict with a prescribed treatment regimen, the client may have difficulty maintaining the plan of care.
    c. Future orientation emphasizes planning and schedules, which is often the value perspective of the dominant American culture and health professionals.

        (1) May have little difficulty following a treatment plan as long as its future benefits are clear.

        (2) May have difficulty dealing with a chronic illness for which no complete cure is known.

  3. Most cultures combine all three time orientations, but one is more likely to dominate.

E. Environmental control (Andrews & Boyle, 2002; Giger & Davidhizar, 2004; Kozier et al., 2000; Spector, 2004).

  1. Ability of members of a particular cultural group to plan activities that control nature or direct environmental factors.

  2. Beliefs about causes of illness, health beliefs, health behaviors, and actions taken when illness or disease (cultural health practices) occurs are influenced by the individual perception of the environment, which is influenced by the individual's culture.

    a. How one experiences and copes with illness is based on individual's explanation of sickness.

    b. Types of health beliefs.

      (1) Magico-religious health belief view in which health and illness are controlled by supernatural forces.

        (a) Illness is the result of being bad or opposing God's will.

        (b) Getting well depends on God's will.

        (c) Use of charms, holy words, holy actions to prevent and cure illnesses.

      (2) Scientific or biomedical health belief.

        (a) Life and life processes are controlled by physical and biochemical processes that can be manipulated by humans.

        (b) Illness is caused by microorganisms or physiologic breakdown of the body.

        (c) Client expects medication, a treatment, or surgery to cure the health problem.

      (3) Holistic health view.

        (a) Forces of nature must be maintained in balance or harmony.

        (b) When the natural balance or harmony is disturbed, illness results.

        (c) Use of natural environment and use of herbs, plants, minerals, animal substances to prevent and treat illnesses.

    c. Folk medicine as a cultural health practice.

      (1) Beliefs and practices relating to health, illness, and prevention that are based on cultural traditions.

        (a) Viewed as more humanistic than Western health care.

      (2) Consistent with holistic health view.

        (a) The body, mind, and spirit are viewed as a whole.

        (b) Healing is viewed as restoration of a person to a state of harmony among the body, mind, and spirit.

      (3) Often involves a healer who prepares a treatment and involves some ritual practice.

        (a) Healer understands the problem within a cultural context, speaks the same language, and shares a similar worldview (the way individuals look at the universe to form values about their lives and the world around them) as the client.

        (b) Healer often is consulted first by client because the healer is heritage consistent.

      (4) Consultation occurs within the community.

(5) May involve the use of herbs, plants, minerals, animal substances to prevent and treat illness.
    (a) Remedies passed down from generation to generation.
    (b) Rituals and customs often involved.
F. Biologic variations (Giger & Davidhizar, 2004; White, 2001).
    1. Differences in skin, mucous membrane, eye, or hair color; amount of body hair; hair texture; facial characteristics (e.g., thickness of lips, eye shape, location of eyelids, shape of ears, size of nose, tooth size); body size and shape.
    2. Enzymatic and genetic variations causing differences in metabolism of drugs and alcohol. For example,
        a. European Americans metabolize and excrete caffeine faster because of liver enzyme differences.
        b. Approximately 60% of the African American population more rapidly metabolize isoniazid (used to treat tuberculosis) and render it inactive more rapidly.
        c. Rapid metabolism of alcohol results in facial flushing and other vasomotor symptoms in Asian Americans and American Indians/Alaskan Natives.
        d. Chinese males tend to need about one half as much propranolol (to treat hypertension) compared with Caucasian males.
    3. Increased susceptibility to certain diseases. For example,
        a. Tay-Sachs disease is more common in people of Jewish ancestry.
        b. Thalassemia is more common among people of Mediterranean descent.
        c. Sickle cell disease is more common among African Americans.
        d. Variations in cancer incidence and mortality discussed in Section V of Theory.
    4. Dietary practices.
        a. Often culturally based in that they are learned during childhood.
            (1) Adults set tone for food patterns that establish the foundation for the child's lifelong eating customs regarding time of meals, number of meals per day, acceptable foods, methods of preparation, likes and dislikes, table manners.
G. Table 4-2 summarizes specific information on the major ethnic minority groups using the six cultural phenomena described above.
    1. This information should be used only as a guideline for practice to avoid generalizations and stereotypes.
        a. As within cultural groups, there are many subgroups that vary in beliefs and practices.
        b. Nursing interventions that consider the cultural background of a client and family must be based on a sound assessment and validation of the role that culture plays in the life of the client and family.
        c. Clients may also vary in the degree to which they identify with their dominant and traditional culture.
            (1) Values and beliefs of the children of immigrants to the United States may be less traditional than their parents.
            (2) Need to determine degree of acculturation, which is the assumption of the values, attitudes, beliefs, or practices of the dominant group (Kozier et al., 2000).
            (3) Heritage consistency is the degree to which a person's lifestyle reflects his/her traditional culture (Estes & Zitzow, 1980).

TABLE 4-2
Cross-Cultural Examples of Cultural Phenomena Affecting Nursing Care

Regions of Origin	Communication	Space	Time Orientation	Social Organization	Environmental Control	Biologic Variations
Asian China Hawaii Philippines Korea Japan Southeast Asia (Laos, Cambodia, Vietnam)	National language preference Dialects, written characters Use of silence Nonverbal and contextual cuing	Noncontact people	Present	Family: hierarchic structure; loyalty Devotion to tradition Many religions, including Taoism, Buddhism, Islam, Christianity Community social organizations	Traditional health and illness beliefs Use of traditional medicines Traditional practitioners: Chinese doctors and herbalists	Liver cancer Stomach cancer Coccidioidomycosis Hypertension Lactose intolerance
African West Coast (as slaves) Many African countries West Indian Islands Dominican Republic Haiti Jamaica	National languages Dialect: Pidgin, Creole, Spanish, French	Close personal space	Present over future	Family: many female, single parent Large, extended family networks Strong church affiliation within community Community social organizations	Traditional health and illness beliefs Folk medicine tradition Traditional healer: root-worker	Sickle cell anemia Hypertension Cancer of the esophagus Stomach cancer Coccidioidomycosis Lactose intolerance

Group	Language	Space/Touch	Time	Social Organizations	Health Beliefs	High-Risk Health Problems
Europe Germany England Italy Ireland Other European countries	National languages Many learn English immediately	Noncontact people Aloof Distant Southern countries: closer contact and touch	Future over present	Nuclear families Extended families Judeo-Christian religions Community social organizations	Primary reliance on modern health care system Traditional health and illness beliefs Some remaining folk medicine traditions	Breast cancer Heart disease Diabetes mellitus Thalassemia
Native American 170 Native American tribes Aleuts Eskimos	Tribal languages Use of silence and body language	Space very important and has no boundaries	Present	Extremely family oriented Biologic and extended families Children taught to respect traditions Community social organizations	Traditional health and illness beliefs Folk medicine tradition Traditional healer: medicine man	Accidents Heart disease Cirrhosis of the liver Diabetes mellitus
Hispanic countries Spain Cuba Mexico Central and South America	Spanish or Portuguese primary language	Tactile relationships Touch Handshakes Embracing Value physical presence	Present	Nuclear family Extended families *Compadrazzo:* godparents (rural Mexico) Community social organizations	Traditional health beliefs Folk medicine tradition Traditional healers: *curandero, espiritista, partera, señora*	Diabetes mellitus Parasites Coccidioidomycosis Lactose intolerance

Modified from Spector RE: Culture, ethnicity, and nursing. In Potter PA, Perry AG, editors: *Fundamentals of nursing: concepts, process, and practice*, ed 5, St Louis, 2001, Mosby.

(a) Exists on a continuum.
(b) A person can possess value characteristics of both a consistent heritage (traditional) and an inconsistent heritage (acculturated).
(c) Factors that demonstrate heritage consistency include the individual (Spector, 2004).
  (i) Grew up in the country of origin or lives in a U.S. neighborhood of like ethnic group.
  (ii) Participates in traditional religious or cultural activities.
  (iii) Makes frequent visits to the country of origin or to the old neighborhood in the United States.
  (iv) Maintains regular contact or lives with the extended family.
  (v) Name has not been Americanized.
  (vi) Was educated in a school with a religious or ethnic philosophy similar to personal background.
  (vii) Participates mainly in social activities with others of the same ethnic background.
  (viii) Demonstrates personal pride about his/her national and ethnic origin.
  (ix) Includes elements of historical beliefs and practices into personal philosophies.

Assessment

I. Accurately assessing a client's culture begins with self-awareness (Kozier et al., 2000; Potter & Perry, 2001).
  A. Understanding that each individual, including the nurse, is unique and a product of past experiences, beliefs, and values that have been learned and passed down from one generation to the next.
  B. Knowledge of the nurse's own culture, which includes the culture of the U.S. health care system.
  C. Recognition of the nurse's prejudices and biases.
  D. Demonstration of respect and appreciation for cultural behaviors based on an understanding of the other person's perspective.
II. Assessing the client's culture (Andrews & Boyle, 2002; Giger & Davidhizar, 2004; ONS, 1999).
  A. Culture.
    1. Does the client identify with a particular ethnic, racial, or cultural group?
    2. Where was the client born?
    3. How long has the client lived in the United States?
  B. Communication.
    1. Can the client communicate in English?
      a. Both spoken and written?
      b. How fluent is the client in use of English?
    2. What language is spoken in the home?
      a. Does the client speak other languages?
    3. Does the client speak for self or defer to another?
      a. Is there a family spokesperson?
    4. What nonverbal communication behaviors are observed (e.g., touching, eye contact, silence)?
      a. What significance do these behaviors have for the nurse-client interaction?

C. Space.
　　1. Observe the client's proximity to other people and objects within the environment.
　　2. How does the client react to the nurse's movement toward the client?
　　3. Assess the client's physical environment (especially important in home health care, community nursing, long-term care nursing).
　　4. What cultural objects within the environment have importance for health promotion and health maintenance?
D. Social organization.
　　1. Who comprises the client's social network (family, friends, peers, etc.)?
　　　　a. What are the client's role and function in the family and the community?
　　2. Is the client the primary decision maker for health care behaviors?
　　　　a. Must the client consult another to make health decisions? If so, who?
　　3. Are there cultural or religious leaders who are important in the client's health decision making?
　　4. Does the client identify with a specific religious group?
　　　　a. How do the beliefs of this group affect practices related to health and illness?
　　　　b. What is the role of religious representatives and beliefs and practices during health and illness?
　　5. What does the client do during free time?
　　6. Who financially supports the family?
　　　　a. How important is work to the client and family (from an economic and value-to-the-client perspective)?
E. Time.
　　1. What is the client's time orientation: past, present, or future?
　　2. What is the significance of time for the client?
　　3. Does the client talk about time in specifics, such as dates or times, or in generalities, such as "a long time" or a "short time"?
F. Environmental control.
　　1. What is the client's view of health beliefs?
　　　　a. What does the client believe to be the cause of the cancer?
　　　　　　(1) Do the client's beliefs affect decisions regarding cancer treatment?
　　　　b. What does the client believe promotes health?
　　2. What cultural healing practices has the client used?
　　　　a. Has the client used the services of a cultural healer?
　　　　b. Are there healing rituals or practices that the client believes can promote well-being or recovery from illness?
　　　　c. Is the client wearing or carrying any amulets or artifacts that are believed to have healing properties?
　　3. How are Western health care providers perceived?
　　4. Does the gender or culture of the health care provider have an impact on client?
G. Biologic variations.
　　1. Are there normal variations in anatomic characteristics (e.g., body structure or size, color of skin and mucous membranes, hair color, hair texture or distribution, facial characteristics)?
　　2. What are the dietary preferences of the client?
　　　　a. Are the dietary preferences related to the client's ethnicity?
　　　　b. What is the meaning of food and mealtimes to the client?

    c. Are there preferences for kinds of food, time of day of eating, or food taboos?

      (1) Do these practices conflict with recommended dietary practices?

  3. Is the client at risk for nutritional deficiencies because of ethnicity (e.g., pernicious anemia, lactose intolerance)?

  4. Are there variations in physiologic functioning related to the client's ethnicity (e.g., drug metabolism, alcohol metabolism)?

  5. Are there illnesses or diseases for which the client is at risk because of ethnicity (e.g., hypertension, diabetes mellitus, sickle cell anemia, specific cancers)?

H. Other cultural assessment tools may be located in the following:

  1. ONS Multicultural Tool Kit (www.ons.org) (ONS, 2001).

  2. Estes, 2002.

  3. Luckmann, 2000.

Nursing Diagnoses

Many nursing diagnoses are appropriate for a client of any cultural group. Based on a complete and valid assessment, the nurse will identify appropriate nursing diagnoses and individualize nursing interventions based on the client's beliefs, values, and practices, as appropriate. The following are selected nursing diagnoses that are likely to have cultural implications.

  I. Impaired verbal communication

 II. Decisional conflict.

III. Compromised family coping

IV. Noncompliance.

Outcome Identification

  I. Client is able to effectively communicate needs.

 II. Client expresses satisfaction with health care decisions that are congruent with his/her beliefs, values and practices.

III. Family able to adapt care for client based on their and the client's beliefs, values, practices.

IV. Client follows the therapeutic plan that is adapted to client's beliefs, values, lifestyle, as appropriate.

Planning and Implementation

  I. Interventions related to the nurse (Giger & Davidhizar, 2004; Harkreader & Hogan, 2000; Kozier et al., 2000; Potter & Perry, 2001; White, 2001).

  A. Recognize that cultural diversity (differences among people that result from racial, ethnic, cultural variations) exists and that culture has a significant impact on health care.

  B. Assess personal beliefs regarding individuals from different cultures.

    1. Review personal beliefs, past experiences, biases, prejudices, stereotypes.

    2. Set aside any values, biases, ideas, attitudes that are judgmental and may negatively affect health care.

      a. As with clients, these values are not likely to change but once identified, their impact on the nurse's behaviors can be minimized.

  C. Analyze personal communication style (e.g., facial expressions, body language) and how these behaviors may be interpreted by others.

   D. Be sensitive to the uniqueness of the client.
      1. Respect the unfamiliar.
   E. Appreciate that each person's cultural values are ingrained and therefore very difficult to change.
   F. Understand that respect for the client and his/her beliefs and practices is central to the therapeutic relationship.
      1. Communicate respect by using a kind and attentive approach.
      2. Adopt an attitude of flexibility, respect, and interest to help bridge barriers imposed by culture.
   G. Do not expect all members of one cultural group to behave in exactly the same way. Expect individual differences.
      1. Many individuals have beliefs, values, and practices from their cultural group as well as the dominant Western culture (see information on heritage consistency in Section VI.G of Theory).
   H. Remember that the color of a client's skin does not always determine the client's culture.
   I. Learn about the different beliefs and values of the major ethnic or cultural groups with whom the nurse is likely to have contact.
      1. Identify sources of discrepancy between the client's and the nurse's concepts of health and illness.
      2. Respect the client's right to have his/her own beliefs and practices even if they differ from the nurse's and the nurse disagrees with them.
   J. Complete a cultural assessment.
      1. Use the data to implement an individualized plan of care incorporating the client's cultural values and beliefs, as appropriate.
II. Interventions related to interacting with clients of different cultures (Harkreader & Hogan, 2000; Kozier et al., 2000; Potter & Perry, 2001; White, 2001).
   A. When meeting a client for the first time, the nurse should introduce himself/herself and explain his/her position.
      1. Be aware of nonverbal cues about space and touch as the nurse approaches the client.
   B. Be honest about the knowledge the nurse lacks about the client's culture.
      1. Do not make assumptions about the client's beliefs, values, practices.
      2. Ask the client about anything the nurse does not understand.
         a. Use the client and family as sources of information whenever possible.
   C. Always address the client by last name (e.g., Mr. Sanchez, Dr. Bonito) until he/she gives the nurse permission to use other names.
   D. Use language that is culturally sensitive (e.g., Latino versus Hispanic, Asian versus Oriental, African American versus black).
   E. Determine if the client's beliefs and practices about health and illness conflict with the dominant culture.
      1. If they are not congruent, determine what impact it will have.
   F. Be willing to modify health care delivery in keeping with the client's cultural background.
   G. Support the client's practices, and incorporate them into nursing practice whenever possible and when they are not contraindicated for health reasons.
      1. Recognize that cultural symbols and practices can often bring a client comfort.
      2. Do not impose a cultural practice on a client without knowing whether it is acceptable, desirable, or important to the client.
   H. Be considerate of reluctance to talk when the subject involves intimate matters.

        1. For example, sexual matters are not freely discussed and especially not with members of the opposite gender in some cultures.

   I. During illness clients may return to their preferred cultural practices.

        1. For example, a client who has learned English as a second language may revert to the primary language.

III. Interventions related to communication (Harkreader & Hogan, 2000; Kozier et al., 2000; Potter & Perry, 2001; Purnell & Paulanka, 2003; White, 2001).

   A. Relate to the client in an unhurried manner that takes into account the social and cultural amenities.

        1. Give time for the client to answer.

        2. Engaging in appropriate social conversation before discussing more intimate personal details may be an effective strategy.

        3. Learn how listening is communicated in the client's culture.

        4. Listen actively and attentively.

   B. Recognize differences in the ways clients communicate, and do not assume the meaning of a specific behavior (e.g., lack of eye contact) without validating its meaning.

   C. Use validating techniques in communication.

        1. Be alert for feedback that the client is not understanding.

        2. Note that big smiles and frequent head nodding or lack of questions may indicate that the client is trying to please, not necessarily that the client understands.

   D. Be aware that in some cultural groups, discussion concerning the client with others may be offensive and may impede the nursing process.

   E. Use interpreters to improve communication.

        1. Use dialect-specific interpreters.

        2. Use interpreters trained in health care, if available.

        3. Avoid interpreters from a rival tribe, state, region, or nation.

        4. Be aware of gender and relationship differences between the interpreter and client.

            a. Same-gender interpreters are preferred.

            b. Caution is needed because the client may be hesitant to reveal personal information if the interpreter is a child, relative, or friend.

        5. Be aware of age differences between the interpreter and client.

            a. Older, more mature interpreter is preferred.

        6. Address questions to the client, not the interpreter.

        7. Ask one question at a time, and allow time for interpretation and a response before asking another question.

        8. Ask the interpreter to translate as closely as possible the words used by the nurse.

        9. Observe the facial expressions and body language of the client and interpreter.

            a. The client is likely very aware of the nurse's body language and verbal communication. Speak slowly in a quiet tone of voice in an unhurried manner.

   F. Adopt special approaches when there is no interpreter (Andrews & Boyle, 2003).

        1. Use a caring tone of voice and appropriate facial expressions to help alleviate client fears.

            a. Proceed in an unhurried manner.

            b. Pay attention to any effort by the client and family to communicate.

        2. Speak slowly and distinctly but not loudly.

            a. Be polite.

3. Greet the person using the last or complete name.
4. Use gestures, pictures, and play acting to help the client understand.
5. Use any words known in the client's language.
   a. Learn key phrases in languages that are commonly encountered in the nurse's community.
6. Ask who among the client's family and friends could serve as an interpreter.
7. Try a third language.
   a. Some Indo-Chinese speak French.
   b. Many Koreans speak Japanese.
8. Keep the message simple, and repeat frequently.
   a. Avoid medical jargon.
9. Validate whether the client understands by having him/her repeat instructions, demonstrate procedure, or act out meaning.

IV. Interventions to enhance access to health care (Black & Ades, 1994; Itano, Clark, & Hussey, 2001).
   A. Involve trusted and respected members of cultural groups in the planning and delivery of health care services to their communities.
   B. Develop culturally sensitive client education materials.
   C. Use the navigator concept to assist individuals in overcoming health care access barriers.
      1. Use of a navigator, often an individual of similar cultural background, who can guide the client around and through the labyrinth of the health care system.
      2. Navigator also provides education and support to the client.

Evaluation

The oncology nurse systematically and regularly evaluates the client's and/or family's responses to interventions to determine progress toward the achievement of expected outcomes. Relevant data are collected, and actual findings are compared with expected findings. Nursing diagnoses, outcomes, and plans of care are reviewed and revised as necessary.

REFERENCES

American Cancer Society (ACS). (1989a). *Cancer in the economically disadvantaged: A special report.* Atlanta: Author.

American Cancer Society (ACS). (1989b). A summary of the American Cancer Society report to the nation: Cancer in the poor. *CA: A Cancer Journal for Clinicians 39,* 263-265.

American Cancer Society (ACS). (2003a). *Cancer facts & figures for African Americans, 2003-2004.* Atlanta: Author.

American Cancer Society (ACS). (2003b). *Cancer facts & figures for Hispanics/Latinos, 2003-2005.* Atlanta: Author.

Andrews, M., & Boyle, J. (2002). *Transcultural concepts in nursing care* (4th ed.). Philadelphia: Lippincott Williams & Wilkins.

Bach, P.B., Schrag, D., Brawley, O.W., et al. (2002). Survival of blacks and whites after a cancer diagnosis. *JAMA 287*(16), 2106-2113.

Black, B.L., & Ades, T. (1994). American Cancer Society urban demonstration projects: Models for successful intervention. *Seminars in Oncology Nursing 10,* 96-103.

Bradley, C.J., Givens, C.W., & Roberts, C. (2001). Disparities in cancer diagnosis and survival. *Cancer 91*(1), 178-188.

Eberhardt, M.S., Ingram, D.D., Makuc, D.M., et al. (2001). *Health, United States, 2001, with urban and rural health chartbook.* Hyattsville, MD: National Center for Health Statistics.

Estes, G., & Zitzow, D. (1980, November). *Heritage consistency as a consideration in counseling Native Americans.* Paper read at the National Indian Education Association Convention, Dallas.

Estes, M. (2002). *Health assessment and physical examination* (2nd ed.). Independence, KY: Delmar Publishing.

Freeman, H.P. (2004). Poverty, culture and social injustice: Determinants of cancer disparities. CA: *A Cancer Journal for Clinicians* 54, 72-77.

Giger, J.N., & Davidhizar, R.E. (2004). *Transcultural nursing: Assessment & intervention* (4th ed.). St. Louis: Mosby.

Giuliano, A.R., Papenfuss, M., Schneider, A. (1999). Risk factors for high-risk type human papillomavirus infection among Mexican-American women. *Cancer Epidemiology, Biomarkers and Prevention 8,* 615-620.

Harkreader, H., & Hogan, M.A. (2000). *Fundamentals of nursing.* Philadelphia: W.B. Saunders.

Hernandez, B. (2003). Highlights of cancer incidence data in Hawaii. *Hawaiian Medical Journal* (62), 17-18.

Itano, J., Clark, F.V., & Hussey, L.O.L. Cancer prevention and early detection in native hawaiians In M. Frank-Stromberg & S.J. Olsen, *Cancer prevention in diverse populations: cultural implications for the multidisciplinary team* (2nd ed.). Pittsburgh: Oncology Nursing Society.

Jemal, A., Murray, T., Samuels, A. et al. (2003). Cancer statistics, 2003. *CA: A Cancer Journal for Clinicians 53*(1), 5-26.

Kagawa-Singer, M. (1996). Cultural systems. In R. McCorkle, M. Grant, & M. Frank-Stromberg (Eds.). *Cancer nursing: A comprehensive textbook* (2nd ed.). Philadelphia: W.B. Saunders.

Keppel, K.G., Pearcy, J.N., & Wagener, D.K. (2002). Trends in racial and ethnic specific rates for the health status indicators: United States, 1990-1998. Atlanta: Centers for Disease Control.

Kozier, B., Erb, G., Berman, A.J., & Burke, K. (2000). *Fundamentals of nursing* (6th ed.). Upper Saddle River, NJ: Prentice Hall Health.

Leininger, M. (1991). Transcultural nursing: The study and practice. *Imprint 38,* 55-66.

Luckmann, J. (2000). *Transcultural communication in nursing.* Independence, KY: Delmar Publishing.

Miller, B.A., Kolonel, L.N., Berstein, L. (Eds.). (1996). *Racial/ethnic patterns of cancer in the United States, 1988-1992* (NIH Publication No. 96-4104). Bethesda, MD: National Cancer Institute.

O'Brien, K., Cokkinides, V., Jemal, A. (2003). Cancer statistics for Hispanics, 2003. *CA: A Cancer Journal for Clinicians 53*(4), 208-226.

Oncology Nursing Society (ONS). (1999). *Multicultural outcomes: Guidelines for cultural competence.* Pittsburgh: Oncology Nursing Press.

Oncology Nursing Society (ONS). (2001). Multicultural tool kit: Moving toward cultural competence. Accessed January 9, 2004 from the World Wide Web: http://www.ons.org/xp6/ONS/Clinical.xml/MulticulturalToolKit.xml

Potter, P.A., & Perry, A.G. (2001). *Fundamentals of nursing* (5th ed.). St. Louis: Mosby.

Purnell, L.D., & Paulanka, B.J. (2003). *Transcultural health care* (2nd ed.). Philadelphia: F.A. Davis Co.

Shavers, V.L., & Brown, M.L. (2002). Racial and ethnic disparities in the receipt of cancer treatment. *Journal of the National Cancer Institute 94*(5), 334-357.

Simmonds, M.A. (2003). Cancer statistics, 2003: Further decrease in mortality rates, increase in persons living with cancer. *CA: A Cancer Journal for Clinicians 53*(5), 4.

Smedley, B.D., Stith, A.Y., & Nelson, A.R. (Eds.). (2002). *Unequal treatment confronting racial and ethnic disparities in health care. Committee on Understanding and Eliminating Racial and Ethnic Disparities in Health Care.* Institute of Medicine. Washington, DC: National Academy Press.

Spector, R. (2004). *Cultural diversity in health and illness* (6th ed.). Upper Saddle River, NJ: Pearson Education.

Survelliance, Epidemiology and End Report (SEER). (2003). All sites age adjusted SEER incidence and US death rates by race and ethnicity, 1996-2000. Retrieved September 1, 2003, from the World Wide Web: http://seer.cancer.gov/csr/1975_2000/results_merged/topic_race_ethnicity.pdf

U.S. Census Bureau. (2001a). Health insurance coverage: 2001. Retrieved August 12, 2003, from the World Wide Web: http://www.census.gov/hhes/hlthins/hlthino01/hlth01asc.html

U.S. Census Bureau. (2001b). Poverty in the United States: 2001. Retrieved August 12, 2003, from the World Wide Web: http://www.census.gov/prod/2002pubs/p60-219.pdf

U.S. Census Bureau. (2003). Asian Pacific American heritage month: May 2003. Retrieved August 13, 2003, from the World Wide Web: http://www.census.gov/press-release/www/2003/cb03-ff05.html

U.S. Department of Commerce. (2001, May). *Profiles of general demographic characteristics, 2000.* Washington, DC: U.S. Census Bureau.

U.S. Department of Commerce. (2002, February). *The Asian population: 2000.* Washington, DC: U.S. Census Bureau.

U.S. Department of Commerce. (2001, December). *The Native Hawaiian and other Pacific Islander population: 2000.* Washington, DC: U.S. Census Bureau.

White, L. (2001). *Foundations of nursing.* Albany, NY: Delmar Thomson Learning.

5 Coping: Survivorship Issues and Financial Concerns

SUSAN LEIGH

Theory

I. Definition.
  A. When cancer was considered an incurable disease, the family members or significant others who lost a loved one to cancer were the original cancer *survivors.*
  B. As curative therapies became available, clinicians and researchers used a 5-year landmark to define cancer survivors—free of disease 5 years from diagnosis or from the completion of therapy (Leigh & Clark, 2002).
  C. Many health care providers today differentiate between *clients* who are receiving therapy and *survivors* who have completed treatment (Leigh & Clark, 2002).
  D. A broader, more philosophical definition of cancer survivor (*"from the time of its discovery and for the balance of life, an individual diagnosed with cancer is a survivor"*) was initially proposed by the National Coalition for Cancer Survivorship (NCCS) in 1986 (Mullan, 1996a, p. 1).
    1. Implications of the NCCS definition for health care providers and the public include the following:
      a. Cancer survival begins at the moment of diagnosis and proceeds along a continuum through and beyond treatment to remissions, recurrences, cure, and the final stages of life.
      b. Survivorship can be seen as a dynamic, evolutionary process rather than a predetermined stage of survival. It is living with, through, or beyond a diagnosis of cancer, regardless of outcome (Leigh & Clark, 2002; Mullan, 1996b).
    2. Survivorship issues also affect persons other than the diagnosed client—family members, significant others, friends, coworkers, health care professionals, social support networks. These supporters can also be considered *secondary survivors* (Aziz, 2002).
II. "Seasons of Survival" (Mullan, 1985)—a dynamic model of life after a cancer diagnosis that consists of three *stages*—the acute, extended, and permanent stages of survival.
  A. Acute stage.
    1. Begins at the moment of diagnosis and extends through the initial treatments.
    2. Individuals may be dealing with the following:
      a. Acute or potential losses.
      b. Fear of dying or impending death.

      c. Acute side effects from treatment.

      d. Disruption in family and social roles.

  B. Extended stage.

    1. Follows the completion of the initial treatment.

    2. Individuals may be in remission or receiving maintenance therapy, or their condition may be terminal.

    3. Individuals may be dealing with the following:

      a. Severing of treatment-based support systems.

      b. Feeling ambiguous about the joy of being alive and feeling fear of recurrence or fear of death.

      c. Adjusting to physical or psychosocial compromise.

      d. Reintegrating and reorganizing individual and family concerns.

      e. Isolating the individual because of external or self-imposed forces.

      f. Seeking community-based support systems.

  C. Permanent stage.

    1. Gradual evolution to a time of diminished probability for disease recurrence.

    2. If cancer is arrested permanently, some survivors may be considered "cured."

    3. Individuals may be dealing with the following:

      a. Discrimination in the workplace.

      b. Procurement or maintenance of adequate insurance coverage.

      c. Adaptation to the physical and psychosocial changes resulting from disease.

      d. Treatment for long-term or late effects of disease and therapy (Tables 5-1 and 5-2) (Ganz, 2001; Loescher et al., 1989; Moore & Hobbie, 2000).

TABLE 5-1
Examples of Common Chemotherapy Agents and Possible Long-Term or Late Effects

Agent	Effect
Actinomycin D (Dactinomycin)	Hepatic fibrosis, cirrhosis
BCNU (Carmustine)	Pulmonary fibrosis, ovarian failure, azoospermia
Bleomycin (Blenoxane)	Pulmonary fibrosis, hyperpigmentation, digital cutaneous ulceration
Chlorambucil (Leukeran)	Progressive germinal aplasia, azoospermia
Cisplatin (Platinol)	Hearing loss, peripheral neuropathy
Cyclophosphamide (Cytoxan)	Progressive germinal aplasia, azoospermia, ovarian failure, chronic hemorrhagic cystitis
Doxorubicin (Adriamycin)	Cardiomyopathy
Etoposide (VP-16)	Testosterone deficiency, peripheral neuropathy
5-Fluorouracil (Adrucil, Efudex, Fluoroplex)	Irreversible tear-duct fibrosis
Ifosfamide (Ifex)	Reduced bladder capacity, tubular dysfunction, chronic hemorrhagic cystitis, ovarian failure
Methotrexate (Mexate, Folex)	Hepatic fibrosis, cirrhosis, leukoencephalopathy, renal failure
Nitrogen mustard (Mustargen)	Azoospermia, oligospermia
Procarbazine (Matulane)	Azoospermia, oligospermia, ovarian failure
Steroids	Cataracts, osteonecrosis, avascular necrosis
Vincristine (Oncovin)	Peripheral neuropathy

BCNU, Bis-chloroethyl-nitrosourea.

TABLE 5-2
Examples of Radiation Sites and Possible Long-Term or Late Effects

Site	Effect
Abdomen/intestines	Adhesions, fibrosis
Bladder	Fibrosis, hypoplasia
Central nervous system	Stroke, blindness, myelitis, focal necrosis, peripheral neuropathy, leukoencephalopathy, neurocognitive deficits
Chest	Breast cancer, soft tissue sarcomas, difficulty swallowing, pulmonary fibrosis
Head and neck	Hypothyroidism, hyperthyroidism, osteonecrosis of mandible, increased dental caries, alopecia, chronic otitis, hearing loss, xerostomia, hoarseness
Heart	Pericarditis, coronary artery disease, cardiomyopathy, pericardial effusion, myocardial infarction
Liver	Fibrosis, cirrhosis
Ovaries	Ovarian failure, premature menopause
Skeletal system	Late fractures, osteonecrosis
Skin	Fibrosis, necrosis, basal cell carcinoma, hyperpigmentation
Testicles	Oligospermia, azoospermia, testosterone deficiency
Urinary tract	Fibrosis, strictures
Vagina	Fibrosis, decreased vaginal secretions

        (1) Long-term effects are chronic sequelae that may develop during or result from treatment and may persist for months to years after the cancer is eradicated and treatment is complete (amputations, hair loss, neuropathies, scarring).

        (2) Late effects are clinically obvious, clinically subtle, or subclinical sequelae that may become apparent months to years after completion of treatment (pulmonary fibrosis, infertility, second malignancies, disease recurrence).

    e. Maintenance of adequate follow-up care.

  D. Death can occur in any one of these stages and should be included as an integral component of the survivorship continuum. It could also be seen as another stage in the above model (i.e., the final stage of survival).

III. Impact of survival.

  A. The impact of cancer survival may be long term or delayed (Leigh, 1998; Moore & Hobbie, 2000).

  B. Multiple factors determine the occurrence, frequency, and severity of actual or potential effects.

    1. Type of cancer.

    2. Location of disease.

    3. Size and extent of the primary tumor.

    4. Type and aggressiveness of therapy.

    5. Age of the individual at diagnosis.

    6. State of general physical and mental health of the individual at diagnosis.

    7. Quantity and quality of psychosocial support available.

    8. Individual coping strategies.

    9. Comorbidities.

    10. Lifestyle factors.

C. Effects can be categorized as physiologic, psychologic, social, or spiritual. Examples include the following:
1. Physiologic effects (Harpham, 1994; Moore & Hobbie, 2000).
    a. Recurrence of disease.
    b. Second malignancies.
        (1) Overall risk is low but remains a serious problem for those affected.
        (2) Risk of second malignancies does not contraindicate therapy for first malignancy.
    c. Functional changes—lymphedema, neuropathies, fatigue, decreased physical stamina.
    d. Cosmetic changes—ostomies, amputations, hair loss or thinning.
    e. System-specific effects.
        (1) Neurologic—neuropathies, delayed radiation necrosis, neuralgias.
        (2) Cardiovascular—cardiomyopathy, pericardial effusion, arterial and venous obstruction or occlusion.
        (3) Pulmonary—fibrosis, pleural effusions, spontaneous pneumo-thorax.
        (4) Urologic—nephritis, tubular atrophy, cystitis, urinary diversions.
        (5) Gastrointestinal—transient liver enzyme elevations, bowel diversions, adhesions, obstruction, hepatic venoocclusive disease.
        (6) Sexual/reproductive—sterility, impotence, testicular atrophy, premature menopause, changes in sexual response times.
        (7) Musculoskeletal—late fractures, muscle atrophy.
2. Psychologic effects (Dow et al., 1999; Harpham, 1994; Welch-McCaffrey et al., 1989).
    a. Fear of recurrence (Damocles syndrome).
    b. Heightened sense of vulnerability.
    c. Recurrent episodes of anxiety during routine health care follow-up or cancer-related anniversaries.
    d. Ambivalence about health care follow-up, ranging from hypochondriacal obsession to complete avoidance.
    e. Changes in body image or self-concept that result in less than satisfactory expression of self and sexuality.
    f. Continued need for psychosocial support after therapy.
3. Social effects (Leigh & Clark, 2002; Welch-McCaffrey et al., 1989).
    a. Social stigma associated with external sources (shunning by others) or internal sources (isolation).
    b. Difficulties with transition from sick role to previous roles or to the development of new roles and responsibilities.
    c. Inconsistent perceptions of the state of health of the survivor among individual, family, and social acquaintances.
    d. Employment-related problems may include avoidance by coworkers; demotion or lack of promotion; job-lock for fear of losing benefits; and dismissal from the job (Hoffman, 2002).
        (1) Legal protection is provided through the Federal Rehabilitation Act of 1973 that prohibits discrimination against the handicapped or those perceived as handicapped by employers who receive federal funding (federal agencies, hospitals, universities).
        (2) Additional protection is provided for workers not protected by the Federal Rehabilitation Act under the Americans with Disabilities Act (ADA) of 1990.

(3) Federal and state laws specifically prohibit cancer-related employment discrimination; contain information on how to file a complaint and with whom; prohibit employers from requiring preemployment examinations; and allow medical questions only after one is offered the job and only if the questions are related specifically to the job.

e. Insurance-related problems may include refusal of new applications, waiver or exclusion of preexisting conditions, extended waiting periods, an increase in premiums and reduction of benefits for the employee and employer, or cancellation of health and life insurance policies (Calder & Pollitz, 2002).

(1) Legal protection includes Consolidated Omnibus Budget Reconciliation Act (COBRA) of 1986, which mandates that employers of more than 20 workers offer group medical coverage to employees (18 months) and their dependents (36 months) if they lose a job or need to work fewer hours.

(2) Other protection includes high-risk insurance pools in some states for the medically uninsurable—insurers share both the risks and expenses with the high-risk population.

(3) Social Security Disability Insurance Program is available to individuals who have paid into the program previously; eligibility begins 6 months after being declared medically or mentally impaired.

(4) Portability of insurance and deletion of preexisting conditions for insurability through recent legislation will be modest improvements in insuring people with histories of cancer. Because there are no limitations on what companies can charge people who have cancer histories, most survivors will be unable to afford the inflated premiums for medical insurance.

4. Spiritual issues (Dow et al., 1999; Welch-McCaffrey et al., 1989).

a. Changes in life priorities and values after critical evaluation and a search for meaning.

b. Deepening sense of spirituality, which may or may not include organized religion.

c. Expressed concerns about the quality of one's life.

d. Increased self-love or self-acceptance.

e. An increased passion or zest for life.

f. Ambivalent feelings about occasional periods of depression.

g. Survivor's guilt, especially experienced during follow-up examinations when confronted with others who are not doing well, who are more debilitated, or whose condition is terminal.

Assessment

I. Identification of stage of survival.

A. Acute—diagnosis and treatment.

B. Extended—at completion of treatment or receiving maintenance therapy.

C. Permanent—long-term survival, "cured."

II. Evaluation of cancer history.

A. Individual diagnosis and treatment plan.

1. Chemotherapy drugs and doses.

2. Radiation fields and doses.

3. Biotherapy treatment.

    4. Surgeries.
  B. Risk or probability for the following:
    1. Recurrence of original disease.
    2. Long-term (chronic) effects or symptoms.
    3. Late (delayed) effects or symptoms.
III. Psychosocial interview.
  A. Client.
    1. Psychologic issues.
    2. Social issues.
    3. Financial issues.
  B. Family and significant others.
    1. Psychologic issues.
    2. Social issues.
    3. Financial issues.

Nursing Diagnoses

  I. Ineffective individual coping.
 II. Compromised family coping.
III. Risk for spiritual distress.
IV. Effective therapeutic regimen management.
  V. Fear.

Outcome Identification

  I. Client identifies and uses available alternative coping strategies and available resources.
 II. Family uses supportive services and effective coping strategies.
III. Client expresses hope and value in his/her own belief system and inner resources.
IV. Client understands need for continued long-term medical follow-up.
  A. Client and family receive appropriate information and referrals to optimize acute and long-term treatment plans.
  V. Client acknowledges and discusses fears and describes a reduction in fear.

Planning and Implementation

  I. Planning and interventions are guided by two beliefs and values.
  A. From diagnosis to death, all people with histories of cancer are survivors.
  B. Cancer survivors are entitled to certain rights (Box 5-1).
    1. Assurance of lifelong medical care, as needed.
    2. Pursuit of happiness.
    3. Equal job opportunities.
    4. Assurance of access to adequate public or private health insurance.
 II. Acute-stage interventions.
  A. Begin to incorporate rehabilitation models of care at the time of diagnosis; for example, referring to local support groups, encouraging appropriate exercise and nutrition plans, assisting with information gathering.
  B. Encourage client and family involvement in treatment decisions and planning for transitions in the level of care and services.
  C. Introduce survivorship potential and support with factual information and available resources.

BOX 5-1
THE CANCER SURVIVORS' BILL OF RIGHTS

The American Cancer Society presents this Survivors' Bill of Rights to call public attention to survivor needs, to enhance cancer care, and to bring greater satisfaction to cancer survivors, as well as to their physicians, employers, families and friends:

1. **Survivors have the right to assurance of lifelong medical care, as needed. The physicians and other professionals involved in their care should continue their constant efforts to be:**
   - Sensitive to the cancer survivors' lifestyle choices and their need for self-esteem and dignity;
   - Careful, no matter how long they have survived, to have symptoms taken seriously, and not have aches and pains dismissed, for fear of recurrence is a normal part of survivorship;
   - Informative and open, providing survivors with as much or as little candid medical information as they wish, and encouraging their informed participation in their own care;
   - Knowledgeable about counseling resources, and willing to refer survivors and their families as appropriate for emotional support and therapy that will improve the quality of individual lives.

2. **In their personal lives, survivors, like other Americans, have the right to the pursuit of happiness. This means they have the right:**
   - To talk with their families and friends about their cancer experience if they wish, but to refuse to discuss it if that is their choice and not to be expected to be more upbeat or less blue than anyone else;
   - To be free of the stigma of cancer as a "dread disease" in all social relations;
   - To be free of blame for having gotten the disease and of guilt for having survived it.

3. **In the workplace, survivors have the right to equal job opportunities. This means they have the right:**
   - To aspire to jobs worthy of their skills, and for which they are trained and experienced, and thus not to have to accept jobs they would not have considered before the cancer experience.
   - To be hired, promoted, and accepted on return to work, according to their individual abilities and qualifications, and not according to "cancer" or "disability" stereotypes;
   - To privacy about their medical histories.

4. **Since health insurance coverage is an overriding survivorship concern, every effort should be made to ensure all survivors adequate health insurance, whether public or private. This means:**
   - For employers, that survivors have the right to be included in group health coverage, which is usually less expensive, provides better benefits, and covers the employee regardless of health history;
   - For physicians, counselors, and other professionals concerned, that they keep themselves and their survivor-clients informed and up-to-date on available group or individual health policy options, noting, for example, what major expenses like hospital costs and medical tests outside the hospital are covered and what amount must be paid before coverage (deductibles);
   - For social policymakers, both in government and in the private sector, that they seek to broaden insurance programs like Medicare to include diagnostic procedures and treatment, which help prevent recurrence and ease survivor anxiety and pain.

Modified from Springarn ND: *The cancer survivors' bill of rights,* Silver Spring, Md, 1999, National Coalition for Cancer Survivorship.

    D. Assess changes in individual and family coping demands and resources throughout the seasons of survivorship.

    E. Establish exit interviews as clients complete initial treatment to assist in the transition to the extended stage.

III. Extended-stage interventions.

    A. Encourage periodic follow-up examinations and continued access to health care.

    B. Make referrals to appropriate supportive services within the treatment center and the community, such as the American Cancer Society, Leukemia & Lymphoma Society, United Ostomy Association, community-based resource and support centers, national advocacy organizations, and vocational rehabilitation programs (see Chapter 8).

    C. Give client, family, and children updated information and keep them informed of changes in the status of the client.

IV. Permanent-stage interventions.

    A. Encourage the development of systematic follow-up programs for long-term survivors for both pediatric and adult oncology.

    B. Encourage participation in activities related to changes in public and private policies affecting cancer survivors.

    C. Assist in the development of guidelines for continued care that transfers to other care providers; for example, algorithms for specific disease follow-up to primary care physicians.

Evaluation

The oncology nurse systematically and regularly evaluates the client's and/or family's responses to interventions to determine progress toward the achievement of expected outcomes. Relevant data are collected, and actual findings are compared with expected findings. Nursing diagnoses, outcomes, and plans of care are reviewed and revised as necessary.

REFERENCES

Aziz, N.M. (2002). Long-term survivorship: Late effects. In A. Berger, R.K. Portenoy, & D.E. Weissman (Eds). *Principles and practice of supportive oncology.* Philadelphia: Lippincott Williams & Wilkins, pp. 1019-1033.

Calder, K.J., & Pollitz, K. (2002). *What cancer survivors need to know about health insurance. A publication of the National Coalition for Cancer Survivorship (NCCS).* Silver Spring, MD. National Coalition for Cancer Survivorship.

Dow, K.H., Ferrell, B.R., Haberman, M.R., & Eaton, L. (1999). The meaning of quality of life in cancer survivorship. *Oncology Nursing Forum 26*, 519-528.

Ganz, P.A. (2001). Late effects of cancer and its treatment. *Seminars in Oncology Nursing 17*, 241-248.

Harpham, W.S. (1994). *After cancer: A guide to your new life.* New York: W.W. Norton & Co.

Hoffman, B. (2002). *Working it out: Your employment rights as a cancer survivor. A publication of the National Coalition for Cancer Survivorship (NCCS).* Silver Spring, MD. National Coalition for Cancer Survivorship.

Leigh, S., & Clark, E.J. (2002). Psychosocial aspects of cancer survivorship. In A. Berger, R.K. Portenoy, & D.E. Weissman (Eds). *Principles and practice of supportive oncology* (2nd ed.). Philadelphia: Lippincott Williams & Wilkins, pp. 1032-1043.

Leigh, S.A. (1998). The long-term cancer survivor: A challenge for nurse practitioners. *Nurse Practitioner Forum 3*, 192-196.

Loescher, L.J., Welch-McCaffrey, D., Leigh, S.A., et al. (1989). Surviving adult cancer. 1. Physiologic effects. *Annals of Internal Medicine 3,* 411-432.

Moore, I.M., & Hobbie, W. (2000). Late effects of cancer treatment. In C.H. Yarbro, M.H. Frogge, M. Goodman, & S.L. Groenwald (Eds.). *Cancer nursing: Principles & practice* (5th ed.) Sudbury, MA: Jones and Bartlett Publishers, pp. 597-615.

Mullan, F. (1985). Seasons of survival: Reflections of a physician with cancer. *New England Journal of Medicine 313,* 270-273.

Mullan, F. (1996a). Survivorship: An idea for everyone. In F. Mullan & B. Hoffman (Eds.). *Charting the journey: An almanac of practical resources for cancer survivors.* Mount Vernon, NY: Consumers Union, p. 1.

Mullan, F. (1996b). Survivorship: A powerful place. In B. Hoffman (Ed). *A cancer survivor's almanac: Charting your journey.* Minneapolis: Chronimed Publishing, pp. XV-XIX.

Welch-McCaffrey, D., Hoffman, B., Leigh, S.A., et al. (1989). Surviving adult cancer. II. Psychosocial implications. *Annals of Internal Medicine 3,* 411-432.

6 Sexuality

PATRICIA W. NISHIMOTO*

Theory

I. Assessing and providing information and holistic care about sexual functioning, and how it is affected by a diagnosis of cancer and its treatment is necessary because of:
   A. Improved treatments and outcomes.
      1. Clients are living longer.
         a. In 2002 there were an estimated 8.9 million cancer survivors in the United States.
         b. Client's sexual dysfunction can increase risk of emotional morbidity.
         c. If health care providers intervene, 70% of clients with cancer can have improved sexual functioning.
         d. Cancer advocacy has resulted in more clients asking questions of how treatment might impact sexual aspects of their lives.
      2. Focus on quality of life (QOL).
         a. QOL includes sexual functioning.
         b. To optimize clients' QOL, nurses must do the following:
            (1) Have evidence-based knowledge of how diagnosis/treatment affects sexual functioning.
            (2) Conduct nursing assessment of client's sexual health before diagnosis.
            (3) Inform clients of possible changes in sexual function because of treatment.
            (4) Educate clients and their partners.
            (5) Provide anticipatory guidance and suggestions for adapting to changes.
            (6) Know available resources and refer when needed.
      3. There is a legal liability if clients are not informed about possible risks to sexual functioning.
   B. World Health Organization (WHO) and Oncology Nursing Society (ONS).
      1. Recognize sexuality as an important aspect of health care.
      2. WHO defines sexual health as integrating the somatic, emotional, intellectual, and social aspects of a sexual being.
      3. ONS has written specific standards of care for this component of nursing care (ANA & ONS, 1996).
   C. Nurses often do not incorporate sexuality into their clinical practice. See Box 6-1 for staff beliefs that prevent intervention with client sexuality (Estes, 2002).
II. Multiple theories have been used to explore the phenomenon of sexuality, with each having strengths and weaknesses.
   A. One theory with the ability to provide direction for appropriate nursing intervention is Johnson's Behavioral Model (JBM) (Newman, 1994).

---

*The views expressed in this chapter are those of the author and do not reflect the official policy or position of the Department of the Army, Department of Defense, or the United States Government.

BOX 6-1
STAFF BELIEFS THAT PREVENT INTERVENTION WITH CLIENT SEXUALITY

Someone else will do it.	They are not worried about it.
They never bring up the subject.	They are too (young, old, sick, etc.).
I do not know how to help.	It will offend them if I ask.
I do not have the time.	There is no privacy.
Only perverts have questions.	I am not married.
I do not believe in sex for single people.	I do not have the specialized education.
They should be grateful to be alive.	

1. Person is seen as a behavioral system, not simply a biologic system.
2. Biologic, psychologic, and sociologic factors considered.
3. Consists of seven subsystems—interrelated, yet open.
    a. Attachment/affiliative.
    b. Dependency.
    c. Ingestive.
    d. Eliminative.
    e. Sexual.
    f. Aggressive.
    g. Achievement.
4. Disturbance in one subsystem affects other subsystems (e.g., when ingestive subsystem is affected by stomatitis from chemotherapy and client cannot eat solid foods, it affects the attachment subsystem by interfering with going to a restaurant for a date).
5. JBM illustrates how treatment of childhood malignancy impacts the sexual subsystem when these children become adults.
    a. Example—survivors may have cardiomyopathy or pulmonary fibrosis, which affects their achievement subsystem by not allowing them to play in sports, which impacts their attachment/affiliative subsystem (Olivo & Woolverton, 2001).
   B. Symbolic interaction theory combined with JBM explains how the individual interpretation of a symbol can affect behavior. For example,
    1. When chemotherapy stops menses, one woman may interpret this as she is "no longer a woman" and stop coitus.
    2. Another woman may have the same side effect but may interpret it as "no more mess" and increase sexual activity based on her interpretation.
III. PLISSIT model for sexuality counseling (Estes, 2002).
   A. Useful model for levels of nursing intervention based on the nurse's comfort with subject of sexuality.
   B. Ability to intervene at an appropriate level based on nurse's expertise.
   C. Nurse may refer to another provider at any level of intervention, but first, it is important to verify the skill of referral source.
    1. P = Permission.
        a. First level of intervention.
            (1) All nurses are able to provide this level of intervention.
            (2) It is permission to discuss the topic, *not* blanket permission for all behaviors.
            (3) Nurses initiate discussion to convey acceptability that discussing sexual changes caused by treatment is appropriate.

(4) Permission includes giving patients permission to not engage in sexual activity.
   b. To effectively intervene, nurses need to know basic information about sexuality.
      (1) Anatomy and physiology.
      (2) How disease affects sexual functioning.
      (3) How treatment affects sexual functioning.
      (4) Sexual response cycle.
   c. Example—when talking with a patient who has recently had a mastectomy, the nurse can note, "Often women wonder how a mastectomy might affect how their husband views them as a woman. Have you wondered about how this might affect your role as a wife?"
2. LI = Limited Information.
   a. Second level of intervention.
      (1) Most nurses are able to intervene at this level.
      (2) Addresses concerns, questions, myths, misconceptions.
   b. Nurses need to know how diagnosis and treatment can affect sexuality.
   c. Example—sometimes men have worried that if they have intercourse with their wife after treatment of cervical cancer with a radiation implant, their penis will "glow in the dark." The nurse would mention that this is a common concern and then explain that it does not happen (LI level).
3. SS = Specific Suggestions.
   a. Third level of intervention.
      (1) Many experienced or advanced practice nurses are able to intervene at this level.
      (2) Suggestions need to be appropriate for the following:
         (a) Cultural and religious beliefs.
         (b) Client's value system.
         (c) Partner's value system.
   b. Opportunity to consider different options but nurse does not impose them.
   c. Example—hormonal therapy can sometimes decrease vaginal lubrication (LI level). Water-soluble lubrication can decrease the risk of vaginal tears or dyspareunia (SS level).
4. IT = Intensive Therapy.
   a. Requires in-depth knowledge level about sexuality and counseling.
   b. Usually needed for long-standing or severe concerns.
   c. Example—if treatment brings up issues of childhood abuse, intensive therapy is needed.

Assessment, Planning, and Implementation

I. Reproductive issues.
   A. Prevention of pregnancy.
      1. Risk factors.
         a. Risk of birth defects, miscarriages.
            (1) Radiation from diagnostic workups and radiation therapy.
            (2) Mutagenic, teratogenic effects of chemotherapy.
            (3) Spontaneous abortion following surgical procedure.
         b. May use unreliable birth control because of the following:
            (1) Cultural beliefs.
            (2) Lack of access to birth control.

(3) Partner may not accept birth control.

(4) Denial the client has cancer.

(5) Desire to get "accidentally" pregnant.

    (a) Yearning for "return to normal."

    (b) Opportunity for adolescent to rebel.

    (c) May worry treatment will cause infertility, so seen as "last chance."

2. Prevention.

  a. Need to assess above risks.

    (1) Work with client to choose appropriate intervention for prevention of pregnancy based on belief system, religious belief, culture, other reasons.

    (2) Assess "meaning" of pregnancy to client.

    (3) Explain to clients the rationale for no conception during the diagnostic workup, treatment, and minimum of 1 year after treatment.

  b. Limited information level of intervention needed.

    (1) Intrauterine device (IUD)—risk of infection if client is neutropenic.

    (2) Diaphragm—need for refitting if weight change; risk of infection if client is neutropenic.

    (3) Hormonal birth control—not appropriate for hormone-dependent tumors; can decrease vaginal lubrication and increase risk of dyspareunia and risk of tears in vaginal mucosa, which increases risk of infection.

    (4) Condoms and foam—allow prevention of sexually transmitted diseases (STDs) and together reduce risk of pregnancy. Foam may irritate vaginal mucosa if female receiving chemotherapy and has decreased vaginal lubrication.

3. Management.

  a. Ensure referral for birth control counseling.

  b. Use PLISSIT model for intervention management.

  c. Discuss importance of not becoming pregnant after treatment (specific time based on type of treatment given and follow-up needed, e.g., scans that have radiation risk).

B. Treatment issues during pregnancy.

  1. Risk factors (depend on trimester).

  a. Diagnostic tests.

    (1) May be risk to the fetus.

    (2) Radioactive iodine contraindicated for staging of pregnant woman.

    (3) Diagnosis of cancer itself may be more difficult because of pregnancy changes.

      (a) Example—1% to 4% of women with breast cancer are pregnant at the time of diagnosis.

      (b) Diagnosis of breast cancer may be delayed because of vascular, lymphatic, and density changes in the breast consequent to pregnancy.

      (c) Diagnostic tests may be delayed owing to pregnancy, which may affect survival of client.

      (d) Needs to make evidence-based decisions; that is, bilateral mammogram causes less than 500 centigray (cGy) of radiation to fetus.

  b. Chemotherapy agents.

        (1) Type of agent affects risk to fetus.
           (a) Avoid antimetabolites (especially methotrexate), alkylating agents, and folic acid antagonists in the first trimester.
           (b) Avoid radiolabeled monoclonal antibodies.
           (c) Teratogenic potential affected by drug dosage, ability of drug to enter fetal circulation, route of administration.
        (2) First trimester is greatest time of risk.
           (a) National Cancer Institute (NCI) set up database in 1985 to examine pregnancy outcomes after use of chemotherapy.
           (b) Consensus is that clients with high-grade lymphoma during first trimester should not delay therapy.
           (c) Slower-growing tumors may allow treatment to be delayed until second trimester or after delivery.
    c. Radiation therapy.
        (1) Usually delayed until after delivery.
        (2) Risk depends on field, amount of cGy.
  2. Prevention of complications during treatment while pregnant.
    a. Considerations with diagnostic tests.
        (1) May adjust diagnostic workup to reduce risk to fetus.
           (a) May order ultrasound instead of radiologic test, if possible.
           (b) Magnetic resonance imaging (MRI) instead of computed tomography (CT) scan so no radiation exposure to fetus.
           (c) If early-stage disease, may omit late-stage workup (e.g., bone scan).
        (2) May be able to modify diagnostic test procedure (e.g., shield fetus).
        (3) Serum tumor markers may not be reliable when client is pregnant.
        (4) Consult obstetrician when making diagnostic decisions.
    b. Chemotherapy agents.
        (1) Usually safer to give chemotherapy during the second or third trimester.
        (2) May increase risk to fetus of the following:
           (a) Low birth weight.
           (b) Mutagenesis.
           (c) Teratogenic effects.
        (3) Weigh risks/benefits of various regimens.
        (4) Consider delay of treatment initiation, if possible.
        (5) Address issue of pregnancy termination, but keep in mind cultural and religious beliefs.
        (6) Be aware of risk to fetus from antiemetics, growth factors, analgesics.
    c. Radiation therapy.
        (1) Shield fetus, if possible.
        (2) Delay therapy until after delivery, if possible.
        (3) Use machine with low leakage; consider target dose, size of radiation therapy field, and the distance the field edges are to fetus.
    d. Surgery.
        (1) Timing of surgery (trimester of pregnancy).
        (2) Type of surgery.
        (3) Anesthetic agent used.
           (a) Relatively safe.
           (b) Compensate for pregnancy-induced physiologic and anatomic changes.

        (4) Length of surgery.

        (5) Ostomy patients may have trouble "pushing" for a vaginal delivery because of removal of muscles.

   3. Management of pregnant client during oncologic treatment.

     a. Review choices concerning continuation of pregnancy.

     b. If the client remains pregnant, provide high-risk prenatal care.

        (1) Risk of thrombocytopenia.

        (2) Risk of disseminated intravascular coagulation.

        (3) Risk of premature delivery because of physical stress of illness, treatment, or side effects.

     c. Evaluate treatment options with client, and discuss one with lowest risk to fetus.

     d. Initiate discussion about which life is a priority if an emergency occurs.

     e. Carefully evaluate each drug for safety.

        (1) Assess if crosses placental barrier.

           (a) Example—lorazepam increases risk of floppy baby syndrome.

        (2) After delivery, need to counsel mother about risk to baby if she breastfeeds while receiving chemotherapy.

           (a) Potential for immunosuppression/neutropenia.

           (b) Unknown effect on growth.

           (c) Possible risk of carcinogenesis.

     f. Counsel mother that breast irradiation may result in little or no breast milk production.

 C. Fertility.

   1. Risk factors.

     a. Type and amount of chemotherapy.

        (1) Lomustine, doxorubicin, and melphalan can suppress gonadal function.

        (2) Cyclophosphamide, cytarabine, and fluorouracil usually have reversible germ cell toxicity.

        (3) Childhood treatment of sarcoma with high-dose cyclophosphamide has high risk of gonadal dysfunction for males because of depletion of germinal epithelium and for females because of fall in estradiol and progesterone levels and elevation in follicle-stimulating hormone (FSH) and luteinizing hormone (LH) (Kenney et al., 2001).

        (4) Eighty percent of men who receive mechlorethamine, Oncovin (vincristine), procarbazine, prednisone (MOPP) combination therapy have fertility affected.

        (5) Fertility affected in 35% of men treated with Adriamycin (doxorubicin), bleomycin, vinblastine, dacarbazine (ABVD) combination therapy; fertility is usually recovered.

        (6) Severity of pretreatment oligospermia and cumulative dose affect spermatogenesis.

        (7) Fertility may reverse as late as 4 years after treatment, so serial measurements of serum FSH and sperm counts need to be done.

        (8) High-dose chemotherapy (i.e., bone marrow transplant) has high rate of permanent sterility (Kant, 2001).

     b. Hormonal therapy.

        (1) Tamoxifen (Nolvadex) will not decrease fertility but may increase risk of pregnancy while taking it.

        (2) Avoid pregnancy while receiving hormone therapy and for at least 2 months after therapy.

    c. Radiation therapy.
      (1) For males receiving pelvic radiation.
        (a) Age of male does not affect risk of sterility.
        (b) Less than 4 cGy results in temporary sterility.
        (c) Greater than 5 cGy results in permanent sterility.
      (2) For females.
        (a) Age and amount of radiation dosage affect risk of sterility.
        (b) Ninety-five percent of women less than the age of 40 years receiving 20 cGy fractionated over 5 to 6 weeks will have sterility.
        (c) More than age 40 years, a dose of only 6 cGy affects sterility.
      (3) Field of radiation therapy (i.e., abdomen or pelvis).
        (a) Twenty-five percent of men and women receiving radiation below diaphragm risk sterility.
    d. Type of surgery.
      (1) Bilateral orchiectomy.
      (2) Total penectomy.
      (3) If surgery affects prostatic nerve plexus or presacral sympathetic nerves.
      (4) Complete removal of prostate and seminal vesicles.
      (5) Hysterectomy.
    e. Age of client at time of treatment.
    f. Type of malignancy.
      (1) Example—many men when diagnosed with Hodgkin's disease or testicular cancer have low sperm count before treatment.
  2. Prevention of infertility.
    a. Choose treatment with least risk to fertility.
    b. Use of oophoropexy reduces ovarian exposure by as much as 50%.
    c. No direct radiation treatment to gonads if possible.
    d. Strategies to preserve male fertility.
      (1) Freezing stem cells from testicular tissues of prepubertal males.
      (2) If adult male without sperm cells in electrically stimulated ejaculate, spinning down urine after orgasm to collect sperm or surgical removal of sperm from epididymis or testicular tissue has been attempted.
    e. Methods to preserve fertility (Box 6-2).
      (1) Experimental fertility preservation methods are being investigated.
        (a) www.fertilehope.org is one source with links to studies being conducted.
      (2) GnRH (gonadotropin-releasing hormone) agonist or cyclic oral contraceptives have been used to try to protect ovaries during chemotherapy but controversial results on effectiveness.

BOX 6-2
PRESERVATION OF FERTILITY

Sperm banking	Shielding of gonads during radiation
Egg retrieval (experimental)	therapy
Zone drilling of egg (experimental)	Retrieval of sperm from retrograde
Careful selection of chemotherapy	ejaculation
agents	Oophoropexy

3. Management.
   a. Grief counseling for loss of fertility.
   b. Treatment for retrograde ejaculation may restore fertility.
      (1) Certain drugs can temporarily close sphincter so the man can ejaculate sperm.
         (a) Example—sympathomimetic phenylpropanolamine.
II. Sexual dysfunction.
   A. Risk factors.
      1. Hormonal.
         a. Effects of hormonal therapy in men.
            (1) Gynecomastia.
            (2) Feminization.
            (3) Erection dysfunction.
            (4) Decreased fertility.
            (5) Penile/testicular atrophy.
            (6) Decrease or loss of libido (Fowler et al., 2002).
         b. Effects of hormonal therapy in women.
            (1) Decreased vaginal lubrication.
            (2) Change in libido.
            (3) Masculinization.
            (4) Amenorrhea that may affect libido based on meaning of menses to woman and her partner.
            (5) Menopause that may include menopausal symptoms of mood swings, hot flushes, sleep disturbance, dyspareunia (Wilmoth & Bruner, 2002).
      2. Radiation therapy.
         a. Effects of radiation therapy.
            (1) Radiation therapy to the pelvis may cause temporary or permanent erectile dysfunction or decreased vaginal lubrication from vascular or nerve damage to pelvis.
            (2) Amount of radiation therapy to bulb of penis correlates to risk of erectile dysfunction because of effect on nitric oxide–producing cells destroyed by radiation.
               (a) Erection of penis during sexual stimulation is mediated by nitric oxide released from nerve endings close to the blood vessels of the penis.
            (3) Radiation-induced sexual dysfunction in cervical cancer ranges from 30% to 90%.
            (4) Prostate brachytherapy causes erectile dysfunction in 6% to 61% of men (Stipetich et al., 2002).
            (5) See Box 6-3 for sexual dysfunction after pelvic radiation in women.
         b. Amount of radiation (cGy).
         c. Type of radiation.
            (1) External radiation to pelvis can cause fibrosis to blood vessels.
            (2) Internal radiation to cervix can cause vaginal stenosis.
      3. Effects of chemotherapy.
         a. Decrease or loss of libido.
         b. Retarded ejaculation, an inhibition of ejaculation.
         c. Erectile dysfunction or loss of vaginal lubrication.
         d. Neuropathies.
            (1) If pain in fingers, affects ability to touch partner.
            (2) If pain in jaw, affects ability to kiss partner.

BOX 6-3
SEXUAL DYSFUNCTION AFTER PELVIC RADIATION THERAPY (FEMALE)

Decreased vaginal lubrication	Change in usual sexual expression
Dyspareunia	Shortening of vaginal vault
Change in vaginal sensation	Decreased elasticity of vagina
Risk of infection because of decreased vaginal lubrication	Increased vaginal irritation

e. Antimetabolites and antitumor antibiotics as single agents do not directly cause sexual dysfunction but may potentiate dysfunction when given with alkylating agents.

f. Chemotherapy side effects of oral or vaginal stomatitis, dry mouth, nausea, fluid retention, fatigue, and others affect sexual functioning (Wilmoth & Bruner, 2002).

g. Alopecia whether partial or complete may affect not only the client but also the partner (Batchelor, 2001).
   (1) Loss of eyelashes may cause "constant blinking," which may affect attractiveness.
   (2) Loss of pubic hair may make the client feel "childlike" and affect sexual desire.

h. May cause premature menopause, which may affect libido, body image, and dyspareunia (Rogers & Krisjanson, 2002).

4. Surgical intervention.
   a. Prostatectomy.
      (1) Retrograde ejaculation.
      (2) Erectile dysfunction if there is damage to autonomic nerve plexus.
      (3) Occasionally, diminished orgasm intensity (Schover et al., 2002).
      (4) Incontinence can affect self-esteem, and odor of urine on clothes can affect libido of client and partner (Maliski et al., 2001).
   b. Orchiectomy.
      (1) No change if only one testicle is removed.
      (2) Bilateral orchiectomy may decrease libido and cause atrophy of the penis.
      (3) Risk of erectile dysfunction, decreased libido, premature ejaculation, decreased orgasm intensity if radical abdominal lymph node dissection is done (Wilmoth & Bruner, 2002).
   c. Cystectomy.
      (1) Loss of vaginal lubrication in women or erectile dysfunction in men because of damage to nerves.
      (2) Change in vaginal diameter and length.
      (3) Retrograde ejaculation (Horenblas et al., 2001).
   d. Mastectomy/lumpectomy.
      (1) Numbness in previously sensitive breast, which may affect sexual pleasure.
      (2) If mastectomy, may have phantom nipple sensations.
      (3) Change in body image.
      (4) May affect usual sexual activity (Wilmoth, 2001).
   e. Head and neck surgery.

(1) Appearance affects body image and the way in which others view client.
(2) Change in speech and ability to whisper during lovemaking.
(3) Removal of spinal accessory nerve affects ability to turn the head.
(4) Change in smell and taste sensations.
(5) Drooling or the sensation of respirations on the neck of partner may affect partner's sexual desire.

f. Ostomy surgery.
(1) Body image changes to include the change in how clothes fit on the client because of appliance.
(2) Decreased blood flow to vagina/penis will affect lubrication/erection.
(3) Concerns regarding odor; can decrease with tight seal of appliance, emptying appliance before sexual activity, avoiding certain foods that cause flatulence or increased odor (Nishimoto, 2001).
(4) Appliance may "stick" to body of client or partner because of sweating so use lingerie, T-shirt, or appliance cover.

g. Hysterectomy.
(1) Can increase or decrease sexual enjoyment.
(2) May have phantom uterine contractions postoperatively.
(3) Decreased libido, vaginal lubrication for some women.
(4) Scar tissue may cause dyspareunia.
(5) Removal of cervix may reduce sexual pleasure.
(6) Body image changes of self as a woman for some clients.

B. Prevention of sexual dysfunction.
1. Education and anticipatory guidance.
a. Explain physiology of sexual functioning and ways in which diagnosis and treatment may affect functioning.
(1) See Box 6-4 for psychologic factors that affect sexual functioning.
(2) See Box 6-5 for physiologic factors that influence sexual functioning.
b. Do not assume that the client knows basic sexuality information.
(1) Use models or drawings.
(2) Provide the American Cancer Society (ACS, 2001a, 2001b) publication on sexuality and the man or woman with cancer.
c. Dispel myths or misconceptions (e.g., fear that anal stimulation caused rectal cancer).
2. Encourage the couple's intercommunications.
a. Serve as a role model for couple by speaking openly when discussing sexual functioning.
b. Use a nonjudgmental approach as they discuss their fears or feelings.

BOX 6-4
PSYCHOLOGIC FACTORS THAT AFFECT SEXUAL FUNCTIONING

Anxiety	Low self-esteem
Fear	Feelings of isolation
Depression	Change in body image
Change in affect/personality	Fear of transmitting cancer
Grief	Heightened sense of vulnerability
Guilt	Withdrawal

BOX 6-5
PHYSIOLOGIC FACTORS THAT AFFECT SEXUALITY

Fatigue	Lymphedema
Pain	Change in skin texture/pigmentation
Sleep deprivation	Decreased vaginal lubrication
Constipation/diarrhea	Weight fluctuations/muscle atrophy
Respiratory compromise	Menopausal symptoms
Alopecia	Decreased complete blood counts
Fistulas/draining wounds	Severity of cancer
Neuropathy	Comorbidity of chronic diseases
Shingles	Phantom uterine contractions after
Availability of partner	hysterectomy

      c. Allow them to conduct role playing in a safe environment demonstrating how they may begin conversation with a partner about changes in sexual functioning.

      d. Encourage attendance at classes or support groups where sexuality is openly discussed.

    3. Be a client advocate.

      a. Be aware of medications that affect sexual functioning (e.g., narcotics, hormones, sedatives).

      b. Suggest medications with fewer side effects.

      c. Be aware of studies that are being done on equipment/devices to decrease sexual dysfunction (i.e., Eros device that mechanically increases blood flow to the clitoris and external genitalia is FDA [U.S. Food and Drug Administration] approved).

      d. Encourage couple to speak with surgeon before surgery about the benefits and risks of sexuality-preserving procedures (Wang et al., 2002).

  C. Management.

    1. Conduct a sexual history.

    2. Intervene using the PLISSIT model (Estes, 2002).

      a. Incorporate client's value system and cultural beliefs into intervention.

      b. Help client expand sexual options to accommodate changes in sexual functioning.

        (1) Massage, fantasy, change in positions, use of sexy lingerie to cover incision site or stoma, use of lubricants, penile stuffing.

        (2) Facilitate referrals for medical intervention for pelvic floor muscle exercise and manometric biofeedback, penile implants, penile injections, vacuum devices, vaginal reconstruction (Dorey et al., 2003).

      c. Provide strategies to enlarge clients' knowledge base.

        (1) Encourage attendance at support groups.

        (2) Inform them of written resources on sexuality and cancer.

        (3) Write a short article on sexuality and cancer for the local support group newsletter or offer to present a class to them.

        (4) Many other factors, such as activity intolerance, anxiety, bowel incontinence, chronic pain, decreased cardiac output, disturbed sleep pattern, fatigue, impaired urinary elimination, impaired oral mucous membrane, nausea, caregiver role strain, and risk for activity intolerance, can affect sexual functioning.

(a) Example—for a client experiencing impaired gas exchange, the client may become easily fatigued during sexual activity.
(b) Use PLISSIT model to intervene.
  (i) **P:** bring up subject that shortness of breath (SOB) may affect sexuality.
  (ii) **LI:** inform couple how SOB can affect stamina.
  (iii) **SS:** help couple explore ways to conserve energy by a change in position.
  (iv) **IT:** refer to sex therapist if above three levels of intervention not effective.

Nursing Diagnoses

I. Disturbed body image.
II. Sexual dysfunction.
III. Ineffective sexuality patterns.
IV. Impaired social interaction.

Outcome Identification

I. Client expresses feelings about alterations (e.g., alopecia, body image changes, altered sexual functioning). (Caution: these outcomes are specific to Western culture.)
II. Client identifies potential or actual alterations in sexuality caused by disease or treatment (e.g., infertility, dry mucous membranes, decreased/lack of libido, erectile dysfunction, premature menopause).
  A. Client identifies personal and community resources to assist with changes in body image and sexuality.
III. Client describes strategies he/she can use in response to actual or potential sexual changes (e.g., change in position to decrease fatigue, penile implant if erectile dysfunction is present).
  A. Client identifies satisfactory alternative methods for expressing sexuality.
IV. Client engages in open communication with partner.

Evaluation

The oncology nurse systematically and regularly evaluates the client's and/or the family's responses to interventions to determine progress toward the achievement of expected outcomes. Relevant data are collected, and actual findings are compared with expected findings. Nursing diagnoses, outcomes, and plans of care are reviewed and revised as necessary.

REFERENCES

American Cancer Society (ACS). (2001a). *Sexuality and cancer for the man who has cancer and his partner* (Publication No. 4658). Atlanta: American Cancer Society.
American Cancer Society (ACS). (2001b). *Sexuality and cancer for the woman who has cancer and her partner* (Publication No. 4657). Atlanta: American Cancer Society.
American Nurses Association (ANA) and Oncology Nursing Society (ONS). (1996). *Statement on the scope and standards of oncology nursing practice.* Washington, DC: American Nurses Publishing.

Batchelor, D. (2001). Hair and cancer chemotherapy: Consequences and nursing care—A literature study. *European Journal of Cancer Care 10*(3), 147-163.

Dorey, G., Feneley, R.C.L., & Speakman, M.J. (2003). Pelvic floor muscle exercises and manometric biofeedback for erectile dysfunction and postmicturition dribble: Three case studies. *Journal of Wound, Ostomy and Continence Nursing 30*(1), 44-52.

Estes, J.P. (2002). Beyond basic ADLs: Sexual expression is an important but often overlooked activity of daily living. *Rehabilitation Management: International Journal of Rehabilitation 15*(3), 36-37.

Fowler, F.J., Collins, M.M., Corkery, E.W., et al. (2002). The impact of androgen deprivation on quality of life after radical prostatectomy for prostate carcinoma. *Cancer 95*(2), 287-295.

Horenblas, S., Meinhardt, W., Ijzerman, W., & Moonen, L.F.M. (2001). Sexuality preserving cystectomy and neobladder: Initial results. *Journal of Urology 166*(3), 837-840.

Kant, L.U. (2001). Sexuality and reproductive issues in nursing management of symptoms associated with chemotherapy. In J.M. Yasko (Ed.). *Nursing management of symptoms associated with chemotherapy* (5th ed.). Conshohocken, PA: Menisus.

Kenney, L.B., Laufer, M.R., Grant, F.D., et al. (2001). High risk of infertility and long term gonadal damage in males treated with high dose cyclophosphamide for sarcoma during childhood. *Cancer 91*(3), 613-621.

Maliski, S.L., Heilemann, M.V., & McCorkle, R. (2001). Mastery of postprostatectomy incontinence and impotence: His work, her work, our work. *Oncology Nursing Forum 28*(6), 985-992.

Newman, M.A. (1994). Theory for nursing practice. *Nursing Science Quarterly 7*(4), 153-157.

Nishimoto, P.W. (2001). Sexuality. In R. Gates & R.M. Fink. *Oncology nursing secrets* (2nd ed.). Philadelphia: Hanley & Belfus.

Olivo, E.L., & Woolverton, K. (2001). Surviving childhood cancer: Disruptions in the developmental building blocks of sexuality. *Journal of Sex Education and Therapy 26*(3), 172-180.

Rogers, M., & Krisjanson, L.J. (2002). The impact of sexual functioning of chemotherapy-induced menopause in women with breast cancer. *Cancer Nursing 25*(1), 57-65.

Schover, L.R., Fouladi, R.T., Warneke, C.L., et al. (2002). Defining sexual outcomes after treatment for localized prostate carcinoma. *Cancer 95*(8), 1773-1785.

Stipetich, R.L., Abel, L.J., Blatt, H.J., et al. (2002). Nursing assessment of sexual function following permanent prostate brachytherapy for patients with early-stage prostate cancer. *Clinical Journal of Oncology Nursing 6*(5), 271-274.

Wang, C., Wang, C., Huang, H., et al. (2002). Fertility-preserving treatment in young patients with endometrial adenocarcinoma. *Cancer 94*(8), 2192-2198.

Wilmoth, M.C. (2001). The aftermath of breast cancer: An altered sexual self. *Cancer Nursing 24*(4), 278-286.

Wilmoth, M.C., & Bruner, D.W. (2002). Integrating sexuality into cancer nursing practice. *Updates in Oncology Nursing 9*(1), 1-7, 11-14.

7 Supportive Care: Dying and Death

MARGARET J. CROWLEY

HOSPICE CARE AND PALLIATIVE CARE

Theory

I. Hospice care and palliative care involve a team-oriented approach to expert medical care, symptom management, and emotional and spiritual support to clients and families facing a life-threatening illness (National Hospice & Palliative Care Organization, 2003).

II. Hospice.
   A. Program of care that provides for the needs of the client and family/significant others as they deal with the client's terminal illness.
   B. Program of care provided across a variety of settings and based on the understanding that death is part of the normal life cycle (Egan & Labyak, 2001).
   C. Program of care that is initiated at the time of referral from primary caregivers secondary to an appropriate prognosis (<6 months to live) and is covered under Medicare, Medicaid, private insurance plans, and managed care organizations.
   D. Imminent death is often the stimulus for hospice referral although earlier referral may allow more appropriate use of this service (Super, 2001).
   E. Provides a variety of caregivers, including client's personal physician, hospice physician, home health aides, nurses, social workers, clergy, trained volunteers and speech, physical, and occupational therapists if needed.
   F. "The nurse coordinates the plan of care with the patient, family, and other members of the team" (Egan & Labyak, 2001, p. 19).
   G. Goals of care are directed by the client and family.
   H. Bereavement care is provided to the family after the death of the client.
   I. "Hospice philosophy emphasizes palliative care, which can be as aggressive as curative care, but with a focus on comfort, dignity, quality of life closure and patient/family choice" (Egan & Labyak, 2001, p. 9).

III. Palliative care.
   A. An approach that improves quality of life of clients and their families facing problems associated with life-threatening illness (WHO, 2003).
   B. Can be initiated at the time of a life-threatening diagnosis for which cure is not available (Super, 2001) and therefore extends the principles of hospice care to a broader population that can benefit from care earlier in their illness (National Hospice & Palliative Care Organization, 2003).
   C. Can be provided in conjunction with other therapies that are intended to prolong life, such as chemotherapy or radiation therapy (WHO, 2003).

    D. Symptom management, comfort, and support to clients and families, which includes psychologic and spiritual aspects of care, are provided.

    E. Care is best provided by an interdisciplinary team (Super, 2001).

IV. Major goal of care at the end of life is to enhance quality of life by decreasing stress from symptoms (Hermann & Looney, 2001).

    A. Symptom management is a primary responsibility of the nurse caring for dying clients (Hermann & Looney, 2001).

    B. "The most commonly reported symptoms and those that cause the greatest patient distress should be addressed first by the hospice interdisciplinary team" (McMillan & Small, 2002, p. 1427).

V. The relationship with the client and family together with the knowledge and skills of the nurse is the essence of palliative care nursing (Coyle, 2001, p. 3).

Assessment

I. Collaborate with the physician to determine the diagnosis, prognosis of the client as well as the treatment plan.

II. Evaluate the client's understanding of the disease trajectory and treatment options.

III. Determine if the client has an advance directive or surrogate decision maker identified.

IV. Evaluate the client's, family's, and medical team's goals for the care of the client.

    A. Symptom management with continued treatment intended to prolong life.

    B. Symptom management with appropriate prognosis to qualify for hospice care.

V. Determine that the client and family chose hospice/palliative care.

VI. Assess existing physical, psychologic, social, and spiritual symptoms.

Nursing Diagnoses

I. Deficient knowledge related to the care of the client who is terminally ill.

II. Readiness for enhanced family coping.

III. Effective therapeutic regimen management.

Outcome Identification

I. Learning needs of client and family related to the care of the client are identified and met.

    A. Symptoms are controlled.

II. Client and family choose a hospice/palliative care program.

    A. Focus on palliative care increases and curative care decreases as the disease progresses (Abrahm, 2000).

    B. Palliative care is integrated with the medical treatments that are used to control or minimize disease.

III. Client receives care that is appropriate for client and family goals.

Planning and Implementation

I. Establish a therapeutic relationship that allows for communication regarding death and dying.

II. Complete holistic assessment of physical, spiritual, social, and psychologic needs.

    III. Consult palliative care team as needed and available.
    IV. Provide symptom management to enhance quality of life.
     V. Ensure client and family recognize the possibility of hospice care with appropriate prognosis.
    VI. Inform client and family of appropriate agencies.
  VII. Complete a referral to agency.
VIII. Obtain informed consent from client for hospice care.

Evaluation

The oncology nurse systematically and regularly evaluates the client's and/or family's response to interventions to determine progress toward the achievement of expected outcomes. Relevant data are collected, and actual findings are compared with expected findings. Nursing diagnoses, outcomes, and plans of care are reviewed and revised as necessary.

PAIN (see also Chapter 1)

Theory

      I. Factors influencing the client's perception of pain include spiritual, psychologic, social, and physical concerns (Easley & Elliot, 2001).
         A. Each factor influences the others, and total assessment includes recognizing the relationships (ELNEC, 2002).
    II. "Undertreatment of pain is often due to clinician's failure or inability to evaluate or appreciate the severity of the client's problem" (Fink & Gates, 2001).
  III. Pain associated with cancer and the terminal phase of the disease occurs in the majority of clients (Fink & Gates, 2001).
  IV. "Cancer pain may be acute, chronic, or intermittent, and it often has a definable etiology, which is usually related to tumor recurrence or treatment" (American Pain Society, 1999, p. 4).
     V. Most pain in advanced cancer is related to the disease or treatment (Abrahm, 2000).
         A. Only 5% to 10% of pain is not related to the cancer.
         B. Ninety-five percent of pain is caused by cancer either from direct tumor involvement (75%) or from treatment of the disease (15% to 29%), such as mucositis from chemotherapy (Abrahm, 2000, p. 80).
         C. Constant monitoring and adjustment of the pain control regimen are required.
  VI. Barriers to adequate pain control are provided in Box 7-1.
      Pharmacologic interventions.
         A. Opioids are the drugs of choice for severe pain.
             1. Oral administration is preferred route.
             2. Drugs are given around the clock.
         B. Adjuvant medications enhance pain control.
             1. Steroids.
             2. Tricyclics.
             3. Anticonvulsants.
             4. Nonsteroidal antiinflammatory drugs (NSAIDs).
             5. Bisphosphonates for bone metastases or multiple bone lesions of multiple myeloma (Abrahm, 2000).
         C. Intraspinal or epidural infusion may be considered.

BOX 7-1
BARRIERS TO OPTIMAL PAIN ASSESSMENT

Health care professional barriers
  Lack of identification of pain assessment and relief as a priority in client care
  Inadequate knowledge about how to perform a pain assessment
  Perceived lack of time to conduct a pain assessment
  Inability of clinician to empathize or establish rapport with client
  Prejudice and bias in dealing with clients
Health care system barriers
  A system that fails to hold health care professionals accountable for pain assessment
  Lack of criteria or availability of instruments for pain assessment in health care settings
  Lack of institutional policies for performance and documentation of pain assessment
Client/family/societal barriers
  The highly subjective and personal nature of the pain experience
  Lack of client and family awareness about the importance of pain assessment
  Lack of client communication with health care professionals about pain
  Presence of unfounded beliefs and myths about pain and its treatment

From Fink R, Gates R: Pain assessment. In Ferrell BR, Coyle N, editors: *Textbook of palliative nursing*, New York, 2001, Oxford University Press, p 54.

    1. When pain not relieved with systemic opioids.
    2. If side effects of systemic opioids limit escalation.
VII. Other invasive interventions may be used for pain as appropriate to the source of the pain.
    A. Radiation for bony metastases (McQuay et al., 2002).
    B. Radiopharmaceuticals for more generalized bone pain from metastases. (e.g., strontium 89) (McQuay et al., 2002).
    C. Neural blockade and neuroablation for pain control not amenable to other modalities (Abrahm, 2000).
VIII. Nonpharmacologic interventions.
    A. Physical and behavioral interventions may be used in addition to pharmacologic therapy.
        1. Cutaneous stimulation (e.g., heat and cold, massage).
        2. Behavioral interventions (e.g., relaxation technique).
        3. Complementary therapies (e.g., healing touch, acupuncture).
        4. Effectiveness of nonpharmacologic strategies is not intended to replace pharmacologic interventions (Sellick & Zaza, 1998).
        5. Evidence of the effectiveness of nonpharmacologic interventions needs to be further studied so that nurses can select appropriate interventions (Sellick & Zaza, 1998).
    B. Physiatric interventions can be helpful in pain management (Coyle & Layman-Goldstein, 2001).
        1. The static positions of debilitated clients may increase pain.
        2. Activity including range of motion exercises helps maintain muscle tone.

Assessment

    I. Evaluate pain status via pain assessment tool (see Chapter 1) (McCaffrey, Pasero, 1999).
    II. Evaluate pain measures (Box 7-2).

BOX 7-2
HIERARCHY OF IMPORTANCE OF BASIC MEASURES OF PAIN INTENSITY

> 1. Patient's self-report using a pain rating scale (0-10)
> 2. Pathologic conditions or procedures that usually cause pain
> 3. Behaviors (e.g., facial expressions, body movements, crying)
> 4. Report of pain from parent, family, or others close to patient: these individuals may be asked to give proxy pain ratings—guesses about the intensity of the patient's pain
> 5. Physiologic measures: these are the least sensitive indicators of pain

Information from Acute Pain Management Guideline Panel: *Acute pain in infants, children, and adolescents: operative and medical procedures. Quick reference guide for clinicians.* AHCPR Publication No. 92-0019, Rockville, Md, 1992, Agency for Health Care Policy and Research, Public Health Service, U.S. Department of Health and Human Services; Acute Pain Management Guideline Panel: *Acute pain management in adults: operative procedures. Quick reference guide for clinicians.* AHCPR Publication No. 92-0019, Rockville, Md, 1992, Agency for Health Care Policy and Research, Public Health Service, U.S. Department of Health and Human Services; McGrath PJ et al: Report of the subcommittee on assessment and methodological issues in the management of pain in childhood cancer, *Pediatrics* 86(suppl 5):814-817, 1990; McCaffrey M, Pasero C: *Pain: Clinical manual,* St. Louis, 1999, Mosby, p 95.

    III. Assess all domains (physical, social, psychologic, spiritual) influencing the client's perception of pain.
    IV. Determine client and family goals for pain control.
     V. Obtain history of drugs used for pain management.
    VI. Obtain history of nonpharmacologic and other noninvasive management techniques employed.
   VII. Continuously evaluate pain control and pain status.
       A. Determine if pain is changing in location or quality.
       B. Determine if pain is not responding to current interventions.
       C. Change pain management program as indicated.
  VIII. Evaluate for side effects of medications.
       A. Opioids.
          1. Constipation.
          2. Nausea and vomiting.
          3. Sedation.
          4. Pruritus.
          5. Mental status changes.
          6. Respiratory depression.
          7. Myoclonus (high doses).
       B. Other medication side effects (i.e., gastrointestinal [GI] upset with NSAIDs).
    IX. Determine barriers to pain control.

Nursing Diagnoses

     I. Acute or chronic pain.
    II. Deficient knowledge related to pain management.
   III. Ineffective role performance.

Outcome Identification

     I. Client and family goals for pain relief are met.
       A. Client is comfortable at the time of death.

II. Client and family have adequate knowledge related to pain regimen.
III. Client participates in activities of daily living (ADLs) for as long as possible.

Planning and Implementation

I. Instruct the client and family on the pain control regimen.
  A. Round-the-clock dosing.
  B. Keeping a log of medication used and client's response to medication.
  C. Proper use of delivery system for intravenous (IV), subcutaneous, or epidural administration of medication.
II. Consult with physician regarding the appropriate titration of medications for pain relief.
III. Assess the client's ability to take oral medications and use alternate route when necessary.
  A. Transdermal.
  B. Sublingual.
  C. Transmucosal.
  D. Rectal suppositories.
  E. Subcutaneous, intermittent.
  F. IV or subcutaneous, continuously.
  G. IV or subcutaneous continuously and with client-controlled bolus dosing as needed.
IV. Consult with physician regarding the use of adjuvant medications for pain.
V. Collaborate with physician regarding nonpharmacologic and other invasive interventions, and ensure client understanding of modalities.
VI. Utilize the interdisciplinary team to ensure appropriate support/interventions for the spiritual, psychologic, and social factors affecting pain.
VII. Collaborate with physician regarding nonresponsive pain, and consider referral to pain team or clinic.
VIII. Teach and evaluate psychologic interventions (guided imagery, relaxation) depending on the client's cognitive functions.
IX. Utilize complementary interventions depending on client wishes and evidence of effectiveness.
X. Position clients to promote normal physiologic function of the musculoskeletal system (Coyle & Layman-Goldstein, 2001).
XI. Consult with physical therapy, and encourage physical activity as long as the client is capable.

Evaluation

The oncology nurse systematically and regularly evaluates the client's and/or family's response to interventions to determine progress toward the achievement of expected outcomes. Relevant data are collected, and actual findings are compared with expected findings. Nursing diagnoses, outcomes, and plans of care are reviewed and revised as necessary.

ELIMINATION (see also Chapter 15)

Theory

I. The most common cause of constipation in clients with cancer is opioid use (Abrahm, 2000).

A. Opioids interfere with normal peristalsis, causing a slowing of the transport of feces, and they cause an increase in the tone and decrease in the sensitivity of the anorectal sphincter (Abrahm, 2000).

B. Additional causes of constipation include low-fiber diet, dehydration, reduced defecation, depression, hypercalcemia, and damage to spinal cord (Economou, 2001).

C. Persons who are not eating continue to produce waste in the bowel.

II. Causes of diarrhea include fecal impaction, malignant intestinal obstruction, laxative imbalance, and loss of sphincter control (Economou, 2001).

III. Urinary retention and/or urinary incontinence may result from spinal cord involvement by tumor, increased weakness and confusion, side effects of medication, urinary tract infection, and dehydration (Gray & Campbell, 2001).

Assessment

I. Obtain history of the bowel problem including those laxatives that have been used.

II. Complete abdominal physical assessment.

A. Examine abdomen for presence of fecal masses and tenderness.

B. Assess bowel sounds.

C. Palpate for full bladder.

D. Perform rectal examination for presence of impacted feces, malignant stenosis, and empty balloon rectum (higher impaction).

III. Obtain history of usual bowel and bladder elimination patterns.

IV. Obtain intake history, and evaluate hydration status.

V. Review medication history for side effects contributing to problems in elimination.

VI. Assess for urinary tract infection—frequency, burning on urination, urgency.

VII. Assess signs of spinal cord involvement.

A. Back pain.

B. Lower extremity weakness.

C. Loss of rectal sensation.

VIII. Assess skin integrity.

Nursing Diagnoses

I. Constipation.

II. Diarrhea.

III. Impaired urinary elimination.

IV. Urinary retention.

V. Risk for impaired skin integrity.

Outcome Identification

I. Client passes soft, formed stool at a frequency perceived as "normal" for the client.

II. Normal bowel elimination pattern for client is achieved.

III. Client is continent of urine or verbalizes satisfactory management.

IV. Client empties bladder completely.

V. Skin remains intact.

BOX 7-3
CONSTIPATION MANAGEMENT

Start all clients on the following:
    Senna (Senokot-S) 2 tabs PO at bedtime
If no bowel movement in any 24-hour period:
    Senna (Senokot-S), 2-4 tabs PO bid or tid
If no bowel movement in any 48-hour period:
    Bisacodyl (Dulcolax) 2-3 tabs PO at bedtime-tid
If no bowel movement in any 72-hour period:
    Nonimpacted
        Magnesium with mineral oil (Haley's MO) 45-60 ml PO
        Magnesium citrate (Citrate of Magnesia), 8 oz PO
        Lactulose (Chronulac, Evalose), 45-60 ml PO
        Dulcolax suppository, 1 PR
        Phosphates (Fleet Phospho-Soda) Enema, 1 PR
    Impacted
        Disimpact
        Enemas until clear
Increase daily Senokot-S and Dulcolax

From Levy MH: Pharmacologic management of cancer pain, *Semin Oncol* 21(6):730, 1994.
tabs, Tablets; *PO,* orally; *bid,* twice daily; *tid,* three times daily; *PR,* per rectum.

Planning and Implementation

    I. Teach constipation management (Box 7-3).
   II. Remove fecal impaction, as needed.
  III. Teach dietary interventions (see Chapter 15).
  IV. Teach use of protective skin barriers and adult incontinence pads.
   V. Teach use of antidiarrheal medications.
 VI. Obtain urine for culture if appropriate.
VII. Institute bladder training program.
VIII. Insert urinary catheter for retention, and teach the family the care of the catheter.
  IX. Encourage increased intake of fluids with care not to overhydrate the client.
   X. Notify physician if spinal cord involvement is suspected.

Evaluation

The oncology nurse systematically and regularly evaluates the client's and/or family's response to interventions to determine progress toward the achievement of expected outcomes. Relevant data are collected, and actual findings are compared with expected findings. Nursing diagnoses, outcomes, and plans of care are reviewed and revised as necessary.

DYSPNEA (see also Chapter 16)

Theory

    I. Dyspnea is one of the most common and distressing symptoms occurring in clients admitted to hospice with advanced cancer (McMillan & Small, 2002).

A. Subjective symptom that can be undetected by an outside observer.
B. Client's report of dyspnea or breathlessness must be accepted without measurable physical signs (Dudgeon, 2001).
C. Dyspnea is accompanied by feelings of anxiety and frustration.

II. Causes of dyspnea in advanced cancer are multiple and may be related to the following:
  A. Primary diagnosis, that is, lung cancer.
  B. Secondary diagnosis, that is, pleural effusion or metastasis to the lungs.
  C. Treatment for the primary disease, that is, as anemia secondary to chemotherapy (Kazanowski, 2001).

III. Dying clients may experience dyspnea in the absence of hypoxia or lung disease because of progressive muscle weakness from cachexia, malnutrition, inanition (Mosenthal & Lee, 2002).

IV. There is evidence to support the use of oral or parental opioids to palliate breathlessness (Jennings et al., 2002).

V. The role of oxygen therapy in nonhypoxic, dyspneic cancer clients is uncertain, but it may increase comfort and a trial of oxygen should be used for each client (Mosenthal & Lee, 2002).

VI. Management should first be directed at treatable underlying causes and then proceed to symptom management.

Assessment

I. Ask client about presence of feelings of breathlessness or shortness of breath with activities (Dudgeon, 2001).

II. Consider the use of a visual analogue scale to measure intensity of dyspnea (Kazanowski, 2001).

III. Assess respiratory status.
  A. Auscultate all lung fields for the following:
    1. Breath sounds.
    2. Crackles or wheezes.
    3. Cough.
    4. Secretions—amount, consistency, color.
  B. Evaluate respiratory pattern.
    1. Rate.
    2. Depth.
    3. Regular or irregular pattern.
  C. Obtain history.
    1. Onset: sudden or gradual.
    2. Impact on activity.
    3. Frequency and duration.
    4. Pulmonary metastases.
  D. Assess for anemia (see Chapter 16).
  E. Assess for congestive heart failure.
    1. Auscultate lungs for rales.
    2. Check for peripheral edema.

IV. Evaluate subjective symptoms.
  A. Weakness.
  B. Suffocation.
  C. Tightness.
  D. Panic or anxiety.

Nursing Diagnoses

  I. Anxiety.
 II. Activity intolerance.
III. Impaired gas exchange.
 IV. Deficient knowledge related to dyspnea.

Outcome Identification

  I. Client reports a reduction in level of anxiety expressed.
    A. Client is relieved of the perception of breathlessness.
 II. Client maintains activity level within capabilities.
III. Client's respiratory rate remains at a comfortable level.
    A. Client is relieved of dyspnea.
 IV. Client is able to manage episodes of dyspnea.

Planning and Implementation

  I. Collaborate with the physician to treat the cause of dyspnea as possible (i.e., thoracentesis for effusions, blood transfusions for anemia).
 II. Collaborate with the physician regarding pharmacologic management, and teach the family and client proper use of medications.
    A. Bronchodilators.
    B. Anxiolytics.
    C. Steroids.
    D. Humidified oxygen as indicated by oxygen saturation or client comfort.
    E. Morphine orally or intravenously
    F. Nebulized morphine has been utilized but according to Jennings et al. (2002) there is no evidence to support the use of nebulized morphine and further studies are needed.
    G. Diuretics for congestive heart failure.
    H. Blood transfusion may provide relief for the client with severe anemia.
III. Teach behavioral interventions (Dudgeon, 2001).
    A. Positioning.
        1. Sitting up, using a table to support the arms and upper body.
        2. Elevating head of bed.
    B. Pacing of activities.
        1. Provide periods of rest between activities.
        2. Change times of activities.
        3. Transfer responsibilities to someone else.
        4. Shower while sitting.
    C. Pursed-lip breathing.
    D. Use of electric fan to create a stream of air against cheek.
 IV. Provide reassurance to reduce anxiety.
    A. Have someone remain with the client during acute attacks.
    B. Instruct the client and family that dyspnea can be controlled.

Evaluation

The oncology nurse systematically and regularly evaluates the client's and/or family's response to interventions to determine progress toward the achievement of

expected outcomes. Relevant data are collected, and actual findings are compared with expected findings. Nursing diagnoses, outcomes, and plans of care are reviewed and revised as necessary.

ANOREXIA/CACHEXIA (see also Chapter 14)

Theory

   I. "Anorexia and cachexia are distinct syndromes but clinically difficult to differentiate" (Kemp, 2001, p. 105).
  II. Anorexia is a decrease in appetite resulting in weight loss and may be reversible (Abrahm, 2000).
 III. Cachexia is a metabolic syndrome associated with cancer that results in loss of fat and muscle and the loss of bone mineral content (Kemp, 2001).
  IV. Enteral feedings are not usually suggested for clients with end-stage disease but may be used in early reversible weight loss (Kemp, 2001).
   V. Parenteral feedings, although used during treatments such as bone marrow transplantation, are not appropriate in end-stage illness (Kemp, 2001).
  VI. Pharmacologic agents to address anorexia/cachexia are not usually indicated in end-stage illness (Kemp, 2001).

Assessment

   I. Explore the meaning of not eating with the client and family.
  II. Identify factors that discourage eating.
 III. Obtain dietary history.

Nursing Diagnosis

   I. Imbalanced nutrition: less than body requirements.

Outcome Identification

   I. Client eats what he/she wishes.
      A. Client and family accept the client's inability to eat.
      B. Inappropriate parenteral or enteral nutrition is avoided.

Planning and Implementation

   I. Help family members understand nutritional limitations of the client with a terminal disease (Kemp, 2001).
      A. Caregiver may feel frustrated with preparation of foods that are not eaten.
      B. Client may feel unable to live up to caregiver expectations.
  II. Explain possible causes of anorexia and/or cachexia.
 III. Inform the caregiver that the client is unable and not unwilling to eat.
  IV. Suggest small meals and liquid supplements.
   V. Treat symptoms such as nausea that may contribute to decreased appetite.
  VI. Consult with physician to determine if appetite stimulants may be appropriate. (e.g., megestrol [Megace]) (Abrahm, 2000).

Evaluation

The oncology nurse systematically and regularly evaluates the client's and/or family's response to interventions to determine progress toward the achievement of expected outcomes. Relevant data are collected, and actual findings are compared with expected findings. Nursing diagnoses, outcomes, and plans of care are reviewed and revised as necessary.

NAUSEA AND VOMITING (see also Chapter 14)

Theory

   I. Multiple causes of nausea and vomiting in terminal illness (Box 7-4).
     A. Attempt should be made to identify underlying etiologies, and corrective measures may be instituted.
     B. Client preferences and prognostic expectations must be weighed when considering therapeutic interventions.
  II. Palliative treatment most often consists of antiemetics, dietary manipulation, and behavioral interventions.
 III. Combining antiemetics from different classes seems to improve efficacy of the individual drugs (King, 2001).
 IV. Bowel obstructions may be treated conservatively with antiemetics, stool softeners, and soft or liquid diets.
     A. Initiation of IV fluids and antiemetics with the use of nasogastric suction may be considered for severe obstruction and vomiting.
     B. Nasogastric tubes are uncomfortable, and medical management without suction may be preferred.
     C. Octreotide may be indicated to reduce gastric secretions (Lublin & Schwartzentruber, 2002).

Assessment

   I. Assess for possible causes of nausea and vomiting as identified in Box 7-4.
  II. Obtain history of occurrences of nausea and vomiting.
 III. Review antiemetics that have been tried.

Nursing Diagnoses

   I. Nausea.
  II. Risk for deficient fluid volume.

Outcome Identification

   I. Nausea and vomiting are controlled.
  II. Adequate hydration is maintained, as appropriate, to promote client comfort.

Planning and Implementation

   I. Treat causes of nausea and vomiting when possible (i.e., relieve bowel obstruction).
  II. Collaborate with physician in selecting antiemetic protocols that combine different classes of drugs.

BOX 7-4
CAUSES OF NAUSEA AND VOMITING

Irritation/Obstruction of Gastrointestinal (GI) Tract	Biochemical Abnormalities
Cancer	Hypercalcemia
Chronic cough	Hyponatremia
Esophagitis	Fluid and electrolyte imbalances
Peptic ulcer	Volume depletion
Gastric distention	Adrenocortical insufficiency
Gastric compression	Liver failure
Delayed gastric emptying	Renal failure
Bowel obstruction	Drugs
Constipation	Chemotherapy
Hepatitis	Opioids
Biliary obstruction	Digoxin
Chemotherapy	Antibiotics
Radiation	Anticonvulsants
Sepsis	Aspirin and nonsteroidal antiinflamma-
Metastases	tory drugs (NSAIDs)
Central nervous system (CNS)	Increased Intracranial Pressure
Brain	Cerebral edema
Meninges	Intracranial tumor
Liver	Intracranial bleeding
Psychologic	Skull metastases
Fear	
Anxiety	

From King C: Nausea and vomiting. In Ferrell BR, Coyle N, editors: *Textbook of palliative care nursing*, New York, 2001, Oxford University Press, p 109.

   III. Teach client and family use of medications.
   IV. Suggest dietary changes.
      A. Cold foods or foods at room temperature (decrease odors).
      B. Clear liquid diet.
      C. Avoidance of sweet, fatty, highly salted, or spicy foods.
    V. Limit sights, sounds, or smells that can induce vomiting.
   VI. Provide fresh air.
  VII. Provide distraction and relaxation techniques.
 VIII. Report signs of bowel obstruction, and consult client, family, and physician if nasogastric suction is appropriate and initiate.

Evaluation

The oncology nurse systematically and regularly evaluates the client's and/or family's response to interventions to determine progress toward the achievement of expected outcomes. Relevant data are collected, and actual findings are compared with expected findings. Nursing diagnoses, outcomes, and plans of care are reviewed and revised as necessary.

DEHYDRATION

Theory

I. Dehydration in terminally ill clients may be considered predictable and "should not always be viewed negatively in palliative care clients" (McAulay, 2001, p. 36).

II. "There is no consensus among experts on whether it is physically, psychologically, socially or ethically appropriate to provide artificial hydration or nutrition to a terminally ill patient" (Kedziera, 2001, p. 156).

III. Major complaint by clients related to dehydration is dry mouth (Matzo & Sherman, 2001).

IV. Positive effects of dehydration may include the following:
  A. Decreased urine output with the effect of less incontinence and less need for urinary catheterization.
  B. Decreased gastric secretions and less vomiting.
  C. Decreased pulmonary secretions and edema with quieter breathing and less need for suctioning.
  D. Decreased ascites and peripheral edema.

V. Negative effects of dehydration may include aggravation of confusion and restlessness (Kedziera, 2001, p. 157).

Assessment

I. Assess client's intake and output.

II. Evaluate client's and family's wishes for intervention.

III. Assess condition of client's mouth.

Nursing Diagnoses

I. Deficient fluid volume.

II. Impaired oral mucous membrane.

Outcome Identification

I. Family recognizes dehydration as predictable event in the dying process.
  A. Client is comfortable at the time of death.
  B. Client and family are comfortable with the decision regarding hydration.

II. Client's oral mucous membranes moist and intact.

Planning and Implementation

I. Recognize the complex issue in determining whether or not to hydrate.

II. Describe possible positive effects of dehydration.

III. Discuss disadvantages of hydration.
  A. Invasive procedures.
  B. Increased pulmonary and cardiac load.
  C. Possible need for urinary catheterization.
  D. May decrease client comfort.

IV. Recognize family needs and respect wishes if the family chooses hydration.

V. Consult with physician, and initiate hydration if appropriate.

VI. Teach oral care every 2 hours to moisten mouth and protect mucous membranes (Kedziera, 2001).

VII. Provide small amounts of fluids or ice chips for comfort.

Evaluation

The oncology nurse systematically and regularly evaluates the client's and/or family's response to interventions to determine progress toward the achievement of expected outcomes. Relevant data are collected, and actual findings are compared with expected findings. Nursing diagnoses, outcomes, and plans of care are reviewed and revised as necessary.

PSYCHOLOGIC: DEPRESSION AND ANXIETY
(see also Chapter 2)

Theory

I. Three areas of concern in the category of psychologic distress include depression, anxiety, and neurocognitive changes (Sivesind & Baile, 2001).

II. Clients at the end of life may experience anxiety related to uncertain future, separation from loved ones, burden on family, and loss of control (Pasacreta et al., 2001).

III. "Depression and anxiety are appropriate to the stress of having a serious illness, and the boundary between normal and abnormal symptoms is often unclear" (Pasacreta et al., 2001, p. 273).

IV. Supportive therapy or cognitive behavioral techniques and medications such as antidepressants or antianxiety medications are useful in the management of psychologic distress in clients with cancer.

Assessment

I. Recognize evidence of depression, such as hopelessness, helplessness, worthlessness, guilt, and sustained suicidal ideation (Block, 2001).

II. Assess for anxiety (Sivesind & Baile, 2001).
   A. Physical symptoms, such as dyspnea, chest tightness, heart palpitations.
   B. Psychologic symptoms, such as irritability, worry, fear.

III. Review medications for drugs that may contribute to anxiety, such as steroids.

IV. Assess for suicide plan.

Nursing Diagnoses

I. Fear.
II. Anxiety.
III. Risk for suicide.

Outcome Identification

I. Client verbalizes a reduction of fear.
   A. Client identifies sources of fear related to dying.

II. Client expresses a reduction in the level of anxiety experienced.

III. Client verbalizes suicidal ideation.
   A. Suicide does not occur.

Planning and Implementation

I. Collaborate with physician to determine use of antidepressants or antianxiety medications.

II. Consider the need for referral to mental health care clinicians for diagnosis and counseling.

III. Collaborate with physician to discontinue medications or change doses of drugs that may contribute to anxiety or depression.

IV. Utilize holistic communication skills, such as active listening, to provide empathic understanding for the client (Klagsbrun, 2001).

V. Seek immediate assistance for the client reporting continued suicidal ideation, especially if the client describes a plan for suicide.

VI. Identify available support systems, and evaluate need for referral to community agencies for additional support services.

Evaluation

The oncology nurse systematically and regularly evaluates the client's and/or family's response to interventions to determine progress toward the achievement of expected outcomes. Relevant data are collected, and actual findings are compared with expected findings. Nursing diagnoses, outcomes, and plans of care are reviewed and revised as necessary.

PSYCHOLOGIC: DELIRIUM

Theory

I. Delirium is present in 25% to 40% of clients with cancer at some point during their lives (Sivesind & Baile, 2001).

II. Delirium is characterized by an alteration in the level of consciousness that may occur abruptly and may fluctuate throughout the day (Sivesind & Baile, 2001).

III. Causes of delirium may include medications such as steroids and opioids, organ failure, infection, metabolic changes, and the effects of disease on the central nervous system (Block, 2001).

IV. Terminal restlessness is a specific form of delirium occurring in the last days or hours before death and may not be reversible (Kuebler et al., 2001).

Assessment

I. Assess for delirium, which may be manifested as agitation and restlessness.

II. Review medications for drugs that may contribute to delirium and agitation.

III. Note degree of agitation and the effects on the family.

   A. Caregivers unable to sleep at night.

   B. Disorganization in the home because of client demands.

IV. Assess for safety.

   A. Client not left alone.

   B. Room is well lit at night.

   C. Room uncluttered.

Nursing Diagnoses

I. Acute confusion.

II. Risk for injury.
III. Caregiver role strain.

Outcome Identification

I. Client is calm and suffers a minimum amount of agitation as death approaches.
II. Client is not injured.
III. Family receives adequate support to care for the client at home or to support the client's death with dignity in an institution.

Planning and Intervention

I. Treat reversible causes if appropriate.
II. Provide a calm environment (i.e., soft music, low lights, familiar objects).
III. Minimize disturbances in the environment.
IV. Teach family safety precautions (i.e., fall precautions, ambulation with assistance, safety rails in bathrooms).
V. Support family with additional help in the home if appropriate.
VI. Provide explanations and support to the family.
VII. Provide respite in a community skilled nursing facility if the client is cared for at home and the family needs relief from stress.
VIII. Consult with physician if drugs, such as haloperidol (Haldol) or chlorpromazine (Thorazine), are needed to control symptoms.

Evaluation

The oncology nurse systematically and regularly evaluates the client's and/or family's response to interventions to determine progress toward the achievement of expected outcomes. Relevant data are collected, and actual findings are compared with expected findings. Nursing diagnoses, outcomes, and plans of care are reviewed and revised as necessary.

IMMINENT DEATH

Theory

I. Pain, dyspnea, restlessness, and agitation are the physical symptoms requiring maximum care in the hours and days before death occurs (Berry et al., 2002).
II. Supporting the family during the dying process is an important nursing function and has been described as an honor and a privilege (Berry & Griffie, 2001).
III. Dying is a continuous process since multiorgan failure occurs and physical signs may occur gradually over weeks or months or rapidly over days (Arnold, 2001).
IV. Emotion, cognition, thinking behavior, and autonomic function all slowly deteriorate, and coma usually occurs before death (Berry & Griffie, 2001).
V. Some clients at the end of life will experience refractory symptoms that are not possible to control without sedation (Coyle & Layman-Goldstein, 2001).
   A. Sedation may occur when medications are titrated for symptom management.

    B. Total sedation (often referred to as terminal sedation) is appropriate when consent has been obtained from the client and family and close attention has been paid to assessment and management of symptoms causing distress (Fine, 2001).

    C. Need for total sedation is uncommon yet has been reported fairly widely in the literature (Fine, 2001).

Assessment

  I. Assess for signs of impending death (Berry & Griffie, 2001; Matzo & Sherman, 2001).

    A. Mental changes such as withdrawal from social interaction, dreaming about or visualizing persons who have died, or talking about going away on a trip or going back home.

    B. Decreased fluid and food intake.

    C. Dysphagia.

    D. Increased sleeping.

    E. Decreased urine output.

    F. Restlessness and agitation.

    G. Changes in breathing pattern.

    H. Noisy or moist breathing.

    I. Decreased circulation with mottling of the skin.

    J. Coma.

 II. Assess caregiver knowledge related to recognition of impending death.

III. Assess for symptom control.

IV. Assess for unrelieved pain and suffering that are not controlled with usual interventions.

Nursing Diagnoses

  I. Death anxiety.

 II. Caregiver role strain.

Outcome Identification

  I. Client dies with dignity.

    A. Symptoms are controlled.

 II. Family demonstrates confidence and competence in performing caregiver role.

    A. Family is prepared for client's death.

Planning and Implementation

  I. Ensure that all comfort measures are provided.

    A. Continue medications via appropriate route for pain, seizures.

    B. Provide mouth care.

    C. Provide preventive skin care.

    D. Ensure proper positioning of client.

 II. Consult with physician for medications, such as anticholinergics for moist breathing and benzodiazepines for restlessness.

III. Discuss with team the need for total sedation, ensure client and family understanding of total or terminal sedation (Fine, 2001), and initiate and maintain sedation if appropriate.
IV. Instruct the family in the symptoms of impending death.
V. Plan with the family for the death event.
  A. Who will be staying with the client?
   1. Will there be adequate caregivers in the home?
   2. Does the family member wish to be with the client in the hospital?
  B. Does the family wish that the nurse, chaplain, or social worker visit at the time of death?
  C. Are funeral arrangements in place?
  D. If the death is at home does the family understand the need to call the hospice nurse at the time of death?
  E. Is the family aware of the local requirements regarding pronouncement at the time of death?
VI. Encourage the family members to say good-bye and to give permission to the dying person to let go.

SOCIAL SUPPORT

Theory

  I. Major family reorganization occurs with the terminal phase of cancer (Davies, 2001).
   A. Seven dimensions are noted in relation to the family and the dying process.
    1. Redefining roles within the family is central to the family experiencing the death of a member.
    2. Dealing with the burden of caring for the family member.
    3. Struggling with the paradox of living and dying.
    4. Contending with change in daily life.
    5. Searching for meaning.
    6. Living day to day and attempting to enjoy the time left.
    7. Preparing for death in concrete ways, such as legal and financial matters.
   B. Assessing the family as a system is an important component of terminal care (Goetschius, 2001).
  II. Families desire a few basic interventions from the nurse (Goetschius, 2001).
   A. Honest, open communication.
   B. Skilled nursing interventions aimed at care and comfort.

Assessment

  I. Assess family functioning.
   A. How are families communicating?
   B. Are they open to accepting support?
   C. Are there financial concerns?
   D. Are there differences in opinions regarding the care for the client?
  II. Assess family structure.
   A. Who is included in the family?
   B. How did the family function before the illness?

III. Assess strengths, such as members with health care training, or weaknesses, such as frail caregiver.
IV. Assess knowledge deficits in end-of-life care.
V. Collaborate with the social worker to complete a family assessment.

Nursing Diagnoses

I. Compromised family coping.
II. Anticipatory grieving.
III. Deficient knowledge related to terminal care needs.

Outcome Identification

I. The family identifies the effect client's illness has on the family unit.
   A. The family uses resources and support services to provide the care that the client requires.
II. The client and family begin the work of anticipatory grief.
III. The client experiences a death with dignity.
   A. The family demonstrates caregiving skills appropriate for the client.

Planning and Implementation

I. Interventions to strengthen the family.
   A. Encourage communication among family members.
      1. Listen to family members and client.
      2. Encourage the family and client to "tell their own stories."
      3. Address fears directly, and provide information to allow the family to deal with fears.
      4. Be prepared to repeat information.
   B. Respect the privacy of the family, and accept the family's coping styles.
   C. Provide access to resources for meeting family needs.
      1. Offer volunteers from the hospice.
      2. Refer to community agencies.
      3. Provide homemaker support.
      4. Provide respite care in a community facility.
   D. Spend time with families of hospitalized clients, and create a safe environment for families within the institution (Goetschius, 2001).
II. Interventions to teach caregiving skills to primary caregiver.
   A. Provide instruction regarding technical skills and comfort measures.
   B. Demonstrate appropriate skills.
   C. Provide 24-hour availability for emergency situations or caregiver questions and concerns.
III. Help the client redefine long-term goals and set more immediate goals, such as seeing friends, listening to music, or completing unfinished business.

Evaluation

The oncology nurse systematically and regularly evaluates the client's and/or family's response to interventions to determine progress toward the achievement of expected outcomes. Relevant data are collected, and actual findings are compared with expected findings. Nursing diagnoses, outcomes, and plans of care are reviewed and revised as necessary.

SPIRITUAL AND CULTURAL (see also Chapters 2 and 4)

Theory

   I. Spiritual beliefs and cultural values influence how individuals view death (Taylor, 2001).

 II. Spiritual needs include the following:
    A. Finding meaning.
      1. Meaning of the illness.
      2. Meaning of life as it was lived.
      3. Meaning of the remaining days.
    B. Finding hope.
      1. Expectation of a good that is yet to come.
      2. Desire not to die alone.
      3. Exploration of belief in afterlife, resurrection, or rebirth.
    C. Defining relatedness.
      1. To God.
      2. To others.
      3. To nature.
    D. Finding forgiveness.
      1. Finding a means of dealing with mistakes or sins.
      2. Acceptance of life, mistakes, suffering.

III. Spirituality and religion are complementary but not identical concepts (Highfield, 2000).

IV. Religion offers a participant a world view and answers questions about ultimate meaning.

 V. Culture identifies a group of people with similar values, norms, lifestyles, rules, language, and beliefs.

VI. Spirituality and culture overlap or are difficult to separate (Taylor, 2001).

Assessment

   I. Assess for spiritual distress, and determine spiritual needs.
    A. What does being in this situation mean to you?
    B. Are there things in your life about which you feel particularly proud? Regret?
    C. What is left undone in your life?
    D. What is your hope for yourself?
    E. What are your spiritual needs?

 II. Identify religious practices that have meaning for the client.
    A. Religious affiliation.
    B. Degree of involvement with church, synagogue, or other institutions.
    C. Rituals or sacraments that are meaningful to the client.

III. Assess for cultural values that may impact the client's terminal care.
    A. Decision making is independent by client or part of family dialogue.
    B. Cultural rituals surrounding death and mourning.

IV. Assess for personal beliefs and practices that the client regards as important.

Nursing Diagnosis

   I. Spiritual distress.

Outcome Identification

I. Client and family/significant other are sustained during the dying process by their own spiritual/cultural values.

Planning and Implementation

I. The nurse should recognize her/his own spiritual-cultural values (Taylor, 2001).
II. Find ways to give client permission to talk about spiritual concerns (Highfield, 2000).
   A. Listen to the client as he/she questions spiritual issues.
   B. Remain nonjudgmental as the client questions as well as finds answers.
   C. Encourage the family to remain present with the client.
III. Share normative information.
   A. Fears, guilt, doubts, and failure of faith are not uncommon.
   B. Virtually everyone involved in this work has similar struggles.
IV. Activate the client's spiritual resources.
   A. Refer to clergy member or hospice chaplain.
   B. Acquire reading material, and read with client.
   C. Pray with the client, if appropriate.
V. Include cultural aspects in providing care to client and family.

Evaluation

The oncology nurse systematically and regularly evaluates the client's and/or family's response to interventions to determine progress toward the achievement of expected outcomes. Relevant data are collected, and actual findings are compared with expected findings. Nursing diagnoses, outcomes, and plans of care are reviewed and revised as necessary.

BEREAVEMENT

Theory

I. Bereavement care is part of a comprehensive palliative/hospice care program.
II. Bereavement is a human experience occurring with the death of a loved one (Corless, 2001).
III. Tasks of bereavement include the following:
   A. Accepting the reality of the loss.
   B. Experiencing the pain of grief.
   C. Adjusting to the new environment.
IV. Manifestations of grief associated with loss of loved one are many and may include the following:
   A. Social withdrawal.
   B. Restlessness.
   C. Loss of weight.
   D. Inability to sleep.
   E. Exhaustion.
   F. Heart palpitations.
   G. Anxiety.
   H. Decreased interest, motivation, or initiative.

V. Complicated grief is manifested by an increased intensity of response and increased length of response (i.e., >1 year) (Corless, 2001).
VI. Risk factors for developing complicated grief may include the following (Potter, 2001):
   A. Reawakening of an old loss.
   B. Multiple losses.
   C. Guilt associated with relationship with deceased.
   D. Angry or ambivalent relationship with deceased.
   E. Social isolation.
   F. Lack of financial support.
   G. History of physical and/or mental illness.

Assessment

I. Assess family for risk factors associated with unresolved grief.
II. Evaluate family members for manifestations of grief.
III. Assess social support available to family.

Nursing Diagnosis

I. Dysfunctional grieving.

Outcome Identification

I. Family completes the tasks of bereavement.

Planning and Implementation

I. Before death occurs, encourage family members and significant others to say good-bye to client.
II. Provide time for family/significant others to relive the traumatic events of the death and "tell their stories."
III. Add to the stability of the family's social world.
   A. Make bereavement visit.
   B. Attend or participate in funeral.
   C. Ensure bereavement follow-up.
      1. Refer to appropriate counseling.
      2. Collaborate with social worker and chaplain in completing referral.
IV. Provide information regarding grief response.

Evaluation

The oncology nurse systematically and regularly evaluates the client's and/or family's response to interventions to determine progress toward the achievement of expected outcomes. Relevant data are collected, and actual findings are compared with expected findings. Nursing diagnoses, outcomes, and plans of care are reviewed and revised as necessary.

REFERENCES

Abrahm, J. (2000). *A physician's guide to pain and symptom management in cancer clients.* Baltimore: Johns Hopkins University Press.

American Pain Society. (1999). *Principles of analgesic use in the treatment of acute pain and cancer pain* (4th ed.). Glenview, IL: American Pain Society.

Arnold, G. (2001). The pathophysiology of the death and dying process. In B. Poor & G.P. Poirries (Eds.). *End of life nursing care.* Sudbury, MA: Jones and Bartlett Publishers.

Berry, P., & Griffie, J. (2001). Planning for the actual death. In B.R. Ferrell & N. Coyle (Eds.). *Textbook of palliative nursing.* New York: Oxford University Press, pp. 382-394.

Berry, P.H., Griffie, J., & Heidrich, D.E. (2002). The dying process. In K. Kuebler, P.H. Berry, & D.E. Heidrich (Eds.). *End of life care clinical practice guidelines.* Philadelphia: W.B. Saunders, pp. 39-50.

Block, S.D. (2001). Psychological considerations, growth, and transcendence at the end of life: The art of the possible. *Journal of the American Medical Association 285*(22), 2898-2905.

Corless, I.B. (2001). Bereavement. In B.R. Ferrell & N. Coyle (Eds.). *Textbook of palliative nursing.* New York: Oxford University Press, pp. 352-362.

Coyle, N. (2001). Introduction to palliative nursing care. In B.R. Ferrell & N. Coyle (Eds.). *Textbook of palliative nursing.* New York: Oxford University Press, pp. 3-6.

Coyle, N., & Layman-Goldstein, M. (2001). Pain assessment and management in palliative care. In M.L. Matzo & D.W. Sherman (Eds.). *Palliative care nursing: Quality care to the end of life.* New York: Springer Publishing Co., pp. 362-461.

Davies, B. (2001). Supporting families in palliative care. In B.R. Ferrell & N. Coyle (Eds.). *Textbook of palliative nursing.* New York: Oxford University Press, pp. 363-378.

Dudgeon, D. (2001). Dyspnea, cough and death rattle. In B.R. Ferrell & N. Coyle (Eds.). *Textbook of palliative nursing.* New York: Oxford University Press, pp. 164-174.

Easley, M.K., & Elliott, S. (2001). Managing pain at the end of life. *Nursing Clinics of North America 36*(4), 779-794.

Economou, D.C. (2001). Bowel management: Constipation, diarrhea, obstruction and ascites. In B.R. Ferrell & N. Coyle (Eds.). *Textbook of palliative nursing.* New York: Oxford University Press, pp. 139-155.

Egan, K.A., & Labyak, M.J. (2001). Hospice care: A model for quality end-of-life care. In B.R. Ferrell & N. Coyle (Eds.). *Textbook of palliative nursing.* New York: Oxford University Press, pp. 7-26.

End of Life Nursing Education Curriculum (ELNEC). (2002). Nursing care at the end of life. In *End of life nursing education curriculum.* Washington, DC: American Association of Colleges of Nursing and City of Hope National Medical Center, pp. 1-79.

Fine, P.G. (2001). Total sedation in end-of-life care: Clinical considerations. *Journal of Hospice and Palliative Nursing 3*(3), 81-87.

Fink, R., & Gates, R. (2001). Pain assessment. In B.R. Ferrell & N. Coyle (Eds.). *Textbook of palliative nursing.* New York: Oxford University Press, pp. 76-98.

Goetschius, S.K. (2001). Caring for families: The other patient in palliative care. In D.W. Sherman & M.L. Matzo (Eds). *Palliative care nursing: Quality care to the end of life.* New York: Springer Publishing Co., pp. 245-274.

Gray, M., & Campbell, F.G. (2001). Urinary tract disorders. In B.R. Ferrell & N. Coyle (Eds.). *Textbook of palliative nursing.* New York: Oxford University Press, pp. 175-191.

Hermann, C., & Looney, S. (2001). The effectiveness of symptom management in hospice clients during the last seven days of life. *Journal of Hospice and Palliative Nursing 3*(3), 86-96.

Highfield, M.E.F. (2000). Providing spiritual care to clients with cancer. *Clinical Journal of Oncology Nursing 4*(3), 115-120.

Jennings A.L., Davies A.N., Higgins J.P.T., Broadley K. (2004). Opioids for the palliation of breathlessness in terminal illness (Cochrane Review). In *The Cochrane Library,* Issue 2. Chichester, UK: John Wiley & Sons, Ltd.

Kazanowski, M.K. (2001). Symptom management in palliative care. In M.L. Matzo & D.W. Sherman. (Eds.). *Palliative care nursing: Quality care to the end of life.* New York: Springer Publishing Co., pp. 327-361.

Kedziera, P. (2001). Hydration, thirst and nutrition. In B.R. Ferrell & N. Coyle (Eds.). *Textbook of palliative nursing.* New York: Oxford University Press, pp. 156-163.

Kemp, C. (2001). Anorexia and cachexia. In B.R. Ferrell & N. Coyle (Eds.). *Textbook of palliative nursing.* New York: Oxford University Press, pp. 101-106.

King, C. (2001). Nausea and vomiting. In B.R. Ferrell & N. Coyle (Eds.). *Textbook of palliative nursing,* New York: Oxford University Press, pp. 107-121.

Klagsbrun, J. (2001). Listening and focusing: Holistic health care tools for nurses. *Nursing Clinics of North America 36*(1), 115-129.

Kuebler, K.K., English, N., & Heidrich, D.E. (2001). Delirium, confusion, agitation, and restlessness. In B.R. Ferrell & N. Coyle (Eds.). *Textbook of palliative nursing.* New York: Oxford University Press, pp. 250-308.

Levy, M.H. (1994). Pharmacologic management of cancer pain. *Seminars in Oncology 21*(6), 718-739.

Lublin, M., & Schwartzentruber, D.J. (2002). Bowel obstruction . In A.M. Berger, R.K. Portenoy, & D.E. Weissman (Eds.). *Principles and practices of palliative care and supportive care.* Philadelphia: Lippincott Williams & Wilkins, pp. 250-263.

Matzo, M.L. & Sherman, D.W. (Eds.). *Palliative care nursing: Quality care to the end of life.* New York: Springer Publishing Co., pp. 118-139.

McAulay, D. (October, 2001). Dehyrdration in the terminally ill patient. *Nurs Stand 16*(4):33-7.

McCaffrey, M., & Pasero, C. (1999). *Pain: Clinical manual.* St. Louis: Mosby.

McMillan, S.C., & Small, B.J. (2002). Symptom distress and quality of life in clients with cancer newly admitted to hospice home care. *Oncology Nursing Forum 29*(10), 1421-1428.

McQuay H.J., Collins S.L., Carroll D., Moore R.A. (2004) Radiotherapy for the palliation of painful bone metastases (Cochrane Review). In: *The Cochrane Library,* Issue 2. Chichester, UK: John Wiley & Sons, Ltd.

Mosenthal, A.C., & Lee, K.F. (2002). Management of dyspnea at the end of life: Relief for clients and surgeons. *Journal of the American College of Surgery 194*(3), 377-386.

National Hospice & Palliative Care Organization. (2003). What is hospice & palliative care. Retrieved January 17, 2004 from the World Wide Web: http://sss.nhpso.org/i4a/pages/index.cfm?pageid=3281

Pasacreta, J., Minarik, P., & Nield-Anderson, L. (2001). Anxiety and depression. In B.R. Ferrell & N. Coyle (Eds.). *Textbook of palliative nursing.* New York: Oxford University Press, pp. 269-389.

Potter, M. (2001). Loss, suffering, bereavement, and grief. In M.L. Matzo & D.W. Sherman (Eds.). *Palliative care nursing: Quality care to the end of life.* New York: Springer Publishing Co., pp. 27-326.

Sellick, S.M., & Zaza, C. (1998). Critical review of 5 nonpharmacologic strategies for managing cancer pain. *Cancer Prevention and Control 2*(1), 7-13.

Sivesind, D., & Baile, W.F. (2001). The psychological distress in clients with cancer. *Nursing Clinics of North America 36*(4), 809-825.

Super, A. (2001). The context of palliative care in progressive illness. In B.R. Ferrell & N. Coyle (Eds.). *Textbook of palliative nursing.* New York: Oxford University Press, pp. 29-36.

Taylor, E.J. (2001). Spirituality, culture, and cancer care. *Seminars in Oncology Nursing 17*(3), 197-205.

World Health Organization. (2003). WHO definition of palliative care. Retrieved January 17, 2004 from the World Wide Web: http://www.who.int/cancer/palliative/definition/en/

Supportive Care: Rehabilitation and Resources

SUE L. FRYMARK

Theory

I. Rationale for rehabilitation.
   A. More than 8.9 million Americans alive today have a history of cancer.
      1. The 5-year survival rate for all cancers combined is now 62% (ACS, 2003).
   B. Increasing need for rehabilitation to improve the quality of life of cancer clients whose lives have been extended with advancement in technology and treatment (Gerber, 2001).
   C. The long-term effects of cancer treatment generate additional rehabilitation issues (Frymark, 1999).
II. Synopsis of *Rehabilitation of People with Cancer: An ONS Position Statement* (ARN & ONS, 2003; Lundgren, 1999).
   A. Definition—rehabilitation is the process by which individuals are assisted, within their environments, to achieve optimal functioning and wellness.
   B. Structure—rehabilitation services available to address the individual's physical, psychologic, spiritual, social, vocational, and educational potential.
   C. Process—services provided according to the individual's preventive, restorative, supportive, or palliative needs.
   D. Outcome—individuals achieve optimal functioning and wellness.
III. Cancer rehabilitation concepts.
   A. The interdisciplinary team of health professionals, volunteers, and, most importantly, the client and family, contributes to the rehabilitation plan (Gerber & Vargo, 1998).
      1. Composition of team varies according to client need and resource availability.
         a. Health professionals involved may include oncology nurse—inpatient, outpatient, home care; physiatrist; social worker; physician; physical therapist; occupational therapist; dietitian; chaplain/minister; psychologist; financial counselor; enterostomal therapist; pharmacist; recreational therapist; dentist; psychiatrist; speech language pathologist; vocational rehabilitation counselor (Lundgren, 1999).
         b. Case manager or other specialist may serve as coordinator of the rehabilitation process (Frymark, 1998).
   B. Continuity of cancer care requires coordinated and comprehensive system of care throughout the health care and community-based settings (Gudas, 2001).

    C. Rehabilitation is enhanced through the process of sharing and developing a common bond with others who have similar problems.

    D. Human needs that include the physiologic, functional, psychosocial, and spiritual dimensions addressed through a holistic approach.

IV. Goals of rehabilitation.

    A. Goal setting requires interaction between the client and family and health professionals.

        1. Validate strengths, limitations, and rehabilitation potential with client.

        2. Identify goals that are realistic and achievable within the context of the client and family situation.

    B. Goals for rehabilitation services.

        1. Preventive rehabilitation.

            a. Reduce impact and severity of disabilities.

            b. Focus is on clients with a disability that can be predicted.

        2. Restorative rehabilitation.

            a. Resume preillness level of functioning with minimal residual disability.

            b. Focus is on clients who are cured.

        3. Supportive rehabilitation.

            a. Reduce cancer-related disability in clients who are receiving treatment for ongoing disease to control cancer.

        4. Palliative rehabilitation.

            a. Reduce and/or eliminate complications, increase autonomy, provide comfort and emotional support when there is increasing disability from progressive disease.

            b. Focus is on terminally ill clients and family training.

V. Barriers to cancer rehabilitation.

    A. Cancer viewed as terminal rather than curable, as compared with other chronic diseases, by both the public and health professionals.

    B. Lack of referrals because of absence of individual assessment of needs across the care continuum.

    C. Control of health care cost in a managed care environment further constrains rehabilitation.

        1. Lack of available and appropriate rehabilitation resources.

        2. Limitations in rehabilitation benefits from health plans.

    D. Fiscal crisis in the federal and state government affects community support and resources for continuity of comprehensive services to clients and families.

VI. Major trends that affect rehabilitation.

    A. Of all cancers, 77% occur in those ages 55 years and older (ACS, 2003).

    B. Growing numbers of elderly, ethnic minorities, and poor who need assistance to do the following:

        1. Enroll in and utilize appropriate hospital and community services.

        2. Meet their basic extramedical needs, such as housing, food, and clothing.

        3. Become well informed to make sound decisions about their treatment.

    C. Increasing use of complementary services to promote mental and physical fitness—diet, exercise, stress reduction (Frymark, 1999).

    D. Increasing consumer awareness related to wellness, prevention, self-determination, and quality of life (Dow, 2003).

    E. Increasing role for rehabilitation services in improving quality of living for those with an advancing cancer (Bunting & Shea, 2001; Cheville, 2001).

F. Shift from inpatient to outpatient care requires increased technologic skills and complex care in the community setting and produces increasing demands on the caregiver (Bedder & Aikin, 1994; Frymark, 1998).

G. National shortage of registered nurses as well as many local shortages of social workers and rehabilitation therapists.

Assessment

I. Data collection.
   A. Use a comprehensive, reliable, and valid tool to assess rehabilitation needs (Box 8-1) (Baker, 1995; Mellette & Blunk, 1994).
   B. On entry to a health care facility, obtain baseline assessment data.
      1. Identify trigger cues for further evaluation by appropriate health professionals (Figure 8-1).
   C. Data should include the following:
      1. Demographic and medical information.
         a. Disease process—type and stage of disease, location of cancer, prognosis.

BOX 8-1
CANCER REHABILITATION: COMPREHENSIVE NEEDS

Functional Needs
- Gait/balance
- Mobility
- Activities of daily living
- Strength and endurance
- Swallowing
- Communication
- Sexual function
- Prosthesis
- Stair climbing
- Transfers: chair, auto, bathroom
- Upper extremity function
- Fine motor skills
- Accessibility

Physiologic Needs
- Symptom control
- Nutrition
- Fatigue
- Ostomy and wound care
- Bowel and bladder
- Skin integrity
- Lymphedema
- Cognition
- Sleep patterns
- Sensory changes

Emotional Needs
- Coping skills
- Fear of recurrence
- Fear of death
- Body image
- Self-esteem
- Intimacy
- Fear of losses
- Impact on roles and relationships

Social Needs
- Communication
- Family relationships
- Role changes
- Workplace/school adjustments
- Legal/financial
- Leisure activities
- Transportation
- Social isolation
- Insurance coverage

Spiritual Needs
- Why me?
- Harmony: God, self, others
- Forgiveness
- Love
- Meaning of life
- Peace

Sample of Admission Database

1.	Activities of daily living:	I = Independent	A = Needs Assist	U = Unable						

		Usual	On Admission		Usual	On Admission		Usual	On Admission
ACTIVITY/EXERCISE	Feeding			Toileting			Ambulating		
	Grooming			Bathing			Climbing Stairs		
	Dressing			Transferring					

2.	Do you exercise regularly? ❏ Yes ❏ No
	Type _____ Frequency _____

❏ No problem
❏ Self-care deficit (OT, PT)
❏ Feeding
❏ Toileting
❏ Bathing/hygiene
❏ Dressing/grooming
❏ Transferring/ambulation

FIGURE 8-1 ■ Sample of an admission database form. *OT*, Occupational therapy; *PT*, physical therapy. (Courtesy St. Francis Medical Center, Honolulu, 1996.)

   b. Type and duration of treatment.
   c. Other comorbidities.
   d. Biographic data—age, occupation, socioeconomic status, ethnic and cultural background, religion, education, marital status, insurance.
   2. Psychosocial.
     a. Personal characteristics—attitudes toward cancer, coping abilities, problem-solving skills, self-concept, motivation to learn, recreational interests.
     b. Family characteristics—perception of cancer; reaction to stress, roles, and relationships.
     c. Support systems.
       (1) Identify available support—spouse or significant other, children, friends, peers, minister, chaplain, church member, school counselor, teacher, employer.
       (2) Assess type of support family member or significant other is able to provide—educational, emotional, instrumental (care and tasks).
   3. Physical assessment.
     a. Body system review for physiologic problems or symptoms that may affect rehabilitation potential.
     b. Functional health patterns—cognition, communication, mobility, activities of daily living (ADLs), nutrition, bowel and bladder functioning, pain and fatigue.
   D. Continue assessment as needs change.

Nursing Diagnoses

   I. Ineffective coping.
   II. Compromised family coping.
   III. Ineffective role performance.
   IV. Disturbed body image.
   V. Deficient knowledge related to the disease process and treatment.

VI. Self-care deficit: feeding, bathing/hygiene, dressing/grooming, toileting.
VII. Activity intolerance.
VIII. Impaired home maintenance.

Outcome Identification

I. Client participates in decision making and care.
II. Client and family demonstrate measures to manage symptoms from disease process and treatment.
III. Client and family use appropriate resources to cope with alterations in roles and lifestyle.
IV. Client and family use appropriate sources of support to cope with alterations in body image.
V. Client and family demonstrate knowledge of disease process and treatment.
VI. Client safely performs self-care activities (feeding, bathing/hygiene, dressing/grooming, toileting) to maximum ability.
VII. Client maintains activity level within capabilities.
VIII. Client and family identify available organizations that can provide assistance at home.

Planning and Implementation

I. Interventions to promote client autonomy and independence.
  A. Encourage client to participate in decisions that affect his/her care.
  B. Based on assessment of needs, provide and reinforce information on cancer, treatment plan, symptom management, rehabilitation, and cancer resources in the community (Holley & Borger, 2001).
  C. Praise client for positive self-care behaviors to build self-confidence and facilitate mastery of technical skills.
  D. Work collaboratively with health care team to identify and control or treat factors that interfere with self-care activities—electrolyte imbalance, fatigue, cognitive changes, malnutrition, situational depression, uncontrolled pain, and so on.
  E. Support family members in their role as coach to encourage the client to assume greater responsibility for self-care.
  F. Empower client and family through education—coping skills, self-care skills, symptom management, community resources.
  G. Explore the cultural expectations of client and family, and adapt care and teaching to meet their needs.
II. Interventions to help cancer clients and their families cope with cancer-associated treatment, losses, and lifestyle changes.
  A. Support client in expression of feelings about changes in appearance, function, and lifestyle.
  B. Encourage open communication between client and family to meet their individual and collective needs (e.g., reassignment of roles, social activities).
  C. Refer client to the local office of the American Cancer Society (ACS) and other cancer-related organizations for support groups, volunteer visitation programs, and educational programs.

    D. Make referrals to mental health professionals and social services for individual and family counseling to resolve issues related to body image, role alterations, coping with uncertainty (Varricchio & Aziz, 1999).

    E. Provide information about prosthetic devices, wigs, cosmetics, and reconstructive surgery to enhance self-esteem in clients facing mastectomy or lumpectomy, amputation, head and neck surgery, chemotherapy- or radiation-associated skin changes and hair loss.

III. Interventions to rehabilitate cancer clients with functional status limitations.

    A. Consult with an occupational therapist, physical therapist, nutritionist, social service worker, and members of other appropriate disciplines to assist with the identification of resources, special equipment, devices, and environmental modifications necessary to permit maximal functioning (Donovan, 2000).

    B. Encourage progressive mobility from active range of motion exercises to functional activities (Sabers et al., 1999).

    C. Coordinate treatment and activities to minimize fatigue.

    D. Provide positive reinforcement for activities out of bed. Avoid immobilization or long confinement in bed.

    E. Maintain normal range of motion and exercises to increase endurance and strength.

    F. Promote a progressive and structured exercise program to enhance quality of life (Young-McCaughan et al., 2003).

IV. Interventions to provide comprehensive care and continuity of services.

    A. Conduct a client and family meeting with appropriate health care professionals before treatment (surgery, chemotherapy, radiation) to do the following:

        1. Clarify myths and misconceptions.

        2. Identify potential and actual problems.

        3. Identify resource availability in the acute care setting and at home.

    B. Initiate site- or treatment-specific client and family education using educational materials appropriate to their level of understanding.

    C. Utilize a language interpreter for non–English-speaking client and family.

    D. Recognize the developmental needs of the young and the elderly cancer clients when planning the rehabilitation goals, interventions, and outcome.

    E. Support family in their role of caregiver through caregiver education programs and by encouraging use of self-help groups, respite care, and volunteers to supplement care.

    F. Refer client to cancer rehabilitation team members to assist with the physical, psychosocial, spiritual, vocational/economic, legal/ethical, and home care/personal care issues (Marciniak et al., 1996) (Table 8-1).

    G. Assist client and family to contact and use the following:

        1. Local agencies for nonmedical needs.

            a. Agencies on aging.

            b. Legal Aid Society.

            c. Social Security Administration.

            d. Veterans Affairs Center.

    H. Refer to local, regional, national, and international organizations for information and support services (Table 8-2).

TABLE 8-1
Comprehensive Rehabilitation: Multidisciplinary Team Resources

Rehabilitation Issues	Resources

Cancer education
    Disease
    Treatment
    Nutrition
    Community resources
    Levels of care
	Individual or group teaching: nurse, physician,
	    dietitian, social worker

Physical—functional status
    Self-care skills
    Technical skills
        Ostomy care
        Incontinence management
        Assistive devices
        Symptom management
          (e.g., pain, nausea, vomiting)
	Physical therapist, occupational therapist, nurse,
	    enterostomal therapist, physical/occupational
	    therapist, pain specialist, clinical pharmacist,
	    nutritionist

Communication/speech	Speech/language pathologist

Psychologic support
    Coping skills
    Lifestyle changes
	Social worker, psychiatric nurse specialist,
	    psychiatrist, sex therapist

Spiritual support, beliefs, practices	Minister, priest

Economic issues
    Financial resources
    Insurance—life and medical
    Disability benefits
    Vocational—employment discrimination
	Social worker, financial counselor

Legal and ethical issues
    Client rights
    Advanced directives: wills, power
      of attorney
	Nurse, client advocate, social worker, attorney

School-related issues
    School reentry and academic
      performance
	Social worker, nurse, school counselor, teacher

Housing	Social worker

Personal care: grooming, bathing, dressing,
    toileting, mobility, meal preparation,
    shopping, household chores, child care,
    transportation, equipment
	Home care nurse, physical therapist, occupational
	    therapist, home health aides

TABLE 8-2
National Cancer Resources

Community Resources	Services Provided
Alliance for Lung Cancer Advocacy, Support, and Education (ALCASE) PO Box 849 Vancouver, WA 98666 (800) 298-2436 www.alcase.org	Provides education, advocacy, and support for those with lung cancer
American Brain Tumor Association 2720 River Road, Suite 146 Des Plaines, IL 60018 (800) 886-2282 (708) 827-9910 www.abta.org	Provides educational material including a "Patient Reference Guide"; lists of support groups and support service referrals
American Cancer Society PO Box 102454 Atlanta, GA 30368-2454 (800) ACS-2345 www.cancer.org	Provides education, advocacy, and support for clients, families, friends, and survivors with cancer
American Foundation for Urologic Disease 1128 North Charles Street Baltimore, MD 21201 (410) 468-1800 www.afud.org	Provides "Prostate Cancer Resource Guide," Prostate Support Group Network
Cancer Care, Inc. 275 7th Avenue New York, NY 10001 (800) 813-HOPE or (212) 712-8080 www.cancercare.org	Provides social work services and counseling; toll-free counseling line for information, support, and referral to local services; on-line educational programs
Cancer Information Service (CIS) (800) 4-CANCER www.cis.nci.nih.gov	National Cancer Institute Program that provides information about cancer, diagnosis, treatment, rehabilitation, and research; information about local resources; PDQ data for public and health care professionals
Cancersource.com 263 Summer Street Boston, MA 02210-1506 (617) 399-4483 www.cancersource.com	Website devoted to up-to-date cancer information including self-care educational materials for cancer survivors; interactive website; information for oncology health care professionals as well
Candlelighters Childhood Cancer Foundation PO Box 498 Kensington, MD 20895-0498 (800) 366-2223 (301) 962-3520 www.candlelighters.org	International organization of parents whose children have or had cancer; provides information, support, referral, and access to survivors of childhood cancers
Encore Plus YWCA of the USA 1015 18th Street, NW, Suite 700 Washington, DC 20036 (800) YWCA-US1 (202) 467-0801 www.ywca.org	Offers postdiagnostic support including a specially designed exercise regimen and peer support

(Continued)

TABLE 8-2
National Cancer Resources—cont'd

Community Resources	Services Provided
International Association of Laryngectomees 8900 Thorton Road, Box 99311 Stockton, CA 95209 (866) 425-3678 www.larnxlink.com	An association with over 230 local groups providing preoperative and postoperative visits to those with cancer of the larynx with support and educational follow-up
Leukemia & Lymphoma Society 1311 Mamaroneck Avenue White Plains, NY 10605 (800) 955-4572 www.leukemia-lymphoma.org	Provides information, education, support groups, and some financial assistance to those with leukemia, lymphoma, or multiple myeloma
National Brain Tumor Association 414 Thirteenth Street, Suite 700 Oakland, CA 94612-2603 (800) 934-2873 or (510) 839-9777 www.braintumor.org	Provides educational materials, network of brain tumor support groups, and support line via phone
The National Coalition for Cancer Survivorship 1010 Wayne Avenue, Suite 770 Silver Spring, MD 20910 (301) 650-9127 www.canceradvocacy.org	Advocates issues related to cancer survivors; provides information and programs for cancer survivors
National Hospice and Palliative Care Association 1700 Diagonal Road, Suite 265 Alexandria, VA 22314 (800) 646-6460 www.nhpco.org	Provides information and education about end-of-life issues and hospice services throughout the United States
National Lymphedema Network Latham Square 1611 Telegraph Avenue, Suite 1111 Oakland, CA 94612-2138 (800) 541-3259 www.lymphnet.org	Provides information about primary and secondary lymphedema, including prevention and management, network of providers, support groups, resource guide
The Oley Foundation 214 Hun Memorial, A-28 Albany Medical Center Albany, NY 12208-3478 (800) 776-OLEY www.oley.org	Provides free information and emotional support to those requiring home nutritional support, including enteral and parenteral nutrition; listing of regional volunteer coordinators for information and support
United Ostomy Association, Inc. 19772 MacArthur Boulevard, Suite 200 Irvine, CA 92612-2405 (800) 826-0826 www.uoa.org	Provides information, education, and support and advocacy to those who have had or will have an intestinal or urinary diversion; visitation program and networks by age-group and language
US TOO! International, Inc. 5003 Fairview Downers Grove, IL 60515 (800) 80-US TOO ([800] 808-7866) www.ustoo.org	Organization devoted to support groups for men with prostate cancer in addition to information about prostate cancer treatment

(Continued)

TABLE 8-2
National Cancer Resources—cont'd

Community Resources	Services Provided
Y-ME National Breast Cancer Organization 212 W. Van Buren, Suite 500 Chicago, IL 60607 (800) 221-2141 (English) (800) 986-9505 (Español) www.y-me.org	National organization for breast cancer support and education; offers counseling, education, and self-help groups for women with breast cancer and their families; local affiliates listed

REFERENCES

American Cancer Society (ACS). (2003). *Cancer facts and figures.* Atlanta: American Cancer Society.

Association of Rehabilitation Nurses (ARN) & Oncology Nursing Society (ONS). (2003). Rehabilitation of people with cancer: ARN & ONS position statement. Pittsburgh: Oncology Nursing Society.

Baker, C. (1995). A functional status scale for measuring quality of life outcomes in head and neck cancer clients. *Cancer Nursing 18,* 452-457.

Bedder, S.M., & Aikin, J.L. (1994). Continuity of care: A challenge for ambulatory oncology nursing. *Seminars in Oncology 10,* 254-263.

Bunting, R.W., & Shea, B. (2001). Bone metastasis and rehabilitation. *Cancer 92*(4, Suppl.), 1020-1028.

Cheville, A. (2001). Rehabilitation of patients with advanced cancer. *Cancer 92*(4, Suppl.) 1039-1048.

Donovan, E.S. (2000). What the rehabilitation therapies can do. In M.L. Winningham & M. Barton-Burke (Eds.). *Fatigue in cancer: A multidisciplinary approach.* Sudbury, MA: Jones and Bartlett Publishers, pp. 339-350.

Dow, K.H. (2003). Challenges and opportunities in cancer survivorship research. *Oncology Nursing Forum 30,* 455-469.

Frymark, S.L. (1999). Cancer rehabilitation: The road to survivorship. *Oncology Issues 14*(6), 16-19.

Frymark, S.L. (1998). Providing cancer rehabilitation services. *Cancer Management 3*(1), 8-13.

Gerber, L. (2001). Cancer rehabilitation into the future. *Cancer 92*(4, Suppl.), 975-979.

Gerber, L., & Vargo, M. (1998). Rehabilitation of patients with cancer diagnosis. In J.A. De Lisa & B.M. Gans (Eds.). *Rehabilitation medicine.* Philadelphia: Lippincott-Raven, pp. 1293-1318.

Gudas, S. (2001). Cancer rehabilitation in the home setting. *Home Care Provider 6,* 172-176.

Holley, S., & Borger, D. (2001). Energy for living with cancer: Preliminary findings of a cancer rehabilitation group intervention. *Oncology Nursing Forum 28,* 1393-1396.

Lundgren, J. (1999). A rehabilitation hospital—services for the oncology patient. *Oncology Issues 14*(6), 20-22.

Marciniak C., Sliwa, J., Spill, G., et al. (1996). Functional outcome following rehabilitation of the cancer patient. *Archives of Physical Medicine and Rehabilitation 77,* 54-57.

Mellette, S.F., & Blunk, K. (1994). Cancer rehabilitation. *Seminars in Oncology 21,* 779-782.

Sabers, S., Kokal, J., Girardi, J., et al. (1999). Evaluation of consultation-based rehabilitation for hospitalized cancer patients with functional impairment. *Mayo Clinic Proceedings 74*(9), 855-861.

Varricchio, C., & Aziz, N. (1999). Rehabilitation and survivorship. In R. Lenhard (Ed.). *Textbook of clinical oncology* (3rd ed.). Atlanta: American Cancer Society.

Young-McCaughan, S., Mays, M., Arzola, S., et al. (2003). Change in exercise tolerance, activity and sleep patterns, and quality of life in patients with cancer participating in a structured exercise program. *Oncology Nursing Forum 30,* 441-452.

9 Supportive Care: Support Therapies and Procedures

JANIS M. PETREE

BLOOD COMPONENT THERAPY

Theory

I. Use of blood component therapy in cancer care has increased because of the following (Cooper & Serpian, 2001; Goodnough et al., 2003; Griffin, 2001; Hoffbrand et al., 2001; Micromedex, 2004a; Schiffer et al., 2001):
   A. Advancement of surgical oncology techniques.
   B. Use of more aggressive single-modality and multimodality cancer therapy and the resulting bone marrow suppression.
   C. Development of donor programs, hemapheresis technology, peripheral stem cell programs, and bone marrow transplantation.
II. Types of blood component therapy (Table 9-1).
III. Sources of blood components.
   A. Homologous blood—blood collected from donors for transfusion to another individual.
   B. Autologous blood—blood collected from the intended recipient.
      1. Self-donation usually made before elective surgery.
      2. Red blood cell (RBC) salvage during surgery by use of automated "cell saver" device or manual suction equipment.
   C. Directly donated blood—blood collected from a donor designated by the intended recipient.
IV. Potential complications of blood component therapy (Demetri & Anderson, 2001; Goodnough et al., 2003; Haire, 2001; Hoffbrand et al., 2001; Micromedex, 2004b; Perrotta & Snyder, 2001; Schiffer et al., 2001).
   A. Allergic reactions.
   B. Febrile reactions.
   C. Hemolytic reactions.
   D. Bacterial contamination.
   E. Volume overload.
   F. Hypothermia.
   G. Air emboli.
   H. Transmission of viruses.

Assessment

I. All clients with a diagnosis of cancer may need some form of blood component therapy during the course of their illness (Goodnough et al., 2003; Perrotta & Snyder, 2001; Schiffer et al., 2001).

TABLE 9-1
Types of Blood Component Therapy

Blood Component	Indication	Consideration
Whole blood	Replacement of blood volume Replacement of RBCs	Rarely used, except in extreme loss of volume
RBCs (packed)	Anemia, for replacement of RBCs	Volume overload
Leukocyte-poor packed RBCs	Prior febrile reactions to packed RBCs May delay alloimmunizations	May use a leukocyte filter to further reduce risk of reaction
Washed or plasma-poor RBCs	Prior urticarial reaction, IgA deficiency, need to avoid complement transfusion	Increased viscosity of blood, thin with normal saline before transfusion
Frozen packed RBCs	Rare blood types, autologous donations; a separation process removes plasma and leukocytes	Used for severe RBC reaction
Platelets, random	Control or prevent bleeding; platelet count <10,000-20,000/mm^3 or client is bleeding or preoperative	Few RBCs present, ABO compatibility not required
Single-donor platelets	May delay alloimmunization, lower risk of infection, exposure to one donor	Poor increase in platelet count.
Leukocyte-poor platelets	Prior febrile reactions to platelets	Febrile reactions, poor increase in platelet count.
HLA-matched platelets	Poor response to prior platelet transfusion because of alloimmunization	Only get increase in platelet count if HLA-matched platelets used.
Granulocytes	Documented infection from bacteria or fungi not responsive to therapy, with severe neutropenia, not expected to recover for several days to 1 wk	Long-term therapeutic effect questionable
Fresh frozen plasma	Increase the level of clotting factors in client with documented deficiency	Plasma compatibility preferred; when thawed must transfuse within 24 hr; watch for fluid overload
Cryoprecipitate	Increase levels of factors VIII and XIII, fibrinogen, and von Willebrand factor	Plasma compatibility preferred; when thawed must transfuse within 6 hr; if pooled, within 4 hr
Factor VIII	Hemophilia A or low ATIII levels	Clients with volume overload problems, plasma cannot be used
Factor IX	Hemophilia B deficiency	Need replacement of factor
Colloid solutions	Expand blood volume	ABO compatibility not required
Plasma substitutes	Chiefly 5% and 25% albumin and PPF	Provide volume expansion and colloid replacement without risk of hepatitis or HIV
Serum immune globulins	Provide passive immunity protection (i.e., against cytomegalovirus) or treat hypogammaglobulinemia	Avoid transfusion for client with allergic reactions to plasma

RBCs, Red blood cells; *IgA,* immunoglobulin A; *HLA,* human leukocyte antigen; *HIV,* human immunodeficiency virus; *PPF,* plasma protein fraction.

II. Factors that increase the likelihood that blood component therapy will be needed.
   A. Cancer treatment—surgery, radiation therapy, chemotherapy.
   B. Cancer that has invaded the bone marrow.
   C. Drugs that suppress bone marrow production.
   D. Chronic infection.
   E. Chronic or acute virus infection.
   F. Aging.
   G. Malnutrition.
   H. Stress.
   I. Chronic immune deficiency.
III. Physical assessment (see sections on neutropenia and thrombocytopenia in Chapter 13 and section on anemia in Chapter 16).
IV. Evaluation of laboratory data (Hoffbrand et al., 2001; Micromedex, 2003a; Perrotta & Synder, 2001).
   A. ABO type.
   B. Hemoglobin: less than 9 g/dl.
   C. Platelet count.
      1. Less than $10,000/mm^3$, with or without bleeding.
      2. Less than $20,000/mm^3$, with active bleeding.
      3. Less than $50,000/mm^3$ and scheduled for surgical procedure.
   D. Neutrophils—less than $500/mm^3$, with an infection unresponsive to antibiotic therapy.

Nursing Diagnoses

I. Deficient knowledge related to need for and risks of blood component therapy.
II. Risk for injury.

Outcome Identification

I. Client discusses the rationale for blood component therapy.
   A. Client describes risk factors for blood component therapy.
II. Client receives blood component therapy without reaction.
   A. Risk of blood component therapy reaction reduced through accurate assessment and early intervention.
   B. Client lists signs and symptoms of reactions to blood component therapy that should be reported to the health care team.

Planning and Implementation (Perrotta & Synder, 2001)

I. Interventions to maximize client safety.
   A. Obtain blood components according to the institutional protocol.
   B. Check blood component type with medical order.
   C. Check blood component type and identification numbers with another registered nurse.
   D. Compare blood component identification information with client identification information before administration.
   E. Examine blood product for clots, bubbles, and discoloration.
   F. Never add medications to blood products.
II. Interventions to monitor for complications of blood component therapy.

   A. Assess for general signs and symptoms—fever, chills, muscle aches and pain, back pain, chest pain, headache, heat at site of infusion or along vessel.

   B. Assess for respiratory signs and symptoms—shortness of breath, tachypnea, apnea, cough, wheezing, rales, and/or air embolism.

   C. Assess for cardiovascular signs and symptoms—bradycardia or tachycardia, hypotension or hypertension, facial flushing, cyanosis of extremities, cool clammy skin, distended neck veins, edema.

   D. Assess for integumentary signs and symptoms—rash, hives, swelling, urticaria, posttransfusion purpura, diaphoresis.

   E. Assess for gastrointestinal (GI) signs and symptoms—nausea, vomiting, abdominal cramping and pain, diarrhea.

   F. Assess for renal signs and symptoms—dark, concentrated, red- to brown-colored urine.

   G. Assess for other delayed complications—delayed hemolytic transfusion reaction, graft-versus-host disease (from nonirradiated blood), iron overload, alloimmunization, infections—hepatitis, human immunodeficiency virus (HIV), cytomegalovirus (CMV), bacterial contamination, parasites.

   H. Assess for changes in laboratory values, such as hypocalcemia and hyperkalemia, resulting from anticoagulants in blood products interacting with electrolytes.

III. Interventions to decrease incidence and severity of side effects (Hoffbrand et al., 2001; Micromedex, 2004a; Perrotta & Snyder, 2001).

   A. Premedicate client with antipyretics and antihistamines as ordered by physician.

   B. Attach appropriate filter and/or blood component set to the blood product.

   C. Use 20-gauge or larger needle for infusion, preferably a needle-free system.

   D. Infuse component over time, according to institutional guidelines.

      1. Packed RBCs—infuse slowly over initial 15 minutes, then remainder over 1 to 2 hours per unit.

      2. Platelets—infuse random donor or single donor platelets over 30 to 60 minutes, or according to volume.

      3. Granulocytes—infuse slowly over 2 to 4 hours; premedicate with acetaminophen (Tylenol) and diphenhydramine (Benadryl).

      4. Fresh frozen plasma—administer each unit slowly or as tolerated by fluid volume.

      5. Cryoprecipitate—infuse rapidly.

      6. Concentrated factor VIII, or factor IX—infuse rapidly.

   E. Observe for signs and symptoms of transfusion reaction—fever, chills, shortness of breath, hives, kidney or back pain, blood in urine, hypotension, tachycardia, chest pain, headache.

      1. If a reaction occurs (Micromedex, 2004b; Perrotta & Synder, 2001):

         a. Stop infusion and keep intravenous (IV) line open with normal saline solution.

         b. Report reaction to the physician and the transfusion service or blood bank.

         c. Check identifying tags and numbers on the blood component at the bedside.

         d. Treat symptoms noted, as ordered.

            (1) Diphenhydramine—administer 25 to 50 mg IV.

            (2) Hydrocortisone—have available 50 to 100 mg.

(3) Meperidine (Demerol), 25 to 50 mg IV, to treat uncontrolled rigors or shaking.

(4) Acetaminophen, 650 to 1000 mg by mouth (PO).

(5) In the future, client should be premedicated with acetaminophen and diphenhydramine.

(6) Oxygen.

   e. Monitor vital signs every 15 minutes.

   f. Send blood bag and attached administration set and labels to the transfusion service or blood bank.

   g. Collect blood and urine samples, and send to the laboratory.

2. Document transfusion reaction.

   a. Date and time noted.

   b. Signs and symptoms observed.

   c. Actions taken.

   d. Response of client after transfusion discontinued.

IV. Interventions to incorporate client and family into care.

   A. Teach the purpose of the transfusion.

   B. Review procedure of administration of transfusion.

   C. Teach the signs and symptoms of transfusion reaction to report to the health care team.

V. Interventions to monitor for response to blood component therapy.

   A. Assess changes in laboratory values.

   B. Monitor changes in subjective responses of clients to blood component therapy.

VI. Pharmacologic interventions (see also Chapter 10) (Griffin, 2001).

   A. For anemia.

   1. Erythropoietin (Epogen, Procrit) administered three times per week to weekly (Micromedex, 2004f).

   2. Darbepoetin (Aranesp) administered every 2 weeks.

   B. Granulocyte colony-stimulating factor (G-CSF) stimulates the myeloid line and increases white cell production after chemotherapy.

   1. Starts 24 hours after chemotherapy for 3 to 14 days.

   2. Pegfilgrastim (Neulasta) is a longer-acting G-CSF given every 21 to 28 days.

   C. Granulocyte-macrophage colony-stimulating factor (GM-CSF) is a multilineage growth factor that increases monocyte, macrophage, and dendritic cell production after bone marrow transplant and chemotherapy.

   D. Thrombopoietin, platelet growth factor, to increase platelets.

   E. Recombinant factor VIIa for clients with existing coagulopathy (Madhu et al., 2004).

   1. Activates factor X to Xa. Activated factor Xa converts prothrombin to thrombin, which then acts to convert fibrinogen to fibrin, forming a hemostatic plug.

   2. U.S. Food and Drug Administration (FDA) approved for the treatment of bleeding episodes in hemophilia A or B clients with inhibitors to factor VIII or factor IX.

   3. Potential use in those with disseminated intravascular coagulation (DIC), severe thrombocytopenia refractory to specific-typed platelets.

   F. Vitamin K is essential for activating factors II, VII, IX, and X, and its deficiency impairs the function of clotting factors.

   G. Warfarin (Coumadin) acts by inhibiting vitamin K-dependent coagulation factors (Micromedex, 2004c; RxList, 2003b).

    H. Heparin (Micromedex, 2004d; RxList, 2003a).
        1. In combination with antithrombin III (heparin cofactor) inhibits thrombosis by inactivating activated factor X and inhibiting the conversion of prothrombin to thrombin.
        2. Inactivates thrombin and prevents the conversion of fibrinogen to fibrin.
        3. Prevents the formation of a stable fibrin clot by inhibiting the activation of the fibrin.
    I. Artificial plasma for treatment of shock, acute liver failure, acute respiratory distress syndrome (ARDS), severe hyponatremia, renal dialysis.

Evaluation

The oncology nurse systematically and regularly evaluates the client's and/or family's responses to interventions to determine progress toward the achievement of expected outcomes. Relevant data are collected, and actual findings are compared with expected findings. Nursing diagnoses, outcomes, and plans of care are reviewed and revised as necessary.

NUTRITION SUPPORT THERAPY

Theory (Angus & Burakoff, 2003; Heyland et al., 2002; Millikan & Millikan, 2003; Nelson & Walsch, 2002)

   I. Nutritional complications.
    A. Poor nutrition is a common consequence of cancer and its treatments. Those with poor nutrition are as follows:
        1. Less able to tolerate therapy and receive optimal benefits from treatment.
        2. More susceptible to infection, debilitation, poor wound healing, skin breakdown, weakness, fatigue, depression, and apathy; poor nutrition impacts quality of life.
    B. Effects of malignant tumors.
        1. Cancer cells compete with normal cells for nutrients needed for cellular division and growth.
        2. Exact demands of the tumor on the host are unknown; the following metabolic changes are proposed:
           a. Altered carbohydrate metabolism—glucose is mobilized for energy and results in glucose intolerance in selected clients, causing the following:
             (1) Anaerobic glycolysis—produces two adenosine triphosphate (ATP) molecules where complete oxidation of glucose yields 36 ATP molecules; thus anaerobic glycolysis is less efficient. Tumors use anaerobic glycolysis.
             (2) Increased rate of gluconeogenesis—an estimated 10% increase in energy expenditure for an individual with cancer.
             (3) Glucose intolerance—evidenced by a delayed clearing of IV or oral glucose, which could be caused by lack of tissue response to insulin or a defect of insulin response to hyperglycemia.
           b. Altered protein metabolism—muscle tissue is mobilized to meet increased metabolic demands and results in muscle wasting, especially

in those clients with cachexia, a severe syndrome of malnutrition (Dell, 2002; Millikan & Millikan, 2003; Nelson & Walsch, 2002; Pfitzenmaier et al., 2003; Rhoney et al., 2002; Strasser & Bruera, 2002).
  (1) Serum albumin is often used to measure protein status.
      (a) Hypoalbuminemia is common in clients with cancer.
          (i) Normal albumin level is 4 g/dl.
          (ii) In a client with cancer, average albumin level is 2.9 g/dl.
  (2) Increased uptake of amino acids by tumor.
  (3) Decreased protein synthesis.
  (4) Increased protein degradation; muscle protein breakdown is accelerated.
  (5) Protein loss by abnormal leakage or exertion leads to depletion of protein stores and decreased muscle mass.
  (6) Use of protein for energy needs (Fearon & Moses, 2002; Nelson & Walsch, 2002).
  (7) In cancer cachexia, protein is wasted despite intake of protein, resulting in the following:
      (a) Weight loss that is often difficult to counteract, despite aggressive feeding.
          (i) Results in negative nitrogen balance.
          (ii) May affect survival and tolerance to treatment.
      (b) Decrease in food intake with partial starvation caused by the conserving lean body mass and host depleting own muscle mass to provide amino acids needed.
      (c) Loss of appetite, alteration in taste and smell, loss of appealing foods.
      (d) Weakness, reduction of strength, decreased functional capacity.
  c. Fluid and electrolyte disturbances (see Chapter 14) (Heyland et al., 2002; Micromedex, 2003b; Millikan & Millikan, 2003).
      (1) Hypercalcemia—high calcium levels in blood caused by certain tumors.
      (2) Hyperuricemia—along with hyperphosphatemia and hyperkalemia is a result of chemotherapy breakdown of cells in some leukemias and lymphomas, leading to tumor lysis syndrome.
      (3) Hyponatremia—common presentation with bronchogenic and small cell carcinoma causing syndrome of inappropriate antidiuretic hormone (SIADH) secretion and causing persistent loss of sodium and excessive retention of water by the kidneys.
      (4) Hypokalemia may be caused by treatment with chemotherapy or antifungal therapy.
3. Cancer cells also produce biochemical substances that affect the desire for food, altering taste, causing anorexia (by central mechanisms or neurotransmitters) (Nelson & Walsch, 2002).
4. Malignant tumors may invade or compress structures and organs vital to the ingestion, digestion, and elimination of food and fluids or may increase metabolic demands.
  a. Fistula formation.
  b. Obstruction.
  c. Decubitus.
  d. Ulcerations.

C. Effects of cancer treatment.
  1. Structural changes in the GI system may result from surgery and result in the following (Angus & Burakoff, 2003; Heyland et al., 2002; Millikan & Millikan, 2003; Stroud et al., 2003):
     a. Inability to feed oneself.
     b. Inability to masticate or swallow.
     c. Inability to move food through the stomach and bowel.
     d. Bowel diversion.
     e. Nausea and vomiting.
  2. Functional changes may occur as a result of surgery, radiation therapy, or chemotherapy and may result in the following (Heyland et al., 2002; Millikan & Millikan, 2003):
     a. Malabsorption of fat.
     b. Gastric hypersecretion of acid.
     c. Water and electrolyte loss.
     d. Dumping syndrome.
     e. Xerostomia.
     f. Mucositis.
     g. Constipation.
     h. Changes in taste and smell.
  3. Metabolic changes may occur as a result of treatment or side effects of treatment, such as increased energy demands that result from fever, stress, diarrhea, vomiting, and cell division or destruction.
II. Nutritional assessment.
  A. Nutritional screening—should be performed before therapy or shortly after starting therapy (Millikan & Millikan, 2003).
    1. Extensive nutrition history and dietary habits taken.
    2. Anthropometric measurements—height, weight, midarm circumference, skinfold thickness, calculation of ideal body weight, body surface area.
    3. Biochemical measurements of protein status—serum albumin (half-life 20 days), transferrin (half-life 8 days), prealbumin (half-life 2 days); assessing long-term, intermediate-term, and short-term protein status.
III. Principles of medical management (Angus & Burakoff, 2003; Heyland et al., 2002; Millikan & Millikan, 2003; Rhoney et al., 2002; Smith & Souba, 2001; Strasser & Bruera, 2002).
  A. Controversies exist in nutritional support for long-term management in clients with cancer because of the following:
    1. Nourishing a client with cancer may enhance tumor growth by improving its nutrient supply.
    2. Beneficial effects of nutritional support are temporary.
  B. Goals of nutritional therapy should be established.
    1. Determine calories needed and calculate basal metabolic rate (BMR).
    2. Increase weight.
    3. Maintain weight.
    4. Maintain fluid and electrolyte balance.
    5. Improve sense of well-being.
    6. Prolong life.
  C. Selection of type of nutritional therapy (enteral or parenteral) depends on the following:
    1. Function of GI tract.
    2. Severity of nutritional problem.
    3. Ability of client to masticate and swallow.

4. Length of proposed therapy and prognosis.
5. Community resources for management at home.
6. Cost.
D. Type of nutritional support (Angus & Burakoff, 2003; Heyland et al., 2002; Micromedex, 2003d; Rhoney et al., 2002; Tisdale, 2002).
   1. Increasing normal intake of food or liquids.
      a. Five or six small meals per day.
      b. High-protein snacks.
      c. High-calorie, low-fat snacks.
      d. Liquids that have calories, such as nutritional shakes, smoothies, or supplements.
      e. Activities to increase appetite, such as light exercise.
      f. Avoid empty calorie food that does not offer nutrition.
      g. Enteral or parenteral therapy is used only if adequate oral intake cannot be maintained.
   2. Enteral therapy—provision of nutritional replacement through the GI tract through an entry other than the mouth, such as a gastrostomy (button), jejunostomy, or nasogastric (temporary) feeding tube or combination gastrostomy and jejunostomy tube in one.
      a. Indicated if the need for nutritional support is anticipated for more than 1 month and attempts at oral intake have been unsuccessful; at least 30 cm of functioning small bowel required.
      b. May require percutaneous endoscopic feeding tube placement.
      c. Potential complications of enteral tube placement and feedings are included in Table 9-2.
      d. Selection of appropriate formula is essential, and different ones may need to be tried (Stroud et al., 2003).
         (1) Choice of formula based on current nutritional requirements, any abnormalities of GI absorption, motility, or diarrhea loss and other coexisting diseases; also considered are laboratory data, amount of protein needed, nitrogen balance and metabolic rate of client; lactose tolerance/intolerance.
         (2) Polymeric formulas contain nitrogen as a whole protein; carbohydrate is partially hydrolyzed starch; and fat contains long-chain triglycerides. Most contain fiber.
            (a) Requires the gut to have some degree of digestive and absorptive capacity.
         (3) Predigested formulas contain nitrogen as short peptides or if elemental formula, proteins are free amino acids; carbohydrates provide much of the energy content and both long-chain and medium-chain triglycerides are present.
            (a) Indicated in presence of significant malabsorption.
         (4) Disease-specific formulas, for example:
            (a) Respiratory failure formulas have low carbohydrate/fat ratio to minimize carbon dioxide production.
            (b) In renal failure, formulas have modified protein, electrolytes, and volume.
      e. Maintenance of gut and maintenance of gut ability (including acid balance and luminal microflora) are first line of defense against invaders into gut.
   3. Parenteral therapy—provision of feeding through an IV route when the GI tract cannot be used for nutritional replacement (Micromedex, 2003d, 2004e; Millikan & Millikan, 2003; Smith & Souba, 2001).

TABLE 9-2
Potential Complications of Enteral Tube Placement and Feedings

Complication	Nursing Intervention
NASOGASTRIC	
Malpositioned tube	Verify proper placement via chest x-ray examination.
	Check placement each time before using tube:
	Aspirate gastric contents.
	Observe for air bubbles by placing distal end of tube in water.
	Inject air and listen with stethoscope over stomach.
	Tape tube securely to nose.
Aspiration	Give bolus feeding rather than continuous feeding.
	Administer no more than 350-400 ml over 20 min every 3-4 hr while client is awake.
	Administer initial volume of 240 ml.
	Keep head of bed elevated 30 degrees during and 1 hr after infusion.
Contaminated equipment, clogged tube	Change feeding bag and tube daily.
	Flush nasogastric tube with 30 ml of water or cranberry juice after each feeding.
	If tube is clogged, flush with 30 ml cranberry juice and 1/4 tsp meat tenderizer.
Abdominal distention, vomiting, cramping, diarrhea	Regulate infusion accurately over 20 min.
	Give formula at room temperature, may need to decrease volume of formula given. Diarrhea may be caused by formula, lactose intolerance, bacterial contamination, osmolality, antibiotics, *Clostridium difficile.*
NASODUODENAL	
Aspiration	Decreased risk of occurrence because tube is in the small bowel.
	Give continuous rather than bolus feeding.
	Small bowel is sensitive to osmolarity; therefore administer at initial rate of 30-50 ml/hr for isotonic formula and increase by 25 ml/hr every 12 hr until desired volume is reached.
Contaminated equipment	Do not allow amount of formula in bag to exceed that which can be administered in 4 hr.
	Change entire administration set every 24 hr, and rinse with hot water every 8 hr.

    a. Requires placement of a central venous line or PICC (peripherally inserted central catheter) line, although peripheral parenteral nutrition (PPN) can be given with lower glucose percentages.

    b. Infusion is a mixture of amino acids, glucose, fluid, vitamins, minerals, electrolytes, and trace elements. Lipid emulsions can be added to increase calories with smaller volume.

    c. Potential complications of parenteral therapy are presented in Table 9-3.

Assessment

  I. Nutritional assessment includes an evaluation of the desire and ability of the client to ingest and process nutritional products (Heyland et al., 2002; Metheny & Stewart, 2002; Rhoney et al., 2002; Strasser & Bruera, 2002).

  A. Ingestion.

TABLE 9-3
Potential Complications of Parenteral Therapy

Complication	Nursing Intervention
TECHNICAL OR MECHANICAL	
Pneumothorax	May occur during insertion of subclavian catheter.
	Observe client during insertion for chest pain, dyspnea, cyanosis.
	Obtain chest x-ray examination after insertion to verify placement.
	Verify blood return before connecting IV tubing to catheter.
Arterial puncture	May occur during insertion.
	Observe for bright red blood, pulsating from catheter.
	Client may complain of pain at site.
	Apply pressure to site for 15 min; may need to apply a sandbag after this.
Malpositioned catheter	Monitor catheter for migration from the superior vena cava to another vein. Note client complaint of neck and shoulder pain, swelling in the surrounding area.
Clotted catheter	NOTE: if unable to infuse solution through catheter and unable to obtain blood return, "declot" according to institutional policy (see Section III of Theory under Vascular Access).
	Infuse 10% dextrose in water solution peripherally or through other lumen of catheter, at the same rates as TPN to prevent hypoglycemia.
Fluid overload	Regulate infusion on a volumetric pump for accuracy.
	Place a time tape on infusion, checking volume infused over each hour.
	Obtain daily weights.
Air emboli	Secure all IV tubing connections with tape to prevent disconnection.
	If air emboli are suspected, clamp tubing immediately and place client on left side in Trendelenburg's position.
METABOLIC	
Hyperglycemia	Increase rate of infusion gradually.
	Check urine for sugar and acetone every 6 hr.
	Monitor serum glucose levels daily.
Hypoglycemia	Observe for signs and symptoms of hypoglycemia.
	Monitor serum glucose levels.
	If sudden cessation of TPN occurs, infuse 10% dextrose in water solution peripherally at same rate as TPN.
	Per physician's order, administer 50 ml of 50% dextrose IV.
INFECTIONS	
Contaminated solution	Do not leave solution unrefrigerated for longer than 4 hr.
	Check each bottle before and during infusion for color and clarity of solution.
Contaminated equipment	Change all IV tubing per institutional/agency procedure, using aseptic technique.
	Do not interrupt TPN for other infusions or blood collecting.
Local site infection	Change dressing, using aseptic technique and following institutional procedure.
	Observe site for redness, tenderness, swelling, exudates.
Fever	Monitor vital signs every 4 hr.
	Obtain both peripheral and central line blood cultures to identify source of infection.

IV, Intravenous; *TPN,* total parenteral nutrition.

   1. Desire to eat.
   2. Patterns of dietary intake.
   3. Ability of client to prepare food and feed self.
   4. Food allergies and preferences.
   5. Dentition.
   6. Ability of client to moisten, chew, and swallow nutrients.
   B. Digestion.
      1. Ability to digest food in stomach and small intestine.
      2. Ability to move digested stomach contents through bowel.
   C. Metabolism.
      1. Presence of abnormal carbohydrate, fat, or protein metabolism.
      2. Presence of vitamin and mineral deficiencies.
   D. Excretion (Eisenberg, 2002).
      1. Bowel elimination patterns.
      2. Urinary elimination patterns.
      3. Characteristics of urine and stool.
II. Nutritional assessment includes evaluation of the effects of dietary intake on the person.
   A. Physical assessment (Heyland et al., 2002).
      1. Skin turgor.
      2. Weight in comparison with ideal body weight.
      3. Muscle mass as measured by the midarm circumference.
      4. Fat stores as measured by triceps skinfold thickness.
   B. Evaluation of laboratory data.
      1. Serum albumin, total protein, and serum transferrin to assess protein stores.
      2. Nitrogen balance to assess energy balance.
      3. Creatinine height index to assess protein stores.
      4. Hemoglobin and hematocrit index.
      5. Electrolyte levels.

Nursing Diagnoses

   I. Imbalanced nutrition: less than body requirements.
  II. Deficient fluid volume or excess fluid volume.
 III. Risk for infection.
  IV. Diarrhea.
   V. Risk for aspiration.
  VI. Deficient knowledge related to nutritional support therapy.

Outcome Identification

   I. Client achieves adequate nutritional status.
  II. Client maintains normal fluid volume.
 III. Client remains free of infection, or infection is recognized early and promptly treated.
  IV. Client does not experience diarrhea during enteral feedings.
   V. Client maintains patent airway and does not aspirate tube feedings.
  VI. Client and family discuss rationale for nutritional support therapy (Strasser & Bruera, 2002).
   A. Client and family demonstrate necessary skills to manage nutritional support therapy.

   B. Client and family list signs and symptoms of complications of nutritional support therapy to report to the health care team.

Planning and Implementation

   I. Interventions to maximize client safety.
      A. Administer nutritional therapy according to institutional protocol.
      B. Examine nutritional supplement for abnormalities in color or clarity.
      C. Check expiration date on nutritional supplement.
      D. Confirm placement of feeding tube or catheter before administering nutritional supplement.
   II. Interventions to monitor for complications of nutritional therapy.
      A. Infection—fever and redness, swelling, pus, pain along feeding tube, catheter tract, or exit site.
      B. Respiratory complications—chest pain, dyspnea, cough, cyanosis.
      C. Fluid overload—weight gain, edema, shortness of breath, distended neck veins.
      D. Hyperglycemia—glucose monitoring every 6 hours, pattern of urinary elimination.
      E. GI—character of stool, bloating, pattern of bowel elimination.
      F. Electrolyte abnormalities—changes in mental status, weakness, fatigue, changes in neurologic examination (restlessness, agitation).
   III. Interventions to decrease the incidence and severity of complications of nutritional support therapy (see Tables 9-2 and 9-3).
   IV. Interventions to incorporate client and family into care.
      A. Teach client and family procedures needed to manage the feeding tube or catheter.
      B. Teach client and family signs and symptoms of complications of nutritional support therapy.
      C. Encourage participation of client and family in decision making about nutritional therapy.

Evaluation

The oncology nurse systematically and regularly evaluates the client's and/or family's responses to interventions to determine progress toward the achievement of expected outcomes. Relevant data are collected, and actual findings are compared with expected findings. Nursing diagnoses, outcomes, and plans of care are reviewed and revised as necessary.

VASCULAR ACCESS: VENOUS, ARTERIAL, AND PERITONEAL DEVICES

Theory

   I. Vascular access devices are essential in the care of clients with cancer because of the following (Alexander, 2001; Camp-Sorrell, 2004; Intravenous Nurses Society, 2002; Jacobsen, 2004; Kuter, 2004; Libutti & Horne, 2001; O'Grady et al., 2002; Otto & Metivier-Johnston, 2001; Rabinowitz-Hirsch & Olsen, 2004; Sansivero & Barton-Burke, 2001; Smith & Souba, 2001; Standiford, 2001; Woods et al., 2000):
      A. Increased use of combination IV therapy in the treatment of cancer.

B. Increased use of supportive therapy (nutritional support, antibiotics, blood component therapy) in cancer care.

C. Increased laboratory monitoring required with aggressive therapy.

II. Types of venous catheters (Moran & Camp-Sorrell, 2002; Smith & Souba, 2001).

   A. Short-term or intermediate-term catheters.

      1. Description—single-lumen or multilumen catheters.

         a. Insertion.

            (1) Peripherally in forearm or antecubital fossa into the cephalic, basilic, or median cubital veins.

            (2) Centrally in the neck or chest into the jugular (external or internal) or subclavian veins.

         b. Made of silicone elastomer, polyurethane, or elastomeric hydrogel.

      2. Types.

         a. Catheter-over-needle or butterflies, inserted into peripheral veins.

         b. Midline catheters 6 to 8 inches long, used for therapy 2 to 6 weeks or longer, considered an intermediate-term device.

         c. Short-term central venous pressure (CVP) lines used for 7 to 10 days.

   B. Long-term venous catheters (Sansivero & Barton-Burke, 2001; Smith & Souba, 2001).

      1. Description—single-lumen or multilumen catheters inserted into jugular, subclavian, feoral veins.

      2. Types.

         a. Tunneled.

            (1) Description—single-lumen or multilumen catheters tunneled subcutaneously into jugular, subclavian, basilic, cephalic, and femoral veins.

            (2) Tip of catheter, which is open or closed, is inserted to the distal superior vena cava and sometimes in the right atrium (for monitoring purposes).

            (3) Dacron cuff along the length of the catheter becomes embedded into the subcutaneous tissue.

              (a) Stabilizes the catheter.

              (b) Minimizes the risk of ascending infections up the tunnel.

            (4) Silver-ion embedded cuff, in a biodegradable collagen matrix, at the exit site to prevent ascending microbes; or chlorhexidine and silver sulfadiazine embedded into polyurethane catheters.

            (5) Made of polyurethane or elastomeric silicone, or Silastic (lower grade material).

         b. Nontunneled.

            (1) Description—catheters placed directly into jugular, femoral, or subclavian veins.

            (2) Long- or short-term catheters depending on catheter materials (silicone, Silastic, polyurethane).

            (3) Catheter tip placement in jugular vein, subclavian vein, superior vena cava, inferior vena cava, or right atrium (depending on entry site).

   C. Implanted ports (Sansivero & Barton-Burke, 2001; Smith & Souba, 2001).

      1. Description—single or double unit implanted surgically.

         a. Port (reservoir with self-sealing septum or reservoir) is sutured into a subcutaneous pocket near the vessel in which the catheter is inserted.

         b. Size of reservoir and gauge of the catheter vary.

     c. Entry to the port may be parallel or perpendicular to the skin (i.e., side or top entry).

     d. Port is reached with a straight or angled noncoring needle or noncoring catheter-over-needle (needle removed and catheter left in port).

  2. Types.

     a. Vascular—venous and arterial (direct administration of chemotherapy into tumor, which results in low systemic toxicity) ports.

     b. Peripheral ports—placed in basilic, cephalic, or median cubital veins with port above or below antecubital fossa.

     c. Epidural or intraspinal ports—for administration of anesthetics, narcotics, or both for pain management.

     d. Intraperitoneal—temporary or permanent placement in abdominal cavity for peritoneal chemotherapy, surgically or percutaneously placed; either a port or catheter.

  3. Made of elastomeric silicone, Silastic, or polyurethane.

  4. Size—various French sizes according to needs of client.

D. Peripherally inserted central catheters (PICCs; Figure 9-1) (Smith & Souba, 2001).

  1. Description—central catheters placed in antecubital fossa in cephalic, basilic, or median cubital veins for short- or intermediate-term therapy.

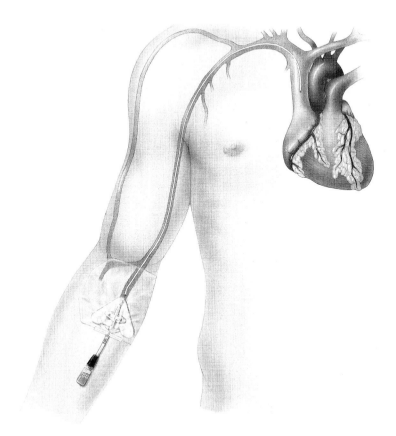

FIGURE 9-1 ■ Peripherally inserted central catheter. (Courtesy of HDC Corporation, San Jose.)

2. Inexpensive access device with low incidence of thoracic complications; major complications: malposition, bleeding at access site, thrombophlebitis.
3. Advantages—decreased risk of infection; decreased risk of insertion complications; decreased costs; increased satisfaction with lack of multiple IV sticks; decreased air embolism, pneumothorax, thrombosis (caused by small catheter size).
4. Types—open or closed ends, single- or double-lumen (staggered ends), made out of silicone, Silastic, or polyurethane materials.

III. Potential complications associated with vascular access devices (Smith & Souba, 2001).
   A. Infection; follow agency policy for changes in dressings, cap, and flushing.
   B. Occlusion techniques.
      1. From medications or lipids.
      2. Mechanical withdrawal occlusions.
         a. Pinch-off syndrome, wherein catheter becomes pinched between the clavicle and the first rib.
         b. Secondary collapse of catheter lumen caused by negative pressure.
         c. Catheter is abutted against a vein wall, such that attempts to aspirate will cause an occlusion.
            (1) These actions can move the catheter off the vein wall: Valsalva's maneuver, cough, deep breath, raising arms, changing position, and lying in Trendelenburg's position.
         d. A fibrin sheath can form at the lumen of the catheter, causing a one-way valve effect, allowing infusion of IV fluids into the client but causing withdrawal occlusion.
   C. Catheter migration.
   D. Catheter constriction by a suture.
   E. Contrast extravasations.
   F. Malpositioned catheter tips.
   G. Catheter leak.
   H. Catheter fracture.
   I. Vascular access device maximal pressure recommendations are exceeded (Conn, 1993).
      1. May lead to catheter rupture, catheter separation, or septum rupture.
      2. Usually occurs when positive or negative force is used to clear an occlusion.
      3. Maximum pressure recommendations.
         a. Ports—usually maximal pounds per square inch (psi) is 40, with most manufacturers recommending that a smaller than 10-ml syringe not be used for flushing.
         b. Silastic catheters open ended or blunt tipped with side slit valves—maximal psi 40, with a 10- to 20-ml syringe for flushing.

Assessment (Sansivero & Barton-Burke, 2001)

I. Identification of potential candidates for venous, arterial, and intraperitoneal access devices (Table 9-4).
II. Physical examination.
   A. Evaluate site of potential insertion.
   B. Evaluate condition of skin over potential insertion site.
   C. Assess patency of vascular access device.

TABLE 9-4
Criteria and Indications for Vascular Access Devices

Type of Device	Clinical Indications	Client Selection Criteria
Short-term venous catheters	Infusions of chemotherapy, antibiotics, TPN, PPN, blood components, and analgesics Infusions of vesicant or irritating agents that may damage peripheral veins Urgent venous access needed	Limited venous access available Frequent venous access required Peripheral lines and midlines: need to consider osmolality of solution infused through vein (dextrose 12.5% or less)
Long-term venous catheters	Infusions of chemotherapy, antibiotics, TPN, blood components, analgesics Collection of blood samples	Limited venous access available, frequent venous access needed for prolonged period of time Long-term catheterization desired by the client; ability to take care of device is necessary
Implanted ports	Infusions of all above agents Collection of blood samples	Limited venous access available for continuous or intermittent therapy anticipated, client/family unable to take care of device (infections are feared)
PICCs	All above therapies Blood collection samples	Client does not desire device in chest, intermediate-term therapy for 4-6 wk or longer
Arterial catheters and implanted ports	Delivery of high concentrations of chemotherapy directly into tumor	Tumor with direct vascular access Tumor sensitive to antineoplastic agents
Intraperitoneal catheters or implanted ports	Delivery of high concentrations of chemotherapy to disease in peritoneal cavity	Metastatic cancer into the abdomen and peritoneum; diagnosis of cancers of the ovary or colon mesothelioma, or malignant ascites

TPN, Total parenteral nutrition; *PPN,* peripheral parenteral nutrition; *PICCs,* peripherally inserted central catheters.

III. Psychosocial examination.
    A. Ability of client/family to care for the catheter or port.
    B. Knowledge of procedures for use of vascular access device for therapy.
    C. Concerns expressed about implications of insertion of device.

Nursing Diagnoses

    I. Risk for infection.
    II. Deficient knowledge related to care of vascular access devices.

Outcome Identification

    I. Client remains free of infection, or infection is recognized early and promptly treated.
    II. Client and family demonstrate appropriate care of vascular access devices.
        A. Client and family describe the rationale, benefits, and risks of vascular access device.

    B. Client and family list the signs and symptoms of complications of vascular access device to report to a member of the health care team.

Planning and Implementation

I. Interventions to maximize safety for the client.
    A. Maintain aseptic technique when entering or manipulating the system.
    B. Teach client and family emergency procedures if the catheter is severed.
    C. Await radiographic confirmation of catheter or port placement before using device (except for midlines, radiographic examination not necessary).
    D. Teach family and client how to care for and maintain vascular access device and flushing techniques according to agency policy and procedure.
        1. Evaluate understanding of care including return demonstration.

II. Interventions to monitor for complications of venous, arterial, or peritoneal devices (Smith & Souba, 2001).
    A. Occlusion—inability to infuse fluids with minimal pressure or inability to withdraw samples of blood or peritoneal fluid (caused by venous thrombosis or drug precipitate).
    B. Air embolism—presence of sudden-onset pallor or cyanosis, shortness of breath, cough, or tachycardia.
    C. Pneumothorax—presence of shortness of breath, chest pain, or tachycardia.
    D. Infection—presence of redness, pain, swelling, warmth, or drainage at exit site or along track or pocket.
        1. Preventive measures.
            a. Catheters coated with chlorhexidine, silver sulfadiazine, or antibiotics are under investigation and may prevent infection.
            b. Antibiotic locks are under investigation; risk is antimicrobial resistance.
            c. Hubs that are coated with antiinfective agents, such as iodinated alcohol.
            d. Removal of catheter should be based on clinical judgment and institutional policy.
    E. Dislodgement—increase in the length of the external catheter, pain during infusion of fluids, swelling along the catheter tract or insertion site, or catheter embolization if shears off or fractures.
    F. Migration—regional discomfort, pain, swelling, or difficulty in using device, or catheter fracture or tear.
    G. Arterial injury—bleeding at exit or entrance site caused by puncture of artery near access site.
    H. Phlebitis—mechanical or chemical irritation that may cause injury to vein.
        1. Treatment involves warm compresses, elevation, rest.
        2. Evaluate using scale of 0 to 4.
            a. 0 = no symptoms.
            b. 1 = erythema at access site with or without pain.
            c. 2 = pain at access site with erythema and/or edema.
            d. 3 = pain at access site with erythema and/or edema, streak formation.
            e. 4 = pain at access site with erythema and/or edema, streak formation, palpable venous cord greater than 1 inch in length, or purulent drainage (Intravenous Nurses Society, 2000).
    I. Extravasation—management depends on drug; consult agency protocols.
    J. Arrhythmias—caused by line placement in right atrium or ventricle.

III. Interventions to minimize risks for complications of venous, arterial, or peritoneal devices (Table 9-5).

TABLE 9-5

Interventions for Complications of Venous, Arterial, and Peritoneal Vascular Access Devices

Complication	Prevention	Restoration
Loss of blood return	Maintain flushing routine, flush with push-stop method causing swirling action in device.	Change client position, roll on to right or left side, sit up, lie flat. Change intrathoracic pressures: have client inhale fully and hold breath or exhale fully and hold breath. Attempt push-pull method using normal saline–filled syringe (avoid using high force or high pressure) or a thrombolytic agent.
Occlusion	Maintain flushing routines, flush with push-stop method causing swirling, prevent clotting. Always flush with normal saline before and after drug administration. Avoid incompatible drugs.	If occlusion the result of clotted blood, urokinase may be instilled with a physician order If drug precipitate, determine type of drug, check with pharmacist for drug to dissolve precipitate. *Lipids* dissolve with ethyl alcohol 70% via 22-mcg filter. Drugs dissolve with *sodium bicarbonate (1 mEq/ml)* or *hydrochloric acid (0.1 N)*.
Pinch-off syndrome	Proper placement by surgeon.	Put client in Trendelenburg's position, with arms raised, and attempt to redraw blood.
Infection	Wash hands thoroughly. Follow strict aseptic techniques when using device.	Administer antibiotic as ordered by the physician. Remove device as ordered by the physician, if allowed by institutional policy.
Dislodgement	Avoid pulling on the catheter. Tape catheters to body. Teach client to avoid manipulation of catheter or port and prevent trauma to catheter.	Refer to physician for resuturing if tip of the catheter remains in the vessel. Remove device if cannot be used safely.
Catheter migration	Protect device from trauma. Anchor device appropriately with sutures.	Refer to physician for repositioning catheter using fluoroscopy. Remove device if cannot be used safely.
Catheter pinholes, tracks, cuts	Avoid use of scissors or sharp objects near the catheter. Clamp properly, moving device up and down length of clamping area.	Repair using appropriate repair kit. Move up and down to prevent areas from being worn with clamp.
Erosion of port through subcutaneous tissue	Maintain adequate nutrition status. Avoid placing port at sites of actual or potential tissue damage (in radiation field). Avoid trauma or pressure over port.	Refer to physician to remove the device.
Port-catheter separation	Avoid trauma and high-pressure infusions, or flushing with 1-ml or 3-ml syringes when clogged.	Refer to physician for removal of device. Use devices that are preconnected by manufacturer, instead of attaching in operating room.
Dislodgement of port access needle	Tape needle securely in place. Avoid tension on the needle or tubing. Place clear dressing over needle, securely fastening.	Remove needle and reaccess the port using a sterile noncoring needle.

Evaluation

The oncology nurse systematically and regularly evaluates the client's and/or family's responses to interventions to determine progress toward the achievement of expected outcomes. Relevant data are collected, and actual findings are compared with expected findings. Nursing diagnoses, outcomes, and plans of care are reviewed and revised as necessary.

INFUSION SYSTEMS

Theory (Alexander, 2001; Metheny & Stewart, 2002)

   I. Infusion systems have become critical in the care of clients with cancer because of the following:
     A. Increased emphasis on timing of antineoplastic therapy.
     B. Increased number of IV therapies.
     C. Need to minimize entry into the infusion system to minimize risk of infection.
  II. Uses for infusion systems.
     A. Controlling the rate of infusions.
     B. Providing positive pressure for infusions.
     C. Providing alarms for early identification of a problem.
 III. Types of infusion systems.
     A. Large volume.
       1. Examples—controllers (computer-controlled infusion pumps), volumetric pumps (mechanical pumps), variable flow systems (systems that allow large flow volumes), multiinfusion devices or pumps.
       2. Used to administer blood components, antibiotics, parenteral nutrition, and IV fluids (including chemotherapy).
     B. Small volume.
       1. Examples—intermittent syringe devices, continuous and intermittent peristaltic devices (fluid released by pressure, from a springlike device), elastomeric (release of fluid by pressure-filled balloonlike device), programmable portable single-infusion or multiinfusion devices (used in home, office, hospital).
       2. Used to administer products similar to those in large-volume systems except in smaller volumes.
     C. Client controlled.
       1. Systems controlled by the client—deliver infusions at continuous, variable, intermittent, and basal rates.
       2. Used to administer antibiotics, antiemetics, and analgesics.
 IV. Potential complications associated with infusion systems.
     A. Occlusion.
     B. Severed or leaking infusion tubing.
     C. Mechanical errors—power failure, error in programming, insufficient fluid volume, error in setting up the system.
     D. Infection.

Assessment

   I. Identification of potential candidates for infusion systems.
     A. Requires long-term or short-term, controlled-rate IV therapy.
     B. Has peripheral or central venous access established.
  II. Physical examination.

    A. Site of venous access—color, temperature, contour, drainage of entry site, exit site, or tunnel of catheter.

    B. Patency of venous access device.

III. Psychologic examination.

    A. Ability of client and family to care for infusion device if intended for home use.

    B. Concerns expressed about infusion device use.

Nursing Diagnoses

  I. Risk for infection.

 II. Risk for injury.

III. Deficient knowledge related to management of infusion systems.

Outcome Identification

  I. Client remains free of infection, or infection is recognized early and promptly treated.

 II. Fluids, medications, or blood components are infused safely and accurately.

III. Client and family demonstrate proper technique in managing infusion systems.

    A. Client and family monitor infusion systems for proper function.

    B. Client and family report signs of potential complications to appropriate health care provider.

Planning and Implementation

  I. Interventions to maximize safety for the client.

    A. Maintain aseptic technique when entering or manipulating the system.

    B. Teach client and family emergency procedures to use if the system is disengaged.

    C. Maintain electrical safety—check all wiring, plugs, and accessory power packs; keep electrical equipment away from water hazards; do not overload electrical outlets.

 II. Interventions to minimize risks of complications from infusion system.

    A. Check patency of system with each system component change.

    B. Assess intactness of system, rate of infusion, remaining volume to be infused, and site of infusion at regular intervals.

    C. Use accessory components designed for the specific system.

    D. Operate infusion systems only for their intended use.

    E. Replace equipment and accessory components at intervals recommended by the manufacturer or institutional policy.

III. Interventions to monitor for complications of infusion system.

    A. Assess for redness, pain, swelling, and pus at infusion site.

    B. Assess client response to fluids being infused.

    C. Assess the system when any alarm sounds.

Evaluation

The oncology nurse systematically and regularly evaluates the client's and/or family's responses to interventions to determine progress toward the achievement of expected outcomes. Relevant data are collected, and actual findings are compared with expected findings. Nursing diagnoses, outcomes, and plans of care are reviewed and revised as necessary.

REFERENCES

Alexander, H.R. (2001). Vascular access and other specialized techniques of drug delivery. In V.T. DeVita, Jr., S. Hellman, & S. Rosenberg (Eds.). *Cancer: Principles and practice of oncology* (6th ed.). Philadelphia: Lippincott Williams & Wilkins, pp. 2753-2766.

Angus, F., & Burakoff, R. (2003). The percutaneous endoscopic gastrostomy tube: Medical and ethical issues in placement. *American Journal of Gastroenterology 98*(2), 272-277.

Camp-Sorrell, D. (Ed.). (2004). *Access device guidelines: Recommendations for nursing practice and education*. Pittsburgh, PA: Oncology Nursing Society.

Conn, C. (1993). The importance of syringe size when using implanted vascular access devices. *Journal of Vascular Access Network 3*(1), 11-18.

Cooper, D.L., & Serpian, S. (2001). Autologous stem cell transplantation. In V.T. DeVita, Jr., S. Hellman, & S. Rosenberg (Eds.). *Cancer: Principles and practice of oncology* (6th ed.). Philadelphia: Lippincott Williams & Wilkins, pp. 2753-2765.

Dell, D.D. (2002). Cachexia in patients with advanced cancer. *Cancer 6*(4), 235-238.

Demetri, G.D., & Anderson, K.C. (2001). Disorders of blood cell production. In M.D. Abeloff, J.O. Armitage, A.S. Lichter, & J.E. Niederhuber (Eds.). *Clinical oncology* (2nd ed.). Philadelphia: Livingston, Division of Harcourt Brace and Co., pp. 628-656.

Eisenberg, P. (2002). An overview of diarrhea in the patient receiving enteral nutrition. *Gastroenterological Nursing 25*(3), 95-104.

Fearon, K., & Moses, A. (2002). Cancer cachexia. *International Journal of Cardiology 85*, 73-81.

Goodnough, L.T., Shander, A., & Brecher, M.E. (2003). Transfusion medicine: Looking to the future. *Lancet 361*, 161-169.

Griffin, J.D. (2001). Hematopoietic growth factors. In V.T. DeVita, Jr., S. Hellman, & S. Rosenberg (Eds.). *Cancer: Principles and practice of oncology* (6th ed.). Philadelphia: Lippincott Williams & Wilkins, pp. 2798-2809.

Haire, W.D. (2001). Thrombotic complications. In M.D. Abeloff, J.O. Armitage, A.S. Lichter, & J.E. Niederhuber (Eds.). *Clinical oncology* (2nd ed.). Philadelphia: Livingston, Division of Harcourt Brace and Co., pp. 657-689.

Heyland, D.K., Drover, J.W., Dhaliwal, R., & Greenwood, J. (2002). Optimizing the benefits and minimizing the risks of enteral nutrition in the critically ill: Role of small bowel feeding. *Journal of Parenteral and Enteral Nutrition 26*(6, Suppl.), 551-557.

Hoffbrand, A.V., Pettit, J.E., & Moss, P.A.H. (2001). *Essential haematology*. Oxford: Blackwell Science, pp. 307-318.

Intravenous Nurses Society. (2000). Infusion nursing standards of practice: Flushing. *Journal of Intravenous Nurse 23*(6S), S53-S54.

Intravenous Nurses Society. (2002). *Policies and procedures for infusion nursing* (2nd ed.). Norwood, MA: Intravenous Nurses Society.

Jacobsen, J. (2004). Vascular access. In V.A. Fahey (Ed.). *Vascular nursing* (4th ed.). St. Louis: Saunders, pp. 429-455.

Kuter, D.J. (2004). Thrombotic complications of central venous catheters in cancer patients. *The Oncologist 9*(2), 207-216.

Libutti, S.K., & Horne, M.K. (2001). Vascular access and specialized techniques and drug delivery. In V.T. DeVita, Jr., S. Hellman, & S. Rosenberg (Eds.). *Cancer: Principles and practice of oncology* (6th ed.). Philadelphia: Lippincott Williams & Wilkins, pp. 760-768.

Madhu, V.M., Mehta, P., Waner, W., & Fink, L.M. (2004). Recombinant factor VIIA in the treatment of bleeding. *American Journal of Clinical Pathology*. Retrieved March 30, 2004 from the World Wide Web: http://www.medscape.com/viewarticle/466983

Metheny, N.A., & Stewart, B.J. (2002). Testing feeding tube placement during continuous tube feeding. *Applied Nursing Research 15*(4), 254-258.

Micromedex. (2003a). Blood products and plasma expanders. In *Martindale. The complete drug reference*. Retrieved April 17, 2004 from the World Wide Web: http://healthcare. micromedex.com/msxcgi/mdxhtml.

Micromedex. (2003b). Electrolytes. In *Physicians' desk reference*. Retrieved April 17, 2004 from the World Wide Web: http://healthcare.micromedex.com/msxcgi/mdxhtml.

Micromedex. (2003c). Erythropoietin. In *Physicians' desk reference*. Retrieved April 17, 2004 from the World Wide Web: http://healthcare.micromedex.com/msxcgi/mdxhtml.

Micromedex. (2003d). TPN, enteral feedings. In *Martindale*: *The complete drug reference.* Retrieved April 17, 2004 from the World Wide Web: http://healthcare.micromedex. com/msxcgi/mdxhtml.

Micromedex. (2004a). Blood products and growth factors in patients with cancer. Healthcare series 115. In *Physicians' desk reference.* Retrieved April 17, 2004 from the World Wide Web: http://healthcare.micromedex.com/msxcgi/mdxhtml.exe?tmp.

Micromedex. (2004b). Cautious use of blood components—FDA Bulletin. In *Physicians' desk reference.* Retrieved April 17, 2004 from the World Wide Web: http://healthcare.micromedex. com/msxcgi/mdxhtml.

Micromedex. (2004c). Coumadin. DrugDex drug evaluation. Retrieved April 17, 2004 from the World Wide Web: http://healthcare.micromedex.com/msxcgi/mdxhtml.

Micromedex. (2004d). Heparin. DrugDex drug evaluation. Retrieved April 17, 2004 from the World Wide Web: http://healthcare.micromedex.com/msxcgi/mdxhtml.

Micromedex. (2004e). Nutritional agents and vitamins. In *Martindale. The complete drug index, enteral and parenteral nutrition, dietary modification.* Retrieved April 17, 2004 from the World Wide Web: http://healthcare.micromedex.com/msxcgi/mdxhtml.

Micromedex. (2004f). Procrit. In *Physicians' desk reference.* Retrieved April 17, 2004 from the World Wide Web: http://healthcare.micromedex.com/msxcgi/mdxhtml.

Millikan, J., & Millikan, K.W. (2003). Nutritional support. In T. J. Saclarides, K.W. Millikan, & C.V. Godellas (Eds.). *Surgical oncology: An alogorithmic approach.* New York: Springer-Verlag, pp. 720-727.

Moran, A., & Camp-Sorrell, D. (2002). Maintenance of vascular access devices in patients with neutropenia. *Clinical Journal of Oncology Nursing 6*(3), 126-130.

Nelson, K.A., & Walsch, D. (2002). The cancer anorexia-cachexia syndrome: A survey of the prognostic inflammatory and nutritional index in advanced disease. *Journal of Pain and Symptom Management 24*(2a), 424-428.

O'Grady, N.P., Alexander, M., Dellinger, E.P., et al. (2002). Guidelines for the prevention of intravascular catheter-related infections. *MMWR: Morbidity and Mortality Weekly Report 51*(rr-10), 1-34. Retrieved from the World Wide Web: www.cdc.gov/MMWR/PDF/ rr/rr5110.pdf

Otto, S.E., & Metivier-Johnston, L.A. (2001). Venous access devices. In S.E. Otto (Ed.). *Oncology nursing* (4th ed.). St. Louis: Mosby (a Harcourt Health Sciences Co.), pp. 589, 814-821.

Perrotta, P.L., & Snyder, E.L. (2001). Transfusion therapy. In V.T. DeVita, Jr., S. Hellman, & S. Rosenberg (Eds.). *Cancer: Principles and practice of oncology* (6th ed.). Philadelphia: Lippincott Williams & Wilkins, pp. 2753-2766.

Pfitzenmaier, J., Vessella, R., Higano, C.S., et al. (2003). Elevation of cytokine levels in cachectic patients with prostate carcinoma. *Cancer 97*(5), 1211-1216.

Rabinowitz-Hirsch, N., & Olsen, M.M. (2004). Venous access devices. In B.K. Shelton, C.R. Ziegfeld, & M.M. Olsen (Eds.). *Manual of cancer nursing.* Philadelphia: Lippincott Williams & Wilkins, pp. 484-500.

Rhoney, D.H., Parker, D., Jr., Formen, C.M., et al. (2002). Tolerability of bolus versus continuous gastric feedings in brain injured patients. *Neurology Research 24*(6), 613-620.

RxList. (2003a). Heparin. Retrieved March 30, 2004 from the World Wide Web: http://www.rxlist.com/cgi/generic/heparin_cp.htm.

RxList. (2003b). Warfarin. Retrieved March 30, 2004 from the World Wide Web: http://www.rxlist.com/cgi/generic/warfarin.htm.

Sansivero, G.S., & Barton-Burke, M. (2001). Chemotherapy administration: General principles for vascular access. In M. Barton-Burke, G.M. Wilkes, & K. Ingwerson. *Cancer chemotherapy: A nursing process approach* (3rd ed.). Sudbury, MA: Jones and Bartlett Publishers, pp. 645-668.

Schiffer, C.A., Anderson, K.C., Bennett, C.L., et al. (2001). Platelet transfusion for patients with cancer: Clinical practice guidelines of the American Cancer Society of Clinical Oncology. *Journal of Clinical Oncology 19*, 1519-1538.

Smith, J.S., & Souba, W.W. (2001). Nutritional support. In V.T. DeVita, Jr., S. Hellman, & S. Rosenberg (Eds.). *Cancer: Principles and practice of oncology* (6th ed.) Philadelphia: Lippincott Williams & Wilkins, pp. 3012-3031.

Standiford, S.B. (2001). Central venous access for chemotherapy. In M.C. Perry (Ed.). *Chemotherapy source book* (3rd ed.). Philadelphia: Lippincott Williams & Wilkins, pp. 559-565.

Strasser, F., & Bruera, E.D. (2002). Update on anorexia and cachexia. *Hematology-Oncology Clinics of North America 16*(3), 589-617.

Stroud, M., Duncan, H., & Nightingale, J. (2003). Guidelines for enteral feedings in adult hospital patients. *Gut 52*(Suppl. VII)L:vii1-vii12.

Tisdale, M.J. (2002). Cachexia in cancer patients. *National Review of Cancer 2*(11), 862-871.

Woods, S.S., Nass, Y., & Deisch, P. (2000). Selection and implementation of a transparent dressing for central vascular access devices. *Nursing Clinics of North America 35*, 385-393.

10 Supportive Care: Pharmacologic Interventions

ROBERT J. IGNOFFO, CAROL S. VIELE, AND ZOE NGO

ANTIMICROBIALS

Theory

I. Rationale/indications.
   A. For use in the treatment of infections.
      1. Infections are a major complication of cancer and cancer therapy.
      2. Infections are the most common cause of death in persons with cancer.
      3. As a result of changes in immune functions, many of the usual signs and symptoms of infection are absent in the client diagnosed with cancer or receiving cancer treatment.
II. Types of antimicrobial drugs (Table 10-1).
Principles of medical management (Freifeld et al., 1997; Gilbert et al., 2002).
   A. At the first sign of temperature greater than 100.4° F (38° C), a fever workup is initiated.
      1. Physical examination.
      2. Blood cultures—peripheral and central.
      3. Central venous catheter or port cultures.
      4. Urine culture, sputum culture.
      5. Chest x-ray examination.
      6. Other cultures from wounds and drainage, if applicable.
   B. Initiation of empiric antimicrobial therapy.
      1. Selection of antibiotics based on the following:
         a. Coverage for common infectious organisms among persons with cancer.
         b. Prevalence rates for microorganisms and the patterns of resistance within the institution.
      2. Most antibiotic regimens are developed using the current information regarding the specific organisms that are predominant in the institution.
      3. Intravenous (IV) doses and schedules are designed to provide bactericidal serum levels for as long as possible between each dose interval.
      4. Duration of treatment is sufficient for the resolution of the fever without exposure to unnecessary side effects of the antimicrobial drug therapy.
         a. Negative culture results—if no organisms were isolated, treatment continues for a minimum of 7 days.
         b. Afebrile for 3 days.
         c. Neutrophil count greater than 500 cells/mm^3.
      5. If fever is unresponsive to initial antibiotic therapy, the risk of nonbacterial cause, infectious organisms resistant to antimicrobial therapy (e.g.,

Text continued on page 178

TABLE 10-1
Types of Antimicrobial Therapy

Antimicrobial Agent	Indications	Potential Side Effects of Group	Nursing Implications
PENICILLINS			
Penicillin G (Bicillin)	*Streptococcus pneumoniae, S. pyogenes, S. viridans, S. bovis, Neisseria,* and most anaerobes (except *Bacteroides fragilis*)	Hypersensitivity reactions, 5%-10% fatal Skin rash hypersensitivity up to 0.05% Dizziness, neuromuscular hyperirritability, seizures Decreased sense of taste and smell, stomatitis, flatulence, diarrhea Pancytopenia	Monitor changes in respiratory status, itching, hives, skin rash, fever, pain, changes in pulse rate, decrease in blood pressure, decrease in urinary output. Neurologic examination. Provide safety measures for clients with dizziness. Implement seizure precautions as needed. Evaluate the effects of changes in taste and smell, nausea, and stomatitis on nutrition, intake and output. Implement strategies to control flatulence and diarrhea. Evaluate the effect of diarrhea on perineal skin and rectum. Monitor CBC test results. Assess for signs and symptoms of infection, bleeding, effects of fatigue. Implement strategies to manage neutropenia, anemia, low platelets (see Chapters 13 and 16).
Methicillin (Staphcillin)	*Staphylococcus aureus,* streptococci	Hypokalemia; changes in liver and kidney function studies	Monitor electrolyte, liver function, and BUN and creatinine test results. Assess for signs of low potassium: paralytic ileus, muscle weakness, arrhythmias. Administer potassium supplement as ordered.
Nafcillin (Nafcil)	Same as Penicillin G + *S. aureus*		
Oxacillin (Bactocil)	Same as Penicillin G + *S. aureus*	Same as Penicillin G + →	Same as Penicillin G + Evaluate laboratory test results.
Ampicillin	*Streptococcus faecalis, Listeria monocytogenes, Haemophilus, Escherichia coli, Salmonella, Proteus*	Nausea and vomiting	Assess for effects of nausea and vomiting on nutrition, fluid and electrolyte balance. Implement strategies to manage nausea and vomiting (see Chapter 14).

Drug	Spectrum/Activity	Side Effects	Nursing Considerations
Ampicillin, sulbactam (Unasyn)	Active against ampicillin-resistant bacteria—S. aureus, B. fragilis, β-lactamase–producing Enterobacteriaceae		→
Ticarcillin and clavulanate (Timentin)	Haemophilus influenzae, Klebsiella spp. and anaerobes, but not against Pseudomonas aeruginosa and Enterobacter cloacae	→	→
Mezlocillin (Mezlin)	P. aeruginosa, Enterobacter, Proteus, Serratia, Acinetobacter, Providencia, Klebsiella spp.		
Piperacillin (Pipracil)	Same as Penicillin G but with increased activity against P. aeruginosa	Same as Penicillin G + Prolonged bleeding	Same as Penicillin G + Monitor sites of invasive procedures for bleeding. Assess for signs and symptoms of internal or external bleeding. Implement strategies to manage bleeding as needed (see Chapter 13). Monitor coagulation laboratory test results.
Azlocillin	Same as Piperacillin sodium		→
Piperacillin/tazobactam (Zosyn)	Increased activity over piperacillin alone against gram-negative rods and anaerobes; better β-lactamase inhibitor	→	→
CEPHALOSPORINS FIRST GENERATION Cephalothin	E. coli, Klebsiella, Proteus, Haemophilus, S. aureus, Staphylococcus epidermidis, streptococci	Cross sensitivity of 5%-15% in clients with history of penicillin allergy; Skin rash without fever and eosinophilia—13%; Neurologic effects in high doses—headache, agitation, dizziness, vertigo; Hypersensitivity reaction	Monitor changes in respiratory status, itching, hives, skin rash, fever, pain, changes in pulse rate, decrease in blood pressure, decrease in urinary output. Monitor for skin rash. Monitor for neurologic changes and headache at regular intervals. Provide safety measures for client experiencing dizziness and vertigo.
Cefazolin (Ancef, Kefzol)	Similar to Cephalothin sodium but more active against Klebsiella and E. coli		Monitor changes in respiratory status, itching, hives, skin rash, fever, pain, changes in pulse rate, decrease in blood pressure, decrease in urinary output.

(Continued)

TABLE 10-1
Types of Antimicrobial Therapy—cont'd

Antimicrobial Agent	Indications	Potential Side Effects of Group	Nursing Implications
		Headache, dizziness, vertigo; seizures in high doses with renal failure	Monitor for neurologic changes at regular intervals. Assess for headache, and administer analgesic as needed. Provide safety measures for client experiencing dizziness and vertigo. Implement seizure precautions.
		Nausea, vomiting, anorexia, abdominal cramping and diarrhea	Abdominal assessment. Evaluate effect of GI adverse effects on nutrition, fluid and electrolyte balance, weight, perineal skin, comfort. Implement strategies to manage these adverse effects (see Chapters 14 and 15).
		Pancytopenia; oliguria; changes in AST, ALT, alkaline phosphatase, BUN, and creatinine clearance	Evaluate CBC, liver and kidney function test results. Monitor intake and output. Assess and manage possible infection, fatigue, bleeding (see Chapters 13 and 16).
SECOND GENERATION Cefamandole	Most active against *Haemophilus, Klebsiella, E. coli, Enterobacter* spp., *Proteus,* less active against gram-positive cocci	Mild BUN and creatinine elevation, especially in the elderly	Monitor serum BUN and creatinine.
Cefoxitin (Mefoxin)	Same as Cephalothin plus *Proteus* spp. and anaerobes	Rare disulfuram reactions with alcohol	Instruct clients to avoid alcoholic intake during therapy.
THIRD GENERATION Cefotaxime (Claforan)	Same as Cephalothin + *Enterobacter* spp., *Proteus, H. influenzae, Citrobacter* spp., *Serratia* spp., some *P. aeruginosa* and *Bacteroides* spp.	Hypersensitivity reactions: maculopapular rash, urticaria, anaphylaxis	Monitor for skin rash and itching. Evaluate condition of skin before initiation of treatment. Implement strategies to minimize symptoms of local skin reactions (see Chapter 12).
		Nausea, vomiting, diarrhea	Monitor changes in respiratory status, itching, hives, skin rash, fever, pain, changes in pulse rate, decrease in blood pressure, decrease in urinary output. Abdominal assessment. Evaluate effect of GI adverse effects on nutrition, fluid and electrolyte balance, weight, perineal skin.

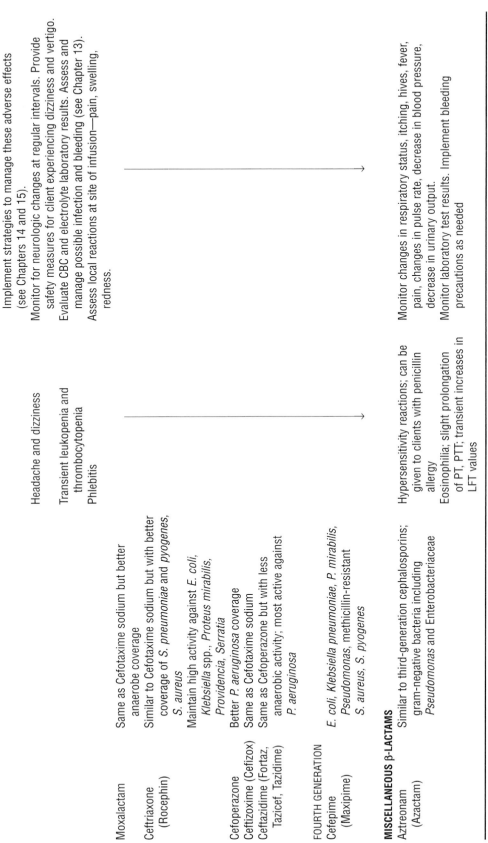

Drug	Coverage	Adverse Effects	Nursing Considerations
Moxalactam	Same as Cefotaxime sodium but better anaerobe coverage	Headache and dizziness Transient leukopenia and thrombocytopenia Phlebitis	Implement strategies to manage these adverse effects (see Chapters 14 and 15). Monitor for neurologic changes at regular intervals. Provide safety measures for client experiencing dizziness and vertigo. Evaluate CBC and electrolyte laboratory results. Assess and manage possible infection and bleeding (see Chapter 13). Assess local reactions at site of infusion—pain, swelling, redness.
Ceftriaxone (Rocephin)	Similar to Cefotaxime sodium but with better coverage of *S. pneumoniae* and *pyogenes*, *S. aureus* Maintain high activity against *E. coli*, *Klebsiella* spp., *Proteus mirabilis*, *Providencia*, *Serratia*		
Cefoperazone	Better *P. aeruginosa* coverage		
Ceftizoxime (Cefizox)	Same as Cefotaxime sodium		
Ceftazidime (Fortaz, Tazicef, Tazidime)	Same as Cefoperazone but with less anaerobic activity; most active against *P. aeruginosa*		
FOURTH GENERATION			
Cefepime (Maxipime)	*E. coli*, *Klebsiella pneumoniae*, *P. mirabilis*, *Pseudomonas*, methicillin-resistant *S. aureus*, *S. pyogenes*		
MISCELLANEOUS β-LACTAMS			
Aztreonam (Azactam)	Similar to third-generation cephalosporins; gram-negative bacteria including *Pseudomonas* and Enterobacteriaceae	Hypersensitivity reactions; can be given to clients with penicillin allergy Eosinophilia; slight prolongation of PT, PTT; transient increases in LFT values	Monitor changes in respiratory status, itching, hives, fever, pain, changes in pulse rate, decrease in blood pressure, decrease in urinary output. Monitor laboratory test results. Implement bleeding precautions as needed

(Continued)

TABLE 10-1
Types of Antimicrobial Therapy—cont'd

Antimicrobial Agent	Indications	Potential Side Effects of Group	Nursing Implications
Imipenem/cilastatin (Primaxin), Meropenem (Merrem IV)	Broad-spectrum gram-negative aerobic, including *Pseudomonas*, Enterobacteriaceae, *Klebsiella* spp. Anaerobic gram-positive and gram-negative anaerobes, including *B. fragilis* and some mycobacteria Gram-positive cocci, including *S. aureus* and *epidermidis, S. pneumoniae* and *pyogenes, Enterococcus*	Rare seizures Nausea, vomiting, diarrhea	Neurologic assessment. Implement seizure precautions as needed. Abdominal assessment. Evaluate effect of GI adverse effects on nutrition, fluid and electrolyte balance, weight, perineal skin, comfort. Implement strategies to manage these adverse effects (see Chapters 14 and 15).
FLUOROQUINOLONES			
Ciprofloxacin (Cipro)	Gram-negative rods, Enterobacteriaceae; most active against *P. aeruginosa, Haemophilus, Chlamydia,* some *Mycoplasma, Legionella;* less active against gram-positive organisms, especially *Streptococcus* and *Staphylococcus* spp.	GI irritation, nausea, vomiting, diarrhea Decreased oral absorption with aluminum, calcium, and magnesium antacids Potential crystalluria in alkaline urine Rare interstitial nephritis CNS changes from mild light-headedness to seizures Phototoxicity	Abdominal assessment. Evaluate effect of GI adverse effects on nutrition, fluid and electrolyte balance, weight, perineal skin. Implement strategies to manage these adverse effects (see Chapters 14 and 15). Do not take with sucralfate or antacids. Administer 1-2 hr before or after these antacids are given. Encourage 8 glasses of water per day while taking these agents. Monitor serum BUN and creatinine; intake and output, serum and urine protein levels. Daily weights. Monitor for neurologic changes at regular intervals. Provide safety measures for client experiencing light-headedness. Avoid prolonged sun exposure.
Norfloxacin (Noroxin) Levofloxacin (Levaquin)	No pseudomonal activity; used in GI and urinary tract infections *Klebsiella, Mycoplasma, Legionella;* less active against *Staphylococcus* and *Streptococcus*		

Moxifloxacin (Avelox)	*Streptococcus pneumoniae, Haemophilus, Klebsiella*		
Ofloxacin (Floxin)	Most active against *Chlamydia*	Changes in blood sugar—hyperglycemia or hypoglycemia ↓	Monitor blood sugars; assess for signs and symptoms of hypoglycemia or hyperglycemia. ↓
AMINOGLYCOSIDES			
Gentamicin (Garamycin)	*P. aeruginosa*, Enterobacter, *Enterococcus*; synergistic use with penicillin/vancomycin for gram-positive cocci (e.g., streptococci)	Vestibular toxicity; hearing loss, loss of balance, high-frequency deafness, peripheral neuritis, numbness, tingling of skin / Granulocytopenia, anemia, thrombocytopenia purpura / Nephrotoxicity—proteinuria, oliguria, changes in BUN and creatinine, especially with elevated serum concentrations	Evaluate neurologic status before initiation of therapy. Assess hearing status before therapy or periodically during prolonged treatment. Assess sensory input. Implement safety measures if dizzy or sensory changes present as needed. Assess and manage effects of low white cell, red cell, and platelet counts (see Chapters 13 and 16). Monitor serum BUN and creatinine levels. Monitor intake and output. Daily weights. Evaluate serum peak/trough or serial troughs with prolonged use.
Tobramycin (Nebcin)	Similar to Gentamicin sulfate except not as active against *Enterococcus*	Nausea and vomiting / Headache, fever, lethargy / Changes in AST, ALT, LDH; pancytopenia, nausea, vomiting, headache, fever, lethargy	Abdominal assessment. Evaluate effect of nausea and vomiting on nutrition, fluid and electrolyte balance. Implement strategies to manage nausea and vomiting (see Chapter 14). Assess for pain, and provide pain medications as needed. Implement measures to manage fever (see Chapter 13). Assist with activities of daily living as needed; implement energy-conserving measures. Evaluate LFT and CBC test results. Assess and manage possible infection, fatigue, and bleeding (see Chapters 13 and 16).
Amikacin (Amikin)	*Serratia, Proteus, Pseudomonas,* Enterobacteriaceae, *Providencia*	Drowsiness, headache, unsteady gait, paresthesias, tremors / Hypotension, tachycardia / Oliguria, hematuria, thirst / Ringing or buzzing in ears, high-frequency hearing loss	Neurologic assessment. Provide assistance with activities of daily living and ambulation as needed. Teach client and family about use of assistive aids for ambulation. Monitor blood pressure and pulse rate at regular intervals. Monitor intake and output and character of urinary output. Assess levels of hearing before and periodically during treatment.

(Continued)

TABLE 10-1
Types of Antimicrobial Therapy—cont'd

Antimicrobial Agent	Indications	Potential Side Effects of Group	Nursing Implications
ANTIFUNGALS			
Amphotericin B (Abelcet, Amphotec)	*Candida, Aspergillus,* Zygomycetes, *Torulopsis, Cryptococcus, Histoplasma*	Bleeding reactions Fever, headache, and shaking chills and rigors may be noted; arrhythmias and hypotension/hypertension Sedation, weakness, paresthesia, flushing, vertigo Tinnitus and hearing loss Nausea, vomiting, diarrhea Coagulation deficits, electrolyte imbalances (decreased potassium, magnesium, sodium) Pancytopenia, hepatic dysfunction, renal failure, increased serum creatinine	Monitor for signs of bleeding (see Chapter 13). Monitor temperature, blood pressure, pulse, and ECG at regular intervals. Assess for fever and shaking chills; most clients require premedication with acetaminophen and diphenhydramine. Meperidine used for rigors. Monitor neurologic changes at regular intervals. Provide safety measures for client experiencing paresthesia, weakness, vertigo. Evaluate changes in sensory perception over time. Assess impact of neurologic changes on ability to accomplish activities of daily living. Assess levels of hearing before and periodically during treatment. Abdominal assessment. Evaluate effect of GI adverse effects on nutrition, fluid and electrolyte balance, weight, perineal skin. Implement strategies to manage these adverse effects (see Chapters 14 and 15). Monitor laboratory test results. Assess and manage effects of coagulation deficits, granulocytopenia, thrombocytopenia (see Chapter 13), anemia (see Chapter 16), electrolyte imbalances (see Chapter 14). Monitor intake and output.
Liposomal amphotericin (L-AMB)	Patients intolerant or hypersensitive to amphotericin B or with compromised renal function	→	→
Flucytosine (Ancobon)	*Cryptococcus, Candida, Torulopsis,* chromomycosis	GI—nausea, vomiting, diarrhea	Abdominal assessment. Evaluate effect of GI adverse effects on nutrition, fluid and electrolyte balance, weight, perineal skin, comfort. Implement strategies to manage these adverse effects (see Chapters 14 and 15).

Drug	Uses	Side Effects	Nursing Interventions
		Hematologic—anemia, leukopenia, thrombocytopenia	Monitor CBC test results. Assess for signs and symptoms of infection, bleeding, effects of fatigue. Implement strategies to manage neutropenia, anemia, low platelets (see Chapters 13 and 16).
		Asymptomatic elevation in SGOT or ALT	Monitor serum liver enzyme laboratory results.
Clotrimazole (Lotrimin)	*Candida* spp., dermatophytes	Erythema, stinging, blistering, peeling, edema, and pruritus with topical application	Evaluate condition of skin before initiation of treatment. Implement strategies to minimize symptoms of local skin reactions (see Chapter 12).
Ketoconazole (Nizoral)	Similar to Clotrimazole	Gynecomastia	Assess changes in volume of breast tissue.
		Adrenal insufficiency	Monitor for signs of adrenal insufficiency—weakness, fever, abdominal pain, nausea, vomiting, diarrhea, decreased blood pressure.
		Nausea, vomiting	Evaluate effect of nausea and vomiting on nutrition, fluid and electrolyte balance. Implement strategies to manage nausea and vomiting (see Chapter 14).
		Increased liver transaminases	Monitor laboratory test results.
		Headache, dizziness, nervousness, photophobia, suicidal tendency	Monitor for neurologic changes at regular intervals. Provide safety measures for client experiencing dizziness. Provide for darkened room if photophobic. Assess for suicidal intent; refer to mental health professional as needed.
		Drug interactions with phenytoin, cyclosporine, and tacrolimus (increased levels and renal toxicity), warfarin (increased bleeding), oral sulfonylureas (enhanced hypoglycemic effect)	Review other medications client is taking to avoid drug interactions.
Fluconazole (Diflucan)	*Candida*, cryptococcal meningitis, coccidiomycosis	Hypersensitivity reaction	Monitor changes in respiratory status, itching, hives, fever, pain, changes in pulse rate, decrease in blood pressure, decrease in urinary output. Assess for headache, and provide pain medication as indicated.
		Headache Nausea, vomiting	Evaluate effect of nausea and vomiting on nutrition, fluid and electrolyte balance. Implement strategies to manage nausea and vomiting (see Chapter 14).

(Continued)

TABLE 10-1
Types of Antimicrobial Therapy—cont'd

Antimicrobial Agent	Indications	Potential Side Effects of Group	Nursing Implications
		Elevated LFTs	LFT test results.
		Skin rash, Stevens-Johnson syndrome, alopecia	Evaluate condition of skin before initiation of treatment. Implement strategies to minimize symptoms of local skin reactions (see Chapter 12). Assess and manage the effect of alopecia on body image (see Chapter 3).
		Drug interactions with phenytoin, cyclosporine, and tacrolimus (increased levels and renal toxicity), warfarin (increased bleeding), oral sulfonylureas (enhanced hypoglycemic effect), zidovudine (increased activity); cimetidine may decrease fluconazole levels	Review other medications client is taking to avoid drug interactions.
Itraconazole (Sporanox)	Aspergillosis: refractory to amphotericin B or intolerant	Nausea, vomiting, diarrhea, abdominal pain	Abdominal assessment. Evaluate effect of GI adverse effects on nutrition, fluid and electrolyte balance, weight, perineal skin, comfort. Implement strategies to manage these adverse effects (see Chapters 14 and 15).
	Plastomycosis—pulmonary and extrapulmonary		
	Histoplasmosis—pulmonary, disseminated nonmeningeal	Rash	Evaluate condition of skin before initiation of treatment. Implement strategies to minimize symptoms of local skin reactions (see Chapter 12).
		Headache, dizziness, malaise, somnolence	Monitor for neurologic changes at regular intervals. Provide safety measures for client experiencing dizziness. Provide pain medication for headache as needed.
		Decreased libido	See Chapter 6 for strategies related to sexual dysfunction.
		Hypertension	Monitor vital signs.
		Hypokalemia, increased LFT values, increased triglycerides	Monitor laboratory test values.
		Drug interactions with phenytoin, cyclosporine, and tacrolimus	Review other medications client is taking to avoid drug interactions.

(increased levels and renal toxicity), warfarin (increased bleeding), oral sulfonylureas (enhanced hypoglycemic effect), digoxin (increased levels), HMG-CoA reductase inhibitors (contraindicated)

Cimetidine, INH, phenytoin, and rifampin may decrease itraconazole levels

Voriconazole (Vfend)	Invasive *Aspergillus, Scedosporium apiospermum, Fusarium* spp.	Headache, hallucinations and dizziness, visual disturbances, photophobia	Monitor for neurologic changes at regular intervals. Provide safety measures for client experiencing dizziness and visual disturbances. Provide for darkened room if photophobic and safety precautions and decreased stimuli if hallucinating.
		Nausea, vomiting, diarrhea	Abdominal assessment. Evaluate effect of GI adverse effects on nutrition, fluid and electrolyte balance, weight, perineal skin, comfort. Implement strategies to manage these adverse effects (see Chapters 14 and 15).
		Rash, Stevens-Johnson syndrome	Evaluate condition of skin before initiation of treatment. Implement strategies to minimize symptoms of local skin reactions (see Chapter 12).
		Acute kidney failure	Assess kidney function—intake and output; vital signs; electrolyte, BUN, and creatinine levels.
		Tachycardia, peripheral edema, chest pain, prolonged QT	Baseline ECG, assess vital signs, assess for edema and skin changes. Evaluate for any medications currently receiving that would prolong QT.
		LFT abnormalities, cholestatic jaundice	Monitor LFTs, bilirubin levels. Assess for signs of jaundice.
		Anemia, leukopenia, thrombocytopenia	Monitor CBC results, and assess and manage possible infection, fatigue, and bleeding (see Chapters 13 and 16). Review other medications client is taking to avoid drug interactions. Monitor for drug interactions with agents listed for other antifungal azoles above.

(Continued)

TABLE 10-1
Types of Antimicrobial Therapy—cont'd

Antimicrobial Agent	Indications	Potential Side Effects of Group	Nursing Implications
Caspofungin (Cancidas)	Invasive *Aspergillus*	Pain/redness at site of injection (phlebitis 15%)	Monitor for pain/redness during drug administration.
		Nausea or vomiting	Assess for GI side effects, fluid and electrolyte balance, weight. Implement antiemetics or other management strategies (see Chapters 14 and 15).
		Flushing	Assess for facial or torso redness. Discontinue therapy if very bothersome or use an antihistamine such as diphenhydramine.
		Anemia (4%)	Causality uncertain because most patients have severe underlying conditions (hematologic malignancy, HIV infection).
		Headache (11%)	Causality uncertain. May use acetaminophen to treat headache.
		Drug interactions	Concurrent use with cyclosporin has been associated with transient elevation of hepatic transaminases possibly due to increased drug concentration of caspofungin by 35%.
ANTIVIRALS			
Acyclovir (Zovirax)	Herpes simplex virus, varicella zoster virus	Renal toxicity, neurotoxicity	Monitor flow rate for infusion and maintain hydration. Monitor for neurologic changes at regular intervals. Monitor blood pressure, pulse rate, respiratory rate, intake and output, BUN, creatinine and electrolyte laboratory values.
		Arthralgias	Assess for joint pain.
Ganciclovir (Cytovene)	CMV retinitis, pneumonia, colitis, CMV pneumonia with IVIG in BMT	Granulocytopenia, thrombocytopenia	Monitor CBC. Assess and manage effects of low white blood cells and platelets (see Chapter 13).
		Fever	Assess temperature; administer antipyretic for elevated temperature.
		Rash	Evaluate condition of skin before initiation of treatment. Implement strategies to minimize symptoms of local skin reactions (see Chapter 12).

Drug	Use	Adverse Effects	Nursing Interventions
Foscarnet (Foscavir)	CMV retinitis, ganciclovir resistance or intolerance, acyclovir-resistant CMV	Increase in LFT values	Monitor LFT laboratory results.
		Headache, fatigue, nausea, fever	Vital signs. Assess for headache, fatigue, nausea, fever. Administer antipyretic, antiemetic, and/or analgesic as needed. Provide for rest periods. Assess for effect of nausea on nutrition and fluid intake.
		Neuropathy, seizures	Monitor for neurologic changes at regular intervals. Implement safety measures and seizure precautions as needed.
		Electrolyte disturbances, increase in serum creatinine, decrease in white cell count	Monitor BUN, creatinine, serum electrolytes, CBC, intake and output. Assess for potential infection.
Valganciclovir (Valcyte)	CMV retinitis	Neutropenia, thrombocytopenia, anemia	Monitor blood counts as ordered. Monitor for signs and symptoms of any infection or bleeding. Check vital signs on a regular basis. Implement strategies to manage these adverse effects (see Chapters 13 and 16).
		Diarrhea, nausea, vomiting, abdominal pain	Abdominal assessment. Evaluate effect of GI adverse effects on nutrition, fluid and electrolyte balance, weight, perineal skin, comfort. Implement strategies to manage these adverse effects (see Chapters 14 and 15).
		Fever, headache, insomnia	Assess for headache, fever, sleep patterns. Administer antipyretic and/or analgesic as needed. Provide for rest periods.
MISCELLANEOUS			
Erythromycin (E-Mycin)	*Legionella, Mycoplasma*	Transient deafness	Assess hearing status before therapy or periodically during prolonged treatment.
		Decreased liver or renal function	Monitor BUN, creatinine, serum electrolytes, liver enzymes, bilirubin, PT/PTT, intake and output. Monitor LFTs. Assess for signs of jaundice.
		Abdominal cramping and distention, diarrhea	Abdominal assessment. Evaluate effect of GI adverse effects on nutrition, fluid and electrolyte balance, perineal skin, comfort. Encourage client to increase activity to promote peristalsis. Implement strategies to manage these adverse effects (see Chapter 15).
		Phlebitis	Assess local reactions at site of infusion—pain, swelling, redness.

(Continued)

TABLE 10-1
Types of Antimicrobial Therapy—cont'd

Antimicrobial Agent	Indications	Potential Side Effects of Group	Nursing Implications
Clindamycin (Cleocin HCL)	*Clostridia, S. pneumoniae, S. viridans, S. pyogenes, S. aureus*	Decreased taste, abdominal pain, bloating, nausea, vomiting, diarrhea	Abdominal assessment. Evaluate effect of GI adverse effects on nutrition, fluid and electrolyte balance, weight, perineal skin. Implement strategies to manage these adverse effects (see Chapters 14 and 15).
		Neutropenia, thrombophlebitis	Monitor CBC results, and assess and manage possible infection, bleeding (see Chapter 13).
		Jaundice, abnormal liver function	Monitor liver enzymes, bilirubin, PT/PTT test results, intake and output. Monitor LFTs. Assess for signs of jaundice.
		Headache, depression, confusion	Monitor for neurologic changes at regular intervals. Implement safety measures and seizure precautions as needed. Assess for suicidal intent; refer to mental health professional as needed.
Chloramphenicol (Chloromycetin)	*Haemophilus, B. fragilis, S. pneumoniae, Neisseria, Salmonella, Klebsiella, Rickettsia,* and most anaerobes	Nausea, vomiting, diarrhea, perianal irritation, stomatitis, xerostomia, abdominal distention	Abdominal assessment. Evaluate effect of GI adverse effects on nutrition, fluid and electrolyte balance, weight, perineal skin, comfort. Encourage client to increase activity to promote peristalsis. Assess rectal area for irritation. Teach perianal hygiene and protective measures. Implement strategies to manage these adverse effects (see Chapters 14 and 15).
		Blotching skin	Evaluate condition of skin before initiation of treatment. Implement strategies to minimize symptoms of local skin reactions (see Chapter 12).
		Cyanosis	Evaluate pulmonary status at least each shift—respiratory rate, effort. Monitor oxygen saturation q2-4 h.
		Hypothermia	Assess temperature. Provide warmth—extra blankets, reduce air drafts, increase room temperature as needed.
		Severe bone marrow depression	Monitor blood counts as ordered. Monitor for signs and symptoms of any infection or bleeding. Check vital signs on a regular basis. Implement strategies to manage these adverse effects (see Chapters 13 and 16).

Drug	Uses/Organisms	Side Effects	Nursing Considerations
Interferons (α, β, γ)	Herpes simplex virus, varicella zoster virus	Local pain, fever, fatigue	Assess local reactions at site of infusion. Assess temperature and administer antipyretic as needed. Evaluate effect of fatigue on activities of daily living.
		Anorexia	Assess appetite. Implement strategies to manage anorexia (see Chapter 14).
		Alopecia Myelosuppression	Assess effect of alopecia on body image (see Chapter 3). Monitor blood counts as ordered. Monitor for signs and symptoms of any infection or bleeding. Check vital signs on a regular basis. Implement strategies to manage these adverse effects (see Chapters 13 and 16).
Metronidazole (Flagyl)	All anaerobes, including *B. fragilis*, *Clostridium difficile* toxin—PO or IV	Metallic taste in mouth, darkened stools	Educate client on effect of medication on taste and stools.
		Headache, dizziness, vertigo, paresthesias; peripheral neuropathy can occur with high doses and prolonged treatment; rare seizures, irritability, depression	Monitor for neurologic changes at regular intervals. Assess for headache, administer pain medications as needed. Implement safety measures if dizzy or peripheral neuropathy present. Implement seizure precautions as needed. Assess for suicidal intent; refer to mental health professional as needed.
		Occasional musculoskeletal pain	Assess for joint/muscle pain. Administer pain medications as needed.
		Skin flushing, rash	Evaluate condition of skin before initiation of treatment. Implement strategies to minimize symptoms of local skin reactions (see Chapter 12).
		Drug interactions: cimetidine enhances metronidazole effects; metronidazole enhances warfarin effect; concurrent alcohol may lead to disulfiram-like reaction	Review other medications client is taking to avoid drug interactions. Avoid alcohol while taking this drug.
Rifampin (Rifadin)	Mycobacteria, most gram-positive and gram-negative bacteria, *Neisseria* meningitis. Used mainly to enhance bactericidal activity of other antistaphylococcal agents in refractory or chronic infections	Flulike syndrome, fatigue	Vital signs. Administer antipyretics as needed. Encourage fluids and rest.

TABLE 10-1
Types of Antimicrobial Therapy—cont'd

Antimicrobial Agent	Indications	Potential Side Effects of Group	Nursing Implications
	Develops resistance quickly if used singly	Discoloration of body fluids	Educate client about changes to urine.
		Headache, somnolence, dizziness, ataxia	Monitor for neurologic changes at regular intervals. Assess for headache, administer pain medications as needed. Implement safety measures if dizzy, ataxic, or asleep. Assist with ambulation.
		Blurred vision, conjunctivitis	Assess vision. Implement safety measures if vision impaired. Administer eye drops as needed.
		Dyspepsia, nausea, vomiting, diarrhea	Abdominal assessment. Evaluate effect of GI adverse effects on nutrition, fluid and electrolyte balance, weight, perineal skin. Assess rectal area for irritation. Teach perianal hygiene and protective measures. Implement strategies to manage these adverse effects (see Chapters 14 and 15).
		Acute renal failure (rare), hematuria, menstrual changes	Monitor intake and output. Assess urine for color, clarity. Monitor BUN and creatinine. Assess and document menstrual changes.
		Transient leukopenia, thrombocytopenia	Monitor CBC results. Assess and manage possible infection and bleeding (see Chapter 13).
		Hepatotoxicity, elevated LFTs	Monitor liver enzymes, bilirubin, PT/PTT, intake and output. Monitor LFTs. Assess for signs of jaundice.
		Pruritus, rash, urticaria	Evaluate condition of skin before initiation of treatment. Implement strategies to minimize symptoms of local skin reactions (see Chapter 12).

Drug	Organisms	Side effects/Drug interactions	Nursing interventions
Trimethoprim-sulfamethoxazole (Bactrim, Septra)	*P. carinii, S. aureus, S. pneumoniae, S. pyogenes, Salmonella, Listeria, E. coli, Proteus, Serratia, Haemophilus, Neisseria*	Drug interactions: rifampin enhances the metabolism of anti-coagulants, digoxin, opiates, cyclosporine, estrogens, oral contraceptives, oral sulfonyl-ureas, phenytoin, quinidine, verapamil, increases INH hepatotoxicity Myelosuppression	Review other medications client is taking to avoid drug interactions. Monitor CBC laboratory results. Assess for signs and symptoms of anemia, infection, or bleeding. Check vital signs on a regular basis. Implement strategies to manage these adverse effects (see Chapters 13 and 16).
Vancomycin (Vancocin)	*C. difficile, S. aureus, S. epidermidis, S. fecalis,* corynebacteria, *S. bovis* Methicillin-resistant *S. aureus,* Oral formil *difficile* toxin	Hypersensitivity reaction Vertigo, dizziness Tinnitus, ototoxicity Increased BUN and creatinine levels Phlebitis Suprainfection	Monitor for hypersensitivity reactions—changes in respiratory status, itching, hives, fever, pain, changes in pulse rate, decrease in blood pressure, decrease in urinary output. Monitor for neurologic changes at regular intervals. Implement safety measures for dizziness. Monitor client responses to change in hearing. Monitor intake and output. Monitor BUN and creatinine laboratory test results. Assess local reactions at site of infusion—pain, swelling, redness. Vital signs. Assess for infection. Administer antibiotics as needed.

Modified from DeVita VT, Jr, Hellman S, Rosenberg S, editors: *Cancer: Principles and practice of oncology,* ed 4, Philadelphia, 1993, Lippincott, pp 2300-2307. Pagana K, Pagana T: *Manual of diagnostic and laboratory tests,* St Louis, 2002, Mosby, pp 40-42, 120-123.

CBC, Complete blood count; *BUN,* blood urea nitrogen; *GI,* gastrointestinal; *AST,* aspartate aminotransferase; *ALT,* alanine aminotransferase; *PT,* prothrombin time; *PTT,* partial thromboplastin time; *LFT,* liver function test; *CNS,* central nervous system; *LDH,* lactate dehydrogenase; *ECG,* electrocardiogram; *SGOT,* serum glutamic-oxaloacetic transaminase; *INH,* isoniazid; *CMV,* cytomegalovirus; *IVIG,* intravenous immune globulin; *BMT,* bone marrow transplant; *PO,* by mouth; *IV,* intravenous.

methicillin-resistant *Staphylococcus aureus,* vancomycin-resistant *Enterococcus*), inadequate serum and tissue levels of antimicrobials, or drug fever should be considered.

   a. Continue current antimicrobials if clinical condition is unchanged and evaluation reveals no new information.
   b. Change antimicrobial program if evidence of progressive infection is present.
   c. Add an antifungal agent to the antimicrobial program.
      (1) One third of febrile neutropenic clients who do not respond to 1 week of antimicrobial therapy have a systemic fungal infection.
      (2) Most common organisms include *Candida* and *Aspergillus.*
   6. Antiviral therapy should be considered if client has a past history of positive titers/positive history of an outbreak during chemotherapy (e.g., herpes simplex, herpes zoster).

III. Potential adverse effects of antimicrobial therapy (see Table 10-1).
   A. Suprainfection.
   B. Renal toxicity—acute renal tubular necrosis, nephritis, electrolyte imbalances.
   C. Hematologic—bleeding, neutropenia, anemia.
   D. Hepatotoxicity—elevated liver function tests.
   E. Cardiovascular—phlebitis, hypotension, arrhythmias, prolonged QT interval.
   F. Gastrointestinal (GI)—nausea, vomiting, anorexia, diarrhea, colitis.
   G. Neurotoxicity—seizures, dizziness, ototoxicity.
   H. Dermatologic—rash, Stevens-Johnson syndrome, thrush, esophagitis, vaginitis.
   I. Fluid and electrolyte imbalances—hypokalemia, hypernatremia, hypomagnesemia, dehydration, fluid volume overload.
   J. Hypersensitivity reactions.

Assessment

I. Assess for presence of risk factors (see Chapter 13) (Wujcik, 1999).
   A. Disruption of primary barriers to organisms.
      1. Surgical disruption of skin.
      2. Invasive procedures (e.g., insertion of central vascular access catheters, indwelling urinary catheters).
      3. Extravasation of vesicant antineoplastic agents.
      4. Stomatitis/mucositis.
      5. Rectal fissures.
      6. Burns.
   B. Alteration in phagocytic defenses.
      1. Neutropenia with granulocyte count less than $1000/mm^3$.
      2. Length of time client has been neutropenic.
      3. Steroid use.
      4. Previous antibiotic therapy.
   C. Concurrent disease states.
      1. Diabetes.
      2. Cardiovascular disease.
      3. Renal disease.
      4. Liver disease.
      5. GI disease.

      6. Fistula, abscesses.
      7. Stress.
    D. Tumor necrosis and invasion.
    E. Previous cancer therapy.
    F. History of drug allergies/drug reaction or intolerance.
  II. Physical examination (see Chapter 13).
 III. Current medications.
 IV. Evaluation of diagnostic and laboratory data.
    A. Culture and sensitivity: blood, urine, sputum.
    B. Chest x-ray examination.
    C. Complete blood count with differential.
    D. Other—computed tomography (CT), spiral CT, magnetic resonance imaging (MRI), ultrasound, esophagogastroduodenoscopy (EGD), bronchoscopy.

Nursing Diagnoses

   I. Risk for infection.
  II. Risk for imbalanced body temperature.
 III. Deficient knowledge related to antimicrobial drug therapy.

Outcome Identification

   I. Client remains free of infection, or infection is recognized early and treated promptly.
    A. Client and family describe personal risk factors for infection.
  II. Client maintains body temperature within normal range.
 III. Client and family discuss the rationale for immediate evaluation of fever.
    A. Client discusses rationale for use of antimicrobial drug therapy, including schedule of administration.
    B. Client describes potential adverse effects of antimicrobial drug therapy.
    C. Client describes measures to manage adverse effects of antimicrobial drug therapy.
    D. Client lists signs and symptoms of adverse effects of antimicrobial drug therapy to report to the health care team.

Planning and Implementation

   I. Implement strategies to manage elevated body temperature and prevent infections (see Chapter 13).
  II. Implement strategies to educate client about the following:
    A. Risk factors for infection (see Assessment).
    B. Signs and symptoms of infection.
    C. Rationale for use of antimicrobial drug therapy and for taking antimicrobials as scheduled.
    D. Adverse effects and strategies to manage adverse effects.
    E. Adverse effects to report to health care team.
 III. Assess client's and family's cultural and ethnic background, particularly health care practices and values and beliefs related to pharmacotherapy.
    A. Assess understanding and compliance to Western/mainstream prescribed therapy.

B. Determine if client and family are also consulting traditional healers and/or taking herbal preparations, megavitamins (potential drug interactions).

C. Determine client's racial group because biologic variations among racial groups may affect drug metabolism rates, clinical drug responses, and side effects of drugs.

IV. Implement strategies to monitor for adverse effects of antimicrobial therapy (see Table 10-1).

V. Implement interventions to decrease the incidence and manage the adverse effects of antimicrobial therapy (see Table 10-1).

VI. Implement measures to monitor for therapeutic response to antimicrobial therapy.

A. Monitor temperature, pulse, respirations, and blood pressure.

B. Discuss with the client and family rationale for immediate evaluation of fever.

C. Assess changes in laboratory values/fluid volume status.

Evaluation

The oncology nurse systematically and regularly evaluates the client's and/or family's responses to interventions to determine progress toward the achievement of expected outcomes. Relevant data are collected, and actual findings are compared with expected findings. Nursing diagnoses, outcomes, and plans of care are reviewed and revised as necessary.

ANTIINFLAMMATORY AGENTS

Theory

I. Rationale/indications (Paice, 1999).

A. To reduce inflammation and pain.

1. Although the inflammatory process is a protective mechanism, in certain situations it may cause harm and pain to the individual.

a. The inflammatory process involves the production of prostaglandins by the action of the enzyme cyclooxygenase (also known as prostaglandin synthetase).

(1) Prostaglandins are particularly associated with the pain that accompanies inflammation.

b. Inhibition of cyclooxygenase by antiinflammatory agents will inhibit production of prostaglandin. This break in the cascade suppresses the inflammatory response of white blood cell and macrophage migration to the site of injury and results in or contributes to symptom relief.

II. Types of antiinflammatory agents.

A. Nonsteroidal antiinflammatory drugs (NSAIDs) (Table 10-2).

B. Corticosteroids (Table 10-3).

III. Principles of medical management.

A. Pain management (see Chapter 1).

1. Treatment of mild to moderate pain.

2. Adjuvant pharmacologic pain management with opiates.

B. Symptom management of tumor lysis fever, bony metastases, nausea and vomiting from chemotherapy (see Chapters 14 and 18).

IV. Potential adverse effects (Table 10-4).

TABLE 10-2
Commonly Used Nonsteroidal Antiinflammatory Drugs in Cancer

Nonsteroidal Drug	Usual Adult Oral Dosages (max. dosage is per 24 hr)	Notable Drug Information
PROPIONIC ACIDS		
Fenoprofen (Nalfon, various generics)	300-600 mg q4-6h (max. 3000 mg)	Prescription; dizziness, GI side effects
Ibuprofen (various generics [OTC])	400-800 mg q4-6h (max. 3200 mg)	200 mg available OTC; GI side effects
Ketoprofen (Orudis)	25-60 mg q6-8h (max. 300 mg)	GI side effects, headache, dizziness
Naproxen (Naprosyn, Aleve [OTC])	250-275 mg q6-8h (max. 1250 mg)	Weight gain; do NOT crush tablets
ACETIC ACIDS		
Diclofenac (Voltaren)	50-75 mg q8-12h (max. 200 mg)	GI side effects, take with food
Etodolac (Lodine, Lodine XL)	200-400 mg q6-8h (max. 1200 mg)	GI side effects, fluid retention
Indomethacin (Indocin)	25 mg q8-12h (max. 200 mg)	Renal toxicity, GI side effects
Ketorolac (Toradol)	10 mg q4-6h (max. 40 mg)	Use lower doses in elderly
Sulindac (Clinoril)	200 mg q12h (max. 400 mg)	Less renal toxicity
Tolmetin (Tolectin)	200-600 mg q8h (max. 1800 mg)	Fewer GI side effects; take on empty stomach
OXICAM		
Piroxicam (Feldene)	20 mg daily (max. 40 mg)	Long half-life allows for once daily dosing; use with caution in elderly; causes fluid retention
SALICYLATES		
Acetylsalicylic acid/ aspirin	325-650 mg q3-4h (max. 6000 mg)	Do not combine with NSAIDs; potent antiplatelet effects
Choline magnesium trisalicylate (Trilisate)	1500 mg q12h (max. 3000 mg)	Has no antiplatelet effect
Salsalate (Disalcid; various generics)	750 mg q8-12h (max. 3000 mg)	Has no antiplatelet effect
CYCLOOXYGENASE-2 SELECTIVE INHIBITORS		GI safety advantages yet to be demonstrated with chronic use
Valdecoxib (Bextra)	10-20mg daily (max. 40mg)	Should not be taken by patients with sulfonamide allergy; well-tolerated with renal failure, use with caution in patients with hepatic failure or edema; can be taken at the same time with antacids (aluminum/ magnesium hydroxide)
Celecoxib (Celebrex)	100-200 mg q12h (max. 400 mg)	Fewer GI and platelet side effects; renal elimination 27%; mostly hepatic metabolism by CYP-2C9; fluconazole may increase concentrations of celecoxib Give antacids 1 hr apart from celecoxib to avoid decreased absorption; inter-acts with warfarin, lithium, and methotrexate to increase levels and toxicity

GI, Gastrointestinal; *OTC,* over the counter; *NSAIDs,* nonsteroidal antiinflammatory drugs.

TABLE 10-3
Corticosteroids Used in the Treatment of Cancer

Corticosteroids	Equivalent Dose	Notable Drug Information
SHORT ACTING (8-12 HR)		
Cortisone (various trade names)	30 mg	Sodium and water retention
Hydrocortisone (various trade names)	20 mg	Sodium and water retention
INTERMEDIATE ACTING (12-36 HR)		
Methylprednisolone (Medrol)	4 mg	Minimal sodium-retaining activity
Prednisolone (various trade names)	5 mg	Minimal sodium-retaining activity
Prednisone (various trade names)	5 mg	Metabolized to prednisolone
LONG ACTING		
Dexamethasone (Decadron)	0.75 mg	No sodium-retaining activities with lower doses

TABLE 10-4
Adverse Effects of Nonsteroidal Antiinflammatory Drugs and Corticosteroids

Adverse Effects	Nursing Implications
NONSTEROIDALS	
GASTROINTESTINAL	
Ulceration, bleeding, gastritis, dyspepsia, abdominal pain, constipation, PUD Risks increase with age, chronic use, concomitant corticosteroid use and history of PUD; misoprostol (Cytotec) can be used to prevent NSAID-induced ulcers	Administer with food or milk. Guaiac stool. Assess for signs/symptoms of GI bleeding.
PANCREAS	
Pancreatitis reported with sulindac	Monitor serum amylase and lipase and urinary amylase results. Monitor for signs/symptoms of pancreatitis (e.g., sudden and intense epigastric pain, nausea and vomiting, low-grade fever, jaundice).
HEPATIC	
Increased ALT, AST, bilirubin; risks for hepatotoxicity include alcoholism, chronic active hepatitis, history of hepatitis, cirrhosis, and CHF	Monitor liver enzymes, bilirubin laboratory results. Assess health history for risk factors.
CENTRAL NERVOUS SYSTEM	
Dizziness, drowsiness, light-headedness/vertigo, somnolence, mental confusion	Neurologic examination for alertness and orientation. Advise clients/families to avoid driving or other hazardous activities that require mental alertness until CNS effects can be determined. Implement measures for client safety as needed (e.g., assist with ambulation, fall precautions). Avoid alcohol and other CNS depressants.
Malaise, fatigue	Assess level of fatigue. Provide for rest periods. Monitor CBC laboratory test results.

TABLE 10-4

Adverse Effects of Nonsteroidal Antiinflammatory Drugs and Corticosteroids—cont'd

Adverse Effects	Nursing Implications
Headache	Assess level of headache, and administer pain medications as needed.
CARDIOVASCULAR CHF, peripheral edema, fluid retention, hypertension	Monitor fluid status, lung sounds, pitting edema, vital signs.
RENAL Acute renal failure, elevated BUN and serum creatinine levels and proteinuria; risks include advanced age, chronic renal disease, CHF	Monitor intake and output. Monitor BUN, creatinine, and urinalysis laboratory test results and blood pressure. Assess for edema. Assess health history for risk factors.
HEMATOLOGIC Neutropenia, leukopenia, thrombocytopenia, decreased hemoglobin/hematocrit levels Exception: choline magnesium trisalicylate (Trilisate)	Monitor CBC results. Assess and implement measures to manage infection, bleeding, fatigue (see Chapters 13 and 16).
PLATELET AGGRESSION Prolonged bleeding time	Monitor platelet levels. No IM shots. Implement bleeding precautions.
SPECIAL SENSES Visual disturbance, blurred vision, photophobia, ocular cataracts, glaucoma, ear pain, tinnitus	Regular eye examinations and hearing tests. Educate client to report blurred vision, eye pain, ear pain, and tinnitus to health care provider. Darken room, wear sunglasses if photophobic.
HYPERSENSITIVITY Asthma and anaphylaxis	Monitor for hypersensitivity reactions—changes in respiratory status, itching, hives, fever, pain, changes in pulse rate, decrease in blood pressure, decrease in urinary output. Assess breath sounds, elevate HOB to ease breathing. Oxygen administration as needed. Administer bronchodilators, antihistamines, or pressor agents as needed. NSAIDs contraindicated in clients with ASA allergy, nasal polyps, bronchospastic disease.
RESPIRATORY Dyspnea, hemoptysis, bronchospasm, shortness of breath	Respiratory assessment; monitor breath sounds. Examine sputum. Elevate HOB to ease breathing. Administer bronchodilators and oxygen as needed.
DERMATOLOGIC AND SKELETAL Rash, erythema, urticaria, photosensitivity, osteoporosis, poor wound healing, skin thinning, growth arrest	Observe for rash, and monitor wounds for prolonged healing. Advise clients to use sunblock, wear protective clothing, protect skin, avoid prolonged exposure to sunlight. Monitor height.

(Continued)

TABLE 10-4
Adverse Effects of Nonsteroidal Antiinflammatory Drugs and Corticosteroids—cont'd

Adverse Effects	Nursing Implications
ELECTROLYTE IMBALANCE Hyperglycemia with glycosuria, hypokalemia, hypernatremia; disturbances can lead to hypertension and possible edema	Monitor blood glucose and electrolyte laboratory test results. Monitor vital signs and presence of peripheral edema.
PITUITARY Adrenal insufficiency caused by prolonged use and rapid withdrawal	Observe for signs of cortisol insufficiency, such as fever, low blood pressure, disorientation, myalgia, arthralgia.
INFECTIOUS DISEASE Immunosuppressive with increased risk of infections—bacterial, fungal, viral; activation of tuberculosis and spread of herpes conjunctivitis	Cultures, dermatologic examination. Administer antimicrobial drugs and antipyretics as needed. Be aware that signs/symptoms of infection may be masked by NSAIDs.
CORTICOSTEROIDS CUSHING'S SYNDROME WITH LONG-TERM USE Central obesity, moon face, buffalo hump, easy bruising, acne, hirsutism, striae, skin atrophy	Assess client's body image concerns. Provide opportunity for client to share concerns and discuss coping strategies. Educate regarding care of skin and safety precautions.
ELECTROLYTE AND METABOLIC IMBALANCES Hyperglycemia, hypernatremia, hypokalemia, and hypocalcemia leading to edema, hypertension, diabetes, osteoporosis	Monitor laboratory results (blood glucose, electrolytes, calcium), vital signs, body weight. Assess for edema.
NEUROMUSCULAR AND SKELETAL Arthralgia, myalgia, fatigue, muscle weakness, myopathy, osteoporosis, muscle wasting, fractures	Monitor muscle strength. Administer pain medication as needed. Encourage regular exercise to promote bone development. Implement safety measures to prevent falls and injuries.
OCULAR EFFECTS Cataracts and glaucoma	Regular eye examinations. Educate client to report any eye pain, blurred vision to health care provider. Those with open-angle glaucoma should avoid corticosteroids.
SUPPRESSION OF PITUITARY-ADRENAL FUNCTION With long-term use, sudden withdrawal may cause acute adrenal insufficiency and dependence; fever, myalgia, arthralgia, malaise; unable to respond to stress	Monitor blood pressure for hypotension. Monitor electrolytes for hyponatremia. Assess for dehydration, fatigue, diarrhea, anorexia. Monitor vital signs and muscle and joint pain; administer pain medication. Educate regarding stressful situations, both physiologic and emotional, and when to contact health professional for assistance.

TABLE 10-4
Adverse Effects of Nonsteroidal Antiinflammatory drugs and Corticosteroids—cont'd

Adverse Effects	Nursing Implications
PSYCHIATRIC DISTURBANCES Paranoia, psychosis, hallucinations	Observe for and report any mental status changes. Suicide precautions, if needed. Refer to mental health professional as needed.
GASTROINTESTINAL Peptic ulcers, GI bleeding	Assess for epigastric pain 1-3 hr after meals. Assess for nausea/vomiting and observe for hematemesis. Monitor CBC and guaiac stools/emesis.
MISCELLANEOUS Poor wound healing, immunosuppression, menstrual irregularities, arrest of growth	Assess any wounds for prolonged healing. Monitor CBC; assess and manage effects of low white cell, red cell and platelet counts (see Chapters 13 and 16). Monitor height.

ALT, Alanine aminotransferase; *ASA,* acetylsalicylic acid; *AST,* aspartate aminotransferase; *BUN,* blood urea nitrogen; *CBC,* complete blood count; *CHF,* congestive heart failure; *CNS,* central nervous system; *GI,* gastrointestinal; *HOB,* head of bed; *IM,* intramuscular; *NSAIDs,* nonsteroidal antiinflammatory drugs; *PUD,* peptic ulcer disease.

Assessment

I. Identification of clients at risk.
   A. For pain (see Chapter 1).
   B. For nausea and vomiting (see Chapter 14).
   C. Clients with cancers that commonly metastasize to bone (e.g., prostate, breast, lung).
   D. Clients with fever from tumor lysis (see Chapter 18).
II. Physical examination.
   A. Vital signs.
   B. Pain assessment (see Chapter 1).
   C. Assess for effects of nausea and vomiting (see Chapter 14).
   D. Assess for effects of tumor lysis (see Chapter 18).
III. Current medications.
IV. Evaluation of diagnostic and laboratory data.
   A. Complete blood count.
   B. Hepatic and renal function.

Nursing Diagnoses

I. Acute or chronic pain.
II. Nausea.
III. Risk for imbalanced body temperature.
IV. Deficient knowledge related to antiinflammatory drug therapy.

Outcome Identification

I. Client states that the pain is reduced or relieved to his/her satisfaction.
II. Client states relief of nausea and has no vomiting episodes.

III. Client maintains body temperature within normal range.

IV. Client discusses the rationale for the use of antiinflammatory drug therapy, including schedule of administration.

    A. Client describes potential adverse effects of antiinflammatory drug therapy.

    B. Client describes measures to manage adverse effects of antiinflammatory drug therapy.

    C. Client lists signs and symptoms of adverse effects of antiinflammatory agents to report to the health care team.

Planning and Implementation

  I. Implement strategies to manage pain (see Chapter 1), nausea and vomiting (see Chapter 14), and fever from tumor lysis (see Chapter 18).

 II. Implement strategies to educate client about the following:

    A. Rationale for use of antiinflammatory drug therapy and for taking antiinflammatory drugs as scheduled.

    B. Adverse effects and strategies to manage adverse effects.

    C. Adverse effects to report to health care team.

III. Assess client's and family's cultural and ethnic background, particularly health care practices and values and beliefs related to pharmacotherapy (see Antimicrobials, Planning and Implementation section).

IV. Implement strategies to monitor for adverse effects of antiinflammatory drug therapy (see Table 10-4).

 V. Implement interventions to decrease the incidence and manage the adverse effects of antiinflammatory drug therapy (see Table 10-4).

    A. Establish client's allergies before administering NSAIDs.

        1. NSAIDs are contraindicated in clients with aspirin allergy or hypersensitivity to acetylsalicylic acid (ASA), nasal polyps, and bronchospastic disease.

        2. Patients allergic to sulfonamides should not receive valdecoxib (Bextra).

    B. Review client's current medications for potential drug interactions.

        1. For example, NSAIDs can increase the effects of phenytoin (Dilantin), sulfonamide, and warfarin (Coumadin).

    C. Review use of complementary therapy that may alter the metabolism of NSAIDs.

VI. Implement measures to monitor for therapeutic response to antiinflammatory drug therapy.

    A. Assess client for adequate symptom relief (e.g., of pain, nausea, vomiting).

    B. Assess client for infection because the antipyretic and antiinflammatory actions of NSAIDs may mask signs and symptoms of infection.

Evaluation

The oncology nurse systematically and regularly evaluates the client's and/or family's responses to interventions to determine progress toward the achievement of expected outcomes. Relevant data are collected, and actual findings are compared with expected findings. Nursing diagnoses, outcomes, and plans of care are reviewed and revised as necessary.

ANTIEMETIC THERAPY

Theory

  I. Rationale/indications (Gralla, 2002; Koeller et al., 2002; NCCN, 2004; Wickham, 1999).

A. For treatment of nausea and vomiting.
   1. Causes of nausea and vomiting.
      a. Chemotherapy with moderate to highly emetogenic potential (Table 10-5).
      b. Radiation therapy alone or in combination with antineoplastic chemotherapy.
      c. Tumor-related problems, such as intestinal obstruction or head and neck metastases.
      d. Concomitant pharmacologic therapy (e.g., opiates, antibiotics).
      e. Concomitant medical complications.
         (1) Fluid and electrolyte disturbances (e.g., hypercalcemia, volume depletion, water intoxication, hypoadrenalism).
         (2) Infection (e.g., septicemia, central nervous system [CNS] infection [meningitis]).
         (3) Constipation and bowel obstruction.
   2. Classifications of nausea and vomiting.
      a. Anticipatory.
         (1) Arises from the cortex and limbic region of the brain.
         (2) Classic pavlovian conditioned response in clients with prior episodes of poorly controlled nausea and vomiting.

TABLE 10-5
Emetogenic Potential, Onset, and Duration of Action of Select Chemotherapeutic Agents

Incidence	Agent	Onset (hr) of Nausea/Vomiting	Duration (hr) of Nausea/Vomiting
VERY HIGH (>90%)			
	Carmustine, 250 mg/m^2*	2-4	4-24
	Cisplatin, >50 mg/m^2*	1-6	24-72+
	Cyclophosphamide, >1500 mg/m^2	4-8	12-24
	Dacarbazine	1-3	1-12
	Mechlorethamine	0.5-2	8-24
	Melphalan (high dose)	3-6	6-12
HIGH (60%-90%)			
	Aldesleukin (IL-2)	2-4	24
	Amifostine	<30 min	0.5-2
	Carboplatin*	4-6	12-24
	Carmustine, <250 mg/m^2*	2-4	4-24
	Cisplatin, <50 mg/m^2*	1-6	24-72+
	Cyclophosphamide†	4-12	12-24
	Cytarabine, ≥1 g/m^2	6-12	3-12
	Dactinomycin	1-2	4-20
	Doxorubicin, ≥60 mg/m^2*	4-6	6-18
	Etoposide†	4-6	24+
	Irinotecan	2-6	24
	Melphalan, >50 mg/m^2	2-4	12-24
	Methotrexate, >1 g/m^2	1-12	24-72
	Oxaliplatin	1-6	24
	Procarbazine	24-27	Variable

(Continued)

TABLE 10-5

Emetogenic Potential, Onset, and Duration of Action of Select Chemotherapeutic Agents—cont'd

Incidence	Agent	Onset (hr) of Nausea/Vomiting	Duration (hr) of Nausea/Vomiting
MODERATE (30%-60%)			
	Alemtuzumab	2-6	24
	Arsenic trioxide	2-6	24
	Capecitabine	4-8	4
	Cytarabine*	6-12	3-12
	Daunorubicin	4-6	4
	Doxorubicin, 20-59 mg/m^2	4-6	6+
	Doxorubicin liposome	4-6	4
	Epirubicin, 60-90 mg/m^2	2-6	24+
	Fluorouracil*	3-6	24+
	Gemcitabine	2-6	24
	Gemtuzumab	2-6	24
	Idarubicin	2 (PO)/15-30 min (IV)	24+
	Ifosfamide	3-6	24-72
	Mitomycin-C*	1-4	48-72
	Mitoxantrone	4-6	6+
	Pentostatin	12-24	24
LOW (10%-30%)			
	Topotecan	2-6	24
	Amifostine (subcutaneous)	0.5-1	2
	Altretamine	2-6	2-24
	Asparaginase	2-4	8-24
	Bexarotene	24-28	24-48
	Bleomycin	3-6	2-4
	Daunorubicin*	1-2	4-6
	Docetaxel	4-8	6-8
	Etoposide[†]	3-8	4-6
	Lomustine*	2-6	2-24
	Melphalan*	6-12	48
	Mercaptopurine	4-8	4-6
	Methotrexate*	4-12	3-12
	Mitomycin-C*	1-4	48-72
	Paclitaxel	4-8	6-8
	Vinblastine	4-8	4
	Vindesine	4-8	4
	Vinorelbine	4-8	4
VERY LOW (<10%)			
	Bacillus Calmette-Guerin (BCG)	n.a.	n.a.
	Chlorambucil	n.a.	n.a.
	Flutamide	n.a.	n.a.
	Goserelin	n.a.	n.a.
	Tretinoin	n.a.	n.a.
	Vincristine	4-8	4

Modified from National Comprehensive Cancer Network (NCCN). Clinical Practice Guidelines in Oncology–v.1.2004. Antiemesis. Version 1.2004, 07-08-2004 © 2004. National Comprehensive Cancer Network, Inc. All rights reserved.
PO, By mouth; *IV,* intravenous; *n.a.,* not applicable.
*Dose related; potential increases with higher doses.
[†]Route and dose related.

(3) Nonthreatening cues (auditory, visual, or sensory) may trigger reaction.

(4) Provoked by anxiety.

b. During and after chemotherapy.

(1) Nausea, mediated through the autonomic nervous system.

(2) Acute vomiting phase.

(a) Occurs within 24 hours of antineoplastic administration.

(b) Stimulation of reflex arc that includes the intestinal tract and release of various neurotransmitters, the chemoreceptor trigger zone (CTZ) located in the area postrema of the brainstem and the vomiting center (VC) located in the medulla oblongata.

(3) Delayed vomiting phase.

(a) Delayed emesis begins 18 to 24 hours after chemotherapy.

(b) This phase is common after cisplatin administration. Vomiting may last up to 7 days, peaking at 48 to 72 hours.

(c) With administration of carboplatin, cyclophosphamide, and doxorubicin, symptoms may persist up to 5 days.

c. Refractory.

(1) Resistant or nonresponsive to antiemetic therapy.

B. Antiemetic drug therapy.

1. Prevents nausea and vomiting by pharmacologically inhibiting neurotransmitters that stimulate the reflex arc of nausea and vomiting.

II. Types of antiemetic drugs (Table 10-6).

III. Principles of medical management (Gralla, 2002; Koeller et al., 2002; NCCN, 2004; Wickham, 1999).

A. Goal is prevention of emesis.

B. Use the lowest effective antiemetic dose before chemotherapy.

C. Selection of appropriate antiemetics (Table 10-6) should be based on the emetogenic potential of the chemotherapy as well as client risk factors.

D. Administer antiemetics prophylactically to cover onset, peak, and duration period of each antineoplastic agent.

E. Assess the client for risk of delayed emesis, and provide prophylactic therapy if indicated.

F. Complete follow-up assessment of outcomes 48 to 72 hours after chemotherapy, and offer advice if indicated.

IV. Potential adverse effects (Gralla, 2002; Koeller et al., 2002; NCCN, 2004; Wickham, 1999).

A. Uncontrolled nausea and vomiting.

1. Fluid and electrolyte imbalance.

2. Anorexia and weight loss.

3. Esophageal tear or hemorrhage.

4. Loss of quality of life.

5. Potential noncompliance with therapeutic regimen.

B. Adverse effects of drug therapy.

1. Adverse effects (see Table 10-6).

2. Administration difficulties.

a. Erratic absorption because of client variables (e.g., gastric resection).

b. Special needs for compounding alternative drug formulations (e.g., suppositories, suspensions).

TABLE 10-6
Antiemetic Therapy: Select Pharmacologic Agents for the Control of Chemotherapy-Induced Nausea and Vomiting, Acute

Classification	Generic Name	Trade Name(s)	Route	Dose/Schedule (Adult)	Adverse Effects of Class	Nursing Implications
Serotonin agonist	Ondansetron	Zofran	IV	8-32 mg × 1 before chemotherapy or 0.15 mg/kg q8h × 3 doses	Headache and fever	Assess for headache and fever. Administer acetaminophen for headache and fever.
					Diarrhea and constipation	Assess for number and consistency of stools. Administer stool softeners (docusate) and stimulants (senna) to prevent constipation. Increase fluids and roughage in diet.
					Transient increases in serum AST/GPT	Monitor liver function test results. Administration: Give higher doses over atleast 30 min to prevent dizziness, headache, hypotension.
	Granisetron	Kytril	PO	8 mg tid or bid	Headache and constipation	Assess for headache and bowel regularity. Acetaminophen, 650 mg, for headache and stool softeners (docusate) and stimulants (senna) to prevent constipation. Increase fluids and roughage in diet.
			IV	10 mcg/kg or 1 mg over 5 min, within 30 min of chemotherapy		
			PO	1-2 mg daily before chemotherapy		
	Dolasetron	Anzemet	IV	100 mg over 5 min within 30 min of chemotherapy	Same as granisetron + prolonged QT interval	Same as granisetron + monitor ECG. If client complains of shortness of breath or skipped heart beats, notify physician.
			PO	100-200 mg within 60 min of chemotherapy		
	Palonosetron	Aloxi	IV	0.25 mg IV push	Same as granisetron.	Same as granisetron.
NK-1 antagonist	Aprepitant	Emend	PO	125 mg day 1 80 mg days 2 and 3	Constipation, diarrhea, hiccups, tiredness	Assess for GI effects. Give stool softeners (docusate) and stimulants (senna) to treat constipation
Substituted benzamide	Metoclopramide	Reglan	IV	2 mg/kg q2h × 4	Sedation	Assess level of sedation. Avoid tasks that require alertness until drug response is established. Avoid alcohol and other CNS depressants.
			PO	0.5-2 mg/kg q3-4h or 20-40 mg q4-6h	Extrapyramidal symptoms (EPSs), e.g., akathisia, acute	Assess for EPS reactions (i.e., involuntary eye, facial, or limb movements). Prophylactic

Class	Generic Name	Trade Name	Route	Dose	Side Effects	Nursing Considerations
Phenothiazines	Prochlorper-azine	Compazine	IM	10 mg q4-6h	dystonic reactions (increased incidence in clients <40 yr)	diphenhydramine to prevent EPSs for high doses; may be used with lower doses if EPSs occur.
			IV	10-40 mg q4-6h		
			PO	10 mg q4-6h	Diarrhea (high doses)	Assess number and consistency of stools. Administration: Do not administer to clients with prior hypersensitivity to procaine or procainamide; epilepsy or pheochromocytoma or where stimulation of GI motility is contraindicated (e.g., mechanical obstruction, GI bleeding).
			Span-sule	15-30 mg q12h		
			PR	25 mg q4-6h	Sedation	Avoid tasks that require alertness until drug response is established. Avoid alcohol and other CNS depressants.
					Blurred vision EPSs, e.g., akathisia	Assess vision and impact on safety. Monitor for and be prepared to treat EPSs with diphenhydramine, 25 mg IV or PO.
					Dry mouth	Suck on ice chips or hard candy. Frequent intake of fluids.
					Orthostatic hypotension	Monitor VS and BP lying and sitting or standing for orthostatic changes. Educate client to rise slowly from lying or sitting position.
					Anticholinergic crisis with overuse	Give benztropine or diphenhydramine for treatment for anticholinergic crisis. See Prochlorperazine.
	Chlorpromazine	Thorazine	IM	12.5-50 mg q4-6h	Dizziness, hypotension, EPSs, e.g., akathisia, dry mouth	See Prochlorperazine. Administration: Do not give IV—causes hypotension.
			IV	12.5-50 mg q4-6h		
			PR	12.5-50 mg q4-6h		
	Thiethylperazine maleate	Torecan	IM	10 mg daily tid	Drowsiness; EPSs, e.g., dystonia, torticollis, akathisia, gait disturbances; hypotension	Torecan injection contraindicated in clients who are allergic to sulfites.
			PO	10 mg daily tid		
			PR	10 mg daily tid		
Corticosteroids	Dexamethasone	Decadron	IV	10-20 mg given ×1 before chemotherapy for preventing acute emesis	Dyspepsia and increased appetite Hiccups Euphoria and insomnia Fluid retention, hyperglycemia, hypokalemia	Take with food or milk. Monitor weight. Assess for prolonged hiccups. Assess emotional status and ability to sleep. Monitor intake and output and weight. Assess for edema. Monitor blood sugar and electrolyte results. Assess for effects of low potassium.

(Continued)

TABLE 10-6
Antiemetic Therapy: Select Pharmacologic Agents for the Control of Chemotherapy-induced Nausea and Vomiting, Acute—cont'd

Classification	Generic Name	Trade Name(s)	Route	Dose/Schedule (Adult)	Adverse Effects of Class	Nursing Implications
		Hexadrol	PO	4-8 mg twice daily × 4 doses on days 2 through 4 for preventing delayed emesis	Adrenal gland suppression	Monitor for fever, hypotension, hyperkalemia, myalgia, arthralgia. Slow IV infusion to prevent perineal itching/burning (see Table 10-4). Give dexamethasone no later than 3 PM
	Methylprednisolone	Solu-Cortef	PO	50-125 mg q4-12h	Dyspepsia, hiccups, increased appetite, euphoria, insomnia, fluid retention, hyperglycemia	See Dexamethasone and Table 10-4.
Butyrophenones	Haloperidol	Haldol	IM	2-5 mg q2h × 3-4 doses/24 hr	Sedation	Assess level of sedation. Avoid tasks that require alertness until drug response is established. Avoid alcohol and other CNS depressants.
			PO	2-5 mg q2h × 3-4 doses/24 hr		
			IV	2 mg × 1	EPSs, e.g., akathisia	Monitor for and be prepared to treat EPS with diphenhydramine, 25 mg IV or PO. Monitor VS and BP lying and sitting or standing for orthostatic changes. Educate client to rise slowly from lying or sitting position.
					Orthostatic hypotension	
	Droperidol (not recommended)	Inapsine	IM	2-5 mg q4-6h	Sedation	Assess level of sedation. Avoid tasks that require alertness until drug response is established. Avoid alcohol and other CNS depressants.
			IV	2-5 mg q4-6h or drip	EPSs, e.g., akathisia	Monitor for and be prepared to tract EPSs with diphenhydramine 25 mg IV or PO. Monitor VS.
					Hypotension	

Category	Drug	Brand	Route	Dose	Side Effects	Nursing Interventions
Cannabinoids	Dronabinol	Marinol	PO	2.5-10 mg 1-3 hr before chemotherapy, then q2h × 4-6 doses/day	Prolongation of QT	Monitor ECG. If client complains of shortness of breath or skipped heart beats, notify physician. Black box warning or sudden depth due to prolonged QT interval.
					Sedation and dizziness	Assess level of sedation. Avoid tasks that require alertness until drug response is established. Avoid alcohol and other CNS depressants.
					Dry mouth	Suck on ice chips or hard candy. Frequent intake of fluids.
						Assess emotional status.
					Euphoria or dysphoria / Orthostatic hypotension	Monitor VS and BP lying and sitting or standing for orthostatic changes. Educate client to rise slowly from lying or sitting position
					CNS adverse reactions more common in the elderly	Administer with caution to the elderly.
Drugs used to augment antiemetics	Diphenhy-dramine	Benadryl	PO / IM / IV	25-50 mg q4h prn / 25-50 mg q4h prn / 25-50 mg q4h prn	Sedation and dizziness	Assess client's level of consciousness and risk for oversedation. Avoid tasks that require alertness until drug response is established. Avoid alcohol and other CNS depressants. Assess vision and impact on safety.
					Blurred vision/diplopia / Dry mouth	Suck on ice chips or hard candy. Regular oral care. Frequent intake of fluids.
	Hydroxyzine	Atarax, Vistaril	PO, IM	25 mg q4-6h prn	Drowsiness	Assess client's level of consciousness and risk for oversedation. Avoid tasks that require alertness until drug response is established. Avoid alcohol and other CNS depressants.
					Dry mouth	Suck on ice chips or hard candy. Regular oral care. Frequent intake of fluids.
					Rare hypersensitivity reactions (IV only)	Never give IV.
						Administration: When administering IM, may cause marked discomfort at injection site; Z-track method is preferred, deep into large muscle mass.

(Continued)

TABLE 10-6
Antiemetic Therapy: Select Pharmacologic Agents for the Control of Chemotherapy-Induced Nausea and Vomiting, Acute—cont'd

Classification	Generic Name	Trade Name(s)	Route	Dose/Schedule (Adult)	Adverse Effects of Class	Nursing Implications
	Lorazepam	Ativan	IV PO SL	0.5-2 mg 0.5-2 mg 0.5-2 mg	Sedation, dizziness, weakness, unsteadiness, disorientation	Assess client's level of consciousness and orientation. Avoid tasks that require alertness until drug response is established. Avoid alcohol and other CNS depressants. Implement measures for client safety. Fall precautions.
					Anterograde amnesia	Assess memory. Refer to mental health professional as needed. Monitor VS.
Miscellaneous	Promethazine	Phenergan and multiple generics	PO	25 mg q4h prn	Hypotension Sedation and disorientation	Assess client's level of consciousness. Avoid tasks that require alertness until drug response is established. Avoid alcohol and other CNS depressants. Monitor elderly clients for confusion, sedation.
			IV, IM	12.5-25 mg q4h prn	Hypotension	Monitor VS, especially during IV administration because hypotension may occur.
					Dry mouth	Suck on ice chips or hard candy. Regular oral care. Frequent intake of fluids.
					Urine retention	Monitor intake and output. Palpate bladder, Catheterize after voiding to measure retention.
					Lower seizure threshold Photo sensitivity	Neuro assessment. Seizure precautions as needed. Avoid bright lights. Darken room, wear sunglasses.
					Rash	Assess skin prior to start of drug treatment and daily. Report to health care provider.

Modified from Cleri LB: Serotonin antagonists: State of the art management of chemotherapy-induced emesis, *Oncol Nurs* 2(1):6-7, 1995.
IV, Intravenous; *AST*, aspartate transaminase; *GPT*, glutamic-pyruvic transaminase; *PO*, by mouth; *tid*, three times daily; *bid*, twice daily; *ECG*, electrocardiogram; *CNS*, central nervous system; *GI*, gastrointestinal; *IM*, intramuscular; *PR*, per rectum; *VS*, vital signs; *BP*, blood pressure; *prn*, as needed; *SL*, sublingual.

Assessment

I. Identification of clients at risk for nausea and vomiting (see Chapter 14).
  A. Current treatments and medical history.
    1. Chemotherapy agent, dose, and schedule.
    2. Radiation therapy, location, and dosage.
    3. Other medical problems.
    4. Current medications.
  B. Client-related factors.
    1. Age less than 50 years old—may have more anticipatory vomiting.
    2. Heavy ethanol intake—may have lower incidence.
    3. Women more than men.
    4. Positive history of prenatal nausea and vomiting.
    5. Positive history of motion sickness.
II. Physical examination (see Chapter 14).
  A. Number and volume of emetic episodes.
  B. Retching.
  C. Lack of oral intake; intake and output.
  D. Fluid balance, signs and symptoms of dehydration—poor skin turgor, concentrated urine, low urine output, orthostatic hypotension.
  E. Presence of blood in vomitus.
  F. Vital signs—orthostatic hypotension.
  G. History of present health problems (e.g., clients with glaucoma should avoid many of the antiemetics).
III. Evaluation of diagnostic and laboratory data.
  A. Serum electrolyte values.

Nursing Diagnoses

I. Nausea.
II. Risk for deficient fluid volume.
III. Deficient knowledge related to antiemetic drug therapy.

Outcome Identification

I. Client states relief of nausea and has no vomiting episodes.
II. Client maintains fluid volume and electrolyte balance.
III. Client discusses the rationale for the use of antiemetic drug therapy and the schedule of administration.
  A. Client describes potential adverse effects of antiemetic drug therapy.
  B. Client describes measures to manage adverse effects of antiemetic drug therapy.
  C. Client lists signs and symptoms of adverse effects of antiemetic drug therapy to report to the health care team.

Planning and Implementation

I. Implement strategies to manage nausea and vomiting (see Chapter 14).
  A. Follow recommended schedules for administration (e.g., administer oral antiemetics 30 to 40 minutes before treatment, IV bolus approximately 10 to 30 minutes before treatment).
II. Implement strategies to educate client about the following:

A. Rationale for use of antiemetic drug therapy and for taking antiemetics as scheduled.
B. Adverse effects and strategies to manage adverse effects.
C. Adverse effects to report to health care team.
III. Assess client's and family's cultural and ethnic background, particularly health care practices and values and beliefs related to pharmacotherapy (see Antimicrobials, Planning and Implementation section).
IV. Implement strategies to monitor for adverse effects of antiemetic drug therapy (see Table 10-6).
A. Implement strategies to maximize client safety.
1. Assess for mental status changes, dizziness, sedation, and implement safety measures (e.g., fall precautions) as needed.
V. Implement interventions to decrease the incidence and manage the adverse effects of antiemetic drug therapy (see Table 10-6).
VI. Implement measures to monitor for response to antiemetic therapy.

Evaluation

The oncology nurse systematically and regularly evaluates the client's and/or family's responses to interventions to determine progress toward the achievement of expected outcomes. Relevant data are collected, and actual findings are compared with expected findings. Nursing diagnoses, outcomes, and plans of care are reviewed and revised as necessary.

ANALGESICS

Theory

I. Rationale/indications (Paice, 1999).
A. To reduce the effect of noxious stimuli caused by heat, cold, or mechanical injury that elicit a response known as pain.
B. Analgesics work by interfering with the pain transmission initiated by the pain receptors, primary afferent neuronal fibers, the spinothalamic tract, collateral fibers, and higher brain centers.
C. Indicated for musculoskeletal, visceral, and neuronal pain.
II. Types of analgesics (Paice, 1999).
A. Opiate agonist compounds.
1. Morphine sulfate (Astramorph, Duramorph).
2. Hydromorphone hydrochloride (Dilaudid).
3. Codeine sulfate and codeine phosphate.
4. Hydrocodone bitartrate.
5. Oxycodone hydrochloride (OxyContin).
6. Oxymorphone hydrochloride (Numorphan).
7. Levorphanol tartrate (Levo-Dromoran).
8. Fentanyl citrate (Fentanyl).
9. Methadone hydrochloride (Dolophine).
10. Meperidine hydrochloride (Demerol).
11. Propoxyphene napsylate (Darvon compounds).
B. Nonopioid analgesics (see Antiinflammatory Agents section).
C. Adjuvant agents (see Psychotropic Drugs: Sedative/Hypnotic and Antianxiety Agents and Antiinflammatory Agents sections).
III. Principles of medical management (Paice, 1999).

A. Selection of appropriate analgesia based on pharmacokinetic factors (Table 10-7) and client's physical needs, age, history of analgesia usage, and organ function.
B. Reassess effectiveness and side effect profile (see Chapter 1).
IV. Potential adverse effects (Paice, 1999).
A. Adverse effect profile of opioid analgesics (Table 10-8).
B. Tolerance and dependence.
C. Opioid withdrawal.
D. Drug interactions with multidrug regimens (Table 10-9).
Other sedative/hypnotic drugs—potentiate sedative properties of opiates and combination opiate substances.

TABLE 10-7
Pharmacokinetic Factors of Opiates and Nonopiates

Drug (Oral)	Equivalent Potency to Morphine Sulfate	Onset of Effect (min)	Peak Effect (min)	Duration of Effect (hr)	Plasma Half-life (hr)
Morphine	10 mg IV	30	30-90	3-7	2-3
controlled or sustained release (MS Contin, Oramorph SR)	30 mg PO	30	30	8-12	8-12
Codeine	100 mg	30	45-90	4-6	3-4
Fentanyl patch (Duragesic)	50 mcg topical	10	20-30	1-2	3-4
Fentanyl (Fentanyl Oralet, Actiq)	400 mcg PO	5-15	Hypoventilation risks; instruct patient to suck, not swallow or chew, for 15 min	10-60 min	
Hydro-morphone (Dilaudid)	1.5 mg IV	30	30-90	4-5	2-4
Levorphanol (Levo-Dromoran)	2 mg PO	30	60-90	4-8	10-12
Meperidine (Demerol)	150 mg IV	15	30-60	2-4	3-4*
Methadone (Dolophine)	10 mg	15	60-120	4-6	22-55*
Oxycodone (immediate release)	15 mg	15	45-60	4-6	2
Oxycodone (delayed release)	30 mg	30	60	12	4
Oxymorphone (Numorphan)	1-1.5 mg IV	10	30-90	3-6	2
	5 mg PR	30	60-90	4-6	2
Acetaminophen	n.a.	15	30-60	4-6	1.25-3

*IV, Intravenous; PO, by mouth; PR, per rectum; n.a., not applicable.
*Active metabolite normeperidine 14-24 h in normal renal function.

TABLE 10-8
Side Effect Profile of Opioid Analgesics

Side Effects	Nursing Implications
GASTROINTESTINAL	
Nausea, vomiting	Monitor nausea and number of vomiting episodes and effect on comfort and fluid balance. Administer antiemetic drug therapy as needed.
Constipation	Assess bowel elimination patterns and compare with client's normal pattern. Stool softeners and/or stimulant cathartics. Increase fluid and dietary fiber intake.
Narcotized bowel	Abdominal assessment; report decreased or absent bowel sounds and increased abdominal pain.
CARDIOVASCULAR	
Arteriolar vasodilation and reduced peripheral resistance; decrease in blood pressure; tachycardia, bradycardia	Monitor vital signs, blood pressure for orthostatic hypotension. Provide for client safety if blood pressure is low.
RESPIRATORY	
Depressant effect on brainstem reduces respiratory rate, minute volume, tidal exchange; irregular and periodic breathing; respiratory arrest	Monitor level of sedation; respiratory rate and depth; arterial blood gases; vital signs, O_2 saturations. Have available narcotic antagonist and measures for respiratory assistance.
Decreased cough reflex	Monitor coughing ability postoperatively. Aspiration precautions.
CENTRAL NERVOUS SYSTEM	
Drowsiness, alteration in mood and mental clouding; visual and auditory hallucinations, euphoria, dizziness, disorientation, paranoia; lethargy, inability to concentrate, apathy; seizure, uncontrollable twitching, myoclonus	Neurologic assessment. Provide for client safety. Institute fall precautions as needed. Monitor for preseizure activity, especially in clients taking meperidine: monitor for twitching. Level of sedation may indicate degree of respiratory depression. Methylphenidate (Ritalin), 5-10 mg PO bid or tid may be helpful for somnolence or mental clouding from opiates.
PUPIL	
Miosis	Monitor pupil size and response to light (contraction).
SMOOTH MUSCLE	
Contraction of gallbladder, bile duct, sphincter of Oddi	Monitor for signs of gastric upset. If present, evaluate liver and pancreatic function tests.
GENITOURINARY	
Urinary retention	Monitor urine output, palpate bladder, catheterize (straight or indwelling) as needed.
DERMATOLOGIC	
Skin rash, cutaneous vasodilation	Monitor skin integrity. Administer antihistamines for allergic reactions. Educate client to avoid scratching. Provide cool environment.

PO, By mouth; *bid,* twice daily; *tid,* three times daily.

TABLE 10-9
Common Drug Interactions of Analgesics

Drug	Effect
ACETAMINOPHEN (APAP) PLUS (+)	
Ethanol (ETOH)	Chronic ETOH causes increased toxicity of APAP overdose
Food	Delayed APAP absorption
Phenytoin (Dilantin)	Increased hepatic metabolism of APAP
Metoclopramide (Reglan)	Increased APAP absorption
Diazepam (Valium)	Decreased diazepam bioavailability
METHADONE +	
Barbiturates, carbamazepine (Tegretol), phenytoin, rifampin (Rifadin)	Reduced methadone plasma levels by enhancing CYP2D6 metabolism
Fluconazole (Diflucan), itraconazole (Sporanox), ketoconazole (Nizoral)	Increased methadone plasma levels by inhibiting CYP3A4 metabolism; enhanced sedation may be observed
OPIOID ANALGESICS +	
Barbiturates	Enhanced CNS depressant effects
Cimetidine (Tagamet)	Enhanced respiratory and CNS depressant effects
Chlorpromazine (Thorazine)	Enhanced CNS depression and hypotension
Ethanol	Enhanced CNS depressant effects
Monoamine oxidase inhibitors	Increased adverse reactions (excitation, sweating, rigidity, hypertension)
Neuromuscular blockers+	Additive respiratory depression
Rifampin	Decreased opioid plasma levels
Tricyclic antidepressants	Enhanced CNS depressant effects
MEPERIDINE +	
Isoniazid (INH)	Potentiates isoniazid
Phenytoin	Reduced meperidine plasma levels
NSAID +	
ACE inhibitors	Reduced antihypertensive effect
β-adrenergic receptor blockers	Reduced antihypertensive effect
Corticosteroids	Increased incidence of GI ulceration
Hydralazine (Apresoline)	Reduced antihypertensive effect
Prazosin (Minipress)	Reduced antihypertensive effect
Potassium-sparing diuretics	Decreased renal function
SALICYLATES +	
Warfarin (Coumadin)	Increased risk of bleeding
Acetazolamide (Diamox)	May enhance renal salicylate excretion and increase salicylate penetration into the brain, causing CNS salicylate toxicity
ETOH	Increased risk of GI blood loss
Heparin (Liquaemin)	Increased risk of bleeding
Methotrexate (Folex, Mexate)	Increased risk of methotrexate toxicity
Probenecid (Benemid)	Inhibits uricosuric effects of probenecid
Sulfinpyrazine (Anturane)	Inhibits uricosuric effects of sulfinpyrazone
Antacids	Reduced salicylate levels; increased renal elimination of salicylates
Antidiabetic agents	Increased response of sulfonylureas; chlorpropamide most likely affected

CYP2D6, Cytochrome P450 enzyme 2D6; *CYP3A4*, cytochrome P450 enzyme 3A4; *CNS*, central nervous system, *NSAIDs*, nonsteroidal antiinflammatory drugs; *ACE*, angiotensin-converting enzyme; *GI*, gastrointestinal.

1. Drugs that lower seizure threshold—increase potential for seizure disorder.
2. Concomitant drugs that alter mental status equilibrium.
3. Other drugs that alter hepatic metabolism, renal excretion.
4. Other drugs that alter bioavailability, absorption, or pharmacokinetics of the administered drug.

E. Abnormalities in drug absorption caused by the following:
   1. GI.
      a. Surgical resections including gastrectomy, jejunectomy, and duodenectomy may increase transit time and/or decrease absorption.
      b. Feeding tubes inserted at various points in the GI tract may not be appropriate point of absorption of individual drug.
         (1) Tube feedings or fluids administered through tubes may increase transit time and decrease absorption.
      c. Pharmacologically induced changes in gut motility (e.g., laxatives, muscarinics, prokinetic agents—cisapride, metoclopramide-antidiarrheal drugs, narcotics).
   2. Topical absorption.
      a. Skin integrity—moisture content, friability, fat/lean body ratio, homogeneous epidermis without ulcerations.
      b. Occlusive dressings increase absorption.
      c. Location of application—areas of high vascularity may have higher absorption.

F. Potential adverse effects caused by compromised organ systems.
   1. Renal insufficiency—may slow rate of elimination of drug and/or metabolites, leading to increased potential for toxicities.
   2. Hepatic insufficiency—may increase amount of drug available to body because of decreased first pass effect, altered enzyme pathways, or other metabolic pathways.
   3. CNS—brain metastases, underlying seizure disorders may predispose to CNS toxicity.
   4. Urinary—benign prostatic hypertrophy may contribute to urinary retention.
   5. Respiratory—underlying lung disorders including emphysema, chronic obstructive pulmonary disease (COPD), lung metastases, asthma; in addition, acute pulmonary distress syndromes may compromise respiratory drive.
   6. GI—history of nausea and vomiting, impaired cough reflex.
   7. Cardiovascular—coronary artery disease, congestive heart failure.

Assessment

I. Identification of clients at risk for pain (see Chapter 1).
   A. Assessment of type of pain—description, etiology, classification, degree of pain.
   B. History of past and current analgesia regimens and their effectiveness.
      1. Time to onset of pain relief.
      2. Duration of time of pain relief.
      3. Quality or rating of decrease of pain.
   C. Assessment of side effects from previous regimens.
      1. Description of side effects.
      2. Onset and duration of side effects.

3. Pharmacologic and/or other interventions to control or alleviate side effects.
4. Severity of side effects.
II. Physical examination.
   A. Review of systems.
   B. Examination of area of pain and/or originating site of pain—redness, temperature changes, atrophy, tenderness (see Chapter 1).
III. Current medications.
IV. Evaluation of diagnostic and laboratory data.
   A. Renal indices—serum creatinine and blood urea nitrogen (BUN), intake and output.
   B. Hepatic indices—aspartate aminotransferase (AST), alanine aminotransferase (ALT), bilirubin, alkaline phosphatase.
   C. Electrocardiogram (ECG), electroencephalogram (EEG) if indicated.
   D. X-ray examination, bone scan, CT, MRI, positron emission tomography (PET) scan, ultrasound.

Nursing Diagnoses

I. Acute or chronic pain.
II. Deficient knowledge related to pharmacologic management of pain.

Outcome Identification

I. Client states pain is relieved or reduced to his/her satisfaction.
II. Client discusses the rationale for the use of analgesics, including the schedule of administration.
   A. Client describes adverse effects of use of analgesics.
   B. Client describes measures to manage adverse effects of use of analgesics.
   C. Client lists signs and symptoms of adverse effects of analgesics to report to the health care team.
   D. Client and family discuss that the risk of addiction is extremely rare.

Planning and Implementation

I. Implement strategies to manage pain (see Chapter 1).
II. Implement strategies to educate client about the following:
   A. Rationale for taking analgesic medications, including schedule of administration.
   B. Adverse effects and strategies to manage adverse effects.
   C. Low risk for addiction.
   D. Adverse effects to report to health care team.
III. Assess client's and family's cultural and ethnic background, particularly health care practices and values and beliefs related to pharmacotherapy (see Antimicrobials, Planning and Implementation section).
IV. Implement strategies to monitor for adverse effects of analgesic agents (see Table 10-8).
V. Implement strategies to decrease the incidence and manage the adverse effects of analgesics.
   A. Assess baseline data (e.g., vital signs, CNS—orientation, alertness, affect; respiratory effort, oxygen saturation, rate, depth, sedation score).

    B. Review client's medical history for existing or previous conditions, such as acute alcoholism, impaired hepatic or renal function, advanced age, increased intracranial pressure.

    C. Assess normal bowel patterns.

    D. Review client's medications for possible drug interactions.

VI. Implement measures to monitor for response to analgesia.

    A. Assess client's pain experience.

    B. Assess for adverse effects, toxicity, and drug interactions.

Evaluation

The oncology nurse systematically and regularly evaluates the client's and/or family's responses to interventions to determine progress toward the achievement of expected outcomes. Relevant data are collected, and actual findings are compared with expected findings. Nursing diagnoses, outcomes, and plans of care are reviewed and revised as necessary.

PSYCHOTROPIC DRUGS: SEDATIVE/HYPNOTIC AND ANTIANXIETY AGENTS

Theory

I. Rationale/indications (Goebel, 1999).

    A. Antianxiety agents are used to do the following:

        1. Reduce behavioral and physiologic abnormalities caused by anxiety disorders.

        2. Control anxiety induced by other medical conditions, psychiatric disorders, or pharmacologic disorders.

        3. As adjuvant pharmacologic management for pain associated with marked anxiety or maniclike symptoms.

        4. Alcohol or narcotic withdrawal.

    B. Sedative/hypnotic agents use.

        1. For sleep disorders (e.g., insomnia).

        2. As adjuvant pharmacologic management for pain associated with marked anxiety or maniclike symptoms.

        3. Alcohol or narcotic withdrawal.

II. Types of psychotropic drugs.

    A. Barbiturates (Table 10-10).

    B. Benzodiazepines (see Table 10-10).

    C. Neuroleptics (Table 10-11).

III. Principles of medical management (Goebel, 1999).

    A. Selection of therapy.

        1. Psychotherapy.

        2. Pharmacologic (see Tables 10-10 and 10-11).

            a. Half-life.

            b. Sedative properties.

            c. Psychomotor and memory impairment.

            d. Dose-response profiles.

            e. Cost.

            f. Duration of therapy.

            g. Dosage conversion.

TABLE 10-10
Common Sedative/Hypnotic and Antianxiety Agents

Drug and Dose	Indications and Notable Pharmacologic Facts	Adverse Effects of Class	Nursing Implications
BARBITURATES		Lethargy, drowsiness	Assess level of consciousness and degree of sedation. Implement measures for client safety as needed (e.g., assist with ambulation, fall precautions). Avoid tasks that require alertness until drug response is established. Avoid alcohol and other CNS depressants.
		Apnea	Monitor respiratory status and oxygen saturation. Report periods of apnea to physician.
		Rash→Stevens-Johnson syndrome	Evaluate condition of skin before initiation and during treatment.
		Risk of overdose, especially in those with liver dysfunction	Monitor liver function. Assess VS and presence of toxicity symptoms.
		Barbiturate toxicity (e.g., hypotension; cold, clammy skin; insomnia; nausea; vomiting; delirium; weakness)	Notify physician if present.
		Rare bone marrow suppression	Monitor RBC, hemoglobin, and hematocrit laboratory test results. Precautions: Give on empty stomach for best absorption. Physical dependency may occur if long-term use. Do not discontinue drug abruptly; taper off over 1-2 wk.

(Continued)

TABLE 10-10
Common Sedative/Hypnotic and Antianxiety Agents—cont'd

Drug and Dose	Indications and Notable Pharmacologic Facts	Adverse Effects of Class	Nursing Implications
Short Acting Secobarbital (Seconal), 100 mg PO hs	Insomnia, basal hypnosis for anesthesia, emergency control of convulsions. Incompatible with several medications (e.g., codeine, cimetidine, diphenhydramine, hydrocortisone, insulin, meperidine, methadone, vancomycin); decreases effect of oral anticoagulants and corticosteroids.	Same as barbiturates Tolerance builds quickly after approximately 2 wk	Same as barbiturates. Administration: Aqueous solutions must be prepared with sterile water for injection. Use solution within 30 min because of instability. Aqueous polyethylene glycol vehicles should be given slowly IV and client monitored closely with emergency equipment available.
Long Acting Phenobarbital, 15-100 mg PO hs (Luminal)	Sedation, grand mal and focal seizures alone or in combination with other antiepileptic drugs. Administered IV in acute convulsive states.	Loss of concentration, mental dulling, depression of affect Skin rashes Folate deficiency possible May increase metabolic activity of liver enzymes and decrease effects of drugs biotransformed by these enzymes Apnea	Neurologic assessment. Assess mental status. Educate client and family of possible effects on client's affect. Evaluate skin before start of therapy and during treatment. Monitor RBC, hemoglobin, and hematocrit laboratory test results. Monitor liver enzyme laboratory test levels. Consult pharmacist regarding possible drug interactions. Respiratory assessment. Monitor serum drug levels. Administration: Administer injection within 30 min after opening vial. Precautions: Long half-life and too frequent dosing can lead to accumulation toxicity.
BENZODIAZEPINES	These agents bind to GABA receptors, inhibiting CNS excitation and	Sedation and difficulty in concentration and information recall are	Assess level of consciousness and degree of sedation. Implement measures for client safety as needed (e.g.,

Drug	Effects	Side Effects / Adverse Reactions	Nursing Interventions
	resulting in CNS depression. Intermediate-acting agents are better tolerated in cancer patients. Lorazepam, oxazepam, alprazolam, and temazepam are preferred over triazolam, flurazepam, and chlordiazepoxide.	most common; rebound anxiety and early morning insomnia may occur with short-acting agents Acute confusional states and increased risk of falls, especially in the elderly Withdrawal symptoms (psychosis, seizures, coma) occur more frequently with short-acting agents	assist with ambulation, fall precautions). Avoid tasks that require alertness until drug response is established. Avoid alcohol and other CNS depressants. Monitor for signs of abnormal behavior, CNS excitability.
Long Acting (Not Recommended) Flurazepam (Dalmane), 15 mg PO hs	Insomnia. Sedation. Longest-acting benzodiazepine hypnotic. Daytime carryover effects are common (e.g., decreased alertness, impaired coordination, confusion, personality changes). Side effects may persist for days after discontinuation of drug.	Lethargy, disorientation, slurred speech, faintness, confusion, nervousness, apprehension, weakness, irritability, short-term memory impairment, depression Palpitations Anorexia Drowsiness, dizziness, headache, ataxia, light-headedness common in elderly	Neurologic assessment. Assess memory. Implement measures to provide for client safety (e.g., emotionally safe environment, fall precautions, assist with ambulation). Avoid tasks that require alertness until drug response is established. Avoid alcohol and other CNS depressants. Educate client and family about possible adverse effects. Refer to mental health professional as needed. Monitor VS. Educate client to report feelings of "racing or pounding heart." Assess appetite and impact on nutrition. Have client select diet, and ask family to provide favorite foods. Use with caution in the elderly.
Intermediate (Recommended) Temazepam (Restoril), 15-30 mg PO hs	Insomnia, sedation. Minimal hangover effect. May take two nights before beneficial effects felt. Sleep disturbances can occur for several nights after discontinuance.	Lethargy, drowsiness, daytime sedation	Assess level of consciousness and degree of sedation. Implement measures for client safety as needed (e.g., assist with ambulation, fall precautions). Avoid tasks that require alertness until drug response is established. Avoid alcohol and other CNS depressants.

(Continued)

TABLE 10-10
Common Sedative/Hypnotic and Antianxiety Agents—cont'd

Drug and Dose	Indications and Notable Pharmacologic Facts	Adverse Effects of Class	Nursing Implications
		Nausea, vomiting, constipation, diarrhea	Assess for effects of nausea and vomiting on nutrition, fluid and electrolyte balance. Administer antiemetics as needed. Assess number and consistency of stools. Administer antidiarrhea drugs, or stool softeners (docusate) and stimulants (senna) to prevent constipation as needed. Increase fluids and roughage in diet.
		Rare bone marrow suppression and hepatic enzyme elevation	Monitor laboratory results (hemoglobin, hematocrit, liver function tests).
Oxazepam (Serax), 10-30 mg PO tid	Insomnia. Sedation. No accumulation of metabolites.	Same as Temazepam	Same as Temazepam.
Short Acting (Recommended) Triazolam (Halcion), 0.125-0.25 mg PO hs	Insomnia. Sedation. Minimal daytime hangover effect. May take two nights before beneficial effects felt. Increased wakefulness during the last third of the night.	Anterograde amnesia possible	Assess memory. Refer to mental health professional as needed.
		Headache	Assess for headache. Administer pain medication as needed.
		Lethargy and drowsiness	Assess level of consciousness and degree of sedation. Implement measures for client safety as needed (e.g., assist with ambulation, fall precautions). Avoid tasks that require alertness until drug response is established. Avoid alcohol and other CNS depressants.
		Rare bone marrow suppression and hepatic enzyme elevation	Monitor laboratory results (hemoglobin, hematocrit, liver function tests).
Short Acting (Not Recommended) Alprazolam (Xanax), 0.5-3 mg PO 1-3 times daily	Anxiety.	Drowsiness and light-headedness common during early stages of therapy	Assess mental status, monitor affect, drowsiness. Implement measures for client safety (e.g., assist with ambulation, fall precautions).

Drug/Dosage	Action/Use	Side Effects	Nursing Considerations
Chlordiazepoxide (Librium), 15-100 mg PO tid	Used in anxiety and for ETOH withdrawal. Less potent than diazepam and less anticonvulsive activity. Excreted slowly by kidneys.	Orthostatic hypotension	Monitor VS. Assess for orthostatic hypotension (BP lying/sitting and standing); if systolic BP drops 20 mm Hg, hold drug, notify prescriber.
		Blurred vision	Assess vision, report blurred vision. Determine impact on client safety.
		Antidepressant activity at higher doses	Assess for depression and suicidal risk. Refer to mental health professional as needed.
Diazepam (Valium), 2.5-5 mg PO tid or 0.5-2 mg IM, IV q4 h	Used in anxiety, acute seizure control, operating procedures.	Dizziness and drowsiness; orthostatic hypotension; blurred vision	See Alprazolam. IM solution prepared immediately before administration. IM solution not to be given IV because of air bubbles from solution. Inject IM slowly and deeply. IV solution to be reconstituted with sterile water or saline. Give IV over 1 min. Do not give IV preparation IM because of pain on injection. Do not add IV dose to IV solution because of instability and quick deterioration.
		Dizziness and drowsiness; orthostatic hypotension; blurred vision	See Alprazolam. Can be given IM or IV. Do not add to IV fluids. When administering IV, use large vein, inject slowly, maximum rate no greater than 5 mg/min. Assess site for phlebitis. Be prepared to provide respiratory assistance.
Lorazepam (Ativan), 0.125-0.5 mg PO hs	Acute anxiety, preoperative sedation, insomnia. Shortest-acting drug used for anxiety and preanesthetic. No active metabolite formed, so less danger of accumulation.	Dizziness and drowsiness; orthostatic hypotension; blurred vision	See Alprazolam.
		May impair short-term memory	Assess memory. Refer to mental health professional as needed.

CNS, Central nervous system; ETOH, ethyl alcohol; VS, vital signs; RBC, red blood cell; PO, by mouth; hs, at bedtime; tid, three times daily; IV, intravenous; GABA, γ-aminobutyric acid; BP, blood pressure; IM, intramuscular.
* These drugs have high abuse potential and have given way to other sedative hypnotics. They are included here to provide complete information.

TABLE 10-11
Neuroleptics[*]

Drug and Usual Dose	Sedation	Anticholinergic effects	Extrapyramidal	Orthostatic Hypotension	Nursing Implications
					Side Effect Frequency
PHENOTHIAZINES	Used in pain management with behavioral problems such as anxiety or psychoses				
Chlorpromazine (Thorazine) 6.25-50 mg PO tid	High	Moderate	Moderate	High	Sedation: Assess mental status: level of consciousness, affect, oversedation. Implement safety measures (e.g., fall precautions, assist with ambulation). Avoid tasks that require alertness until drug response is established. Avoid alcohol and other CNS depressants. EPSs: Assess and be prepared to treat EPSs with anticholinergic therapy (benztropine or diphenhydramine). Orthostatic hypotension: Monitor VS; assess BP, pulse lying and standing/sitting. Constipation: Prevent constipation (e.g., stool softeners/stimulants, increase bulk/fluids, increase ambulation). Administration: Dilute IV solution to 1 mg/ml in saline and administer at 1 mg/min.
Fluphenazine (Prolixin, Permitil) 0.5-10 mg bid PO, IM	Low	Low	Very high	Low	EPSs: Assess and be prepared to treat EPSs with anticholinergic therapy (benztropine or diphenhydramine). Rare aplastic anemia—monitor CBC. Rare liver or hepatic dysfunction—monitor serum creatinine and liver function tests. Constipation: See Chlorpromazine. Precautions: Because of impaired GI absorption, avoid antacids with oral forms of fluphenazine. Educate client/family on what adverse effects to report immediately. Educate client/family that urine may turn pink to reddish brown. Administration: Protect solution from light. Moisture may cloud solution so use dry syringe and needle for injection.
Perphenazine (Trilafon) 4-16 mg tid PO, IM	Low	Low	High	Low	EPSs: Assess and be prepared to treat EPSs. Rare aplastic anemia—monitor CBC. Rare liver or hepatic dysfunction—monitor serum creatinine and liver function tests. Administration: Monitor BP/pulse when administering IV because hypotension can occur. For oral concentrate, dilute (60 ml diluent/5 ml concentrate) in water, fruit juices except apple; no caffeinated beverages.

Drug					Nursing Considerations
Thioridazine (Mellaril), 10-75 mg tid PO	High	High	Low	Low	Sedation: See Chlorpromazine. EPSs: Assess and be prepared to treat EPSs with anticholinergic therapy (benztropine or diphenhydramine). Constipation: Prevent constipation (e.g., stool softeners/stimulants, increase bulk/fluids, increase ambulation). Prolonged QT interval: Monitor ECG and cardiac status. Urinary retention: Monitor urine output; palpate bladder; check for residual urine. Rare pancytopenia: Monitor CBC. Rare hepatic dysfunction: Monitor liver function tests. Potential impotence: Educate client regarding this possibility. Offer suggestions to manage impotence (see Chapter 6). Administration: For oral concentrate, dilute immediately before use with fruit juice or water. After IM injection, instruct client to remain lying for 30 min.
BUTYROPHENONE					
Haloperidol (Haldol)	Very low	Very low	Very high	Very low	EPSs: Assess for and be prepared to treat EPSs. May lower seizure threshold: Use cautiously in individuals with epilepsy, neurologic assessment, seizure precautions as needed. Constipation: See Chlorpromazine. Orthostatic hypotension: See Chlorpromazine. Rare pancytopenia: Monitor CBC. Rare liver dysfunction: Monitor liver function tests. May prolong QT interval: Monitor ECG and cardiac status. Urinary retention: Monitor urine output; palpate bladder and check for residual urine. Dose reduction in the elderly. Administration: IM injection into deep muscle mass, client to remain lying for 30 min after injection. Do not mix oral concentrate in coffee or tea.

PO, By mouth; *tid*, three times daily; *CNS*, central nervous system; *EPSs*, extrapyramidal symptoms; *VS*, vital signs; *BP*, blood pressure; *IV*, intravenous; *bid*, twice daily; *CBC*, complete blood count; *GI*, gastrointestinal; *IM*, intramuscular; *ECG*, electrocardiogram.

*Neuroleptics are used for several psychiatric problems, including anxiety, delirium, and acute confusional states (hallucinations, nightmares from opiates, terminal dyspnea).

      h. Routes of administration.
      i. Compromised organ function.
      j. Age-related alterations.
IV. Potential adverse effects (see Tables 10-10 and 10-11).
    A. Dependence and withdrawal.
    B. Drug interactions.
    C. Respiratory depression.
    D. Inappropriate behavior.
    E. Noncompliance.

Assessment

  I. Identify clients at risk for anxiety disorders (see Chapter 2), pain or sleep disorders (see Chapter 1).
    A. Assess for signs and symptoms of anxiety, pain, or sleep disorders.
  II. Physical examination (see Chapters 1 and 2).
  III. Current medications.
  IV. Evaluation of diagnostic and laboratory data.
    A. Electrolyte abnormalities and blood glucose levels.
    B. Drug level abnormalities.

Nursing Diagnoses

  I. Anxiety.
  II. Disturbed sleep pattern.
  III. Acute or chronic pain.
  IV. Deficient knowledge related to use of psychotropic drugs.

Outcome Identification

  I. Client describes a reduction in anxiety.
  II. Client achieves adequate amount of sleep.
  III. Client states pain is relieved or reduced to his/her satisfaction.
  IV. Client discusses the rationale for the use of psychotropic drugs, including schedule of administration.
    A. Client describes adverse effects of use of psychotropic drugs.
    B. Client describes measures to manage adverse effects of psychotropic drugs.
    C. Client lists signs and symptoms of adverse effects of psychotropic drugs to report to the health care team.

Planning and Implementation

  I. Implement strategies to manage pain or sleep disorders (see Chapter 1) and anxiety (see Chapter 2).
  II. Implement strategies to educate client about the following:
    A. Rationale for use of psychotropic drug therapy and taking psychotropics as scheduled.
    B. Adverse effects and strategies to manage adverse effects.
    C. Adverse effects to report to health care team.
  III. Assess client's and family's cultural and ethnic background, particularly health care practices and values and beliefs related to pharmacotherapy (see Antimicrobials, Planning and Implementation section).

A. Determine client's racial group because biologic variations among racial groups may affect drug metabolism rates, clinical drug responses, and drug side effects. For example, Asians may require lower doses of neuroleptics; Chinese may require lower doses of benzodiazepines and may be more sensitive to the sedative effects of this class of drugs.

IV. Implement strategies to monitor for adverse effects of psychotropic drugs (see Tables 10-10 and 10-11).

V. Implement interventions to decrease the incidence and manage the adverse effects of psychotropic drugs (see Tables 10-10 and 10-11).
   A. Assess baseline data (e.g., vital signs, CNS—orientation, alertness, affect; respiratory effort, rate, depth).
   B. Review client's medical history for existing or previous conditions.
   C. Review client's medications for potential drug interactions.

VI. Implement measures to monitor for response to psychotropic drugs.
   A. Psychiatric/psychologic consult as needed.
   B. Assess for level of anxiety, pain, and amount of restful sleep.

Evaluation

The oncology nurse systematically and regularly evaluates the client's and/or family's responses to interventions to determine progress toward the achievement of expected outcomes. Relevant data are collected, and actual findings are compared with expected findings. Nursing diagnoses, outcomes, and plans of care are reviewed and revised as necessary.

ANTIDEPRESSANTS

Theory

I. Rationale/indications (Barsevick & Much, 1999).
   A. For treatment of depression.
      1. Depression is a commonly identified response of cancer patients to the cancer experience.
      2. Depression can range from minor mood changes to major emotional responses of suicidal ideation.
      3. Types of depression.
         a. Bipolar—with manic phase.
         b. Major depression—unipolar only.
         c. Situational depression.
         d. Drug- or food-induced depression.
   B. Antidepressants used.
      1. To treat clinical unipolar or bipolar depression.
      2. In depression associated with chronic pain.
      3. As adjuvant pharmacologic pain management in pain conditions, including postherpetic neuralgia, migraine and chronic tension headaches, sundowner syndrome.
      4. To treat insomnia.

II. Types of antidepressants (Table 10-12).
   A. Tricyclic antidepressants.
   B. Selective serotonin reuptake inhibitors (SSRIs).

III. Principles of medical management (Barsevick & Much, 1999).
   A. Selection of therapy.

TABLE 10-12
Common Antidepressants

Drug and Indications	Sedation	Anticholinergic	Orthostatic Hypotension	Side Effect Frequency — Nursing Implications
TRICYCLIC ANTIDEPRESSANTS				
Amitriptyline (Elavil, Endep) Used in endogenous depressions accompanied with anxiety; adjuvant treatment for pain	High	High	High	Sedation: Assess mental status (e.g., excessive sedation, affect, suicidal tendencies). Give at bedtime to minimize daytime drowsiness. Avoid tasks that require alertness until drug response is established. Avoid alcohol and other CNS depressants. EPSs: Assess and be prepared to treat EPSs with anticholinergic therapy (benztropine or diphenhydramine). Orthostatic hypotension: Monitor VS. Assess for orthostatic hypotension—if systolic BP drops 20 mm Hg, hold drug, notify practitioner. Institute safety precautions; teach client to avoid rapid position changes. Rare pancytopenia: Monitor CBC. Urinary retention: Monitor urinary output; palpate bladder, check for residual urine.
Imipramine (Tofranil) Used in endogenous depression and in reducing enuresis in children	Moderate	Moderate	Moderate	Sedation: Assess mental status (e.g., excessive sedation, affect, suicidal tendencies). Give at bedtime to minimize daytime drowsiness. Avoid tasks that require alertness until drug response is established. Avoid alcohol and other CNS depressants. EPSs: Assess and be prepared to treat EPSs with anticholinergic therapy (benztropine or diphenhydramine). Orthostatic hypotension: Monitor VS. Assess for orthostatic hypotension—if systolic BP drops 20 mm Hg, hold drug, notify practitioner. Institute safety precautions; teach client to avoid rapid position changes. Constipation: Assess client's normal bowel pattern. Implement interventions to prevent constipation: stool softeners/stimulants, increase bulk/fluid in diet, ambulation. Rare arrhythmias: Take VS q4h for clients with CV disease. Monitor ECG and cardiac status. Rare pancytopenia: Monitor CBC. Rare hepatic dysfunction: Monitor liver function tests. Changes in affect; risk for suicide: Monitor mental status, complete suicide assessment. Precautions: If client consumes alcohol, hold dose.

				Nursing Considerations
Desipramine (Norpramin) Active metabolite of imipramine with same uses	Low	Low	Moderate	Orthostatic hypotension: Monitor VS. Assess for orthostatic hypotension—if systolic BP drops 20 mm Hg, hold drug, notify practitioner. Institute safety precautions; teach client to avoid rapid position changes. Rare arrhythmias: Take VS q4h for clients with CV disease. Monitor ECG and cardiac status. Rare pancytopenia: Monitor CBC. Rare hepatic dysfunction: Monitor liver function tests. Risk for suicide: Complete suicide assessment. Urinary retention: Monitor urinary output; palpate bladder, check for residual urine. Precautions: If client consumes alcohol, hold dose.
TRIAZOLOPYRIDINE Trazodone (Desyrel) Used in depression exhibited as persistent, prominent dysphoria (occurring nearly every day for at least 2 weeks with at least 4 of the following 8 symptoms: appetite change, sleep pattern change, increased fatigue, impaired concentration, feelings of guilt or worthlessness, loss of interest in usual activities, psychomotor agitation or retardation, suicidal ideation. Also to treat neurogenic pain.	High	Very low	Moderate	Sedation: Assess mental status (e.g., excessive sedation, affect, suicidal tendencies). Give at bedtime to minimize daytime drowsiness. Avoid tasks that require alertness until drug response is established. Avoid alcohol and other CNS depressants. Orthostatic hypotension: Monitor VS. Assess for orthostatic hypotension—if systolic BP drops 20 mm Hg, hold drug, notify practitioner. Institute safety precautions; teach client to avoid rapid position changes. Rare arrhythmias: Take VS q4h for clients with CV disease. Monitor ECG and cardiac status. Rare pancytopenia: Monitor CBC. Rare hepatic dysfunction: Monitor liver function tests. Changes in affect; risk for suicide: Monitor mental status, complete suicide assessment. Urinary retention: Monitor urinary output; palpate bladder, check for residual urine. Precautions: If client consumes alcohol, hold dose.

(Continued)

TABLE 10-12
Common Antidepressants—cont'd

Drug and Indications	Sedation	Anticholinergic	Orthostatic Hypotension	Nursing Implications
SELECTIVE SEROTONIN REUPTAKE INHIBITORS (SSRIS)				
Citalopram hydrobromide (Celexa) Same uses as Trazodone except for pain control.	Low	Low	Low	Constipation: Assess client's normal bowel pattern. Implement interventions to prevent constipation: stool softeners/stimulants, increase bulk/fluid in diet, ambulation. Rare arrhythmias: Take VS q4h for clients with CV disease. Monitor ECG and cardiac status. Drug interactions: Avoid cimetidine, carbamazepine, MAO inhibitors, nefazodone, metoprolol. Precautions: Use with caution in the elderly and clients with renal or hepatic dysfunction. If client consumes alcohol, hold dose.
Fluoxetine hydrochloride (Prozac) Same as Trazodone except for pain control; also for OCD, panic disorder, premenstrual dyphoric, bulimia.	None	Very low	None	Constipation: Assess client's normal bowel pattern. Implement interventions to prevent constipation: stool softeners/stimulants, increase bulk/fluid in diet, ambulation. Rare arrhythmias: Take VS q4h for clients with CV disease. Monitor ECG and cardiac status. Anorexia: Assess appetite. Monitor effect on nutrition and weight. Have client select own diet. Have family bring in favorite foods. Rare pancytopenia: Monitor CBC. Rare hepatic dysfunction: Monitor liver function tests. Changes in affect; insomnia, risk for suicide: Monitor mental status; assess sleep patterns; complete suicide assessment. Urinary retention: Monitor urinary output; palpate bladder, check for residual urine. Precautions: If client consumes alcohol, hold dose.
Paroxetine hydrochloride (Paxil) Same as Fluoxetine and social anxiety disorder and	Low	Low	Low	Constipation: Assess client's normal bowel pattern. Implement interventions to prevent constipation: stool softeners/stimulants, increase bulk/fluid in diet, ambulation. Changes in affect, risk for suicide: Monitor mental status; complete suicide assessment. Urinary retention: Monitor urinary output; palpate bladder, check for residual urine.

Drug				Nursing Implications
generalized anxiety disorder.	None	None		Rare arrhythmias: Take VS q4h for clients with CV disease. Monitor ECG and cardiac status. Precautions: If client consumes alcohol, hold dose. Same as Paroxetine.
Sertraline (Zoloft) Same as Trazodone except for pain control. Psychotherapy augments therapeutic result. Used for major depressive disorders, OCD, post traumatic stress disorder.	None	None		
Venlafaxine (Effexor) Inhibits both serotonin and norepinephrine uptake	Low	Low to none	Low to moderate	Orthostatic hypotension: Monitor VS. Assess for orthostatic hypotension—if systolic BP drops 20 mm Hg, hold drug, notify practitioner. Institute safety precautions; teach client to avoid rapid position changes. Sustained hypertension may occur in clients receiving doses >350 mg: Monitor cardiac status, take VS q4h for clients with CV disease. Rare pancytopenia: Monitor CBC. Rare hepatic dysfunction: Monitor liver function tests. Changes in affect, risk for suicide: Monitor mental status; complete suicide assessment.

CNS, Central nervous system; *EPS,* extrapyramidal symptom; *VS,* vital signs; *BP,* blood pressure; *CBC,* complete blood count; *CV,* cardiovascular; *ECG,* electrocardiogram; *MAO,* monoamine oxidase; *OCD,* obsessive-compulsive disorder.

    1. Depression.
      a. Psychotherapy.
      b. Pharmacologic therapy (see Table 10-12).
    2. Pain (see Analgesics section above).
  IV. Potential adverse effects (see Table 10-12).
    A. Drug interactions.
    B. Dietary restrictions.

Assessment

  I. Identification of clients at risk for depression (see Chapter 2).
    A. Age—younger more than older persons.
    B. Health conditions (e.g., advanced stage of disease), negative body image.
    C. Mental health history—family or individual history of depression or substance abuse.
    D. Disease recurrence, treatment failure.
    E. Unrelieved symptoms, especially pain.
    F. Interactions with other medications.
      1. Antihypertensive and cardiovascular drugs: guanethidine (Ismelin), methyldopa (Aldomet), reserpine (Serpalan, Serpasil), propranolol (Inderal), metoprolol (Lopressor), prazosin (Minipress), clonidine (Catapres), digitalis.
      2. Sedative/hypnotic agents: alcohol, chloral hydrate (Noctec), benzodiazepines, barbiturates, meprobamate (Equanil).
      3. Antiinflammatory agents and analgesics: indomethacin (Indocin), phenylbutazone, opiates, pentazocine (Talwin).
      4. Steroids: corticosteroids, oral contraceptives, estrogen withdrawal.
      5. Miscellaneous: antiparkinsonian drugs, antineoplastic agents (interferon aldesleukin [Interleukin-2]), ethambutol (Myambutol), neuroleptics, stimulant withdrawal.
    G. Concomitant medical diseases.
      1. Endocrine disorders: hypothyroidism, hyperthyroidism, diabetes mellitus, hyperparathyroidism, Cushing's disease, Addison's disease.
      2. CNS disorders: brain tumors, Parkinson's disease, multiple sclerosis, Alzheimer's disease, Huntington's disease.
      3. Cardiovascular disorders: myocardial infarction (MI), cerebral vascular accident (CVA), congestive heart failure (CHF).
      4. Miscellaneous disorders: rheumatoid arthritis, pancreatic disease, carcinoma, systemic lupus erythematosus, infectious disease, metabolic abnormalities, pernicious anemia, malnutrition.
  II. Identification of clients at risk for pain (see Chapter 1).
  III. Assess for signs and symptoms (see Chapters 1 and 2).
  IV. Physical examination (see Chapters 1 and 2).
  V. Evaluation of diagnostic and laboratory data.
    A. Electrolyte disorders.
    B. Fluid imbalances.

Nursing Diagnoses

  I. Ineffective coping.
  II. Risk for violence: self-directed.
  III. Acute or chronic pain.
  IV. Deficient knowledge.

Outcome Identification

I. Client experiences adequate management of his/her depression with minimal adverse effects from medications.
II. Client verbalizes suicidal ideations and agrees to contract not to act on impulse.
III. Client states that the pain is reduced or relieved to his/her satisfaction.
IV. Client discusses rationale for use of antidepressant drug therapy, including schedule of administration.
   A. Client describes potential adverse effects of antidepressants.
   B. Client describes measures to manage adverse effects of antidepressants.
   C. Client lists signs and symptoms of adverse effects of antidepressants to report to the health care team.

Planning and Implementation

I. Implement strategies to manage effects of depression (see Chapter 2) and pain (see Chapter 1).
II. Implement strategies to educate client about the following:
   A. Rationale for use of antidepressant drug therapy and taking antidepressants as scheduled.
   B. Adverse effects and strategies to manage adverse effects.
   C. Adverse effects to report to health care team.
III. Assess client's and family's cultural and ethnic background, particularly health care practices and values and beliefs related to pharmacotherapy (see Antimicrobials, Planning and Implementation section).
IV. Implement strategies to monitor for adverse effects of antidepressants (see Table 10-12).
V. Implement interventions to decrease the incidence and manage the adverse effects of antidepressants (see Table 10-12).
VI. Implement measures to monitor for therapeutic response to antidepressants.
   A. Monitor client for emotional changes, suicidal ideation.
      1. Obtain psychiatric/psychologic consultation as needed.
   B. Monitor client for response pain management.
   C. Assess for adverse effects, toxicity, and drug interactions.

Evaluation

The oncology nurse systematically and regularly evaluates the client's and/or family's responses to interventions to determine progress toward the achievement of expected outcomes. Relevant data are collected, and actual findings are compared with expected findings. Nursing diagnoses, outcomes, and plans of care are reviewed and revised as necessary.

ANTICONVULSANTS

Theory

I. Rationale/indications.
   A. For prophylaxis and treatment of seizure activity.
   B. As adjuvant pharmacologic therapy for pain with neurologic etiology (trigeminal neuralgia, phantom limb pain, thalamic syndrome or lightning tabetic pain).
II. Types of anticonvulsants (Table 10-13).

TABLE 10-13
Common Anticonvulsants and Adjunct Therapy

Drug	Indications and Notable Pharmacologic Facts	Usual Adult Oral Maintenance Dosage	Potential Adverse Effects of Class	Nursing Implications
Phenytoin (Dilantin)	Grand mal and partial complex seizures	300-400 mg; increase to 600 mg may be required; therapeutic drug level 10-20 mcg/ml	Drowsiness, dizziness Hypotension Ventricular fibrillation Hepatitis, nephritis Hematologic disorders Systemic lupus erythematosus (SLE) Stevens-Johnson syndrome	Assess level of consciousness and level of sedation. Implement safety measures as needed (e.g., assist with ambulation, fall precautions). Avoid tasks that require alertness until drug response is established. Avoid alcohol and other CNS depressants. Monitor VS. Initiate CPR. Monitor liver enzymes, BUN and creatinine laboratory test results. Intake and output. Monitor CBC results. Assess for signs and symptoms of SLE (butterfly rash, joint pains, kidney and blood cell abnormalities, etc.). Assess for skin changes before start of therapy and during therapy. Monitor serum drug levels. Precautions: Administer IV slowly, and monitor VS. Do not exceed rate of 50 mg/min; avoid continuous infusion. Phenytoin suspension has erratic GI absorption.
Carbamazepine (CBZ, Tegretol)	Spectrum of action similar to that of phenytoin; also for treatment of trigeminal neuralgia and neuropathic pain in those with cancer	800-1600 mg in 2-4 divided doses; therapeutic drug level 4-12 mcg/ml	Blood dyscrasias (e.g., aplastic anemia, leukopenia, thrombocytopenia, eosinophilia, leukocytosis) Hyponatremia, drowsiness, dizziness, ataxia, nausea, blurred vision, diplopia with too rapid titration of dose	Monitor CBC laboratory test results for abnormalities. Report to physician. Manage possible anemia/fatigue, neutropenia/infection, and thrombocytopenia/bleeding (see Chapters 13 and 16). Educate client about side effects to report to health care providers. Monitor electrolyte laboratory test results and intake and output. Assess mental status, vision, ability to work, and nausea. Implement measures to provide for client safety as needed. Anticipate change in medication order. Precaution: Administer drug with meals to decrease GI upset.

Drug	Uses/Notes	Dose	Side Effects	Nursing Interventions
Oxcarbazepine (Trileptal)	Spectrum of activity similar to CBZ	1200–2400 mg in 2 divided doses	Hyponatremia Headache Ataxia, dizziness, drowsiness Stevens-Johnson syndrome	Monitor electrolyte laboratory test values and intake and output. Assess intensity of headache. Administer pain medication as needed. Assess mental status and ability to ambulate. Implement measures to provide for client safety as needed. Avoid tasks that require alertness until drug response is established. Avoid alcohol and other CNS depressants. Assess for skin changes before start of therapy and during therapy.
Ethosuximide (Zarontin)	Petit mal seizures Long half-life that can lead to cumulative toxicity	500–1500 mg in 2 divided doses	Drowsiness, dizziness, ataxia Headache Hiccoughs Rash GI distress with too rapid dosing titration (e.g., nausea, cramping, diarrhea)	Assess mental status and ability to ambulate. Implement measures to provide for client safety as needed. Avoid tasks that require alertness until drug response is established. Avoid alcohol and other CNS depressants. Assess intensity of headache. Administer pain medication as needed. Monitor for prolonged hiccoughs. Monitor skin before start of treatment and during therapy. Administer drug with meals to decrease GI upset.
Gabapentin (Neurontin)	Neuropathic pain	900–3600 mg in 3 divided doses	Discoloration of urine Drowsiness, dizziness, blurred vision, tremor, slurred speech Fatigue Weight gain Skin rash Nausea, vomiting	Educate client that urine may turn pink to reddish brown from drug. Neurologic assessment. Assess mental status; level of sedation; vision; speech; sensory, and motor function. Implement measures to provide for client safety as needed. Avoid tasks that require alertness until drug response is established. Avoid alcohol and other CNS depressants. Assess level of fatigue. Provide for periods of rest. Monitor CBC. Monitor weight and food intake. Assess skin before the start of treatment and during therapy for changes. Assess for nausea and episodes of vomiting. Monitor effect on comfort and fluid balance. Administer antiemetics as needed. Precaution: Discontinue drug gradually.
Lamotrigine (Lamictal)	Partial seizures, Lennox-Gastaut syndrome	200–500 mg in 2 divided doses	Stevens-Johnson syndrome/toxic epidermal necrolysis Fatigue	Discontinue drug immediately at first sign of rash. Assess level of fatigue. Provide for periods of rest. Monitor CBC.

(Continued)

TABLE 10-13
Common Anticonvulsants and Adjunct Therapy—cont'd

Drug	Indications and Notable Pharmacologic Facts	Usual Adult Oral Maintenance Dosage	Potential Adverse Effects of Class	Nursing Implications
			Dizziness, headache, blurred or double vision	Assess mental status, level of sedation, vision. Implement measures to provide for client safety as needed. Avoid tasks that require alertness until drug response is established. Avoid alcohol and other CNS depressants.
Levetiracetam (Keppra)	Partial seizures	1000-3000 mg in 2 divided doses	Drowsiness, dizziness	Assess level of headache. Administer pain medication as needed. Assess level of sedation. Avoid tasks that require alertness until drug response is established. Avoid alcohol and other CNS depressants. Assess mental status.
			Weakness	Monitor activity tolerance. Implement measures to ensure safety of client as needed. Monitor VS, especially temperature. Monitor CBC laboratory test results. Assess
			Infection	skin, lungs, urine for possible infection.
Phenobarbital (Luminal)	Sedation, grand mal and focal seizures alone or in combination with other antiepileptic drugs; IV in acute convulsive states	60-200 mg in 2-3 divided doses	Loss of concentration, mental dulling, depression of affect	Neurologic assessment. Assess mental status. Educate client and family of possible effects on client's affect.
			Skin rashes Folate deficiency possible May increase metabolic activity of liver enzymes and decrease effects of drugs biotransformed by these enzymes	Evaluate skin before start of therapy and during treatment. Monitor RBC, hemoglobin, and hematocrit laboratory test results. Monitor liver enzyme laboratory test levels. Consult pharmacist regarding possible drug interactions.
Tiagabine (Gabitril)	Partial seizures	32-56 mg in 2-4 divided doses	Drowsiness, dizziness, nervousness	Assess level of sedation, dizziness, and nervousness and effect on daily activities. Avoid tasks that require alertness until drug response is established. Avoid alcohol and other CNS depressants.
			Weakness	Monitor activity tolerance. Implement measures to ensure safety of client as needed.

Medication	Uses	Dosage	Side Effects	Nursing Considerations
Topiramate (Topamax)	Partial onset seizures, grand mal seizures, Lennox-Gastaut syndrome	400-1600 mg in 2 divided doses	Drowsiness, dizziness, cognitive dysfunction; Fatigue; Ocular impairment; Weight loss; Kidney stones	Assess level of sedation and cognitive ability. Avoid tasks that require alertness until drug response is established. Avoid alcohol and other CNS depressants. Provide for periods of rest. Monitor CBC laboratory test results. Assess level of fatigue and effect on daily living. Provide for periods of rest. Monitor CBC laboratory test results. Assess vision. Report abnormalities to physician. Monitor weight, food intake, and intake and output. Force fluids, 2-3 L/day, if not contraindicated. Strain urine for stones. Provide pain medication as needed. Precaution: Do not break tablets because of bitter taste.
Valproate/valproic acid (Depakene, Depakote)	Simple and complex absence seizures; adjunct in treatment of multiple seizure types	Initial 10-15 mg/kg/day; increase by 5-10 mg/kg/wk max of 60 mg/kg/day; therapeutic drug level 50-100 mcg/ml	Nausea, vomiting; diarrhea and abdominal cramps at initiation of therapy; Sedation, ataxia, tremor, behavioral disturbances more predominant if taken with other anticonvulsants; Elevated serum transaminase and hepatic failure	Abdominal assessment. Assess GI symptoms and effect on comfort, fluid balance, perineal skin. Administer antiemetics, pain medication, antispasmodtics, or antidiarrhea medications as needed. Assess level of sedation, ability to walk/maintain balance, sensory and motor functions and behavior. Avoid tasks that require alertness until drug response is established. Avoid alcohol and other CNS depressants. Refer to mental health professional as needed. Monitor serum liver enzyme test results, bilirubin, ammonia levels as needed. Precautions: Administer with meals to decrease stomach upset. Do not break or crush the tablet or capsule; can cause irritation of mouth and throat.
Zonisamide (Zonegran)	Partial seizures	300-600 mg daily or in 2 divided doses	Drowsiness, ataxia; Fatigue; Kidney stones; Agranulocytosis, aplastic anemia	Assess mental status and ability to ambulate. Assess level of fatigue and effect on daily living. Provide for periods of rest. Monitor CBC laboratory test results. Force fluids, 2-3 L/day, if not contraindicated. Strain urine for stones. Provide pain medication as needed. Monitor serum creatinine and BUN. Monitor CBC laboratory test results. Assess and manage possible neutropenia/infection, anemia/fatigue, and thrombocytopenia/bleeding (see Chapters 13 and 16). Precaution: Contraindicated in clients with hypersensitivity to sulfonamides.

CNS, Central nervous system; VS, vital signs; CPR, cardiopulmonary resuscitation; BUN, blood urea nitrogen; CBC, complete blood count; IV, intravenous; GI, gastrointestinal; RBC, red blood cell.

   III. Principles of medical management.
      A. Diagnosis of appropriate seizure activity.
      B. Diagnosis of appropriate pain syndrome.
      C. Selection of appropriate pharmacologic therapy (see Table 10-13).
   IV. Potential adverse effects (see Table 10-13).

Assessment

   I. Identification of clients at risk for seizure activity.
      A. Underlying seizure disorder.
         1. Previous seizure history.
      B. Drugs that lower seizure threshold, e.g., phenobarbital (Luminal), ethanol, benzodiazepines, amphetamines, antibiotics, immunosuppressants (cyclosporine [Neoral, Sandimmune], tacrolimus [Prograf, Protopic]) and salicylate toxicity.
      C. Medical conditions that lower seizure threshold.
         1. Trauma.
         2. Febrile episodes.
         3. Tumor pressure within brain.
   II. Identification of clients at risk for neurologic pain.
   III. Physical examination.
      A. Neurologic examination (Lewis et al., 2000).
         1. Mental status—general appearance, level of consciousness, mood and affect, thought content and intellectual capacity.
         2. Cranial nerve assessment.
         3. Sensory function.
         4. Motor function.
         5. Assessment of reflexes.
   IV. Evaluation of diagnostic and laboratory data (Lewis et al., 2000).
      A. Anticonvulsant serum levels.
      B. Serum electrolytes values.
      C. Analysis of cerebrospinal fluid.
      D. EEG, CT scan, MRI, PET.

Nursing Diagnoses

   I. Risk for injury.
   II. Acute or chronic pain.
   III. Deficient knowledge related to use of anticonvulsant drug therapy.

Outcome Identification

   I. Client incurs no injuries during a seizure.
      A. Client experiences adequate seizure control with minimal side effects.
   II. Client states pain is relieved or reduced to his/her satisfaction.
   III. Client discusses the rationale for the use of anticonvulsants, including schedule of administration.
      A. Client describes potential adverse effects of anticonvulsants.
      B. Client describes measures to manage adverse effects of anticonvulsants.
      C. Client and family list the signs and symptoms of adverse effects of anticonvulsants to report to the health care team.

Planning and Implementation

I. Implement strategies to ensure client safety in the event of a seizure (Lewis et al., 2000).
   A. Institute seizure precautions.
   B. Provide safe environment free of physical hazards.
   C. Assess for injuries after completion of the seizure activity.
      1. Vital signs.
      2. Neurologic examination.
II. Implement strategies to manage pain (see Chapter 1).
III. Implement strategies to educate client about the following:
   A. Rationale for use of anticonvulsant drug therapy and taking anticonvulsants as scheduled.
   B. Adverse effects and strategies to manage adverse effects.
   C. Adverse effects to report to health care team.
IV. Assess client's and family's cultural and ethnic background, particularly health care practices and values and beliefs related to pharmacotherapy (see Antimicrobials, Planning and Implementation section).
V. Implement strategies to monitor for adverse effects of anticonvulsants (see Table 10-13).
VI. Implement strategies to decrease the incidence and manage the adverse effects of anticonvulsants (see Table 10-13).
   A. Assess baseline data (e.g., neurologic status).
   B. Review client's medical history for existing or previous conditions.
   C. Review client's medications for potential drug interactions.
   D. Conduct client/family teaching (e.g., good oral hygiene; avoiding driving or other potentially hazardous activity that requires mental alertness).
VII. Implement measures to monitor for a therapeutic response to anticonvulsant drug therapy.
   A. Assess neurologic status and pain level.
   B. Assess for adverse effects, toxicity, and drug interactions.

Evaluation

The oncology nurse systematically and regularly evaluates the client's and/or family's responses to interventions to determine progress toward the achievement of expected outcomes. Relevant data are collected, and actual findings are compared with expected findings. Nursing diagnoses, outcomes, and plans of care are reviewed and revised as necessary.

HEMATOPOIETIC GROWTH FACTORS

Theory

I. Rationale/indications (Wilkes et al., 2003).
   A. Hematopoietic growth factors are glycoproteins that stimulate the proliferation of bone marrow progenitor cells and their maturation into fully differentiated circulating blood cells.
      1. Provide initiation, modification, and/or restoration of the hematopoietic and immune system and its various cell lines by exerting the following:
         a. Direct antitumor activity via cytotoxic or antiproliferative mechanisms of action.

      b. Biologic effects, such as enhancing differentiation or maturation of immunologic cell lines, thus decreasing neutropenia and risk of infection; decreasing thrombocytopenia and risk of bleeding and decreasing anemia, fatigue, and activity intolerance.

  B. For primary treatment of cancer (e.g., hairy cell leukemia, Kaposi's sarcoma, renal cell carcinoma).

  C. For supportive treatment (Table 10-14).

    1. To shorten the duration of neutropenia following chemotherapy, radiation therapy, or bone marrow transplant.

    2. To increase red blood cell count, neutrophil and macrophage cell count, and platelet levels.

II. Types of growth factors (Langer et al., 2002; Wilkes et al., 2003).

  A. Single lineage factors.

    1. Granulocyte colony-stimulating factors (G-CSF, pegfilgrastim).

      a. Stimulate target cells that include a late precursor committed to the neutrophil lineage and the mature neutrophil.

      b. Increase phagocytic activity.

      c. Increase antimicrobial killing.

      d. Enhance antibody-dependent cell-mediated cytotoxicity.

    2. Erythropoietin (r-HuEPO), darbepoetin alfa (Aranesp) (Glaspy & Tchekmedyian, 2002; Littlewood et al., 2001).

      a. Naturally produced by the kidneys.

      b. Production in normal hosts is regulated by a feedback mechanism involving the perception of decreased oxygen tension in tissue.

      c. Interacts with specific receptors on erythroid burst-forming units and erythroid colony-forming units.

      d. Binding of the stimulating factor and these units leads to erythropoiesis and subsequent production and differentiation of erythrocytes, or red blood cells.

    3. Platelet growth factors.

      a. Isolation of hormone thrombopoietin (TPO) thought to regulate platelet production or megakaryocytopoiesis, a function similar to erythropoiesis.

      b. Megakaryocyte growth and development factor under study in vitro.

      c. Interleukin-11: a thrombopoietin growth factor that stimulates the bone marrow stem cells and megakaryocytic progenitor cells so platelet production is increased.

    4. Stem cell factor (SCF)—also known as mast cell factor, steel factor, and c-kit ligand.

      a. Mechanism of action—works on primitive and mature progenitor cells. Murine SCF enhances erythropoietin-dependent colony-forming unit—granulocyte, erythrocyte, megakaryocyte, monocyte (CFU-GEMM) and burst-forming unit erythrocyte colony formation.

  B. Multilineage factors.

    1. Granulocyte-macrophage colony-stimulating factor (GM-CSF)—receptors exist on myeloid cell lines.

      a. Major effect stimulates the proliferation and differentiation of the cells destined for the neutrophil and macrophage lines.

      b. Enhances functional activities of neutrophils and monocytes/macrophages, leading to enhanced activity in clearing bacterial and fungal organisms.

TABLE 10-14
Growth Factors

Drug	Indications	Side Effects	Nursing Implications
GM-CSF or sargramostim (Leukine)	Myeloid recovery after autologous BMT BMT graft failure or engraftment delay Following induction chemotherapy for acute myelogenous leukemia; use if bone marrow hypoplastic with <5% blasts on day 10	Low dose: bone pain, local skin reaction, fever, flulike symptoms, headache, arthralgias, myalgias High dose: pericardial effusions, capillary leak syndrome, third spacing Phlebitis with peripheral IV administration	Low dose: monitor level of pain; acetaminophen for bone/joint/muscle pain, headache, fever; monitor VS, especially temperature; encourage fluids and rest High dose: cardiovascular assessment, VS, monitor fluid balance and edema, intake and output, breath sounds; monitor electrolyte and CBC laboratory test results Monitor IV site for pain and redness; discontinue IV if present Monitor CBC laboratory test results for return of granulocytes and monocytes Administration: subcutaneous administration standard; IV administration may require albumin in IV carrier
Pegfilgrastim (Pegylated G-CSF, Neulasta)	Antineoplastic chemotherapy-induced neutropenia	Bone pain Adult respiratory distress syndrome (rare) Splenic rupture (rare)	Monitor level of pain; administer acetaminophen for bone pain Assess respiratory status (breath sounds, rate, pattern and depth of respirations, oxygen saturation); notify physician of worsening symptoms Abdominal assessment and pain; notify physician Monitor CBC laboratory test results for return of neutrophils Precautions: Contraindicated in patients with known hypersensitivity to *Escherichia coli*–derived proteins; *do not* administer sooner than 24 hr after chemotherapy and in the case of pegfilgrastim must be no sooner than 14 days before chemotherapy
G-CSF or filgrastim (Neupogen)	Antineoplastic chemotherapy-induced neutropenia	Bone pain	Monitor level of pain; administer acetaminophen for bone pain Monitor CBC for increase in neutrophils Precautions: Contraindicated in clients with known hypersensitivity to *Escherichia coli*–derived products; do not shake vial vigorously if giving subcutaneous injection

(Continued)

TABLE 10-14
Growth Factors

Drug	Indications	Side Effects	Nursing Implications
Erythropoietin (Epogen, Procrit)	Cancer patients receiving chemotherapy	Hypertension	Monitor blood pressure
	Anemia of chronic cancer	Thrombotic events	Assess for possible emboli in lower extremities or lungs
	Zidovudine-treated HIV-infected patients	Seizures	Assess for seizure activity; implement seizure precautions as needed
		Headaches	Assess level of headache; administer pain medication as needed
	Chronic renal failure	Skin rashes, urticaria; transient rash at injection site	Assess skin before the start of treatment and during treatment; rotate injection sites
			Monitor CBC laboratory test results for increase in red blood cell count
Darbepoetin, NESP, (Aranesp)	Renal failure	Hypertension	Contraindicated in patients with uncontrolled hypertension; closely monitor blood pressure of all patients; rotate injection sites; monitor blood counts
	Chemotherapy-induced anemia in clients with nonmyeloid malignancies, chronic renal failure not on dialysis	Fatigue	Assess level of fatigue; provide for periods of rest between activities; educate about energy-conserving strategies
		Edema	Assess skin for edema; elevate lower extremities; protect skin from damage; intake and output; assess breath sounds
		Vascular access thrombosis and thrombotic events	Assess for possible emboli in lower extremities or lungs and in vascular access devices; report positive evidence to physician
		Fever, pneumonia, dyspnea, sepsis	Monitor VS; monitor respiratory status (breath sounds: rate, depth, ease, and pattern of respirations; dyspnea/shortness of breath; oxygen saturation, etc.); administer antipyretics and antimicrobials as needed
		Seizures	Assess for seizure activity; implement seizure precautions as needed
		Nausea, vomiting, diarrhea, dehydration	GI assessment and effect of nausea, vomiting, and diarrhea on comfort, fluid balance, perineal skin; intake and output; administer antiemetic and antidiarrhea drugs as needed; encourage fluids if tolerated; monitor signs of dehydration (dry skin and mucous membranes, concentrated urine, thirst, fever)
			Monitor CBC laboratory test results for increase in red blood cell count

GM-CSF, Granulocyte-macrophage colony-stimulating factor; *BMT,* bone marrow transplant; *VS,* vital signs; *CBC,* complete blood count; *IV,* intravenous; *G-CSF,* granulocyte colony-stimulating factor; *HIV,* human immunodeficiency virus; *GI,* gastrointestinal.

      c. Stimulates production of secondary cytokines such as tumor necrosis factor (TNF), interleukin-1, and macrophage colony-stimulating factor (M-CSF).

III. Principles of medical management (Wilkes et al., 2003).

    A. History of antineoplastic use, radiation therapy, surgery, or biotherapy.

    B. History of other medication use known to cause immunosuppression, neutropenia, anemia, and/or thrombocytopenia.

      1. Immunosuppressants—corticosteroids.

      2. H_2 antagonists—cimetidine, ranitidine.

      3. Aspirin-containing products, nonsteroidal antiinflammatory agents.

    C. Assessment of concurrent disease state or chronic illnesses contributing to neutropenia or anemic state.

      1. Human immunodeficiency virus (HIV) infection.

      2. Immunosuppressive disorders: systemic lupus erythematosus, multiple sclerosis, rheumatoid arthritis.

    D. Assessment of chronic illnesses that may be exacerbated by use of growth factors.

      1. Cardiac—congestive heart failure, pericardial effusion, hypertension.

      2. Endocrine—hyperthyroid, diabetes.

      3. Neurologic or psychiatric disorders—seizure disorders or depressive disorders.

    E. Appropriate time from chemotherapy and nadir recovery.

      1. Colony-stimulating factor (CSF) to start no sooner than 24 hours after chemotherapy and in the case of pegfilgrastim (Neulasta) must be no sooner than 14 days before chemotherapy (Wilkes et al., 2003).

    F. Appropriate supportive therapy.

      1. Blood product support.

      2. Antimicrobial therapy.

      3. Side effect management—nutrition, pain management, electrolyte and fluid balance, dermatologic and mucosal support.

IV. Potential adverse effects.

    A. Side effects (see Table 10-14).

Assessment

  I. Identification of clients at risk for the following:

    A. Neutropenia—absolute neutrophil count less than $500/mm^3$ (see Chapter 13).

    B. Anemia—hemoglobin level less than 10 mg/dl (see Chapter 16).

    C. Thrombocytopenia—platelet count less than 75,000 cells/mm^3 (see Chapter 13).

 II. Physical examination (see Chapters 13 and 16).

III. Current medications.

IV. Evaluation of diagnostic and laboratory data (see Chapters 13 and 16).

Nursing Diagnoses

  I. Risk for infection.

 II. Fatigue.

III. Ineffective protection.

IV. Deficient knowledge related to hematopoietic growth factor drug therapy.

Outcome Identification

I. Client remains free of infection, or infection is recognized early and treated promptly.

    A. Client and family describe personal risk factors for infection.

II. Client achieves adequate activity tolerance.

    A. Client establishes pattern of rest/sleep to achieve optimal performance of desired/required activities.

III. Client has reduced risks of bleeding.

IV. Client and family demonstrate self-care skills required to administer HGF, as applicable (e.g., subcutaneous injections).

    A. Client identifies the type of and describes the rationale for treatment with HGFs, including schedule of administration.

    B. Client describes potential adverse effects of hematopoietic growth factor therapy.

    C. Client describes measures to manage adverse effects of hematopoietic growth factor therapy.

    D. Client lists signs and symptoms of adverse effects of hematopoietic growth factor therapy to report to the health care team.

Planning and Implementation

I. Implement strategies to manage neutropenia/infection, thrombocytopenia/bleeding (see Chapter 13), and anemia/fatigue (see Chapter 16).

II. Assess client's and family's cultural and ethnic background, particularly health care practices and values and beliefs related to pharmacotherapy (see Antimicrobials, Planning and Implementation section).

III. Implement strategies to educate client about the following:

    A. Rationale for need of medications and taking as scheduled.

    B. Administration of hematopoietic growth factor (e.g., subcutaneous injection).

    C. Adverse effects and strategies to manage adverse effects.

    D. Adverse effects to report to health care team.

IV. Implement strategies to monitor for adverse effects of hematopoietic growth factors (see Table 10-14).

V. Implement strategies to decrease the incidence and manage the adverse effects of hematopoietic growth factors (see Table 10-14).

    A. Assess baseline data (e.g., vital signs, neurologic status).

    B. Review client's medical history for existing or previous conditions.

    C. Review client's medications for potential drug interactions.

    D. Conduct client/family teaching (e.g., on side effects and self-management; medication administration).

VI. Implement measures to monitor for response to hematopoietic growth factors.

    A. Monitor laboratory results (e.g., complete blood count).

    B. Assess activity level, presence of infection and bleeding, as applicable.

    C. Assess for adverse effects, toxicity, and drug interactions.

Evaluation

The oncology nurse systematically and regularly evaluates the client's and/or family's responses to interventions to determine progress toward the achievement of expected outcomes. Relevant data are collected, and actual findings are compared

with expected findings. Nursing diagnoses, outcomes, and plans of care are reviewed and revised as necessary.

REFERENCES

Barsevick, & Much, J.K., A.M. (2004). Depression. In C. Yarbro, M. Frogge, & M. Goodman (Eds.). *Cancer symptom management.* Sudbury, MA: Jones and Bartlett, pp. 668-672.

Freifeld, A., Walsh, T., & Pizzo, P. (1997). Infection in the cancer patient. In V. Devita, S. Hellman, & S. Rosenberg, (Eds.). *Cancer principles and practice of oncology* (5th ed.). Philadelphia: Lippincott, pp. 2659-2704.

Gilbert, D., Moellering, R., & Sande, M. (2002). *Sanford guide to antimicrobial therapy.* Hyde Park, VT: Antimicrobial Therapy.

Glaspy, J., & Tchekmedyian, N. (2002). Darbepoietin alfa administered every 2 weeks alleviates anemia in cancer patients receiving chemotherapy. *Oncology (Huntington NY) 16*(Suppl. 11), 23-29.

Goebel, A. (1999). Anxiety. In C. Yarbro, M. Frogge, & M. Goodman (Eds.). *Cancer symptom management.* Sudbury, MA: Jones and Bartlett, pp. 680-693.

Gralla, R. (2002). New agents, new treatments and antiemetic therapy. *Seminars in Oncology 29,*119-124.

Koeller, J.M., Aspro, M.S., Gralla, R.J., et al. (2002). Antiemetic guidelines: Creating a more practical treatment approach. *Support Care in Cancer 10,* 519-522.

Langer, C.J., Choy, H., Glaspy, J.A., & Colowick, A. (2002). Standards of care for anemia management in oncology. *Cancer 95,* 613-623.

Lewis, S.M., Heitkemper, M.M., & Direksen, S.R. (2000). *Medical-surgical nursing* (5th ed.). St. Louis: Mosby.

Littlewood, T.J., Bajetta, E., Nortier, J.W.R., et al. (2001). Effects of epoetin alfa on hematologic parameters and quality of life in cancer patients receiving non-platinum chemotherapy: Results of a randomized, double-blind, placebo-controlled trial. *Journal of Clinical Oncology 19,* 2865-2874.

National Comprehensive Cancer Network (NCCN). Clinical Practice Guidelines in Oncology–v.1.2004. Antiemesis. Version 1.2004, 07-08-04 © 2004. National Comprehensive Cancer Network, Inc. All rights reserved.

Paice, J. (1999). Pain. In C. Yarbro, M. Frogge, & M. Goodman (Eds.). *Cancer symptom management.* Sudbury, MA: Jones and Bartlett, pp. 118-148.

Wickham, R. (1999). Nausea and vomiting. In C. Yarbro, M. Frogge, & M. Goodman (Eds.). *Cancer symptom management.* Sudbury, MA: Jones and Bartlett, pp. 228-263.

Wilkes, G.M., Ingwersen, K., & Barton-Burke, M.B. (2003). *Oncology nursing drug handbook.* Sudbury, MA: Jones and Bartlett.

Wujcik, D. (1999). Infection. In C. Yarbro, M. Frogge, & M. Goodman (Eds.). *Cancer symptom management.* Sudbury, MA: Jones and Bartlett, pp. 307-327.

11 Supportive Care: Nonpharmacologic Interventions

DENISE MURRAY EDWARDS

Theory

I. Definition.
   A. Interventions that are supportive in nature and focused on increasing well-being, healing, or management of symptoms.
   B. Terminology in this field has changed frequently in the past few years.
      1. Definitions used in this section (Theory) are developed by the National Center for Complementary and Alternative Medicine (NCCAM) at the National Institutes of Health (NIH).
   C. Most often used in conjunction with conventional medical treatment.
      1. Conventional medicine is medicine practiced by medical doctors (MDs), doctors of osteopathy (DOs), or other allied health professionals, such as physical therapists, psychologists, and registered nurses. Some medical practitioners are also practitioners of complementary and alternative medicine (CAM).
      2. Other terms for conventional medicine include allopathy; Western, mainstream, orthodox, or regular medicine; and biomedicine.
   D. Often categorized as CAM, which includes therapies that may be used in place of (alternative) or together with (complementary) conventional medical therapy.
      1. Integrative medicine combines mainstream medical therapies and CAM therapies for which there is some high-quality scientific evidence of safety and effectiveness (NCCAM, 2003).
   E. Ultimately, the client's worldview determines what he/she considers mainstream or complementary.
   F. May be categorized as those that focus on the following:
      1. The mind, body, and spirit connection.
      2. Manual and energy healing and physical touch techniques, including manipulation, movement, or touching the body and energy fields (NCCAM, 2003).
II. Characteristics of users of CAM.
   A. According to Sparber et al. (2000), in a study of 100 clients with cancer,
      1. Forty-four percent reported use of one or two CAM therapies.
      2. More women used CAM.
      3. Eighty-one percent were between the ages of 21 and 60 years.
      4. Forty-seven percent reported an annual income above $50,000.
      5. Forty-two percent reported use of CAM therapies within 1 year of the diagnosis of cancer.

B. Reasons given by clients for using CAM.
  1. Helps to cope more effectively with stress.
  2. Decreases discomforts of treatment.
  3. Gives increased sense of control.
  4. Improves quality of life.
  5. Relieves symptoms (e.g., pain, nausea, fatigue, insomnia).
III. Health problems for which clients identified CAM therapies as helpful (Table 11-1).
IV. Types of CAM nonpharmacologic interventions (not all-inclusive).
  A. Mind-body-spirit techniques.
    1. Imagery uses the power of the imagination to access physical, emotional, and spiritual dimensions to affect changed perceptions or sense of well-being (Post-White, 2002).
      a. Images employ six senses: visual, aural, tactile, olfactory, proprioceptive, kinesthetic.
      b. Often referred to as visualization; however, also includes imagining through any sense and not just being able to see something in the "mind's eye."
      c. Wealth of material available to create images for relaxation or distraction (Murray Edwards, 2002).
      d. Imagery-induced relaxation can decrease a variety of symptoms including pain, nausea, and insomnia (Rusy & Weisman, 2000; Van Fleet, 2000).
      e. In guided imagery, the listener is given directions to activate his/her imagination in a way that appeals to the senses, distracts the listener from stressful stimuli, and connects the listener with concepts that may be helpful. An example of guided imagery is provided in Box 11-1.
    2. Meditation—a state of poised, highly directed concentration focused on a clearly defined thought or stimulus (LeShan, 1988).
      a. Can be defined as a "training of attention" or a "stilling of the mind."
      b. Can be used to develop powers of concentration, promote relaxation, enhance self-understanding and well-being, and enrich personal and spiritual growth.
      c. Specific approaches to meditation vary with individual instructors.

TABLE 11-1
Complementary and Alternative Medicine Therapies Identified as Helpful by Clients with Cancer

Therapy	Helpful*	Number
Spiritual	94%	34
Relaxation	50%	22
Exercise	67%	12
Imagery	86%	8
High-dose vitamins	14%	8
Self-help groups	100%	7
Herbal/botanical	20%	5
Lifestyle diet	60%	5
Massage	80%	5

From Sparber A et al: Use of complementary medicine by adult patients participating in cancer clinical trials, Oncol Nurs Forum 27(4):628, 2000.
*Percentage reflects answers given as helpful/very helpful.

BOX 11-1
SAMPLE GUIDED IMAGERY

Hope Kindled*
KATHERINE BROWN-SALTZMAN, RN, MA
Taking a deep breath you stand at night's edge surrounded by darkness, tilting your head up to the sky above you. There amongst the dark void are endless stars. Light carried across the universe. You steady yourself, feeling your feet firmly planted on the ground, as you take in the endless number, letting your eyes settle on the great distance. Filling you up with those small twinkling lights.

There too is the sliver of a moon, a fraction of its real size, you remind yourself. For the moon is full, as full as it has ever been, just now beyond your reach. You become aware that all of this darkness is a mere shadow, for on the other side of the world the sun's brightness fills the other half. Never is there total darkness, only the narrowed perception of light. Now you lie down on the field of grass letting the ground hold you, the sky above so immense that you open yourself to the awe and beauty. You allow yourself to expand into the space; you allow your breath to rise up in greeting. And then you watch as one star falls across the sky, gently tumbling through time and dipping down into your chest, where your heart opens to it. A gift filled with wishes and light, hope kindled and restored.

Little by little you become present to the room, with a slow deep breath and an awareness of the gift, now within you. Forever settled within you.

*Reprinted from Murray Edwards D, editor: *Voice massage: Scripts for guided imagery*, Pittsburgh, 2002, Oncology Nursing Society.

3. Mindfulness meditation, a popular form of meditation, involves maintaining awareness of body sensations and thoughts without passing judgments on them.
   a. Focus is on being truly present in the moment.
   b. Has been successful in symptom management for clients experiencing pain and chronic obstructive pulmonary disease.
4. Yoga, an East Indian discipline, has been practiced as a way to bring the body, mind, and spirit into harmony with a higher consciousness (Groves, 1995).
   a. The word *yoga* means union.
   b. Several schools of yoga, which range from a rigorous workout to slow-motion relaxation.
      (1) All are centered on a series of carefully crafted postures, called *asanas*, that develop balance, flexibility, and strength.
   c. In a typical yoga class, participants are guided through a series of sitting, standing, and prone poses, relaxing into the poses and focusing on breathing and how the body feels.
      (1) Many classes end with a meditation or deep relaxation exercise.
   d. Although yoga is not a religion, many find the classes promote a union of body, mind, and spirit, leaving them energized and peaceful.
   e. Yoga promotes relaxation, improves flexibility, and improves concentration.
5. Aromatherapy, one of the earliest forms of medicine, historically involves burning aromatic plants in order to "smoke" the illness out of the client (Lavabre, 1990).

    a. Fragrant plants and oils have had a role in medicine throughout the centuries for use in healing via the skin and fumigating the air to ward off disease.

    b. Scents are also used to evoke positive memories and enhance moods.

    c. Studies have supported the use of aromatherapy to decrease anxiety, but conclusive research is lacking for further indications (Cooke & Ernst, 2000).

6. Biofeedback—mechanism for external feedback of an internal process (e.g., muscle tension or skin temperature).

    a. Can be very helpful in teaching clients to relax.

    b. External device or signal (e.g., lowering the pitch of a sound) keeps the attention focused on a changing physical parameter until the person is skilled enough to achieve the goal independently.

    c. Used successfully to manage hypertension, decrease muscle tension, control incontinence, prevent anticipatory nausea and vomiting, reduce pain, and decrease anxiety (Benson & Stuart, 1992).

7. Hypnosis—an artificially induced alteration of consciousness characterized by increased suggestibility and receptivity to direction.

    a. It has been used to reduce anxiety, nausea, vomiting, and pain and to promote healing (Ginandes & Rosenthal, 1999; Pelletier, 2000).

8. Music is considered a universal language and is used in combination with many approaches to enhance relaxation (Halstead & Roscoe, 2002; White, 1997).

    a. Music therapists represent a specific discipline with a bachelor's degree in music therapy and a supervised internship.

    b. Studies support the effectiveness of music as a nonpharmacologic method of pain reduction by stimulating the release of endorphins.

    c. May be of benefit in moderating anxiety during radiation therapy and is a simple, low-cost intervention (Smith et al., 2001).

    d. In addition to the more melodic forms of music, chanting has had a long traditional association with healing.

9. Humor.

    a. Ability to see the humor in situations in life is a valuable health asset and can be cultivated even during a serious illness such as cancer.

    b. Laughing relaxes the nervous system, and the diaphragm moves up and down vigorously, emptying the lungs more completely than usual.

    c. Reading positive books, watching funny movies, and surrounding themselves with supportive people help clients avoid the "bleak brigade" according to Cousins (1979).

    d. Humor is an effective coping mechanism in the adjustment to a diagnosis of cancer and can assist survivors to find meaning and purpose in their lives (Johnson, 2002).

    e. Use of humor by nurses can help in establishing a trustworthy relationship.

10. Reiki—an ancient form of energy healing that originated in Japan (Stein, 1995).

    a. "Rei" means universal life intelligence, and "Ki" means that which animates all living things and is equivalent to the concept of Qi/Chi.

    b. Healers use the energy of the universe to help others heal themselves.

    c. Students receive attunements or energy transfers from Reiki masters and are taught specific hand positions to use to channel energy. The person being helped uses it where it is needed most.

    d. Is also a spiritual and philosophic approach to living, one that brings the healer's mind, body, and spirit into harmony.

    e. Clients receiving Reiki treatments remain fully clothed.

11. Traditional Chinese medicine (TCM) is the contemporary version of the centuries-old medical practices of China (Kaptchuk, 2000).

    a. Is a comprehensive theoretic and therapeutic system including carefully formulated techniques, such as acupuncture, herbal remedies, nutrition, and Qi Gong.

    b. Difference between TCM and Western medicine is the focus.

       (1) TCM focuses on the client, identifying patterns of disharmony and imbalance that may ultimately lead to disease.

       (2) Western medicine focuses on different organ systems and symptoms.

    c. Central concept in Chinese medicine is the concept of Qi (pronounced "chee"), which is the vital energy or life force that animates all living beings and the universe.

    d. A balanced, harmonious flow of Qi is important because it naturally maintains a state of health.

    e. When flow is blocked or unbalanced, illness will be the result.

    f. Also essential in this balance is the concept of yin and yang, the feminine and masculine entities.

       (1) Yin is associated with the feminine, with passive, dark, and inner qualities.

       (2) Yang is associated with the masculine, with active, light, and outer qualities.

       (3) For health to be present, yin and yang must be in balance.

    g. A modality that seeks to balance yin and yang, thus influencing the flow of Qi through the body, is acupuncture.

12. Qi Gong is an ancient Chinese system of exercise combining physical movement with controlled breathing.

    a. TCM theory regards a healthy individual as having a full and flowing supply of Qi, or vital energy, similar to the blood and lymph systems.

    b. Body can be compared to a battery, which can hold, increase, or decrease its energy.

    c. Stress, disease, and poor health habits can challenge the Qi system.

    d. Helps to dissipate the effects of stress and prescribes tools for self-care.

    e. Intent is to promote health by directing the internal flow of Qi.

    f. Has been studied in China for its impact on arthritis, hypertension, cancer, heart disease, and gastrointestinal (GI) problems, but there are few evidence-based studies in the United States.

    g. Has become a popular form of exercise for increasing flexibility and promoting relaxation.

13. Tai Chi involves a precise sequence of slow, graceful movements, accompanied by deep breathing and mental attentiveness.

    a. Goal is to achieve balance between the body and the mind and to focus the Qi.

    b. Essence of Tai Chi is the relaxed state of the performer, who is aware of the present moment and feels a sense of balance and inner peace.

c. Usually performed while standing, but persons with physical limitations can participate while seated in a chair.
   (1) Elderly participants have gained balance and strength from this form of exercise (Adler et al., 2000; Wolfson, 1996).
d. The combination of slow rhythmic breathing and relaxed circular movements assists in initiating and maintaining the mind/body response of physical and psychologic relaxation.
   (1) Heart rate, blood pressure, and muscle tension are lowered.
   (2) A sense of well-being, inner peace, and alertness is increased.
e. No equipment or special clothing is required so it can be practiced by anyone, anywhere, at any time.
f. Frequently practiced in groups in a natural setting.
   (1) A casual observer walking through San Francisco's Chinatown on a Saturday morning may see many people in a school yard practicing Tai Chi.

B. Manual or energy healing techniques (not all-inclusive).
1. Acupressure is based on the Eastern concept that Qi, or energy, flows through the body in defined pathways called meridians (Dibble et al., 2000).
   a. This energy can be blocked or stuck and pressing on specific points along the meridians or channels through which Qi is thought to flow can improve the flow and relieve the imbalance.
   b. Eastern practitioners, for example, practitioners of TCM, assess and treat the whole person.
      (1) A more Western explanation would include evaluating the release of neurotransmitters and neurohormones as well as activation of the opioid system.
2. Applied kinesiology (AK) is a system of manual healing used to diagnose and treat a variety of health problems, based on a belief that weakness in a complementary group of muscles will correspond to specific diseases or body imbalances (Valentine et al., 1987).
   a. Developed by a chiropractor, George Goodheart, Jr., in the 1960s.
   b. The International College of Applied Kinesiology (ICAK), founded in the 1970s, has established standards of practice for assessment.
   c. This approach is thought to be free of direct harmful effects but could be indirectly harmful by causing delay in diagnosis.
   d. There is limited research available at this point.
3. Healing touch (HT) is an energy-based therapeutic approach to healing that works with the body's energy (Brennan, 1993; Bruyere, 1994).
   a. Can involve movement of a practitioner's hands over a client's body and/or use of a specific healing technique on the surface of the body.
   b. Used to influence the energy system, thus affecting physical, emotional, mental, and spiritual health and healing.
   c. Client is fully clothed during the treatment.
   d. Goal is to restore harmony and balance in the energy system to help the person to self-heal.
   e. Certification of HT practitioners and instructors available from Healing Touch International.
   f. HT has been found helpful in reducing anxiety, depression, and fatigue (Rexillius et al., 2002).
4. Therapeutic touch (TT) is an intervention developed in the 1970s (Krieger, 1997).

      a. May not involve any actual touching of the physical body.

      b. Based on the conscious use of the hands to direct or modulate select nonphysical human energies that activate the physical body.

      c. Practitioner assumes a meditative state of awareness called "centering" and places his/her hands 2 to 4 inches from the client's skin.

         (1) Practitioner uses his/her hands to "scan," determining areas of tension.

         (2) Then places his/her hands over areas of accumulated tension, and these energies are redirected to promote healing.

      d. Nurse Healers Professional Associates, Inc. is a training organization for therapeutic touch.

         (1) There are standardized techniques but no formal certification or competency-based assessment for therapy providers.

      e. The client is fully clothed during the treatment.

      f. Research studies supported efficacy in reducing anxiety, relieving pain, and accelerating wound healing (O'Mathuna, 2000; Winstead-Fry & Kijek, 1999).

  5. Acupuncture regulates the flow of Qi (Kaptchuk, 2000).

      a. Underlying belief is that deficiency or stagnation of Qi causes most health problems.

      b. Symptoms and medical history, qualities of the tongue, and six radial wrist pulses determine the diagnosis and treatment.

      c. Treatments involve leaving thin, sterile acupuncture needles in the skin for 20 minutes (longer if one is doing Japanese acupuncture to rebalance Qi).

      d. Effects of treatment are cumulative, and several treatments may be needed to correct the problem.

      e. A common use is for the relief of chronic pain and for problems attributed to stress and tension, such as muscular disorders, digestive problems, urinary problems, sinus problems, asthma, headaches, and premenstrual syndrome (PMS).

      f. An expert panel convened by the NIH published a consensus statement in November 1997 (NIH, 1997). Among their findings are the following:

         (1) Clear evidence that needle acupuncture is efficacious for nausea and vomiting in the adult caused by chemotherapy or after surgery and is probably efficacious for nausea related to pregnancy.

         (2) Evidence of efficacy for postoperative dental pain.

      g. Additional studies show relief of pain with acupuncture on diverse pain conditions, such as menstrual cramps, tennis elbow, and fibromyalgia (Lewis, 1999).

  6. Polarity therapy is based on the theory that energy flows through the body along five predictable pathways.

      a. Touch is used at specific points to influence the energy flow.

      b. Lifestyle changes, including diet and exercise, are incorporated into a treatment plan.

      c. Anecdotal reports of improvement in pain, anxiety/stress, and side effects from surgery, chemotherapy, radiation therapy (including nausea, hair loss, neuropathy/nerve pain, radiation burns, hardening/scarring of tissue in mastectomy clients) (CancerSource, 2003).

      d. At present, there are no systematic scientific studies in humans on the effects of this therapy.

C. Physical touch techniques.
 1. Chiropractic is derived from the Greek words "praxis" and "cheir" meaning "practice by hand" (Chapman-Smith, 2000).
    a. Based on the philosophy that the body is intelligent and has an innate ability to heal itself.
    b. Proper spinal alignment allows the nervous system to operate in a healthy, balanced state as it was designed to do.
    c. Treats subluxation, a joint problem that affects the function of nerves and can therefore affect the body's musculoskeletal system, organs, and general health.
    d. Historically, chiropractic research has been largely anecdotal; however, recent research supports chiropractic as a viable treatment for acute low back pain, cervicogenic and tension-type headache (Carey et al., 1995).
 2. Craniosacral therapy is based on the theory that any blow or trauma to the head could interfere with the craniosacral rhythmic flow of cerebrospinal fluid and natural expansion and contraction (Upledger & Vredevoogd, 1983).
    a. This light and gentle movement of the head, which may be barely perceptible to the client, may prove helpful in treating headaches, pains originating in the temporomandibular (jaw) joint, neck pain, and other facial pain.
 3. Massage—systematic manipulation of the body's soft tissues that promotes healing and relaxation.
    a. Brings fresh nutrients to the body's impoverished cells and activates the body's natural relaxation response.
    b. Within the first few minutes of massage, most people experience reduced blood pressure; reduced heart rate; endorphin release (the body's natural pain killers); slower, deeper, more effective breathing; and reduction of muscular tension.
    c. Common types of massage are Swedish massage, deep tissue massage, and shiatsu acupressure.
    d. Therapeutic massage for relaxation and symptom management can be incorporated into the treatment plan in any setting, including home care (Grealish et al., 2000; Rexillius et al., 2002).
 4. Reflexology—a form of foot massage designed to harmonize body functions.
    a. Based on the concept that the whole person is interconnected and that imbalance in one part of the body is reflected in changes elsewhere.
    b. Techniques can be learned by professionals and laypeople.
    c. Research by Stephenson et al. (2000) indicates foot reflexology is successful in reducing anxiety and pain in some clients with cancer.
 5. Temperature—the use of hot and/or cold to provide comfort or symptom management or assist in purification rituals has a long-established tradition.
    a. Cold.
       (1) Is indicated in acute trauma since cold causes vasoconstriction, decreases muscle fatigue, and decreases edema (Lewis et al., 2000).
       (2) Naturopaths recommend the use of cold compresses, left on the body for a few hours to promote sweating and detoxification, to promote self-healing (Woodham & Peters, 1997).

    b. Heat.

        (1) Promotes increased rate of removal of local tissue products.

        (2) Causes vasodilation of capillaries and increases arterial and venous circulation, lowering blood pressure.

        (3) This results in improved circulation, helps remove waste products from the body, sends more oxygen and nutrients to the tissues to repair damage and boost the immune system.

    c. Cold and heat.

        (1) Some therapies use cold and hot water alternately to stimulate the hormonal system, reduce circulation congestion caused by muscle spasm, and reduce inflammation.

        (2) This treatment may be used for sprains or swollen joints.

Assessment

  I. Assess client's health history.

    A. Medical.

      1. Cancer history.

        a. Type and current stage of cancer.

        b. Past and current medical treatments.

        c. Presence and management of side effects.

      2. Other health problems.

    B. Psychosocial.

      1. Emotional response to cancer experience.

      2. Coping of client and family.

      3. Culture and spiritual/religious beliefs on health since CAM practices may be an integral part of these beliefs.

  II. Use of CAM practices.

    A. Current use of CAM therapies.

      1. Nonpharmacologic and pharmacologic/biologically based (see Chapter 41) approaches.

        a. Client is often important source of knowledge regarding CAM therapies and their uses.

      2. Client's perception of effect of these therapies (positive and negative) on self and how they impact current conventional treatment.

Nursing Diagnoses

  I. Disturbed energy field.

  II. Effective therapeutic regimen management.

  III. Deficient knowledge related to cancer treatment and CAM practices.

  IV. Decisional conflict.

Outcome Identification

  I. Client reports relief of symptoms after energy healing session.

  II. Client manages his/her treatment regimen.

  III. Client describes prescribed conventional treatment and its effects.

    A. Client identifies CAM practices and its effect to health care providers.

  IV. Client verbalizes positive and negative aspects of choices and alternative actions related to health.

    A. Client expresses satisfaction with choices made.

Planning and Implementation

I. Interventions for client collaboration.
   A. Include a section on CAM practices on health history/physical examination form.
      1. Frequently clients do not share this information unless asked by their health care providers.
      2. Encouraging this exchange early in the relationship, in an open and non-judgmental way, can build rapport necessary for further discussion.
      3. Clients are an excellent source of learning about CAM therapies in a positive way and can also alert health care providers to potentially dangerous practices in the community.
   B. Emphasize the client's right to become an informed consumer and to choose among the therapeutic options.
      1. Examine health care providers' beliefs about nonconventional therapy and respect for client's choice in seeking CAM therapies.
   C. Remove barriers to communication.
      1. Clients may fear sharing use of CAM therapies with health care providers.
      2. Recognize that pleading ignorance or dismissing CAM practices may shut down communication.
      3. Provide planned opportunities to share this information by asking if client:
         a. Is curious or interested in exploring "unconventional" options.
         b. Has any questions "you've been hesitant to ask."
         c. Has any information "you've been hesitant to tell your doctor."
      4. Being knowledgeable about CAM practices by health care providers.
         a. Difficult to be current on all CAM practices; may consult the following:
            (1) Web-based resources (see Table 41-1).
            (2) The hospital/clinic may have available a list of licensed/certified CAM clinicians to refer clients.
            (3) Some oncology practices have successfully developed relationships with local pharmacy schools who serve as resources for questions about herbs or supplements.

Evaluation

The oncology nurse systematically and regularly evaluates the client and/or family's response to interventions to determine progress toward the achievement of expected outcomes. Relevant data are collected, and actual findings are compared with expected findings. Nursing diagnoses, outcomes, and plans of care are reviewed and revised as necessary.

REFERENCES

Adler, P., Good, M., Roberts, B., & Snyder, S. (2000). The effects of tai chi on older adults with chronic arthritis pain. *Image: The Journal of Nursing Scholarship* 32(4), 377.

Benson, H., & Stuart, E. (1992). *The wellness book: The comprehensive guide to maintaining health and treating stress-related illness.* New York: Simon & Schuster.

Brennan, B. (1993). *Light emerging: The journey of personal healing.* New York: Bantam Books.

Bruyere, R. (1994). *Wheels of light: Chakras, auras and the healing energy of the body.* New York: Simon & Schuster.

CancerSource. (2003). Polarity therapy. Retrieved July 3, 2003 from the World Wide Web: http://cit.cancersource.com/LearnAbout/monograph.cfm.

Carey, T., Garrett, J., Jackman, A., et al. (1995). The outcomes and costs of care for low back pain among patients seen by primary care practitioners, chiropractors, and orthopedic surgeons. *New England Journal of Medicine 333*, 913-917.

Chapman-Smith, D. (2000). *The chiropractic profession.* West Des Moines, IA: NCMIC Group.

Cooke, B., & Ernst, E. (2000). Aromatherapy: A systematic review. *British Journal of General Practice 50*, 493-496.

Cousins, N. (1979). *Anatomy of an illness as perceived by the patient: Reflections on healing and regeneration.* New York: W.W. Norton & Co.

Dibble, S., Chapman, J., Mack, A., & Shih, A. (2000). Acupressure for nausea: Results of a pilot study. *Oncology Nursing Forum 27*(1), 41-47.

Ginandes, C., & Rosenthal, D. (1999). Using hypnosis to accelerate healing of bone fractures; a randomized controlled pilot study. *Alternative Therapies in Health and Medicine 5*(2), 67-75.

Grealish, L., Lomasney, A., & Whiteman, B. (2000). Foot massage: A nursing intervention to modify distressing symptoms of pain and nausea in patients hospitalized with cancer. *Cancer Nursing 23*(3), 237-243.

Groves, D. (1995). *Yoga for busy people.* Novato, CA: New World Library.

Halstead, M., & Roscoe, S. (2002). Restoring the spirit at the end of life: Music as an intervention for oncology nurses. *Clinical Journal of Oncology Nursing 6*(6), 332-336.

Johnson, P. (2002). Use of humor and its influences on spirituality and coping in breast cancer survivors. *Oncology Nursing Forum 29*(4), 691-695.

Kaptchuk, T. (2000). *The web that has no weaver.* Chicago: Contemporary Books.

Krieger, D. (1997). *Therapeutic touch: Inner workbook.* Rochester, VT: Bear & Co.

Lavabre, M. (1990). *Aromatherapy workbook.* Rochester, VT: Healing Arts Press.

LeShan, L. (1988). *How to meditate: A guide to self-discovery.* New York: Bantam Books.

Lewis, L. (1999). Acupuncture: Another therapeutic choice? *Patient Care.* Available on the World Wide Web: www.patientcare.com.

Lewis, S.M., Heitkemper, M.M., & Dirksen, S.R. (2000). *Medical-surgical nursing* (5th ed.). St. Louis: Mosby.

Murray Edwards, D. (Ed.). (2002). *Voice massage: Scripts for guided imagery.* Pittsburgh: Oncology Nursing Society.

National Center for Complementary and Alternative Medicine (NCCAM): What is complementary and alternative medicine (CAM)? Accessed July 3, 2003 from the World Wide Web: http://nccam.nih.gov/health/whatiscam/.

National Institutes of Health (NIH) Acupuncture. NIH Consensus Statement Online (1997 Nov 3-5). 15(5):1-34. Accessed June 17, 2004 from the World Wide Web: http://consensus.nih.gov/cons/107/107_statement.htm.

O'Mathuna, D. (2000). Evidence-based practice reviews of therapeutic touch. *Image: The Journal of Nursing Scholarship 32*(3), 279-285.

Pelletier, K. (2000). *The best alternative medicine.* New York: Simon & Schuster.

Post-White, J. (2002). Clinical indications for use of imagery in oncology practice. In D. Murray Edwards (Ed.). *Voice massage: Scripts for guided imagery.* Pittsburgh: Oncology Nursing Society, pp. 3-14.

Rexillius, S., Mundt, C., Erickson, M., & Agrawal, S. (2002). Therapeutic effects of massage therapy and healing touch on caregivers of patients undergoing autologous hematopoietic stem cell transplant. *Oncology Nursing Forum 29*(3), 1-15. Retrieved from the World Wide Web: www.ons.org.

Rusy, L., & Weisman, S. (2000). Complementary therapies for acute pediatric pain. *Pediatric Clinics of North America 47*, 589-599.

Smith, M., Casey, L., Johnson, D., et al. (2001). Music as a therapeutic intervention for anxiety in patients receiving radiation therapy. *Oncology Nursing Forum 28*(5), 855-862.

Sparber, A., Bauer, L., Curt, G., et al. (2000). Use of complementary medicine by adult patients participating in cancer clinical trials. *Oncology Nursing Forum 27*(4), 623-630.

Stein, D. (1995). *Essential Reiki: A complete guide to an ancient healing art.* Berkeley, CA: The Crossing Press.

Stephenson, N., Weinrich, S., & Tavakoli, A. (2000). The effects of foot reflexology on anxiety and pain in patients with breast and lung cancer. *Oncology Nursing Forum 27*(1), 67-72.

Upledger, J., & Vredevoogd, J. (1983). *Craniosacral therapy.* Seattle, Washington: Eastland Press.

Valentine, T., Valentine, C., & Hetrick, D. (1987). *Applied kinesiology: Muscle response in diagnosis, therapy & preventive medicine.* Rochester, VT: Healing Arts Press.

Van Fleet, S. (2000). Relaxation and imagery for symptom management: Improving patient assessment and individualizing treatment. *Oncology Nursing Forum 27,* 501-507.

White, J. (2001). Music as an intervention: A notable endeavor to improve patient outcomes. *Nursing Clinics of North America 36,* 83-92.

White, P.F. (1997). Are nonpharmacologic techniques useful alternatives to antiemetic drugs for the prevention of nausea and vomiting? *Anesthesia Analgesia 84,* 712-714.

Winstead-Fry, P., & Kijek, J. (1999). An integrative review and meta-analysis of therapeutic touch research. *Alternative Therapeutic Medicine 5*(6), 58-67.

Wolfson, L. (1996). Balance and strength training in older adults: Intervention gains and tai chi maintenance. *Journal of American Geriatric Society 44,* 498-506.

Woodham, A., & Peters, D. (1997). *Encyclopedia of healing therapies.* London: Dorling Kindersley.

PART TWO

PROTECTIVE
MECHANISMS

12 Alterations in Mobility, Skin Integrity, and Neurologic Status

JENNIFER DOUGLAS PEARCE

ALTERATIONS IN MOBILITY

Theory

I. Impaired physical mobility (immobility)—a state in which the individual experiences or is at risk for experiencing limitation in independent, purposeful physical movement of the body or of one or more extremities (NANDA, 2003).

II. Physiology.
  A. Frequent muscle contractions that occur during movement maintain muscle strength (Armstrong, 2003).
  B. Inactivity and limited use or disuse of muscle groups can decrease the muscles' ability to contract and can lead to decreased muscle size, muscle atrophy, and weakness.
  C. Motor impairment (spasticity, muscle weakness, paralysis, hemiparesis, ataxia) may occur in primary cancer (brain tumors) or as a secondary effect in metastatic disease (spinal cord compression), infections, and cancer therapy or in nonmalignant conditions in clients with cancer.

III. Risk factors.
  A. Disease related.
    1. Primary or metastatic tumors to the skeletal system (Flounders & Ott, 2003).
    2. Primary and metastatic tumors of the brain and spinal cord.
    3. Obstruction in lymphatic or systemic circulation.
    4. Bone pain.
    5. Physical response to disease: pain, stiffness, fatigue.
    6. Spinal cord compression.
    7. Sensory-perceptual alterations.
    8. Nonmalignant conditions: herniated disks, vertebral fractures secondary to osteoporosis.
    9. Complications of bed rest.
    10. Complications of cardiopulmonary disorders.
  B. Treatment related.
    1. Side effects of corticosteroid therapy.
    2. Side effects of radiation therapy.
    3. Side effects of chemotherapy.
    4. Residual effects of surgical intervention: nerve and muscle damage.
  C. Lifestyle related.
    1. Changes in physical activity level.

      2. High or low stress level.

      3. Independent versus dependent personality.

   D. Psychologic and social issues.

      1. Presence or absence of social support.

      2. Depression.

Assessment

  I. History.

    A. Presence of risk factors.

    B. Recent treatment and anticipated side effects.

    C. Decreased activity level.

    D. Functional level evaluation (NANDA, 2003).

    E. Presence of pain (neck, back), muscle weakness, and fatigue.

    F. Presence of dyspnea, activity intolerance.

    G. Evaluation of fall risk.

    H. History of alcohol or drug use.

    I. Current exercise practice.

    J. Current therapy.

 II. Physical examination.

    A. Changes in muscle tone, strength, and muscle mass.

    B. Unintentional weight loss.

    C. Strength and motor function.

    D. Mobility function.

    E. Sensory function.

    F. Functional health assessment.

    G. Change in sexual function.

    H. Changes in bowel and bladder function.

    I. Incontinence and loss of sphincter control.

    J. Range of joint motion.

    K. Positive Babinski's sign.

    L. Reflexes (Zembrzuski, 2001).

    M. Observe alignment, balance, gait, and joint structure.

    N. Observe muscle mass, tone, and strength.

III. Psychosocial examination.

    A. Depression.

    B. Anxiety.

    C. Lack of motivation.

IV. Laboratory data.

    A. Hypercalcemia.

    B. Electrolyte abnormalities.

    C. Lumbar puncture results.

Nursing Diagnoses

   I. Impaired physical mobility.

  II. Activity intolerance.

 III. Risk for injury.

 IV. Risk for impaired skin integrity.

  V. Acute pain.

Outcome Identification

I. Client will actively participate in measures to maintain optimal physical function.
   A. Client will participate in activities to prevent complications of immobility.
   B. Client and family will demonstrate appropriate use of adaptive devices to increase mobility.
II. Client maintains activity level within capabilities.
III. Client and family will verbalize and use safety measures to minimize risk for injury.
IV. Client's skin remains intact.
V. Client verbalizes adequate relief of pain.

Planning and Implementation

I. Interventions to increase physical functioning, mobility, and activity (Armstrong, 2003).
   A. Perform active range of motion (AROM) exercises on unaffected limbs at least three or four times per day and passive range of motion (PROM) on affected limbs.
   B. Monitor progress from AROM to functional activities.
   C. Maintain the client's body alignment while in bed.
   D. Change the client's position every 2 hours.
   E. Observe client before, during, and after activity/exercise.
   F. Obtain appropriate assistive devices (e.g., splints, walker, cane, overhead trapeze).
   G. Consult with rehabilitation services for physical and occupational therapy.
II. Interventions to decrease risk of further complications of immobility.
   A. Establish a routine for activities of daily living.
   B. Provide adaptive devices as needed.
   C. Provide assistance and supervision as needed.
   D. Place call light within reach if the client is alone.
III. Interventions to maximize safety for the client.
   A. Protect areas of decreased sensation from extremes of heat and cold.
   B. Teach the client with decreased perception of lower extremities to check where the limb is placed when changing positions.
   C. Place the bed in low position and the two side rails at the head of bed (HOB) up.
   D. Clear pathways in room and hallways.
IV. Interventions to enhance adaptation and rehabilitation.
   A. Positive reinforcement for behaviors that contribute to positive outcomes.
   B. Have the client and family responsible for aspects of care according to their capabilities.
   C. Initiate and follow up with referrals to rehabilitation services.
V. Interventions to incorporate client and family in care.
   A. Instruct client and family about signs and symptoms to report to health team.
   B. Discuss risk factors for impaired mobility.
VI. Interventions to decrease pain.
   A. Pharmacologic interventions (see Chapter 1).
   B. Nonpharmacologic interventions (see Chapter 11).

1. Instruct client on use of guided imagery.
2. Use of massage therapy.
3. Use of meditation.

Evaluation

The oncology nurse systematically and regularly evaluates the client's and/or family's responses to interventions in order to determine progress toward the achievement of expected outcomes. Relevant data are collected, and actual findings are compared with expected findings. Nursing diagnoses, outcomes, and plans of care are reviewed and revised as necessary.

ALTERATIONS IN SKIN INTEGRITY

Theory

I. Physiology.
  A. The skin is composed of three layers: the epidermis, the dermis, and the subcutaneous tissue.
    1. The epidermis is the avascular, outer layer, which serves as a barrier to prevent water loss and renews itself continuously through cell division.
    2. The dermis, the inner connective tissue layer, is highly vascular with afferent sensory nerve receptors, which provide nutritional support to the avascular epidermal layer.
    3. The subcutaneous tissue is composed of adipose tissue, which serves as a cushion to physical trauma, an insulator to temperature changes, and an energy reservoir.
  B. Intact skin protects the body from bacteria, temperature changes, physical trauma, and radiation.
  C. Skin regulates fluid and electrolyte balance and plays a role in vitamin synthesis (Haisfield-Wolfe & Rund, 2000).
II. Risk factors.
  A. Disease related.
    1. Thrombocytopenia.
    2. Cutaneous metastases (late manifestation in the course of the illness for solid tumors of the breast and lung, squamous cell carcinoma of the head and neck, malignant melanoma, lymphoma, Kaposi's sarcoma).
    3. Cutaneous paraneoplastic syndromes: acanthosis nigricans; acquired ichthyosis; Paget's disease; telangiectasia; hypertrichosis; lanuginosa acquisita; erythroderma (Weiss, 2000).
    4. Primary malignant skin cancer (melanoma, basal cell carcinoma, squamous cell carcinoma, Kaposi's sarcoma).
    5. Mycosis fungoides (slow progressive cutaneous T-cell lymphoma).
    6. Premalignant lesions (actinic keratosis, leukoplakia, dysplastic nevus syndrome).
  B. Treatment related.
    1. Desquamative skin reaction (radiation enhancement, radiation recall, combined modality therapy) as a result of chemotherapy in association with radiation therapy.
    2. Fragile skin from steroid therapy.
    3. Erythema multiforme (widespread, scattered, cutaneous vesicles) associated with multiple drug therapy (Haisfield-Wolfe & Rund, 2000).

4. Erythema nodosum (tender, subcutaneous, anterior leg nodules) hypersensitivity reaction to penicillin or sulfonamides (Haisfield-Wolfe & Rund, 2000).
5. Graft-versus-host disease (skin reactions related to bone marrow transplantation).
6. Side effects of biologic response modifiers.
7. Side effects of chemotherapy: mucositis, compromised nutritional status.
8. Side effects of radiation therapy: immunosuppression, compromised nutritional status, diarrhea.
9. Extravasation of chemotherapy.
10. Adhesive dressings (central and peripheral intravenous [IV] access).
11. Tubes.
    a. Chest tubes, Foley catheter, biliary catheters.
    b. Feeding tubes—gastrostomy, jejunostomy.
    c. Tubes for decompression and drains.
12. Malnutrition: decreased protein stores.
13. Other effects—alopecia; pressure ulcers; edema; pruritus; jaundice; incontinence; infection.

Assessment

I. History.
   A. Presence of risk factors.
   B. Client's age.
   C. General health status.
   D. Exposure to infection.
   E. Recent treatment and anticipated side effects.
   F. Current drug therapy.
   G. Past and current skin conditions.
   H. Review of personal hygiene practices.
   I. Nutritional status.
   J. Smoking habits.
   K. Incontinence of bowel or bladder.
II. Physical examination.
   A. Skin: color, integrity, temperature, texture, turgor, presence of sloughing.
   B. Presence of redness, petechiae, purpura, ecchymosis, jaundice.
   C. Presence of erythema, dry desquamation, moist desquamation.
   D. Local inflammation at injection site (erythema, induration, blisters).
   E. Ulcerations of mouth; dry, cracked mucous membranes and lips.
   F. Presence of alopecia.
   G. Presence of stomatitis.
   H. Presence of pruritus.
   I. Integrity of tube sites, perirectal tissue, perineal tissue.
   J. Presence of pressure ulcers.
   K. Presence of pain.
III. Psychosocial examination.
   A. Social isolation.
   B. Anxiety.
   C. Depression.
IV. Laboratory data.
   A. Complete blood count (CBC).
   B. Blood chemistries.

    C. Platelet count.
    D. Serum albumin: total protein.

Nursing Diagnoses

    I. Impaired skin integrity.
   II. Impaired oral mucous membranes.
  III. Situational low self-esteem.
  IV. Social isolation.
   V. Imbalanced nutrition, less than body requirements.
  VI. Risk for infection.
 VII. Risk for pain.

Outcome Identification

    I. Client and family verbalize strategies involved in routine and preventive skin management.
       A. Client actively participates in routine and preventive skin care management.
   II. Client verbalizes strategies to minimize the risk of and to manage mucositis.
  III. Client and family discuss effects of skin alterations on self-concept and body image.
  IV. Client engages in strategies to be more involved with others.
   V. Client increases and/or maintains adequate dietary and fluid intake.
  VI. Client does not develop an infection.
       A. Client identifies the risk factors and initial signs and symptoms of infection to report to a member of the health care team.
 VII. Client does not report any pain.

Planning and Implementation

    I. Assess knowledge of risk factors and side effects of therapy.
   II. Interventions to increase or maintain dietary and fluid intake.
       A. Offer small frequent meals with increased protein and calories.
       B. Moisten foods with liquids, sauces, and gravy.
       C. Increase fluid intake to 3 L/day if not medically contraindicated.
       D. Rinse the oral cavity with normal saline or a nonalcoholic mouthwash.
  III. Interventions to decrease inflammation of mucous membranes (see Chapter 14).
  IV. Interventions to teach self-care techniques and prevent complications.
       A. Teach the client and family to assess the skin every 4 hours.
       B. Teach client and family tube and drain management.
       C. Assist with turning and positioning every 2 hours.
       D. Massage uninjured areas gently.
       E. Use a therapeutic mattress, specialty bed, or a water mattress for high-risk persons.
       F. Instruct on gentle skin cleansing with mild pH-balanced skin cleanser.
       G. Rinse soap thoroughly off skin, and pat dry.
       H. Moisturize and lubricate skin.
       I. Use dry, clean, wrinkle-free linens and devices such as an egg crate mattress.
       J. Use specialty beds.

V. Interventions to protect skin integrity.
  A. Teach effects of treatments on skin.
  B. Teach use of protective film, skin barriers, or collection devices around drains and tubes with copious drainage.
  C. Teach use of sterile technique for invasive procedures, such as insertion of tubes.
  D. Teach hand washing.
  E. Keep client's fingernails smooth and short.
  F. Teach reportable signs and symptoms of infection.
  G. Recommend use of cotton clothing and avoidance of restrictive clothing.
  H. Report changes in skin color, integrity, pain, increased pruritus, drainage (amount, odor, color, consistency) to health care provider.
VI. Interventions for oral, perineal, and general hygiene practices (Haisfield-Wolfe & Rund, 2000).
  A. Use soft toothbrush or oral sponges.
  B. Apply moisturizers to oral mucosa.
  C. Cleanse the perineal area with mild soap, rinsing thoroughly, patting the area dry, and applying a skin barrier after each bowel movement.
  D. Apply adhesive perineum pad or panty liner without deodorant to the undergarment.
  E. Gently clean skin with mild soap and tepid water, and pat dry with soft cloth.
VII. Nonpharmacologic interventions.
  A. Add emollients to bath water; skin lubricants to skin other than to irradiated sites.
  B. Oatmeal baths.
  C. Application of cool or warm compresses.
  D. Avoid alcohol-based skin lotions.
VIII. Interventions to adapt and cope with hair loss (see Chapter 3).
  IX. Interventions to care for acute and chronic skin reactions to radiation therapy (see Chapter 36).

Evaluation

The oncology nurse systematically and regularly evaluates the client's and/or family's responses to interventions in order to determine progress toward the achievement of expected outcomes. Relevant data are collected, and actual findings are compared with expected findings. Nursing diagnoses, outcomes, and plans of care are reviewed and revised as necessary.

NEUROPATHIES

Theory

I. Physiology.
  A. Neuropathies describe any functional disturbances and/or pathologic changes in the peripheral nervous system (PNS)—cranial, sensory, and motor nerves, and portions of the autonomic nervous system.
  B. Neuropathies of the central nervous system (CNS) include seizures, encephalopathy, cerebellar dysfunction, ophthalmologic toxicities and ototoxicities, mental status changes, and peripheral neuropathies with sensory and motor dysfunction.

    C. The incidence and severity of neuropathies may vary depending on the administration of immunosuppressive therapy.

    D. Toxicities may be dose related and reversible on discontinuation of therapy.

II. Risk factors.

    A. Disease related.

        1. Effects of cancer.

        2. Postherpetic neuralgia (PHN) (Bush & Hartkopf Smith, 2002).

        3. Presence of infiltrative emergencies (i.e., spinal cord compression).

        4. Other diseases (i.e., history of hepatic or neurologic dysfunction).

        5. Preexisting neuropathies as a result of diabetes mellitus, human immunodeficiency virus (HIV) infection, preexisting vitamin B complex deficiency (Boyle, 2002).

    B. Treatment related.

        1. Side effects of high-dose chemotherapy (e.g., cerebellar dysfunction, "strokelike reaction," generalized weakness, gait disturbance, numbness of feet, loss of proprioception).

        2. Peripheral neuropathies: tingling of fingers and toes, jaw pain, footdrop, wristdrop, muscular atrophy (Landier, 2001).

        3. Side effects of radiation therapy (e.g., ataxia, dysarthria, nystagmus, radicular pain).

        4. Age: older than 60 years.

        5. Preexisting neuropathy related to radiation therapy.

    C. Situational related.

        1. Psychologic issues.

        2. Social issues.

Assessment

I. History.

    A. Presence of risk factors.

    B. Posttraumatic stress disorder (PTSD) (Kwekeboom & Seng, 2002).

    C. Psychiatric and current life problems.

    D. Acute herpes zoster.

    E. Recent chemotherapy treatment and anticipated side effects.

    F. Presence of weakness.

    G. Presence of burning, numbness, tingling in feet and hands, perioral numbness, paresthesias—stocking-glove distribution (Sweeney, 2002).

    H. Presence of paresthesia of hands and feet, constipation, loss of deep tendon reflex.

    I. Presence of cerebellar involvement (e.g., tremors, loss of balance and fine motor movement).

    J. Inability to perform activities of daily living.

    K. Performance of occupational and recreational activities.

    L. Current medication therapy.

    M. Presence of anxiety, low self-esteem.

II. Physical examination (Table 12-1).

    A. Vital signs.

    B. Baseline sensory, mobility, and motor function.

    C. Baseline autonomic function.

    D. Baseline cranial nerve assessment.

    E. Baseline cerebellar function.

TABLE 12-1
Assessment Skills Used to Evaluate Neuropathy

Function	Procedure
Cerebellar and proprioception	▪ Evaluate rapid alternating movement of hands. ▪ Observe for accurate movement of extremities. ▪ Evaluate balance using Romberg's test: Have client stand with feet together, arms at side with eyes closed. A slight sway is normal. ▪ Observe gait for stride and stance.
Sensory function	▪ Test for response to touch and pain. ▪ Check vibration sense using a tuning fork. ▪ Evaluate position sense: Move a finger or great toe up and down while client's eyes are closed; have client identify position of the digit. ▪ Assess for discrimination between sharp and dull sensations. ▪ Evaluate the ability to distinguish the body part being touched. ▪ Evaluate for stereognosis, the ability to distinguish a common object, such as a coin. ▪ Evaluate for graphesthesia, the ability to identify a common letter or number drawn on the hand.
Deep tendon reflexes	▪ Test deep tendon reflexes (biceps, brachioradial, triceps, patellar, Achilles). ▪ Check for clonus.

From Marrs J., Newton S. Updating your peripheral neuropathy "know how," *Clini J Oncol Nurs* 7(3):299-303, 2003.

    F. Speech or language ability.
    G. Sight-related changes (i.e., blurred vision, impaired color perception).
  III. Psychologic examination.
    A. Anxiety management strategies.
    B. Coping style and ability.
  IV. Laboratory data.
    A. Nerve conduction studies (i.e., electromyogram).
    B. Muscle or nerve biopsy.

Nursing Diagnoses

    I. Risk for injury.
   II. Risk for impaired skin integrity.
  III. Impaired physical mobility.
  IV. Pain.
   V. Constipation.
  VI. Anxiety.

Outcome Identification

    I. Client verbalizes measures to maximize safety and manage self-care.
   II. Client's skin remains intact.
  III. Client maintains or increases mobility.
  IV. Client verbalizes a satisfactory relief of pain.
   V. Client maintains regular bowel function.
  VI. Client verbalizes concerns related to treatment and issues related to the unknown.

Planning and Implementation

I. Interventions to increase participation in care.
  A. Assess knowledge of early signs and symptoms of peripheral and other neuropathies.
  B. Teach side effects of chemotherapy.
  C. Teach hand and foot care (use of massage and lotions).
  D. Refer to occupational and rehabilitation services.
  E. Before start of chemotherapy, instruct about potential neurologic side effects.
  F. Instruct on how to maintain a safe environment both at home and at work.
  G. Give positive feedback and honest reassurance.

II. Interventions to maximize safety for the client (see Alterations in Mobility, Planning and Implementation section).

III. Interventions to promote stool softening.
  A. Monitor and record stools.
  B. Use stool softeners.
  C. Increase fluid intake to 3000 ml/day unless medically contraindicated.
  D. Modify diet to include gradual increase of high-fiber foods.

IV. Interventions to minimize diminished sensations.
  A. Protect hands and feet from cold through use of gloves and socks.
  B. Avoid excess stimulation of skin; avoid tight clothing.
  C. Wear gloves for gardening activities.
  D. Teach inspection of affected areas for burns, cuts, abrasions.

V. Interventions for pain reduction.
  A. Use of capsaicin (over the counter [OTC]) topical cream three or four times daily (Marrs & Newton, 2003).
    1. Education regarding the application and use of topical cream.
  B. Pharmacologic treatment (Marrs & Newton, 2003).
    1. Mild analgesics: acetaminophen (Tylenol) and nonsteroidal antiinflammatory drugs.
    2. Antidepressants: amitriptyline (Elavil), imipramine (Tofranil), nortriptyline (Pamelor).
    3. Anticonvulsants: gabapentin (Neurontin), phenytoin (Dilantin), carbamazepine (Tegretol).
    4. Opioids.
    5. Amifostine (Ethyol).
    6. Glutamine.

VI. Interventions to promote self-care and decrease mobility impairment.
  A. Collaborate with physical and occupational rehabilitation services.
  B. Develop an exercise and muscle-strengthening program.
  C. Use assistive devices.
  D. Assist in performance of activities of daily living, as needed.

VII. Nonpharmacologic interventions to manage pain, anxiety, depression (Gorman, 2002; Marrs & Newton, 2003).
  A. Exercise.
  B. Transcutaneous electrical nerve stimulation (TENS).
  C. Acupuncture and acupressure.
  D. Relaxation techniques: yoga, meditation, guided imagery.
  E. Biofeedback.
  F. Art and music therapy.

Evaluation

The oncology nurse systematically and regularly evaluates the client's and/or family's responses to interventions to determine progress toward the achievement of expected outcomes. Relevant data are collected, and actual findings are compared with expected findings. Nursing diagnoses, outcomes, and plans of care are reviewed and revised as necessary.

ALTERATIONS IN MENTAL STATUS

Theory

I. Physiology.
   A. With alterations in mental status, there may be changes in general appearance, cognition (process that involves perception, memory, and thinking; changes in behavior/personality), and changes in self-care skills (Sakallaris, 2002).
   B. Components of behavior/personality involve a person's presence or consciousness noted in thoughts, emotions, and actions.
   C. An alteration in mental status can also result in a loss of the ability to carry out activities of daily living and meet self-care needs.
II. Risk factors.
   A. Disease related.
      1. CNS neoplasm, primary or metastatic disease.
      2. Metabolic emergencies (e.g., hypercalcemia, hyperuricemia, sodium or potassium imbalances).
      3. Uncontrolled pain.
      4. Head injury.
      5. Preexisting depression.
      6. HIV-related dementia.
      7. Opportunistic infections (e.g., toxoplasmosis, encephalitis, cryptococcal meningitis).
      8. Liver disease.
   B. Treatment related.
      1. Side effects of chemotherapy (e.g., sleep disturbance, headache, hyperkinesis).
      2. Side effect of biologic response modifier therapy (e.g., lethargy, somnolence, disturbance in recent memory).
      3. Side effect of steroid therapy (e.g., depression, psychotic reactions).
      4. Analgesics.
      5. Dehydration.
      6. Electrolyte imbalance (e.g., hyperuricemia, hyponatremia, hypokalemia).
   C. Situation related.
      1. Emotionally traumatic situations.
      2. Significant loss.
      3. Depression with melancholia, anxiety, anger.
      4. Rejection and abandonment.
      5. Hopelessness.
      6. Powerlessness.

Assessment

I. History.
   A. Presence of risk factors.

    B. Analgesics.
    C. Recent head injury, trauma, falls.
    D. Medication history.
    E. Allergy to steroids.
    F. High-dose meperidine (Demerol).
    G. Narcotic use.
    H. Alcohol abuse.
    I. Reported confusion at night.
    J. Uncontrolled pain.
  II. Physical examination.
    A. Neurologic examination results.
    B. Cognitive mental status screening.
    C. Impaired memory, recent and remote.
    D. Impaired problem solving.
    E. Impaired communication and language.
 III. Psychosocial examination.
    A. Changes in emotional and behavioral affect.
    B. Mood swings.
    C. Anxiety.
    D. Hallucinations, illusions.
    E. Impaired judgment.
    F. Decreased level of consciousness.
    G. Agitation, restlessness, seizures, shakiness.
    H. Tremors, confusion, grand mal seizures, coma, death.
    I. Influence of culture.
    J. Obtain information on baseline status from family members or caregivers.
 IV. Laboratory data.
    A. CBC.
    B. Serum electrolyte levels.
    C. Thyroid and liver function.

Nursing Diagnoses

   I. Disturbed thought processes.
  II. Bathing/hygiene self-care deficit, dressing/grooming self-care deficit, feeding self-care deficit, toileting self-care deficit.
 III. Risk for injury.
 IV. Anxiety.

Outcome Identification

   I. Client demonstrates improvement or adjustment to altered orientation, behavioral patterns, or mood states.
  II. Client participates in activities of daily living and self-care activities to the limits of his/her ability.
 III. Client remains free from injury related to cognitive impairment.
 IV. Client demonstrates a reduction in anxiety experienced.

Planning and Implementation

   I. Interventions to maintain or regain client's cognitive functions.
    A. Assess degrees of altered attention and concentration.

    B. Reorient the client to time, place, and reason for hospitalization.

    C. Provide clear, concise information, using simple terms, with face-to-face interaction with client.

    D. Provide a structured, organized environment.

    E. Provide cues for orientation: clock, calendar, personal items.

    F. Maintain a quiet environment; approach the client in a slow, unhurried manner.

    G. Provide structure in routine activities: specific time for breakfast, hygiene, medications, lunch, visitors.

    H. Clarify distortion in feelings and thoughts.

    I. Allow time for response to questions and decisions.

  II. Psychoeducational interventions (Barsevick et al., 2002).

    A. Use of counseling and psychotherapy.

    B. Use of behavior therapy.

    C. Provide education about disease process, self-care management.

    D. Encourage attendance at a support group.

 III. Interventions to involve client and family in care.

    A. Assess the family's understanding and educate family members about potential cognitive dysfunction.

    B. Engage client and/or family in discussion of illness from their perspective, including influence of culture.

    C. Discuss appropriate cultural interventions that may complement the medical regimen.

    D. Provide opportunities for family members to ask questions and obtain information.

    E. Teach the family to monitor changes in cognitive status.

    F. Instruct client and family about signs and symptoms to report to health team.

    G. Reinforce information that the health care provider discussed during visits.

    H. Teach avoidance of alcohol and unessential medications.

 IV. Interventions to ensure a safe environment (Craven & Hirnle, 2003).

    A. Maintain the bed in the lowest position with wheels locked; have the call light within reach.

    B. Provide sufficient light so client can see surroundings, especially if in a new, strange environment.

    C. Use a chair as a barrier, to inhibit client from wandering out of room or area.

    D. Use an alarm system to alert nurse or nurses' station when client is attempting to get out of bed or chair.

    E. Request a sitter if client is considered unsafe.

    F. Use side rails as a last resort.

       1. If client has a tendency to climb out of bed, side rails may increase the risk to safety.

       2. If any form of restraint is used, consider relevant (Joint Commission on Accreditation of Healthcare Organizations (JCAHO) regulations.

    G. Provide a rocking chair during the day to help client use up some energy.

    H. Assess limitations in and assist with activities of daily living, as needed.

    I. Assess for the presence of pharmacologic agents that can alter cognitive function.

    J. Assess the person's thoughts and feelings toward staff and the need for hospitalization.

    K. Discuss the client's fears and concerns.

  V. Nonpharmacologic interventions to manage anxiety and depression.

    A. Cognitive distraction: imagery, music therapy.

    B. Psychoeducation.

C. Art therapy.
D. Massage therapy.
E. Pet therapy.

Evaluation

The oncology nurse systematically and regularly evaluates the client's and/or family's responses to interventions to determine progress toward the achievement of expected outcomes. Relevant data are collected, and actual findings are compared with expected findings. Nursing diagnoses, outcomes, and plans of care are reviewed and revised as necessary.

REFERENCES

Armstrong, G.E. (2003). Mobility and body mechanics. In R.F. Craven & C.J. Hirnle (Eds.). *Fundamentals of nursing: Human health and function* (4th ed.). Philadelphia: Lippincott Williams & Wilkins, pp. 753-809.

Barsevick, M.A., Sweeney, C., Haney, E., & Chung, E. (2002). A systematic qualitative analysis of psychoeducational interventions for depression in patients with cancer. *Oncology Nursing Forum 29*(1), 73-82.

Boyle, D.M. (2002). Peripheral neuropathy. In D. Camp-Sorrell & R.A. Hawkins (Eds.). *Clinical manual for the oncology advanced practice nurse.* Pittsburgh: Oncology Nursing Society, pp. 751-757.

Bush, N.J., & Hartkopf Smith, L. (2002). Neuropathic pain. *Oncology Nursing Forum 29*(3), 457-459.

Craven, R.F., & Hirnle, C.J. (2003). *Safety in fundamentals of nursing: Human health and function* (4th ed.). Philadelphia: Lippincott Williams & Wilkins, pp. 649-677.

Flounders, J., & Ott, B.B. (2003). Oncologic emergency modules: Spinal cord compression. *Oncology Nursing Forum 30*(1). Retrieved February 23, 2003 from the World Wide Web http://www.ons.org/xp6/ONS/Library.xlm/ONSPublications.xml/ONF.xml/ONF200/FebJan03/Mem.

Gorman, L. (2002). In N. Bush & L. Hartkopf Smith. Neuropathic pain. *Oncology Nursing Forum 29*(3), 457-459.

Haisfield-Wolfe, M., & Rund, C. (2000). A nursing protocol for the management of perineal-rectal skin alterations. *Clinical Journal of Oncology Nursing 4*(1), 15-21.

Kwekeboom, L.J., & Seng, S.J. (2002). Recognizing and responding to post-traumatic stress disorder in people with cancer. *Oncology Nursing Forum 29*(4), 643-649.

Landier, W. (2001). Continuing education: Childhood acute lymphoblastic leukemia: Current perspectives. *Oncology Nursing Forum 28*(5). Retrieved February 23, 2003 from the World Wide Web http://www.ons.org/xp6/ONS/Library,xml/ONS_Publications.xml/ONF2001.xml/June2001

Marrs, J., & Newton, S. (2003). Updating your peripheral neuropathy "know how." *Clinical Journal of Oncology Nursing 7*(3), 299-303.

North American Nursing Diagnosis Association (NANDA). (2003). *Nursing diagnoses: Definitions and classification 2003-2004.* Philadelphia: NANDA.

Sakallaris, B.R. (2002). Mental status and neurological techniques. In M.A. Zator-Estes. *Health assessment and physical examination* (2nd ed.). Clifton Park, NY: Delmar Learning.

Sweeney, C. (2002). Understanding peripheral neuropathy in patients with cancer: Background and patient assessment. *Clinical Journal of Oncology Nursing 6*(3), 163-166.

Weiss, P. (2000). Cutaneous paraneoplastic syndromes. *Clinical Journal of Oncology Nursing 4*(6), 257-262.

Zembrzuski, C.D. (2001). *Neurological assessment: Clinical companion for assessment of the older adult.* Albany, NY: Delmar.

13 Myelosuppression

DAWN CAMP-SORRELL

Theory

I. Myelosuppression is a reduction in bone marrow function that results in a reduced production of red blood cells (RBCs), white blood cells (WBCs), and platelets into the peripheral circulation (Ezzone, 2000).
  A. Decreased RBC production results in anemia (see Chapter 16) and problems of fatigue (see Chapter 1).
  B. Decreased WBC production results in neutropenia and risk for infection and sepsis.
  C. Decreased platelets result in thrombocytopenia and risk for bleeding or hemorrhage.

NEUTROPENIA

Theory

I. Definition—a decrease in number of circulating neutrophils in the blood evidenced by an absolute neutrophil count (ANC) less than 1000/mm³ (Boxer & Dale, 2002; Lynch, 2000a).
  A. Neutrophils are the first line of the body's defense against bacterial infection by localizing and neutralizing bacteria (Barber, 2001).
  B. Normal range of neutrophil counts is 2500 to 6000 cells/mm³ accounting for 50% to 60% of the total number of WBCs.
II. Physiology (Boxer & Dale, 2002; Lynch, 2000a).
  A. Neutrophils arise from the myeloid stem cells as well as eosinophils, basophils, and monocytes.
  B. Collectively, neutrophils, eosinophils, and basophils are called *granulocytes*.
  C. Lymphocytes (B and T cells) are produced from the lymphoid stem cells.
III. Risk factors (Barber, 2001; Dale, 2002; Koh & Pizzo, 2002; Lynch, 2000a).
  A. Client related.
    1. Older clients, who have more fat and less cellular marrow than younger counterparts.
    2. Tumor cell invasion into the bone marrow.
    3. Poor nutritional status (Rust et al., 2000).
    4. High negative nitrogen balance compromising the marrow.
    5. Certain diseases, such as aplastic anemia, have a decreased production of neutrophils.
    6. Interruption of the integrity of normal barriers, such as from open wounds, mucositis, or vascular access devices.
    7. Comorbid diseases, such as diabetes mellitus, chronic obstructive pulmonary disease, heart failure.
    8. Hematologic malignancies.

    B. Treatment related.

        1. Chemotherapy—destruction of the rapidly dividing hematopoietic cells, which results in decreased production of neutrophil precursors as well as other WBCs with eventual destruction of the mature neutrophil cells.

        2. Radiation therapy—treatment fields that receive 20 Gy or more that involve the major bone marrow production sites of the ilia, vertebrae, ribs, skull, sternum, and metaphyses of the long bones.

        3. Biotherapy—because these agents modulate the immune system, the potential for alteration exists.

        4. Steroids—prevent migration of neutrophils to the bacteria and the process of phagocytosis.

        5. Prior treatment with chemotherapy, radiation therapy, or multimodal therapy.

        6. Combined modality therapies are more likely to produce myelosuppression.

IV. Principles of medical management (Adams, 2000; Dale, 2002; Koh & Pizzo, 2002).

    A. Antibiotic, antifungal, antiviral medications for the organism isolated (see Chapter 10).

        1. Antibiotics are continued for a minimum of 7 days.

        2. Antibiotics are continued until there is clinical, microbiologic, and radiologic resolution of infection (Barber, 2001).

        3. Antibiotics are usually continued until the ANC is greater than 500/mm^3.

        4. Antibiotic therapy initially consists of broad-spectrum antibiotics directed at both gram-positive and gram-negative organisms (Koh & Pizzo, 2002).

            a. Monotherapy with an extended-spectrum cephalosporin or a fluoroquinolone.

            b. Combination therapy with a penicillin, fluoroquinolone, and/or cephalosporin.

            c. Duotherapy with the addition of vancomycin.

            d. Therapies differ among institutions and geographic locations.

        5. If fever continues after the client has been receiving antibiotics for 3 days without a known cause, an antifungal agent is initiated.

        6. Antiviral drugs are recommended if mucosal lesions or viral disease is suspected.

    B. Hematopoietic growth factors are glycoprotein hormones that act as a natural regulator of hematopoiesis to promote the proliferation and differentiation of hematopoietic progenitor cells along multiple pathways (see Chapter 10) (Boxer & Dale, 2002; Buchsel et al., 2002; Dale, 2002; Ozer et al., 2000).

        1. Used to shorten the duration and/or severity of neutropenia.

        2. Dramatically reduces the occurrence of morbidity and mortality associated with infections as a result of neutropenia.

            a. Granulocyte colony-stimulating factor (G-CSF) predominantly enhances the growth of granulocyte colonies by affecting the proliferation and differentiation of neutrophil progenitor and precursor cells.

            b. Granulocyte-macrophage colony-stimulating factor (GM-CSF) is a multilineage hematopoietic growth factor that stimulates neutrophils, macrophages, monocytes, and eosinophils.

        3. Recommended dose for CSF is to be administered daily.

            a. G-CSF dose is 5 mcg/kg/day subcutaneous injection for up to 14 days or until the ANC is greater than 10,000/mm^3. Once discontinued, a precipitous drop in ANC occurs.

       b. GM-CSF dose may be given by subcutaneous injection or intravenously (IV) in doses of 250 mcg/m^2/day and up to 300 mcg/m^2/day if the patient has not engrafted by 21 days.

       c. Long-acting form of G-CSF is administered once per chemotherapy cycle at a dose of 6 mg subcutaneously 24 hours after chemotherapy and no sooner than 14 days before next cycle (*The Medical Letter,* 2002).

    4. Growth factors are started if the client is at a high risk for febrile neutropenia, such as after receiving high-dose chemotherapy or bone marrow transplant and in the following situations (Ozer et al., 2000):

       a. Prophylaxis with dose-intensive chemotherapy associated with increased incidence of febrile neutropenia.

       b. Previous febrile neutropenic episode with a course of cancer treatment.

       c. If a dose reduction or delay is not recommended to treat the cancer.

V. Potential sequelae of prolonged neutropenia.

  A. Infectious organism resistant to antibiotics.

  B. Sepsis and septic shock.

    1. Infections increase in frequency and severity as the ANC decreases.

    2. When the nadir persists for more than 7 to 10 days, the risk for severe infection increases.

  C. Death.

  D. Delay in administering treatment on time or dose delays; dose reductions.

Assessment

  I. History (Barber, 2001; Lynch, 2000a).

    A. Review of previous cancer therapy, such as chemotherapy, radiation therapy, biotherapy, or multimodal therapy.

    B. Review of current antibiotic regimen, such as trimethoprim-sulfamethoxazole (Bactrim) or amphotericin B, that can decrease the neutrophil count.

    C. Review of current hematopoietic growth factor use.

    D. Review of comorbid conditions and current medications.

  II. Physical examination (Boxer & Dale, 2002; Lynch, 2000a).

    A. Assess access device and other catheter exit sites for swelling, drainage, erythema, or tenderness.

    B. Assess nutritional status—protein-calorie malnutrition causes lymphopenia, diminished levels of the complement system, and a decrease of certain immunoglobulins (Rust et al., 2000).

    C. Assess vital signs—fever may be the only response to an infection.

      1. A fever of 100.5° F (38.1° C) is significant in a client with an ANC less than 500/mm^3. Fever is the most common and important sign of infection.

      2. If the client's pulse is over 100 beats/min and the blood pressure is dropping, the client may be developing sepsis (see Sepsis, Chapter 18).

    D. Assess for signs of infection, which may not be apparent with the inhibition of phagocytic cells; therefore redness, inflammation, and drainage may be minimal or absent.

      1. Most commonly infected sites include the respiratory tract, gastrointestinal (GI) tract, genitourinary tract, perineum, anus, and skin.

      2. Assess all indwelling catheter sites.

    E. Assess for abnormal breath sounds.

    F. Assess the oral cavity for thrush, plaque, redness, infected ulcerations.

    G. Assess for abdominal tenderness, stiffness, guarding.

    H. Assess for change in mental status.

   III. Laboratory data.
      A. Complete blood count (CBC) with differential.
      B. Calculate the ANC (Box 13-1).
      C. Culture and sensitivity testing of urine, blood, stool, sputum, cerebrospinal fluid, wound, drainage tubes or bags.

Nursing Diagnoses

   I. Risk for imbalanced body temperature.
   II. Risk for infection.
   III. Deficient knowledge related to infection precautions.

Outcome Identification

   I. Client's ANC is greater than $1000/mm^3$.
   II. Client does not develop major complications as a result of neutropenia.
   III. Client accurately describes appropriate infection precautions.

Planning and Implementation

   I. Pharmacologic—see Section IV of Theory.
   II. Nonpharmacologic (Barber, 2001; Ellerhorst-Ryan, 2000; Rust et al., 2000).
      A. Interventions to minimize the occurrence of infection.
         1. Employ strict hand washing technique.
         2. Restrict fresh fruits and vegetables in the client's diet.
         3. Restrict fresh flowers or other sources of stagnant water.
         4. Encourage client to bathe daily with meticulous personal hygiene and perineal care.

BOX 13-1
CALCULATION OF ABSOLUTE NEUTROPHIL COUNT

The absolute neutrophil count (ANC) is calculated as follows:

$$ANC = \frac{\% \text{ neutrophils} + \% \text{ bands}}{100} \times \text{white blood cell (WBC) count}$$

The example shows how to calculate the ANC of a client with the following counts: neutrophils = 50%, bands = 8%, WBCs = 4000.

$$ANC = \frac{(50\% + 8\%)}{100} \times 4000$$

$$ANC = (.50 + .08) \times 4000$$

$$ANC = 2320$$

Infection Risk

Not significant	ANC = 1500-2000
Minimal	ANC = 1000-1500
Moderate	ANC = 500-1000
Severe	ANC = <500

From Liebman MC, Camp-Sorrell D: *Multimodal therapy in oncology nursing,* St. Louis, 1996, Mosby, p 377.

5. Limit visitors to those without communicable illness. Avoid having children visit.

6. Give meticulous care to all catheters, such as venous access devices, urinary or feeding tubes.

7. Use aseptic technique for all nursing interventions.

8. Change water in pitchers, denture cups, and nebulizers daily.

B. Interventions to monitor for complications.

1. Monitor for nadir (the lowest point of the blood cell levels after cancer treatment).

a. As immature cells in the marrow and mature cells in the bloodstream are destroyed, the nadir becomes apparent.

(1) Usually 7 to 14 days after chemotherapy, except for the nitrosourea agents, in which nadir occurs in 3 to 4 weeks, and except for cases employing radiation to the large bones.

(2) Occasional occurrence after biotherapy.

(3) Usually after multimodal treatment, the nadir occurs sooner and more severely than from single-modality therapy.

b. Nadir resolves within 3 to 4 weeks when the cells in the bone marrow mature and are released into the peripheral blood. With the exception of cases involving the administration of nitrosourea agents, the nadir resolves in 6 to 8 weeks.

c. Cancer treatment is usually held for an ANC less than 1000 to 1500/mm^3.

2. Monitor for risk of infection according to ANC and other factors (Koh & Pizzo, 2002; Lynch, 2000a).

a. 1000/mm^3 or less—low risk of infection.

b. 500/mm^3 or less—moderate risk of infection.

c. 100/mm^3 or less—severe risk of infection.

d. Risk is greater when patient experiences neutropenia of longer than 7 days' duration or from prolonged neutropenia.

e. Comorbid diseases present.

3. Obtain cultures from the blood, urine, stool, and wound drainage immediately as prescribed and before starting antibiotic therapy (Boxer & Dale, 2002; Koh & Pizzo, 2002; Lynch, 2000a).

a. Approximately 85% of infections arise from endogenous microbial flora from the GI and respiratory tracts.

b. Bacteremia is principally caused by aerobic gram-negative bacilli (*Escherichia coli, Klebsiella pneumoniae, Pseudomonas aeruginosa*) and gram-positive cocci (coagulase-negative staphylococci, pneumococci, *Enterococcus, Streptococcus* species, *Staphylococcus aureus*).

c. Fungal infections commonly occur from *Candida albicans*.

4. Obtain chest x-ray as ordered.

III. Report critical changes in client assessment parameters to physician.

A. Signs and symptoms of infection.

B. Temperature greater than 100.5° F (38.1° C).

IV. Interventions to incorporate client and family in care.

A. Teach personal hygiene measures to minimize the occurrence of infection, such as wiping the perineal area from front to back after voiding and after a stool; daily bathing.

B. Teach infection precautions and how to minimize the risk of infection, such as strict hand washing.

C. Teach subcutaneous administration of hematopoietic growth factors.

D. Teach the symptoms for which to call the physician or nurse, such as temperature greater than 100.5° F (38.1° C) , productive cough, painful urination, or sore throat.

Evaluation

The oncology nurse systematically and regularly evaluates the client's and/or family's responses to interventions to determine progress toward the achievement of expected outcomes. Relevant data are collected, and actual findings are compared with expected findings. Nursing diagnoses, outcomes, and plans of care are reviewed and revised as necessary.

THROMBOCYTOPENIA

Theory

I. Definition—decrease in the circulating platelets below 100,000/mm^3 (McCullough, 2000).
  A. Normal count is 150,000 to 400,000/mm^3.
  B. Life span of platelets is 8 to 10 days.
II. Physiology (Lynch, 2000b).
  A. Platelets are developed from megakaryocytes in the bone marrow.
  B. Major function of platelets is to maintain vascular hemostasis and prevent blood loss through platelet adhesion to block small breaks in blood vessels and initiate clotting mechanisms.
III. Risk factors (Lynch, 2000b).
  A. Disease related.
    1. Idiopathic thrombocytopenia purpura or thrombotic thrombocytopenia purpura: accelerated destruction of platelets. Platelet sequestration in spleen.
    2. Hypocoagulation disorders, such as liver disease or vitamin K deficiency, alter the development of prothrombin and several clotting factors.
    3. Hypercoagulation disorders, such as paraneoplastic syndromes, disseminated intravascular coagulation, and thrombosis, increase the use of platelets.
    4. Invasion of tumor cells in the bone marrow.
    5. Cancers involving the bone marrow, such as multiple myeloma, lymphoma, and leukemia, alter platelet production.
  B. Treatment related.
    1. Chemotherapy—destruction of the rapidly dividing hematopoietic cells, which results in a decrease of the production of platelet precursors with eventual destruction of mature platelets.
      a. Platelet count usually decreases in 7 to 14 days after administration or sooner with multimodal treatment.
      b. Platelet count usually decreases after the drop in WBCs.
      c. Recovery usually occurs within 2 to 6 weeks.
    2. Radiation therapy—treatment field that receives 20 Gy or more that involves the major bone marrow production sites of the ilia, vertebrae, ribs, skull, sternum, and metaphyses of the long bones.
    3. Endotoxins released from bacteria during an infection can damage platelets and alter platelet aggregation.

    4. Some medications can alter platelet development, such as aspirin, digoxin (Lanoxin), furosemide (Lasix), heparin, phenytoin (Dilantin), quinidine, sulfonamides (Bactrim), and tetracycline.

IV. Principles of medical management.

  A. Administer platelets when platelet count is less than 10,000 cells/mm^3 or in presence of bleeding to increase the peripheral blood level approximately 10,000 to 12,000 cells/mm^3 per unit or to control bleeding (McCullough, 2000).

    1. Single-donor platelets (or pheresis) are taken from one donor.

    2. Random-donor platelets are harvested from whole blood from several different donors. The client is exposed to multiple-donor antigens.

    3. Human leukocyte antigen (HLA)–matched platelets are indicated if the client's platelet count fails to increase after repeated transfusion from non–HLA-matched products.

    4. Leukocyte-depleted filters or irradiated products may be used to eliminate WBCs from the product, which prevents alloimmunization.

  B. Platelet growth factors promote maturation of the megakaryocyte (Begley & Basser, 2000; Demetri, 2000; Lynch, 2000b).

    1. Investigational agents include thrombopoietin, interleukin-1, interleukin-3, and interleukin-6.

      a. Thrombopoietin is thought to be the hormone responsible for the production and maturation of megakaryocytes.

      b. No other biotherapeutic agent acts specifically on the megakaryocyte.

    2. Interleukin-11 is approved for chemotherapy-induced thrombocytopenia.

      a. Indirectly promotes proliferation and maturation of megakaryocytes.

      b. Dose is 50 mcg/kg administered subcutaneously until the platelet count is greater than 50,000 cells/mm^3 or discontinued 2 days before next chemotherapy cycle.

  C. Administer plasma to replenish clotting factors when client is actively bleeding and becomes refractory to platelets.

  D. Progestational agents may be prescribed to decrease menstrual bleeding.

  E. Drug induced or disease related may be treated with steroids.

V. Potential sequelae of prolonged thrombocytopenia (McCullough, 2000).

  A. Refractory to platelet transfusion.

  B. Internal bleeding, such as intracranial, GI, or respiratory tract bleeding.

  C. Transfusion reaction or transmitted disease.

  D. Death.

  E. Delay in administering treatment on time or dose delays; dose reductions.

Assessment

I. History.

  A. Previous cancer treatment, such as chemotherapy, radiation therapy, or multimodal therapy.

  B. Current medications that could alter platelet production.

  C. Social history of alcohol intake and illicit drug use.

II. Physical examination (Lynch, 2000b; McCullough, 2000).

  A. Assess for bleeding such as from rectum, nose, ears, oral cavity.

    1. Platelet levels between 40,000 and 60,000/mm^3 are associated with an increased risk of postsurgical and traumatic bleeding.

    2. Platelet level less than 20,000/mm^3 is a major risk for spontaneous bleeding not caused by trauma.

    3. Platelet level lower than 10,000/mm^3 is associated with fatal central nervous system (CNS) bleeding or massive GI tract or respiratory tract hemorrhage.

  B. Assess for petechiae, which usually appear initially on the upper and lower extremities, then on pressure points, elbows, and the oral palate.

  C. Assess all stool, urine, and vomitus for blood.

  D. Assess the skin for ecchymosis, purpura, or oozing of puncture sites.

  E. Assess for conjunctiva hemorrhage and sclera injection.

  F. Assess for menstrual bleeding and the number of sanitary napkins or tampons used.

  G. Assess for changes that indicate intracranial bleeding, such as changes in level of consciousness, restlessness, headache, seizures, pupil changes, ataxia.

III. Laboratory data.

  A. Platelet count.

  B. Coagulation values—fibrinogen, prothrombin time, partial thromboplastin time.

Nursing Diagnoses

  I. Deficient knowledge related to bleeding precautions.

  II. Risk for injury.

III. Risk for impaired skin integrity.

Outcome Identification

  I. Client has resolution of thrombocytopenia.

  II. Client does not develop any complications as a result of thrombocytopenia.

III. Client accurately describes appropriate bleeding precautions.

Planning and Implementation

  I. Pharmacologic—see Section IV of Theory.

  II. Nonpharmacologic (Gobel, 2000; Lynch, 2000b).

    A. Interventions to minimize the occurrence of bleeding.

      1. Avoid using/overinflating a blood pressure cuff or using a tourniquet when the platelet count is less than 20,000/mm^3.

      2. Avoid invasive procedures, such as enemas, rectal temperatures, suppositories, bladder catheterization, venipunctures, finger sticks, nasogastric tubes, subcutaneous or intramuscular injections.

      3. Prepare environment to avoid trauma, for example, pad side rails, arrange furniture to eliminate sharp corners, clear walkways.

      4. Apply firm direct pressure to venipuncture site for 5 minutes.

      5. Encourage client to wear shoes during ambulation to maintain skin integrity.

      6. Encourage client to avoid sharp objects, such as a straight-edge razor.

      7. If bleeding is not controlled, absorbable gelatin sponges or liquid thrombin can be applied.

        a. For nosebleeds, the client should be placed in high Fowler's position and pressure applied to the nose.

        b. Ice packs may help to decrease the bleeding.

    8. Implement a bowel regimen to prevent constipation.
    9. Use soft toothbrushes to avoid gingival trauma.
    10. Avoid physical activity that may lead to trauma.
III. Monitor platelet levels.
    A. Cancer treatment is usually held for platelet count less than 50,000 to 100,000/mm³.
    B. Platelets are usually administered if the count is 10,000 to 20,000/mm³ or if the client is actively bleeding.
IV. Implement strategies to incorporate client and family in care.
    A. Teach the family and client bleeding precautions.
    B. Teach the family and client signs of bleeding that should be called to attention of the physician or nurse.
    C. Teach safety measures to decrease the occurrence of bleeding when performing activities of daily living.

Evaluation

The oncology nurse systematically and regularly evaluates the client's and/or family's responses to interventions to determine progress toward the achievement of expected outcomes. Relevant data are collected, and actual findings are compared with expected findings. Nursing diagnoses, outcomes, and plans of care are reviewed and revised as necessary.

INFECTION

Theory (Ellerhorst-Ryan, 2000; Ezzone, 2000)

  I. When the body or a part of the body is invaded by a microorganism or virus, an infection develops, depending on three factors.
    A. Source of infectious organism (Barber, 2001; Koh & Pizzo, 2002).
      1. Endogenous organisms are within the body's normal flora and help to prevent colonization of microorganisms.
      2. Exogenous organisms are found in the environment.
    B. Methods of transmission include direct contact, indirect contact, and airborne.
    C. Susceptible host, which refers to the ability to prevent or fight infection.
      1. Intact mechanical barriers, such as the skin and mucous membranes.
      2. Chemical barriers, such as the pH of the tissues.
      3. Intact inflammatory and immune responses.
 II. Physiology (Boxer & Dale, 2002; Ellerhorst-Ryan, 2000).
    A. Most important physical barrier against invasion of organism is the skin. Breakdown in the skin is a portal entry for organisms.
    B. Mucociliary action in mucous membranes is an important barrier.
    C. WBCs, particularly neutrophils, are an important defense against infection.
III. Risk factors (Barber, 2001; Ellerhorst-Ryan, 2000; Rust et al., 2000).
    A. Disease related.
      1. Hematologic/lymphoid malignancy.
      2. Altered skin and mucosal barriers.
      3. Recent exposure to an infectious organism.
      4. Human immunodeficiency virus (HIV).
      5. Chronic neutropenic conditions (Glauser, 2000).

    B. Treatment related.

        1. Myelosuppression induced from cancer treatment.

        2. Prolonged use of antibiotics or steroids.

        3. Multimodal cancer treatment.

IV. Principles of medical management (Adams, 2000; Koh & Pizzo, 2002).

    A. Administer antibiotics according to organism isolated.

    B. Employ meticulous wound care.

    C. Administer WBC line growth factors as appropriate (Buchsel et al., 2002).

V. Potential sequelae of prolonged infection.

    A. Septic shock.

    B. Resistance to antibiotics or superinfection.

    C. Death.

Assessment

I. History (Ezzone, 2000).

    A. Review previous cancer therapy, such as chemotherapy, radiation therapy, biotherapy, or multimodal therapy.

    B. Review known allergies to medications, especially antibiotics.

    C. Review immunosuppressive therapy.

II. Physical examination (Barber, 2001; Ellerhorst-Ryan, 2000; Ezzone, 2000).

    A. Comprehensive assessment every 4 to 8 hours or more often as indicated, with special attention to access device sites, lungs, integument, oral cavity, and perineum for drainage, open wounds, erythema.

    B. Assess vital signs every 4 to 8 hours or more often as indicated for trends or deviations from the normal.

    C. Assess the character of the urine for sediment, color, odor, blood.

    D. Assess the mental status for orientation, confusion, memory recall, alertness.

III. Laboratory data.

    A. CBC with differential.

    B. Culture and sensitivity testing of the urine, stool, blood, sputum, wounds, drainage bags or tubes.

Nursing Diagnoses

I. Risk for imbalanced body temperature.

II. Risk for infection.

III. Deficient knowledge related to infection precautions.

IV. Risk for impaired skin integrity.

V. Impaired oral mucous membrane.

Outcome Identification

I. Client accurately describes appropriate infection precautions.

II. Client does not develop major complications from the infectious process.

Planning and Implementation

I. Pharmacologic—see Section IV of Theory.

II. Nonpharmacologic (Barber, 2001; Ezzone, 2000).

    A. Interventions to minimize infections.

1. Employ strict hand washing before and after all contacts with client.
2. Promote and encourage daily meticulous personal hygiene, oral hygiene, perineal care.
3. Avoid unnecessary invasive procedures, such as enemas, rectal temperatures, bladder catheterization, venipunctures.
4. Administer vaccinations, such as a flu shot, to prevent communicable infections.
5. Use aseptic technique when performing nursing interventions.
6. Maintain adequate hydration and a high-calorie, high-protein diet (Rust et al., 2000).
   B. Interventions to locate source of infection by obtaining appropriate cultures, such as blood, sputum, stool, urine, and wounds, as indicated.
   C. Educate the client/family about signs and symptoms of infection and when to call the physician or nurse.

Evaluation

The oncology nurse systematically and regularly evaluates the client's and/or family's responses to interventions to determine progress toward the achievement of expected outcomes. Relevant data are collected, and actual findings are compared with expected findings. Nursing diagnoses, outcomes, and plans of care are reviewed and revised as necessary.

HEMORRHAGE

Theory

I. Definition—the occurrence of abnormal internal or external discharge of blood.
II. Physiology (Gobel, 2000).
   A. Hemostasis is the process of a solid clot forming in the blood from a fluid component.
   B. Coagulation is the mechanism of forming a stable fibrin clot.
   C. Hemorrhage occurs in cancer patients from alterations in hemostasis or coagulation mechanisms.
III. Risk factors (Adams, 2000).
   A. Disease related.
      1. Cerebral hemorrhage can occur with severe thrombocytopenia or with brain metastases.
      2. Myeloproliferative disorders, such as polycythemia vera, myelofibrosis, and thrombocythemia, can cause hemorrhage phenomena.
      3. Disseminated intravascular coagulation from prostate cancer or acute promyelocytic leukemia.
      4. Paraneoplastic syndromes can stimulate bleeding.
      5. Splenomegaly.
   B. Treatment related.
      1. Bone marrow or hematopoietic stem cell transplantation can cause a diffuse alveolar hemorrhage clinically characterized by cough, dyspnea, hypoxemia.
      2. Disseminated intravascular coagulation as a result of cancer treatment.

3. High-dose chemotherapy, such as cyclophosphamide (Cytoxan), can cause hemorrhagic cystitis or myocardial hemorrhage.

4. All types of surgical procedures have the risk for hemorrhage, especially if the tumor is embedded within arteries or veins.

IV. Principles of medical management (Gobel, 2000).

   A. Administer appropriate blood products (McCullough, 2000).

   B. Administer oxygen.

   C. Give vasopressor drugs, which may control severe bleeding.

   D. Lavage iced saline through a nasogastric tube, which may control gastric bleeding.

V. Potential sequelae of prolonged hemorrhage.

   A. Viral disease from numerous blood transfusions.

   B. Shock.

   C. Transfusion reaction.

   D. Death.

Assessment

I. History (Gobel, 2000, McCullough, 2000).

   A. Review previous cancer therapy, such as chemotherapy, radiation therapy, or multimodal treatment.

   B. Ascertain recent traumatic events.

   C. Review the cancer disease.

      1. Evidence of metastasis to the brain or bone marrow.

      2. Leukemia, especially nonlymphocytic leukemia, can cause hemorrhage as a result of a paraneoplastic process.

   D. Review past medical history for the occurrence of peptic/gastric ulcer disease or esophageal varices.

II. Physical examination (Lynch, 2000b).

   A. Assess for signs of hemorrhage complications, such as weak pulse, irregular pulse, pale skin, cold and moist skin.

   B. Assess all urine, stool, vomitus, and sputum for blood.

   C. Assess vital signs.

   D. Assess for neurologic deficits, such as reduced level of alertness or orientation.

III. Laboratory data.

   A. CBC.

   B. Coagulation factors.

   C. Occult stool test.

   D. Bleeding time.

Nursing Diagnoses

I. Decreased cardiac output.

II. Risk for deficient fluid volume.

III. Ineffective tissue perfusion.

Outcome Identification

I. Client does not develop complications as a result of hemorrhage.

II. Client does not have compromise of the tissue as a result of hemorrhage.

III. Client has resolution of hemorrhage.

Planning and Implementation

I. Pharmacologic—see Section IV of Theory.
II. Nonpharmacologic (Gobel, 2000; Lynch, 2000b).
   A. Interventions to minimize the bleeding.
      1. Apply occlusive dressings to open bleeding wounds after cleansing the area.
      2. If applicable, elevate the body part above the heart level and apply firm pressure over the area.
      3. Administer plasma and other blood components as ordered (McCullough, 2000).
   B. Interventions to monitor for complications.
      1. Hemodynamic measurements—decrease in cardiac output and decrease in blood pressure.
      2. Strict intake and output records to detect negative fluid balance.
   C. Report critical changes in the client's assessment parameters to the physician, such as change in mental status, decrease in blood pressure, increase in bleeding.

Evaluation

The oncology nurse systematically and regularly evaluates the client's and/or family's responses to interventions to determine progress toward the achievement of expected outcomes. Relevant data are collected, and actual findings are compared with expected findings. Nursing diagnoses, outcomes, and plans of care are reviewed and revised as necessary.

FEVER AND CHILLS

Theory

I. Definition—elevation of body temperature above 100.4° F (38° C) to 101.3° F (38.5° C) orally (Barber, 2001; Ezzone, 2000).
   A. Chills (shivering) occur as a body's response to heat loss when the body's temperature abruptly increases, such as with fever or drug reaction.
      1. During shivering the body produces involuntary contractions of the skeletal muscles.
      2. The internal body temperature is maintained by shivering, which is a thermoregulatory mechanism.
      3. A subjective feeling of cold.
   B. Fever is initiated by the release of endogenous pyrogens from phagocytic WBCs.
      1. Vasodilation and sweating are the physiologic mechanisms used to increase heat loss.
      2. Vasoconstriction and shivering are the body's mechanisms for conserving or producing heat.
      3. Production of fever occurs as a response to the elevation of the set point in the temperature-regulating center in the hypothalamus.
      4. Results in an increase in metabolic activity and oxygen consumption brought about by an increase in muscle tone and shivering.
      5. Skin temperature drops because of vasoconstriction, which decreases heat loss.

    C. Each degree of temperature Fahrenheit results in a 7% increase in metabolic rate and increases the demands on the heart (Ezzone, 2000).

  II. Physiology (Ezzone, 2000).

    A. Normally the thermoregulatory center in the hypothalamus controls body temperature.

    B. Various heat loss mechanisms help return the temperature to normal levels during fevers.

  III. Risk factors (Barber, 2001).

    A. Disease related.

      1. Tumor involving the hypothalamus, where the temperature control for the body is located.

      2. Paraneoplastic syndrome.

        a. Pyrogens are released by the tumor cells producing a fever, especially in the presence of uncontrolled tumor growth.

        b. Most common tumors associated with tumor-induced fever include Hodgkin's disease, osteogenic sarcoma, lymphoma, liver metastasis.

    B. Treatment related.

      1. Neutropenia following cancer treatment.

      2. Chemotherapy side effects from agents that can cause a drug fever or flu-like syndrome (e.g., bleomycin [Blenoxane], daunorubicin [Cerubidine], thiotepa [Thioplex], methotrexate [Mexate], dacarbazine (DTIC-Dome), plicamycin [Mithracin]).

      3. Blood transfusion reaction.

      4. Biotherapy side effect from interferon, monoclonal antibody, or interleukin.

      5. Steroid-induced adrenal insufficiency.

      6. Drug induced, such as vancomycin or amphotericin B.

      7. Invasive procedure.

  IV. Principles of medical management (Barber, 2001; Ezzone, 2000).

    A. Administer acetaminophen alternated with ibuprofen every 2 hours to decrease fever and drug toxicity. Use with caution in clients with thrombocytopenia.

    B. Administer nonsteroidal antiinflammatory drugs (NSAIDs) for tumor-induced fever. Use with caution in clients with thrombocytopenia.

    C. Administer meperidine (Demerol) to relieve chills.

    D. Administer antimicrobial therapy as indicated (Koh & Pizzo, 2002).

  V. Potential sequelae of prolonged fever and chills.

    A. Increase in fatigue, muscle weakness, myalgia; reducing quality of life.

    B. Death.

Assessment

  I. History (Barber, 2001; Ezzone, 2000).

    A. Previous cancer treatments.

    B. Previous exposure to infections.

    C. Type of cancer and extent of disease.

    D. Previous blood transfusions.

    E. Current medications.

  II. Physical examination (Barber, 2001; Ezzone, 2000).

    A. Assess vital signs frequently.

    B. Perform a complete physical examination to ascertain the source of fever.

III. Laboratory data.
   A. CBC.
   B. Appropriate cultures and sensitivities.

Nursing Diagnoses

   I. Risk for imbalanced body temperature.
   II. Risk for imbalanced fluid volume.
   III. Risk for infection.
   IV. Ineffective thermoregulation.

Outcome Identification

   I. Client's fever and chills resolve.
   II. Client does not develop complications as a result of fever and chills.
   III. Client participates in strategies to maximize comfort.

Planning and Implementation

   I. Pharmacologic—see section IV of Theory.
   II. Nonpharmacologic.
      A. Interventions to locate the source of infection.
         1. Obtain cultures from the blood, throat, urine, stool, sputum, and wounds when an infection is suspected.
         2. Obtain cultures from all access devices.
   II. Interventions to provide comfort.
      A. Promote slow cooling of the skin and mucous membranes.
         1. Tepid sponge baths.
         2. Reduced amount of client clothing.
         3. Mechanical cooling blankets.
         4. Reduction of the environmental temperature.
      B. Avoid rapid reduction in body temperature that can cause chilling by providing warm blankets or heating pads at the first sign of chilling.
      C. Change damp clothing immediately to prevent chilling.
      D. Administer acetaminophen to reduce fever every 4 hours, not to exceed 4000 mg in a 24-hour period, which can be alternated with aspirin and NSAIDs. Use acetaminophen with caution in clients with liver disease; use aspirin and NSAIDs with caution in clients with thrombocytopenia.
      E. Increase fluid intake to prevent dehydration.
      F. Patient education as to self-care measures for fever/chills including medication management.
   III. Interventions to minimize the occurrence of infection in common sites.
      A. Encourage coughing and deep breathing every 4 to 8 hours while awake.
      B. Encourage oral hygiene every 4 hours while awake.
      C. Encourage client to void frequently.
      D. Avoid the use of douches or tampons.
      E. Encourage the client to eat well-balanced meals and increase fluid intake.

Evaluation

The oncology nurse systematically and regularly evaluates the client's and/or family's responses to interventions to determine progress toward the achievement of

expected outcomes. Relevant data are collected, and actual findings are compared with expected findings. Nursing diagnoses, outcomes, and plans of care are reviewed and revised as necessary.

REFERENCES

Adams, V.R. (2000). Adverse events associated with chemotherapy for common cancers. *Pharmacotherapy 20*, 96-103.

Barber, F.D. (2001). Management of fever in neutropenic patients with cancer. *Nursing Clinics of North America 36*, 631-644.

Begley, C.G., & Basser, R.L. (2000). Biologic and structural differences of thrombopoietic growth factors. *Seminars in Hematology 37*(Suppl. 4), 19-27.

Boxer, L., & Dale, D.C. (2002). Neutropenia: Causes and consequences. *Seminars in Hematology 39*, 75-81.

Buchsel, P.C., Forgey, A., Grape, F.B., & Hamann, S.S. (2002). Granulocyte macrophage colony-stimulating factor: Current practice and novel approaches. *Clinical Journal of Oncology Nursing 6*, 198-205.

Dale, D.C. (2002). Colony-stimulating factors for the management of neutropenia in cancer patients. *Drugs 62*(Suppl. 1), 1-15.

Demetiri, G.D. (2000). Pharmacologic treatment options in patients with thrombocytopenia. *Seminars in Hematology 37*(Suppl. 4), 11-18.

Ellerhorst-Ryan, J.M. (2000). Infection. In C.H. Yarbro, M.H. Frogge, M. Goodman, & S. Groenwald (Eds.). *Cancer nursing principles and practice* (5th ed.). Sudbury, MA: Jones and Bartlett Publishers, pp. 691-708.

Ezzone, S.A. (2000). Fever. In D. Camp-Sorrell & R. Hawkins (Eds.). *Clinical manual for the oncology advanced practice nurse*. Pittsburgh: Oncology Nursing Press, pp. 813-824.

Glauser, M.P. (2000). Neutropenia: Clinical implications and modulation. *Intensive Care Medicine 26*, S103-S110.

Gobel, B.H. (2000). Bleeding. In C.H. Yarbro, M.H. Frogge, M. Goodman, & S. Groenwald (Eds.). *Cancer nursing principles and practice* (5th ed.). Sudbury, MA: Jones and Bartlett Publishers, pp. 709-736.

Koh, A. & Pizzo, P.A. (2002). Empirical oral antibiotic therapy for low risk febrile cancer patients with neutropenia. *Cancer Investigation 20*, 420-433.

Liebman, M.C., & Camp-Sorrell, D. (1996). *Multimodal therapy in oncology nursing*. St. Louis: Mosby, p. 377.

Lynch, M.P. (2000a). Neutropenia. In D. Camp-Sorrell & R. Hawkins (Eds.). *Clinical manual for the oncology advanced practice nurse*. Pittsburgh: Oncology Nursing Press, pp. 693-698.

Lynch, M.P. (2000b). Thrombocytopenia. In D. Camp-Sorrell & R. Hawkins (Eds.). *Clinical manual for the oncology advanced practice nurse*. Pittsburgh: Oncology Nursing Press, pp. 703-707.

McCullough, J. (2000). Current issues with platelet transfusion in patients with cancer. *Seminars in Hematology 37*(Suppl. 4), 3-10.

The Medical Letter. (2002). Pegfilgrastim (Neulasta) for prevention of febrile neutropenia. *The Medical Letter 44*, 44-45.

Ozer, H., Armitage, J.O., Bennett, C.L., et al. (2000). 2000 update of recommendations for the use of hematopoietic colony-stimulating factors: Evidence-based, clinical practice guidelines. *Journal of Clinical Oncology 18*, 3558-3585.

Rust, D.M., Simpson, J.K., & Lister, J. (2000). Nutritional issues in patients with severe neutropenia. *Seminars in Oncology Nursing 16*, 152-162.

PART THREE

GASTROINTESTINAL AND URINARY FUNCTION

14 Alterations in Nutrition

MARILYNN BERENDT AND SHERRI D'AGOSTINO

DYSPHAGIA

Theory

I. Definition—difficulty in swallowing, pain; usually accompanied by a sensation of material lodging in the esophagus (Turnkel et al., 2000).
II. Pathophysiology, etiology, and risk factors.
   A. Neurologic impairment.
      1. Loss of innervation (i.e., of cranial nerves V, VII, IX, X, XI, and/or XII, thus loss of swallow reflex).
      2. Loss of vocal cord control.
   B. Tumor infiltration and impingement of the esophagus and mouth by tumor and/or treatment-related effects.
      1. Major surgery that impairs the ability to hold food in mouth, lateralize, masticate, form a bolus, and move a bolus through the oropharynx and esophagus.
      2. Radiation therapy (RT) to the site causing fibrosis or stenosis.
      3. Mucositis.
      4. Aphthous ulceration.
      5. Candidiasis.
      6. Chemotherapy effects (e.g., fluorouracil [5-fluorouracil, 5-FU]) on the oral cavity and esophagus.
      7. Changes in character of oral secretions as a result of RT and chemotherapy.
   C. Iatrogenic factors.
      1. Psychotropic medications that impair gag reflex and swallowing.
      2. Anticholinergic drugs.
   D. Lifestyle-related effects (e.g., emotional responses to disease and treatment).
III. Progression of dysphagia.
   A. Usually insidious and slowly progressive.
   B. Usually manifested as difficulty swallowing solids progressing to difficulty swallowing liquids, including saliva, causing fluids and foods to flow into the lungs, increasing the risk for aspiration and/or pneumonia.
   C. Usually associated with weight loss, anorexia, nausea, dehydration, protein-calorie malnutrition, cachexia, muscle wasting, and negative nitrogen wasting.
   D. Elderly at increased risk, as well as clients with certain cancer types—head and neck cancer, esophageal and lung carcinomas with lymph node involvement.
IV. Principles of medical management.
   A. Treatment for underlying disease—nodal radiation, laser surgery, antifungal and antibiotic medications.
   B. Endoscopic laser therapy.

    C. Alternate method for feedings, which may require short- or long-term interventions.

    D. Use of thickening agents (e.g., Thick-It, Nutra-Thik, Thick'N Easy) to lessen the risk for flow of liquids into the airway causing choking and aspiration.

    E. Medications—steroids, expectorants, bronchodilators, pain and anxiety medications to relieve symptoms related to dysphagia.

    F. Swallowing therapy and/or direct swallowing exercise.

Assessment

    I. History.

      A. Previous treatments for cancer.

      B. Presence of underlying systemic disease—infection, cardiac, or stroke.

      C. Patterns of dysphagia—incidence; pattern; alleviating, aggravating, and precipitating factors.

      D. Impact on lifestyle, comfort, activities of daily living, and quality of life (QOL).

    II. Physical examination.

      A. Observe for presence of facial droop, drooling, oral retention, choking, coughing after swallowing, and gurgling voice quality.

      B. Determine ability to masticate, hold food in mouth, and propel food to oropharynx using tongue.

      C. Elicit client's subjective report of pain or discomfort; weakness of lips, tongue, or jaw; "lump in the throat."

      D. Assess lungs.

Nursing Diagnoses

    I. Impaired swallowing.

    II. Risk for aspiration.

    III. Disturbed sensory perception: gustatory.

    IV. Risk for imbalanced fluid volume.

    V. Imbalanced nutrition: less than body requirements.

    VI. Fear.

    VII. Ineffective coping.

    VIII. Anxiety.

Outcome Identification

    I. Client states goals for therapy and rehabilitation for dysphagia.

    II. Client participates in measures to minimize the risk of occurrence, severity, and complications of dysphagia.

    III. Client and family state signs and symptoms of dysphagia and techniques for minimizing these signs and symptoms.

    IV. Client and family demonstrate competence in emergency techniques related to aspiration, regurgitation, and airway obstruction related to dysphagia.

    V. Client and family identify resources in the community to assist with rehabilitation.

    VI. Client and family list symptoms or changes that require professional assistance and management.

      A. Aspiration.

B. Airway obstruction.

C. Weight loss greater than 5% of body weight.

D. Dehydration.

E. Any change that constitutes a concern for client safety or well-being.

Planning and Implementation

I. Nonpharmacologic interventions that minimize the risk of occurrence or complications of dysphagia.

    A. Manage the underlying cause of dysphagia.

    B. Consult with speech or occupation therapy to perform a swallow test to determine extent of problem.

    C. Perform and teach client/family methods to facilitate the effectiveness and ease of swallowing. According to the Institute of Compensatory Swallowing Techniques (Turnkel et al., 2000), the following have been found to be useful:

        1. Head posture.

           a. Chin tuck.

           b. Turn head to weaker side.

           c. Tilt head to stronger side.

           d. Tilt head backward.

        2. Body posture.

           a. Upright at 90 degrees.

           b. Lying on one side.

        3. Manner of oral intake.

           a. Decrease rate of intake.

           b. Multiple swallows per bolus.

           c. Alternate solids with liquids.

           d. Decrease bolus size.

           e. Liquids by spoon.

           f. Liquids or puree by syringe.

    D. Provide appropriate assist devices—straws, plunger spoon, Asepto syringe, and/or pastry tube.

    E. Maintain adequate food and calorie intake with high-calorie, high-protein foods and/or enteral feedings, throughout the day—eight small feedings.

    F. Institute and teach client/family other measures to decrease pain with swallowing—ice chips, soft or pureed foods, semisolid foods, avoidance of hot and spicy foods, use of local anesthetics.

II. Interventions to maximize safety.

    A. Prevent aspiration by mechanical techniques.

        1. Elevate head of bed 45 to 90 degrees, with head slightly forward while eating and maintain position for 45 to 60 minutes after oral intake.

        2. Assist with moving food from front of tongue to posterior area using a long-handled spoon or a syringe as needed.

    B. Minimize swallowing difficulty by avoiding milk and milk products, alternating solids with liquids, and encouraging chewing thoroughly using the strongest side of the mouth.

    C. Explain all procedures before occurrence to decrease fear or anxiety associated with attempts to swallow and stay with client during feedings.

    D. Avoid small pieces of solids that can become lost in the mouth.

    E. Consult with dietitian to provide thickening agents to minimize aspiration.

    F. Utilize a variety of foods served in an appetizing way, in a progressive manner—pureed to ground to soft textured to all textures.

   III. Interventions to monitor complications related to dysphagia.
      A. Maintain daily food record.
      B. Weigh daily or at least every other day if daily weights upset client.
      C. Assess for signs and symptoms—dehydration, aspiration, increased/decreased secretions.
      D. Explore the need for alternative methods for providing nutrition, such as total parenteral nutrition (TPN); enteral feedings via percutaneous endoscopic gastrostomy (PEG); nasogastric (NG), low-profile gastrostomy; or percutaneous endoscopic jejunal access devices if oral intake is not possible via oral route.
      E. Elicit client's subjective reports of changes in patterns of dysphagia and measures that enhance or aggravate swallowing—room temperature foods versus cold or hot foods, consistency.
   IV. Interventions to involve client/family in care.
      A. Determine willingness of significant other to assist with care.
      B. Teach client/family all aspects of care, including emergency measures, pulmonary hygiene, oral hygiene, and appropriate time to report complications to a member of the health care team.
   V. Interventions to enhance adaptation.
      A. Provide ongoing support to client in a situation that may potentially cause fear, anxiety, and inability to cope.
      B. Provide detailed written and/or audiovisual materials.
      C. Initiate early referral to speech therapist and dietitian for nutritional advice and suggestions.
   VI. Interventions patients may use in addition to, or instead of, conventional treatments.
      A. Explore patient's awareness of and/or use of complementary/alternative medicine (CAM), such as mind/body control interventions, homeopathy, acupuncture, and vitamins or herbal products.
      B. Identify which methods are practiced, if they were used before cancer diagnosis or after diagnosis, and their feelings about effectiveness (see Chapters 11 and 41).

Evaluation

The oncology nurse systematically and regularly evaluates the client's and/or family's responses to interventions to determine progress toward the achievement of expected outcomes. Relevant data are collected, and actual findings are compared with expected findings. Nursing diagnoses, outcomes, and plans of care are reviewed and revised as necessary.

ANOREXIA

Theory

   I. Definition—loss of appetite accompanied by decreased food intake (Grant & Kravitz, 2000). May be insidious and may not be accompanied by obvious manifestations of disease other than progressive weight loss (Stepp & Pakiz, 2001).
   II. Etiology of anorexia.
      A. Physiologic factors (Grant & Kravitz, 2000).
         1. Presence of concurrent symptoms, including nausea/vomiting, early satiety, pain, dysphagia, mucositis, ascites, alterations in taste.

      2. Structural problems, such as abdominal tumor, structural changes caused by surgery and/or dental involvement.

      3. Metabolic disturbances, such as hypercalcemia, hypokalemia, uremia, hyponatremia.

      4. Medication side effects associated with narcotics, antibiotics, iron, and so on.

      5. Treatment-related effects from chemotherapy, RT, surgery, and biotherapy.

  B. Psychologic factors.

      1. Anxiety, depression, fear (Grant & Kravitz, 2000).

      2. Loss of previous pleasure associated with food (McGrath, 2002).

  C. Social factors (Grant & Kravitz, 2000).

      1. Changes in eating environment.

      2. Changes in companionship during eating.

III. Principles of medical management.

  A. Early detection and ongoing evaluation of nutritional status (Finley, 2000).

  B. Correct underlying cause, such as uncontrolled pain, mucositis, nausea/vomiting, gastroesophageal reflux (Stepp & Pakiz, 2001).

  C. Support with nutritional supplementation or replacement.

  D. Employ nursing interventions to minimize occurrence and severity.

IV. Sequelae of prolonged anorexia.

  A. Contributes to decreased calorie and protein intake with subsequent weight loss, weakness, fatigue (Stepp & Pakiz, 2001).

  B. Can lead to cachexia, which can affect prognosis by making client less tolerant of therapy, causing dose/schedule changes that may diminish treatment effectiveness (Stepp & Pakiz, 2001).

  C. Results in abnormalities of carbohydrate, protein, and fat metabolism.

  D. Visceral and lean body mass depletion—muscle atrophy, visceral organ atrophy, hypoalbuminemia (Stepp & Pakiz, 2001).

  E. Leads to compromised humoral and cellular immune function—impaired neutrophil function (chemotaxis, fungicidal, bactericidal) and delayed bone marrow replenishment of cells (Cunningham & Bell, 2000).

  F. Protein-calorie malnutrition interferes with the delivery of oncologic therapy and enhances the severity of side effects of treatment (Stepp & Pakiz, 2001).

Assessment

  I. History.

    A. Previous dietary patterns, food preferences, eating habits, and history of anorexia with client/family.

    B. Patterns of anorexia: onset, frequency, severity; associated symptoms—food intolerances, taste abnormalities, mouth/throat pain, dysphagia; other factors—precipitating, aggravating, alleviating factors.

    C. Previous self-care strategies.

      1. Ability to implement interventions to relieve anorexia.

      2. Use of food, nutritional supplements, and other remedies.

      3. Use of alternative or complementary nutritional products (Foltz, 2000).

    D. Current or recent treatment for cancer and anticipated side effects.

  II. Physical examination.

    A. Determine present weight and amount of total weight loss.

    B. Assess for presence of dehydration and/or electrolyte imbalances—dry mouth, poor skin turgor, decreased urinary output.

    C. Assess client for associated ethnic, socioeconomic, emotional, and motivational factors that may affect the loss of weight or decreased oral intake.

D. Assess psychosocial responses to fear, anxiety, depression and to noxious stimuli in the environment.

Nursing Diagnoses

I. Imbalanced nutrition: less than body requirements.
II. Risk for imbalanced fluid volume.
III. Risk for impaired skin integrity.
IV. Fatigue.
V. Deficient knowledge related to, for example, personal risk for complications caused by loss of appetite and adverse effects of cancer therapies on nutritional reserves.
VI. Risk for spiritual distress.
VII. Powerlessness.
VIII. Risk for caregiver role strain.

Outcome Identification

I. Client states the goals of interventions related to anorexia.
II. Client states the personal risk for complications related to loss of appetite and ways in which various cancer therapies may adversely affect nutritional reserves.
III. Client and family participate in measures to minimize risk of occurrence, severity, and complications of anorexia.
IV. Client's nutritional intake increases to appropriate calories needed to maintain weight.
V. Client states the changes in condition that require professional assistance and/or intervention.
  A. Weight loss of greater than 5% of body weight.
  B. Dehydration and/or inability to eat or drink.
  C. Changes in skin integrity and wound healing.
  D. Fever over 98.6° F (37° C), which increases the need for additional calories.
  E. Any other area of concern for client's well-being related to lack of food intake.
VI. Client and family state awareness of resources in the community to assist with nutrition.

Planning and Implementation

I. Implement nonpharmacologic interventions to increase calorie and nutritional value of oral intake. As noted by Finley (2000)—teach client/family to attempt the following:
  A. Consume nutritionally dense foods such as cottage cheese, puddings, oatmeal; eat frequently, in small portions throughout the day.
  B. Maximize food intake during periods of greatest strength and appetite, usually early in the day.
  C. Increase the kilocalorie (kcal) protein content of foods by adding instant nonfat dry milk powder or instant breakfast powders to gravies, puddings, other foods.
  D. Maximize food preferences and access to favorite foods within dietary restrictions.

   E. Choose high-protein, high-calorie, healthy snacks between meals.
   F. Try cold, room-temperature, and soft foods to improve intake.
   G. Give oral supplements to increase protein/calorie intake between meals and/or at bedtime.
   H. Limit liquids at mealtime because they may cause early satiety and nausea.
 II. Interventions to promote maximal comfort and ease while eating. Teach client/family to do the following:
   A. Administer pain medications, if needed, 30 to 60 minutes before meals.
   B. Assist with oral care, as needed, before and after meals.
   C. Plan activities according to client's activity level.
      1. Adequate rest period before meals.
      2. Encourage a short walk and fresh air before a meal to stimulate appetite.
   D. Minimize noxious stimuli in the environment.
III. Interventions to monitor complications related to anorexia. Stress the importance of the following:
   A. Maintaining a daily dietary intake record and weighing regularly.
   B. Assessing for signs and symptoms of electrolyte imbalances and dehydration.
   C. Assessing overall skin and nail condition for adverse effects of poor nutrition or intake—skin breakdown, dehiscence, or poor wound healing.
IV. Interventions to incorporate client/family in care.
   A. Encourage family to provide foods within dietary restrictions and to explore necessity of dietary restrictions when calorie/nutritional requirements are not being met as a result of restrictions (Bloch, 2000).
   B. Teach family methods to enhance calorie/protein content of foods and methods to enhance food intake.
      1. Provide a list of high-calorie, high-protein foods.
      2. Offer suggestions for supplementing nutritional value by adding powders and supplements.
      3. Use medications as ordered by physician—pain medications, vitamin supplements, medications that may stimulate appetite (e.g., megestrol acetate [Megace]).
      4. Plan mealtimes that are relaxed, unhurried, and pleasant.
      5. Encourage maintaining a positive eating environment by setting table attractively and avoiding eating from cartons or cans (Wickham, 2001).
      6. Utilize a variety of foods to avoid taste fatigue.
      7. Avoid fixating on intake to the point that it may become counterproductive.
   C. Teach client/family signs and symptoms of dehydration (dry skin and mucous membranes, poor skin turgor, decreased urinary output), delayed wound healing, malnutrition (wasting of skeletal mass, body fat decrease, weight loss, sepsis, decreased energy) and when to report critical symptoms to the treatment team.
   D. Develop a nurse/client contract for increasing the intake of calories/protein each day.
 V. Interventions to enhance adaptation and rehabilitation.
   A. Provide written and/or audiovisual materials on nutrition at the client's level of education and understanding.
   B. Initiate early referral to a dietitian for nutritional assessment/intervention, as indicated.
VI. Interventions patients may use in addition to or instead of conventional treatments (see Dysphagia, Planning and Implementation section, VI.).

Evaluation

The oncology nurse systematically and regularly evaluates the client's and/or family's responses to interventions to determine progress toward the achievement of expected outcomes. Relevant data are collected, and actual findings are compared with expected findings. Nursing diagnoses, outcomes, and plans of care are reviewed and revised as necessary.

MUCOSITIS/ESOPHAGITIS

Theory

I. Definition—a general term that describes the biologic response of the gastrointestinal (GI) mucosa to a physical or chemical assault that can occur on all surfaces of the GI tract from the mouth to the rectum. The mucosal tissue injury can result in changes in function, thinning, erythema, bleeding, exudate, inflammation, tissue sloughing, necrosis, and ulceration (Fulton et al., 2002). These cells readily renew when exposed to normal wear and tear but are unable to do so when toxicity (mucositis) results from cancer treatments.
- A. *Stomatitis* is mucositis or an inflammation and ulcerative reaction of the oral cavity (Miller & Kearney, 2001).
- B. *Esophagitis* is mucositis in the esophagus.
- C. *Gastroenteritis* is mucositis in the intestine.

II. Pathophysiology.
- A. Drugs interfere with DNA, RNA, or protein synthesis and cause destruction of cells that are rapidly proliferating. Cellular proliferation rates differ throughout the GI tract, which explains the difference in onset of symptoms related to toxicity.
  1. Small intestine proliferation rate is approximately 4 days versus 34 days for the dermis. Esophageal tissue is somewhere between these two (McGuire, 2002).
- B. As the host's marrow function becomes more suppressed, the damage is greater.
- C. Incidence and prevalence of tissue injury depend on many factors, including the diagnosis and treatment regimens for cancer.

III. Risk factors.
- A. Disease or host related.
  1. Infiltration of mucosal membranes of the GI tract by primary or metastatic tumor, contributing to the mucositis.
  2. Age of the patient, with those less than 20 years old having a higher risk than older patients.
  3. Type and location of tumor—frequency of oral problems two to three times higher in hematologic malignancies than solid tumors (Miller & Kearney, 2001).
- B. Treatment related.
  1. Damage is directly related to the dose and may be so severe that the cancer therapy must be stopped or interrupted.
  2. Can be acute, manifested by mucosal inflammation, ulceration, infection, and mucosal hemorrhage. Small intestine will show damage within a few days of cytotoxic exposure and large intestine a short while later (McGuire, 2002).

3. Can be chronic, manifested by changes in healthy tissues resulting from xerostomia, taste alterations, trismus (spasms and muscular fibrosis), and soft tissue and bone necrosis.
4. Drug administration—antineoplastic therapies exert both direct and indirect effects on the GI mucosal tissue.
   a. Chemotherapy attacks the stratified squamous nonkeratinizing epithelium of the oral mucosa. According to Miller and Kearney (2001), this results from one of two mechanisms: direct effects of a treatment on the oral mucosa, through interference with the proliferative ability of mucosal cells, called direct somatotoxicity, or indirect effect on salivary glands that causes damage to the permeable barrier that helps protect the mucosa from the invasion of microorganisms, called indirect somatotoxicity.
      (1) Mainly antimetabolites, antitumor antibiotics, and other miscellaneous drugs such as methotrexate (Mexate), fluorouracil (5-fluorouracil, 5-FU), cisplatin (Platinol), cytarabine (araC, cytosine arabinoside, Cytosar-U), etoposide (VP-16, Etopophos, VePesid), cyclophosphamide (Cytoxan), mechlorethamine (nitrogen mustard, Mustargen) vinblastine (Velban), vincristine (Oncovin), hydroxyurea (Hydrea, Mylocel), and procarbazine (Matulane), in which effects are dose related and cumulative. Oral mucositis occurs in approximately 40% of patients receiving "standard" dose chemotherapy and up to 70% in patients receiving higher doses seen with bone marrow transplantation (Borbasi et al., 2002).
      (2) Depends on the method of infusion; for example, continuous infusion schedules have greater negative effect than short infusions.
      (3) Correlates directly with the white blood cell nadir.
   b. Radiation therapy (RT)—according to Miller and Kearney (2001), radiation-induced damage to the mucosa differs from chemotherapy-induced damage in that the tissues from RT remain in jeopardy throughout the life of the patient.
      (1) Effects are greater when chest, abdomen, head and neck, and intestines are in the field, and
      (2) Are dose related; that is, higher doses of RT given to larger volumes over shorter periods increase the severity of mucositis.
      (3) Severity of mucositis is also related to the daily dose of RT, the total cumulative dose, and the volume of irradiated tissue (Loprinzi et al., 2000).
   c. Medications, such as antimicrobials and steroids.
   d. Oral graft-versus-host disease.
   e. Immunosuppression—cancer and cancer treatments decrease the body's immune system and alter protective barriers, such as oral mucous membranes.
C. Lifestyle related.
   1. Inadequate oral hygiene; periodontal disease.
   2. Exposure to irritants—chemical (citrus, spicy, mouthwashes, tobacco, alcohol) or physical (temperature extremes, poor-fitting prosthesis).
   3. Dehydration.
   4. Malnutrition.
   5. Age—frequency greater in younger than older age.
   6. Renal and hepatic dysfunction both alter drug metabolism.
   7. QOL, how well the patient is functioning.

IV. Principles of medical management.

A. Antimicrobial agents, growth factors, cytokines, coating agents, and antiinflammatory agents are the main modalities used in the treatment of radiation-induced oral mucositis (Shih et al., 2002). Antifungal and antiviral drugs are controversial.

B. Research is being directed at studying systems of drug delivery that can target specific regions or cells (McGuire, 2002).

C. The type of treatment needed to improve a cancer patient's nutrition is chosen based on the following factors:

1. Presence of a working GI tract.

2. Type of cancer therapy, such as where and how much surgery was done, type of chemotherapy, location and dose of RT, use of biologic response modifiers, and combinations of therapies used.

3. QOL and the expected outcome of the cancer.

D. Systemic therapy such as with acetaminophen or narcotics (e.g., opioids) and/or topical analgesics (e.g., lidocaine [Xylocaine] solutions, dyclonine [Cepacol, Sucrets], UlcerEase, sucralfate [Carafate], vitamin E).

E. Systemic and/or local antiinflammatory agents, such as nonsteroidal antiinflammatory agents and/or antacids.

F. Topical protective and coating agents, such as sucralfate suspension (Carafate), benzocaine (Orabase, Oratect-gel, Hurricaine), and lidocaine (Zilactin).

G. Cryotherapy (ice) before and during administration of specific chemotherapy agents serves as a prevention method to decrease drug exposure to the oral mucosa (Loprinzi et al., 2000).

H. Dietary and vitamin supplements, such as oral liquid supplements that contain soy proteins, have been found to improve total energy/protein consumption (Brown, 2002).

I. Biologic response modifiers—prostaglandin E_2, interleukin, fibronectin, immunoglobulin, β-carotene, and epidermal growth factors. Antidiarrheal medications, Tucks, compresses, and sitz baths.

J. Problem-specific approaches—xerostomia, taste changes, anorexia, hemorrhage (thrombin-soaked collagen gauzes with ice and/or vasoconstricting agents).

V. Potential sequelae of prolonged mucositis/esophagitis.

A. Impaired integrity of the mucous membranes.

B. Infection, pain, ulceration, bleeding.

C. Difficulty swallowing and speaking.

D. Inadequate nutritional intake and/or absorption leading to nutritional deficits, weight loss, and potential malnutrition and wasting. Complications related to nutritional replacement can occur.

E. Diarrhea.

F. Bleeding/hemorrhage.

Assessment

Distinguish between drug-induced mucositis and infection.

I. History.

A. Previous therapy for cancer.

B. Medications that affect nutrition.

C. Chemical and/or physical exposure.

D. Routine oral hygiene practices.

E. Assessment of weight history, such as measuring the percentage (%) of weight change from usual body weight (by dividing the current measured weight by the usual weight and multiplying by 100). This percent should be evaluated for difference from the preillness, prediagnosis, and after-diagnosis weights. Weight loss of 2% to 5% is considered severe (McMahon & Brown, 2000).

F. Changes in eating/drinking and how long changes have lasted.

G. Symptoms affecting eating/drinking, for example, nausea/vomiting, diarrhea, constipation, sores in the mouth, dry mouth, taste and smell changes.

H. Other illness that can affect nutrition.

I. Assess likes and dislikes.

J. Patterns of mucositis—incidence; frequency; precipitating, alleviating, and aggravating factors.

K. Overall pattern of mucositis along the entire GI tract.

L. Impact of stomatitis/mucositis on lifestyle, comfort, nutrition, activities of daily living, QOL, and mental attitude.

M. Assess patient's level of functioning.

N. Assess if there is prolonged neutropenia where metabolic needs may increase 25% with a body temperature of 102° F (38.9° C) (National Cancer Institute [NCI], 2002b).

II. Physical examination.

A. Utilize an oral assessment tool and grading scale on an ongoing basis so that changes can be consistently qualified as they occur and compared with the baseline assessment. Approach depends on severity. According to McGuire (2002), there are, however, no instruments for the assessment of GI mucosal injury.

1. As many as 12 different tools to assess the oral cavity exist in the literature.

2. Institutions should choose one and use it exclusively and consistently, at least every 24 hours.

3. The National Cancer Institute has adopted a Common Toxicity Criteria scale (Rogers, 2001). In general the grades are as follows:

Grade 0   None.
Grade 1   Soreness and erythema of oral mucosa. No ulcers.
Grade 2   Painful erythema, edema, or ulcers but able to eat.
Grade 3   Painful erythema, edema, or ulcers but only able to drink.
Grade 4   Severe ulceration and unable to eat or drink, requiring parenteral or enteral nutritional support or prophylactic intubation.

B. Be alert to timing of complications in relation to the chemotherapy and/or RT.

1. For example, complaints of mucous membrane burning by client within 3 to 10 days of chemotherapy frequently precede objective signs. May develop erythema and progress to erosion/ulceration over the next 3 to 5 days.

2. Neutropenic patients frequently are found to have mucosal ulcerations infected by *Candida* sp. throughout the GI tract but are often asymptomatic (Bodkey, 2000).

C. Examine and palpate the oral cavity and throat for redness, swelling, presence of white patches, shiny appearance, pain or burning, decreased or increased salivation, and presence of sensation changes.

D. Observe for inflammation of all mucous membranes—anorectal area, stomal, vaginal.

  E. Assess weight loss, loss of fat under skin, muscle wasting, fluid collection in the legs, and the presence of ascites.
  F. Be alert to the timing of complications in relation to the chemotherapy and/or RT treatments.

Nursing Diagnoses

See diagnoses listed in Xerostomia section. Nursing diagnoses related to mucositis/esophagitis in addition to those listed in Xerostomia section include the following:
  I. Deficient fluid volume.
  II. Diarrhea.
  III. Acute pain.
  IV. Anxiety.
  V. Disturbed body image.

Outcome Identification

  I. Client describes personal risk factors for mucositis/esophagitis.
  II. Client and family list signs, symptoms, and complications of mucositis/esophagitis to observe for and to report to the health care team.
  III. Client discusses measures to minimize risk of occurrence, severity, complications of mucositis, and the importance of daily assessment and an oral care regimen that fits the condition of the oral cavity.
  IV. Client and family list situations that require professional assistance and intervention.
    A. Temperature elevations greater than 101° F (38.3° C).
    B. Significant decrease in oral intake.
    C. Poorly controlled pain or diarrhea, such as more than five stools per day.

Planning and Implementation

  I. Provide information before cancer treatments in order to optimize the efficiency in managing oral mucositis. Stress importance of the following:
    A. Regular dental care.
    B. Consistent oral assessments.
    C. Initiation of a standardized oral hygiene program.
  II. Interventions to minimize the risk of occurrence and severity of mucositis.
    A. Nonpharmacologic measures to decrease inflammation of mucous membranes.
      1. Encourage oral and perineal hygiene measures.
      2. Encourage fluid intake of greater than 3000 ml/day, if tolerated.
      3. Avoid exposures to chemical and physical irritants.
    B. Measures to increase comfort.
      1. Use topical protective agents, such as a benzocaine magnesium hydroxide rinse.
      2. Increase frequency of oral hygiene, depending on grade of mucositis, use of appropriate cleansing devices according to extent of mucosal involvement/pain.
      3. Use rinses (normal saline, salt and baking soda [½ teaspoon each in 1 cup of warm water], hydrogen peroxide [3% solution], antimicrobial solutions [e.g., Peridex]).
      4. Give systemic or topical analgesics, such as viscous lidocaine, local diphenhydramine hydrochloride suspension, and/or benzydamine

hydrochloride, a nonsteroidal antiinflammatory agent that possesses analgesic, anesthetic, antiinflammatory, and antimicrobial properties (Loprinzi et al., 2000).
    5. Encourage sitz baths.
  C. Measures to decrease risk of complications of mucositis/esophagitis.
    1. Modify intake to bland, soft, liquid, high-calorie, high-protein foods.
    2. Use of amifostine (Ethyol) (acts as a radioprotector), as appropriate, when RT is used.
    3. Encourage oral assessment daily and a systematic oral care regimen consisting of cleansing, lubricating, and coating, because systematic performance (compliance) is of more value than the actual agents used.
    4. Discourage sexual intercourse and douching during the inflammatory stage of mucositis, and encourage meticulous perineal care.
III. Interventions to monitor client response to symptom management.
  A. Monitor client's subjective reports of changes in the pattern of mucositis.
  B. Monitor changes in level of comfort.
  C. Monitor changes in integrity of the mucous membranes.
  D. Monitor compliance with measures to decrease severity of mucositis and to reduce the incidence of complications.
IV. Interventions to incorporate client/family in care.
  A. Teach oral and perineal hygiene measures.
  B. Teach signs and symptoms of infection, impaired skin integrity, and complications to report to the health care team.
    1. Temperature elevations above 101° F (38.3° C).
    2. Significant changes in nutritional intake.
    3. Poorly controlled symptom management—diarrhea, discomfort.
  C. Explore ways to enhance QOL issues that affect patient comfort, appetite, communication, and general well-being (Shih et al., 2002).
 V. Interventions patients may use in addition to or instead of conventional treatments (see Dysphagia, Planning and Implementation section, VI.).

Evaluation

The oncology nurse systematically and regularly evaluates the client's and/or family's responses to interventions to determine progress toward the achievement of expected outcomes. Relevant data are collected, and actual findings are compared with expected findings. Nursing diagnoses, outcomes, and plans of care are reviewed and revised as necessary.

XEROSTOMIA

Theory

  I. Definition—a subjective sensation of dryness in the mouth characterized by a decrease in composition and physical properties in the quality and quantity of saliva (Miller & Kearney, 2001).
 II. Pathophysiology—result of cytotoxic therapy on the oral mucosa that causes atrophy and fibrosis of the salivary glands (Miller & Kearney, 2001).
III. Risk factors and etiology.
  A. Disease related.
    1. Primary tumor involvement of the salivary/parotid glands.
    2. Metastatic tumor involvement of salivary glands.

3. Other diseases or conditions—diabetes, infection, candidiasis, Sjögren's syndrome, obsessive-compulsive and anxiety states.
B. Treatment related.
   1. Surgical removal of salivary glands.
   2. Pharmacologic therapy for symptom management, such as antihistamines, decongestants, anticholinergics, diuretics, antidepressants, opioids, and phenothiazines, that can contribute to the problem.
   3. RT effects.
      a. Can be transient or prolonged, leading to dental caries, taste dysfunction, mucosal lesions, pain, and *Candida* or other fungal infections.
      b. Symptoms develop within first to second week of therapy, causing the mouth to become dry with thick, ropy saliva that is directly proportional to the amount of radiation dose (Gy) given. As dose and percentage of tissue irradiated increase, damage to tissues increases. As dose increases, there is a reduction in salivary flow rates, pH, and secretory immunoglobulin A (IgA) (Turnkel et al., 2000).
C. Lifestyle related—alcohol, caffeine, nicotine ingestion, and ingestion of drugs that may also decrease the flow of saliva. Examples may include anorexic agents, anticholinergics, antidepressants, antihistamines, antihypertensives, antipsychotics, antiparkinson agents, diuretics, hypnotics, and sedatives (Turnkel et al., 2000).
D. Age—young are more likely to recover salivary flow than older adults.
IV. Principles of medical management.
   A. Artificial saliva/lubricants.
   B. Surgical interventions—salivary reservoirs and reconstruction with a mandibular denture.
   C. Dental prophylaxis with frequent cleaning and fluoride treatments before, during, and after radiation treatments.
   D. Prophylactic oral antimicrobial therapy.

Assessment

I. History.
   A. Previous therapy for cancer.
   B. Prescription and nonprescription medications and supplements (e.g., vitamins and mineral supplements).
   C. Pattern of xerostomia—incidence, frequency, alleviating and aggravating factors.
   D. Impact of xerostomia on food taste, intake, swallowing, digestion, and communication as well as psychosocial response to condition.
II. Physical examination.
   A. Dry, shiny mucous membranes of oral cavity.
   B. Thick, ropy, and/or scant saliva.
   C. Difficulty swallowing, chewing, and communicating.
III. Laboratory findings—decreased pH of oral secretions.
IV. Psychosocial examination—presence of fear and/or anxiety.

Nursing Diagnoses

I. Impaired oral mucous membrane.
II. Ineffective protection.
III. Impaired swallowing.

   IV. Risk for infection.
    V. Impaired verbal communication.
  VI. Disturbed sensory perception: gustatory.
 VII. Imbalanced nutrition: less than body requirements.

Outcome Identification

    I. Client describes personal risk factors for development of xerostomia.
   II. Client states signs, symptoms, and complications of xerostomia and participates in interventions that may prevent or alter severity of symptoms/complications.
 III. Client and family list changes that require professional assistance in management—infection, lesions or ulcerations of the oral cavity, dental caries, and unintentional weight loss greater than 5% of body weight.

Planning and Implementation

  I. Interventions to minimize the risk of occurrence and severity of xerostomia.
    A. Measures to increase salivary flow by stimulating residual parenchyma.
      1. Offer sialagogues (agents that affect salivary glands).
        a. Tart sugar-free lemon candies, ice, fresh pineapple.
        b. Salivary enzyme products (e.g., Biotene sugarless gum, toothpaste and mouthwash containing xylitol).
        c. Pilocarpine (Salagen), a systemic parasympathomimetic, has been studied and used to reduce the severity of xerostomia and salivary dysfunction by stimulating remaining salivary gland function. Doses of 5 mg orally three or four times daily, up to 10 mg three times per day maximum (Loprinzi et al., 2000).
    B. Measures to provide moisture to the oral mucosa.
      1. Moisten foods with liquids, milk, or gravies.
      2. Sip liquids with and between meals at frequent intervals.
      3. Increase intake to 8 glasses of liquid per day unless contraindicated.
      4. Use artificial saliva that contains mucin (e.g., Mouthkote, Xerlube, Mostir, Salivert).
      5. Ice chips, Popsicles, effervescent vitamin C, citric acid (except when receiving RT) malic acid, pilocarpine (Miller & Kearney, 2001).
      6. Use room humidifier and/or humidified face mask at night. Use of hyperthermic humidification may show some promise (Criswell & Sinha, 2001).
      7. Utilize protective enzymes present in some foods.
        a. Papain, which is found in papaya juice.
        b. Amylase, present in pineapples (use frozen to minimize stinging).
        c. Meat tenderizer, which helps dissolve and break up thick saliva (swab mouth before meals).
      8. Lubricate mucosa with ⅛ teaspoon of butter or vegetable or corn oil before meals, starting 2 to 3 weeks after radiation is complete.
      9. Use lip balm.
    10. Nonpharmacologic measures.
        a. Acupuncture has been shown to increase salivary flow and feelings of well-being (Miller & Kearney, 2001).
        b. Acupressure. Application of physical techniques tailored to client preference, such as neck massage and/or pressure on the sternal notch.

        c. Psychotherapy to aid in pain relief.

        d. Hypnosis.

        e. Relaxation techniques.

        f. Imagery training.

        g. Therapist's support.

  C. Measures to decrease risk of complications of xerostomia.

     1. Make frequent assessments because early detection and prevention are key.

     2. Encourage meticulous oral hygiene with mechanical and chemical debridement of accumulated plaque and microorganisms at regular intervals at least before and after each meal—every 2 hours is ideal.

     3. Avoid physical, chemical, and thermal irritants, such as poorly fitting dental prosthetics, hydrogen peroxide, alcohol, tobacco, commercial mouthwashes, and food items such as dry, bulky, spicy, and acidic foods.

 II. Interventions to monitor for complications related to xerostomia.

  A. Examine oral cavity daily. Observe lips, tongue, buccal area membranes, throat/swallow, roof/floor of mouth, saliva, and voice quality.

  B. Encourage periodic dental examinations.

  C. Seek prompt and appropriate medical treatment if infection develops.

III. Interventions patients may use in addition to or instead of conventional treatments (see Dysphagia, Planning and Implementation section, VI).

Evaluation

The oncology nurse systematically and regularly evaluates the client's and/or family's responses to interventions to determine progress toward the achievement of expected outcomes. Relevant data are collected, and actual findings are compared with expected findings. Nursing diagnoses, outcomes, and plans of care are reviewed and revised as necessary.

NAUSEA

Theory

  I. Definition—a highly subjective, unobservable phenomenon of an unpleasant sensation experienced in the back of the throat and the epigastrium that may or may not culminate in vomiting. One of the most feared side effects of cancer treatment (Finley, 2000). Nausea and/or vomiting occurs when the vomiting center (VC), a group of neurons in the brainstem, is stimulated by various incoming pathways (Wickham, 2001). The chemoreceptor trigger zone (CTZ) is located near the VC in the fourth ventricle, outside of the blood-brain barrier. The CTZ detects drugs and other substances in the blood and central nervous system (CNS), causing release of neurotransmitters that stimulates the VC (Wickham, 2001).

 II. The following risk factors represent many ways that the VC becomes activated.

  A. Disease related.

     1. Primary or metastatic tumor of the CNS that includes the VC, or increased intracranial pressure (Grant & Kravitz, 2000).

     2. Delayed gastric emptying (Grant & Kravitz, 2000).

     3. Obstruction of a portion of the GI tract.

     4. Food toxins, infection, or motion sickness.

5. Metabolic abnormalities, such as hyperglycemia, hyponatremia, hypercalcemia, and/or renal or hepatic dysfunction (Grant & Kravitz, 2000).
- **B.** Treatment related.
    1. Stimulation of the receptors of the labyrinth in the inner ear.
    2. Obstruction, irritation, inflammation, and delayed gastric emptying stimulating the GI tract through vagal visceral afferent pathways.
    3. Stimulation of the VC through mucosal injury causing release of serotonin associated with chemotherapy (Hesketh, 2000).
    4. Stimulation of the VC through afferent pathways from RT of the GI tract.
    5. Side effects of medications, such as digitalis, morphine, antibiotics, iron, vitamins, and antineoplastic agents, such as cisplatin (Platinol), mechlorethamine (nitrogen mustard, Mustargen), and dacarbazine (DTIC-Dome).
    6. Side effects of concentrated nutritional supplements.
- **C.** Situational.
    1. Younger age; increased incidence in those less than 50 years (Marchioro et al., 2000).
    2. Experienced by females more than males (Marchioro et al., 2000).
    3. Increased levels of stress, emotions, and/or anxiety (Marchioro et al., 2000).
    4. Noxious odors or visual stimuli.
    5. Conditioned (anticipatory) responses to previous cancer treatment and/or other stressful experiences (Finley, 2000). Occurs in 25% of chemotherapy patients.
- **III.** Principles of medical management.
    - **A.** Treatment of underlying disease.
    - **B.** Antiemetic therapy (Rosenthal, 2001).
        1. Serotonin antagonists (e.g., ondansetron [Zofran], granisetron [Kytril], dolasetron [Anzemet]); used alone or in combination with steroids.
        2. Dopamine receptor antagonists, such as metoclopramide (Reglan), haloperidol (Haldol), droperidol (Inapsine).
        3. Phenothiazines, such as prochlorperazine (Compazine), chlorpromazine (Thorazine).
        4. Corticosteroids, such as dexamethasone (Decadron); most effective when paired with serotonin antagonists.
        5. Benzodiazepines, such as lorazepam (Ativan); most effective when combined with other agents.
        6. Cannabinoids, such as dronabinol (Marinol) and nabilone (Cesamet).
    - **C.** Nonpharmacologic interventions.
        1. Relaxation and distraction techniques, including guided imagery and music therapy (Finley, 2000).
        2. Acupressure—may decrease symptom experience and/or intensity of nausea (Dibble et al., 2000).
        3. Acupuncture (Finley, 2000).
        4. Hypnosis—Marchioro et al. (2000) found a complete response to anticipatory nausea and a major response to chemotherapy-induced nausea.
        5. Foot massage—Grealish et al. (2000) found that foot massage had a significant impact on reducing feelings of nausea.
        6. Deep breathing (Grant & Kravitz, 2000).
        7. Exposure to fresh air and elimination of odors (Grant & Kravitz, 2000).

8. Herbal supplements—ginger (dried or fresh) has been known to have an effect on decreasing nausea associated with chemotherapy (Wickham, 2001).
9. Aromatherapy—the use of scented candles, essential oils, and sachets is currently being researched (Ott, 2002).
    D. Management of concurrent symptoms, such as fatigue and pain (Grant & Kravitz, 2000).
IV. Potential sequelae of prolonged nausea.
    A. Vomiting.
    B. Taste changes, development of food aversions (Wickham, 2001).
    C. Anorexia with resultant weight loss, fluid and electrolyte imbalances, dehydration.
    D. Noncompliance or refusal to complete treatment plan (Hesketh, 2000).
    E. Altered QOL (Hesketh, 2000).

Assessment

I. History.
    A. Presence of risk factors for nausea, including a history of motion sickness or pregnancy-induced nausea (Grant & Kravitz, 2000).
    B. Presence of defining characteristics of nausea.
    C. Present symptoms, client's perception of possible correlation between occurrence of nausea and distress; and perceived meaning of nausea to the client and family, work, role responsibilities, and mood.
    D. Patterns of nausea—onset, frequency, associated symptoms, precipitating factors, aggravating factors, and alleviating factors. Assess client's previous experiences with nausea (Grant & Kravitz, 2000).
II. Physical examination.
    A. Signs of sweating, tachycardia, dizziness, pallor, excessive salivation, and weakness.
    B. Laboratory reports to assess for other causes—serum electrolytes, liver and renal function tests.
    C. Weight.
III. Psychosocial assessment.
    A. Explore anxiety-producing events and coping abilities.
    B. Attempt to identify strengths of client/family.

Nursing Diagnoses

I. Nausea.
II. Imbalanced nutrition: less than body requirements.
III. Risk for imbalanced fluid volume.
IV. Ineffective coping.
V. Risk for spiritual distress.

Outcome Identification

I. Client describes personal risk for nausea.
II. Client participates in measures to minimize the risk of occurrence of nausea.
III. Client demonstrates competence in self-care techniques for management of nausea.
IV. Client and family list changes in the condition of the client that require professional assistance in management.

    A. Presence of unrelieved nausea and/or inability to eat and drink.

    B. Weight loss greater than 5% of body weight.

    C. Presence of signs and symptoms of dehydration.

Planning and Implementation

  I. Interventions to minimize the risk of occurrence, severity, or complications of nausea.

    A. Individualize drug regimen according to emetic potential of chemotherapy, expected duration of nausea and vomiting, and current pattern of symptoms.

    B. Modify the environment—cool, well ventilated, lowered lighting and noise levels, absence of noxious sights and smells (Rosenthal, 2001).

    C. Modify diet to include bland, chilled foods with liquids served separately.

    D. Avoid movement and reclining within first 30 minutes after eating.

    E. Replace fluids with Popsicles, sports drinks (e.g., Gatorade), and frozen fruit or yogurt bars.

    F. Administer antiemetics around the clock until the nausea cycle is broken.

    G. Encourage nonpharmacologic treatments, such as those listed in the treatment section.

  II. Interventions to maximize safety.

    A. Position during vomiting episodes, if they occur, to reduce risk of aspiration.

    B. Anticipate needs as a result of weakness and/or sedative effects of antiemetics and provide assistance with ambulation, using raised side rails and emesis basin within reach.

 III. Interventions to monitor for complications of nausea.

    A. Observe for signs of dehydration, electrolyte imbalance, and profound loss of weight in a short time frame.

    B. Observe for side effects that may be associated with antiemetic therapy.

  IV. Interventions to incorporate client/family in care.

    A. Teach positioning techniques to decrease risk of aspiration.

    B. Teach home management techniques to avoid or minimize emetic events, including use of medications around the clock, portable infusion devices, and combining medications for maximal effect.

    C. Encourage the use of self-care diaries and logs to record frequency and severity of nausea and response to therapies.

    D. Teach importance of reporting critical changes in client condition to the treatment team, including presence of adverse or intensified pattern of vomiting; signs and symptoms of aspiration, dehydration, or other pathologic condition.

    E. Instruct client/family on use of nonpharmacologic interventions, such as those listed in the treatment section.

    F. Instruct client/family to recognize concurrent symptoms, such as pain or fatigue, that may increase the experience of nausea.

  V. Interventions patients may use in addition to or instead of conventional treatments (see Dysphagia, Planning and Implementation section, VI).

Evaluation

The oncology nurse systematically and regularly evaluates the client's and/or family's responses to interventions to determine progress toward the achievement of expected outcomes. Relevant data are collected, and actual findings are compared with expected findings. Nursing diagnoses, outcomes, and plans of care are reviewed and revised as necessary.

VOMITING

Theory

I. Definition—a somatic process performed by the respiratory muscles causing a forceful oral expulsion of gastric, duodenal, or jejunal contents through the mouth.
   A. With chemotherapy treatment: can be acute, within 24 hours of chemotherapy; delayed, begins 24 hours after chemotherapy; or anticipatory, a conditioned response associated with prior chemotherapy administration (Hesketh, 2000).

II. Pathophysiology—the VC, located in the brainstem, is directly activated by the visceral and vagal afferent pathways from the GI tract, the CTZ, vestibular apparatus, and the cerebral cortex. Chemotherapy, RT, and other toxins cause cellular damage to the GI mucosa. The damaged mucosa causes the enterochromaffin cells in the GI tract to release serotonin locally, resulting in activation of 5HT3 receptors on the visceral afferent fibers in the vagus nerve, which in turn induces impulses to areas in the medulla responsible for vomiting (Hesketh, 2000).

III. Risk factors.
   A. Disease related.
      1. Primary or metastatic tumor of the CNS.
      2. Increased intracranial pressure from tumor or hemorrhage.
      3. GI or biliary obstruction.
      4. Metabolic abnormalities such as hypercalcemia, hyponatremia.
      5. Renal or hepatic dysfunction.
      6. Food toxins, infection, or motion sickness.
   B. Treatment related.
      1. Stimulation of the VC and the CTZ by cancer therapies.
      2. Cellular damage to the enterochromaffin cells by chemotherapy (Hesketh, 2000).
      3. RT to the intradiaphragmatic area.
      4. Severity of vomiting is influenced by the emetic potential of the chemotherapy drugs that are administered.
      5. Side effects of medications—digitalis, morphine, antibiotics, vitamins, iron, narcotics.
      6. Side effects of concentrated nutritional supplements.
   C. Situational.
      1. Increased levels of tension, stress, and/or anxiety.
      2. Noxious odors or visual stimuli.
      3. Conditioned (anticipatory) responses to poor previous emetic control.
      4. Being young, less than 50 years old (Marchioro et al., 2000).
      5. Being female (Marchioro et al., 2000).
      6. History of motion sickness and/or pregnancy-induced nausea/vomiting (Wickham, 2001).

IV. Principles of medical management (see Nausea, Theory section).

V. Potential sequelae of prolonged vomiting.
   A. Fluid and electrolyte imbalances.
   B. Anorexia with resultant weight loss.
   C. Esophageal tears and/or aspiration.
   D. Noncompliance or refusal to complete treatment plan (Hesketh, 2000).
   E. Altered QOL (Hesketh, 2000).

Assessment

I. History.
   A. Presence of risk factors for vomiting or actual episodes of emesis.
   B. Character of emesis.
   C. Present symptoms, client's perception of possible correlation between occurrence of vomiting and stress, and the perceived meaning of vomiting to the client/family, work, role responsibilities, and mood.
   D. Patterns of vomiting—onset, frequency, associated symptoms, precipitating factors, aggravating factors, alleviating factors.
II. Physical examination.
   A. Observe for sweating, tachycardia, dizziness, pallor, excessive salivation, weakness, increased blood pressure, and decreased muscle strength.
   B. Monitor laboratory reports to assess other causes—serum electrolytes, liver and renal function tests.
   C. Monitor weight.
III. Psychosocial assessment.
   A. Explore anxiety-producing events and coping abilities.
   B. Attempt to identify strengths of client and significant others.

Nursing Diagnoses

See Nausea, Nursing Diagnoses section. Nursing diagnoses related to vomiting in addition to those listed for nausea include the following:
I. Risk for aspiration.
II. Fatigue.
III. Risk for injury.

Outcome Identification

I. Client describes personal risk for vomiting related to potential causes and timing of episodes related to chemotherapy and RT.
II. Client self-medicates with antiemetics to minimize the risk of occurrence, severity, and complications of vomiting.
III. Client performs safety measures to avoid injury related to the effects of vomiting.
IV. Client and family list changes in the condition of the client that require professional assistance in management.
   A. Changes in amount or presence of blood, or lack of relief from antiemetics.
   B. Weight loss greater than 5% of body weight.
   C. Presence of signs and symptoms of dehydration.
V. Family or significant others involve themselves in distraction and relaxation techniques, including guided imagery, to assist client (Finley, 2000).

Planning and Implementation

See Nausea, Planning and Implementation section.

Evaluation

The oncology nurse systematically and regularly evaluates the client's and/or family's responses to interventions to determine progress toward the achievement of

expected outcomes. Relevant data are collected, and actual findings are compared with expected findings. Nursing diagnoses, outcomes, and plans of care are reviewed and revised as necessary.

TASTE ALTERATIONS

Theory

   I. Definition—an actual or perceived change in taste sensation or loss of taste.

     A. Hypogeusesthesia—a decrease in the acuity of the taste sensation.

     B. Dysgeusia—an unusual taste perception, perceived as unpleasant.

     C. Ageusia—an absence of the taste sensation, "mouth blindness."

   II. Pathophysiology, etiology, and risk factors.

     A. Disease related.

       1. Excretion of amino acid–like substances from the tumor cells, which changes taste bud sensations (sweet, sour, bitter, salty).

       2. Invasion of tumor into the oral cavity or salivary glands.

       3. Oral infections—for example, candidiasis.

     B. Treatment related.

       1. Specific surgical sites—oral cavity, tongue, salivary glands, pathway of the olfactory nerve, tracheostomy.

       2. Radiation induced—changes in salivation usually precede mucositis.

         a. Destruction of the taste buds occurs at doses greater than 1 Gy at about day 10 to 14 and persists for 14 to 21 days. Taste is nonexistent by the third or fourth week and may never return to normal (Loprinzi et al., 2000).

         b. Saliva can become thick/tenacious early, and membranes may become dry at about day 10 to 14; condition may continue for 2 to 4 months. Club soda has been shown to be effective in thinning viscous secretions.

       3. Chemotherapy induced.

         a. Certain drugs have greater effect on taste sensation than others—for example, cisplatin (Platinol), cyclophosphamide (Cytoxan), dacarbazine (DTIC-Dome), dactinomycin (actinomycin D, Cosmegen), mechlorethamine (nitrogen mustard, Mustargen), methotrexate (Mexate), vincristine (Oncovin), and fluorouracil (5-FU, 5-fluorouracil).

         b. Taste alterations include the following:

           (1) Constant or intermittent metallic and bitter taste sensations.

           (2) Increased or decreased threshold for the sweetness sensation, increased threshold for salty and sour tastes, usually decreased threshold for bitter taste.

           (3) Aversion to meats.

     C. Lifestyle related.

       1. Poor oral hygiene.

       2. Nutritional deficiencies—zinc, copper, nickel, niacin, vitamin A.

     D. Developmental.

       1. Age-induced degeneration of the taste buds.

       2. Learned aversions.

         a. Taste changes or aversions that develop when a food is in association with unpleasant symptoms, such as nausea and vomiting and pain.

         b. Seem to develop most rapidly to new or novel foods.

  III. Principles of medical management.

    A. Nutritional replacement supplements.

    B. Experimentation with different combinations to mask or improve taste.

IV. Potential consequences to taste alterations.

    A. Anorexia—mainly caused by decreased intake, decreased quality of foods consumed, decreased volume of saliva and gastric secretions, which are necessary for effective digestion to take place.

    B. Decreased intake because of food aversion that can persist up to 1 year after therapy.

    C. Altered or perverted sense of taste, causing many clients to refuse meats, fish, poultry, eggs, tomatoes, and fried foods, which can lead to protein-calorie malnutrition and weight loss.

Assessment

I. History.

    A. Presence of hypogeusesthesia, ageusia, or dysgeusia.

    B. History of risk factors, including degree and duration of taste alterations.

    C. Subjective description of changes in taste and impact of taste alterations on the nutritional status and usual lifestyle patterns.

II. Physical examination.

    A. Oral assessment.

        1. Evaluate oral cavity and throat for presence of erythema, desquamation, dryness or excess saliva, and/or ulceration.

        2. Observe for signs and symptoms of secondary oral infection.

    B. Weight.

    C. Presence of other physical problems associated with altered intake.

III. Laboratory findings associated with compromised nutritional status.

    A. Decreased levels of albumin, transferrin, and total lymphocytes.

    B. Decreased levels of zinc, copper, and nickel.

    C. Decreased levels of niacin and vitamin A.

Nursing Diagnoses

I. Imbalanced nutrition: less than body requirements.

II. Impaired oral mucous membranes.

III. Disturbed sensory perception: olfactory, gustatory.

IV. Dysfunctional grieving.

Outcome Identification

I. Client states the goal of interventions related to taste alterations.

II. Client describes the personal risk for changes in taste sensations.

III. Client reports signs and symptoms related to taste alterations to health care team.

IV. Client uses the appropriate interventions to achieve and maintain optimal nutrition.

V. Client uses interventions to minimize the degree and duration of taste alterations.

Planning and Implementation

I. Interventions to minimize risk of occurrence and severity of taste alterations.

    A. Institute measures to increase sensitivity of taste buds.

        1. Experiment with spices and flavorings to enhance taste.

    2. Use the aroma of foods to stimulate taste.

    3. Increase fluid intake with meals.

    4. Encourage oral hygiene before and after meals.

    5. Use amifostine (Ethyol) with RT, as appropriate, to possibly prevent taste loss caused by RT.

  B. Institute nonpharmacologic measures to decrease aversion to certain foods.

    1. Add increased sweeteners to foods; marinate meats in sweet juices.

    2. Substitute other sources of protein for poorly tolerated foods.

    3. Avoid the sight and smell of foods causing unpleasantness.

    4. Consume candies such as lemon drops and/or chew gum to change taste before meals and before chemotherapy treatment to reduce metallic taste.

  C. Institute nonpharmacologic measures to increase salivation.

    1. Increase water or juices at frequent intervals—for example, several times per hour.

    2. Spray water, saline, or artificial saliva on the mucous membranes.

    3. Have client suck on smooth flat tart candies or lozenges to stimulate saliva.

    4. Have client avoid alcohol, commercial mouthwashes, and smoking.

    5. Humidify the environmental air.

II. Interventions to monitor for complications related to taste alterations.

  A. Weigh at regular intervals.

  B. Maintain a daily diet record.

  C. Teach clients the importance of diligent oral care and inspection and in which situations they should access the health care team.

III. Interventions to incorporate client and family in care (see Anorexia, Planning and Implementation section).

IV. Interventions patients may use in addition to or instead of conventional treatments (see Dysphagia, Planning and Implementation section, VI).

Evaluation

The oncology nurse systematically and regularly evaluates the client's and/or family's responses to interventions to determine progress toward the achievement of expected outcomes. Relevant data are collected, and actual findings are compared with expected findings. Nursing diagnoses, outcomes, and plans of care are reviewed and revised as necessary.

ELECTROLYTE IMBALANCES

Theory

  I. Tumor or treatment-related metabolic disturbances frequently occur in clients with cancer.

  II. Calcium (Ca^{++}) imbalances.

    A. Usual reference range: 4.5 to 5.5 mEq/L, or 8.5 to 10.5 mg/dl.

    B. Calcium is the fifth most abundant inorganic element in body, found in bone and teeth, with 99% in the form of insoluble crystals and 1% distributed between the body's intracellular and extracellular fluids; 45% to 50% is ionized in the serum (the active form), 40% bound by protein, and 10% to 15% found in insoluble complexes (Wickham, 2000).

      1. Ionized Ca^{++}—necessary for excitation of nerves, action of voluntary skeletal muscles, cardiac muscle, and involuntary muscles of the gut.

a. If the body has too much ionized Ca^{++}, there is decreased excitability of these tissues (hypercalcemia: serum calcium >11 mg/dl).
   b. If there is too little ionized Ca^{++}, there is increased excitability of nerves and muscles (hypocalcemia: serum calcium <8.5 mg/dl).
2. Since 40% of the Ca^{++} outside the bone and teeth is bound to albumin, it is important to correct value of ionized Ca^{++} in the serum if albumin is low.
C. Pathophysiology of calcium imbalances.
   1. Hypercalcemia—most frequently seen with cancers of the breast, lung, and multiple myeloma (Wickham, 2000). Can be caused by secretion of parathyroid-related protein by tumor, secretion of other bone-resorbing substances by the tumor, decreased ability of the kidneys to clear Ca^{++} from the blood, and increased Ca^{++} absorption from the gut (also see Chapter 18).
   2. Hypocalcemia.
      a. General causes: hypoparathyroidism, vitamin D deficiency, multiple citrated blood transfusions, hyperphosphatemia, magnesium deficiency, chronic renal failure (Kaplow, 2002).
      b. Cancer-related causes: cisplatin-based chemotherapy (Kintzel, 2001), osteoblastic bone metastasis and oncogenic osteomalacia, metastatic spread into the parathyroid glands, tumor lysis syndrome (Lydon, 2000), adjuvant tamoxifen (Nolvadex) therapy for breast cancer (Kailajarvi et al., 2000).
D. Clinical symptomatology of calcium imbalances depends on blood levels.
   1. Hypercalcemia.
      a. Calcium level 10 to 12 mg/dl—fatigue, lethargy, impaired concentration, mild confusion, constipation, anorexia, nausea/vomiting, polyuria.
      b. Calcium level higher than 12 mg/dl—stupor, altered mental status, coma, decreased deep tendon reflexes, increased cardiac contractility, oliguria, renal failure.
   2. Hypocalcemia.
      a. Early—increased neuromuscular irritability, paresthesias of fingers and toes and perioral region.
      b. Late—clinical course varies from tetany of facial muscles in response to stimulation (Chvostek's sign) and carpopedal spasm (Trousseau's sign) to CNS abnormalities, seizures; from emotional disturbances to impairment of cognitive functions to hallucinations; from laryngospasm and bronchospasms to possible death.
      c. Electrocardiogram (ECG) changes: inverted T wave, lengthening of the QT interval, ventricular arrhythmias, heart block, cardiac arrest (Kaplow, 2002).
E. Treatment of calcium imbalances.
   1. Hypercalcemia (Wickham, 2000).
      a. Pharmacologic interventions: fluid repletion with saline solutions, bisphosphonates including pamidronate (Aredia), calcitonin, corticosteroids, plicamycin (Mithracin), gallium nitrate (Ganite), antitumor treatment.
      b. Nonpharmacologic interventions: increased mobility/exercise to help maintain bone mass; dialysis.
   2. Hypocalcemia.
      a. If severe—intravenous (IV) calcium (calcium chloride or calcium gluconate), institute seizure precautions, and monitor ECG (Lydon, 2000).
      b. If chronic—oral calcium supplements with vitamin D.

III. Magnesium (Mg^{++}) imbalances.
  A. Usual reference range: 1.8 to 2.4 mg/dl.
  B. Second most abundant intracellular cation, with liver and muscle cells having highest concentration; 30% to 40% of dietary intake absorbed through the GI tract with the bulk of the remainder found in the urine.
  C. Mg^{++} is a critical cofactor in regulating cellular calcium, hydrogen, sodium, and potassium pumps and in the phosphorylation of glucose.
  D. Pathophysiology of magnesium imbalances.
    1. Hypermagnesemia (>3 mg/dl) can be caused by renal failure and/or adrenal insufficiency.
    2. Hypomagnesemia (<1.7 mg/dl) can be caused by the following:
      a. Cisplatin- and carboplatin-induced renal wasting of Mg^{++} (Kintzel, 2001).
      b. Use of diuretics, especially mannitol diuresis.
      c. Some antibiotics, especially aminoglycosides and amphotericin B.
      d. Any condition (e.g., liver failure) that potentiates nephrotoxicity.
      e. Other electrolyte abnormalities that contribute to, or are associated with, hypomagnesemia.
        (1) Hypercalcemia and hyperaldosteronism.
        (2) Hypomagnesemia frequently (40%) causes decreases in potassium and sodium levels.
        (3) Hypophosphatemia is associated with decreased magnesium.
  E. Clinical symptomatology of magnesium imbalances.
    1. Hypermagnesemia: lethargy, flushing, diaphoresis, decreased blood pressure and decreased rate and depth of respirations, diminished deep tendon reflexes.
    2. Hypomagnesemia: neuromuscular and CNS symptoms comparable with those of hypocalcemia, including seizures.
  F. Treatment for magnesium imbalance.
    1. Hypermagnesemia—diuretics; volume expansion with saline and mannitol diuresis potentiates Mg^{++} wasting.
    2. Hypomagnesemia—magnesium sulfate given orally or IV, and amifostine (Ethyol) administered before cisplatin (Platinol) therapy to help minimize renal tubular wasting of magnesium (Camp-Sorrell, 2000).
IV. Sodium (Na$^+$) imbalances.
  A. Usual reference range: 135 to 145 mEq/L.
  B. Sodium is the major cation in the plasma and extracellular fluid. Regulated indirectly by alterations in the total body water content, accompanied by sensory receptors (osmoreceptors) that promote either the uptake of water or the excretion of urine.
  C. Serum osmolality is physiologically maintained between 286 and 294 mOsm and is accomplished through coordination with the central thirst mechanism, antidiuretic hormone (ADH), and renal sodium and water excretion.
  D. Sodium is the major determinant of serum osmolarity and tonicity.
  E. Pathophysiology of sodium imbalances.
    1. Hypernatremia (>160 mEq/L). Seen less frequently in clients with cancer. Can be caused by inadequate intake of water and/or diabetes insipidus, impaired renal function, dehydration, increased insensible water loss, some medications (e.g., corticosteroids, antihypertensives [e.g., methyldopa (Aldomet), hydralazine (Apresoline), reserpine (Serpalan, Serpasil)]).
    2. Hyponatremia (<130 mEq/L). Most common electrolyte disorder in cancer. Can be caused by the following:

      a. Syndrome of inappropriate antidiuretic hormone (SIADH) associated with lung cancer, occurs in more than 50% of cases (DeMichele & Glick, 2001).

      b. Abrupt withdrawal of steroids (DeMichele & Glick, 2001), diuretic therapy including the use of mannitol, chemotherapeutic drugs (e.g., cyclophosphamide (Cytoxan), vincristine (Oncovin).

F. Clinical symptomatology of sodium imbalances.

  1. Hypernatremia: polydipsia, low-grade fevers, dry/sticky mucous membranes, flushed/dry skin, muscle weakness, diminished reflexes, restlessness (irritability, disorientation), depression, lethargy, intracranial bleeding, convulsions, stupor, coma.

  2. Hyponatremia.

      a. Mild (125 to 134 mEq/L)—vague symptoms that often go unnoticed, including anorexia, headache, nausea and vomiting, myalgias, subtle neurologic symptoms.

      b. Moderate (115 to 124 mEq/L)—nausea, weakness, anorexia, fatigue, muscle cramps (Stewart-Haapoja, 2000).

      c. Severe (<115 mEq/L)—seizures, alterations in the mental status ranging from confusion to psychotic behavior to coma and death (DeMichele & Glick, 2001).

G. Treatment of sodium imbalances (dependent on the degree/duration).

  1. Hypernatremia should be corrected slowly over 2 to 3 days.

      a. IV desmopressin (DDAVP).

      b. If chronic, desmopressin by nasal route.

  2. Hyponatremia.

      a. Correct cause (e.g., SIADH), which resolves the underlying cause of excessive ADH production (e.g., chemotherapy for lung cancer and RT for brain metastasis).

      b. Water restriction of 500 to 1000 ml/day.

      c. For severe, acute-onset hyponatremia, administer IV hypertonic saline over 24 hours and furosemide (to aid water excretion) (Stewart-Haapoja, 2000).

      d. Demeclocycline (Declomycin)—an oral antibiotic used to treat SIADH (Stewart-Haapoja, 2000).

      e. Administration of urea, which produces osmotic diuresis (Stewart-Haapoja, 2000).

V. Potassium (K^+) imbalances.

A. Usual reference range: 3.5 to 5 mEq/L.

B. Reciprocal relationship between K^+ and Na^+; a substantial intake of one element causes a corresponding decrease in the other. Body has no efficient method for conserving potassium.

C. Pathophysiology of potassium imbalances.

  1. Hyperkalemia (>6 mEq/L) can be caused by dehydration; compromised renal function from renal disease or renal tubular acidosis (Kaplow, 2002); acidosis; myocardial infarction (MI); burns; tumor lysis syndrome; adrenal insufficiency (as steroids are tapered); medications (e.g., angiotensin-converting enzyme [ACE] inhibitors, β-blockers, potassium-sparing diuretics, nonsteroidal antiinflammatory drugs [NSAIDs]) (Kaplow, 2002).

  2. Hypokalemia (<3 mEq/L)—usually results from multiple factors. Those with hypertension and congestive heart failure are at higher risk. Can be caused by decreased dietary intake and potassium-free IV fluids;

increased renal loss; increased GI losses—vomiting/gastric suction, ileostomy, or diarrhea, which can result from antibiotic therapy; antacids, lactose intolerance, supplemental feedings, and infectious agents (*Clostridium difficile,* GI candidiasis); drug therapies—insulin and glucose administration, loop and thiazide-type diuretics, mineralocorticosteroids, some antibiotics (penicillin, ampicillin, carbenicillin, ticarcillin), and some nephrotoxic antineoplastic agents (streptozocin [Zanosar], carmustine [BCNU], cisplatin).

  D. Clinical symptomatology of potassium imbalances.
   1. Hyperkalemia: muscle weakness, tingling, twitching, malaise, paresthesias (face, tongue, feet, hands), muscle cramps, ascending flaccid paralysis, syncope; bradycardia, arrhythmias, ECG changes—prolonged PR interval, wide QRS, tall T wave, flat P wave (Kaplow, 2002); increased bowel sounds, diarrhea, nausea and vomiting.
   2. Hypokalemia: decreased reflexes, muscle weakness, paresthesias, anorexia, rapid/weak/irregular pulse, hypotension, mental confusion; if severe—ventricular fibrillation, respiratory paralysis, and cardiac arrest, ECG changes—flattened T wave, ST depression, U wave elevation.
  E. Treatment for potassium imbalances.
   1. Hyperkalemia.
    a. Simultaneous hydration and diuresis with loop diuretics (Gobel, 2002).
    b. Sodium polystyrene sulfonate (Kayexalate) administered by mouth or retention enema (does not have an immediate effect) (Gobel, 2002).
    c. Hypertonic glucose solution and insulin given IV to cause extracellular K^+ to move back into the intracellular space (Gobel, 2002).
    d. Sodium polystyrene sulfonate (orally/rectally) to promote excretion of K^+ through the feces.
   2. Hypokalemia—care given when receiving digitalis; may enhance its sensitivity.
    a. IV potassium chloride supplementation—watch cardiac and renal function.
    b. Oral supplementation with medication and/or diet—fruits (e.g., raisins, dates, cantaloupe, bananas, apricots), vegetables (e.g., avocado, potato, tomato, carrots), orange juice, milk.

Assessment

  I. Identification of clients at risk for electrolyte imbalances of potassium, sodium, magnesium, and calcium.
  A. Determine risk for specific electrolyte imbalance.
  B. Establish patterns of occurrence—onset (rapid or slow), frequency, associated symptoms, precipitating factors, aggravating factors, alleviating factors.
  C. Collaborate with treatment team as to etiology or causes of specific electrolyte imbalance.
  D. Be alert to medications that can potentiate specific electrolyte imbalances.
  E. Assess for the use of complementary and alternative therapies that may interfere with electrolyte balance.
  II. Physical examination.
  A. System review for clinical symptomatology of appropriate imbalance.
   1. Cardiovascular—heart rate (pattern/regularity), blood pressure, ECG if indicated.

    2. Neuromuscular—presence of fatigue, weakness, lethargy, cramping, myalgias and arthralgias, tremors, paresthesias and numbness, bone pain, changes in mentation, personality, concentration; confusion and/or seizures.

    3. Renal—changes in elimination (increase or decrease in amount or frequency), weight gain/loss, calculi, or edema.

    4. GI—changes in appetite, food intake (amount/type), presence of nausea, vomiting, anorexia, diarrhea, and/or other insensible losses.

  B. Monitor laboratory data specific to electrolyte imbalance (may include other tests not listed as ordered by physician) (Table 14-1).

    1. Calcium imbalances—serum calcium, corrected serum calcium, albumin, blood urea nitrogen (BUN), creatinine levels, serum potassium, sodium phosphorus, blood coagulation levels.

    2. Magnesium imbalances—serum/urine magnesium, BUN, creatinine levels, potassium, calcium, phosphorus, sodium.

    3. Sodium imbalances—serum/urine sodium, serum/urine osmolality, BUN, creatinine levels, thyroid function tests, potassium, chloride, serum pH, ADH level.

    4. Potassium imbalances—potassium, chloride, pH, sodium, serum glucose, BUN, creatinine levels.

 III. Psychosocial assessment.

  A. Explore anxiety-producing events and coping abilities.

  B. Attempt to identify strengths of client/family.

Nursing Diagnoses

    I. Imbalanced nutrition: less than body requirements.

   II. Deficient fluid volume.

  III. Excess fluid volume.

  IV. Fatigue.

   V. Impaired memory.

  VI. Ineffective tissue perfusion (renal, cerebral, cardiopulmonary).

 VII. Risk for injury.

VIII. Acute confusion.

TABLE 14-1
Serum Electrolyte Values

Electrolyte	Usual Reference Range	Low Values	High Values
Calcium	8.5-10.5 mg/dl	Hypocalcemia: <8.5 mg/dl	Mild hypercalcemia: 10-12 mg/dl Moderate to severe: >12 mg/dl
Magnesium	1.8-2.4 mg/dl	Hypomagnesemia: <1.7 mg/dl	Hypermagnesemia: >3 mg/dl

Sodium	135-145 mEq/L	Mild hyponatremia:
		  125-134 mEq/L
		Moderate hyponatremia:
		  115-124 mEq/L
		Severe hyponatremia:
		  <115 mEq/L
			Hypernatremia: >160 mEq/L

Potassium	3.5-5 mEq/L	Hypokalemia: <3 mEq/L	Hyperkalemia: >6 mEq/L

Outcome Identification

I. Client describes personal risk for specific electrolyte imbalances related to type of cancer and other conditions that may influence imbalance.

II. Client participates in measures to minimize the risk of occurrence, severity, and complications of imbalances.

III. Client consumes foods and drinks that are indicated for specific electrolyte imbalance.

IV. Client and family list changes in the condition of the client that require professional assistance in management.
  A. Presence of new symptomatology and/or change in present condition.
  B. Weight loss or gain greater than 5% of body weight.
  C. Presence of signs and symptoms appropriate to the particular imbalance.

Planning and Implementation

I. Interventions to minimize the risk of occurrence, severity, or complications of electrolyte imbalances.
  A. Individualize client/family teaching according to risk of specific imbalance and according to changes that need to be initiated by client/family in the plan of care.
  B. Modify diet accordingly—increasing or decreasing foods and drinks that may alter electrolyte level.
  C. Encourage compliance with the medication and diet regimen.
  D. Reinforce the need for frequent laboratory sampling.
  E. Provide written instructions and a list of signs and symptoms that need to be observed for and reported.

II. Interventions to maximize safety.
  A. Assist client with ambulation, use of side rails or assistive devices and appropriate exercise as ordered (e.g., active/passive range of motion, isometrics).
  B. Recommend discontinuation of all over-the-counter medications that may interfere with therapeutic plan.

III. Interventions to monitor for complications of electrolyte imbalances.
  A. Observe for signs of dehydration, tremors, personality changes, and profound loss or gain in weight in a short time frame.
  B. Observe for untoward side effects that may be associated with rapid reversal or rebound of electrolyte imbalance.

IV. Interventions to incorporate client/family in care.
  A. Teach home management techniques to avoid or minimize electrolyte imbalances.
  B. Encourage the use of self-care diaries or logs.
  C. Teach importance of reporting critical changes in client condition to the physician, including presence of adverse or intensified pattern of vomiting and diarrhea, presence of mental changes, pain, dehydration, or other pathologic conditions.

V. Interventions that patients use in addition to or instead of conventional treatments (see Dysphagia, Planning and Implementation section, VI).

Evaluation

The oncology nurse systematically and regularly evaluates the client's and/or family's responses to interventions to determine progress toward the achievement of expected outcomes. Relevant data are collected, and actual findings are compared

with expected findings. Nursing diagnoses, outcomes, and plans of care are reviewed and revised as necessary.

WEIGHT CHANGES

Theory

I. The effects of cancer and cancer treatments can cause overnutrition and undernutrition (weight gain and weight loss), which can negatively impact morbidity, survival, and QOL (Foltz, 2000).

II. Etiology of weight gain.
   A. Disease related.
   1. Clients with breast cancer often experience weight gain as a result of multiagent chemotherapy regimens and/or regimens containing steroids (Cunningham & Bell, 2000).
   2. Effusions—pleural, pericardial, abdominal.
   3. Obstruction.
   4. Inactivity.
   5. Electrolyte imbalances.
   B. Treatment related.
   1. Effects of hormonal drugs.
   2. Steroids.
   3. Electrolyte imbalances.
   4. Adjuvant chemotherapy for breast cancer patients (Cunningham & Bell, 2000).
   5. Biologic medications, such as interleukin-2 (IL-2).

III. Etiology of weight loss.
   A. Disease related.
   1. Protein-calorie malnutrition caused by the metabolic effects of the tumor.
   2. Location of the tumor—increased weight loss associated with upper respiratory and gastric tumors (Foltz, 2000).
   B. Surgery related, especially with esophageal, gastric, pancreatic, colorectal, or esophageal surgeries (McGuire, 2000).
   1. May cause alterations in ability to eat (McGuire, 2000).
   2. May cause disrupted absorption of nutrients (Foltz, 2000).
   3. Postprandial dumping syndrome associated with gastric resections (McGuire, 2000).
   4. Surgical oncology patients usually require frequent tests that may limit intake and/or include dietary restrictions (Foltz, 2000).
   5. There is increased calorie expenditure and energy needs during the perioperative period (Foltz, 2000).
   C. Treatment related.
   1. Loss resulting from vomiting associated with chemotherapy and radiation.
   2. Loss resulting from acute or chronic diarrhea caused by drugs (e.g., antibiotics, chemotherapy), dietary alterations, infectious processes (e.g., *Clostridium difficile*), intestinal ischemia, fecal impaction, irritable bowel disease, laxative abuse, endocrine disorders, malabsorption, surgery, and radiation colitis (Cope, 2001).
   3. Presence of concurrent symptoms related to cancer treatment, including taste alterations, mucositis, pain, anxiety, depression, fatigue.
   4. Side effects of medications, including antacids, antibiotics, narcotics, biologic response modifiers.

    D. Insensible losses, such as perspiration, gastric suction, surgical drains, fistulas, wounds.

Assessment

  I. History.
    A. Previous dietary patterns, food preferences, eating habits, and history of weight changes with client/family.
    B. Patterns of weight changes, including type, onset, duration, severity; associated symptoms—food intolerances, taste abnormalities, mouth and throat pain, dysphagia, vomiting, diarrhea; other factors—precipitating, aggravating, alleviating factors.
    C. Previous self-care strategies.
      1. Ability to carry out interventions to maintain weight.
      2. Use of food, nutritional supplements, and other remedies.
    D. Current or recent treatment for cancer and experienced side effects.
  II. Physical examination.
    A. Determine present weight and amount of total weight loss or gain.
    B. Assess for presence of dehydration and/or electrolyte imbalances.
    C. Assess client for associated cultural, socioeconomic, emotional, and motivational factors that may affect weight loss or gain.

Nursing Diagnoses

See Anorexia, Nursing Diagnoses section. Nursing diagnoses related to weight changes in addition to those listed in Anorexia section include the following:
  I. Disturbed body image.
  II. Diarrhea.
  III. Nausea.

Outcome Identification

  I. Client states the goals of interventions related to weight change.
  II. Client states the personal risk for complications related to weight loss or gain and ways in which various cancer therapies may affect nutrition.
  III. Client participates in measures to minimize risk of occurrence, severity, and complications of weight changes.
  IV. Client states the changes in condition that require professional assistance and/or intervention.
    A. Weight loss or gain of greater than 5% of body weight.
    B. Dehydration, increased insensible losses, edema.
    C. Changes in skin integrity, wound healing, respiratory or cardiovascular status, presence of infection.
    D. Inability to eat or drink.
    E. Any area of concern for client's well-being related to intake or lack of intake.
  V. Client and family state awareness of resources in the community to assist with nutrition.

Planning and Implementation

  I. See Anorexia, Planning and Implementation section.
  II. Interventions to incorporate client/family into care (in addition to those listed in Anorexia section).

TABLE 14-2
Body Weight Formulas

Body Type	Formula	Example
For underweight adults	Multiply their weight in pounds × 18 = calories/day	100 lb × 18 = 1800 calories/day
For normal weight adults	Multiply their weight in pounds × 16 = calories/day	140 lb × 16 = 2240 calories/day
For overweight adults	Multiply their weight in pounds × 13 = calories/day	180 lb × 13 = 2340 calories/day

Protein gram requirements per day can be calculated by multiplying the client's weight × 0.5 (National Cancer Institute: PDQ. (2002a). Nutrition, pp. 1-14. Last modified October 2002 from CIS: http://www.cancer.gov/cancerinfo/pdq/supportivecare/nutrition/healthprofessional/).

    A. Assist client/family with calculating individualized calorie and protein requirements so that realistic goals can be set for weight changes. The formulas in Table 14-2 can be used to determine how many calories are needed to maintain a cancer patient's body weight (assuming light activity).

    B. Employ proper quantities of foods from the food groups that provide a balanced, nutritious diet for weight control.

    C. Engage in regular exercise if able. May need to consult with a nutritionist.

    D. Encourage consultation with a dietitian.

Evaluation

The oncology nurse systematically and regularly evaluates the client's and/or family's responses to interventions to determine progress toward the achievement of expected outcomes. Relevant data are collected, and actual findings are compared with expected findings. Nursing diagnoses, outcomes, and plans of care are reviewed and revised as necessary.

CACHEXIA

Theory

    I. Definition—"Cachexia refers to progressive deterioration with muscle wasting that occurs when protein and/or calorie requirements are not met" (Cunningham & Bell, 2000, p. 92).

    II. Pathophysiology. May be primary or secondary.

        A. Primary cachexia—also known as the anorexia-cachexia syndrome.

            1. Complex process, involving anorexia, metabolic alterations, release of cytokines and other catabolic factors that lead to skeletal muscle wasting (Cunningham & Bell, 2000).

            2. Appears to be mediated by proinflammatory cytokines, including tumor necrosis factor (TNF), interleukin (IL)-1, IL-6, interferon (IFN)-α, and IFN-γ, which may be produced by the tumor itself or by the immune system in response to the tumor (Mantovani et al., 2001).

            3. Some of the metabolic alterations include decreased gluconeogenesis; alterations in glucose metabolism; increased metabolic rate; and changed lipid, protein, and carbohydrate metabolism.

    B. Secondary cachexia—defined as involuntary weight loss and inanition based on mechanical factors, such as obstruction or malabsorption; or treatment-induced toxicities, such as nausea/vomiting or alterations in taste (Cunningham & Bell, 2000).

III. Risk factors.

    A. Disease related: cancer, acquired immunodeficiency syndrome (AIDS), infections, septic states, inflammatory diseases (Finley, 2000).

    B. Treatment related: chemotherapy; biotherapy; RT; surgery of the head, neck, stomach, pancreas, and/or bowel (Finley, 2000).

    C. Situational.

        1. Psychologic aspects of nutritional intake—cancer cachexia is viewed by some to be the hallmark of terminal illness; thus clients frequently "give up."

        2. Depression, inactivity, absence of an appetite, and poor performance status all affect the client's QOL.

IV. Principles of medical management.

    A. Treatment of the underlying disease (Finley, 2000).

    B. Pharmacologic interventions.

        1. Megestrol acetate (Megace)—has a dose-response effect and is thought to cause inhibition of TNF (Finley, 2000).

        2. Metoclopramide (Reglan) at low doses to stimulate GI motility and decrease early satiety (Finley, 2000).

        3. Cannabinoid derivatives such as dronabinol or delta-9-tetrahydro-cannabinol (THC) (Marinol) to stimulate appetite (Finley, 2000).

        4. Metabolic inhibitors to induce anabolism.

        5. Dexamethasone (Decadron) and prednisolone (Delta-Cortef, Prelone) to stimulate appetite and sense of well-being (Mantovani et al., 2001).

        6. Other drugs currently being studied with uncertain efficacy: pentoxifylline (Trental), thalidomide (Thalomid), cyproheptadine (Periactin), eicosapentanoic acid, hydrazine sulfate (Finley, 2000).

    C. TPN to replace nutritional deficiencies.

    D. Enteral feedings—oral or tube feedings will help maintain normal GI flora and prevent atrophy of GI mucosa (Finley, 2000).

V. Potential sequelae of cachexia.

    A. Increased morbidity and mortality, present in 80% at death (Nelson, 2000).

    B. Alterations in carbohydrate, protein, and lipid metabolism (Mantovani et al., 2001).

    C. Decreased tissue sensitivity to insulin and decreased insulin response to glucose (Mantovani et al., 2001).

    D. Impairment of immunocompetence: humoral, cellular, secretory, and mucosal immunity (Cunningham & Bell, 2000).

    E. Poor wound healing and increased infection rates (Stepp & Pakiz, 2001).

    F. Protein-calorie malnutrition with resultant weight loss, visceral and somatic protein depletion that compromises enzymatic, structural, and mechanical functions.

    G. Impaction caused by lack of food and fluid intake (Tuchmann, 2001) and the effects of cancer treatments.

Assessment

I. History.

    A. Previous dietary patterns, food preferences, eating habits, type and quantity of food consumed, history of anorexia with client/family.

B. Patterns of anorexia and presence of fatigue and malaise. Assess for onset, frequency, severity; associated symptoms—food intolerances, taste abnormalities, pain, dysphagia; other factors—precipitating, aggravating, alleviating factors.

C. Previous self-care strategies: ability to provide for own interventions to relieve anorexia, use of food, nutritional supplements, and other remedies.

D. Current or recent treatment for cancer and experienced side effects.

E. Associated cultural, socioeconomic, emotional, and motivational factors that may affect the loss of weight.

II. Physical examination.

   A. Determine present weight and amount of total and recent weight loss.

   B. Assess for presence of dehydration and/or electrolyte imbalances.

   C. Assess for muscle atrophy, loss of fat deposits, presence of edema.

   D. Perform anthropometric measurements, or consult a nutritionist.

      1. Triceps skinfolds and midarm muscle circumference.

      2. Height and weight (weight loss >10% in previous 3 months is significant for diagnosis of protein-calorie malnutrition).

   E. Review biochemical measurements.

      1. Visceral protein stores—serum albumin, prealbumin, total iron-binding capacity, transferrin, electrolytes, nitrogen balance (Finley, 2000).

      2. Lean body mass—collect 24-hour urine for creatinine clearance (Finley, 2000) and urinary urea nitrogen (Foltz, 2000).

      3. Degree of anemia.

      4. Deficiencies in trace metals and vitamins, and glucose intolerance.

Nursing Diagnoses

See Anorexia, Nursing Diagnoses section. Nursing diagnoses related to cachexia in addition to those listed in Anorexia section include the following:

  I. Adult failure to thrive.

 II. Disturbed body image.

Outcome Identification

   I. Client consumes frequent small feedings throughout the day by mouth or by alternative route as tolerated.

  II. Client states the personal risk for complications related to cachexia and ways in which various cancer therapies may adversely affect nutritional reserves.

 III. Family/significant other participates in measures to minimize risk of occurrence, severity, and complications of cachexia.

 IV. Client states the changes in condition that require professional assistance and/or intervention.

   A. Weight loss of greater than 5% of body weight.

   B. Dehydration.

   C. Changes in skin integrity and wound healing, and infection.

   D. Inability to eat or drink.

   E. Any other area of concern for client's sense of well-being related to food intake.

  V. Client and family state awareness of resources in the community to assist with nutrition and caregiving support.

Planning and Implementation

See Anorexia, Planning and Implementation section.

Evaluation

The oncology nurse systematically and regularly evaluates the client's and/or family's responses to interventions to determine progress toward the achievement of expected outcomes. Relevant data are collected, and actual findings are compared with expected findings. Nursing diagnoses, outcomes, and plans of care are reviewed and revised as necessary.

ASCITES

Theory

I. Definition—abnormal accumulation of fluid in the abdominal cavity that is not reabsorbed into the systemic circulation.
II. Pathophysiology/risk factors.
  A. Tumor, IL-2, TNF, vascular endothelial growth factors (VEGFs), lymphatic destruction/obstruction leading to decreased outflow from the peritoneal cavity, immune modulators, vascular permeability factors, and metalloproteinases all contribute to the process (Aslam & Marino, 2001). Malignant ascites accounts for 10% of all cases of ascites.
  B. Disease-related risk factors.
    1. Association with various tumors, mainly intraabdominal malignancies: ovarian (accounts for 30% to 54%), endometrial, uterine (Maghfoor et al., 2000).
    2. Breast, lung, and lymphatic system are the most common extraabdominal sites.
    3. Colon, gastric, pancreatic, and to a lesser extent mesothelioma, testicular, and sarcoma.
    4. As a result of liver metastasis.
  C. Treatment-related risk factors—previous radiation to the abdomen and/or surgical modification of venous or lymphatic channels.
III. Principles of medical management.
  A. Treatment of underlying cause. Rule out nonneoplastic causes.
  B. Diet (salt and water restrictions) and diuresis—usually only helpful when cause is cirrhosis.
  C. Repeated therapeutic removal of fluid by paracentesis leads to protein depletion.
  D. Intracavitary therapy—obliteration of the intraperitoneal space using chemotherapy (belly bath) and/or instillation of radioactive colloids (when symptomatic). New approaches under study include intraperitoneal injections of streptococcal antigen, OK-432, anti-VEGFs, and metalloproteinase inhibitors (Aslam & Marino, 2001).
  E. Systemic chemotherapy.
  F. Peritoneovenous shunting (LeVeen or Denver shunts, which divert fluid from the abdomen into the blood circulation).
  G. External drains used but have a high incidence of infection (43%) (Aslam & Marino, 2001).

H. Radiocolloid [32]P (Maghfoor et al., 2000).

I. Parenteral interferon.

J. Ultrasonically guided insertion of a peritoneogastric shunt (from peritoneal cavity to a gastrostomy tube).

IV. Potential sequelae of progressive ascites.

A. Discomfort, anorexia, early satiety, decreased bladder capacity, bowel obstruction, electrolyte imbalance, nausea and vomiting, infection, shortness of breath, respiratory compromise, ankle edema, impaired skin integrity, abdominal distention, fatigue, weight gain.

B. The appearance of ascites in advanced disease means a grim prognosis. Palliation is usually all that can be offered, and palliative draining needs to be done each time fluid reaccumulates.

C. Survival is measured in weeks to months, with 1-year survival being less than 10%. Overall is approximately 20 weeks. Prognosis is somewhat better in ovarian cancer (30 to 35 weeks) and lymphoma (58 to 78 weeks) (Maghfoor et al., 2000).

Assessment

I. History.

A. Presence of risk factors, such as symptoms with a malignancy known to be associated with malignant ascites.

B. Pattern of ascites.

1. Elicit subjective indicators—increasing abdominal girth, indigestion, early satiety, swollen ankles, easy fatigability, shortness of breath, constipation, reduced bladder capacity.

2. Objective indicator is weight gain.

3. Review previous treatment strategies for ascites and current or recent treatment for cancer and anticipated side effects.

C. Presence of self-care strategies.

1. Ability to perform interventions to relieve or minimize effects of ascites.

2. Willingness to self-monitor weight, girth, record keeping.

II. Physical examination.

A. Determine present weight and amount of weight gain, presence of distended abdomen, fluid wave, shifting dullness, bulging flanks, everted umbilicus, stretched skin, and presence of lower extremity edema and increased abdominal girth (approximately 50 ml is the normal net volume in the peritoneal cavity in healthy persons).

B. Assess laboratory indicators for presence of high level of carcinoembryonic antigen (>12 mg/ml), total protein, LDH cell count, differential albumin, fibronectin, cholesterol level, cytologic confirmation of the presence of malignant cells of the ascitic fluid from paracentesis, chemistry confirmation, immunohistochemical staining, cytology examination result, and character of transudate (usually bloody or serosanguineous).

C. Radiologic studies such as ultrasound (can detect as little as 100 ml of fluid) and computed tomography examinations of abdomen (plain x-ray shows a ground-glass appearance with a loss of detail [Maghfoor et al., 2000]).

D. Assess client for associated ethnic, socioeconomic, emotional, and motivational factors that may influence care.

Nursing Diagnoses

   I. Imbalanced nutrition: less than body requirements.
   II. Excess fluid volume.
   III. Risk for impaired skin integrity.
   IV. Risk for activity intolerance.
   V. Impaired urinary elimination.
   VI. Ineffective breathing pattern.
   VII. Decreased cardiac output.
   VIII. Disturbed body image.
   IX. Impaired physical mobility.
   X. Fatigue.

Outcome Identification

   I. Client states the goals of interventions related to ascites.
   II. Client states the personal risk for potential recurrence of ascites and early symptoms that need to be reported to lessen extent of fluid accumulation and discomfort.
   III. Client participates in measures to minimize the discomfort associated with ascites, including positioning and pain control.
   IV. Client and family state the changes in condition that require professional assistance and/or intervention.
      A. Weight gain of more than 2 pounds per day and/or increased abdominal girth.
      B. Acute respiratory distress, fever, or changes in level of pain.
      C. Edema noted in other body parts, such as lower legs and feet.
   V. Client and family state awareness of resources in the community to assist with long-term care and client/family support.

Planning and Implementation

   I. Nonpharmacologic interventions to minimize the risk of occurrence, severity, or complications of ascites.
      A. Teach client/family to decrease sodium and increase protein intake.
      B. Maximize measures to promote comfort.
         1. Teach client/family to maintain high Fowler's position.
         2. Employ positions to reduce edema.
         3. Avoid restrictive clothing.
         4. Remind of need to employ nonpharmacologic techniques for pain relief (e.g., relaxation, imagery, music, distraction, healing touch).
         5. Use methods to assist with activities as needed.
   II. Interventions to incorporate client/family in care.
      A. Encourage family to provide foods within dietary restrictions.
      B. Teach family methods to enhance calorie/protein content of foods and methods to enhance food intake.
      C. Teach family signs and symptoms of dehydration, infection, respiratory distress, and malnutrition.
      D. Teach family how to measure abdominal girth and weigh daily and how to assess changes such as fullness, bloating, and abdominal pressure.
   III. Interventions to enhance adaptation and rehabilitation.
      A. Provide written and audiovisual materials on care issues at client's level of education and understanding.

B. Encourage importance of self-care record keeping, such as diaries and logs.
IV. Interventions patients use in addition to or instead of conventional treatments (see Dysphagia, Planning and Implementation section, VI).

Evaluation

The oncology nurse systematically and regularly evaluates the client's and/or family's responses to interventions to determine progress toward the achievement of expected outcomes. Relevant data are collected, and actual findings are compared with expected findings. Nursing diagnoses, outcomes, and plans of care are reviewed and revised as necessary.

ADDITIONAL RESOURCES FOR INFORMATION ON ALTERATIONS IN NUTRITION

American Cancer Society: www.cancer.org
National Cancer Institute: www.cancer.gov
National Institutes of Health: www.nih.gov
Oncology Nursing Society: www.ons.org

REFERENCES

Aslam, N., & Marino, C. (2001). Malignant ascites: New concepts in pathophysiology, diagnosis, and management. *Archives of Internal Medicine 161*, 2733-2737.

Bloch, A. (2000). Nutrition support in cancer. *Seminars in Oncology Nursing 16*(2), 122-127.

Bodkey, G.P. (2000). Fever in the neutropenic patient. In M. Abelhoff, J. Armitage, A. Licter, & J. Niederbuber (Eds.). *Clinical oncology* (2nd ed.). New York: Churchill Livingstone, pp. 690-706.

Borbasi, S., Cameron, K., Quested, B., et al. (2002). More than a sore mouth: Patient's experience of oral mucositis. *Oncology Nursing Forum 29*(7), 1051-1057.

Brown, J. (2002). A systematic review of the evidence on symptom management of cancer-related anorexia & cachexia. *Oncology Nursing Forum 29*(3), 517-532.

Camp-Sorrell, D. (2000). Chemotherapy: Toxicity management. In C.H. Yarbro, M.H. Frogge, M. Goodman, & S.L. Groenwald (Eds.). *Cancer nursing: Principles and practice* (5th ed.). Sudbury, MA: Jones and Bartlett Publishers, pp. 444-486.

Cope, D. (2001). Management of chemotherapy induced diarrhea and constipation. *Nursing Clinics of North America 36*(4), 695-707.

Criswell, M., & Sinha, C. (2001). Hyperthermic, supersaturated humidification in the treatment of xerostomia. *Laryngoscope 111*(6), 992-996.

Cunningham, R., & Bell, R. (2000). Nutrition in cancer: An overview. *Seminars in Oncology Nursing 16*(2), 90-98.

DeMichele, A., & Glick, J. (2001). Cancer related emergencies. In R. Lenhard, R. Osteen, & T. Gansler (Eds.). *Clinical oncology*. Atlanta: American Cancer Society, pp. 733-764.

Dibble, S., Chapman, J., Mack, K., & Shih, A. (2000). Acupressure for nausea: Results of a pilot study. *Oncology Nursing Forum 27*(1), 41-47.

Finley, J. (2000). Management of cancer cachexia. *AACN Clinical Issues 11*(4), 590-603.

Foltz, A. (2000). Nutritional disturbances. In C.H. Yarbro, M.H. Frogge, M. Goodman, & S.L. Groenwald (Eds.). *Cancer nursing: Principles and practice* (5th ed.). Sudbury, MA: Jones and Bartlett Publishers, pp. 754-775.

Fulton, J., Middleton, G., & McPhail, J. (2002). Management of oral complications. *Seminars in Oncology Nursing 18*(1), 28-35.

Gobel, B. (2002). Management of tumor lysis syndrome: Prevention and treatment. *Seminars in Oncology Nursing 18*(3), 12-16.

Grant, M., & Kravitz, K. (2000). Symptoms and their impact on nutrition. *Seminars in Oncology Nursing 16*(2), 113-121.

Grealish, L., Lomasney, A., & Whiteman, B. (2000). Foot massage. *Cancer Nursing 23*(3), 237-243.

Hesketh, P. (2000). Comparative review of 5-HT3 receptor antagonists in the treatment of acute chemotherapy-induced nausea and vomiting. *Cancer Investigation 18*(2), 163-173.

Kailajarvi, M., Ahokoski, O., Virtanen, A., et al. (2000). Early effects of adjuvant tamoxifen therapy on serum hormones, proteins and lipids. *Anticancer Research 20,* 1323-1328.

Kaplow, R. (2002). Pathophysiology, signs, and symptoms of acute tumor lysis syndrome. *Seminars in Oncology Nursing 18*(3), 6-11.

Kintzel, P. (2001). Anticancer drug induced kidney disorders. *Drug Safety 24*(1), 19-38.

Loprinzi, C., Gastineau, D., & Foote, R. (2000). Oral complications. In M. Abelhoff, J. Armitage, A. Licter, & J. Niederbuber (Eds.). *Clinical oncology* (2nd ed.). New York: Churchill Livingstone, pp. 965-979.

Lydon, J. (2000). Tumor lysis syndrome. In C.H. Yarbro, M.H. Frogge, M. Goodman, & S.L. Groenwald (Eds.). *Cancer nursing: Principles and practice* (5th ed.). Sudbury, MA: Jones and Bartlett Publishers, pp. 920-930.

Maghfoor, I., Doll, D., & Yarbro, J. (2000). Effusions. In M. Abeloff, J. Armitage, A. Licter, & J. Niederbuber (Eds.). *Clinical oncology* (2nd ed.). New York: Churchill Livingstone, pp. 922-946.

Mantovani, G., Maccio, A., Massa, E., & Madeddu, C. (2001). Managing cancer related anorexia/cachexia. *Drugs 61*(4), 499-514.

Marchioro, G., Azzarello, G., Viviani, F., et al. (2000). Hypnosis in the treatment of anticipatory nausea and vomiting in patients receiving cancer chemotherapy. *Oncology 59*, 100-104.

McGrath, P. (2002). Reflections on nutritional issues associated with cancer therapy. *Cancer Practice 10*(2), 94-101.

McGuire, D. (2002). Mucosal tissue injury in cancer therapy; more than mucositis and mouthwash. *Cancer Practice 10*(4), 179-191.

McGuire, M. (2000). Nutritional care of surgical oncology patients. *Seminars in Oncology Nursing 16*(2), 128-134.

McMahon, K., & Brown, J. (2000). Nutritional screening and assessment. *Seminars in Oncology Nursing 16*(2), 106-112.

Miller, M., & Kearney, N. (2001). Oral care for patients with cancer: A review of the literature. *Cancer Nursing 24*(4), 241-253.

National Cancer Institute: PDQ. (2002a). Nutrition, pp. 1-14. Last modified October 2002 from CIS: http://www.cancer.gov/cancerinfo/pdq/supportivecare/nutrition/healthprofessional/

National Cancer Institute: PDQ. (2002b). Oral complications of chemotherapy and head/neck radiation, pp. 1-36. Last modified September 2002 from CIS: http://www.cancer.gov/cancerinfo/pdq/supportivecare/oralcomplications/healthprofessional/

Nelson, K. (2000). The cancer anorexia cachexia syndrome. *Seminars in Oncology 27*(1), 64-68.

Ott, M. (2002). Complementary and alternative therapies in cancer symptom management. *Cancer Practice 10*(3), 162-166.

Rogers, B. (2001). Mucositis in the oncology patient. *Nursing Clinics of North America 36*(4), 745-760.

Rosenthal, P. (2001). Complications of cancer and cancer treatment. In R. Lenhard, R. Osteen, & T. Gansler (Eds.). *Clinical oncology*. Atlanta: American Cancer Society, pp. 231-249.

Shih, A., Miaskowski, C., Dodd, M., et al. (2002). A research review of current treatments for radiation-induced oral mucositis in patients with head and neck cancer. *Oncology Nursing Forum 29*(7), 1063-1077.

Stepp, L., & Pakiz, T. (2001). Anorexia and cachexia in advanced cancer. *Nursing Clinics of North America 36*(4), 735-744.

Stewart-Haapoja, I. (2000). Syndrome of inappropriate antidiuretic hormone. In C. Yarbro, M.H. Frogge, M. Goodman, & S. Groenwald (Eds.). *Cancer nursing: Principles and practice* (5th ed.). Sudbury, MA: Jones and Bartlett Publishers, pp. 913-919.

Tuchmann, L. (2001). Constipation. In R. Gates & R. Fink (Eds.). *Oncology nursing secrets* (2nd ed.). Philadelphia: Hanley & Belfus, Inc., pp. 298-309.

Turnkel, R., Lachmann, E., Boland, P., & Ho, M. (2000) Physical rehabilitation. In M. Abelhoff, J. Armitage, A. Licter, & J. Niederbuber (Eds). *Clinical oncology* (2nd ed.). New York: Churchill Livingstone, pp. 2771-2817.

Wickham, R. (2000). Hypercalcemia. In C.H. Yarbro, M.H. Frogge, M. Goodman, & S.L. Groenwald (Eds.). *Cancer nursing: Principles and practice* (5th ed.). Sudbury, MA: Jones and Bartlett Publishers, pp. 776-791.

Wickham, R. (2001). Nausea and vomiting. In R. Gates & R. Fink (Eds.). *Oncology nursing secrets* (2nd ed.). Philadelphia: Hanley & Belfus, Inc., pp. 353-364.

15 Alterations in Elimination

ANNETTE W. KUCK AND ELISA RICCIARDI

URINARY AND BOWEL INCONTINENCE

Theory

I. Physiology.
  A. Definition.
  1. Urinary incontinence—involuntary loss of urine that is sufficient to be a problem.
    a. Stress—involuntary loss of urine during laughing, coughing, sneezing, or other physical activities that increase abdominal pressure.
    b. Urge—involuntary loss of urine associated with an abrupt and strong desire to void.
    c. Reflex—involuntary loss of urine with no sensation of urge voiding or bladder fullness.
    d. Functional—state in which an individual experiences incontinence because of difficulty in reaching or inability to reach the toilet before urination.
    e. Total—continuous loss of urine without distention or awareness of bladder fullness.
    f. Urinary retention—chronic inability to void followed by involuntary voiding (overflow incontinence) caused by overdistention of the bladder (AHCPR, 1996).
  2. Bowel incontinence—a change in normal bowel habits characterized by involuntary passage of stool at an inappropriate time and place (Schiller, 2002).
  B. Mechanisms.
  1. Bladder incontinence.
    a. Urinary incontinence is a voiding dysfunction and can be classified as storage (stress, urge, total, functional), emptying (urinary retention), and combination of storage and emptying (reflex) problems (AHCPR, 1996).
    b. Storage problems.
      (1) Bladder contracts involuntarily during filling.
      (2) Reduced compliance of bladder wall.
      (3) Sensory urgency.
      (4) Loss of bladder neck and proximal urethra support.
      (5) Intrinsic sphincter dysfunction.
    c. Emptying problems.
      (1) Loss of or impaired contractility.
      (2) Urethral or prostatic obstruction.

    d. Storage and emptying problems.
      (1) Loss of voluntary control of voiding.
      (2) Loss of bladder-sphincter coordination (AHCPR, 1996).
    e. Postprostatectomy incontinence.
      (1) Sphincter competence depends primarily on integrity of the rhabdosphincter (Robinson, 2000).
      (2) Incompetence of the rhabdosphincter is the primary cause and may result from reduced sphincter mobility from scarred or atrophied tissue, tissue injury caused by ischemia during surgery, pudendal nerve injury, and shortening of the urethra.
      (3) Urge is caused by bladder muscle (detrusor) instability, low bladder wall compliance, or both.
      (4) Combination of stress and urge incontinence results from damage to the rhabdosphincter along with detrusor instability.
      (5) With advancing age, there is evidence of atrophy of the rhabdosphincter and neural degeneration (Carlson & Nitti, 2001).
    f. Female.
      (1) Loss of estrogen during menopause can cause urethral epithelium thinning.
      (2) Obstruction can be due to severe genital prolapse (Flessir & Blarvis, 2002).
  2. Rectal incontinence.
    a. Diminished rectal sensation and perception.
    b. Internal anal sphincter relaxation causing diminished anal canal closure.
    c. External anal sphincter and puborectalis muscle tone weakness.
    d. Defect in rectal accommodation (Schiller, 2002).
II. Risk factors.
  A. Disease related.
    1. Loss of ability to inhibit bladder or rectal contractions in clients with lesions in the cortex as a result of a cerebrovascular accident, multiple sclerosis, Parkinson's disease, or primary or metastatic tumor (Robinson, 2000).
    2. Loss of bladder and bowel reflex contractions, which can occur in clients with suprasacral lesions of the spinal cord, spinal cord tumors, compression following radical pelvic surgery, or diabetic neuropathy (Schiller, 2002).
    3. Loss of sphincter competency, which affects the bladder's ability to store urine. May be acquired after radical prostatectomy, radiation treatment, trauma, or sacral cord lesions (Carlson & Nitti, 2001).
    4. Impaired or lost sensation of the bladder caused by inflammation, chronic infection, prolonged bladder distention.
    5. Obstruction of the bladder caused by tumor, prostatic hyperplasia, or fecal impaction.
    6. Immobility commonly associated with chronic degenerative disease.
    7. Endocrine conditions that cloud the sensorium and induce diuresis, such as hyperglycemia and diabetes insipidus.
    8. Loss of functional ability, which often accompanies cognitive impairment in clients with central nervous system (CNS) metastases, Alzheimer's disease, dementia.
    9. Previous transurethral resection of the prostate, anastomotic stricture, stage of disease, surgical technique, experience of the surgeon (Carlson & Nitti, 2001).

10. Inadequate rectal capacity or compliance.
11. Dulled rectal sensation caused by dementia, spinal cord lesions, peripheral nerve problems (Schiller, 2002).
12. Fecal impaction.
B. Treatment related.
1. Surgical intervention that disrupts neural pathways, which may occur with abdominal perineal resection or radical prostatectomy.
2. Inflammatory reaction from the effects of radiation therapy (RT) on bladder and bowel, which may result in fibrosis or stenosis.
3. Chemotherapy agents, such as vincristine (Oncovin) and ifosfamide (Ifex), that cause neurotoxic side effects.
4. Fistula formation as a complication of surgery or RT.
5. Cryosurgery can cause urinary incontinence, urethral sloughing, bladder neck obstruction (O'Rourke, 2000).
6. Medications, including anticholinergics, diuretics, narcotics, sedatives, hypnotics, tranquilizers, laxatives.
7. Complications associated with indwelling catheters include urinary tract infections, urinary stones, epididymitis, scrotal abscess, urethritis, urethral erosion, fistula formation, bladder cancer (Carlson & Nitti, 2001).
III. Principles of medical management.
A. Treatment of underlying condition affecting incontinence.
B. Surgical treatment is considered for postprostatectomy incontinence if incontinence persists 6 to 12 months following radical prostatectomy.
C. Surgical treatment, such as bladder neck suspension, pubovaginal sling, artificial urinary or rectal sphincter, rectal sphincter repair, augmentation cystoplasty, or fecal or urinary diversion.
D. Drug therapy.
E. Bulking agents for bowel incontinence.
F. Dietary modifications by increasing fiber and fluid intake.
G. Bladder and/or bowel training programs (Robinson, 2000).
IV. Potential sequelae of prolonged incontinence.
A. Perianal skin irritation and excoriation.
B. Changes in role relationship and lifestyle.
C. Embarrassment that may prevent seeking needed health care.

Assessment

I. History.
A. Personal history.
1. Cognitive ability.
2. Neurologic disease or symptoms.
3. Motivation to self-care in toileting.
4. Manual dexterity and mobility.
5. Living arrangements.
6. Identification of caregiver and degree of caregiver involvement.
7. Prescription and nonprescription medications.
8. Impact of incontinence on self-esteem and interpersonal relationships.
B. Past and present patterns of elimination.
1. Precipitants of incontinence—caffeine and alcohol consumption, physical activity, surgery, trauma, recent illnesses.
2. Daily fluid intake.

    3. Urinary tract symptoms—nocturia, dysuria, hesitancy, enuresis, straining, poor stream.

    4. Duration of incontinence.

    5. Frequency and amount of continence and incontinence.

    6. Previous treatments and its effects.

    7. Bowel habits and laxative use.

    8. Bladder diary for 3 days (Gormley, 2002).

  II. Physical findings.

    A. Presence of abdominal masses.

    B. Palpation of full bladder.

    C. Pelvic organ prolapse.

    D. Rule out fecal impaction.

    E. Neurologic assessment, including balance, gait, deep tendon reflexes, sphincter tone, external anal sphincter contraction, perineal sensation.

    F. Presence of incontinence, odor, perineal skin irritation or breakdown.

 III. Diagnostic testing.

    A. Urinalysis, culture and sensitivity to assess for hematuria, bacteruria, glucosuria.

    B. Cough stress test.

    C. Presence and amount of postvoiding residual urine (Robinson, 2002).

    D. Urodynamic and imaging studies (e.g., cystometrogram; voiding cystourethrogram; electromyogram to evaluate micturition, bladder filling, and storing function).

    E. Cystoscopy to identify site of obstruction (Carlson & Nitti, 2001).

    F. Stool culture and sensitivity to rule out infection and *Clostridium difficile* infection.

    G. Sigmoidoscopy, colonoscopy, barium enema, three-dimensional endoanal ultrasonography, and anorectal physiology testing to examine the colon and rectum for the presence of disease and to test sphincter control (Schiller, 2002).

Nursing Diagnoses

    I. Impaired urinary elimination.

      A. Reflex urinary incontinence.

      B. Stress urinary incontinence.

      C. Urge urinary incontinence.

      D. Functional urinary incontinence.

      E. Total urinary incontinence.

  II. Urinary retention.

 III. Bowel incontinence.

 IV. Impaired skin integrity.

  V. Social isolation.

Outcome Identification

    I. Client is continent of urine or verbalizes management.

      A. Client and family contact appropriate health care team members to determine etiology of incontinence.

  II. Client empties bladder completely.

 III. Client is continent of stool or reports decreased episodes of bowel incontinence.

    A. Client identifies and implements appropriate measures for managing bowel incontinence.

IV. Client's skin remains intact.
V. Client becomes actively involved with others and participates in activities at level of ability or desire.

Planning and Implementation

I. Interventions to minimize the risk of occurrence, severity, or complications of incontinence.
   A. Determine cause of or contributing factors of incontinence.
   B. Reduce environmental barriers to using toileting facilities.
II. Nonpharmacologic interventions.
   A. Supportive techniques.
      1. Assess perianal skin daily.
      2. Clean area after every voiding or bowel movement with soft washcloth and perianal cleanser, rinse thoroughly, and pat dry.
      3. Apply moisture barrier ointment or skin barrier after each incontinent episode.
      4. Use absorbent pads or briefs (Gormley, 2002).
      5. Penile compression devices and pessaries (Robinson, 2000).
      6. Apply a fecal drainage pouch if there are continuous or frequent episodes of bowel incontinence (Schiller, 2002).
      7. Use external (condom) and internal catheters as a last method to manage incontinence (Robinson, 2000).
   B. Implement appropriate behavioral techniques.
      1. Establish a routine schedule for voiding, such as every 2 to 3 hours (habit training).
      2. Ask the client on a regular basis about voiding (prompt voiding).
      3. Teach the client to suppress the urge to void to rebuild bladder capacity (bladder retraining).
      4. Teach the client to exercise pelvic muscles twice per day.
   C. Design a bowel-training program.
      1. Establish a consistent time for elimination each day.
      2. Use techniques to stimulate bowel evacuation, such as digital stimulation, suppository.
      3. Monitor bowel elimination daily.
      4. Remove fecal impaction if present.
      5. Recognize that bowel evacuation should occur when there is a sensation of rectal distention.
   D. Electrostimulation is delivered by means of electrodes attached to a portable stimulator to stimulate muscle contraction for 30 minutes daily (Gormley, 2002).
   E. Urology consultation for evaluation of voiding problems, appropriate treatment, and behavioral modification or bladder retraining.
III. Pharmacologic interventions.
   A. Urinary incontinence.
      1. α-Adrenergic agonists (e.g., phenylpropanolamine [Rhindecon]).
      2. Anticholinergics and antispasmodics (e.g., oxybutynin [Ditropan]).
      3. Tricyclic antidepressants (e.g., imipramine [Tofranil]).
      4. Calcium antagonists.
      5. Potassium channel openers (Wein & Rovner, 2002).
   B. Fecal incontinence.
      1. Opiate antidiarrheal agents (e.g., loperamide [Imodium A-D]).
      2. Bulking agents (Schiller, 2002).

IV. Interventions to maintain optimal hydration and adequate nutrition.
   A. Increase fluid intake to 2000 to 3000 ml/day unless contraindicated.
   B. Decrease fluid intake after 7:00 PM, and provide minimal fluids during the night.
   C. Reduce intake of caffeine beverages, such as coffee, tea, and colas, and reduce intake of alcohol and other bladder irritants.
   D. Avoid foods that provide a laxative effect or are gas producing (Robinson, 2000).
   E. Include foods that increase the bulk of the stool (Schiller, 2002).
 V. Interventions to monitor the response of the client to symptom management.
   A. Monitor subjective reports of the client and family of changes in the pattern of incontinence.
   B. Monitor the client's compliance to the incontinence management program.
   C. Monitor effectiveness of measures implemented to manage incontinence.
   D. Monitor client's interactions with others and activities of daily life.
VI. Interventions to incorporate client and family in care.
   A. Teach pelvic muscle exercises.
   B. Teach proper use of devices to control incontinence.
   C. Teach toileting programs (e.g., prompted voiding, bladder retraining).
   D. Teach appropriate use of stool softeners, suppositories, enemas.
   E. Discuss the importance of increasing bulk and fluid intake in the diet (Bliss et al., 2001).
   F. Instruct on critical factors that need to be reported to the physician.
      1. Signs and symptoms of urinary tract infections and fecal impaction.
      2. Changes in patterns of elimination.

Evaluation

The oncology nurse systematically and regularly evaluates the client's and/or family's responses to interventions to determine progress toward the achievement of expected outcomes. Relevant data are collected, and actual findings are compared with expected findings. Nursing diagnoses, outcomes, and plans of care are reviewed and revised as needed.

CONSTIPATION

Theory

 I. Definition.
   A. Infrequent passage of hard stool often associated with abdominal cramping and rectal pain.
   B. May also be associated with a feeling of incomplete evacuation following defecation or bloating.
   C. With a fecal impaction, liquid stool can continuously ooze around the impaction and cause fecal incontinence.
II. Physiology. Slowing of intestinal mobility by one of the following mechanisms:
   A. Primary—results from extrinsic factors that slow peristalsis, such as decreased physical activity, lack of time or privacy for defecation, or low-fiber diet.
   B. Secondary—results from pathologic processes, such as bowel obstruction and spinal cord compression or metabolic effects of hypercalcemia, hypokalemia, and hypothyroidism.

    C. Iatrogenic—follows use of pharmacologic agents such as analgesic opiates, chemotherapeutic agents, anticonvulsants, and some psychotropic medications (Yasko, 2002).

III. Risk factors.

    A. Disease related.

        1. Internal or external obstruction of bowel by tumor.

        2. Fluid and electrolyte imbalances—dehydration, hypercalcemia, hypokalemia.

        3. Decreased physical activity and/or immobility.

        4. Spinal cord compression at T8-L3 (levels that control bowel innervation).

        5. Anorexia causing decreased food and fluid intake.

        6. Pressure from ascites.

        7. Neurologic disorders, such as multiple sclerosis, Parkinson's disease, chronic idiopathic intestinal pseudoobstruction, or stroke.

        8. Metabolic and endocrine disorders, such as diabetes, hypothyroidism or hyperthyroidism, or uremia.

        9. Systemic disorders, such as amyloidosis, lupus, or scleroderma.

    B. Treatment related.

        1. Manipulation of intestines during surgery.

        2. Surgical trauma to neurogenic pathways to intestines and/or rectum.

        3. Neurotoxic effects of cancer chemotherapeutic agents such as vincristine (Oncovin, Vincasar PFS) and vinblastine (Velban).

        4. Nutritional deficiencies, such as decreased fiber, roughage, and fluid intake.

        5. Side effects of pharmacologic agents such as narcotics, analgesics, cholinergics, antacids.

    C. Situational.

        1. Lack of privacy.

        2. Interference with usual bowel program.

        3. Failure to respond to defecation reflex because of pain, fatigue, social activities, or inability to reach the toilet.

        4. Depression, decreased physical activity, treatment with anticholinergic medications (Yasko, 2002).

IV. Principles of medical management.

    A. Surgical correction of obstructive disease.

    B. Correction of fluid and electrolyte imbalances.

    C. Enemas or irrigations.

    D. Medications such as laxatives, stool softeners, fiber supplements.

    E. Increased fiber in diet (Yasko, 2002).

V. Potential sequelae of constipation.

    A. Fecal impaction (also called dyschezia or terminal reservoir syndrome).

    B. Paralytic ileus.

    C. Intestinal obstruction.

    D. Laxative dependence (Yasko, 2002).

Assessment

    I. History.

        A. Presence of risk factors.

        B. History of defining characteristics of constipation.

            1. Change in usual patterns of bowel elimination, such as decreased frequency, hard stool, abdominal cramping, increased use of laxatives.

2. Date of last bowel movement.
3. Change in factors contributing to bowel elimination, such as activity level, fluid intake, dietary fiber intake, and/or laxative use.
4. History of constipation and/or chronic laxative use.
5. Anxiety regarding bowel patterns.
6. Perception of incomplete evacuation following defecation.
7. Rectal pain associated with inability to defecate.
8. Sudden onset of diarrhea (can be a symptom of severe impaction).
C. Gastrointestinal (GI) symptoms—nausea, vomiting, anorexia.
D. Pattern of occurrence of constipation—onset; frequency; severity-associated symptoms; precipitating, aggravating, and alleviating factors.
E. Perceived effectiveness of self-care measures to relieve constipation.
F. Perceived impact of constipation on comfort, activities of daily living, mood.
G. History of rectal fissures or abscesses.
II. Physical findings.
A. Inspection of abdomen.
1. Symmetry.
2. Contour.
3. Distention.
4. Bulges.
5. Peristaltic waves.
B. Auscultation of character, frequency, and presence or absence of bowel sounds in the four quadrants of the abdomen.
C. Palpation of abdomen.
1. Masses or stool in the colon.
2. Areas of increased resistance or tenderness.
D. Rectal examination to check for fecal impaction, hemorrhoids, or fissures (Yasko, 2002).

Nursing Diagnoses

I. Constipation.
II. Risk for constipation.
III. Perceived constipation.

Outcome Identification

I. Client reports normal pattern of bowel functioning.
A. Client and family identify and manage factors that may affect constipation, such as diet, stress, physical activity, neurogenic conditions.
B. Client and family contact an appropriate health team member when unable to relieve constipation through self-care measures.
C. Client manages constipation through titration of laxatives.
II. Client does not experience adverse effects or complications of constipation.
III. Client becomes actively involved with others and participates in activities at level of ability or desire.

Planning and Implementation

I. Interventions to minimize risk and severity of constipation.
A. Nonpharmacologic interventions.
1. Encourage at least 3000 ml of fluid intake per day unless contraindicated.

   2. Modify diet as tolerated to include high-fiber foods and roughage, with fresh fruits, vegetables, whole grains, and dried beans to 20 to 35 g of fiber per day.
   3. Maintain or increase physical activity level.
   4. Establish a daily bowel program.
   B. Effective interventions usually used by client to alleviate constipation that are not contraindicated by health status.
   C. Pharmacologic interventions.
      1. Stimulant laxatives—chemically stimulate the smooth muscles of the bowel to increase contractions.
         a. Bisacodyl (Dulcolax).
         b. Cascara (various generics).
         c. Senna (Senokot).
      2. Osmotic laxatives—increase the bulk of the stools by retaining water.
         a. Magnesium salts.
         b. Sodium phosphate.
         c. Polyethylene glycol (MiraLax).
      3. Bulk-forming laxatives—nondigestible substances that pass through the stomach and increase the bulk of the stools.
         a. Methylcellulose.
         b. Psyllium.
      4. Emollient and lubricant laxatives—agents that soften hardened feces and facilitate the passage through the lower intestine.
         a. Docusate.
         b. Mineral oil.
      5. Miscellaneous laxatives.
         a. Glycerin suppositories.
         b. Lactulose.
   D. Initiate a prophylactic bowel regimen with narcotic or vinca alkaloid therapy.
II. Interventions to maximize client safety.
   A. Check for impaction if symptoms warrant, such as decreased or absent bowel sounds, abdominal distention, loss of appetite.
   B. Avoid digital rectal examinations if client is neutropenic and/or thrombocytopenic.
III. Interventions to monitor for complications related to constipation.
   A. Assess for interference with deep breathing related to abdominal distention.
   B. Monitor indicators of social withdrawal related to flatulence and a focus on bowel elimination.
   C. Monitor untoward responses to symptom management.
      1. Abdominal cramping or diarrhea with laxatives.
      2. Rectal emptying and aggravation of constipation with enemas.
      3. Dehydration or decreased fluid intake, which reduces the effectiveness of stool softeners.
   D. Report critical changes to the physician.
      1. Abdominal distention.
      2. Fecal impaction.
      3. Bleeding.
      4. Absence of bowel sounds.
IV. Implement strategies to enhance adaptation and rehabilitation.
   A. Encourage avoidance of laxative abuse with a combination of laxatives and stool softeners.
   B. Emphasize dietary control of constipation with foods high in fiber, such as celery, bran, whole wheat breads.

    C. Advise adoption of a daily fluid intake of 3000 ml, unless contraindicated.

    D. Advise adoption of a daily bowel program.

        1. Daily schedule for evacuation, such as after meals when gastrocolic reflexes are active.

        2. Privacy.

        3. Medications such as stool softeners or expanders or natural laxative mixtures: avoidance of pharmaceutical laxatives if possible.

        4. Enemas or irrigation procedures if necessary.

 V. Interventions to incorporate client and family in care.

    A. Teach to control constipation through fluid intake, dietary control, activity level.

    B. Inform of hazards of laxative dependence.

    C. Instruct to limit use of gas-producing foods, such as cabbage, beans, green peppers, and onions, in meal planning (Yasko, 2002).

Evaluation

The oncology nurse systematically and regularly evaluates the client's and/or family's responses to interventions to determine progress toward the achievement of expected outcomes. Relevant data are collected, and actual findings are compared with expected findings. Nursing diagnoses, outcomes, and plans of care are reviewed and revised as necessary.

DIARRHEA

Theory

 I. Definition—an increase in the quantity, frequency, or fluid content of stool that is different from the usual pattern of bowel elimination. It is often accompanied by a sudden urge to defecate, sense of bloating, and/or cramping abdominal pain.

    A. Classifications.

        1. By volume.

            a. Large volume—results from a larger-than-usual amount of water, intestinal secretion, or both in the intestine.

            b. Small volume—results from excessive intestinal mobility.

        2. By acuity, acute or chronic, depending on underlying pathologic condition.

    B. Physiology.

        1. Osmotic—unabsorbable substances in intestine draw water into intestinal lumen by osmosis, increasing the weight and volume of stool.

            a. Lactose intolerance.

            b. Enteral tube feedings.

            c. Intestinal hemorrhage.

        2. Secretory—intestinal mucosa secretes excessive amounts of fluid and electrolytes.

            a. Bacteria, such as *Escherichia coli* or *C. difficile.*

            b. Laxatives.

            c. Neuroendocrine tumors.

        3. Hypermotility—limited absorption because of increased motility of intestines.

            a. Inflammatory bowel disease.

            b. Radiation proctitis.

       c. Chemotherapy drugs.

       d. Graft-versus-host disease (Yasko, 2002).

  II. Risk factors.

    A. Disease related.

      1. Obstruction of bowel from intrinsic or extrinsic tumor.

      2. Intestinal bacteria or viruses.

      3. Graft-versus-host disease in which immunocompetent cells of the allogeneic donor marrow recognize the normal GI cells as "foreign" and initiate an immune reaction that leads to cell destruction of target tissues in the gut.

      4. Intestinal neuroendocrine tumors with liver metastases.

      5. Food intolerance or allergies.

    B. Treatment related.

      1. Surgical resection of significant portions of bowel can cause fluid malabsorption syndrome.

      2. RT to abdominal area causes increased cellular destruction in bowel lumen and increased intestinal motility.

      3. Chemotherapeutic agents can cause increased cellular destruction on bowel lumen and can heighten intestinal motility (Viele et al., 2002).

      4. Medications such as antibiotics, antacids, or laxatives.

      5. Nutritional therapies such as tube feedings and dietary supplements.

      6. Fecal impaction can create paradoxical diarrhea (Yasko, 2002).

    C. Lifestyle related.

      1. Increased stress and anxiety in presence of inadequate coping strategies.

      2. Changes in usual dietary habits, such as increases in dietary fiber or other foods containing natural laxative properties.

 III. Principles of medical management.

    A. Pharmacologic management of symptoms.

    B. Modification of associated therapy, such as radiation, chemotherapy, nutritional supplements, or antibiotics.

    C. Treatment of associated conditions such as *C. difficile* infection or graft-versus-host disease.

    D. Decompression or surgery for bowel obstruction.

    E. Manual disimpaction if white blood cell (WBC) and platelet counts permit.

    F. Hormone inhibition therapy such as octreotide (Depot, Sandostatin) (Yasko, 2002).

 IV. Potential sequelae of prolonged diarrhea.

    A. Dehydration.

    B. Electrolyte imbalances, such as hypokalemia or hyponatremia.

    C. Impaired skin integrity of perineal area.

    D. Decreased social interaction.

    E. Fatigue (Yasko, 2002).

Assessment

  I. History.

    A. Review of previous and current therapy for cancer.

    B. Review of prescription and nonprescription medications.

    C. Usual bowel pattern—frequency, color, amount, odor, consistency of stool.

    D. Recent changes in factors contributing to usual bowel elimination patterns.

   1. Increased levels of stress.
   2. Dietary changes that increase bowel motility, such as addition of fiber and roughage, fruit juices, coffee, alcohol, fried foods, or fatty foods.
   3. Recent course of antibiotic therapy.
 E. Known food or medication intolerance or allergies.
 F. Presence of flatus, cramping, abdominal pain, urgency to defecate, recent weight loss, decreased urinary output of 500 ml less than intake.
 G. Fluid intake.
 H. Weight loss greater than 1% to 2% in 1 week (Yasko, 2002).
II. National Cancer Institute Grading Criteria.
 A. Grade 1: increase of fewer than 4 stools/day over pretreatment.
 B. Grade 2: increase of 4 to 6 stools/day or nocturnal stools.
 C. Grade 3: increase of 7 or more stools/day or incontinence or need for parenteral support for dehydration interfering with normal activity.
 D. Grade 4: physiologic consequences requiring intensive care; hemodynamic collapse.
III. Physical examination.
 A. Hypotension.
 B. Tachycardia.
 C. Hyperactive bowel sounds.
 D. Hard stool in rectum.
 E. Perineal skin irritation.
 F. Poor skin turgor.
 G. Dry mucous membranes (Yasko, 2002).
IV. Psychosocial examination.
 A. Presence of fear.
 B. Presence of anxiety.
 C. Complaints of isolation (Yasko, 2002).
 V. Diagnostic studies.
 A. Stool culture for *C. difficile*.
 B. Serum electrolytes.
 C. Daily weights.

Nursing Diagnoses

 I. Diarrhea.
 II. Impaired skin integrity.
III. Deficient fluid volume.
IV. Risk for social interaction.

Outcome Identification

 I. Client reestablishes and maintains a normal pattern of bowel function.
 A. Client and family identify and manage factors that may affect diarrhea, such as diet, stress, physical activity, neurogenic conditions.
 B. Client and family contact an appropriate health care team member when diarrhea is severe, prolonged (12 to 24 hours), uncontrollable with self-care measures, interfering with quality of life, or accompanied by fever, nausea, vomiting, or reduced urine output.
 II. Client's skin remains intact.
III. Client experiences adequate fluid volume and electrolyte balance.

IV. Client becomes actively involved with others and participates in activities at level of ability or as desired.
  A. Client performs activities of daily living safely and as independently as possible.

Planning and Implementation

I. Interventions to minimize risk of occurrence and severity of diarrhea.
  A. Pharmacologic interventions.
    1. Antidiarrheals.
      a. Loperamide (Imodium A-D).
      b. Diphenoxylate (Lomotil).
    2. Antispasmodic: atropine.
    3. Antiinflammatory: mesalamine.
    4. Antibiotics.
      a. Metronidazole (Flagyl).
      b. Neomycin (Kehrer et al., 2001).
  B. Nonpharmacologic interventions.
    1. Modify dietary plan to avoid foods the client cannot tolerate.
    2. Decrease fiber and roughage.
    3. Encourage smaller meals eaten more frequently (Yasko, 2002).
II. Implement strategies to decrease bowel motility.
  A. Pharmacologic interventions.
    1. Narcotics: tincture of opium.
    2. Octreotide (Sandostatin).
    3. Bulk forming: methylcellulose (Citrucel), psyllium (Metamucil) (Murphy et al., 2000).
  B. Nonpharmacologic.
    1. Serve foods and liquids at room temperature.
    2. Avoid coffee and alcohol.
    3. Avoid spicy, fried, or fatty foods and food additives.
    4. Teach strategies such as relaxation, distraction, or imagery to modify stress response.
    5. Low-residue diet for clients with bowel irritation.
    6. Low-lactose diet for clients with known or temporary lactose intolerance.
      a. Diet is maintained for 2 weeks after diarrhea subsides.
      b. Dairy products may then be reintroduced slowly into diet (Yasko, 2002).
III. Interventions to maximize client safety.
  A. Monitor level of weakness and fatigue.
  B. Provide assistance with ambulation and activities of daily living as indicated.
IV. Interventions to monitor for complications related to diarrhea.
  A. Assess the character of bowel movement at each stool or with a change in symptoms.
  B. Assess the perineal area every 8 hours or with a change in symptoms.
  C. Monitor intake and output ratio; electrolyte, creatinine, and blood urea nitrogen (BUN) levels.
  D. Monitor for subtle changes in client affect, neuromuscular responses, activity level, and cognitive status as cues for potential electrolyte imbalances.
  E. Weigh daily.
  F. Report significant changes in condition to the physician.

    G. Implement rectal skin care regimen.

    H. Monitor changes in skin turgor and mucous membranes.

  V. Interventions to improve social interactions.

    A. Determine impact of diarrhea on social interactions and activities.

    B. Teach client interventions to minimize impact of diarrhea in social situations and daily living.

  VI. Interventions to incorporate the client and family in care.

    A. Teach a perineal hygiene program to include cleansing perineal area with mild soap, rinsing thoroughly, patting area dry, and applying a skin barrier after each bowel movement.

    B. Teach dietary modifications to minimize diarrhea and replace electrolytes.

    C. Teach signs and symptoms related to complications of diarrhea to report to a member of the health care team (Yasko, 2002).

Evaluation

The oncology nurse systematically and regularly evaluates the client's and/or family's responses to interventions to determine progress toward the achievement of expected outcomes. Relevant data are collected, and actual findings are compared with expected findings. Nursing diagnoses, outcomes, and plans of care are reviewed and revised as necessary.

BOWEL OBSTRUCTION

Theory

  I. Definition—narrowing of the intestinal lumen or interference with peristalsis.

  II. Physiology.

    A. Mechanical obstruction—occurs in small intestines and accounts for 90% of all obstructions.

      1. Causes.

        a. Extrinsic lesions—adhesions of the peritoneum, hernias, volvulus (twisting of the intestines).

        b. Intrinsic lesions—benign or malignant tumors; intussusception (telescoping of the intestines); an ischemic or inflammatory process that involves the bowel wall (e.g., inflammatory bowel disease, diverticulitis) and produces strictures, narrows the intestinal lumen, and impairs transit.

        c. Objects blocking the intestinal lumen, such as foreign bodies and fecal or barium impaction.

      2. Types.

        a. Simple—lumen is occluded in only one place, and blood flow to abdomen is unchanged.

        b. Closed loop—lumen is blocked in two places.

        c. Strangulation—lumen is blocked, and blood flow to some or all of the obstructed segment is restricted.

    B. Nonmechanical obstruction.

      1. Intestinal lumen is patent, but neuromuscular dysfunction or a lack of intestinal blood flow inhibits peristalsis.

        a. Condition also called ileus or functional or adynamic obstruction.

      2. Causes.

      a. Intraabdominal.

        (1) Reflex inhibition associated with laparotomy and other abdominal surgeries or with trauma. The more the bowel is manipulated in surgery, the longer an ileus lasts. The length of surgery is not a factor in the development of ileus.

        (2) Inflammatory conditions, such as peritonitis and pancreatitis.

        (3) Bowel ischemia as a result of mesenteric artery emboli or venous thrombosis.

      b. Extraabdominal.

        (1) Reflex inhibition related to fractures of the ribs, spine, or pelvis; kidney surgery; myocardial infarction; pneumonia; pulmonary embolus; electrolyte imbalances; metabolic imbalances, such as septicemia.

        (2) Pharmacologic reflex inhibition can be caused by anticholinergics, ganglionic blockers, opiates, chemotherapeutic agents.

        (3) Hypokalemia can cause slowed peristalsis leading to ileus.

  C. Location.

    1. Small intestine obstructions occur because of the following:

      a. Postoperative intraabdominal adhesions. They can entrap a loop of intestine and contract, causing an obstruction and possibly strangulation. Adhesions can develop a few days postoperatively or many years later.

      b. Nonsurgical adhesions following an infection such as peritonitis or following RT. Nonsurgical adhesions can occur at any time following the infection or completion of RT.

      c. Hernias.

      d. Miscellaneous conditions, such as cancer, telescoping, inflammatory bowel disease.

    2. Large bowel obstructions occur most often in the sigmoid colon and are caused by the following:

      a. Cancer.

      b. Volvulus.

      c. Diverticulitis (Waldman, 2001).

III. Risk factors.

  A. Disease related.

    1. Obstruction of bowel by tumor. Most common tumors are ovarian cancer and colorectal cancers.

    2. Hernia.

    3. Inflammatory bowel disease.

    4. Gallstones.

    5. Peptic ulcers.

    6. Pancreatitis.

    7. Diverticular disease.

  B. Treatment related.

    1. Manipulation of intestines during surgery.

    2. Surgical trauma to neurogenic pathways to intestines and/or rectum.

    3. Previous intestinal obstruction.

    4. RT to abdominal area.

  C. Situational—ingestion of a foreign body (Waldman, 2001).

IV. Principles of medical management.

  A. Surgical options.

    1. Resection and reanastomosis.

    2. Decompression with a colostomy or ileostomy.

  3. Bypass of an obstructing lesion.
  4. Lysis of adhesions.
  B. Nothing by mouth (NPO).
  C. Abdominal decompression.
  1. Nasogastric suction.
  2. Percutaneous gastrostomy.
  3. Enema.
  4. Rectal tube.
  5. Intestinal stenting—a large-caliber stent placed using fluoroscopic and endoscopic guidance (Aviv et al., 2002; Carter et al., 2002).
  D. Correction of fluid and electrolyte imbalances.
  E. Parenteral nutrition (Waldman, 2001).
  V. Potential sequelae of bowel obstruction.
  A. Dehydration.
  B. Peritonitis.
  C. Bowel perforation.
  D. Hypotension.
  E. Hypovolemic or septic shock (Waldman, 2001).

Assessment

  I. History.
  A. Presence of risk factors.
  B. Symptoms.
  1. Abdominal pain and intestinal colic from intestinal stretching and pressure of peristalsis as the bowel tries to push its contents past the obstruction; can help identify the obstruction's type and severity.
  a. Small intestine obstructions—intermittent, cramping pain in the middle to upper abdomen that is temporarily relieved by vomiting.
  b. Large intestine obstructions—persistent cramping pain in the lower abdomen.
  c. Mechanical obstructions—cramping and spasmodic.
  d. Nonmechanical obstructions—diffuse, constant, and less intense pain that can be described as pressure or fullness.
  e. Partial obstructions—cramping pain after eating along with mild to moderate hypomotility.
  f. Complete bowel obstruction—pain intensifies and comes in waves or spasms as the bowel tries to push the intestinal contents past the obstruction.
  (1) Peristalsis may stop when bowel becomes exhausted.
  g. Strangulation—constant, intense pain that is intensified with movement.
  2. Nausea and vomiting.
  a. Gastric outlet obstruction—sour emesis that is not bile colored and often contains undigested food.
  b. Proximal small intestine obstruction—rapid-onset, bitter, bile-stained emesis that may be projectile.
  c. Distal small intestine obstruction or colonic obstruction with an incompetent ileocecal valve—orange-brown malodorous feculent emesis.
  3. Anorexia.
  4. Constipation.
  a. May experience lack of bowel movements and flatus or may have paradoxical diarrhea (if partial blockage exists).

        b. Bowel may evacuate below an obstruction, and then the client may develop obstipation.

    C. Past and present patterns of elimination.

        1. Any recent changes in stool consistency or bowel habits.

        2. Date and time of last bowel movement.

        3. Use of antacids, laxatives, or enemas.

    D. Miscellaneous.

        1. Current medications.

        2. Endocrine history.

        3. Immunologic history.

        4. Diet (Waldman, 2001).

II. Physical findings.

    A. Abdominal distention.

        1. The lower the obstruction, the longer it lasts.

           a. The more complete it is, the more severe the distention will be.

        2. Baseline measurement of abdominal girth should be obtained.

        3. Boardlike abdomen may indicate peritonitis.

    B. Abnormal bowel sounds.

        1. Intermittent borborygmi (loud prolonged gurgles of hyperperistalsis).

        2. Mechanical obstruction.

           a. Proximal to obstruction, high-pitched, tinkling, or hyperactive bowel sounds that may be heard in clusters or rushes.

           b. Distal to the obstruction, bowel sounds are hypoactive or absent.

        3. Nonmechanical.

           a. Hypoactive, low-pitched gurgles or weak tinkles may be heard.

           b. Absent bowel sounds may indicate a paralytic ileus (Waldman, 2001).

III. Diagnostic tests.

    A. Abdominal radiographs.

    B. Computed tomography (CT) scans of the abdomen (Ahn et al., 2002).

    C. Contrast media studies.

        1. Oral barium is not used if bowel perforation is suspected or until colonic obstruction is ruled out.

        2. Barium enema is used to evaluate colonic obstruction.

    D. Endoscopy.

    E. Magnetic resonance imaging (MRI) (Matsuoka et al., 2002; Waldman, 2001).

Nursing Diagnoses

   I. Acute pain.

  II. Risk for deficient fluid volume.

 III. Risk for infection.

 IV. Imbalanced nutrition: less than body requirements.

Outcome Identification

   I. Client reports adequate pain relief.

  II. Client safety is maintained through nursing intervention and appropriate communication.

 III. Client experiences adequate fluid volume and electrolyte balance.

    A. Client and family contact an appropriate health care team member when symptoms of bowel obstruction occur.

IV. Client remains free of infection.
    A. Infection is recognized early and treated promptly.

Planning and Implementation

    I. Interventions to minimize risk and severity of bowel obstruction.
      A. Promote comfort.
        1. Pharmacologic interventions.
          a. Opiate analgesics.
          b. Analgesic adjuncts.
          c. Smooth muscle relaxants.
          d. Antiemetics.
          e. Corticosteroids.
        2. Nonpharmacologic interventions.
          a. Relaxing environment.
          b. Back rubs or massage.
          c. Position on side and support with pillows.
      B. Administer fluid and electrolyte replacement therapy.
      C. Provide frequent oral care.
        1. Use moistened sponge sticks.
        2. Avoid lemon or glycerin swabs.
      D. Ambulate early and to the client's tolerance.
      E. Encourage deep breathing exercises (Waldman, 2001).
   II. Interventions to maximize client safety.
      A. Elevate head of bed 45 degrees to improve ventilation and avoid aspiration.
      B. Provide care of nasogastric tube.
        1. Assess pressure around nostrils every shift.
        2. Apply a water-soluble lubricant to nasal mucosa.
        3. Irrigate the tube with normal saline.
      C. Report critical changes in client assessment parameters to the physician.
        1. Fever and chills.
        2. Local intense constant pain.
        3. Absence of bowel sounds after full 5 minutes of auscultation.
        4. Muscle guarding, rigidity, rebound tenderness.
        5. Sudden worsening of client's condition (Waldman, 2001).
  III. Interventions to monitor for complications related to bowel obstruction.
      A. Assess for signs and symptoms of dehydration—dry mouth and lips, poor skin turgor, decreased urinary output.
      B. Assess for interference with deep breathing related to abdominal distention.
      C. Assess for signs and symptoms of peritonitis—boardlike abdomen, increased pain on movement, shallow respirations, tachycardia.
      D. Measure abdominal girth every shift.
      E. Monitor intake/output ratio, including gastric output.
      F. Monitor key laboratory values.
        1. Electrolytes—sodium, potassium, chloride levels.
        2. Renal function tests—BUN, creatinine levels.
        3. Complete blood count (CBC)—hemoglobin, hematocrit levels.
        4. Arterial blood gases—bicarbonate level, arterial blood pH.
        5. Serum enzymes—amylase, alkaline phosphatase, creatine kinase, lactate dehydrogenase (LDH) levels.
  IV. Interventions to incorporate the client and family in care.

    A. Explain all treatments and their rationale.

    B. Instruct the client on deep breathing exercises.

    C. Instruct the client on interventions that reduce anxiety and provide comfort, such as relaxation techniques, mental imagery, music.

    D. Instruct the client to breathe through the nose to decrease the amount of air swallowed.

    E. Teach signs and symptoms of bowel obstruction to report to the health care team.

    F. Teach signs and symptoms of infection to report to the health care team.

Evaluation

The oncology nurse systematically and regularly evaluates the client's and/or family's responses to interventions to determine progress toward the achievement of expected outcomes. Relevant data are collected, and actual findings are compared with expected findings. Nursing diagnoses, outcomes, and plans of care are reviewed and revised as necessary.

OSTOMIES AND URINARY DIVERSIONS

Theory

I. Diversions.

    A. Fecal.

        1. Colostomy is a surgical creation of an opening between the colon and the abdominal wall.

            a. Surgical considerations.

                (1) Created in situations in which there is muscle-invasive cancer and locally advanced cancer in the pelvis (i.e., gynecologic and rectal malignancies).

                (2) Extent of colonic resection is determined by blood supply and distribution of lymph nodes.

                (3) Distal sigmoid, rectosigmoid, rectum, and anus are removed through an abdominal and perineal approach resulting in a permanent colostomy.

                (4) Wide excision is done in cancer of the low rectum to remove lymph nodes, remove bulky tumor in the pelvis, and obtain adequate margins.

                (5) Potency and continence are preserved as nerves are spared because of dissection around hypogastric and pelvic plexus (Bresalier, 2002).

            b. Types.

                (1) Temporary—indicated for bowel decompression in the presence of an obstructing tumor or fistulas involving the colon or rectum or to allow for bowel to heal following surgery.

                (2) Permanent—indicated when the distal bowel, rectum, and anus are removed because of rectal cancer.

            c. Location of colostomy determines consistency and volume of output.

                (1) Cecostomy or ascending type produces semifluid to mushy stool that contains residual enzymes and occurs throughout the day.

                (2) Transverse ostomies drain mushy stool at irregular intervals, usually after meals, and contain no enzymes.

        (3) Descending or sigmoid type produces soft to formed stool and can be regulated by irrigation.

    d. Stomas may be identified by the type of surgical construction: end, loop, or double-barrel.

        (1) End stoma is constructed by dividing the bowel and bringing the proximal end of the bowel through an opening in the abdominal wall.

            (a) Distal bowel segment is removed in abdominal perineal resection.

            (b) Distal bowel segment is sutured closed and left in place, called Hartmann's pouch, and continues to produce mucus from the rectum.

        (2) Loop stoma is constructed by bringing a loop of bowel out through an incision and stabilizing it on the abdomen.

            (a) Usually created in the transverse loop.

            (b) Temporary procedure to relieve an obstruction or as palliation in terminal cancer.

        (3) Double-barrel indicates two stomas side by side or apart from one another.

            (a) Distal stoma often referred to as a mucous fistula and produces mucus.

            (b) Proximal stoma produces stool (Potter, 2000).

B. Urinary.

  1. Urinary diversions are surgically created to divert the urine stream away from the original lower urinary tract.

    a. Performed in situations in which the bladder is removed, that is, radical cystectomy or radical cystoprostatectomy for cancer of the bladder.

    b. Involves removal of the bladder, pelvic lymph nodes, prostate (in men) and uterus, fallopian tubes, ovaries, and anterior vaginal wall, possibly urethra (in women).

    c. Sexual dysfunction is common because of neural damage from surgery (Krupski & Theodorescu, 2001).

  2. Types.

    a. Ileal conduit.

        (1) Created from segment of small bowel. As the proximal end is sutured closed, the distal end is brought out through the abdominal wall. Stoma is created, and the ureters are implanted into the small bowel segment.

        (2) Urine is produced almost continuously.

        (3) Requires an external collection device.

        (4) As a freely refluxing system, there is high risk for chronic urinary tract infections, which increases the risk of stone formation (Colwell et al., 2001).

    b. Continent diversions.

        (1) Reservoir constructed from ileum or large intestine, which stores up to 800 ml of urine.

        (2) Continence is maintained by the construction of the reservoir via a one-way flap valve (Krupski & Theodorescu, 2001).

        (3) External collection device not needed.

    c. Orthoptic neobladder.

        (1) Newer urinary reconstructive procedure in which a surgically constructed bladder is created from intestine or stomach and attached to the urethra.

        (2) Intermittent catheterization may be necessary.

(3) Voiding is accomplished by relaxation of the urinary sphincters and a simultaneous practice of Valsalva's maneuver.

(4) Factors that would exclude creation of neobladder include cancer extending in urethra, past history of inflammatory bowel disease, radiation, or short gut syndrome from previous bowel resection (Krupski & Theodorescu, 2001).

II. Risk factors.
  A. Low rectal cancers.
  B. Ulcerative colitis (Bresalier, 2002).
  C. Pelvic radiation.
  D. Chemotherapy.
  E. Bladder cancer with muscle invasion (Colwell et al., 2001).
III. Effects of treatment.
  A. Pelvic exenteration can result in a urinary diversion, fecal diversion, or both.
  B. Pelvic and abdominal radiation causes damage to the mucosa resulting in diarrhea and cystitis.
  C. Mucosal damage can occur when the stoma is located in the field of radiation treatment (Potter, 2000).
  D. Antineoplastic agents, such as 5-fluorouracil (5-FU), mitomycin C, and vincristine (Oncovin), can cause stomatitis, diarrhea, constipation (Yarbro et al., 2000).

Assessment

I. Pertinent personal history.
  A. Type of surgery and stoma.
  B. Previous pelvic or abdominal radiation or chemotherapy treatments.
  C. Changes in patterns of elimination.
  D. Recurrent or chronic urinary tract infections.
  E. Difficulty in catheterizing a continent diversion.
  F. Diet habits and fluid consumption.
  G. History of chronic ulcerative colitis (Krupski & Theodorescu , 2001).
II. Physical findings.
  A. Characteristics of stoma and peristomal skin.
  B. Presence of leakage of urine from a continent diversion.
  C. Effectiveness of pouching system.
  D. Characteristics of effluent, that is, volume, consistency, color (Colwell et al., 2001).

Nursing Diagnoses

I. Deficient knowledge related to management of fecal or urinary diversions.
II. Disturbed body image.
III. Impaired skin integrity.
IV. Social isolation.
V. Sexual dysfunction.

Outcome Identification

I. Client manages care of ostomy/urinary diversion within his/her lifestyle.
  A. Client contacts the wound/ostomy/continence nurse for ongoing evaluations and maintaining up-to-date equipment.

II. Client verbalizes feelings about the ostomy or urinary diversion and effect on body image.
III. Client's stoma remains red and moist.
   A. Skin surrounding stoma is intact.
IV. Client becomes more actively involved with others.
   A. Client is aware of available support groups, such as the United Ostomy Association.
V. Client and significant other demonstrate confidence in their ability to resume previous sexual activities.

Planning and Implementation

I. Interventions to minimize incidence and severity of complications associated with diversions.
   A. Stoma care.
      1. Stoma placement.
         a. Scars, bony prominences, skin creases, or belt line is avoided.
         b. Site is marked while client is lying, standing, and sitting.
         c. Site is located within the borders of the rectus muscle (Colwell et al., 2001).
      2. Appliance selection is based on type of effluent, abdominal contour, manual dexterity, patient preference, cost.
      3. Change appliance every 5 days and as needed for leakage or complaint of peristomal skin discomfort.
      4. Cut pouch opening so barrier clears stoma by ⅛ inch and protect exposed skin with skin barrier paste if needed.
      5. Gently remove pouch by pushing down on the skin while lifting up on the pouch.
      6. Cleanse peristomal skin with water, and pat dry.
      7. Assess stoma and skin around stoma for erythema, dermatitis, bleeding, infection, stomal protrusion, retraction, mucoseparation, prolapse, herniation, and stenosis with each appliance change.
      8. Empty pouch when one third to one half full and before chemotherapy treatment.
      9. Protect stoma from injury (Colwell et al., 2001).
   B. Management of diversion.
      1. Monitor volume, color, and consistency of effluent.
      2. Monitor functioning of new colostomies, which usually commences 3 to 5 days after surgery.
      3. Catheterize new continent diversions beginning about 3 to 4 weeks after surgery (Potter, 2000).
II. Interventions to monitor for side effects of treatment.
   A. Nonpharmacologic interventions.
      1. Cease irrigating colostomy until radiation or chemotherapy has been completed.
      2. Protect stomal mucosa from trauma between daily radiation treatments (Potter, 2000).
      3. Increase dietary fiber and fluid intake (Floruta, 2001).
   B. Pharmacologic interventions.
      1. Encourage use of stool softeners if constipated.
      2. Use silver nitrate sticks to stop bleeding of stoma (Potter, 2000).
III. Implement strategies to enhance adaptation and rehabilitation and decrease social isolation.

    A. Teach the client how to irrigate the colostomy as a management option for regulating function of a descending and sigmoid colostomy.

    B. Teach the client measures to control gas and odor.

    C. Teach ways to manage constipation and diarrhea.

    D. Teach about the importance of adequate dietary fiber and fluid intake.

    E. Discuss the signs and symptoms of urinary tract infections and the time at which to seek medical attention.

    F. Inform about service resources available, such as the United Ostomy Association.

    G. Refer to the wound, ostomy, continence nurse for stoma marking and follow-up care (Colwell et al., 2001).

    H. Teach the client about management of Foley and Malecot catheters on discharge following the initial orthoptic neobladder surgery (Krupski & Theodorescu, 2001).

 IV. Implement strategies to improve sexual functioning (see Chapter 6).

    A. Assess for presence of sexual dysfunction.

    B. Refer patient and partner to appropriate resource for sexual counseling and treatment.

Evaluation

The oncology nurse systematically and regularly evaluates the client's and/or family's responses to interventions to determine progress toward the achievement of expected outcomes. Relevant data are collected, and actual findings are compared with expected findings. Nursing diagnoses, outcomes, and plans of care are reviewed and revised as necessary.

RENAL DYSFUNCTION

Theory

  I. Physiology.

    A. Kidneys regulate fluid and electrolyte balance by filtering essential substances from the blood, selectively reabsorbing needed fluid and electrolytes, and excreting those not needed in the urine (Schollwerth & Gehr, 2000).

    B. Mechanism of chemotherapy-induced renal dysfunction generally includes damage to vasculature or structures of the kidneys, intrarenal damage, hemolytic-uremic syndrome (consists of anemia, thrombocytopenia, acute renal failure), prerenal perfusion deficits, postrenal obstruction from tumor lysis syndrome, and development of obstructive stones.

    C. Severe and prolonged renal hypoperfusion can promote intrinsic renal damage.

    D. Damage to the renal tubules, renal blood vessels, the interstitium or glomerulus of the kidney leads to kidney dysfunction.

    E. Injury to the renal tubules causes electrolyte loss, renal tubular acidosis, loss of urine concentrating ability, and reduction of glomerular filtration rate (Kintzel, 2001).

 II. Risk factors.

    A. Effects of disease.

      1. Compression of ureters by metastatic tumor of the surrounding lymph nodes can cause obstruction, resulting in hydronephrosis.

      2. Loss of ability by the kidneys to concentrate urine occurs in hypercalcemia of malignancy.

    a. Kidneys are attempting to excrete all of the calcium in the blood and hence the diuresis and accompanying electrolyte disturbances, such as hypophosphatemia.

    b. Hypercalcemia of malignancy occurs more commonly in cancers such as breast cancer with metastases; multiple myeloma; squamous cell cancer of the lung, and head and neck; renal cell cancer; lymphomas; leukemia (Kintzel, 2001).

  3. Advanced prostate or cervical cancer renal problems are related to postrenal obstructive uropathy (Yarbro et al., 2000).

B. Treatment related.

  1. Radiation to renal structures can lead to permanent fibrosis and atrophy.

  2. Precipitation of uric acid or calcium phosphate crystallization from lysis of tumor cells may result in obstruction or formation of stones.

  3. Fluid and electrolyte imbalances caused by chemotherapy agents can have an indirect effect on kidney function and can lead to renal failure.

  4. Direct effect by nephrotoxic agents, such as antineoplastic agents cisplatin [Platinol], carboplatin [Paraplatin], ifosfamide [Ifex], gemcitabine [Gemzar], high-dose methotrexate [MTX], carmustine [BiCNU], semustine [Lomustine], pentostatin [Nipent], diaziquone [AZQ], interferon-α [Alferon-N], mitomycin-C [Mutamycin], streptozocin [Zanosar], aminoglycoside antibiotics, amphotericin B [Fungizone].

Assessment

I. Pertinent personal history to identify risk factors.

  A. Advanced age.

  B. Diuretics, cardiac and nephrotoxic medications.

  C. Type of malignancy.

  D. Comorbidities such as hypertension, diabetes insipidus.

  E. Previous pelvic or abdominal radiation or chemotherapy treatments.

  F. Renal stones.

  G. Preexisting renal impairment.

II. Physical findings.

  A. Cardiovascular—arrhythmias, rapid thready pulse, orthostatic hypotension.

  B. Neurologic—lethargy, confusion.

  C. Poor skin turgor, dry mucous membranes.

  D. GI—nausea, vomiting, polydipsia, splenomegaly.

  E. Genitourinary—nocturia, polyuria, oliguria, flank pain, dysuria.

III. Laboratory data.

  A. Serum creatinine and BUN levels reflect renal function.

  B. Creatinine clearance study is often done before implementing chemotherapy to assess renal function.

  C. Elevation of serum uric acid and calcium levels and a decrease in potassium and magnesium levels may suggest renal impairment (Schoolwerth & Gehr, 2000).

Nursing Diagnoses

I. Excess fluid volume.

II. Ineffective tissue perfusion, renal.

III. Deficient knowledge related to effects of disease process and treatment on the kidneys.

Outcome Identification

I. Client maintains adequate fluid volume and electrolyte balance.
II. Client and family identify and manage factors that may affect renal function, such as diet, medications, physical activity.
III. Client and family report development of symptoms or signs of renal dysfunction to the health care provider.

Planning and Implementation

I. Interventions to monitor for incidence and risk of renal toxicity.
  A. Verify baseline renal function.
  B. Nonpharmacologic interventions.
   1. Monitor intake and output closely.
     a. Observing urine output of less than 30 ml/hr may indicate renal impairment.
     b. Maintain adequate fluid intake.
     c. If client is receiving diuretics, maintain a greater intake than output unless contraindicated.
     d. Ensure aggressive hydration before, during, and after cisplatin (Platinol-AQ) administration.
     e. Maintain adequate fluid intake.
     f. Monitor for obstructive diuresis (urine output of greater than 2000 ml in 8 hours) following the removal of obstruction.
     g. Strain urine for stones, if indicated.
   2. Monitor vital signs and postural blood pressure.
   3. Monitor laboratory data: serum creatinine, BUN, phosphorus, potassium, magnesium, sodium, uric acid, and creatinine clearance levels.
   4. Record daily weights.
   5. Maximize mobility.
     a. Change position every 2 hours.
     b. Perform passive range of motion exercises for patients on bed rest.
     c. Encourage weight bearing and ambulation if able (Schoolwerth & Gehr, 2000).
  C. Pharmacologic interventions.
   1. Saline hydration with appropriate diuretic to maintain fluid balance (Kintzel, 2001).
   2. Oral sodium bicarbonate to maintain alkaline urine.
   3. Amifostine and sodium thiosulfate for cisplatin nephrotoxicity (Kintzel, 2001).
II. Interventions to incorporate client and family in care.
  A. Instruct the client on importance of maintaining adequate hydration and safe weight-bearing activity.
  B. Teach the client and family the signs and symptoms of hypercalcemia, dehydration, and obstruction and the appropriate time to seek medical attention.
  C. Explain properties of medications prescribed.

Evaluation

The oncology nurse systematically and regularly evaluates the client's and/or family's responses to interventions to determine progress toward the achievement of expected outcomes. Relevant data are collected, and actual findings are compared

with expected findings. Nursing diagnoses, outcomes, and plans of care are reviewed and revised as necessary.

REFERENCES

Agency for Health Care Policy and Research (AHCPR). (1996). *Managing acute and chronic incontinence: Quick reference guide for clinicians* (AHCPR Publication No. 96-0686). Rockville, MD: U.S. Department of Health and Human Services.

Ahn, S.H., Mayo-Smith, W.W., Murphy, B.L., et al. (2002). Acute nontraumatic abdominal pain in adult patients: Abdominal radiography compared with CT evaluation. *Radiology 225*(1), 159-164.

Aviv, R.I., Shymalan, G., Watkinson, A., et al. (2002). Radiological palliation of malignant colonic obstruction. *Clinical Radiology 57*(5), 347-351.

Bliss, D., Jung, H.J., Savik, K., et al. (2001). Supplementation with dietary fiber improves fecal incontinence. *Nursing Research 50*(4), 203-213.

Bresalier, R. (2002). *Sleisinger and Fordtran's gastrointestinal and liver disease, volume* II (7th ed.). Philadelphia: W.B. Saunders.

Carlson, K., & Nitti, V. (2001). Prevention and management of incontinence following radical prostatectomy. *Urologic Clinics of North America 28*(3), 595-609.

Carter, J., Valmadre, S., Dalyrmple, C., et al. (2002). Management of large bowel obstruction in advanced ovarian cancer with luminal stents. *Gynecological Oncology 84*(1), 176-179.

Colwell, J., Goldberg, M., & Carmel, J. (2001). The state of the standard diversion. *Journal of Wound, Ostomy, & Incontinence Nursing 28*(1), 6-17.

Flessir, A., & Blarvis, J. (2002). Evaluating incontinence in women. *Urologic Clinics of North America 29*(3), 515-526.

Floruta, C. (2001) Dietary choices of people with ostomies. *Journal of Wound, Ostomy, & Incontinence Nursing 28*(1), 28-31.

Gormley, E. (2002). Biofeedback and behavioral therapy for the management of female urinary incontinence. *Urologic Clinics of North America 29*(3), 551-558.

Kehrer, D.F.S., Sparreboom, A., Verweij, J., et al. (2001). Modulation of irinotecan-induced diarrhea by cotreatment with neomycin in cancer patients. *Clinical Cancer Research 7*, 1136-1141.

Kintzel, P. (2001). Anticancer drug-induced kidney disorders: Incidence, prevention, and management. *Drug Safety 24*(1), 19-38.

Krupski, T., & Theodorescu, D. (2001). Orthotopic neobladder following cystectomy: Indications, management, and outcomes. *Journal of Wound, Ostomy, & Incontinence Nursing 28*(1), 37-46.

Matsuoka, H., Takahara, T., Masaki, T., et al. (2002). Preoperative evaluation by magnetic resonance imaging in patients with bowel obstruction. *American Journal of Surgery 183*(6), 614-617.

Murphy, J., Stacey, D., Crook, J., et al. (2000). Testing control of radiation-induced diarrhea with a psyllium bulking agent: A pilot study. *Canadian Oncology Nursing Journal 10*(3), 96-100.

O'Rourke, M. (2000). Urinary incontinence as a factor in prostate cancer treatment selection. *Journal of Wound, Ostomy, & Incontinence Nursing 27*(5), 146-154.

Potter, K. (2000). Surgical oncology of the pelvis: Ostomy planning and management. *Journal of Surgical Oncology 73*(4), 237-242.

Robinson, J. (2000). Managing urinary incontinence following radical prostatectomy. *Journal of Wound, Ostomy, & Incontinence Nursing 27*(5), 138-145.

Schiller, L. (2002). *Sleisinger and Fordtran's gastrointestinal and liver disease, volume* I (7th ed.). Philadelphia: W.B. Saunders.

Schoolwerth, A., & Gehr, T. (2000). Clinical assessment of renal function. In Shoemaker, W.C. Ayres S.M., Grenvik, A.N., & Holbrook, P.R. (Eds.). *Textbook of critical care* (4th ed.). Philadelphia: W.B. Saunders.

Viele, C.S., Stern, J.M., Ippoliti, C., & Rosenoff, S.H. (2002). Symptom management of chemotherapy-induced diarrhea: A multidisciplinary approach. *ONS 2002 Annual Congress Symposia Highlights*, 17-20.

Waldman, A.R. (2001). Bowel obstruction. *Clinical Journal of Oncology Nursing 5*(6), 281-282, 286.

Wein, A., & Rovner, E. (2002). Pharmacologic management of urinary incontinence in women. *Urologic Clinics of North America 29*(3), 537-550.

Yarbro, C., Goodman, M., Frogge, M., & Groenwald, S. (2000). *Cancer nursing: Principles and practice* (5th ed.). Sudbury, MA: Jones and Bartlett Publishers.

Yasko, J.M. (2002). *Nursing management of symptoms associated with chemotherapy.* West Conshohocken, PA: Meniscus Healthcare Communications.

PART FOUR

CARDIOPULMONARY FUNCTION

16 Alterations in Ventilation

LESLIE V. MATTHEWS

ANATOMIC OR SURGICAL ALTERATIONS

Theory

I. Definition—inadequate ventilation or oxygenation because of anatomic or surgical alterations (Braunwald et al., 2001).
  A. Anatomic alterations.
    1. Space-occupying lesions within the lung itself or in the pleural space.
      a. Primary or metastatic cancer of the lung.
      b. Abnormal accumulation of material within lung or pleural space (Braunwald et al., 2001).
        (1) Pneumothorax—abnormal accumulation of air within the pleural space.
        (2) Hemothorax—abnormal accumulation of blood within the pleural space.
        (3) Empyema—abnormal accumulation of infected fluid or pus in the pleural space caused by recent chest surgery, immunocompromise, or lung infections.
    2. Obstruction of tracheobronchial tree from primary or metastatic tumors or enlarged lymph nodes causing atelectasis.
    3. Compression of tracheobronchial tree from bronchospasm or laryngeal swelling from hypersensitivity reactions related to chemotherapy treatments or superior vena cava syndrome (SVCS).
  B. Surgical alterations.
    1. Thoracic surgery with closed chest drainage for removal of primary or metastatic cancer of the lung (Yarbro et al., 2000).
      a. Pneumonectomy—surgical removal of an entire lung.
      b. Lobectomy—removal of a lobe of the lung.
      c. Segmental resection—removal of one or more segments of a lung lobe.
      d. Wedge resection—removal of a small wedge-shaped localized area near the lung surface.
    2. Tracheostomy following head and neck surgery, laryngectomy.
II. Risk factors.
  A. Primary or metastatic cancer of the lung.
  B. Recent surgery (especially thoracic or abdominal), immobility, or situations in which hypoventilation is likely.
  C. Chemotherapy with drugs known to cause allergic reactions (see Chapter 38).
  D. Cancers in which SVCS is associated (see Chapter 19).
  E. Thoracic or head and neck surgery.
    1. Primary or adjuvant tracheobronchial surgeries.
    2. Surgery for palliation, tumor debulking.
  F. History of obstructive or restrictive pulmonary disease.
  G. History of cardiovascular disease.

III. Principles of medical management.
  A. Diagnostic tests (Camp-Sorrell & Hawkins, 2000; DeGowin, 2000).
    1. Chest x-ray examinations, computed tomography (CT) scans, magnetic resonance imaging (MRI), positron emission tomography (PET) scan.
    2. Arterial blood gases.
    3. Pulmonary function tests (PFTs).
    4. Ventilation-perfusion scans.
    5. Bronchoscopy.
    6. Thoracentesis.
  B. Treatment strategies (Johnson & Gross, 1998; Yarbro et al., 2000).
    1. Supplemental oxygen administration to facilitate adequate uptake of oxygen into the blood.
    2. Treatment aimed at the underlying disease process.
      a. Radiation therapy (RT) or chemotherapy for primary or metastatic cancer of the lung or to reduce obstruction of the tracheobronchial tree.
      b. Thoracentesis to remove abnormal accumulated contents in pleural space; systemic antibiotic treatment for empyema.
      c. Treatment for anaphylactic/allergic reactions: stop drug, assess airway, give epinephrine, oxygen, vasopressors, and intravenous (IV) fluid.

Assessment

  I. History (Yarbro et al., 2000).
    A. Cough, very common.
    B. Dyspnea, very common.
    C. Pain in chest.
    D. Ability to carry out activities of daily living.
    E. Tobacco use.
    F. Exercise/activity tolerance.
    G. Number of pillows used for sleep and comfort.
    H. Anxiety and apprehension.
  II. Presence of risk factors.
  III. Physical examination (Camp-Sorrell & Hawkins, 2000; DeGowin, 2000).
    A. Abnormal/altered breathing patterns.
      1. Tachypnea.
      2. Pursed-lip breathing.
      3. Use of accessory muscles of respiration.
    B. Abnormal breath sounds.
      1. Wheezes.
      2. Decreased or absent breath sounds.
    C. Sputum—amount, color, presence of blood.
    D. Cyanosis.
      1. Hypoxemia.
      2. Chronic obstructive pulmonary disease (COPD).
    E. Vital signs and pulse oximetry.
    F. Evaluate airway swelling, oropharyngeal swelling.
    G. Presence of enlarged lymph nodes or other masses in the head and neck area.

Nursing Diagnoses

  I. Impaired gas exchange.
  II. Ineffective breathing patterns.

III. Activity intolerance.
IV. Pain.
 V. Deficient knowledge related to self-care management.

Outcome Identification

  I. Client maintains optimal gas exchange.
 II. Client's breathing pattern is regular in rate and pattern.
III. Client maintains activity level within capabilities.
   A. Client utilizes measures to reduce or conserve energy expenditure.
IV. Client reports adequate relief of pain.
 V. Client and family identify correct procedures and precautions for oxygen use.
   A. Client and family identify critical symptoms or changes in current status to report to health care providers.

Planning and Implementation (Johnson & Gross, 1998)

  I. Interventions to minimize the risk of occurrence, severity, or complications of respiratory distress.
   A. Employ measures to increase the ease and effectiveness of breathing and to promote physical comfort (use of pillows).
   B. Incorporate measures to minimize the pain experience.
   C. Utilize activity limitation and conservation of energy strategies.
 II. Interventions to maximize safety.
   A. Encourage use of assistive devices as needed for ambulation, activities of daily living.
     1. Cane.
     2. Walker.
     3. Wheelchair.
   B. Utilize activity limitation and conservation of energy strategies.
   C. Use bedside rails as appropriate.
III. Interventions to monitor for complications.
   A. Assess level of consciousness, mental status.
   B. Assess heart rate and rhythm, respiratory effort, vascular perfusion.
   C. Report critical changes to the physician.
IV. Interventions to monitor response to management.
   A. Assess respiratory rate, rhythm, effort.
   B. Assess for signs of respiratory impairment.
     1. Dyspnea.
     2. Dry persistent cough.
     3. Basilar rales.
     4. Tachypnea.
   C. Monitor for adequate relief of symptoms.
     1. Subjective reports of client and family of the following:
       a. Changes in the respiratory pattern.
       b. Psychologic responses to respiratory distress.
 V. Interventions to educate client and family regarding the following:
   A. Activity limitation and conservation of energy strategies.
     1. Frequent rest periods.
     2. Easy-to-prepare meals.
     3. Often-used items within reach.

    B. Emergency care, available community resources.

    C. Signs and symptoms to report to the health care team.

Evaluation

The oncology nurse systematically and regularly evaluates the client's and/or family's responses to interventions to determine progress toward the achievement of expected outcomes. Relevant data are collected, and actual findings are compared with expected findings. Nursing diagnoses, outcomes, and plans of care are reviewed and revised as necessary.

PULMONARY TOXICITY RELATED TO CANCER THERAPY

Theory

  I. Definition—parenchymal pulmonary disease caused by antineoplastic therapy, radiation, chemotherapy.

  II. Classification.

    A. Radiation-induced pneumonitis (Stover & Kaner, 2001).

      1. Subacute inflammatory response to radiation exposure to the lung.

      2. Toxic effects are proportionate to the following:

        a. Total radiation dose.

        b. Volume of lung tissue irradiated.

        c. Fractionation schedule.

        d. Concomitant administration of bleomycin (Blenoxane).

    B. Chemotherapy-induced pulmonary fibrosis.

      1. Direct injury to parenchymal endothelial cell membranes of lung.

      2. Hypersensitivity reaction or immune complex–related reaction.

      3. Associated chemotherapy agents (Table 16-1).

  III. Risk factors (Stover & Kaner, 2001; Yarbro et al., 2000).

    A. Radiation therapy.

      1. Occurs in 5% to 15% of all patients receiving RT.

      2. Chemotherapy given at the same time as RT.

      3. Previous RT.

      4. Steroid withdrawal.

      5. Tends to be more severe in the elderly.

    B. Chemotherapy induced.

      1. Age more than 60 years old.

      2. Bleomycin cumulative dose higher than 400 units.

      3. Preexisting pulmonary disease (i.e., COPD).

      4. Smoking history.

      5. Concomitant or prior RT to lungs.

      6. Oxygen therapy at high concentration (>35%).

  IV. Principles of medical management.

    A. RT induced (Stover & Kaner, 2001).

      1. Exclude other causes of pulmonary infiltrates—infection, recurrent tumors, or lymphangitic carcinomatosis.

      2. Mild symptoms managed with cough suppressants, antipyretics, rest.

      3. Severe symptoms and impaired gas exchange.

        a. Administer glucocorticoid therapy until symptoms improve, then taper slowly; pneumonitis may flare if taper is too rapid.

        b. Generally, only 50% respond to glucocorticoid therapy.

TABLE 16-1
Chemotherapy-Induced Pulmonary Toxicity

Drug	Risk Factors	Mechanism	Treatment
Bleomycin (Blenoxane)	Synergism with: Cisplatin (Platinol-AQ) Oxygen (>35%) RT Cumulative dose >400 units Age >60 yr	Endothelial swelling Pulmonary fibrosis Hypersensitivity reactions Direct injury from release of proteins	Assess for risk factors. Monitor and limit cumulative dose. Discontinue drug. Steroids (indicated for bleomycin hypersensitivity). Assess pulmonary status.
Carmustine (BCNU)	Dose related (>1500 mg/m^2) Increased risk with pre-existing lung disease, smoking history	Pulmonary fibrosis Direct injury with toxic oxidant molecules	Assess for risk factors. Discontinue drug. Steroids not usually beneficial. Assess pulmonary status.
Mitomycin (Mutamycin)	Previous cyclophospha-mide or methotrexate administration Increased toxicity with RT High-concentration O$_2$	Hypersensitivity reaction	Assess for risk factors. Discontinue drug. Steroids of some benefit. Assess pulmonary status.
Busulfan (Busulfex, Myleran)	Not considered dose dependent Increased toxicity with RT/alkylating agents	Direct toxicity to epithelial lining Pulmonary fibrosis	Assess for risk factors. Discontinue drug. High-dose steroids. Assess pulmonary status.
Cyclophosphamide (Cytoxan, Neosar)	Increased toxicity with: Cisplatin O$_2$ administration	Pulmonary damage from reactive oxygen metabolites	Assess for risk factors. Discontinue drug. Steroids of some benefit. Assess pulmonary status.
Methotrexate (Folex, Mexate, Rheumatrex)	Synergism with other agents possible	Direct damage unclear Hypersensitivity reaction	Discontinue drug. Assess for capillary leak syndrome. Steroids beneficial. Assess pulmonary status.
Gemcitabine (Gemzar)	Prolonged infusion time >60 min Not dose dependent	Direct cause unknown Drug-induced pneumonitis	Assess for risk factors. Discontinue drug. Steroids may be of some benefit.

Data from Stover DE: Pulmonary toxicity. In De Vita Jr, VT, Hellman S, Rosenberg SA, editors: *Cancer: principles and practice of oncology*, ed 4, Philadelphia, 1993, Lippincott-Raven; Vander Els N, Miller V: Successful treatment of gemcitabine toxicity with a brief course of corticosteroid therapy, *Chest* 114:1179, 1998; Chu E, DeVita Jr, VT, editors: *Physician's cancer chemotherapy drug manual 2002*, Sudbury, Mass, 2002, Jones and Bartlett Publishers.
RT, Radiation therapy.

   B. Chemotherapy induced (DeVita et al., 2001).
       1. Prevention is the best treatment by monitoring baseline PFTs and limiting cumulative dose of bleomycin to less than 400 units.
       2. Discontinuation of drug if dyspnea develops.
       3. Attempt to control symptoms with glucocorticoid therapy.

Assessment

I. History (Stover & Kaner, 2001).
  A. RT-induced pulmonary toxicity.
    1. Early, nonspecific symptoms include cough, dyspnea, low-grade temperature.
    2. Occurs 6 to 12 weeks after completion of RT, although symptoms can range from 1 to 6 months after RT.
  B. Chemotherapy-induced pulmonary toxicity.
    1. Dyspnea is the cardinal symptom; also nonproductive cough, malaise, fatigue, fever.
    2. Generally develops over weeks to months, but it can also develop quickly (within hours).
II. Physical examination (Stover & Kaner, 2001).
  A. RT induced.
    1. Physical examination.
      a. Moist rales.
      b. Pleural friction rub.
      c. Evidence of pleural fluid heard over the area of irradiation.
      d. Tachypnea, cyanosis (late).
    2. Radiographic changes.
      a. Early—diffuse haziness.
      b. Late—infiltrates corresponding to the region of radiation exposure.
  B. Chemotherapy induced.
    1. Physical examination.
      a. Results may be normal.
      b. End-inspiratory basilar rales.
      c. Tachypnea.
    2. Radiographic changes.
      a. Classic diffuse reticular pattern.
      b. Results may also be normal.
  C. Diagnostic tests and findings.
    1. PFTs.
      a. Decreased lung volume.
      b. Decreased diffusion capacity.
    2. Arterial blood gases.
      a. Hypoxia.
      b. Hypocapnia, respiratory alkalosis.

Nursing Diagnoses

I. Impaired gas exchange.
II. Ineffective breathing pattern.
III. Activity intolerance.

Outcome Identification

I. Client maintains optimal gas exchange.
  A. Client and family identify critical symptoms or changes in current status to report to health care providers.
II. Client's breathing pattern is regular in rate and pattern.
III. Client maintains activity level within capabilities.
  A. Client utilizes measures to reduce or conserve energy expenditure.

Planning and Implementation

I. Interventions to monitor client status (Yarbro et al., 2000).
   A. Ensure that PFTs are performed before treatment.
   B. Assess respiratory rate, rhythm, effort.
   C. Monitor cumulative doses of bleomycin and limit cumulative doses of bleomycin to less than 400 units.
   D. Assess for signs of pulmonary toxicity—dyspnea, dry persistent cough, basilar rales, tachypnea.
   E. Monitor activities to minimize energy expenditure.
      1. Frequent rest periods.
      2. Easy-to-prepare meals.
      3. Often-used items within reach.
   F. Monitor for adequate relief of symptoms.
      1. Decreased pain.
      2. Increased comfort of breathing.

Evaluation

The oncology nurse systematically and regularly evaluates the client's and/or family's responses to interventions to determine progress toward the achievement of expected outcomes. Relevant data are collected, and actual findings are compared with expected findings. Nursing diagnoses, outcomes, and plans of care are reviewed and revised as necessary.

DYSPNEA

Theory

I. Definition—a subjective sensation of difficulty breathing, the feeling of inability to get enough air, and the reaction to the sensation (Inzeo & Tyson, 2003).
II. Risk factors.
   A. Disease related.
      1. Tumors that impinge on respiratory structures and decrease the flow of air in and out of the lungs.
      2. Conditions that increase metabolic demands, such as fever, anemia, or infection.
      3. Cerebral metastasis that affects the respiratory center or stimulates the central and peripheral chemoreceptors.
      4. Metastatic effusions in the pleural space, cardiac space, or abdominal cavity that compromise lung expansion, gas exchange, or blood flow to the lungs.
      5. Coexisting pulmonary or cardiac disease that compromises lung expansion or blood flow to the lungs.
   B. Treatment related (Cooley et al., 2002).
      1. Incisional pain that may compromise lung expansion.
      2. Immediate (pneumonitis) and long-term (fibrosis) effects of RT to the lung fields.
      3. Antineoplastic agents that can cause pulmonary toxicity.
         a. For bleomycin (Blenoxane), busulfan (Busulfex, Myleran), nitrosoureas (Carmustine, Lomustine), toxicity is dose related.
         b. For methotrexate (Folex, Mexate, Rheumatrex), toxicity is idiosyncratic and reversible.

4. Anaphylactic reactions to antineoplastic agents and biologic response modifiers.
5. Pneumothorax related to placement of vascular access catheters, fine-needle aspirations, or thoracentesis.
C. Lifestyle related (Sarna et al., 2003).
1. Strong emotional responses, particularly anxiety or anger, contribute to the sensation of dyspnea.
2. Tobacco use.
3. Exposure to environmental toxic substances—asbestos, chromium, coal products, ionizing radiation, vinyl chloride, chloromethyl ethers.
III. Principles of medical management (Michelson & Hollrah, 1999).
A. Treatment of underlying disease with thoracentesis, RT, chemotherapy, antimicrobial medications.
B. Pharmacologic agents.
1. Bronchodilators—increase air flow to the lungs.
2. Glucocorticoids—decrease local inflammation.
3. Narcotics and anxiolytics—decrease pain and anxiety.
4. Diuretics—decrease fluid overload.
C. Supplemental oxygen as indicated.
D. Activity limitation, bronchial hygiene measures, appropriate positioning, relaxation training, exercise as tolerated.
E. Behavior modification, psychosocial support (Inzeo & Tyson, 2003).

Assessment

I. History (Camp-Sorrell & Hawkins, 2000; Gillespie, 2002; Michelson & Hollrah, 1999).
A. Presence of risk factors, such as smoking, chemical exposure.
B. Subjective complaints of shortness of breath, "can't catch breath," "smothering," uncomfortable breathing, anxiety, or panic.
C. Pattern of dyspnea—onset, frequency, severity, associated symptoms, aggravating or alleviating factors.
D. Impact of dyspnea on activities of daily living, lifestyle, relationships, role responsibilities.
II. Physical findings (Camp-Sorrell & Hawkins, 2000; Michelson & Hollrah, 1999).
A. Tachypnea.
B. Increased respiratory excursion.
C. Use of accessory muscles with breathing.
D. Retraction of intercostal spaces.
E. Flaring of nostrils.
F. Clubbing of digits caused by chronic hypoxemia.
G. Cyanosis, pallor.
III. Psychologic signs and symptoms (Inzeo & Tyson, 2003).
A. Concentration and/or memory difficulties.
B. Confusion.
C. Restlessness.
IV. Diagnostic tests and findings (Camp-Sorrell & Hawkins, 2000; Inzeo & Tyson, 2003).
A. Since the symptom is a subjective response, the client may not have abnormal findings or results.
B. Complete blood count (CBC)—hemoglobin deficiencies.
C. Pulse oximetry—severity of hypoxia.

    D. Chest x-ray and CT—structural abnormalities.
    E. PFTs.
    F. Bronchoscopic examination.
    G. Sputum or bronchial cultures.
    H. Arterial blood gas.

Nursing Diagnoses

    I. Impaired gas exchange.
   II. Ineffective breathing pattern.
  III. Activity intolerance.
   IV. Pain.
    V. Anxiety.
  VI. Deficient knowledge related to strategies to manage dyspnea.

Outcome Identification

    I. Client maintains optimal gas exchange.
   II. Client's breathing pattern is regular in rate and pattern.
  III. Client maintains activity level within capabilities.
    A. Client utilizes measures to reduce or conserve energy expenditure.
   IV. Client reports adequate relief of pain.
    V. Client describes a decrease in anxiety.
  VI. Client describes strategies to increase ease of breathing.
    A. Client and family identify correct procedures and precautions for oxygen use.
    B. Client and family identify critical symptoms or changes in current status to report to health care providers.

Planning and Implementation (Johnson & Gross, 1998; Yarbro et al., 2000)

    I. Interventions to increase the ease and effectiveness of breathing and promote comfort.
    A. Utilize upright position with pillows as necessary.
    B. Lean forward with elbows on knees, table, or pillows.
    C. Perform diaphragmatic breathing with slow exhalation; however, this type of breathing is not effective and may be harmful in clients with a history of pulmonary restrictive disease.
    D. Incorporate measures to minimize the pain experience.
    E. Utilize activity limitation and conservation of energy strategies.
    F. Encourage systematic relaxation techniques.
   II. Interventions to maximize safety.
    A. Encourage use of assistive devices as needed for ambulation, activities of daily living, such as cane, walker, or wheelchair.
    B. Utilize activity limitation, conservation of energy strategies.
      1. Frequent rest periods.
      2. Use of ready-made meals.
      3. Often-used items within reach.
    C. Use bedside rails as appropriate.
  III. Interventions to monitor for complications.
    A. Assess level of consciousness and mental status.
    B. Monitor intake and output.

    C. Assess heart rate and rhythm, respiratory effort, vascular perfusion.

    D. Report critical changes to the physician.

       1. Unresponsiveness.

       2. Tachypnea, tachycardia.

       3. Acute pain.

IV. Interventions to monitor response to management.

    A. Observe and report physical symptoms, such as decreased shortness of breath, increased energy, ease of breathing.

    B. Monitor subjective reports of the client and family regarding the following:

       1. Changes in the pattern of dyspnea.

       2. Psychologic responses to dyspnea.

 V. Interventions to educate patient and family.

    A. Teach activity limitation, conservation of energy strategies.

    B. Instruct in emergency care, available community resources.

    C. List signs and symptoms to report to the health care team.

       1. Increased pain.

       2. Increased difficulty in breathing.

       3. Nasal flaring.

       4. Skin changes (pallor, cyanosis).

VI. Behavioral interventions to decrease the sense of dyspnea and enhance psychosocial well-being (Inzeo & Tyson, 2003; Wickham, 2002).

    A. Encourage systematic relaxation techniques.

    B. Use language that the patient can understand (trouble breathing, short of breath).

    C. Complementary and alternative therapies.

       1. Acupuncture and acupressure.

       2. Nondrug self-care therapies.

       3. Prayer and meditation, aromatherapy.

Evaluation

The oncology nurse systematically and regularly evaluates the client's and/or family's responses to interventions to determine progress toward the achievement of expected outcomes. Relevant data are collected, and actual findings are compared with expected findings. Nursing diagnoses, outcomes, and plans of care are reviewed and revised as necessary.

PLEURAL EFFUSIONS

Theory

  I. Definition—presence of abnormal amounts of fluid in the pleural space.

 II. Classification (Ahya & Lee, 2001; Braunwald et al., 2001).

    A. Pleural effusion (benign) may be caused by the following:

       1. Increased hydrostatic pressure (congestive heart failure).

       2. Increased permeability in the microvascular circulation (infection, trauma).

       3. Increased negative pressure in the pleural space (atelectasis).

       4. Decreased oncotic pressure in the microvasculature (nephrotic syndrome, cirrhosis, hypoalbuminemia).

    B. Malignant pleural effusion, the presence of malignant cells in the pleura, may be caused by the following:

1. Direct extension of primary lung tumor to the pleura or mediastinum or mesothelioma involving the pleura.
2. Impaired lymphatic drainage from the pleural space resulting from obstruction caused by tumor.
3. Increased permeability caused by inflammation or disruption of the capillary endothelium.
4. Altered mucosal lung or mediastinal tissue resulting from RT.

III. Risk factors (Chernecky & Sarna, 2000).
  A. Primary tumors of lung, breast, hematopoietic system.
  B. Prior pleural effusion.
  C. Radiation to the chest, thorax, or abdomen.
  D. Surgical modification of venous or lymphatic vessels.

IV. Principles of medical management (Ahya & Lee, 2001; Braunwald et al., 2001).
  A. Diagnostic tests.
    1. Chest x-ray examination—blunting of costophrenic angle.
    2. Fluid accumulation.
    3. Thoracentesis—pleural fluid withdrawal of approximately 25 to 50 ml for accurate cytology testing and culture (to rule out infectious cause).
    4. Pleural biopsy—increases diagnostic yield when combined with cytologic studies.
  B. Treatment strategies.
    1. Thoracentesis.
       a. May improve client comfort and relieve dyspnea.
       b. Reaccumulation of fluid is common.
       c. Potential for hypoproteinemia, pneumothorax, empyema, fluid loculation.
       d. Effective procedure for palliation, relief of acute respiratory distress.
    2. Complete drainage via chest tube to continuous underwater-seal suction—promotes adherence of the visceral and parietal pleural surfaces by removal of accumulated fluid.
    3. Sclerotherapy—instillation of sclerosing agents intrapleurally to produce mesothelial fibrosis using the following:
       a. Tetracycline (Achromycin, Actisite, Panmycin, Robitet, Sumycin, Topicycline), doxycycline (Adoxa, Periostat, Vibra-Tabs, Vibramycin).
       b. Nitrogen mustard (Mustargen), bleomycin (Blenoxane).
       c. Talc.
       d. Lidocaine (LidoPen, Xylocaine) in the sclerosing agent solution helps decrease discomfort associated with procedure.
    4. Parietal pleurectomy.
    5. Open pleurectomy—historically has required thoracotomy.
    6. Videothoracoscopic pleurectomy—using hydrodissection with an irrigation device entering into the pleural space; minimally invasive.
    7. Chemotherapy and mediastinal radiation—may be effective in responsive tumors (lymphoma, small cell lung cancer [SCLC]).

Assessment

I. History (Camp-Sorrell & Hawkins, 2000).
  A. Presence of risk factors.
    1. Breast or lung cancer.
    2. Previous treatment modalities.

    B. Symptoms—severity related to the speed of accumulation, not amount, and usually caused by pulmonary compression.
       1. Dyspnea.
       2. Cough usually dry and nonproductive.
       3. Chest pain.
  II. Physical examination (DeGowin, 2000).
    A. Tachypnea.
    B. Restricted chest wall expansion.
    C. Dullness to percussion.
    D. Diminished or absent breath sounds.
    E. Egophony on the affected side.
    F. Pleural friction rub.
    G. Fever.
    H. General manifestations.
       1. Compression atelectasis.
       2. Mediastinal shift, if pleural effusion severe.

Nursing Diagnoses

  I. Impaired gas exchange.
  II. Ineffective breathing pattern.
  III. Activity intolerance.
  IV. Pain.
  V. Deficient knowledge related to the care of pleural effusions.

Outcome Identification

  I. Client maintains optimal gas exchange.
  II. Client's breathing pattern is regular in rate and pattern.
  III. Client maintains activity level within capabilities.
    A. Client utilizes measures to reduce or conserve energy expenditure.
  IV. Client reports adequate relief of pain.
  V. Client and family identify correct procedures and precautions for oxygen use.
    A. Client and family identify critical symptoms or changes in current status to report to health care providers.

Planning and Implementation (Johnson & Gross, 1998; Yarbro et al., 2000)

  I. Interventions to decrease the severity of symptoms associated with pleural effusion.
    A. Teach measures to increase the ease and effectiveness of breathing and to promote physical comfort.
       1. Utilize upright position with pillows as necessary.
       2. Lean forward with elbows on knees, table, or pillows.
    B. Incorporate measures to minimize the pain experience (narcotic analgesia before chest tube insertion and as needed).
    C. Utilize relaxation techniques as indicated for anxiety.
  II. Interventions to maximize safety.
    A. Encourage use of assistive devices as needed for ambulation, activities of daily living.
    B. Utilize activity limitation and conservation of energy strategies.
    C. Instruct family in use of and precautions related to oxygen therapy.

III. Interventions to monitor the consequences of therapy.
   A. Assess respiratory rate and rhythm, respiratory effort, adventitious breath sounds.
   B. Assess characteristics of pain and relief measures.
   C. Monitor subjective response to drainage and rate of fluid reaccumulation.
   D. Report critical changes to the physician.
      1. Chest pain.
      2. Fever.
      3. Change in character of respiration.
IV. Interventions to educate client and family regarding the following:
   A. Activity limitation, conservation of energy strategies.
   B. Emergency care, available community resources.
   C. Signs and symptoms to report to the health care team.
V. Interventions to enhance adaptation or rehabilitation.
   A. Assist the patient to maintain a safe level of independence within the limitation of symptoms.
   B. Encourage the patient and family to express concerns.

Evaluation

The oncology nurse systematically and regularly evaluates the client's and/or family's responses to interventions to determine progress toward the achievement of expected outcomes. Relevant data are collected, and actual findings are compared with expected findings. Nursing diagnoses, outcomes, and plans of care are reviewed and revised as necessary.

ANEMIA

Theory

   I. Definition—symptom of abnormally low red blood cells (RBCs), quality of hemoglobin (Hgb), and/or volume of packed cells (Ahya & Lee, 2001).
      A. World Health Organization (WHO) definition.
         1. Males—Hgb level less than 13 g/dl; hematocrit (Hct) less than 42%.
         2. Females—Hgb level less than 12 g/dl; Hct less than 36%.
   II. Classification (Braunwald et al., 2001).
      A. Red cell morphology—size of RBC (microcytic, normocytic, or macrocytic).
      B. Amount of hemoglobin pigment (hypochromic, normochromic, or hyperchromic).
   III. Risk factors (Braunwald et al., 2001).
      A. Disease related.
         1. Slow or persistent blood loss (gastrointestinal [GI] neoplasms, esophageal varices, peptic ulcer disease, acetylsalicylic acid/nonsteroidal antiinflammatory drug [ASA/NSAID] ingestion) causing decreased RBC volume.
         2. Primary malignancies of the marrow, tumor invasion of the marrow, or genetically transmitted RBC deficiencies (thalassemias) causing decreased quantity/quality of RBC production.
         3. Impaired absorption (postgastrectomy, celiac disease), inadequate intake (cachexia, alcoholism), or decreased utilization of iron, folic acid, vitamin K, or vitamin B_{12} causing decreased maturity and function of RBCs.
         4. Autoimmune disorders associated with malignancy (multiple myeloma, chronic leukemias) causing increased destruction or sequestration of RBCs.

    5. Conditions that lead to decreased erythropoietin (EPO) production, decreased sensitivity to EPO, or a reduction in erythrocyte progenitor cells, such as acute or chronic renal disease, hemolysis (Gillespie, 2002).
- **B.** Treatment related (Camp-Sorrell & Hawkins, 2000; Gillespie, 2002).
  - **1.** Chemotherapy—destruction of rapidly dividing normal hematopoietic cells results in decreased production of RBC precursors and mature RBCs.
  - **2.** RT—destruction of RBC precursors in the radiation field.
  - **3.** Pharmacologic agents—inhibit RBC production or cause decreased mineral and vitamin levels (oral contraceptives, estrogen, phenytoin (Dilantin), phenobarbital (Luminal).
- **IV.** Principles of medical management (Ahya & Lee, 2001; Camp-Sorrell & Hawkins, 2000).
  - **A.** Once the diagnosis is established, underlying cause must be identified and, if possible, corrected.
  - **B.** Supplements such as iron, vitamins, folic acid.
  - **C.** RBC transfusions are indicated for the following:
    - **1.** Symptomatic anemia (dyspnea, tachycardia) occurs, regardless of the hematocrit.
    - **2.** Client is actively bleeding.
    - **3.** Hemoglobin level drops below 8 g/dl.
  - **D.** Erythropoietin administration (Gillespie, 2002).
  - **E.** Cessation of pharmacologic agents that interfere with RBC production or maturation.

Assessment

- **I.** History (Richer, 1997).
  - **A.** Signs and symptoms depend on the following:
    - **1.** Rate at which anemia develops.
    - **2.** Age of the individual.
    - **3.** Individual's compensatory mechanisms.
    - **4.** Activity level.
  - **B.** Review history of the following:
    - **1.** All medications, prescription and over-the-counter agents.
    - **2.** Acute or chronic blood loss.
    - **3.** Previous therapy for cancer.
    - **4.** Signs and symptoms of anemia.
    - **5.** Impact of anemia on activities of daily living, activity level, lifestyle.
  - **C.** General manifestations of anemia (Loney & Chernecky, 2000).
    - **1.** Easily fatigued.
    - **2.** Dyspnea on exertion.
    - **3.** Pallor (conjunctiva, nail beds, sclera).
    - **4.** Weakness, listlessness.
    - **5.** Headache.
    - **6.** Hypotension.
    - **7.** Tachycardia.
    - **8.** Tachypnea.
- **II.** Physical findings (Ahya & Lee, 2001; Braunwald et al., 2001).
  - **A.** General appearance—pale, lethargic, or no overt signs, if anemia is mild.
  - **B.** Vital signs—pulse and respiration may be increased in moderate to severe anemia; postural hypotension in severe anemia.

    C. Integument—pallor and dryness of the skin and mucous membranes; brittle, flattened, ridged, concave, or spoon-shaped nails (koilonychia); brittle, fine hair.

    D. Head, eyes, ears, nose, and throat (HEENT)—atrophy of the papillae of the tongue, smooth, shiny, beefy-red appearance; angular stomatitis or cheilitis; pale conjunctiva or sclera.

    E. Cardiovascular—tachycardia, mild cardiac enlargement; in severe anemia, functional systolic murmurs.

    F. Abdominal—hepatomegaly, splenomegaly.

    G. Neurologic—usually within normal limits; in severe anemia, confusion.

III. Diagnostic tests and findings (Braunwald et al., 2001; Richer, 1997; Chernecky & Berger, 2004).

    A. Routine CBC (with peripheral smear).

      1. Hgb level decreased.

      2. Hct level decreased.

      3. Mean corpuscular volume (MCV).

        a. Less than 80—microcytic.

        b. 80 to 100—normocytic.

        c. More than 100—macrocytic.

      4. Mean corpuscular hemoglobin concentration (MCHC).

        a. Low—hypochromic.

        b. Normal—normochromic.

      5. Reticulocyte count decreased.

      6. Chemistries.

        a. Iron level, total iron-binding capacity (TIBC); ferritin, folate, vitamins B_{12} and K levels.

        b. Bilirubin level.

Nursing Diagnoses

  I. Fatigue or activity intolerance.

 II. Deficient knowledge related to management of anemia and impact on activities of daily life.

Outcome Identification

  I. Client achieves adequate activity tolerance.

    A. Client establishes pattern of rest/sleep to achieve optimal performance of desired/required activities.

    B. Client and/or family describes strategies to conserve energy.

 II. Client and/or family describes interventions to aid in client safety.

    A. Client lists signs and symptoms that should be reported to the health care team.

Planning and Implementation (Johnson & Gross, 1998; Yarbro et al., 2000)

  I. Interventions to decrease risk of complications of anemia.

    A. Institute safety precautions.

      1. Avoid sudden changes in position, such as from lying to sitting, sitting to standing.

      2. Assist with ambulation and self-care activities as needed.

      3. Teach patient to avoid hazardous activities, such as driving, if syncopal episodes are present.

> **4.** Assist client to conserve energy.
> **5.** Provide a nutritionally balanced diet and/or supplements.
>
> **B.** Educate the client and family regarding the following:
>> **1.** Cause of anemia and treatment plan.
>> **2.** Purpose, dosage, side effects, toxic effects of medication.
>> **3.** Nutrition—counsel regarding specific needs.
>> **4.** Activity—frequent rest periods as needed.
>> **5.** Signs and symptoms related to complications of anemia or treatment to report to a member of a health care team.
>>> **a.** Change in mental status.
>>> **b.** Increased shortness of breath.
>>> **c.** Onset of active bleeding.
>
> **II.** Interventions to monitor for complications related to anemia.
>> **A.** Assess skin for evidence of inadequate oxygenation, such as pallor, decreased capillary refill, or prolonged redness.
>> **B.** Assess blood pressure in lying, standing, and sitting positions.
>> **C.** Assess patient for evidence of side effects of therapy for anemia.
>> **D.** Monitor occurrence of constipation or diarrhea related to iron supplements.

Evaluation

The oncology nurse systematically and regularly evaluates the client's and/or family's responses to interventions to determine progress toward the achievement of expected outcomes. Relevant data are collected, and actual findings are compared with expected findings. Nursing diagnoses, outcomes, and plans of care are reviewed and revised as necessary.

REFERENCES

Ahya, S.N., & Lee, H. (Eds.). (2001). *The Washington manual of medical therapeutics* (30th ed.). Boston: Lippincott Williams & Wilkins.

Braunwald, E., Fauci, A.S., Hauser, S.L., et al. (Eds.). (2001). *Harrison's principles of internal medicine* (15th ed.). New York: McGraw-Hill.

Camp-Sorrell, D., & Hawkins, R.A. (Eds.). (2000). *Clinical manual for the oncology advanced practice nurse.* Pittsburgh: Oncology Nursing Press.

Chernecky, C., & Berger, B. (2004). *Laboratory test and diagnostic procedures* (4th ed.). St. Louis, MO: Elsevier, Inc.

Chernecky, C., & Sarna, L. (2000). Pulmonary toxicities. *Critical Care Nursing Clinics of North America 12(3)*, 281-295.

Chu, E., & DeVita, Jr., V.T. (Eds.). (2002). *Physician's cancer chemotherapy drug manual 2002.* Sudbury, MA: Jones & Bartlett Publishers.

Cooley, M.E., Short, T.H., Moriarty, H.J. (2002). Patterns of symptom distress in adults receiving treatment for lung cancer. *Journal of Palliative Care 18(3)*, 150-159.

DeGowin, R.L. (2000). *DeGowin's diagnostic examination* (7th ed.). New York: McGraw-Hill.

DeVita, Jr., V.T., Hellman, S., & Rosenberg, S.A. (Eds.). (2001). *Cancer: Principles and practice of oncology* (6th ed.). Philadelphia: Lippincott.

Gillespie, T.W. (2002). Effects of cancer-related anemia on clinical and quality-of-life outcomes. *Clinical Journal of Oncology Nursing 6(4)*, 206-211.

Inzeo, D., & Tyson, L. (2003). Nursing assessment and management of dyspneic patients with lung cancer. *Clinical Journal of Oncology Nursing 7(3)*, 332-333.

Johnson, B.L., & Gross, J. (1998). *Handbook of oncology nursing* (3rd ed.). Sudbury, MA: Jones and Bartlett Publishers.

Loney, M., & Chernecky, C. (2000). Anemia. *Oncology Nursing Forum 27(6)*, 951-966.

Michelson, E., & Hollrah, S. (1999). Evaluation of the patient with shortness of breath: An evidence-based approach. *Emergency Medicine Clinics of North America 17*(1), 221-237.

Richer, S. (1997). A practical guide for differentiating between iron deficiency anemia and anemia of chronic disease in children and adults. *Nurse Practitioner 22*(4), 82-103.

Sarna, L., Cooley, M., Danao, L. (2003). The global evidence of tobacco and cancer. *Seminars in Oncology Nursing 19(4)*, 233-243.

Stover, D.E., & Kaner, R.J. (2001). Pulmonary toxicity. In V.T. DeVita, Jr., S. Hellman, & S.A. Rosenberg (Eds.). *Cancer: Principles and practice of oncology* (6th ed.). Philadelphia: Lippincott, pp. 2894-2904.

Vander Els, N., & Miller, V. (1998). Successful treatment of gemcitabine toxicity with a brief course of corticosteroid therapy. *Chest 114,* 1179.

Wickham, R. (2002). Dyspnea: Recognizing and managing an invisible problem. *Oncology Nursing Forum 29*(6), 925-333.

Yarbro, C.H., Frogge, M.H., Goodman., M., & Groenwald, S.L. (Eds.) (2000). *Cancer nursing principles and practice* (5th ed.). Sudbury, MA: Jones and Bartlett Publishers.

17 Alterations in Circulation

KRISTINE TURNER STORY

LYMPHEDEMA

Theory

I. Definition—obstruction of the lymphatic system that causes overload of lymph fluid in interstitial spaces.

II. Physiology (National Lymphedema Network [NLN], 2002).
  A. Occlusion or damage to either the venous side of capillaries or the lymphatic system decreases reabsorption of lymph vessel drainage of fluid and protein, causing lymphedema (Ridner, 2002).
  B. Primary lymphedema.
    1. Classified according to age of onset.
      a. Congenital—present at birth.
      b. Praecox—onset at puberty.
      c. Tarda—onset in adulthood.
    2. Often unknown cause.
    3. May be associated with vascular abnormality.
  C. Secondary lymphedema caused by damage or destruction of the lymphatic system.

III. May be associated with the following (Cope, 2000):
  A. Lymph node dissection.
  B. Radiation therapy (RT), which leads to scarring and fibrosis.
  C. Infection, leading to fibrosis.
  D. Scarring from vesicant extravasation.
  E. Local burns.
  F. Lymph node metastasis.

IV. Incidence.
  A. Upper limb lymphedema.
    1. Occurs in 5% to 10% of women undergoing modified radical mastectomy.
    2. There is a 15% to 28% overall incidence in breast cancer survivors (Chapman & Goodman, 2000; Ridner, 2002).
    3. Usually occurs within 1 year following surgery.
    4. Can occur as late as 20 years after surgery.
    5. Most common in women who have had axillary lymph node dissection and RT in excess of 4600 cGy (Chapman & Goodman, 2000).
  B. Lower limb lymphedema.
    1. There is an 80% occurrence within 5 years of lymph node dissection in the groin (Martin, 2000).
    2. May be underreported or misdiagnosed as edema (Ryan et al., 2003).
    3. In a recent study, 100% of patients who had clinical diagnosis of lower limb lymphedema had lymph node dissection of groin (Ryan et al., 2003).
    4. May extend to include genitalia.

5. May be associated with intraabdominal compression of pelvic or inguinal lymph nodes caused by tumor extension, especially with lymphomas, ovarian tumors, and prostate tumors.
C. Incidence may decrease with increased use of sentinel lymph node dissection (Martin, 2000).

Assessment (Cope, 2000; Martin, 2000; Ridner, 2002; Ryan et al., 2003)

I. Risk factors.
   A. Extent of surgical resection.
   B. Infection of affected extremity.
   C. Diabetes mellitus.
   D. Obesity.
   E. Air travel with suboptimal cabin pressure, long distance travel.
   F. Traumatic injury to affected extremity.
   G. Excessive physical use of affected extremity.
   H. Prolonged standing (lower extremity).
II. Subjective findings.
   A. Tightness of clothing, shoes, watch, jewelry.
   B. Visible puffiness, lumps.
   C. Weakness of affected extremity.
   D. Pain, stiffness, numbness, paresthesia of affected extremity.
   E. Redness, warmth of affected extremity.
III. Objective findings.
   A. Tends to occur distal to proximal.
   B. Thickening, pitting, and erythema of skin; peau d'orange changes.
   C. Increased pigmentation/superficial veins.
   D. Stasis dermatitis.
   E. Induration with nonpitting edema.
   F. Secondary cellulitis.
   G. Extremity measurements.
      1. Arm measured 5 and 10 cm above and below the olecranon process.
      2. Leg measured at the level of the calf.
      3. Classification (Martin, 2000; NLN, 2002).
         a. Stage 1—spontaneously reversible.
            (1) Less than 3-cm difference between extremities.
            (2) Skin smooth textured with pitting edema.
         b. Stage 2—spontaneously irreversible.
            (1) 3- to 5-cm difference between extremities.
            (2) Skin stretched, shiny, with nonpitting edema.
         c. Stage 3—lymphostatic elephantiasis.
            (1) 5-cm difference between extremities.
            (2) Skin discolored, stretched, firm; nonpitting edema.
IV. Laboratory and diagnostic tests.
   A. Venous duplex scan negative.
   B. Computed tomography (CT) or magnetic resonance imaging (MRI) of soft tissue to rule out mass.

Nursing Diagnoses

I. Chronic pain.
II. Impaired physical mobility.

   III. Disturbed body image.
   IV. Risk for infection.
    V. Risk for impaired skin integrity.

Outcome Identification

     I. Client reports acceptable level of pain control.
    II. Client maintains adequate mobility.
   III. Client verbalizes and demonstrates acceptance of body image.
   IV. Infection is identified and treated promptly.
    V. Client maintains intact skin.

Planning and Implementation

     I. There is no known cure for lymphedema; therefore prevention is critical (Box 17-1).
    II. Treatment is mostly symptomatic in nature (Chapman & Goodman, 2000; Cope, 2000; Ridner, 2002; Ryan et al., 2003).
       A. Nonpharmacologic.
          1. Compression garment.
          2. Manual lymphatic drainage.

BOX 17-1
PREVENTION OF UPPER EXTREMITY LYMPHEDEMA

- Report any swelling in the affected extremity.
- Never allow an injection or a blood draw in the affected extremity. Wear a Lymphedema Alert bracelet (available from the National Lymphedema Network).
- Have blood pressure checked on the unaffected arm or on the thigh.
- Keep the affected extremity clean and dry, and lubricate with lotion.
- Avoid vigorous, repetitive movements against resistance with the affected extremity.
- Avoid heavy lifting with the affected extremity. Never carry heavy handbags or bags with over-the-shoulder straps on your affected side.
- Do not wear tight jewelry or elastic bands around the affected extremity.
- Avoid extreme temperature changes when bathing or washing dishes. Avoid saunas and hot tubs. Protect the extremity from the sun at all times.
- Avoid any type of trauma to the extremity, and watch for signs of infection.
- Wear gloves while doing housework, gardening, or any type of work that could result in even a minor injury.
- When manicuring your nails, avoid cutting your cuticles.
- Exercise is important, but consult with your therapist. Do not overtire an extremity at risk.
- When traveling by air, wear a well-fitted compression sleeve. Additional bandages may be required on a long flight. Increase fluid intake while in the air.
- Use a light-weight breast prosthesis and a well-fitted bra with no under wire.
- Use an electric razor to remove hair from the armpits or lower extremities.
- If you have lymphedema, wear a well-fitted compression sleeve during all waking hours.
- If you notice a rash, itching, redness, pain, increase of temperature or fever, see your health care provider immediately.
- Maintain your ideal weight through a well-balanced, low-sodium, high-fiber diet. Avoid smoking and alcohol.

Modified from National Lymphedema Network: *18 steps to prevention*, 2003. Author: Oakland, CA.

3. Pneumatic compression device.
4. Aerobic exercise of extremity with strength training.
5. Extremity elevation.
6. Skin care program with proper bathing, drying, lubrication.
7. Avoid prolonged standing.
   B. Pharmacologic.
      1. Early antibiotic treatment for suspected cellulitis.
      2. Diuretics not helpful (Martin, 2000).
   C. Client education (Chapman & Goodman, 2000).
      1. Preventive measures (see Box 17-1).
      2. Signs and symptoms to report (e.g., high risk for infection).
      3. Requires lifelong follow-up.
      4. Low-sodium, high-fiber, weight control diet.

Evaluation

The oncology nurse systematically and regularly evaluates the client's and/or family's responses to interventions in order to determine progress toward the achievement of expected outcomes. Relevant data are collected, and actual findings are compared with expected findings. Nursing diagnoses, outcomes, and plans of care are reviewed and revised as necessary.

EDEMA

Theory

I. Definition—accumulation of fluid in interstitial spaces.
II. Physiology (Grannis et al., 2002; Winokur, 2000).
   A. Caused by an imbalance between the forces containing fluid within the vasculature and those forcing fluid through the vascular wall.
   B. Increased hydrostatic pressure, increased capillary permeability, decreased plasma oncotic pressure, and lymphatic or venous obstruction forces fluid to move through the blood vessel wall into the tissue, referred to as "second spacing" of fluid (Works & Maxwell, 2000).
   C. Is a problem of fluid distribution, not always fluid overload.
III. May be associated with the following (Works & Maxwell, 2000):
   A. Local inflammation or lymphatic obstruction by tumor.
   B. Systemic conditions—congestive heart failure (CHF), nephrotic syndrome, liver failure.
   C. Medications—hormones, nonsteroidal antiinflammatory drugs (NSAIDs), calcium channel blockers, tricyclic antidepressants, steroids, interleukin-2 (IL-2) therapy.
   D. Allergic response or septic shock, which leads to histamine release.
   E. Hypoproteinemia, hypoalbuminemia.
   F. Iatrogenic causes—plasma expanders, intravenous (IV) fluid overload, blood component therapy.
   G. Deep vein thrombosis.
IV. Incidence.
   A. Unknown because usually not reported.
   B. May be increasing because of longer survival rates (Works & Maxwell, 2000).

Assessment (Grannis et al., 2002; Winokur, 2000)

I. Risk factors.
   A. Preexisting cardiac, renal, or liver disease.
   B. Decreased mobility.
   C. Long distance travel.
   D. Prior history of edema.
II. Subjective findings.
   A. Tightness of clothing, shoes, jewelry, watch.
   B. Pain or stiffness.
   C. Weight gain.
   D. Shortness of breath, dyspnea on exertion, orthopnea, paroxysmal nocturnal dyspnea.
   E. Frequent or decreased urination.
III. Objective findings.
   A. Presence of S_3 or S_4 heart sound.
   B. Increased jugular venous pressure.
   C. Increased blood pressure and heart rate.
   D. Rales.
   E. Ascites, hepatomegaly.
   F. Dependent edema (extremities, sacrum), skin thickening.
   G. Decreased peripheral pulses.
IV. Laboratory and diagnostic tests.
   A. Serum albumin and protein may be decreased.
   B. Creatinine, blood urea nitrogen (BUN), and liver functions may be increased.
   C. Chest x-ray (CXR)—evidence of fluid overload, increased size of heart shadow.
   D. Echocardiogram—decreased ejection fraction (EF) in CHF.

Nursing Diagnoses

I. Risk for impaired skin integrity.
II. Excess fluid volume.
III. Acute or chronic pain.
IV. Ineffective tissue perfusion, peripheral.
V. Impaired mobility.

Outcome Identification

I. Client maintains intact skin.
II. Client maintains baseline weight.
III. Client reports acceptable level of pain control.
IV. Client maintains adequate tissue oxygenation and peripheral perfusion.
V. Client maintains baseline level of mobility.

Planning and Implementation

I. Nonpharmacologic (Winokur, 2000).
   A. Elevate extremities above level of heart.
   B. Compression stockings.
   C. Maintain lubrication of skin.
   D. Bed rest to promote diuresis; reposition every 2 hours.

  E. Fluid restriction.

  F. Treatment of underlying cause.

  G. Monitor intake and output, electrolytes, serum albumin.

 II. Pharmacologic (Grannis et al., 2002; Winokur, 2000).

  A. Diuretics.

  B. Angiotensin-converting enzyme (ACE) inhibitors.

  C. β-Blockers.

 III. Client education.

  A. Low-sodium (<1 g/day), low-potassium diet.

  B. There is no consensus on the optimal protein content of the diet, but normal protein levels are preferred as high levels have no effect on serum albumin and may worsen renal function (Brady, O'Meara, & Brenner, 2004)

  C. Skin care.

  D. Avoidance of prolonged standing.

  E. Avoidance of hepatotoxic drugs and alcohol.

Evaluation

The oncology nurse systematically and regularly evaluates the client's and/or family's responses to interventions in order to determine progress toward the achievement of expected outcomes. Relevant data are collected, and actual findings are compared with expected findings. Nursing diagnoses, outcomes, and plans of care are reviewed and revised as necessary.

PERICARDIAL EFFUSION

Theory

 I. Definition—excess fluid accumulation in the pericardial sac that interferes with cardiac function, resulting in decreased cardiac output.

 II. Physiology (Ruckdeschel & Jablons, 2001; Shelton, 2000).

  A. Normal cardiac pressures are subatmospheric, allowing inflow of venous blood into the right side of the heart.

  B. An imbalance of pressure, production, and clearance of normal fluid in the pericardial space results in the development of an effusion.

  C. The primary pathologic condition is obstruction of lymphatic and venous drainage of the heart because obstruction disturbs the intrapericardial pressure.

  D. When ventricular filling is more severely restricted by fluid in the pericardial sac, cardiac output decreases.

 III. May be associated with the following (Grannis et al., 2002; Warren, 2000):

  A. Primary tumors of the pericardium; mesothelioma most common.

  B. Direct tumor invasion of the myocardium; more common with lung tumors, thymoma, esophageal tumors, lymphoma.

  C. Obstruction of mediastinal lymph nodes by tumor.

  D. Hematogenous spread of tumor; more common with breast cancer, melanoma, lung cancer.

  E. Fibrosis secondary to RT.

  F. May be exacerbated by hypoproteinemia and concurrent infection.

 IV. Incidence.

  A. 10% to 30% of all malignancies (Grannis et al., 2002; Warren, 2000).

  B. Probably underreported since symptoms can be vague.

    C. Mean life expectancy after diagnosis of malignant pericardial effusion is 2 to 5 months (Shelton, 2000).

Assessment

  I. Risk factors (Ruckdeschel & Jablons, 2001; Shelton, 2000).
    A. Coexisting cardiac disease, systemic lupus erythematosus, bacterial endocarditis.
    B. RT of 3000 cGy to more than 33% of heart or fraction sizes of more than 300 cGy/day.
    C. High-dose chemotherapy or biotherapy agents that cause capillary permeability.
      1. Cytarabine (Ara-C, cytosine arabinoside, Cytosar-U).
      2. Cyclophosphamide (Cytoxan, Neosar).
      3. Interferon.
      4. Interleukin-2 (aldesleukin [Proleukin] IL-2), and Interleukin-11 (Oprelvekin [Neumega], rIL-11)
      5. Granulocyte-macrophage colony-stimulating factor.
    D. Rare causes include hemorrhagic tamponade from direct injury or an infectious etiology.
  II. Subjective findings (Grannis et al., 2002).
    A. Symptoms reflect chronicity.
      1. Slowly developing effusions may have little or no symptoms to as much as 4 L of fluid.
      2. Rapidly developing effusions may be symptomatic at 50 to 80 ml (normal pericardial fluid volume = 15 to 50 ml) (Shelton, 2000).
    B. Fatigue, malaise.
    C. Dyspnea at rest and with exertion.
    D. Dull, nonpositional chest pain.
    E. Nonproductive cough.
    F. Tachycardia.
    G. Anxiousness, restlessness.
 III. Objective findings.
    A. Jugular venous distention.
    B. Distant, muffled heart sounds are a late finding.
    C. Pericardial friction rub more likely to occur with radiation-induced or nonmalignant effusions.
    D. Point of maximal impulse shifted to left.
    E. Decreased peripheral pulses.
    F. Moderately increased central venous pressure (15 to 18 cm of H_2O or 8 to 12 mm Hg).
    G. 2 to 3+ pedal edema with slowly developing effusions; may be none with rapid development of effusion.
    H. Narrowing pulse pressure, pulsus paradoxus greater than 13 mm Hg (Warren, 2000).
 IV. Laboratory and diagnostic tests.
    A. CXR indicating cardiac enlargement, widened mediastinum, "water bottle" shape of heart.
    B. Electrocardiogram (ECG) changes including low-voltage QRS, tachycardia, nonspecific ST-T changes; electrical alternans rare finding.
    C. Echocardiogram is a definitive test for effusion and cardiac function.
    D. CT of chest especially helpful if there is a large tumor burden.
    E. May evaluate pericardial fluid for lactate dehydrogenase and protein.

    F. Cardiac catheterization may be indicated if the diagnosis is in question (Warren, 2000).

Nursing Diagnoses

  I. Chronic or acute pain.
  II. Decreased cardiac output.
 III. Ineffective tissue perfusion, cardiopulmonary.
 IV. Activity intolerance.
  V. Disturbed sleep pattern.

Outcome Identification

  I. Client reports acceptable level of pain control.
  II. Client maintains EF within 5% of baseline.
 III. Client demonstrates normal vital signs and oxygen saturation level.
 IV. Client demonstrates tolerance of activities of daily living.
  V. Client reports adequate restful sleep.

Planning and Implementation

  I. Nonpharmacologic interventions (Grannis et al., 2002).
    A. Pericardial drainage (Table 17-1).
    B. RT may be indicated, but not common.
    C. Elevate head of bed to relieve dyspnea.
    D. Minimize activities to conserve energy.
    E. May elect no treatment with close follow-up if asymptomatic.
 II. Pharmacologic interventions.
    A. Chemotherapy may be indicated if tumor responsive (i.e., lymphoma, leukemia, breast cancer) (Grannis et al., 2002).
    B. Administration of sclerosing agents into pericardial space.
    C. Oxygen therapy.
    D. Diuretics probably not beneficial (Grannis et al., 2002).
 III. Client education.
    A. Preparation for pericardial drainage.
    B. Energy conservation methods.

Evaluation

The oncology nurse systematically and regularly evaluates the client's and/or family's responses to interventions in order to determine progress toward the achievement of expected outcomes. Relevant data are collected, and actual findings are compared with expected findings. Nursing diagnoses, outcomes, and plans of care are reviewed and revised as necessary.

CARDIOVASCULAR TOXICITY RELATED TO CANCER THERAPY

Theory

  I. Definition—alteration in cardiac function related to cancer treatment.
 II. Physiology.

TABLE 17-1
Treatment of Neoplastic Cardiac Tamponade

Treatment	Indications	Methodology
Pericardial catheter—may use to drain and remove or leave in for several days	Short-term emergent removal of slowly or rapidly developing effusions	Fluoroscopic-directed pericardial catheter with drainage and/or sclerosis (bleomycin [Blenoxane], doxycycline [Vibramycin], talc)
Balloon pericardiotomy	Short-term emergent removal of slowly or rapidly developing effusions	Catheter inserted into pericardial sac and balloon inflated to open a hole in the pericardial sac; catheter is immediately removed, and pericardial fluid drains into mediastinum
Pericardio-peritoneal shunt	Palliative management of recurrent malignant effusions, particularly with limited life expectancy	Local anesthesia used for percutaneous subxiphoid insertion of a Denver shunt that drains pericardial fluid into the abdomen
Pericardial window	Chronic, severe effusions in a patient with otherwise good performance status; must be able to tolerate a thoracoscopic procedure	Thoracotomy with resection of lower section of pericardial sac; screenlike grid placed to allow pericardial drainage into mediastinum
Pericardectomy	Chronic, severe effusions in a patient with otherwise good performance status; must be able to tolerate a thoracoscopic procedure; used only after catheter or balloon fluid removal and pericardial window have failed	Pericardial resection or stripping so there is no place for pericardial fluid to accumulate
Pericardiocentesis	Life-threatening cardiac tamponade in presence of moderate to large pericardial effusion when open procedure cannot be performed promptly	Emergency bedside insertion of a needle into pericardial sac for removal of fluid; needle inserted subxiphoid and pointed toward left shoulder; needle backed off and fluid aspirated

Modified from Shelton B: Pericarditis/pericardial effusion/cardiac tamponade. In Camp-Sorrell D, Hawkins RA, editors: *Clinical manual for the oncology advanced practice nurse,* Pittsburgh, 2002, Oncology Nursing Press, pp 313-314.

A. Cardiotoxic drugs and RT can cause abnormalities in cardiac conduction and/or function by various mechanisms.

B. DNA intercalators (anthracyclines) cause progressive cardiomyopathy from release of free radicals that result in myocardial cell loss, fibrosis, and loss of contractility (Keefe, 2000; Loerzel & Dow, 2003).

C. High-dose 5-fluorouracil (5-FU) can cause coronary artery spasm, resulting in angina, arrhythmia, myocardial infarction, cardiac arrest, and sudden death (Keefe, 2000).

1. Capecitabine, an oral pro-drug of 5-FU, has been associated with reversible cardiac side effects (Loerzel & Dow, 2003).

D. High-dose cyclophosphamide (Cytoxan, Neosar) is associated with acute myopericarditis, which may cause pericardial effusions, CHF, and cardiac tamponade (Keefe, 2000).

E. Trastuzumab (Herceptin) can cause acute heart failure when used concomitantly or following doxorubicin (Adriamycin, Doxil, Rubex) and epirubicin (Ellence) (Keefe, 2000).

F. All-trans retinoic acid (ATRA) causes a syndrome of fever, dyspnea, weight gain, pulmonary infiltrates, and pleural and pericardial effusions (Keefe, 2000).

G. Paclitaxel (Paxene, Taxol) causes asymptomatic bradycardia in approximately 30% of patients with ovarian cancer.
    1. May also cause atrioventricular conduction blocks, left bundle branch block, ventricular tachycardia, cardiac ischemia (Camp-Sorrell, 2000).

H. RT to areas near the heart can cause subacute myopericarditis with pericardial effusions, tamponade, and late sequelae such as valvular insufficiency, constrictive pericarditis, or acute myocardial infarction (Keefe, 2000).

I. Acridinyl anisidide (m-AMSA, Amsacrine), an alkylating agent, is associated with atrial arrhythmias and QT prolongation (Loerzel & Dow, 2003).

J. IL-2 has been associated with syncopal episodes and atrial arrhythmias associated with fluid retention and increased plasma volume (Loerzel & Dow, 2003).

K. Within 24 hours of rituximab (Rituxan) infusion, deaths from acute myocardial infarction, ventricular fibrillation, or cardiogenic shock have occurred.
    1. Approximately 80% occurred in association with the first infusion (Rituxan Product Information, 2003).

III. Incidence (Camp-Sorrell, 2000; Wilkes, 2001).
    A. Acute reactions—infrequent.
        1. Occur within 24 hours of drug administration.
        2. Usually self-limiting and cease when the drug is stopped.
        3. May not require discontinuation of the drug.
    B. Subacute reactions—infrequent.
        1. Occur several weeks after treatment.
        2. Usually reversible.
        3. Not usually an indication to discontinue use of the drug.
    C. Chronic reactions—dose dependent.
        1. Occurs with cumulative doses of drugs; incidence increases after specific dose levels.
        2. Treatment must be discontinued.
        3. Usually poorly responsive to treatment, progressive, and has a 60% mortality rate (Camp-Sorrell, 2000).
    D. Childhood and adolescent cancer survivors who live more than 5 years after treatment are 8.8 times more likely to die from cardiac-related events (Loerzel & Dow, 2003).

Assessment

I. Risk factors (Camp-Sorrell, 2000; Wilkes, 2001).
    A. Preexisting heart disease, hypertension.
    B. History of smoking.
    C. Age younger than 4 years or advanced age.
    D. Multiple cardiotoxic drugs.
    E. Exceeding recommended total doses or high dose in short period.
    F. RT to the chest.
II. Subjective findings.
    A. Palpitations.
    B. Chest pain.

   C. Shortness of breath, dyspnea, orthopnea.
   D. Exercise intolerance, fatigue.
   E. Weight gain, extremity swelling.
   F. Nonproductive cough.
III. Objective findings.
   A. Tachycardia—early sign in anthracycline toxicity.
   B. Arrhythmias.
   C. Jugular vein distention.
   D. Hypotension.
   E. Bilateral pedal edema.
   F. Presence of S_3 or S_4.
   G. Murmurs with valvular abnormalities.
IV. Laboratory and diagnostic tests.
   A. ECG changes.
      1. Premature atrial contractions, premature ventricular contractions.
      2. Nonspecific ST-T changes.
   B. Echocardiogram or radionuclide cardiac scan (MUGA scan).
      1. Decreased EF.
         a. Decrease of EF to less than 45% or decrease of more than 5% over base-line requires drug discontinuation.
      2. Pericardial effusion.
      3. Left ventricular hypertrophy (Camp-Sorrell, 2000).
   C. Laboratory changes that may impact cardiac function—potassium, magnesium, calcium, renal function, cardiac enzymes.

Nursing Diagnoses

   I. Decreased cardiac output.
  II. Ineffective tissue perfusion, cardiopulmonary.
 III. Impaired gas exchange.
  IV. Activity intolerance.
   V. Chronic pain.

Outcome Identification

   I. Client maintains EF within 5% of baseline.
  II. Client demonstrates normal vital signs and oxygenation level.
 III. Client reports absence of dyspnea.
  IV. Client demonstrates tolerance of activities of daily living.
   V. Client reports pain at acceptable level of control.

Planning and Implementation

   I. Prevention is key.
   A. Document total cumulative dose of drug, discontinue when maximum dose is achieved (Camp-Sorrell, 2000).
      1. Doxorubicin: 550 mg/m^2.
      2. Daunorubicin (Cerubidine, DaunoXome): 600 mg/m^2.
      3. Mitoxantrone (Novantrone): 160 mg/m^2.
      4. High-dose cyclophosphamide: 144 mg/kg for 4 days.
   B. Monitor baseline and interval echocardiogram or MUGA scan.

    C. Administer as weekly low-dose infusions rather than boluses, and avoid drug interactions (Keefe, 2000).

    D. Use of liposomal doxorubicin decreases cardiotoxicity (Camp-Sorrell, 2000).

II. Nonpharmacologic interventions.

    A. Bed rest to promote diuresis and energy conservation.

    B. Valvular surgery may be indicated with radiation-induced valvular disease (Keefe, 2000).

III. Pharmacologic interventions.

    A. Diuretics.

    B. Vasodilators.

    C. β-Blockers.

    D. ACE inhibitors.

    E. Calcium channel blockers.

    F. Digoxin (Lanoxin, Lanoxicaps).

    G. Administration of cardiac protective iron chelating agents, such as dexrazoxane (Zinecard), to prevent doxorubicin-induced cardiotoxicity in clients with metastatic breast cancer who require more than 300 mg/m^2 of drug (Camp-Sorrell, 2000).

IV. Client education.

    A. Signs and symptoms to report.

    B. Low-sodium, low-fat diet.

    C. Avoid isometric exercises, which may be a late cause of heart failure in patients who received anthracyclines (Camp-Sorrell, 2000).

Evaluation

The oncology nurse systematically and regularly evaluates the client's and/or family's responses to interventions in order to determine progress toward the achievement of expected outcomes. Relevant data are collected, and actual findings are compared with expected findings. Nursing diagnoses, outcomes, and plans of care are reviewed and revised as necessary.

THROMBOTIC EVENTS

Theory

    I. Definition—venous thrombus or arterial embolus obstructing arterial blood flow or interfering with venous drainage.

    II. Physiology (Blinder & Behl, 2002; Story, 2000).

        A. A thrombus starts as a clot nidus in the setting of stasis, endothelial injury, and a hypercoagulable state (Virchow's triad).

        B. The clot nidus, composed of red blood cells, fibrin, and platelets, fills the vessel lumen, causing partial or complete obstruction of blood flow, or may shed emboli, causing pulmonary embolus or cerebrovascular accident.

        C. The thrombus may float freely in the blood vessel, leading to embolization where it lodges in a blood vessel, causing partial or complete obstruction of blood flow.

    III. May be associated with the following (Blinder & Behl, 2002; Dell, 2002; Story, 2000):

        A. Thrombocytosis (platelet count over 400,000/mm^3).

        B. Metastatic cancer.

    C. Presence of venous access device.

    D. Disseminated intravascular coagulation.

    E. Cancer treatments, particularly tamoxifen (Nolvadex) therapy and other hormonal agents.

    F. Sepsis.

    G. Cardiac disease.

    H. Clotting abnormalities (factor V Leiden, protein C and protein S deficiency, antiphospholipid antibodies)—less likely in persons with cancer.

    I. Microangiopathic hemolytic anemia (MAHA) associated with thrombotic thrombocytopenic purpura (TTP).

    J. Smoking, obesity, immobility.

    K. Heparin-induced thrombocytopenia.

    L. Disseminated intravascular coagulation (DIC).

IV. Tumor cells may be associated with procoagulant activities (Dell, 2002; Viale, 1999).

    A. Tumor cells deposit fibrin in tissues and act late in clotting cascade, providing a surface for prothrombinase assembly.

    B. Microvasculature becomes hyperpermeable, allowing clotting proteins to leak into extravascular space.

    C. Procoagulants released from cancer cells initiate the clotting cascade.

V. Incidence is 15% to 40% of persons with cancer. More common with the following (Blinder & Behl, 2002; Dell, 2002; Viale, 1999):

    A. Cancers of the breast, lung, and GI tract.

    B. Leukemias.

    C. Hodgkin's and non-Hodgkin's lymphoma.

VI. Deep vein thrombosis (DVT) and/or pulmonary emboli (PE) is the presenting symptom in 5% to 10% of all persons diagnosed with cancer.

    A. In idiopathic DVT/PE, the risk of cancer diagnosis is 4% to 14% in the next 2 years (Blinder & Behl, 2002).

Assessment (Dell, 2002; Story, 2000; Viale, 1999)

  I. Risk factors.

    A. Estrogen, tamoxifen use.

    B. Smoking.

    C. Recent surgery.

    D. Bed rest or decreased activity status.

    E. Recent long distance plane or car travel.

    F. Obesity.

    G. Advanced age.

  II. Subjective findings.

    A. Venous occlusion.

      1. Dull ache, tight feeling, or frank pain in the calf, especially with walking.

      2. Tenderness over involved vein.

    B. Arterial embolus.

      1. Severe pain in involved extremity.

      2. Extremity coolness.

    C. Pulmonary embolus.

      1. Chest pain.

      2. Dyspnea.

      3. Sudden onset of anxiety.

      4. Cardiopulmonary arrest.

   D. Clotting abnormalities.
      1. Easy bruising.
      2. Bleeding from mucous membranes, in urine or stool.
III. Objective findings.
   A. Venous occlusion.
      1. Unilateral edema of involved extremity.
      2. Distention of superficial collateral veins.
      3. Tenderness over involved vein, palpable venous cord.
      4. Homans' sign positive in fewer than 50% of cases with DVT and has a high incidence of false-positive findings (Story, 2000).
   B. Arterial embolus.
      1. Extremity coolness, pallor.
      2. Absent or decreased pulse.
   C. Pulmonary embolus.
      1. Shallow respirations, tachypnea.
      2. Decreased pulse oximetry.
      3. Decreased breath sounds with pleural friction rub.
   D. Clotting abnormalities.
      1. Excessive bruising, bleeding.
IV. Laboratory and diagnostic tests.
   A. Platelet count—thrombocytosis; platelets more than $400,000/mm^3$.
   B. D-dimer—a negative test has a high negative predictive value for DVT but does not exclude DVT in patients with cancer (ten Wolde et al., 2002).
   C. Abnormal venous duplex scan or venogram with venous thromboembolism.
   D. Abnormal arteriogram with arterial embolus.
   E. Abnormal spiral CT or ventilation-perfusion scan with pulmonary embolism.
   F. Abnormal clotting factors.

Nursing Diagnoses

   I. Ineffective tissue perfusion, cardiopulmonary/peripheral.
   II. Risk for impaired skin integrity.
   III. Impaired gas exchange (PE).
   IV. Activity intolerance.
   V. Acute pain.

Outcome Identification

   I. Client's extremities are of normal warmth and color.
   II. Client maintains intact skin.
   III. Client maintains normal respiratory rate.
   IV. Client demonstrates tolerance of physical activity.
   V. Client reports acceptable level of pain control.

Planning and Implementation

   I. Prevention in high-risk patients (Blinder & Behl, 2002; Dell, 2002; Story, 2000; Viale, 1999).
   A. Nonpharmacologic.
      1. Frequent ambulation, leg exercises if bedridden.
      2. Elevation of foot with knee flexed.
      3. Use of elastic stockings, pneumatic compression device.

   B. Pharmacologic.

      1. Acetylsalicylic acid (aspirin, ASA), 81 to 325 mg daily.

      2. Low-dose subcutaneous heparin.

      3. Low-molecular weight heparin (LMWH).

      4. Low-dose warfarin (Coumadin) in patients with long-term indwelling central venous catheters.

  II. Treatment of existing embolus (Blinder & Behl, 2002; Dell, 2002; Story, 2000; Viale, 1999).

   A. Nonpharmacologic.

      1. Placement of inferior vena cava filter.

      2. Arterial embolectomy.

      3. Monitor laboratory parameters—prothrombin time (PT), international normalizing ratio (INR), partial thromboplastin time (PTT).

   B. Pharmacologic.

      1. Heparin infusion.

      2. LMWH.

      3. Warfarin.

      4. Oxygen for pulmonary embolism.

 III. Client education.

   A. Medication administration.

   B. Preventive measures.

   C. Bleeding precautions if client taking anticoagulant.

   D. Dietary restrictions—avoid foods high in vitamin K.

   E. Smoking cessation.

Evaluation

The oncology nurse systematically and regularly evaluates the client's and/or family's responses to interventions in order to determine progress toward the achievement of expected outcomes. Relevant data are collected, and actual findings are compared with expected findings. Nursing diagnoses, outcomes, and plans of care are reviewed and revised as necessary.

REFERENCES

Blinder, M.A., & Behl, M.A. (2002). Coagulation disorders in cancer. In R. Govindan (Ed.). *The Washington manual of oncology.* Philadelphia: Lippincott Williams & Wilkins, pp. 441-447.

Brady, H.R., O'Meara, Y.M., & Brenner, B.M. (2003). The major glomerulopathies, Harrison's Online, Chapter 274. Retrieved 7-2-2004 from *http://www.harrisons.accessmedicine.com/server-java/Arknoid/amed/harrisons/co_chapters/ch274/ch274_p19.html.*

Camp-Sorrell, D. (2000). Chemotherapy: Toxicity management—cardiotoxicity. In C.H. Yarbro, M.H. Frogge, M. Goodman, & S.L. Groenwald (Eds.). *Cancer nursing: Principles and practice* (5th ed.). Sudbury, MA: Jones and Bartlett Publishers, pp. 472-474.

Chapman, D.D., & Goodman, M. (2000). Breast cancer—chronic lymphedema. In C.H. Yarbro, M.H. Frogge, M. Goodman, & S.L. Groenwald (Eds.). *Cancer nursing: Principles and practice* (5th ed.). Sudbury, MA: Jones and Bartlett Publishers, pp. 1038-1039.

Cope, D.G. (2000). Lymphedema. In D. Camp-Sorrell & R.A. Hawkins (Eds.). *Clinical manual for the oncology advanced practice nurse.* Pittsburgh: Oncology Nursing Press, pp. 649-652.

Dell, D.D. (2002). Deep vein thrombosis in the patient with cancer. *Clinical Journal of Oncology Nursing 6,* 43-46.

Grannis, F.W., Wagman, L.D., Lai, L., & Curcio, L.D. (2002). Fluid complications. In R. Pazdur, L.R. Coia, W.J. Hoskins, & L.D. Wagman (Eds.). *Cancer management: A multidisciplinary approach.* Mellville, NY: PRR, Inc., pp. 943-958.

Keefe, D.L. (2000). Cardiovascular emergencies in the cancer patient. *Seminars in Oncology 27,* 244-255.

Loerzel, V.W., & Dow, K.H. (2003). Cardiac toxicity related to cancer treatment. *Clinical Journal of Oncology Nursing 7,* 557-562.

Martin, V. (2000). Ovarian cancer—lymphedema. In C.H. Yarbro, M.H. Frogge, M. Goodman, & S.L. Groenwald (Eds.). *Cancer nursing: Principles and practice* (5th ed.). Sudbury, MA: Jones and Bartlett Publishers, pp. 1390-1391.

National Lymphedema Network (NLN). (2002). Lymphedema: A brief overview. Retrieved February 3, 2003 from the World Wide Web: http://www.lymphnet.org/prevention.html

National Lymphedema Network (NLN). (2003). Prevention. Retrieved June 29, 2004 from the World Wide Web: http://www.lymphnet.org/prevention.html.

Ridner, S.H. (2002). Breast cancer lymphedema: Pathophysiology and risk reduction guidelines. *Oncology Nursing Forum 29,* 1285-1293.

Rituxan Rituximab Product Information. (2003). Warning section, para 1. Retrieved February 7, 2004 from the World Wide Web: http://www.rituxan.com/rituxan/pi/#warnings.

Ruckdeschel, J.C., & Jablons, D. (2001). Malignant effusions in the chest. In J.M. Kirkwood, M.T. Lotze, & J.M. Yasko (Eds.). *Current cancer therapeutics* (4th ed.). Philadelphia: Current Medicine, pp. 334-339.

Ryan, M., Stainton, M.C., Jaconelli, C., et al. (2003). The experience of lower limb lymphedema for women after treatment for gynecologic cancer. *Oncology Nursing Forum 30,* 417-423.

Shelton, B.K. (2000). Pericarditis/pericardial effusion/cardiac tamponade. In D. Camp-Sorrell & R.A. Hawkins (Eds.). *Clinical manual for the oncology advanced practice nurse.* Pittsburgh: Oncology Nursing Press, pp. 307-316.

Story, K.T. (2000). Deep vein thrombosis. In D. Camp-Sorrell & R.A. Hawkins (Eds.). *Clinical manual for the oncology advanced practice nurse.* Pittsburgh: Oncology Nursing Press, pp. 235-243.

ten Wolde, M., Kraaijenhagen, R.A., Prins, M.H., & Buller, H.R. (2002). The clinical usefulness of d-dimer testing in cancer patients with suspected deep venous thrombosis. *Archives of Internal Medicine 162,* 1880-1884.

Viale, P.H. (1999). Management of thromboembolism in patients with cancer. *Oncology Nursing Forum 26,* 1625-1632.

Warren, W.H. (2000). Malignancies involving the pericardium. *Seminars in Thoracic and Cardiovascular Surgery 12,* 119-129.

Wilkes, G.M. (2001). Potential toxicities and nursing management—cardiotoxicity of antineoplastic drugs. In M. Barton-Burke, G.M. Wilkes, & K. Ingwerson (Eds.). *Cancer chemotherapy: A nursing process approach* (3rd ed.). Sudbury, MA: Jones and Bartlett Publishers, pp. 149-154.

Winokur, M.A. (2000). Peripheral edema. In D. Camp-Sorrell & R.A. Hawkins (Eds.). *Clinical manual for the oncology advanced practice nurse.* Pittsburgh: Oncology Nursing Press.

Works, C., & Maxwell, M.B. (2000). Malignant effusions and edemas. In C.H. Yarbro, M.H. Frogge, M. Goodman, & S.L. Groenwald (Eds.). *Cancer nursing: Principles and practice* (5th ed.). Sudbury, MA: Jones and Bartlett Publishers, pp. 813-830.

PART FIVE

ONCOLOGIC EMERGENCIES

18 Metabolic Emergencies

BARBARA HOLMES GOBEL

DISSEMINATED INTRAVASCULAR COAGULATION

Theory

I. Definition: disseminated intravascular coagulation (DIC) is the inappropriate, accelerated, and systemic activation of the coagulation cascade, resulting in thrombosis and, subsequently, bleeding and hemorrhage.

II. Physiology of hemostasis.
  - **A.** Hemostasis is maintained through a balanced system of thrombosis (clot formation) and fibrinolysis (clot breakdown) (Figure 18-1).
    - **1.** The process of thrombosis is initiated through disruption of the endothelial membrane and/or tissue injury.
      - **a.** Disruption of the endothelial membrane activates a cascade of clotting factors in the intrinsic pathway of this cascade, resulting in coagulation.
      - **b.** Tissue injury causes the release of tissue thromboplastin into the circulation and the activation of the extrinsic pathway, resulting in coagulation.
      - **c.** Reactions that occur in the intrinsic and extrinsic pathways of coagulation are combined in a final "common pathway."
      - **d.** The final product of hemostasis is a stable fibrin clot.
    - **2.** Fibrinolysis is the process that functions to break down stable fibrin clots (Mammen, 2000).
      - **a.** Plasmin is an enzyme that digests the components of the fibrin clot (Mammen, 2000).
      - **b.** Thrombin is the central proteolytic enzyme that is necessary for both coagulation and fibrinolysis.
      - **c.** The products of this reaction, fibrin split products (FSPs) or fibrin degradation products (FDPs), are released into the circulation and function as powerful anticoagulant substances.
      - **d.** FDPs are gradually cleared from the circulation in the reticuloendothelial system (RES).

III. In the presence of an underlying condition such as infection, malignancy, or trauma, the intrinsic and/or extrinsic pathway of the clotting cascade is triggered, resulting in excess circulating thrombin.
  - **A.** Excess thrombin results in multiple fibrin clots in the circulation.
  - **B.** Excess clots trap platelets, which leads to microvascular and macrovascular thrombosis.
  - **C.** The lodging of clots leads to ischemia, impaired organ perfusion, and end-organ damage (Bick, 2002; Staudinger et al., 1996).

IV. The consumption of coagulation factors is greater than the ability of the body for replacement, which contributes to the bleeding seen with DIC.

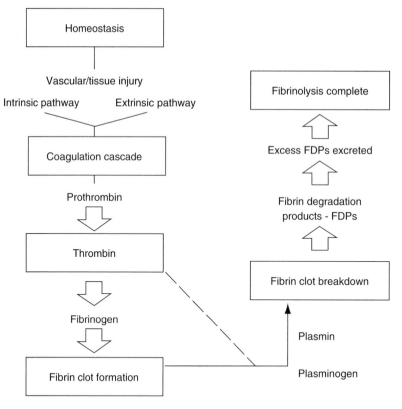

FIGURE 18-1 ■ Normal hemostasis.

V. In addition, fibrinolysis is initiated; FDPs are not removed effectively from the circulation (because there is an excess of FDPs), and an accumulation of these anticoagulant substances occurs, contributing to the bleeding seen with DIC (Gobel, 1999).

VI. Excess plasmin activates the complement and kinin systems; this leads to symptoms such as shock, hypotension, and increased vascular permeability (Gobel, 2000).

VII. Principles of medical management.
   A. Diagnostic tests (Table 18-1).
      1. General tests done to assist in the diagnosis of DIC (Mammen, 2000).
         a. Platelet count.
         b. Fibrinogen level.
         c. D-dimer assay (often done in combination with the FDP titer) (Yu et al., 2000).
         d. FDP titer (often done in combination with the D-dimer assay) (Yu et al., 2000).
      2. Tests done to determine accelerated coagulation (if available).
         a. Antithrombin III level (Wada et al., 1999).
         b. Fibrinopeptide A level.
         c. Prothrombin activation peptides (F1 and F2).
         d. Thrombin-antithrombin complexes.
      3. Tests done to determine accelerated fibrinolysis (Staudinger et al., 1996).
         a. Plasminogen level.
         b. Plasmin α_2-antiplasmin complex levels.

TABLE 18-1
Laboratory Results with Disseminated Intravascular Coagulation

Laboratory Test	Results
Platelet count	Decreased
Fibrinogen level	Decreased
D-dimer assay	Increased
FDP titer	Increased
Antithrombin III level	Decreased
Fibrinopeptide A	Increased
Prothrombin activation peptides	Increased
Thrombin-antithrombin complex	Increased
Plasminogen level	Decreased
Plasmin α_2-antiplasmin complex	Decreased

FDP, Fibrin degradation product.

B. Medical management of DIC is targeted to the treatment of the underlying, predisposing condition or conditions causing the DIC; supporting the patient's hemodynamic status; and managing the bleeding or thrombotic manifestations that are clinically present.

1. Treatment of the underlying, predisposing condition, such as chemotherapy for malignancy or antibiotics for infection.
2. Hemodynamic support.
   a. Fluid replacement to treat hypotension and treat proteinuria (Letsky, 2001).
   b. Oxygen therapy to treat hypoxia and associated acidosis caused by hemorrhage (Gobel, 2002).
3. Blood component therapy for abnormal hematologic parameters or active bleeding (see Chapter 9).
   a. Platelet concentrate if platelet count is less than 20,000/mm³ or if the patient is actively bleeding.
   b. Packed red blood cells (RBCs) if the hemoglobin is less than 8 g/dl or if the patient is actively bleeding.
   c. Fresh frozen plasma provides plasma, fibrinogen, and other clotting factors; use of fresh frozen plasma may aggravate DIC since fibrinogen and new clotting factors are added to the circulation (Bick, 2002).
   d. Cryoprecipitate provides fibrinogen and factor VIII in cases of extreme hyperfibrinolysis.
4. Plasmapheresis to replace coagulation factors.
5. Management of intravascular clotting.
   a. Plasmapheresis removes triggers of coagulation.
   b. Heparin interferes with thrombin production.
      (1) Use is considered controversial except in acute promyelocytic leukemia (APL).
      (2) Heparin is given intravenously (IV) or subcutaneously, using low-dose heparin (Bick, 1996; DeSancho & Rand, 2001).
      (3) Goal is to maintain activated partial thromboplastin time (aPTT) at 1 to 2 times normal levels.
      (4) Primary side effect is bleeding.

(5) Heparin therapy is contraindicated in patients with central nervous system (CNS) compromise (e.g., headache or recent cerebrovascular accident), open wounds, or recent surgery (Gobel, 2000).

6. Management of excessive bleeding (in spite of other measures to control the DIC) with fibrinolytic inhibitor medications (Arkel, 2000).
   a. ε-Aminocaproic acid (EACA) inhibits fibrinolysis.
      (1) Usually given after heparin therapy.
      (2) Primary side effect is clotting and can lead to widespread fibrin deposition.
   b. Antithrombin III inhibits procoagulants and fibrinolytic process.
   c. Tranexamic acid.
      (1) Usually given after heparin therapy.
      (2) Can lead to widespread fibrin deposition.
      (3) Medication can cause severe hypotension, severe hyperkalemia, ventricular arrhythmias (Seto & Dunlap, 1996).

Assessment

I. Identification of clients at risk for DIC.
   A. Acute leukemias, particularly APL.
   B. Solid tumors—mucin-producing adenocarcinomas, such as lung, breast, prostate, pancreas, ovarian, and biliary tract malignancies (Murphy-Ende, 1998).
   C. Infection and sepsis (most common cause of DIC).
   D. Presence of liver disease, including both primary liver disease and secondary metastasis from malignancy (Bick, 1998).
   E. Presence of peritoneovenous shunts—ascitic fluid contains a number of procoagulant substances.
   F. Hemolytic transfusion reaction or massive transfusions of whole blood (Bick, 1998).
   G. Transplant rejection.
   H. Trauma, burns, or shock.
   I. Pregnancy and obstetric complications.

II. Physical examination—early recognition of the signs and symptoms of DIC is critical to prompt intervention and treatment (Gobel, 2000).
   A. Skin—pallor, petechiae, jaundice, ecchymosis, hematomas, acral cyanosis (irregularly shaped blue/gray discolored areas on extremities), and bleeding from any site of invasive procedures.
      1. Bleeding from at least three unrelated sites is not uncommon in DIC.
         a. Bleeding may range from oozing of blood from any site to frank hemorrhage.
         b. Intracranial hemorrhage, gastrointestinal (GI) bleeding, and hemoptysis pose life-threatening events for the client.
   B. GI—tarry stools, hematemesis, abdominal pain, abdominal distention, positive results of guaiac stool test.
   C. Genitourinary—hematuria (burning, dysuria, frequency and pain on urination are associated with hematuria), decreased urinary output.
   D. Respiratory—dyspnea, tachypnea, hypoxia, hemoptysis, cyanosis, shortness of breath.
   E. Neurologic—headache, restlessness, confusion, lethargy, altered level of consciousness, obtundation, seizures, coma.

    F. Musculoskeletal—joint pain and stiffness.

    G. Cardiovascular—tachycardia, hypotension, diminished peripheral pulses, changes in color and temperature of extremities.

III. Evaluation of laboratory data.

    A. Decreased platelet count (not specific or sensitive for DIC) (Gobel, 2003).

    B. Decreased fibrinogen level (not specific or sensitive for DIC) (Gobel, 2003).

    C. Increased D-dimer assay reflects the microangiopathy of DIC (Yu et al., 2000).

    D. Increased FDP titers reflect the microangiopathy of DIC (Yu et al., 2000).

    E. D-dimer assays and FDP titers have been found to be sensitive, specific, and efficient in the diagnosis of DIC (Yu et al., 2000).

    F. Decreased antithrombin III level.

    G. Elevated fibrinopeptide A level.

    H. Elevated prothrombin activation peptides (F1 and F2).

    I. Elevated thrombin-antithrombin complexes.

    J. Decreased plasminogen levels.

    K. Decreased plasmin α_2-antiplasmin complex levels.

Nursing Diagnoses

    I. Ineffective tissue perfusion (renal, cerebral, peripheral, cardiopulmonary, GI).

  II. Risk for injury.

 III. Deficient fluid volume.

  IV. Decreased cardiac output.

   V. Impaired gas exchange.

  VI. Impaired skin integrity.

 VII. Acute pain.

VIII. Acute confusion.

  IX. Anxiety.

   X. Fear.

Outcome Identification

  I. Client and family identify personal risk factors for development of DIC.

 II. Client and family list critical signs and symptoms of DIC that should be reported immediately to the health care team.

III. Client describes self-care measures to maximize personal safety.

Planning and Implementation

  I. Interventions to maximize safety for the client.

    A. Place bed in low position with side rails up.

    B. Clear pathways in room and hallways.

    C. Provide assistance as needed for activities of daily living.

    D. Minimize activities that trigger bleeding.

    E. Minimize activities that contribute to clotting.

      1. No tight or constrictive clothing.

      2. Client not to dangle feet on the side of bed.

      3. No use of knee gatch or pillows under knees.

 II. Interventions to decrease severity of symptoms associated with DIC.

    A. Monitor all bleeding sites frequently.

    B. Monitor red, tender, indurated areas over multiple organ sites (Gobel, 2002).

C. Apply direct pressure to sites of active bleeding.
D. Elevate sites of active bleeding if possible.
E. Apply pressure dressings or sandbags to sites of active bleeding.
F. Administer pain medication as needed.
G. Administer IV fluids as needed.
H. Administer oxygen as needed.

III. Interventions to monitor for sequelae of DIC and treatment.
    A. Monitor for signs and symptoms of progressive DIC.
        1. Fever.
        2. Tachycardia; hypotension.
        3. Cool, clammy, cyanotic skin.
        4. Proteinuria, anuria.
        5. Decreased mental status progressing to coma.
        6. Changes in location, severity, and responses to pain interventions.
        7. Changes in rate, depth, or difficulty of respirations; hypoxia.
        8. GI bleeding.
        9. Ongoing bleeding despite measures to control clotting and bleeding.
    B. Monitor intake and output every hour during acute DIC.
    C. Monitor for signs and symptoms of fluid overload.

IV. Interventions to monitor response of client to medical management.
    A. Monitor sites and amount of bleeding.
        1. Count peripads.
        2. Weigh affected dressings.
        3. Measure bloody drainage.
        4. Hematest stool, urine, emesis.
        5. Measure abdominal girth every 4 hours if abdominal bleeding is suspected.
    B. Monitor changes in laboratory values, and report significant changes to physician.
    C. Assess tissue perfusion parameters—color, temperature, peripheral pulses.
    D. Monitor psychosocial responses of the client and family to critical illness.

V. Interventions to enhance adaptation and rehabilitation.
    A. Provide information about planned therapy and response to treatment on a regular basis.
    B. Listen to fears and concerns of the client and family.

VI. Interventions to incorporate the client and family in care.
    A. Instruct the client and family about critical signs and symptoms to report to the health care team—new sites of bleeding, changes in color of stool or urine, subjective changes in respiratory effort and effectiveness, changes in mental status.
    B. Instruct the client and family to save all stool, urine, and emesis for nurse to check for blood.
    C. Instruct the client and family in measures to prevent bleeding (see Chapter 13).

Evaluation

The oncology nurse systematically and regularly evaluates the client's and/or family's responses to interventions to determine progress toward the achievement of expected outcomes. Relevant data are collected, and actual finding are compared with expected findings. Nursing diagnoses, outcomes, and plans of care are reviewed and revised as necessary.

SEPSIS

Theory

   I. Definition: sepsis is the systemic inflammatory response to a documented infection.

  II. Physiology of sepsis.
   A. Sepsis is a systemic inflammatory response to pathogenic microorganisms and associated endotoxins in the blood.
   1. Sepsis usually presents with two or more of the following parameters (Bone et al., 1992):
   a. Temperature greater than 100.4° F (38° C).
   b. Heart rate greater than 90 beats/min.
   c. Respiratory rate greater than 20 breaths/min.
   d. White blood cell (WBC) count greater than 12,000, or less than 4000, or greater than 10% bands.
   B. Septic shock is manifested by hemodynamic instability and alterations in cellular metabolism caused by sepsis (Figure 18-2). It occurs when the body fails to initiate an adequate immune response.
   1. Septic shock is characterized by fever, chills, tachycardia, tachypnea, mental status changes, and hypoperfusion/hypotension that persist despite aggressive fluid challenge (Petersen, 2000).
   2. Standardized definitions of the phases of septic shock include infection, bacteremia, systemic inflammatory response syndrome (SIRS), sepsis, severe sepsis, septic shock, and multiple organ dysfunction syndrome (MODS) (American College of Chest Physicians [ACCP], 1992).
   3. Because MODS is so severe, homeostasis cannot be maintained without prompt and exact intervention (Segal et al., 2001).

 III. Infectious agents.
   A. Bacterial organisms are the most common source of infection-related sepsis.
   1. Gram-negative bacteria *(Escherichia coli, Klebsiella pneumoniae, Pseudomonas aeruginosa)* have historically accounted for 50% to 60% of all septic shock cases (Rangel-Frausto & Wenzel, 1997).
   2. Currently gram-negative bacteria account for 40% of all septic shock cases (Pelletier, 2003).
   3. Gram-positive bacteria *(Streptococcus pneumoniae, Staphylococcus aureus)* account for 5% to 10% of septic shock cases (Stapczynski, 2002).
   a. The incidence of gram-positive bacteria is increasing rapidly because of extensive use of vascular access devices and mucosal toxicity of cytotoxic regimens (Marchetti et al., 2001).
   4. Other organisms include fungi *(Candida, Aspergillus),* anaerobes, viruses, and protozoa.
   a. Fungal infections are associated with prolonged hospitalization and significant mortality.
   5. Most infections arise from endogenous flora of the client.

 IV. Prognosis.
   A. Untreated bacteremia in clients with associated neutropenia is fatal; septic shock is associated with a 50% to 70% mortality rate.
   B. Mortality is associated with causative organism, site of infection, and the level and duration of neutropenia.

  V. Principles of medical management.
   A. Prevention of infection.

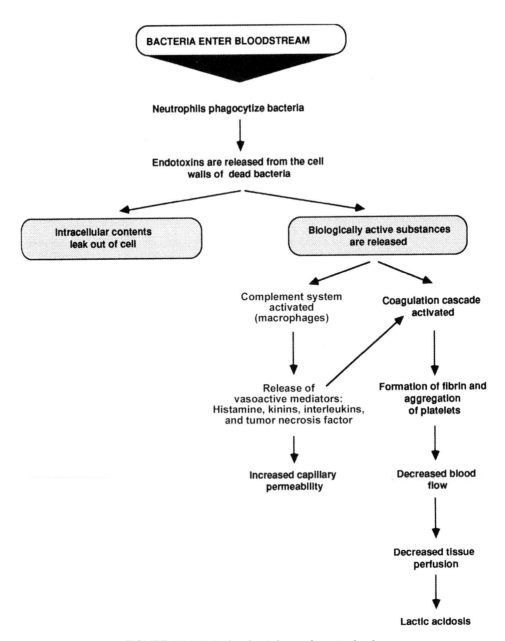

FIGURE 18-2 ■ Pathophysiology of septic shock.

1. Basic infection control precautions (Ellerhorst-Ryan, 2000).
   a. Hand hygiene of clients and health care team.
   b. Good oral care, perineal care.
   c. Identification of clients at risk for infection.
   d. Avoidance of practices that promote colonization of bacteria.
   e. Avoidance of invasive procedures.
2. Multidisciplinary approach.
B. Diagnostic tests—done baseline and repeated every 24 hours if signs and symptoms of sepsis persist (Petersen, 2000).

1. Blood cultures—aerobic and anaerobic, drawn from two separate sources (two venipuncture sites or one venipuncture site and one central venous catheter site).
2. Chest x-ray examination.
3. Cultures of throat, stool, urine, central venous catheters, and any other site of exudates—should be obtained before starting antibiotic therapy to properly identify the pathogen.
4. Complete blood count.
5. Chemistries—electrolytes, liver function tests (LFTs).
6. Prothrombin time (PT), activated partial thromboplastin time (aPTT), coagulation profile.
7. Pulse oximetry, arterial blood gases (ABGs).
8. Electrocardiogram (ECG).
C. Other tests to further evaluate organ dysfunction and detect the infectious source (Aarons & Wheeler, 1997).
   1. Echocardiogram.
   2. Computed tomography (CT) scan.
   3. Ventilation-perfusion scan.
   4. Angiography.
D. Hemodynamic support.
   1. Fluid resuscitation—studies have not demonstrated the superiority of crystalloids or colloid solutions (Koscove, 1998; Krau, 1998).
      a. Crystalloid solutions (normal saline, lactated Ringer's) are used most commonly during early stabilization of septic shock.
      b. Colloid solutions (dextran, albumin, plasma protein fraction).
      c. Fluid resuscitation complications include peripheral and pulmonary edema and hemodilution.
   2. Blood component therapy.
      a. RBCs to raise the hemoglobin to 10 to 12 g/dl, and the hematocrit to 30% to 35%.
   3. Vasopressors and inotropic support.
      a. Dopamine (Intropin)—first-line therapy for its vasopressor and inotropic effects (Petersen, 2000).
      b. Norepinephrine (Levophed)—can add if dopamine alone is not effective; added for increased vasopressor support.
      c. Dobutamine (Dobutrex)—added for increased inotropic effects.
   4. Oxygen therapy.
      a. Oxygen therapy should be started as soon as septic shock is suspected (Rivers et al., 2001).
      b. Early intubation and mechanical ventilation are recommended to increase oxygen delivery and to decrease the oxygen demand until septic shock can be reversed.
E. Treatment of infection.
   1. Empiric antibiotics are started at first suspicion of sepsis (after blood cultures are collected).
      a. Broad-spectrum antibiotic coverage against common gram-negative and gram-positive organisms.
         (1) The antimicrobial regimen is usually not changed for 72 hours, unless clients exhibit signs and symptoms of impending shock (Volker, 1998).
   2. Empiric antifungal therapy is started when the patient remains febrile for 5 to 7 days after the empiric therapy is begun.

       a. Amphotericin B has been the drug therapy of choice for years.

       b. Side effects of amphotericin B include fever, chills, rigors, headache, anorexia, nausea, vomiting, diarrhea, anemia, nephrotoxicity, hypotension, and anaphylaxis (Dismukes, 2000).

       c. New formulations of amphotericin B exist and may be warranted if the serum creatinine starts at or rises to greater than 2.5 mg/dl (Rex et al., 2000).

    F. Supportive therapies.

      1. Nutrition.

      2. Management of coagulopathies.

      3. Electrolyte replacement.

      4. Thermoregulation.

Assessment

  I. Identification of clients at risk.

    A. Granulocytopenia is the single most important risk factor in the development of sepsis (Sachdeva, 2002).

      1. Duration of the granulocytopenia increases the risk for sepsis.

    B. Malignancy-related immunosuppression.

      1. Humoral immunity is modified in patients with chronic lymphocytic leukemia or multiple myeloma because there is bone marrow infiltration of these cells.

      2. Cellular immunity is modified in patients with Hodgkin's disease, acute leukemia, advanced lung cancer, and intravascular tumors and in patients undergoing stem cell transplant (Ellerhorst-Ryan, 2000).

    C. Recent cancer treatment including chemotherapy, radiation therapy (RT), surgery (Safdar & Armstrong, 2001).

    D. Comorbid conditions in patients with cancer including the following (Shelton, 1999):

      1. Diabetes.

      2. Organ-related disease—renal, hepatic, cardiovascular, GI, pulmonary.

    E. Age over 65 years (Stapczyinski, 2002).

    F. Central venous catheters (Hachem & Raad, 2002) and other devices such as feeding tubes, tracheostomy tubes, Foley catheters.

    G. Long intensive care stays (Velasco et al., 1997).

    H. Loss of skin or mucosal integrity.

 II. Physical examination.

    A. Early signs and symptoms of sepsis.

      1. Typical signs and symptoms of infection may be absent because of decreased WBCs.

      2. General—fever or hypothermia and shaking chills.

      3. Central nervous system—earliest signs include confusion, anxiety, restlessness, decreased level of consciousness.

      4. Pulmonary—cough, rales, rhonchi, wheezes, tachypnea.

      5. Cardiovascular—tachycardia, hypotension, widening pulse pressure.

      6. GI—nausea, vomiting, anorexia, decreased GI motility.

      7. Renal—decreased urine output.

      8. Integument—warm, flushed skin.

    B. Late signs and symptoms of sepsis.

      1. CNS—lethargy and disorientation progressing to obtundation and coma.

   2. Pulmonary—dyspnea, hypoxia, cyanosis, increased pulmonary congestion progressing to acute respiratory distress syndrome and respiratory failure.
   3. Cardiovascular—tachycardia, thready pulse, hypotension, narrowing pulse pressure.
   4. GI—stress ulcers, GI bleed.
   5. Renal—decreased urine output progressing to anuria and acute renal failure.
   6. Integument—cool, pale, clammy skin.
III. Evaluation of laboratory data.
   A. Positive blood cultures.
   B. Pulmonary infiltrates seen on chest x-ray, presence or progression of pulmonary edema.
   C. Increased WBC count in the presence of infection, decreased WBC count with sepsis and related treatment of cancer with many chemotherapy agents.
   D. Increased blood urea nitrogen (BUN) and increased creatinine reflect dehydration; initial increase in glucose with subsequent decrease in glucose in prolonged shock (Petersen, 2000); increase in transaminase and bilirubin with septic shock; increased serum lactate levels.
   E. Prolonged PT and aPTT.
   F. Respiratory alkalosis followed by metabolic acidosis.
   G. Tachycardia and arrhythmias on ECG.

Nursing Diagnoses

   I. Ineffective tissue perfusion (renal, peripheral, cardiopulmonary, GI).
   II. Risk for imbalanced fluid volume.
   III. Deficient fluid volume.
   IV. Decreased cardiac output.
   V. Ineffective breathing pattern.
   VI. Risk for injury.
   VII. Acute pain.
   VIII. Hyperthermia, hypothermia.
   IX. Impaired skin integrity.
   X. Impaired urinary elimination.

Outcome Identification

   I. Client and family describe personal risk factors for septic shock.
   II. Client and family list critical signs and symptoms of septic shock that should be reported to a member of the health care team.
   III. Client and family discuss strategies to decrease the risks of septic shock.

Planning and Implementation

   I. Interventions to maximize safety for the client.
   A. Assess environment for safety—bed in low position and side rails up.
   B. Orient client to time, place, and person.
   C. Maintain infection control measures—hand hygiene, oral care, perineal care, limitation of invasive procedures, and care of invasive equipment.
   D. Institute bleeding precautions as needed.

II. Interventions to decrease the severity of symptoms associated with septic shock.
  A. Identify and report early signs and symptoms of septic shock to primary care provider immediately (Reigle & Dienger, 2003).
  B. Obtain critical elements of diagnostic workup as ordered within a limited time frame.
  C. Initiate fluid resuscitation as ordered.
  D. Initiate antibiotic or antifungal therapy immediately after ordered.
  E. Encourage client to turn, cough, and deep breathe to mobilize pulmonary secretions.
  F. Prepare for possible intubation.
  G. Explain procedures, treatments, monitoring activities, and significance of changes in condition to decrease client and family anxiety.
III. Interventions to monitor for sequelae of septic shock.
  A. Monitor vital signs (pulse, blood pressure, respirations, central venous pressure [CVP], pulmonary artery [PA] pressure) at intervals directed by clinical condition.
  B. Monitor pulse oximetry, and administer oxygen as needed.
  C. Assess skin color, temperature, capillary refill.
  D. Monitor intake and output.
  E. Weigh client daily.
  F. Assess potential sites of infection, and obtain order for cultures of suspicious areas.
  G. Assess peripheral pulses.
  H. Monitor for signs and symptoms of complications of septic shock (e.g., DIC, acute respiratory distress syndrome).
IV. Interventions to monitor response to medical management.
  A. Monitor vital signs every 4 hours or more often as clinically indicated; report significant changes in vital signs (marked increase or decrease in temperature, blood pressure, or pulse pressure; marked increase in pulse or respiratory rate).
  B. Monitor changes in laboratory values, and report significant changes (growth in cultures, increase in WBC count).
  C. Monitor for signs and symptoms of fluid overload (rales, edema, weight gain).
  D. Monitor pulse oximetry and patient's response to oxygen therapy.
  E. Monitor strict intake and output.
V. Interventions to enhance adaptation and rehabilitation.
  A. Maintain bed rest for acutely ill client.
  B. Encourage range of motion and isometric exercises.
  C. Organize care activities to minimize energy expenditure and oxygen consumption.
  D. Reinforce principles of infection prevention and control in preparation for discharge.

Evaluation

The oncology nurse systematically and regularly evaluates the client's and/or family's responses to interventions to determine progress toward the achievement of expected outcomes. Relevant data are collected, and actual findings are compared with expected findings. Nursing diagnoses, outcomes, and plans of care are reviewed and revised as necessary.

TUMOR LYSIS SYNDROME

Theory/Physiology

   I. Definition: tumor lysis syndrome is a potentially life-threatening metabolic imbalance that occurs with the rapid release of intracellular potassium, phosphorus, and nucleic acid into the blood as a result of rapid tumor cell kill (Figure 18-3) (Flombaum, 2000).

  II. The syndrome includes the following:

     A. Hyperkalemia.

     B. Hyperphosphatemia.

     C. Hyperuricemia—results from conversion of nucleic acid to uric acid.

     D. Hypocalcemia—results from increased phosphorus binding to calcium to form calcium phosphate salts.

 III. Potential effects of tumor lysis syndrome include the following:

     A. Cardiac arrhythmias.

     B. Renal failure—kidneys are the primary route of elimination for phosphorus, uric acid, and potassium (Van Der Klooster et al., 2000).

     C. Multisystem organ dysfunction.

 IV. Principles of medical management.

     A. Diagnostic tests (Kaplow, 2002).

        1. Liver function tests—lactate dehydrogenase (LDH).

        2. Renal function studies—BUN, creatinine.

        3. Serum electrolytes (potassium, phosphorus, calcium), uric acid.

           a. Above tests should be monitored baseline before cytotoxic therapy is started.

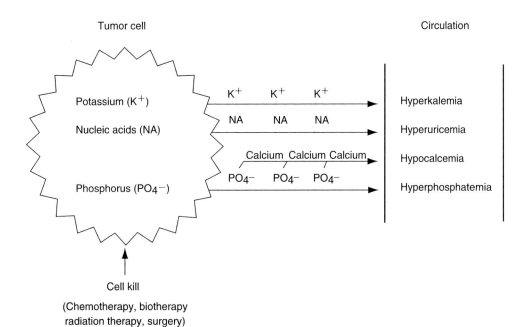

FIGURE 18-3 ■ Metabolic consequences of cell death.

        b. Monitor every 6 to 8 hours daily during first 48 to 72 hours of treatment.

        c. Monitor more often based on client risk.

    4. ECG in clients with identified hyperkalemia.

B. Pharmacologic interventions (Jeha, 2001; Sallan, 2001).

    1. IV hydration.

        a. Ensure adequate hydration of the patient to maintain a urine flow of more than 150 to 200 ml/hr (Feusner & Farber, 2001).

        b. Pretreatment and posttreatment hydration.

        c. Use of normal saline or dextrose 5% in water (D5W) (Gobel, 2002).

    2. Alkalinization of urine.

        a. Sodium bicarbonate to maintain urine pH above 7 and to decrease the solubility of uric acid (Sallan, 2001).

        b. Potential side effects—metabolic alkalosis, hypocalcemia.

    3. Decrease production of uric acid.

        a. Allopurinol (Zyloprim, Aloprim).

            (1) Blocks the enzyme xanthine oxidase to decrease uric acid production and to decrease subsequent deposits of uric acid in the kidney (Heffner & Polman, 1998).

            (2) May be given orally or IV (Aloprim) (Smalley et al., 2000).

            (3) Potential side effects—rash, fever, diarrhea, GI upset, renal failure and insufficiency.

        b. Rasburicase (Elitek).

            (1) Used to treat high uric acid levels in pediatric cases involving tumor lysis syndrome (Goldman et al., 2001).

            (2) Converts circulating uric acid into a by-product excreted by the kidneys.

            (3) Contraindicated in individuals deficient in glucose-6-phosphate dehydrogenase (G6PD).

            (4) Alkalinization of urine is not indicated with rasburicase (Sanofi-Synthelabo Inc., 2002).

            (5) Potential side effects—rash, fever, nausea, vomiting, headaches, abdominal pain, constipation, diarrhea, mucositis, anaphylaxis (Sanofi-Synthelabo Inc., 2002).

    4. Forced diuresis.

        a. Loop diuretics.

            (1) Maintains urinary output if urine flow not achieved by hydration alone (Sallan, 2001).

            (2) Potential side effect—dehydration.

        b. Mannitol may be given if urine flow not achieved with hydration and loop diuretics.

            (1) Potential side effect—dehydration.

    5. Management of hyperphosphatemia, hypocalcemia.

        a. Phosphate-binding aluminum-containing antacids (Robinson, 1998).

            (1) Correction of hyperphosphatemia will usually self-correct the hypocalcemia.

            (2) Binds dietary phosphate from small bowel.

            (3) Potential side effect—constipation.

        b. Hypertonic glucose and insulin if phosphate levels are of great concern.

    6. Management of hyperkalemia.

        a. Exchange resins such as sodium polystyrene sulfonate (Kayexalate) to treat mild hyperkalemia (potassium less than 6.5 mEq/L) (Ezzone, 1999).

(1) Decrease potassium levels.

(2) Potential side effects—hypokalemia, hypomagnesemia, constipation.

b. Severe hyperkalemia (potassium more than 6.5 mEq/L and/or ECG changes) (Gobel, 2002).

(1) Calcium gluconate if ECG changes are apparent.

(2) Hypertonic glucose plus insulin.

(3) Sodium bicarbonate.

(4) Loop diuretics.

C. Nonpharmacologic interventions.

  1. Dialysis—type will depend on patient's condition (Haas et al., 1999).

    a. Hemodialysis (Schelling et al., 1998).

      (1) Preferred method of treatment.

      (2) Rapid ability to correct life-threatening electrolyte abnormalities.

    b. Hemofiltration.

    c. Peritoneal dialysis.

D. Other prevention strategies.

  1. Review of concomitant medications to minimize an increase in the patient's serum potassium and phosphorus (Gobel, 2002).

  2. Avoid medications that are known nephrotoxins.

  3. Avoid exogenous sources of potassium and phosphorus.

    a. Oral supplements of potassium and phosphorus.

    b. Enteral/parenteral nutrition.

    c. Dietary sources of potassium—for example, bananas, oranges, orange juice, tomatoes (Ezzone, 1999).

    d. Dietary sources of phosphorus—for example, meat, eggs, fish, nuts, cheese, bread, poultry, legumes, cereals, carbonated beverages (Ezzone, 1999).

Assessment

I. Identification of clients at risk (Flombaum, 2000; Kalemkerian et al., 1997).

  A. Diagnosis of hematologic tumors with a high growth fraction and large bulky tumors.

    1. Leukemia.

    2. Lymphoma.

    3. Solid tumors.

      a. Small cell lung cancer.

      b. Breast cancer.

      c. Neuroblastoma.

  B. Recent chemotherapy for highly proliferative tumors.

  C. Patients with large tumor burdens combined with lymphadenopathy, splenomegaly, elevated LDH counts.

  D. Recent RT, surgery, or spontaneous induced tumor lysis syndrome (Altman, 2001).

  E. Concurrent renal or cardiac disease.

II. Physical examination.

  A. Manifestations will depend on the degree of abnormality (Reid-Finlay & Kaplow, 2001).

    1. Hyperkalemia—signs and symptoms typically manifested when serum levels exceed 6.5 mEq/L (Altman, 2001; Reid-Finlay & Kaplow, 2001; Sherman, 1999).

        a. ECG changes—for example, bradycardia, ventricular tachycardia, ventricular fibrillation, asystole, cardiac arrest.

        b. Nausea, vomiting, diarrhea.

        c. Muscle weakness, cramps, tingling, twitching, paresthesia, paralysis.

    2. Hyperphosphatemia (Kaplow, 2002).

        a. Edema.

        b. Oliguria.

        c. Anuria.

        d. Renal insufficiency.

        e. Azotemia.

        f. Acute renal failure.

    3. Hypocalcemia.

        a. Hypotension.

        b. ECG changes—for example, ventricular arrhythmias, cardiac arrest.

        c. Muscle cramps.

        d. Twitching.

        e. Paresthesias.

        f. Seizures.

        g. Tetany.

        h. Altered mental status.

    4. Hyperuricemia—signs and symptoms typically manifested when serum uric acid levels exceed 10 mg/dl (Kaplow, 2002).

        a. Oliguria.

        b. Anuria.

        c. Azotemia.

        d. Edema.

        e. Acute uric acid nephropathy.

        f. Flank pain.

        g. Nausea, vomiting, diarrhea.

        h. Hematuria.

        i. Lethargy, somnolence.

        j. Seizure.

Nursing Diagnoses

    I. Ineffective protection.

   II. Risk for injury.

 III. Self-care deficit (e.g., feeding, bathing/hygiene, dressing/grooming, toileting).

 IV. Decreased cardiac output.

    V. Impaired urinary elimination.

 VI. Excess fluid volume.

Outcome Identification

    I. Client and family describe personal risk factors for tumor lysis syndrome.

   II. Client and family participate in strategies to decrease the risk and severity of tumor lysis syndrome.

 III. Client and family describe signs and symptoms of tumor lysis syndrome or side effects to report to the health care team.

 IV. Client and family identify emergency resources in the community.

Planning and Implementation

I. Interventions to maximize safety for the client.
   A. Recognize clients at risk before initiation of treatment (Doane, 2002).
   B. Institute safety measures for changes in level of consciousness.
      1. Place call light within reach.
      2. Evaluate client at regular intervals.
      3. Maintain bed in low position with side rails up.
   C. Institute patient safety measures for patients with seizures as calcium levels warrant (Box 18-1).
   D. Place emergency equipment within access if severe hyperkalemia or hypocalcemia is present.

II. Interventions to decrease incidence and severity of symptoms associated with tumor lysis syndrome.
   A. Teach the client and family about strategies to decrease the incidence of tumor lysis syndrome.
      1. Maintain adequate oral fluid intake.
      2. Review of medications before treatment to minimize exogenous intake of potassium and phosphorus.
      3. Take allopurinol as ordered by physician.
      4. Maintain diet restrictions for potassium and phosphorus as needed and for any preexisting renal dysfunction (Ezzone, 1999).
      5. Teach client and family how to measure intake and output as needed.
      6. Report signs and symptoms of tumor lysis syndrome to the health care team.
   B. Administer allopurinol or rasburicase per order.
   C. Alkalinize urine to maintain urine pH of greater than 7.
      1. Report a urine pH of less than 7.
      2. Alkalinization is not required with the use of rasburicase (Sanofi-Synthelabo Inc., 2002).
   D. Monitor urinary output—may require the use of forced diuresis to force excretion of uric acid.
   E. Consult with dietitian to modify diet if renal dysfunction is present.

III. Interventions to monitor for sequelae of tumor lysis syndrome or treatment.
   A. Assess for symptoms of cardiac arrhythmias (Kaplow, 2002).
      1. Decrease in blood pressure.
      2. Increase in pulse rate.
      3. Irregular pulse, ECG changes.
      4. Chest pain.
      5. Shortness of breath.

BOX 18-1
PATIENT SAFETY MEASURES FOR PATIENTS WITH SEIZURES

- Remain with patient.
- Loosen tight clothing.
- Turn client's head to side.
- Monitor for respiratory distress.
- Alter environment to promote safety.
- Monitor for another seizure before complete recovery from previous seizure.

    B. Assess for symptoms of renal failure.
       1. Decrease in urinary output to less than 600 ml/day.
       2. Changes in mental status.
       3. Nausea, vomiting, anorexia.
       4. Diarrhea.
       5. Increase in weight.
    C. Assess for side effects of treatment.
IV. Interventions to monitor response to medical management.
    A. Maintain strict intake and output. (Urine output should be greater than or equal to 150 to 200 ml/hr.)
    B. Weigh patient daily.
    C. Assess urine pH, color, clarity.
    D. Monitor for further signs of renal impairment: edema, shortness of breath, elevated blood pressure.
    E. Report changes in clinical condition and laboratory values.

Evaluation

The oncology nurse systematically and regularly evaluates the client's and/or family's responses to interventions to determine progress toward the achievement of expected outcomes. Relevant data are collected, and actual findings are compared with expected findings. Nursing diagnoses, outcomes, and plans of care are reviewed and revised as necessary.

HYPERCALCEMIA

Theory

  I. Definition: hypercalcemia is a metabolic disorder that can occur in persons with cancer as a result of increased bone resorption caused either by bone destruction related to tumor invasion or by increased levels of parathyroid hormone, osteoclast-activating factor, or prostaglandin produced by the cancer (Wickham, 2000).
 II. Calcium is essential for forming and maintaining bones and teeth; contractility of muscles (smooth, cardiac, skeletal); transmission of nerve impulses; and maintaining normal clotting mechanisms (Barnett, 1999).
    A. Physiology of serum calcium.
      1. Homeostasis of normal levels of calcium is regulated by a balance of several body processes, including bone remodeling, renal calcium reabsorption, GI absorption, and hormonal influences (Figure 18-4).
        a. The hormonal substances that primarily regulate calcium homeostasis include parathyroid hormone (PTH), 1,25-dihydroxyvitamin D (vitamin D), and calcitonin.
          (1) PTH prevents serum calcium from falling too low by enhancing bone resorption; this process causes an increase in the amount of calcium in the extracellular fluid (Barnett, 1999).
          (2) PTH also increases renal tubular reabsorption of calcium (Struthers et al., 1998).
          (3) PTH indirectly increases vitamin D production, resulting in increased dietary calcium absorption from the GI tract (Schaffer, 1997).
        b. Bone remodeling undergoes constant remodeling activity, yet little transfer of calcium occurs between bone and plasma in a normal state.

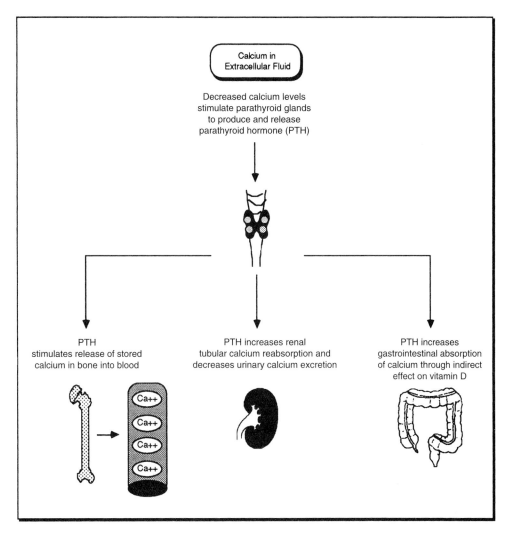

FIGURE 18-4 ■ Regulation of calcium levels.

      c. Extracellular calcium levels are primarily influenced by the ability of the kidneys to reabsorb calcium.

III. Hypercalcemia is defined as a serum calcium level greater than 11 mg/dl.

IV. Hypercalcemia is the most common metabolic complication of malignancy and can be life threatening in some patients (Bayne & Illidge, 2001).

    A. Hypercalcemia occurs in 10% to 20% of patients with cancer (Flombaum, 2000), but in 10% to 40% of patients with cancer it is a late complication of malignancy.

    B. Incidence of hypercalcemia varies widely by tumor type (Heys et al., 1998; National Cancer Institute, 2002).

    C. Greater than 90% of patients who develop hypercalcemia have primary hyperparathyroidism or cancer.

       1. Breast cancer.

       2. Lung cancer.

       3. Head and neck cancer.

       4. Multiple myeloma.

    5. Renal cancer.

    6. Lymphoma.

  D. Other causes of hypercalcemia include drug effects, immobility, congenital problems, and thyroid or renal dysfunction (National Cancer Institute, 2002).

V. The two mechanisms that are the primary causes of hypercalcemia are humoral hypercalcemia of malignancy (HHM) or local osteolytic hypercalcemia (LOH).

  A. HHM is the most common mediator of hypercalcemia.

  B. Patients with HHM (who may or may not have bone metastasis) have tumors that secrete humoral factors (hormones, cytokines) that act locally or systemically to induce excessive calcium resorption from bone with resultant hypercalcemia (Warrell, 1992).

    1. Parathyroid hormone–related protein (PTH-rP) is one of the most common systemic mediators of hypercalcemia in patients with solid tumors (Warrell, 2001).

    2. The release of both PTH and PTH-rP is associated with increased osteoclast bone resorption, decreased bone function, and increased tubular resorption of calcium (National Cancer Institute, 2002).

    3. Tumor-produced mediators of HHM include interleukins, transforming growth factor α– and β–, tumor necrosis factor (TNF), α– and β–interleukin-6, and epidermal growth factor (EGF) (De la Mata et al., 1995; National Cancer Institute, 2002).

      a. These factors can stimulate osteoclastic bone resorption and can potentiate the effects of PTH-rP on osteoclastic activity and calcium homeostasis (National Cancer Institute, 2002).

      b. Renal tubular calcium resorption occurs, which results in renal insufficiency if the patient is also dehydrated; sodium and calcium are conserved to improve extravascular fluid volume (Barnett, 1999; Wickham, 2000).

      c. Vitamin D is another (although uncommon) mediator of cancer-related hypercalcemia seen in human T-cell leukemia virus, related T-cell lymphomas, and Hodgkin's lymphoma (Schweitzer et al., 1994).

  C. Increased bone resorption can also occur secondary to direct tumor invasion (metastatic tumor cells) of the bone.

    1. This process occurs most often late in the disease with extensive osteolytic bone metastasis and is called local osteolytic hypercalcemia (LOH) (Roodman, 1997).

    2. LOH occurs most frequently in relation to breast cancer and multiple myeloma.

    3. Tumor cells release cytokines and other regulatory factors that stimulate the osteoclasts, resulting in hypercalcemia (Guise & Mundy, 1998).

    4. The osteoclasts migrate to the tumor site, which leads to an "uncoupling" of bone formation and bone destruction (Heatly, 2001).

VI. Principles of medical management.

  A. Diagnostic tests.

    1. Serum calcium, potassium, magnesium, sodium, albumin.

    2. Corrected serum calcium levels consider the effect of altered albumin concentration on the calcium level:

$$\text{Corrected serum calcium} = \text{Measured serum calcium} + (0.8 \times [4 - \text{serum albumin concentration}])$$

    3. BUN and creatinine if dehydration is present.

    4. Serum phosphorus and alkaline phosphatase in patients suspected of bony involvement.

    5. Immunoreactive parathyroid hormone (iPTH).
        a. iPTH concentration is increased or rarely normal in hyperparathyroid disease.
        b. iPTH is generally decreased or undetectable in cancer-related hypercalcemia (National Cancer Institute, 2002).
    6. ECG depending on potassium level.
  B. Nonpharmacologic interventions.
    1. Exercise and weight-bearing activity are essential to maintaining bone mass.
    2. Treat symptoms (e.g., pain, nausea and vomiting) to increase the patient's ability to be mobile.
    3. Active or passive range of motion for patients who are bedridden.
  C. Pharmacologic interventions.
    1. Hydration and normal saline diuresis to correct dehydration and to increase renal excretion of calcium.
        a. Mild or asymptomatic hypercalcemia may be managed with oral fluids.
        b. The rate of hydration depends on the severity of dehydration and the cardiovascular status of the client.
        c. Severe hypercalcemia (14 to 16 mg/dl) is considered to be a medical emergency that requires vigorous hydration of up to 4 to 6 L of normal saline per day for up to 48 hours.
        d. The effect of hydration alone is temporary.
    2. Administer antineoplastic therapy (chemotherapy or RT) for primary and metastatic tumors (Esbrit, 2001).
    3. Antiresorptive therapy.
        a. The agent of choice to treat cancer-induced hypercalcemia is a bisphosphonate, because bisphosphonates are the most effective and the least toxic agents to treat hypercalcemia (Body et al., 1998).
           (1) Bisphosphonates bind to mineralized bone matrix and prevent calcium phosphate crystal dissolution (Russell et al., 1999).
           (2) Bisphosphonates have low oral availability and are given IV.
        b. Pamidronate (Aredia) is a common bisphosphonate used to treat hypercalcemia and to maintain normal serum calcium levels after the hypercalcemia is normalized (Russell et al., 1999)
        c. A newer bisphosphonate, zoledronic acid (Zometa), is now available to treat cancer-related hypercalcemia (Berenson, 2001; Saad et al., 2002).
        d. Corticosteroids may be used to treat hypercalcemia associated with steroid-sensitive malignancies, such as lymphoma and multiple myeloma.
        e. Dialysis (peritoneal or hemodialysis) may be instituted to treat severe hypercalcemia in a patient with acute renal insufficiency or congestive heart failure who cannot safely be given a saline load (Flombaum, 2000).

Assessment

  I. Identification of clients at risk for hypercalcemia.
    A. Primary hyperparathyroidism and malignancy account for 90% of all cases of hypercalcemia.
    B. Patients with skeletal metastasis account for 80% of all patients with cancer who develop hypercalcemia (e.g., patients with a diagnosis of breast cancer or lung cancer).

   C. Diagnosis of squamous cell cancer of the lung, head and neck, esophagus
   D. Diagnosis of lymphoma, leukemia, multiple myeloma.
   E. Hormone manipulation with estrogens and antiestrogens for breast cancer (Wickham, 2000).
 II. Identification of contributing factors.
   A. Immobility.
   B. Dehydration.
   C. Older age.
   D. Renal dysfunction.
   E. Total parenteral nutrition.
   F. Vitamin A and D intoxication.
   G. History of lithium and thiazide diuretic therapy, antacids.
III. Physical examination—symptomatology is related to the calcium level and the rapidity of onset (see Table 18-2) (Flombaum, 2000).
   A. Neuromuscular.
     1. CNS.
     2. Peripheral neuromuscular.
   B. GI.
   C. Renal.
   D. Cardiovascular.
   E. Miscellaneous—pruritus, muscle pain.
IV. Evaluation of laboratory data.
   A. Elevated serum calcium levels.
     1. Mild: greater than 11 mg/dl.
     2. Moderate: 12 to 14 mg/dl.
     3. Severe: 14 to 16 mg/dl.
     4. Life threatening: greater than 16 mg/dl.
   B. Decreased potassium (inverse relationship with calcium) and magnesium.
   C. Elevated phosphorus generally in patients with breast cancer and renal dysfunction.
   D. ECG changes (Table 18-2).

Nursing Diagnoses

   I. Deficient fluid volume.
  II. Excess fluid volume.
 III. Acute confusion.
  IV. Risk for injury.
   V. Risk for constipation.
  VI. Impaired urinary elimination.
 VII. Impaired physical mobility.
VIII. Risk for peripheral neurovascular dysfunction.
  IX. Imbalanced nutrition: less than body requirements.
   X. Nausea.
  XI. Acute pain.

Outcome Identification

   I. Client and family identify personal risk factors for the development of hypercalcemia.

TABLE 18-2
Manifestations of Cancer-Related Hypercalcemia

Organ System	Signs and Symptoms of Hypercalcemia
NEUROMUSCULAR	
Central nervous	*Early:* fatigue, apathy, confusion, restlessness, irritability, drowsiness/lethargy, altered personality, altered mental status
	Late: seizure, obtundation, coma
Peripheral neuromuscular	*Early:* muscle weakness, hypotonia
	Late: decreased respiratory muscle, decreased or absent deep tendon reflexes
GASTROINTESTINAL	*Early:* constipation, anorexia, nausea/vomiting
	Late: obstipation, ileus
RENAL	*Early:* polyuria, polydipsia, dehydration, renal calculi
	Late: nephrogenic diabetes insipidus, renal failure
CARDIOVASCULAR	*Early:* bradycardia, bundle branch block, increased sensitivity to digitalis, prolonged PR and QRS intervals
	Late: heart block, widened T waves, ventricular arrhythmias, asystole

Data compiled from Flombaum CD: Metabolic emergencies in the cancer patient, *Semin Oncol* 27:322-334, 2000; National Cancer Institute: Hypercalcemia, 2002. Retrieved March 15, 2003, from the World Wide Web: http://www.cancergov/cancerinfo/pdq/supportivecare/hypercalcemia/HealthProfessional/101k; Warrell RP: Metabolic emergencies. In DeVita VT, Hellman S, Rosenberg SA, editors: *Cancer: principles and practice of oncology,* ed 6, Philadelphia, 2001, Lippincott Williams & Wilkins, pp 2633-2644; Wickham RS: Hypercalcemia. In Yarbro CH, Frogge MH, Goodman H, Groenwald SL, editors: *Cancer nursing: principles and practice,* ed 5, Sudbury, MA, 2000, Jones and Bartlett Publishers, pp 776-791.

II. Client and family describe signs and symptoms of hypercalcemia to report to the health care team (e.g., nausea and vomiting, constipation, fatigue, weakness, changes in mental status or personality).

III. Client and family participate in strategies to decrease the risk or severity of hypercalcemia (e.g., hydration, continued or increased mobility and weight-bearing activity as allowed, altering or stopping medications that may contribute to the hypercalcemia as identified by the health care team).

IV. Client and family understand the importance of adequate pain management to stay physically active.

Planning and Implementation

I. Interventions to maximize safety for the client.
  A. Place call light within reach.
  B. Encourage the client to use assistive personnel or devices with ambulation as needed.
  C. Maintain bed in low position with side rails up for clients with changes in mental status.
  D. Use transfer devices and strategies for immobile clients to decrease risk of pathologic fractures.
  E. Client and family to assess for safety in the home (e.g., remove throw rugs, clutter).
  F. Implement seizure precautions if calcium level greater than 12 mg/dl (Box 18-1).

II. Interventions to decrease the incidence and severity of symptoms associated with hypercalcemia.
   A. Maintain level of mobility consistent with disease status and presenting symptoms.
      1. Full range of activity with assistive personnel or devices.
      2. Active range of motion exercises as appropriate.
      3. Passive range of motion exercises as appropriate.
      4. Weight-bearing activities, such as standing at the bedside as appropriate.
      5. Isometric exercise.
      6. Footboard for bedridden patients.
      7. Monitor skin integrity of bedridden patients.
   B. Encourage oral fluid intake.
   C. Implement measures to control pain (see Chapter 1).
   D. Recommend discontinuance of multivitamin preparations and antacids.
III. Interventions to monitor response to medical management.
   A. Daily weight.
   B. Maintain strict intake and output regimen every 2 hours for first 24 hours, then every 4 to 8 hours as needed.
   C. Maintain urine output within prescribed range (usually 100 to 150 ml/hr with IV fluids and diuretics as ordered).
   D. Observe for neck vein distention.
   E. Observe for edema of sacrum or lower extremities.
   F. Auscultate lungs for breath sounds: rales, shortness of breath.
IV. Interventions to monitor for sequelae of hypercalcemia or treatment.
   A. Monitor for changes in cardiac output related to fluid volume depletion—for example, bradycardia, prolonged PR and shortened QRS intervals, bundle branch block.
   B. Evaluate changes in neurovascular status—reorient client frequently to person, place, time.
   C. Evaluate for changes in nausea, vomiting, constipation—administer antiemetics as ordered, rehydration, bowel regimen.
   D. Evaluate for changes in pain—assess severity, location, effect on activities of daily living; utilize both pharmacologic and nonpharmacologic interventions for bone pain, assess for effectiveness of interventions.

Evaluation

The oncology nurse systematically and regularly evaluates the client's and/or family's responses to interventions to determine progress toward the achievement of expected outcomes. Relevant data are collected, and actual findings are compared with expected findings. Nursing diagnoses, outcomes, and plans of care are reviewed and revised as necessary.

SYNDROME OF INAPPROPRIATE SECRETION OF ANTIDIURETIC HORMONE

Theory

I. Definition: the syndrome of inappropriate secretion of antidiuretic hormone (SIADH) is an endocrine paraneoplastic syndrome resulting from the nonphysiologic release of antidiuretic hormone (ADH) from either the posterior pituitary gland or from an ectopic source leading to impaired renal (free-water) excretion.

II. Physiology of ADH.
   A. ADH (also known as arginine vasopressin [AVP]) is synthesized in the hypothalamus and secreted from the pituitary gland into the bloodstream, based on the response to changes in plasma osmolality or volume (Guyton, 1991).
   B. ADH regulates water reabsorption in the renal tubules based primarily on the following:
      1. Increased plasma osmolality.
      2. Decreased plasma volume.
III. Physiology of SIADH.
   A. SIADH is classified as an endocrine paraneoplastic syndrome primarily caused by abnormal production and secretion of ADH by tumors resulting in the following (Haapoja, 2000):
      1. Dilutional serum hyponatremia.
      2. High urine osmolality (concentrated urine).
      3. Plasma hypoosomolality (excessive water retention in the kidneys).
      4. Elevated urine sodium concentration.
      5. Intracellular edema, which leads to cerebral edema.
   B. SIADH may also result from the ectopic production of atrial natriuretic peptide (ANP) in some patients with small cell lung cancer (SCLC) (Arnold et al., 2001).
      1. ANP arises from cardiac atrial tissue.
   C. SIADH may also result from the ectopic secretion of both ADH and ANP in some patients.
IV. SIADH is a rare emergency in the general oncology population, occurring in only 1% to 2% of patients with cancer (Keenan, 1999).
   A. SCLC accounts for over 75% of all tumors associated with SIADH.
   B. A number of nonmalignant causes of SIADH may also occur in the oncology population (see Assessment).
V. Principles of medical management.
   A. Diagnostic tests.
      1. Serum sodium.
      2. Serum (plasma) osmolality.
      3. Urine osmolality.
      4. Urine specific gravity.
      5. Urine sodium.
      6. Check for euvolemia—normal water body volume.
      7. Electrolytes—uric acid, BUN, creatinine (De Michele & Glick, 2001).
      8. Thyroid, adrenal, cardiac, hepatic, and renal function tests.
      9. Imaging studies (Foster, 2001).
         a. Chest x-ray may identify underlying causes, such as lung cancer or pulmonary disease.
         b. CT of head may identify underlying cause, such as brain tumor, or show evidence of cerebral edema.
   B. Treatments are directed at the underlying cause of SIADH (e.g., cancer treatment or treatment of infectious causes) and correction of hyponatremia.
   C. The severity of the hyponatremia and the presenting symptoms determine treatment of SIADH.
      1. Emergency treatment of SIADH may be required if significant neurologic symptoms are present, which can lead to an irreversible neurodegenerative disorder called central pontine myelinolysis (CPM) (Arnold et al., 2001).
   D. Nonpharmacologic interventions.

1. Fluid restriction (free water) of 500 to 1000 ml/day.
   a. Initial treatment of choice for mild hyponatremia (serum sodium between 125 and 134 mEq/L) (Flombaum, 2000).
   b. Corrects decreased plasma sodium level over 3 to 5 days (Keenan, 1999).
2. The rate of initial correction of hyponatremia should be no faster than 0.5 mEq/L/hr.
   a. Active treatment should stop when the client becomes mildly hyponatremic (serum sodium between 125 and 130 mEq/L).
   b. Correcting the sodium level too rapidly may cause brain damage from brain cell dehydration.
   c. A faster rate of sodium correction may be tolerated in patients experiencing life-threatening neurologic symptoms.
E. Pharmacologic interventions.
   1. Discontinue agents that contribute to SIADH, such as morphine, diuretics, antidepressants, or offending chemotherapy agent.
   2. Oral medications (Table 18-3).
      a. Used for mild to moderate hyponatremia.
      b. Demeclocycline (Declomycin) (600 to 1200 mg/day) in divided doses (Arnold et al., 2001; Foster, 2001).
         (1) Used if fluid restriction cannot be maintained or hyponatremia persists.
         (2) Fluid restriction not required during treatment.
         (3) Inhibits action of ADH on renal tubules, thus stimulating diuresis.
         (4) Onset of action is 3 to 5 days.
      c. Urea (carbamide) (1 to 1.5 g/kg/day as 3% isotonic solution; 0.5 to 1 g/kg/day for refractory SIADH) (Foster, 2001).
      d. Lithium (900 to 1200 mg/day) (Keenan, 1999).

TABLE 18-3
Pharmacologic Agents Used to Treat SIADH

Agent	Action	Nursing Implications
Demeclocycline	Interferes with antidiuretic hormone (ADH) action on tubules	Avoid offering medications with meals. Assess female clients for pregnancy. Assess clients for history of renal or liver disease. Monitor urinary output. Monitor for complaints of nausea or episodes of vomiting. Teach clients to use sunglasses, sunscreen, long-sleeved clothing, and hats and to avoid the sun to decrease risks of photosensitivity. Monitor for symptoms of diabetes insipidus. Monitor for signs and symptoms of infection.
Lithium	Interferes with ADH action	Monitor for complaints of nausea, vomiting, anorexia. Assess neurologic status—presence of tremors or weakness. Assess cardiac status—pulse rate, regularity.
Urea	Causes osmotic diuresis	Monitor for complications of nausea, vomiting, anorexia.

SIADH, Syndrome of inappropriate secretion of antidiuretic hormone.

3. Hypertonic (3% to 5%) saline solution.
   a. Used for severe, symptomatic, acute hyponatremia (serum sodium concentration <110 to 115 mEq/L) (*Merck Manual of Geriatrics,* 2000).
   b. When given as an infusion should increase serum sodium by 6 to 8 mmol/L/day (Foster, 2001).
   c. Furosemide (Lasix) may be given concurrently to increase fluid excretion.
   d. Eliminates threat of serious neurologic consequences.
   e. Hypertonic saline solutions are done only in carefully controlled situations, such as in intensive care settings.
4. Novel pharmacologic agents.
   a. Nonpeptide vasopressin V2 receptor antagonists.
      (1) Selectively blocks effect of ectopic ADH on the collecting duct system.
      (2) Currently in clinical trials (Ishikawa & Toshikazu, 1998).

Assessment

I. Identification of clients at risk (Table 18-4).
   A. Cancer-related causes.

TABLE 18-4
Causes of SIADH

Cancer Related	Non–Cancer-Related
Lung cancer	*Infectious*
Small cell lung cancer*	Pneumonia, tuberculosis, empyema, abscesses
Non–small cell lung cancer	*Antineoplastic agents*
Head and neck cancer	Cyclophosphamide , vincristine, vinblastine, cisplatin,
Breast cancer	ifosfamide, melphalan
Brain cancer	*Medications*
Skin cancer	Morphine/narcotics, general anesthesia, diuretics, NSAIDs,
Prostate cancer	tricyclic antidepressants, SSRIs
Pancreatic cancer	*Central nervous system*
Ovarian cancer	Meningitis/encephalitis, head trauma, intracranial hemorrhage,
GI cancer	positive pressure ventilation, Guillain-Barré syndrome
Genitourinary cancer	*Miscellaneous*
Hematologic cancers	Pain, stress, nausea, surgery (postoperative period),
Hodgkin's disease	idiopathic
Non-Hodgkin's lymphoma	
Acute myelogenous leukemia	
Chronic lymphocytic leukemia	
Sarcoma	

Data compiled from Craig S: Hyponatremia. eMedicine.com, 2001. Retrieved April 1, 2003 from the World Wide Web: http://www.emedicine.com/emerg/topic275.htm; Foster J: Syndrome of inappropriate antidiuretic hormone. eMedicine.com, 2001. Retrieved April 1, 2003 from the World Wide Web: http://www.Emedicine.com/emerg/topic784.htm; Haapoja IS: Paraneoplastic syndromes. In Yarbro CH, Frogge MH, Goodman M, Groenwald SL, editors: *Cancer nursing: principles and practice,* ed 5, Sudbury, MA, 2000, Jones and Bartlett Publishers, pp 792-811; Keenan AM: Syndrome of inappropriate secretion of antidiuretic hormone in malignancy, *Semin Oncol Nurs* 15:160-167, 1999.
SIADH, Syndrome of inappropriate secretion of antidiuretic hormone; *NSAIDs,* nonsteroidal antiinflammatory drugs; *SSRIs,* selective serotonin reuptake inhibitors; *GI,* gastrointestinal.
*Most frequent cause of SIADH.

      1. Primarily associated with SCLC.

      2. Also seen in patients with non–small cell lung cancer (NSCLC) and head and neck cancers (DeMichele & Glick, 2001).

      3. Case reports of SIADH in patients with breast, brain, skin, prostate, ovarian, pancreatic, GI, genitourinary, and hematologic malignancies (Sorensen et al., 1995).

   B. Non–cancer-related causes.

      1. Presence of infection such as pneumonia, tuberculosis, abscesses.

      2. Treatment with medications such as cyclophosphamide (Cytoxan), vincristine (Oncovin), cisplatin (Platinol), thiazide diuretics, morphine, antidepressants, general anesthesia.

      3. CNS disorders, such as CNS infections, head trauma, intracranial hemorrhage.

      4. Miscellaneous—pain, nausea, emotional distress.

II. Physical examination.

   A. Signs and symptoms of SIADH relate to the severity of hyponatremia and its rapidity of development (*Merck Manual of Geriatrics*, 2000).

      1. Rapid-onset hyponatremia (<48 hours) and/or serum sodium of less than 115 mEq/L is associated with the most significant symptomatology (DeMichele & Glick, 2001).

   B. Signs and symptoms of SIADH are directly related to neurologic dysfunction caused by cerebral edema (Flombaum, 2000).

      1. Early signs and symptoms.

         a. Mild hyponatremia may be asymptomatic, or patients may experience nausea, anorexia, malaise, fatigue, weakness, and muscle cramps.

         b. Moderate hyponatremia may be evidenced by thirst, headache, confusion, vomiting, lethargy, weight gain, combativeness, or psychotic behavior.

      2. Late signs and symptoms.

         a. Severe hyponatremia is associated with delirium, obtundation, refractory seizures, coma, and death (*Merck Manual of Geriatrics*, 2000).

III. Evaluation of laboratory data.

   A. Serum sodium less than 130 mEq/L.

      1. Serum sodium concentration in range of 125 to 130 mEq/L is defined as mild hyponatremia.

      2. Serum sodium concentration less than 115 mEq/L is defined as severe hyponatremia (Gross et al., 1998).

   B. Serum osmolality less than 280 mOsm/kg of water to confirm water excess.

   C. Urine osmolality greater than 300 mOsm/L (urine osmolality greater than serum osmolality).

   D. Urine specific gravity greater than 1.015.

   E. Urine sodium greater than 25 mEq/L.

   F. Clinical euvolemia.

      1. Total body water is increased.

      2. Extracellular fluid volume is increased to a minimal or moderate degree, but no edema is present (Craig, 2001).

   G. Decreased levels of BUN, creatinine, uric acid (DeMichele & Glick, 2001).

   H. Normal thyroid, adrenal, cardiac, hepatic, and renal function.

Nursing Diagnoses

  I. Excess fluid volume.

 II. Disturbed thought processes.

III. Risk for injury.
IV. Imbalanced nutrition: less than body requirements.
V. Acute pain.
VI. Acute confusion.
VII. Impaired urinary elimination.
VIII. Impaired mucous membranes.

Outcome Identification

I. Client and family discuss personal risk factors for the development of SIADH.
II. Client participates in measures to decrease the severity of symptoms associated with SIADH.
III. Client and family describe signs and symptoms to report to the health care team—nausea/vomiting, headaches, weight gain greater than 5 pounds in 1 day, decrease in urinary output, mental status changes, any seizure activity.
IV. Client demonstrates self-care skills related to monitoring and treatment of SIADH—for example, weighing self, administering medications, measuring urinary output.
V. Client and family list community resources available for emergency care.

Planning and Implementation

I. Interventions to maximize safety for the client.
   A. Bed in low position with the side rails up.
   B. Bed check device if client is confused.
   C. Call light and personal items within reach.
   D. Use of infusion pump for IV infusions.
   E. Assistance with activities of daily living as needed.
II. Interventions to decrease the severity of symptoms associated with SIADH.
   A. Neurologic changes.
      1. Assess level of consciousness and mental status every 4 hours and as needed.
      2. Orient to person, time, and place as needed.
      3. Use environmental cues, such as calendars and clocks.
      4. Implement seizure precautions as appropriate (see Box 18-1).
   B. Thirst secondary to fluid restriction.
      1. Monitor IV fluid intake.
      2. Rinse mouth with water at least every 2 hours.
      3. Offer sugar-free candy or gum to stimulate salivation.
      4. Assist the client to divide amount of fluids among day, evening, and night hours.
III. Interventions to monitor for sequelae of SIADH or treatment.
   A. Observe for fluid overload, especially with use of hypertonic solutions.
      1. Weigh client daily.
      2. Auscultate lung sounds.
      3. Test urine for specific gravity every 4 to 8 hours.
      4. Maintain strict intake and output records every 4 to 8 hours.
   B. Monitor for electrolyte abnormalities.
      1. Monitor vital signs every 4 hours.
      2. Evaluate for changes in mental status.
      3. Assess for signs and symptoms of hypokalemia.
      4. Assess for signs and symptoms of hyponatremia.

5. Monitor laboratory data (electrolyte values and osmolality of serum and urine) as ordered by the physician.
C. Monitor for side effects of pharmacologic therapy (see Table 18-3).
D. Monitor for rate of correction of serum sodium (Haapoja, 2000).
   1. Rate of sodium correction should be no faster than 0.5 mEq/L/hr.
   2. Discontinue initial therapy when patient becomes mildly hyponatremic (125 to 130 mEq/L).

Evaluation

The oncology nurse systematically and regularly evaluates the client's and/or family's responses to interventions to determine progress toward the achievement of expected outcomes. Relevant data are collected, and actual findings are compared with expected findings. Nursing diagnoses, outcomes, and plans of care are reviewed and revised as necessary.

ANAPHYLAXIS

Theory

I. Definition: anaphylaxis is an immediate, overwhelming, and systemic hypersensitivity reaction that usually occurs within seconds to minutes after the administration of a foreign protein and can be life-threatening. (It is also known as a type I reaction.)
   A. Anaphylaxis is a medical emergency and can result in respiratory failure, cardiovascular collapse, and possibly death.
   B. Anaphylactic reactions are unpredictable.
   C. Certain classes of chemotherapy agents are more commonly associated with hypersensitivity reactions, including the taxanes, platinum compounds, asparaginases, and the epipodophyllotoxins (Camp-Sorrell, 2000; Shanholtz, 2001).
II. Physiology of anaphylaxis.
   A. Immediate hypersensitivity reactions are mediated by immunoglobulin E (IgE), which is produced by B lymphocytes (Figure 18-5).
      1. Factors that influence the development of anaphylaxis (Labovich, 1999).
         a. Route of entry of the antigen.
         b. Amount of antigen introduced.
         c. Rate of antigen absorption.
         d. Client's degree of hypersensitivity to a particular agent.
   B. The antigen-specific IgE (the chemotherapy agent, the chemotherapy agent's metabolite, or the vehicle within which the agent is dissolved) binds to mast cells and sensitizes them to the antigen.
   C. On subsequent exposure of the sensitized mast cell to the antigen, a series of reactions occurs that results in degranulation of the mast cell and release of mediators of the hypersensitivity reaction (Zanotti & Markman, 2001).
      1. Mediators of hypersensitivity reactions include histamine, leukotrienes, eosinophil chemotactic factors of anaphylaxis, neutrophil factors of anaphylaxis, mast cell marker tryptase, and platelet-activating factor (Drain & Volcheck, 2001) (Table 18-5).
      2. These mediators cause systemic effects, including bronchospasm, inflammation, smooth muscle spasm, increased capillary leak, and mucosal edema (Drain & Volcheck, 2001).

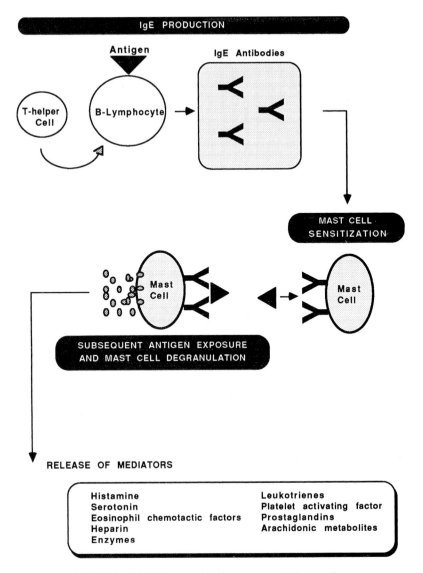

FIGURE 18-5 ■ Immediate hypersensitivity reaction.

III. Signs and symptoms of the immediate hypersensitivity reaction are a result of the effects of the mediators on target organs of the skin, lung, cardiovascular system, and GI tract.
  A. Classic signs and symptoms of anaphylaxis include the following (Freeman, 1998):
    1. Urticaria, pruritus, angioedema.
    2. Dizziness.
    3. Hypotension, tachycardia, shock.
    4. Nausea and vomiting.
    5. Cramping abdominal pain.
    6. Flushing.
    7. Headache.
    8. Chest tightness, substernal chest pain.
    9. Feeling of "impending doom."

TABLE 18-5
Mediators of the Immediate Hypersensitivity Reaction

Mediator	Action
Histamine	Contraction of smooth muscle
	Increased permeability of vessels
	Modulation of chemotaxis and prostaglandins
Serotonin	Contraction of smooth muscle
	Increased permeability of vessels
Eosinophil chemotactic factors	Attraction and deactivation of eosinophils and neutrophils
Heparin	Anticoagulation
Enzymes	Proteolysis, hydrolysis, cleavage
Leukotrienes	Contraction of smooth muscle
	Increased permeability of vessels
	Modulation of histamine, prostaglandins, chemotaxis
Platelet-activating factor	Promotion of platelet aggregation, adhesion
Prostaglandins, arachidonic metabolites	Contraction and relaxation of smooth muscle
	Chemotaxis

IV. Principles of medical management.
  A. Diagnostic tests.
    1. Intradermal skin tests.
      a. Testing done for agents with a high suspicion for hypersensitivity reactions.
      b. Testing done for agents with a prior history of allergy or drug exposure.
      c. Test dose of agents.
        (1) Administer small dose of agent (e.g., one tenth of dose).
        (2) Keep line open if agent given IV.
        (3) Monitor for signs and symptoms of a positive reaction or of anaphylaxis (see Assessment section, II, Physical examination), and stay with patient for at least 15 minutes.
        (4) If no reaction occurs within 1 hour, administer total dose as ordered.
      d. Nonpharmacologic interventions.
    2. Have emergency equipment available for resuscitation (Table 18-6).
    3. Prepare for ABCs of resuscitation as needed.
      a. Airway.
        (1) Maintain open airway.
        (2) Prepare to intubate as needed.
        (3) Prepare for emergency tracheostomy as needed.
      b. Breathing.
        (1) Oxygen as needed.
      c. Circulation.
        (1) Lie head flat.
        (2) Compression as needed.
    4. Hemodynamic monitoring.
  B. Pharmacologic interventions.
    1. IV fluid replacement.
      a. Stop infusion of offending agent at first sign of anaphylaxis.
      b. Administer normal saline rapidly.
      c. Continue crystalloid IV infusion.

TABLE 18-6
Initial Equipment and Pharmacologic Agents Recommended to Manage Hypersensitivity Reactions

Equipment	Pharmacologic Agents
Oxygen, with mask and nasal cannula	Epinephrine 1:1000
Suction machine with catheters	Diphenhydramine
Ambu bag, oral airway	Corticosteroids
	Histamine H_2 antagonists (e.g., famotidine)
IV catheter insertion kits	Dopamine
In acute care areas, add the following:	Atropine
CPR board	
Laryngoscope	
Endotracheal tube	
Defibrillator with ECG leads	
Tracheostomy equipment	Metaproterenol
	Lidocaine
	Calcium gluconate
	Aminophylline
	Sodium bicarbonate
	Crystalloid solution for IV infusion

IV, Intravenous; *ECG,* electrocardiogram.

    2. Prophylactic regimens.
      a. No standard prophylactic regimen exists, particularly since many chemotherapy regimens are now being given weekly or biweekly (Burris, 1998; Trivedic et al., 2000).
      b. Commonly used medications for prophylaxis of anaphylaxis include corticosteroids, H_1 blockers (antihistamines such as diphenhydramine [Benadryl]), H_2 blockers (e.g., famotidine [Pepcid]), and an antipyretic (e.g., acetaminophen).
    3. Medication management (Table 18-6).
      a. Respiratory manifestations (Shanholtz, 2001; Zanotti & Markman, 2001).
        (1) β-Agonist for bronchospasm (e.g., metaproterenol [Alupent]).
        (2) Epinephrine (Adrenalin) for angioedema or laryngeal edema.
        (3) Corticosteroids.
      b. Cardiovascular manifestations (Drain & Volcheck, 2001).
        (1) Crystalloid solution IV for hypotension (e.g., normal saline or lactated Ringer's).
        (2) Diphenhydramine (Benadryl) to antagonize histamines.
        (3) Epinephrine for hypotension.
        (4) Vasopressors for hypotension (e.g., dopamine [Intropin]).
        (5) Antiarrhythmic medications.

Assessment

  I. Identification of clients at risk.
    A. Receiving antineoplastic/biotherapy agents such as L-asparaginase (Elspar), cisplatin (Platinol), paclitaxel (Taxol), or rituximab (Rituxan).
      1. All chemotherapy/biotherapy agents have the potential to cause allergic reactions.

    B. Risk for anaphylaxis increases when agents are as follows:
       1. Given at high doses.
       2. Given IV.
       3. Derived from bacteria such as L-asparaginase.
       4. Crude preparations of the agent, such as those used in phase I studies.
    C. Previous exposure to agent.
    D. Previous allergic reactions to agents such as foods, insulin, opiates, penicillins, bee stings (Grosen et al., 2000) blood products, and radiographic contrast media.
  II. Physical examination.
    A. Early signs and symptoms usually occur within 15 to 30 minutes.
       1. Integumentary—pruritus, urticaria, erythema, angioedema.
       2. Respiratory—dyspnea, wheezing.
       3. Cardiovascular—warmth, flushing, dizziness, hypotension, chest tightness.
       4. GI—nausea, vomiting, diarrhea, abdominal discomfort.
       5. Neurologic—anxiety, dizziness, agitation, feeling of doom.
    B. Late signs and symptoms.
       1. Respiratory—stridor, bronchospasm, laryngeal edema.
       2. Cardiovascular—hypotension, tachycardia, arrhythmias, chest pain.
       3. Neurologic—loss of consciousness.
 III. Evaluation of laboratory data.
    A. Positive or negative test dose.
    B. Arterial blood gases may reflect an altered respiratory or cardiovascular status.

Nursing Diagnoses

    I. Decreased cardiac output.
   II. Deficient fluid volume.
  III. Ineffective breathing pattern.
  IV. Impaired gas exchange.
   V. Fear.
  VI. Anxiety.

Outcome Identification

    I. Client and family identify personal risk factors for anaphylactic reaction.
   II. Client and family describe signs and symptoms of anaphylaxis to the health care team: hives, itching, difficulty breathing, anxiety.
  III. Client participates in strategies to decrease risk of severity of anaphylaxis.
    A. Avoids allergen.
    B. Wears Medic-Alert jewelry.
    C. Informs providers of allergy.
    D. Maintains emergency kit in environment in which potential exposure to an allergen may occur.
  IV. Client and family list the location and telephone numbers of available community emergency resources.

Planning and Implementation

    I. Interventions to maximize safety for the client.
    A. Obtain baseline vital signs.
    B. Document allergy history in medical record.

    C. Remain with the client for 15 to 30 minutes after administering agent.
    D. Maintain a free-flowing IV infusion when administering a potential allergen.
    E. If a reaction occurs, ask the client to stay in the bed and lower the head to a supine position.
    F. Have emergency agents and equipment within reach during administration of high-risk agents.
  II. Interventions to decrease severity of symptoms associated with anaphylaxis.
    A. At first sign of reaction.
      1. Stop the flow of the offending agent.
      2. Maintain IV infusion.
      3. Evaluate patency of airway, and maintain patent airway.
      4. Take vital signs.
      5. Notify primary care provider of signs and symptoms observed and actions taken.
      6. Administer emergency medications (see Table 18-6) as ordered or per institutional protocol.
    B. Position patient in supine position to perfuse vital organs.
    C. Administer cardiopulmonary resuscitation (CPR) as needed.
 III. Interventions to monitor for sequelae of anaphylaxis or treatment.
    A. Observe for symptoms of respiratory distress.
      1. Presence of adventitious breath sounds.
      2. Increase in respiratory rate, rhythm, effort.
      3. Changes in arterial blood gas values.
    B. Observe for signs of fluid overload.
      1. Jugular neck vein distention.
      2. Changes in intake/output ratio.
      3. Changes in weight greater than 5 pounds per day.
    C. Observe for cardiovascular impairment or collapse.
      1. Increase in heart rate.
      2. Cardiac arrhythmias.
      3. Decrease in blood pressure.
    D. Observe for signs of anxiety.
      1. Remain with client during acute reaction.
      2. Explain the process and rationale for each procedure.
      3. Be calm and demonstrate confidence while implementing emergency procedures.

Evaluation

The oncology nurse systematically and regularly evaluates the client's and/or family's responses to interventions to determine progress toward the achievement of expected outcomes. Relevant data are collected, and actual findings are compared with expected findings. Nursing diagnoses, outcomes, and plans of care are reviewed and revised as necessary.

REFERENCES

Disseminated Intravascular Coagulation

Arkel, T.S. (2000). Thrombosis and cancer. *Seminars in Oncology 27*, 362-374.

Bick, R.L. (1996). Disseminated intravascular coagulation: Objective clinical and laboratory diagnosis, treatment, and assessment of therapeutic response. *Seminars in Thrombosis and Hemostasis 22*, 69-88.

Bick, R.L. (1998). Disseminated intravascular coagulation: Pathophysiological mechanisms and manifestations. *Seminars in Thrombosis and Hemostasis 24*, 3-18.

Bick, R.L. (2002). Disseminated intravascular coagulation: A review of etiology, pathophysiology, diagnosis, and management: Guidelines for cancer. *Clinical Application of Thrombosis and Hemostasis 8*(1), 1-31.

DeSancho, M.T., & Rand, J.H. (2001). Bleeding and thrombotic complications in critically ill patients with cancer. *Critical Care Clinics 17*, 599-622.

Gobel, B.H. (1999). Disseminated intravascular coagulation. *Seminars in Oncology Nursing 15*, 174-182.

Gobel, B.H. (2000). Disseminated intravascular coagulation. In C.H. Yarbro, M.H. Frogge, M. Goodman, & S.L. Groenwald (Eds.). *Cancer nursing: Principles and practice* (5th ed.). Sudbury, MA: Jones and Bartlett Publishers, pp. 869-875.

Gobel, B.H. (2002). Disseminated intravascular coagulation in cancer: Providing quality care. *Topics in Advanced Practice Nursing eJournal.* Retrieved October 14, 2002 from the World Wide Web: http://www.medscape.com/viewarticle/442737.

Gobel, B.H. (2003). Disseminated intravascular coagulation. *Clinical Journal of Oncology Nursing 7*, 339-340.

Letsky, E.A. (2001). Disseminated intravascular coagulation. *Best Practice and Research in Obstetrics and Gynaecology 4*, 623-644.

Mammen, E.F. (2000). Disseminated intravascular coagulation (DIC). *Clinical Laboratory Science 13*, 239-245.

Murphy-Ende, K. (1998). Disseminated intravascular coagulation. In C.C. Chernecky & B.J. Berger (Eds.). *Advanced and critical care oncology nursing: Managing primary complications.* Philadelphia: W.B. Saunders, pp. 119-139.

Seto, A.H., & Dunlap, D.S. (1996). Tranexamic acid in oncology. *Annals of Pharmacotherapy 30*, 868-870.

Staudinger, T., Locker, G.J., & Frass, M. (1996). Management of acquired coagulation disorders in emergency and intensive care medicine. *Seminars in Thrombosis and Hemostasis 22*, 93-104.

Wada, H., Sakuragawa, N., Mori, Y., et al. (1999). Hemostatic molecular markers before the onset of disseminated intravascular coagulation. *American Journal of Hematology 60*, 273-278.

Yu, M., Nardella, A., & Pechet, L. (2000). Screening tests of disseminated intravascular coagulation: Guidelines for rapid and specific diagnosis. *Critical Care Medicine 28*, 1777-1780.

Sepsis

Aarons, M.M., & Wheeler, A.P. (1997). Imaging in sepsis. In A.M. Fein, E.M. Abraham, R.A. Balk, et al. (Eds.). *Sepsis and multiorgan failure.* Baltimore: Williams & Wilkins, pp. 327-336.

American College of Chest Physicians (ACCP): American College of Chest Physicians/Society of Critical Care Medicine Consensus Conference. (1992). Definitions for sepsis and organ failure and guidelines for use in innovative therapies in sepsis. *Critical Care Medicine 6*, 867-874.

Bone, R.C., Balk, R.A., Cerra, F.B., et al. (1992). Definition for sepsis and organ failure and guidelines for the use of innovative therapies in sepsis. *Chest 101*, 1644-1655.

Dismukes, W.E. (2000). Introduction to antifungal drugs. *Clinical Infectious Diseases 30*, 653-657.

Ellerhorst-Ryan, J.M. (2000). Infection. In C.H. Yarbro, M.H. Frogge, M. Goodman, & S.L. Groenwald (Eds.). *Cancer nursing: Principles and practice* (5th ed.). Sudbury, MA: Jones and Bartlett Publishers, pp. 691-708.

Hachem, R., & Raad, I. (2002). Prevention and management of long-term catheter related infections in cancer patients. *Cancer Investigation 20*, 1105-1113.

Koscove, E.M. (1998). Sepsis and septic shock. In J.C. Brillman & R.W. Quenzer (Eds.). *Infectious disease in emergency medicine* (2nd ed.). Philadelphia: Lippincott-Raven, pp. 129-152.

Krau, S.D. (1998). Selecting and managing fluid therapy. *Critical Care Nursing Clinics of North America 10*, 401-410.

Marchetti, O., Cometta, A., & Calandra, T. (2001). Fluoroquinolone prophylaxis in granulocytopenic cancer patients: Pro's and con's. 5th International Symposium on Febrile Neutropenia. Retrieved March 2, 2003 from the World Wide Web: http://www.febrileneutropenia.org/abstract/e-caland.htm.

Pelletier, L.L. (2003). Microbiology of the circulatory system. MicroMed, chapter 94. Retrieved March 2, 2003 from the World Wide Web: http://gsbs.utmb.edu/microbook/ch094.htm.

Petersen, J. (2000). Septic shock. In C.H. Yarbro, M.H. Frogge, M. Goodman, & S.L. Groenwald (Eds.). *Cancer nursing: Principles and practice* (5th ed.). Sudbury, MA: Jones and Bartlett Publishers, pp. 876-886.

Rangel-Frausto, M.S., & Wenzel, R.P. (1997). The epidemiology and natural history of sepsis. In A.M. Fein, E.M. Abraham, R.A. Balk, et al. (Eds.). *Sepsis and multiorgan failure*. Baltimore: Williams & Wilkins, pp. 27-34.

Reigle, B.S., & Dienger, M.J. (2003). Sepsis and treatment-induced immunosuppression in the patient with cancer. *Critical Care Nursing Clinics of North America 15*(1), 109-118.

Rex, J.H., Walsh, T.J., Filler, S.G., et al. (2000). Practice guidelines for the treatment of candidiasis. *Clinical Infectious Diseases 30*, 662-678.

Rivers, E., Nguyen, B., Havstad, S., et al. (2001). Early goal-directed therapy in the treatment of severe sepsis and septic shock. *New England Journal of Medicine 345*, 1368-1377.

Sachdeva, K. (2002). Granulocytopenia. eMedicine.com. Retrieved March 3, 2003 from the World Wide Web: http://www.eMedicine.com./MED/topic927.htm.

Safdar, A., & Armstrong, D. (2001). Infectious morbidity in critically ill patients with cancer. *Critical Care Clinics 17*, 531-570.

Segal, B.H., Walsh, T.J., & Holland, S.T. (2001). Infections in the cancer patient. In V.T. DeVita, S. Hellman, S.A. Rosenberg (Eds.). *Cancer: Principles and practice of oncology* (6th ed.). Philadelphia: Williams & Wilkins, pp. 2815-2868.

Shelton, B.K. (1999). Sepsis. *Seminars in Oncology Nursing 15*, 209-221.

Stapczynski, J.S. (2002). Septic shock. eMedicine.com. Retrieved March 1, 2003 from the World Wide Web: http://www.eMedicine.com/EMERG/topic533.htm-101k.

Velasco, E., Thuler, L.C., Martins, C.A., et al. (1997). Nosocomial infections in an oncology intensive care unit. *American Journal of Infection Control 25*, 458-462.

Volker, D. (1998). Fever of unknown origin. *Nurse Practice Forum* 9:170-176.

Tumor Lysis Syndrome

Altman, A. (2001). Acute tumor lysis syndrome. *Seminars in Oncology 28*(Suppl. 5), 3-8.

Doane, L. (2002). Overview of tumor lysis syndrome. *Seminars in Oncology Nursing 18*(Suppl. 3), 2-5.

Ezzone, S.A. (1999). Tumor lysis syndrome. *Seminars in Oncology Nursing 15*, 202-208.

Feusner, J., & Farber, M.S. (2001). Role of intravenous allopurinol in the management of acute tumor lysis syndrome. *Seminars in Oncology 28*(Suppl. 5), 13-18.

Flombaum, C.D. (2000). Metabolic emergencies in the cancer patient. *Seminars in Oncology 27*, 322-334.

Gobel, B.H. (2002). Management of tumor lysis syndrome: Prevention and treatment. *Seminars in Oncology Nursing 18*(Suppl. 3), 12-16.

Gobel, B.H. (2003). Disseminated intravascular coagulation. *Clinical Journal of Oncology Nursing 7*, 339-340.

Gobel, B.H. (2003). Disseminated intravascular coagulation. *Clinical Journal of Oncology Nursing 7*, 339-340.

Goldman, S.C., Holcenberg, J.S., Finklestein, J.Z., et al. (2001). A randomized comparison between rasburicase and allopurinol in children with lymphoma or leukemia at high risk for tumor lysis. *Blood 97*, 2998-3003.

Haas, M., Ohler, L., Watze, H., et al. (1999). The spectrum of acute renal failure in tumour lysis syndrome. *Nephrology, Dialysis, and Transplant 14*, 776 -779.

Heffner, M., & Polman, L.S. (1998). Hyperuricemia. In C.C. Chernecky & B.J. Berger (Eds.). *Advanced and critical care oncology nursing*. Philadelphia: W.B. Saunders, pp. 314-325.

Jeha, S. (2001). Tumor lysis syndrome. *Seminars in Oncology 38*(Suppl. 10), 4-8.

Kalemkerian, G.P., Darwish, B., & Varterasian, M.L. (1997). Tumor lysis syndrome in small cell carcinoma and other solid tumors. *American Journal of Medicine 103*, 363-367.

Kaplow, R. (2002). Pathophysiology, signs, and symptoms of acute tumor lysis syndrome. *Seminars in Oncology Nursing 18*(Suppl. 3), 6-11.

Sanofi-Synthelabo Inc. (2002). Rasburicase (ELITEK). *Prescribing information*. New York: Author.

Reid-Finlay, M., & Kaplow, R. (2001). Leukemia and bone marrow transplantation. In H.M. Schell & K. Puntillo (Eds.). *Critical care nursing secrets.* Philadelphia: Hanley & Belfus, pp. 209-215.

Robinson, J.G. (1998). Tumor lysis syndrome. In C.C. Chernecky & B.J. Berger (Eds.). *Advanced and critical care oncology nursing.* Philadelphia: W.B. Saunders, pp. 637-659.

Sallan, S. (2001). Management of acute tumor lysis syndrome. *Seminars in Oncology 28*(Suppl. 5), 9-12.

Schelling, J.R., Ghandour, F.Z., Strickland, T.J., & Sedor, J.R. (1998). Management of tumor lysis syndrome with standard continuous arteriovenous hemodialysis: Case report and a review of the literature. *Renal Failure 20*, 635-644.

Sherman, M.B. (1999). Renal disorders. In A. Gawlinski & D. Hamwi (Eds.). *Acute care nurse practitioner. Clinical curriculum and certification review.* Philadelphia: W.B. Saunders, pp. 438-475.

Smalley, R.V., Guaspari, A., Haase-Statz, S., et al. (2000). Allopurinol: Intravenous use for prevention and treatment of hyperuricemia in patients with leukemia or lymphoma. *Journal of Clinical Oncology 18*, 1758-1763.

Van Der Klooster, J.M, Van Der Wiel, H.E., Van Saase, J.L., & Grootendorst, A.F. (2000). Asystole during combination chemotherapy for non-Hodgkin's lymphoma: The acute tumor lysis syndrome. *Netherlands Journal of Medicine 56*, 147-152.

Hypercalcemia

Barnett, M.L. (1999). Hypercalcemia. *Seminars in Oncology Nursing 15*, 190-201.

Bayne, M.C., & Illidge, T.M. (2001). Hypercalcemia, parathyroid hormone-related protein and malignancy. *Clinical Oncology 13*, 372-377.

Berenson, J.R. (2001). Hypercalcemia. *Seminars in Hematology 38*(Suppl. 3), 15-20.

Body, J.J., Bartl, R., Burckhardt, P., et al. (1998). Current use of bisphosphonates in oncology. *Journal of Clinical Oncology 16*, 3890-3899.

De la Mata, J., Uy, H.L., Guise, T.A., et al. (1995). Interleukin-6 enhances hypercalcemia and bone resorption mediated by parathyroid hormone-related in vivo. *Journal of Clinical Investigation 95*, 2846-2852.

Esbrit, P. (2001). Hypercalcemia of malignancy—new insights into an old syndrome. *Clinical Laboratory 47*, 67-71.

Flombaum, C.D. (2000). Metabolic emergencies in the cancer patient. *Seminars in Oncology 27*, 322-334.

Guise, T.A., & Mundy, G.R. (1998). Cancer and bone [review]. *Endocrinology Review 19*, 18-54.

Heatly, S. (2001). Metastatic bone disease and tumour-induced hypercalcemia: The role of bisphosphonates. *International Journal of Palliative Nursing 7*, 301-307.

Heys, S.D., Smith, I.C., & Eremin, O. (1998). Hypercalcemia in patients with cancer: Aetiology and treatment. *European Journal of Surgical Oncology 24*, 139-142.

National Cancer Institute. (2002). Hypercalcemia. Retrieved March 15, 2003 from the World Wide Web: http://www.cancergov/cancerinfo/pdq/supportivecare/hypercalcemia/HealthProfessional/101k.

Roodman, G.D. (1997). Mechanisms of bone lesions in multiple myeloma and lymphoma. *Cancer 80*, 1557-1563.

Russell, R.G., Croucher, P.I., & Rogers, M.J. (1999). Bisphosphonates: Pharmacology, mechanisms of action and clinical uses. *Osteoporosis International 9*(Suppl. 2), S66-S80.

Saad, F, Gleason, D.M., Murray, R., et al. (2002). A randomized, placebo-controlled trial of zoledronic acid in patients with hormone-refractory metastatic prostate carcinoma. *Journal of the National Cancer Institute 94*, 1458-1468.

Schweitzer, D.H., Hamdy, N.A.T., Frolich, M., et al. (1994). Malignancy-associated hypercalcemia: Resolution of controversies over vitamin D metabolism by a pathophysiological approach to the syndrome. *Clinical Endocrinology 41*, 251-256.

Struthers, C., Mayer, D., & Fisher, G. (1998). Nursing management of the patient with bone metastasis. *Seminars in Oncology Nursing 14*, 199-209.

Warrell, R.P. (1992). Etiology and current management of cancer-related hypercalcemia. *Oncology 6*, 37-43.

Warrell, R.P. (2001). Metabolic emergencies. In V.T. DeVita, S. Hellman, & S.A. Rosenberg (Eds.). *Cancer: Principles and practice of oncology* (6th ed.). Philadelphia: Lippincott Williams & Wilkins, pp. 2633-2644.

Wickham, R.S. (2000). Hypercalcemia. In C.H. Yarbro, M.H. Frogge, M. Goodman, & S.L. Groenwald (Eds.). *Cancer nursing: Principles and practice* (5th ed.). Sudbury, MA: Jones and Bartlett Publishers, pp. 776-791.

Syndrome of Inappropriate Secretion of Antidiuretic Hormone

Arnold, S.M., Patchell, R., Lowy, A.M., & Foon, K.A. (2001). Paraneoplastic syndromes. In V.T. DeVita, S. Hellman, & S.A. Rosenberg (Eds.).*Cancer: Principles and practice of oncology* (6th ed.). Philadelphia: Lippincott Williams & Wilkins, pp. 2511-2536.

Craig, S. (2001). Hyponatremia. eMedicine.com. Retrieved April 1, 2003 from the World Wide Web: http://www.eMedicine com/emerg/topic275.htm.

DeMichele, A., & Glick, J.H. (2001). Cancer-related emergencies. In R.E. Lenhard, R.T. Osteen, & T. Gansler (Eds.). *The American Cancer Society's clinical oncology.* Atlanta: The American Cancer Society, pp. 733-764.

Flombaum, C.D. (2000). Metabolic emergencies in the cancer patient. *Seminars in Oncology 27,* 322-334.

Foster, J. (2001). Syndrome of inappropriate antidiuretic hormone secretion. eMedicine.com. Retrieved April 1, 2003 from the World Wide Web: http://www.eMedicine.com/emerg/topic784.htm.

Gross, P. Reimann, D., Neidel, J., et al. (1998). The treatment of severe hyponatremia. *Kidney International 53*(Suppl. 64), s6-s11.

Guyton, A.C. (1991). Renal and associated mechanisms for controlling extracellular fluid osmolality and sodium concentration. In A.C. Guyton (Ed.). *Textbook of medical physiology.* Philadelphia: W.B. Saunder, pp. 308-319.

Haapoja, I.S. (2000). Paraneoplastic syndromes. In C.H. Yarbro, M.H. Frogge, M. Goodman, & S.L. Groenwald (Eds.). *Cancer nursing: Principles and practice* (5th ed.). Sudbury, MA: Jones and Bartlett Publishers, pp. 792-811.

Ishikawa, S., & Toshikazu, S. (1998). Therapeutic efficacy of vasopressin receptor antagonists. *Internal Medicine 37,* 217-219.

Keenan, A.M. (1999). Syndrome of inappropriate secretion of antidiuretic hormone in malignancy. *Seminars in Oncology Nursing 15,* 160-167.

Merck manual of geriatrics (3rd ed.). (2000). Whitehouse Station, NJ: Merck Research Laboratories.

Sorenson, J.B., Andersen, M.K., & Hansen, H.H. (1995). Syndrome of inappropriate secretion of antidiuretic hormone (SIADH) in malignant disease. *Journal of Internal Medicine 238,* 97-110.

Anaphylaxis

Burris, H. (1998). Weekly schedules of docetaxel. *Seminars in Oncology 13*(Suppl. 25), 21-23.

Camp-Sorrell, D. (2000). Chemotherapy: Toxicity management. In C.H. Yarbro, M.H. Frogge, M. Goodman, & S.L. Groenwald (Eds.). *Cancer nursing: Principles and practice* (5th ed.). Sudbury, MA: Jones and Bartlett Publishers, pp. 444-486.

Drain, K.L., & Volcheck, G.W. (2001). Preventing and managing drug-induced anaphylaxis. *Drug Safety 24,* 843-853.

Freeman, T.M. (1998). Anaphylaxis: Diagnosis and treatment. *Primary Care: Clinics in Office Practice 25,* 809-817.

Grosen, E., Sittari, E., Larrison, E., et al. (2000). Paclitaxel hypersensitivity reactions related to bee stings allergy (letter). *Lancet, 354,* 288-289.

Labovich, T.M. (1999). Hypersensitivity reactions to chemotherapy. *Seminars in Oncology Nursing 15,* 222-231.

Shanholtz, C. (2001). Acute life-threatening toxicity of cancer treatment. *Critical Care Clinics 17,* 483-502.

Trivedic, C., Redman, B., Flaherty, L.E., et al. (2000). Weekly 1-hour infusion of paclitaxel: Clinical feasibility and efficacy in patients with hormone-refractory prostate carcinoma. *Cancer 89,* 431-436.

Zanotti, K.M., & Markman, M. (2001). Prevention and management of antineoplastic-induced hypersensitivity reactions. *Drug Safety 24,* 767-779.

19 Structural Emergencies

JANE C. HUNTER

INCREASED INTRACRANIAL PRESSURE

Theory

I. Definition: increased intracranial pressure (ICP) can occur when there is an increase in brain tissue, vascular tissue, and/or cerebrospinal fluid (CSF) in the intracranial cavity and can result in nerve cell damage and death.

II. Pathophysiology.
   A. The intracranial cavity is a nonexpandable chamber that contains the following (Myers, 2001):
      1. Brain tissue.
      2. Vascular tissue.
      3. CSF.
   B. An increase in ICP can result when the volume of any of the three components increases (Belford, 2000).
   C. Primary or metastatic tumors within the intracranial cavity can result in increased ICP by the following mechanisms (Belford, 2000):
      1. Displacement of brain tissue.
      2. Edema of brain tissue.
      3. Obstruction of CSF flow.
      4. Increased vascularity associated with tumor growth.

III. Principles of medical management.
   A. Diagnostic tests.
      1. Computed tomography (CT) scan is quick and may be first test.
      2. Magnetic resonance imaging (MRI) is superior imaging modality (Quinn & DeAngelis, 2000). Other MRI techniques can provide additional information.
      3. Cerebral angiography—determines if impression from CT scan or MRI is a vascular abnormality or tumor. Use has decreased if less invasive magnetic resonance angiography (MRA) available.
      4. Myelography—determines if drop metastases are present.
      5. CT-guided or MRI-directed stereotactic biopsy—obtains a tissue diagnosis without open craniotomy. Accurate and simple approach (Levin et al., 2001).
      6. Positron emission tomography (PET)—can distinguish between tumor recurrence and radiation necrosis (Pomper, 2001).
      7. Single photon emission computed tomography (SPECT) is effective in differentiating infiltrating tumor from solid tumor.
   B. Nonpharmacologic interventions.
      1. Surgery.
         a. Emergent surgery is necessary for life-threatening increased ICP. Partial or complete removal of a tumor is necessary if tumor is growing rapidly (Myers, 2001).
            (1) Provides symptomatic relief.

(2) Radiation therapy (RT) or chemotherapy may then be used if tumor is sensitive to these modalities.
   b. Shunt placement—provides an alternate pathway for CSF (Myers, 2001).
2. Hyperventilation is the most rapid method to decrease ICP. Requires patient to be sedated, intubated, and ventilated to a PCO_2 between 25 and 30 mm Hg. This causes vasoconstriction, which decreases cerebral blood volume and ICP. Its short duration requires supplementation by more definitive therapy (Quinn & DeAngelis, 2000).
3. Radiation therapy (RT).
   a. Primary treatment or palliative treatment for metastatic disease, depending on radiosensitivity of tumor. RT should never be started if elevation of ICP is uncontrolled since this can cause acute herniation and death (Quinn & DeAngelis, 2000).
   b. Adjuvant treatment with either surgery or chemotherapy.
   c. Specialized RT approaches for brain metastases.
      (1) Stereotactic external radiation uses a modified linear accelerator, gamma knife unit, or cyclotron to deliver high radiation dose to tumor without significant radiation to surrounding tissues (Ciezki et al., 2000; Wen et al., 2001).
      (2) Brachytherapy (Wen et al., 2001).
C. Pharmacologic interventions.
   1. Chemotherapy.
      a. Most antineoplastic agents do not cross blood-brain barrier; nitrosoureas and procarbazine are exceptions (Wen et al., 2001).
      b. Regional drug delivery, such as intraarterial, intrathecal/intraventricular (via CSF), or intratumor drug administration, circumvents blood-brain barrier.
      c. Some adjuvant chemotherapy regimens are showing effectiveness in the treatment of some metastatic tumors (Wen et al., 2001).
   2. Corticosteroids (Quinn & DeAngelis, 2000; Wen et al., 2001).
      a. Used to decrease inflammation—60% to 80% of clients show decrease in symptoms.
      b. Begins before RT and may be tapered.
      c. May require maintenance doses for residual tumor and dependence may develop from long-term use.
   3. Osmotherapy.
      a. Reduces intracellular water of brain and total water of body.
      b. Mannitol is most often used hyperosmotic agent (Myers, 2001; Quinn & DeAngelis, 2000).
      c. Loop diuretics (Myers, 2001).
   4. Fluid restriction.
   5. Anticonvulsants—when appropriate (Myers, 2001).
      a. Phenytoin (Dilantin)
      b. Carbamazepine (Tegretol).
      c. Phenobarbital.
      d. Valproic acid (Depakote).

Assessment

I. Identification of clients at risk (Myers, 2001).
   A. Clients with cancers of the lung, breast, testes, thyroid, stomach, or kidney or those with melanoma.

    B. Clients with primary tumors of brain or spinal cord.

    C. Clients with a diagnosis of leukemia or neuroblastoma.

    D. Oncology patients with thrombocytopenia or platelet dysfunction may have bleeding that can cause increased ICP.

  II. Physical examination—signs and symptoms depend on volume and location of abnormality.

    A. Early signs and symptoms (Belford, 2000).

      1. Headaches.

        a. Early-morning headache—may be bilateral and located in occipital, temporal, or frontal areas.

        b. Headache may be initiated or aggravated by Valsalva's maneuver, coughing, or bending over.

        c. Pain may be described as dull, sharp, or throbbing. May be described as "uncomfortable feeling in the head."

        d. May increase in severity, frequency, and duration over time.

      2. Neurologic.

        a. Blurred vision.

        b. Diplopia.

        c. Decreased visual fields.

        d. Extremity drifts.

        e. Lethargy, apathy, confusion, restlessness.

        f. Level of consciousness—sensitive index of the patient's neurologic status.

      3. Gastrointestinal (GI).

        a. Loss of appetite.

        b. Nausea.

        c. Occasional vomiting; may be projectile, sudden, and unexpected. Vomiting is not related to food intake.

    B. Late signs and symptoms.

      1. Cardiovascular—bradycardia, widening pulse pressure.

      2. Respiratory—slow, shallow respirations; tachypnea; Cheyne-Stokes respirations.

      3. Neurologic—decreased ability to concentrate; decreased level of consciousness; personality changes; hemiplegia; hemiparesis; seizures; pupillary changes; papilledema (considered cardinal sign of increased ICP).

      4. Abnormal posturing.

      5. Temperature elevations.

      6. Cushing's triad (combination of hypertension, bradycardia, and abnormal respirations) is a very late sign of increased ICP. The patient is usually comatose with this triad.

Nursing Diagnoses

    I. Ineffective tissue perfusion: cerebral.

   II. Disturbed sensory perception.

  III. Disturbed thought processes.

  IV. Ineffective breathing pattern.

   V. Impaired verbal communication.

  VI. Impaired physical mobility.

 VII. Risk for injury.

VIII. Acute pain.

IX. Anxiety.
 X. Deficient knowledge related to signs and symptoms of increased ICP to report for early intervention.

Outcome Identification (Hickman, 1998; Myers, 2001)

I. Client or family identifies signs and symptoms of increased ICP to report to health care team.
II. Client participates in strategies to maximize safety and comfort within the acute care setting and at home.
III. Client participates in decision making regarding treatment and subsequent care needs.
IV. Client describes community resources available for rehabilitation and support.

Planning and Implementation (Belford, 2000; Hickman, 1998; Myers, 2001)

I. Interventions to maximize safety for the client.
 A. Maintain bed rest with increasing ICP and progressive symptoms; elevate head of bed.
 B. Keep bed in lowest position and side rails elevated.
 C. Develop a daily schedule of activities with appropriate rest periods.
 D. Use assistive devices as needed.
II. Interventions to decrease severity of symptoms associated with increased ICP.
 A. Instruct the client to avoid Valsalva's maneuver.
    1. Administer stool softeners as ordered to prevent constipation and straining.
    2. Administer antiemetics as ordered to relieve nausea and vomiting.
 B. Implement measures to control discomfort from headaches.
 C. Instruct client to be passive during turning and repositioning.
 D. Implement measures to decrease stress.
    1. Maintain a calm environment.
    2. Minimize external stimulation—light, noise, touch, temperature extremes.
    3. Encourage calmness during interactions between the client and others.
    4. Teach stress reduction strategies to client and family.
 E. Monitor activities and positioning to minimize increased ICP.
    1. Elevate head of bed 30 degrees to promote venous drainage.
    2. Avoid isometric muscle contractions.
    3. Avoid positions that rotate the head or extend or flex the neck.
    4. Avoid lying in prone position or activities that exert pressure on the abdomen.
III. Interventions to monitor for sequelae of increased ICP.
 A. Monitor blood pressure for widening pulse pressure; pulse for decrease in rate; and respirations for changes in rate, pattern, or effort.
 B. Assess for changes in levels of consciousness with each client contact.
 C. Monitor for sensory or motor changes—changes in visual acuity, pupil reactions, verbal expression; decrease in muscle strength, coordination, movement.
 D. Assess for presence of associated symptoms such as nausea, vomiting, headache.
IV. Interventions to enhance adaptation and rehabilitation.
 A. Assist the client and family to set realistic goals to maintain optimal activity and self-care levels within limitations imposed by disease.

    B. Assist the client and family to assess physical environment in acute care setting and home and make appropriate changes to promote safety.

        1. Encourage having major living area on ground level in the home.

        2. Remove scatter rugs from floors.

        3. Encourage use of rubber-soled, tie shoes and assistive devices as needed.

        4. Orient the client to person, time, and place as needed.

        5. Reinforce safe management and safe environment needs should seizures occur.

    C. Refer to appropriate supportive services.

        1. Physical therapy for activity program and use of assistive devices.

        2. Social services for support, financial evaluation, and community services.

Evaluation

The oncology nurse systematically and regularly evaluates the client's and/or family's responses to interventions to determine progress toward the achievement of expected outcomes. Relevant data are collected, and actual findings are compared with expected findings. Nursing diagnoses, outcomes, and plans of care are reviewed and revised as necessary.

SPINAL CORD COMPRESSION

Theory

    I. Definition: compression of the spinal cord is a neurologic emergency that occurs when primary tumors within the cord or vertebral metastases compress neural tissue and its blood supply, resulting in compromised neurologic function if not treated promptly.

    II. Pathophysiology.

    A. Spinal cord is a cylindric body of nervous tissue that occupies the upper two thirds of the vertebral canal (Flounders, 2003b).

    B. Spinal cord has motor, sensory, and autonomic functions.

    C. Compression of the spinal cord may occur as a result of tumor invasion of the vertebrae and subsequent collapse on the spinal cord; tumor invasion of the spinal canal and resulting increased pressure; or primary tumors of the spinal cord (Fuller et al., 2001).

    D. Compression of the spinal cord can result in minor changes in motor, sensory, and autonomic function to complete paralysis. Spinal cord compression is the second most frequent neurologic complication of metastatic cancer (Myers, 2001).

    III. Principles of medical management.

    A. Emergent treatment required since negative outcomes of deterioration in motor and autonomic function have been associated with delays in initiating treatment (Fuller et al., 2001).

    B. Diagnostic tests (Brigden, 2001; Fuller et al., 2001).

        1. Spinal x-ray examinations—show bone abnormalities or soft tissue masses.

        2. Bone scan—identifies metastases to vertebral bodies.

        3. MRI—diagnostic procedure of choice for evaluating spinal cord compression.

        4. CT scan—exceeds MRI in evaluation of vertebral stability and bone destruction (Fuller et al., 2001).

  5. Myelogram—used with or without CT scan when MRI is nondiagnostic (Flaherty, 2000).
  6. PET—being studied. Its current role not completely defined. PET has been a tool used to evaluate metabolic changes in the cervical spinal cord following mechanical cord compression (Fuller et al., 2001).
  7. Plain x-rays help with identification of the level of deformity and collapse of vertebrae (Manglani et al., 2000).
C. Nonpharmacologic interventions.
  1. RT (Fuller et al., 2001).
      a. Used as most common treatment for epidural metastases and cord compression.
      b. Used alone when no evidence of spinal instability is present and tumor is known to be radiosensitive.
      c. Given over several weeks to a total dose of 3000 to 4000 cGy.
  2. Surgery (Fuller et al., 2001; Myers, 2001).
      a. Used if tumor is not responsive to RT.
      b. Used if recurrent tumor is in an area previously treated with RT (maximal safe RT dose has already been received by spinal cord).
      c. Used to decompress area by laminectomy or resection of a vertebral body. "Immediate surgical decompression should be considered for any patient with neurological progression during radiotherapy" (Fuller et al., 2001, p. 2627).
      d. Initiated soon after corticosteroids.
  3. Surgery followed by RT.
D. Pharmacologic interventions (Fuller et al., 2001).
  1. Corticosteroids.
      a. Reduce spinal cord edema and pain.
      b. May have oncolytic effect on certain tumors.
  2. Chemotherapy.
      a. Used as an adjuvant treatment to radiation and/or surgery for tumors responsive to antineoplastics, such as lymphomas, germ cell tumors, and neuroblastoma.
      b. Used if recurrence of tumor is at a site of previous surgery or RT.
      c. Greater emphasis on use of chemotherapy in children because of greater chemosensitivity of most pediatric cancers; avoids second cancers and spinal deformities in children that can occur after RT (Fuller et al., 2001).
  3. Analgesics—more than 95% of patients with spinal cord compression have pain (see Chapter 10).
      a. Adjunct to opioids helps with neuropathic pain (Flaherty, 2000).
          (1) Anticonvulsants.
          (2) Antidepressants.

Assessment (Flaherty, 2000)

 I. Identification of clients at risk.
  A. Cancers that have a natural history for metastasizing to the bone—breast, lung, prostate, renal, melanoma, myeloma.
  B. Cancers that metastasize to the spinal cord—lymphoma, seminoma, neuroblastoma.
  C. Primary cancers of the spinal cord—ependymoma, astrocytoma, glioma.

   II. Pertinent history.

      A. Type of primary tumor. Identification of histology of tumor can optimize treatment. Responses to treatment and survival following treatment vary among types of cancer.

      B. Time since onset of symptoms, and level and degree of compression.

  III. Physical examination—presenting signs and symptoms vary with the location and severity of the compression. Ask patient to point to site of back pain. Gently percuss this and surrounding areas.

      A. Early signs and symptoms (Fuller et al., 2001).

         1. Neck or back pain always requires prompt evaluation in a client with cancer. Back pain is first symptom in 96% of patients. May be local, radicular, or both.

            a. Local—constant, dull, aching; usually progressive.

            b. Radicular—may be constant or initiated with movement. May be "shooting" in nature. Radiates along the dermatome of the affected nerve root.

            c. Pain usually worse when in supine position.

            d. Pain exacerbated by straining, coughing, or flexion of neck.

         2. Motor weakness or dysfunction. May present as heaviness, stiffness, or weakness of extremities and lead to loss of coordination and ataxia.

         3. Sensory loss for light touch, pain, or temperature.

      B. Late signs and symptoms (Brigden, 2001; Flaherty, 2000; Myers, 2001).

         1. Loss of sensation for deep pressure, vibrations, position.

         2. Incontinence or retention of urine or stool.

         3. Sexual impotence.

         4. Paralysis.

         5. Muscle atrophy.

Nursing Diagnoses

     I. Acute pain.

    II. Impaired physical mobility.

   III. Disturbed sensory perception: tactile.

   IV. Constipation.

    V. Impaired urinary elimination.

   VI. Sexual dysfunction.

  VII. Impaired skin integrity.

 VIII. Disturbed body image.

   IX. Ineffective role performance.

    X. Deficient knowledge related to early signs and symptoms of spinal cord compression and care after spinal cord compression.

   XI. Risk for injury.

  XII. Toileting self-care deficit.

Outcome Identification (Myers, 2001)

   I. Client lists signs and symptoms that should be reported to the health care team.

      A. Changes in bowel or bladder patterns.

      B. Characteristics of pain, sensory and motor function.

      C. Changes in skin integrity.

      D. Changes in sexual function.

II. Client describes strategies to minimize sequelae of spinal cord compression and treatment.
  A. Achieves acceptable pain control.
  B. Maintains optimum level of physical mobility.
  C. Carries out acceptable programs of bowel and urinary elimination.
III. Client and family participate in rehabilitation program designed to promote adaptation to residual limitations associated with spinal cord compression.
IV. Client and family identify community resources available for assistance and support.
  V. Client and family identify complementary or integrative health programs or approaches to care (e.g., pain management, relaxation therapy).

Planning and Implementation (Flaherty, 2000; Forster, 1998; Myers, 2001)

  I. Interventions to maximize safety for the client.
  A. Mobilize the client according to findings of stable or unstable spine (Table 19-1).
  B. Instruct the client and family to assess pressure and temperature of objects coming in contact with the client's areas of compromised feeling or sensation.
 II. Interventions to decrease the severity of symptoms associated with spinal cord compression.
  A. Assist the client to positions of comfort with maintenance of proper body alignment.
  B. Institute nonpharmacologic methods of pain control (see Chapter 1).
  C. Institute a bowel and bladder program (Table 19-2).
III. Interventions to monitor for sequelae of spinal cord compression or treatment.
  A. Monitor for progression of motor or sensory deficits every 8 hours (Table 19-3).
    1. Decrease in muscle strength.
    2. Decrease in coordination.
    3. Decrease in perception of temperature, touch, position.
  B. Monitor bowel and bladder elimination patterns and effectiveness.
    1. Record intake and output every 8 hours.
    2. Palpate for bladder distention if interval between voidings increases.
    3. Record frequency and characteristics of stool with each bowel movement.

TABLE 19-1
Mobility Interventions

Unstable Spine	Stable Spine
Place sandbags on either side of the head to limit movement.	Initiate range of motion exercises after physical therapy evaluation and with a physician order.
Use cervical collar to support cervical spine.	Instruct client/family in isometric exercises.
Support head and neck during all movement.	Provide personal assistance with ambulation.
Use no pillows.	Instruct client/family in use of assistive devices with ambulation.
Maintain alignment when turning or positioning.	Maintain proper alignment while in bed, turning, or positioning.
Use a log roll, pull sheet, or transfer board when turning or positioning.	
Place client on special bed as indicated: Stryker frame or CircOlectric bed.	

TABLE 19-2
Elements of a Bowel and Bladder Program

Bowel Program	Bladder Program
Provide high-fiber diet: fiber, 15-30 g/day.	Include foods in diet to maintain urinary pH of less than 7.
Offer oral fluid intake of 3000 ml/day.	Avoid foods that produce alkaline urine, such as citrus fruits.
Use bedside commode or toilet for all bowel movements.	
Schedule bowel movement at same time each day.	Schedule time for voiding—every 2-3 hr.
Offer a hot drink 30 min before scheduled bowel movement.	Palpate bladder after voiding to evaluate retention.
Use stool softeners, such as mineral oil or dioctyl sodium sulfosuccinate (DSS) (Colace).	Monitor fluid intake.
Monitor for signs and symptoms of fecal impaction.	Decrease fluid intake after 7:00 PM.
	Monitor for signs and symptoms of urinary tract infection.
If Laxatives Are Needed	*If Catheterization Is Needed*
Use stimulant to defecation, such as bisacodyl (Dulcolax), castor oil, senna concentrate (Senokot), or cascara.	Teach client/family intermittent self-catheterization.

TABLE 19-3
Assessment of Motor and Sensory Functions

Function	Assessment Techniques
Muscle strength	Upper extremities: ask client to grip your finger as firmly as possible.
	Lower extremities: ask client to resist plantar flexion of his/her feet.
Coordination of hands and feet	Ask client to touch each finger to his/her thumb in rapid sequence.
	Ask client to turn hand over and back as quickly as possible.
	Ask client to tap your hand as quickly as possible with the ball of each foot.
Sensory perception	Touch client along length of extremities and trunk with the blunt and sharp end of a safety pin, and ask client to identify as either "sharp" or "dull."
	Ask client to report the sensation of touch when touched with a wisp of cotton.
	Move one of the client's fingers, and ask if the finger is being moved up or down.
	Touch skin of client with test tube of hot water and then cold water; ask the client to describe the temperature.

      4. Conduct gentle digital rectal examination to check for impaction if no bowel movement within 3 days.
   C. Assess changes in location, character, and associated aggravating and alleviating factors of pain.
  IV. Interventions to enhance adaptation and rehabilitation.
    A. Inform client and family of changes in the condition of the client.
    B. Initiate a consultation with physical and occupational therapy as soon as the spine has been stabilized.
    C. Assist client to maintain a safe level of independence within the limitations imposed by the cord compression.
    D. Encourage client and family to express concerns about the effect of residual limitations on activities of daily living and lifestyle.
    E. Use PLISSIT (*p*ermission, *l*imited *i*nformation, *s*pecific *s*uggestions, *i*ntensive *t*herapy) model to address changes in sexual function (see Chapter 6).

Evaluation

The oncology nurse systematically and regularly evaluates the client's and/or family's responses to interventions to determine progress toward the achievement of expected outcomes. Relevant data are collected, and actual findings are compared with expected findings. Nursing diagnoses, outcomes, and plans of care are reviewed and revised as necessary.

SUPERIOR VENA CAVA SYNDROME

Theory

I. Definition: superior vena cava syndrome is a result of compromised venous drainage of the head, neck, upper extremities, and thorax through the superior vena cava (SVC) because of compression or obstruction of the vessel by, for example, tumor or thrombus.

II. Pathophysiology.
  A. The SVC is a thin-walled major vessel that carries venous drainage from the head, neck, upper extremities, and upper thorax to the heart (Yahalom, 2001).
  B. The SVC is located in the mediastinum and is surrounded by the rigid structures of the sternum, trachea, and vertebrae, and the aorta, right bronchus, lymph nodes, and pulmonary artery (Yahalom, 2001).
  C. The SVC is a low-pressure vessel that is easily compressed; compression can occur from direct tumor invasion, enlarged lymph nodes, or a thrombus within the vessel (Myers, 2001).
  D. When obstruction of the SVC occurs, venous return to the heart from the head, neck, thorax, and upper extremities is impaired (Myers, 2001; Yahalom, 2001).
    1. Venous pressure increases.
    2. Cardiac output decreases.

III. Principles of medical management.
  A. Goals of treatment include treatment of the underlying cause and of presenting symptoms (Yahalom, 2001).
  B. Treatment and prognosis are determined by the histologic diagnosis of the primary tumor. An attempt to obtain histologic diagnosis should be made so that the primary tumor can get specific treatment (Brigden, 2001; Ciezki et al., 2000).
  C. Diagnostic tests (Sitton, 2000; Yahalom, 2001).
    1. Chest x-ray examination—positive findings associated with superior vena cava syndrome (SVCS) include mass, pleural effusion, and superior mediastinal widening.
    2. CT scan of the thorax (especially with contrast) determines anatomy of mediastinal mass.
    3. MRI is very sensitive for SVCS but may be complicated by inability to tolerate supine position.
    4. Additional tests to determine the histologic diagnosis of the primary condition—bronchoscopy, bone marrow biopsy, mediastinoscopy, thoracentesis, sputum specimen, needle biopsy of palpable lymph nodes (Sitton, 2000).
  D. Nonpharmacologic interventions.
    1. RT—the primary treatment for SVCS if client has non–small cell cancer of the lung. RT may also be used as initial treatment if a histologic diagnosis

cannot be made or the clinical status of the client is deteriorating (Sitton, 2000; Yahalom, 2001).
2. Removal of central venous catheter in catheter-induced SVCS should be combined with anticoagulation to avoid embolization (Yahalom, 2001). Thrombolytic therapy or tissue plasminogen activators may be used to treat a thrombosis that is catheter induced (Flounders, 2003c).
3. Oxygen therapy (Myers, 2001; Yahalom, 2001).
4. Percutaneous transluminal angioplasty using balloon technique (Yahalom, 2001).
5. Insertion of expandable wire stents to open and maintain patency of SVC (Sitton, 2000; Yahalom, 2001).
6. Surgical reconstruction of SVC (Yahalom, 2001).
E. Pharmacologic interventions (Aurora et al., 2000; Myers, 2001).
1. Antineoplastic therapy alone in clients who have had previous maximum mediastinal RT.
2. Antineoplastic therapy in conjunction with RT.
3. Corticosteroids—used at presentation of SVCS.
4. Diuretics—used at presentation of SVCS.
5. Thrombolytic therapy.

Assessment

I. Identification of clients at risk.
   A. Presence of lymphoma involving the mediastinum, germ cell tumors, cancers of the lung and breast, Kaposi's sarcoma (Aurora et al., 2000; Sitton, 2000).
   B. Presence of central venous catheters and pacemakers (Sitton, 2000).
   C. Previous RT to the mediastinum.
   D. Associated conditions, such as histoplasmosis, benign tumors, and aortic aneurysm.
II. Physical examination. Progression of physical signs can be slow or acute. Slow progression allows collateral blood flow to develop.
   A. Early signs and symptoms of SVCS (Aurora et al., 2000; Flounders, 2003c; Sitton, 2000).
      1. Facial swelling on arising in the morning.
      2. Redness and edema in conjunctivae and around the eyes.
      3. Swelling of the neck, arms, hands. Men may have problems buttoning shirt collars (Stoke's sign).
      4. Neck and thoracic vein distention.
      5. Dyspnea—most common symptom.
      6. Nonproductive cough.
      7. Hoarseness.
      8. Cyanosis of upper torso.
      9. Facial erythema.
      10. Nasal stuffiness, epistaxis.
      11. Visible collateral veins on the chest and/or breast. Women may experience swelling of their breasts.
   B. Late signs and symptoms of SVCS (Sitton, 2000).
      1. Severe headache.
      2. Irritability.
      3. Visual disturbances, blurred vision.
      4. Dizziness, syncope.

      5. Changes in mental status.
      6. Stridor.
      7. Tachycardia.
      8. Congestive heart failure.
      9. Decreased blood pressure.
     10. Horner's syndrome.
     11. Dysphagia.
     12. Hemoptysis.
III. Evaluation of laboratory data—assess available laboratory data against previous and normal values.
    A. Arterial blood gases.
    B. Electrolytes.
    C. Kidney function.
    D. Complete blood count (CBC).
    E. Coagulation studies.

Nursing Diagnoses

  I. Ineffective airway clearance.
 II. Decreased cardiac output.
III. Ineffective tissue perfusion: cardiopulmonary and cerebral.
IV. Anxiety.
 V. Deficient knowledge related to signs and symptoms to report for intervention.
VI. Disturbed body image.

Outcome Identification (Myers, 2001; Sitton, 2000)

  I. Client identifies critical signs and symptoms to report to the health care team.
 II. Client describes plans for continued follow-up care.
III. Client participates in decision making about care, discharge planning, life activities.
IV. Client identifies community resources and services for assistance and support.

Planning and Implementation

  I. Interventions to maximize safety for the client.
    A. Provide for environmental safety—bed in low position, side rails up, call light and personal items within reach.
    B. Avoid venipunctures, intravenous (IV) fluid administration, or measurement of blood pressure in the upper extremities.
    C. Take blood pressure in lower extremities.
    D. Assist client with ambulation as needed.
    E. Remove rings and restrictive clothing.
 II. Interventions to decrease severity of symptoms associated with SVCS (Myers, 2001).
    A. Elevate head of bed to decrease dyspnea.
    B. Instruct the client to avoid Valsalva's maneuver or other activities that cause straining.
    C. Apply pressure to sites of invasive procedures in the upper body.
    D. Space care activities to decrease energy expenditure.
    E. Maintain lower extremities in a dependent position.
    F. Explain care procedures in clear, simple terms to decrease anxiety.

    G. Reassure the client that close monitoring will occur.

    H. Encourage client to ask questions about care measures and/or changes in condition.

  III. Interventions to monitor the sequelae of SVCS or treatment (Myers, 2001; Sitton, 2000).

    A. Assess for progressive respiratory distress.

      1. Increased respiratory rate with stridor.

      2. Increased anxiety.

      3. Presence of adventitious breath sounds.

      4. Increased subjective complaints of difficulty breathing.

    B. Monitor for signs of progressive edema.

      1. Increased swelling in face, arms, or neck.

      2. Increased venous distention of neck or thorax.

    C. Monitor for changes in tissue perfusion.

      1. Decreased or absent peripheral pulses.

      2. Decrease in blood pressure—systolic pressure less than 90 mm Hg.

      3. Pale or cyanotic skin of the face, extremities, or nail beds.

    D. Assess for changes in neurologic/mental status.

      1. Decrease in orientation to person, place, time.

      2. Increased confusion.

      3. Presence of lethargy.

      4. Increased dizziness or blurred vision.

      5. Increase in severity of headaches.

    E. Monitor for signs and symptoms of side effects of anticoagulant therapy—petechiae; ecchymoses; bleeding of gums, nose, urinary tract, or GI system.

    F. Monitor for signs and symptoms of steroid therapy—weakness of involuntary muscles, mood swings, steroid-induced glycosuria, dyspepsia, insomnia.

  IV. Interventions to enhance adaptation and rehabilitation from SVCS (Sitton, 2000).

    A. Reassure the client that changes in physical appearance will subside as SVCS resolves.

    B. Assist the client to plan activities that include continued treatment of disease and management of possible side effects of treatment.

    C. Explain changes in status to client and family after each assessment.

Evaluation

The oncology nurse systematically and regularly evaluates the client's and/or family's responses to interventions to determine progress toward the achievement of expected outcomes. Relevant data are collected, and actual findings are compared with expected findings. Nursing diagnoses, outcomes, and plans of care are reviewed and revised as necessary.

CARDIAC TAMPONADE

Theory

  I. Definition: cardiac tamponade can be a life-threatening complication of cancer that occurs because of excess accumulation of fluid in the pericardial sac, resulting in decreased cardiac output and compromised cardiac function.

  II. Pathophysiology.

    A. The pericardium is a two-layered sac surrounding the heart (Miaskowski, 1999; Myers, 2001).

       1. The space between the two layers is the pericardial cavity.

       2. The cavity normally is filled with 50 ml of fluid (Kaplow, 2000). This fluid between opposing layers of the heart allows the heart to move without friction.

  B. An increase in the intrapericardiac pressure may occur because of the following:

       1. Fluid accumulation in the pericardial sac (Myers, 2001).

       2. Direct or metastatic tumor invasion to the pericardial sac (Keefe, 2000).

       3. Fibrosis of the pericardial sac related to RT.

  C. As intrapericardiac pressure increases, the following occur (Kaplow, 2000):

       1. Left ventricular filling decreases.

       2. The ability of the heart to pump decreases.

       3. Cardiac output decreases.

       4. Impaired systemic perfusion occurs.

III. Principles of medical management.

  A. Diagnostic tests.

       1. Chest x-ray examination—enlarged pericardial silhouette. Chest x-ray is not a definitive diagnostic tool (Kaplow, 2000).

       2. CT scan can reveal pleural effusion, masses, or pericardial thickening. The CT scan is limited as a diagnostic tool because of cardiac motion that causes blurring of the pericardial contents (Kaplow, 2000).

       3. Echocardiography (ECHO)—most precise diagnostic test; two echoes are seen with tamponade (Flounders, 2003a; Kaplow, 2000).

       4. Electrocardiography (ECG)—findings are nonspecific. Tachycardia, premature contractions, atrial fibrillation, and electrical alternans are findings on ECG that are consistent with the diagnosis of cardiac tamponade (Kaplow, 2000).

       5. Pericardiocentesis and cytology testing of fluid.

          a. Bloody fluid associated with positive cytology test result.

          b. Cytology testing has a significant false-negative rate.

  B. Nonpharmacologic interventions (Flounders, 2003a).

       1. Pericardiocentesis—temporary removal of excess pericardial fluid.

       2. Pericardial window—surgical opening of the pericardium to allow fluid drainage.

       3. Total pericardectomy—removal of the pericardial sac for clients with constrictive or chronic pericarditis.

       4. RT—radiation to radiosensitive tumors of the pericardium (Miaskowski, 1999). RT is contraindicated in radiation pericarditis and when area involved has previously received radiation (Flounders, 2003a).

  C. Pharmacologic interventions.

       1. Pericardial sclerosis—instillation through a pericardial catheter of chemicals (e.g., doxycycline [Doxy 100], thiotepa (Thioplex), bleomycin (Blenoxane), mitomycin C (Mitomycin), sterile talc) that cause inflammation and subsequent fibrosis (Flounders, 2003a; Kaplow, 2000; Schrump & Nguyen, 2001).

       2. Systemic antineoplastic therapy may be used for chemotherapy-sensitive malignancies, such as lymphoma, breast cancer, or small cell lung cancer (Myers, 2001).

       3. Corticosteroids may be used in cases of mild neoplastic cardiac tamponade (Myers, 2001). These may offer temporary reduction of inflammation of constrictive pericarditis.

Assessment

I. Identification of clients at risk (Kaplow, 2000).

   A. Clients with primary tumors of the heart, including mesothelioma and sarcomas (rare).

   B. Clients with metastatic tumors to the pericardium—lung, breast, GI tract, leukemia, Hodgkin's or non-Hodgkin's lymphoma, sarcoma, melanoma.

   C. Clients who have received more than 4000 cGy of radiation to a field in which the heart is included.

   D. Clients with acquired immunodeficiency syndrome (AIDS)–related Kaposi's sarcoma.

II. Physical examination.

   A. Early signs and symptoms (Flounders, 2003a).

      1. Retrosternal chest pain relieved by leaning forward and intensified when lying supine.

      2. Dyspnea.

      3. Cough.

      4. Muffled heart sounds.

      5. Weak or absent apical pulse.

      6. Anxiety and agitation.

      7. Hiccoughs.

   B. Late signs and symptoms (Flounders, 2003a).

      1. Tachycardia.

      2. Tachypnea.

      3. Decreased systolic pressure and rising diastolic pressure (narrow pulse pressure).

      4. Pulsus paradoxus greater than 10 mm Hg—classic for cardiac tamponade.

      5. Increased central venous pressure (CVP).

      6. Altered levels of consciousness.

      7. Oliguria.

      8. Peripheral edema.

      9. Diaphoresis.

      10. Cyanosis.

      11. Beck's triad forms the classic signs of cardiac tamponade: elevated CVP, hypotension, and distant heart sounds. All three of these signs occur only in advanced cardiac tamponade (Kaplow, 2000).

III. Evaluation of laboratory data—review laboratory data and compare results with previous values and normal parameters.

   A. Arterial blood gas values if client has respiratory distress (Dragonette, 1998).

   B. Electrolyte values.

Nursing Diagnoses

I. Decreased cardiac output.

II. Ineffective breathing pattern.

III. Ineffective tissue perfusion: cardiopulmonary and cerebral.

IV. Acute pain.

V. Anxiety.

VI. Deficient knowledge related to cardiac tamponade and its management.

VII. Fatigue.

Outcome Identification (Myers, 2001)

I. Client identifies signs and symptoms to be reported to the health care team.
II. Client describes the effects of cardiac tamponade or treatment on activities of daily living and lifestyle.
III. Client discusses need and plans for continued follow-up.

Planning and Implementation (Kaplow, 2000; Myers, 2001)

I. Interventions to maximize safety for the client.
   A. Assist the client with activities of daily living and ambulation as needed.
   B. Keep bed in low position and with side rails up.
II. Interventions to decrease severity of symptoms associated with cardiac tamponade.
   A. Elevate head of bed to position of comfort to minimize shortness of breath.
   B. Monitor response to oxygen therapy as ordered by the physician.
   C. Institute nonpharmacologic measures to relieve pain (see Chapter 1).
   D. Plan care activities to minimize energy expenditure and allow for rest periods.
   E. Explain procedures to the client and family to decrease anxiety.
III. Interventions to monitor for sequelae of cardiac tamponade.
   A. Monitor blood pressure, pulse, respirations for narrowing pulse pressure, paradoxical pulse, arrhythmias, and respiratory distress.
   B. Maintain an accurate intake and output record.
   C. Assess level of consciousness for changes in behavior, orientation, awareness.
   D. Monitor subjective complaints of the client about pain and shortness of breath.
   E. Assess character and amount of drainage from pericardial catheter, if present.
   F. Assess catheter site for signs and symptoms of infection.
   G. Evaluate extremities for peripheral edema.
IV. Interventions to enhance adaptation and rehabilitation.
   A. Encourage the client and family to communicate concerns about condition and treatment to a member of the health care team.
   B. Include the client and family in planning and implementation of care if health status permits and participation is not stressful to client and family.

Evaluation

The oncology nurse systematically and regularly evaluates the client's and/or family's responses to interventions to determine progress toward the achievement of expected outcomes. Relevant data are collected, and actual findings are compared with expected findings. Nursing diagnoses, outcomes, and plans of care are reviewed and revised as necessary.

REFERENCES

Aurora, R., Milite, F., & Vander Els, N.J. (2000). Respiratory emergencies. *Seminars in Oncology* 27(3), 256-269.

Belford, K. (2000). Central nervous system cancers. In C.H. Yarbro, M. Goodman, M.H. Frogge, & S.L. Groenwald (Eds.). *Cancer nursing: Principles and practices* (5th ed.). Sudbury, MA: Jones and Bartlett Publishers, pp. 1048-1096.

Brigden, M.L. (2001). Hematologic and oncologic emergencies: Doing the most good in the least time. *Postgraduate Medicine 109*(3), 143-158.

Ciezki, J.P., Komurcu, S., & Macklis, R.M. (2000). Palliative radiotherapy. *Seminars in Oncology 27*(1), 90-93.

Dragonette, P. (1998). Malignant pericardial effusion and cardiac tamponade. In C.C. Chernecky & B.J. Berger (Eds.). *Advanced and critical care oncology nursing: Managing primary complications.* Philadelphia: W.B. Saunders, pp. 425-443.

Flaherty, A.M. (2000). Spinal cord compression. In C.H. Yarbro, M. Goodman, M.H. Frogge, & S.L. Groenwald (Eds.). *Cancer nursing: Principles and practice* (5th ed.). Sudbury, MA: Jones and Bartlett Publishers, pp. 887-899.

Flounders, J.A. (2003a). Cardiovascular emergencies: Pericardial effusion and cardiac tamponade (electronic version). *Oncology Nursing Forum.* Retrieved March 17, 2003 from the World Wide Web: http://ons.org/.

Flounders, J.A. (2003b). Oncology emergency modules: Spinal cord compression (electronic version). *Oncology Nursing Forum.* Retrieved March 17, 2003 from the World Wide Web: http://ons.org.

Flounders, J.A. (2003c). Oncology emergency modules: Superior vena cava syndrome (electronic version). *Oncology Nursing Forum.* Retrieved October 6, 2003 from the World Wide Web: http://ons.org.

Forster, D.A. (1998). Spinal cord compression. In C.C. Chernecky & B.J. Berger (Eds.). *Advanced and critical care oncology: Managing primary complications.* Philadelphia: W.B. Saunders, pp. 566-579.

Fuller, B.G., Heiss, J.D., & Oldfield, E.H. (2001). Oncologic emergencies: Spinal cord compression. In V.T. DeVita, Jr., S. Hellman, & S.A. Rosenberg (Eds.). *Cancer: Principles and practice of oncology* (6th ed.). Philadelphia: Lippincott Williams & Wilkins, pp. 2617-2633.

Hickman, J.L. (1998). Increased intracranial pressure. In C.C. Chernecky & B.J. Berger (Eds.). *Advanced and critical care oncology nursing: Managing primary complications.* Philadelphia: W.B. Saunders, pp. 371-383.

Kaplow, R. (2000). Cardiac tamponade. In C.H. Yarbro, M. Goodman, M.H. Frogge, & S.L. Groenwald (Eds.). *Cancer nursing: Principles and practice* (5th ed.). Sudbury, MA: Jones and Bartlett Publishers, pp. 857-868.

Keefe, D.L. (2000). Cardiovascular emergencies in the cancer patient. *Seminars in Oncology 27*(3), 244-255.

Levin, V.A., Leibel, S.A., & Gutin, P.H. (2001). Neoplasms of the central nervous system. In V.T. DeVita, Jr., S. Hellman, & S.A. Rosenberg (Eds.). *Cancer: Principles and practice of oncology* (6th ed.). Philadelphia: Lippincott Williams & Wilkins, pp. 2100-2160.

Manglani, H.H., Marco, R.A.W., Picciolo, A., & Healey, J.H. (2000). Orthopedic emergencies in cancer patients. *Seminars in Oncology 27*(3), 299-310.

Miaskowski, C. (1999). Oncologic emergencies. In C. Miaskowski & P. Buchsel (Eds.). *Oncology nursing: Assessment and clinical care* (1st ed.). St. Louis: Mosby, pp. 221-243.

Myers, J.S. (2001). Oncologic complications. In S.E. Otto (Ed.). *Oncology nursing* (4th ed.). St. Louis: Mosby, pp. 498-527.

Pomper, M.G. (2001). Functional and metabolic imaging. In V.T. DeVita, Jr., S. Hellman, & S.A. Rosenberg (Eds.). *Cancer: Principles and practice of oncology* (6th ed.). Philadelphia: Lippincott Williams & Wilkins, pp. 679-689.

Quinn, J.A., & DeAngelis, L.M. (2000). Neurologic emergencies in the cancer patient. *Seminars in Oncology 27*(3), 311-321.

Schrump, D.S., & Nguyen, D.M. (2001). Oncologic emergencies: Malignant and pericardial effusions. In V.T. DeVita, Jr., S. Hellman, & S.A. Rosenberg (Eds.). *Cancer: Principles and practice of oncology* (6th ed.). Philadelphia: Lippincott Williams & Wilkins, pp. 2729-2752.

Sitton, E. (2000). Superior vena cava syndrome. In C.H. Yarbro, M. Goodman, M.H. Frogge, & S.L. Groenwald (Eds.). *Cancer nursing: Principles and practice* (5th ed.). Sudbury, MA: Jones and Bartlett Publishers, pp. 900-912.

Wen, P.Y., Black, P.M., & Loeffler, J.S. (2001). Treatment of metastatic cancer. In V.T. DeVita, Jr., S. Hellman, & S.A. Rosenberg (Eds.). *Cancer: Principles and practice of oncology* (6th ed.). Philadelphia: Lippincott Williams & Wilkins, pp. 2655-2670.

Yahalom, J. (2001). Oncologic emergencies: Superior vena cava syndrome. In V.T. DeVita, Jr., S. Hellman, & S.A. Rosenberg (Eds.). *Cancer: Principles and practice of oncology* (6th ed.). Philadelphia: Lippincott Williams & Wilkins, pp. 2609-2616.

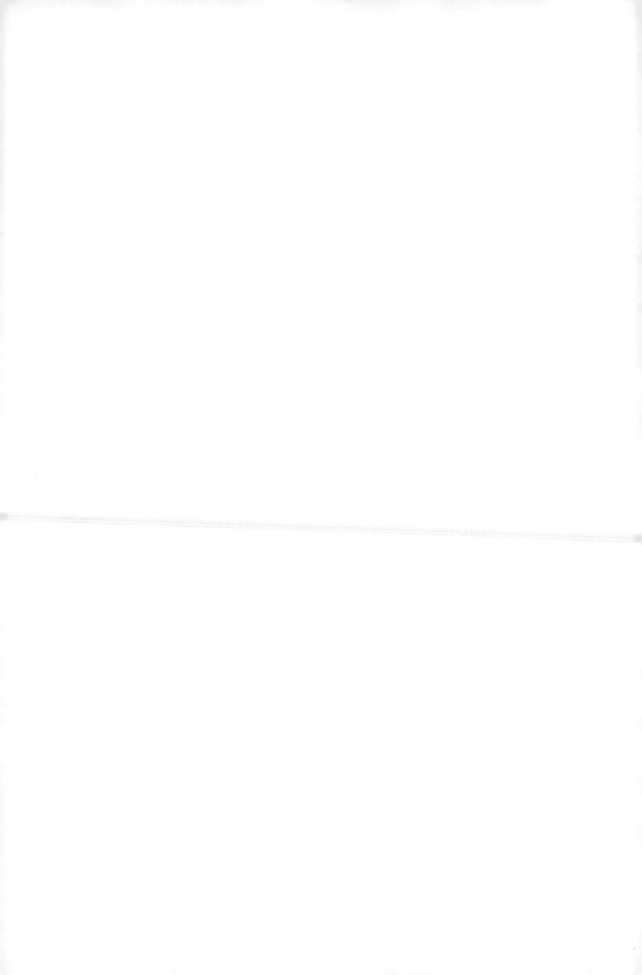

PART SIX

SCIENTIFIC BASIS FOR PRACTICE

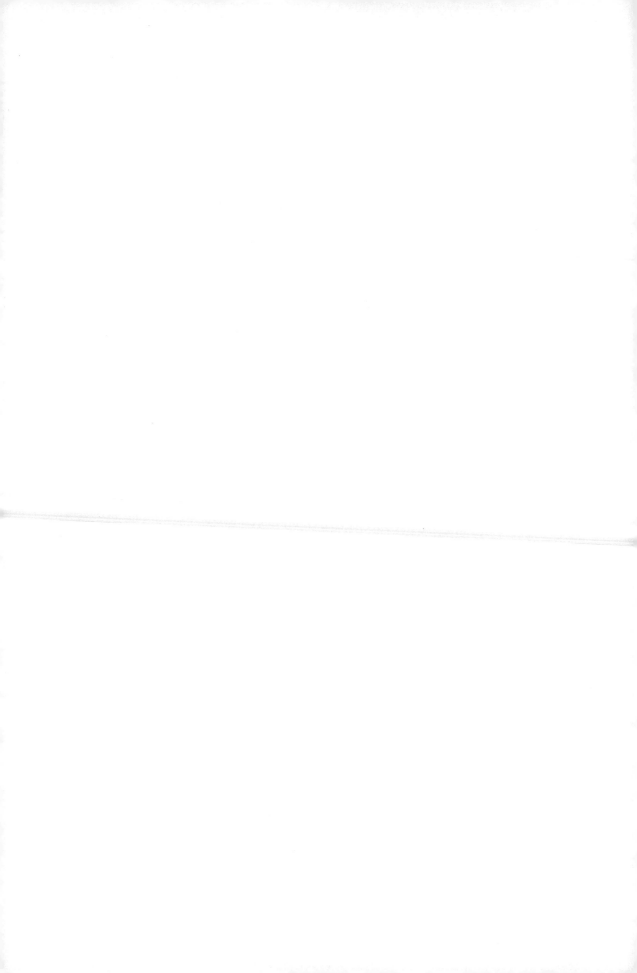

20 Biology of Cancer and Carcinogenesis

DEBORAH L. VOLKER

Theory

I. What is cancer?
   A. Definition—a malignant disease characterized by the following:
   1. A series of cellular, genetic aberrations that cause abnormal cell proliferation.
   2. Unchecked local growth (tumor formation) and invasion of surrounding tissue.
   3. Ability to metastasize (e.g., spread in a noncontiguous fashion to form secondary sites).
   B. Pathology—cancer arises because of multiple sequential alterations in a cell's genes.
   1. Different types of altered genes may interact to ultimately give rise to cancer. The same altered genes may give rise to both inherited and noninherited versions of the same tumor type (Kinzler & Vogelstein, 2002).
      a. Proto-oncogenes—the genetic portion of deoxyribonucleic acid (DNA) that regulates normal cell growth and repair; mutation may allow cells to proliferate beyond normal body needs.
      b. Tumor suppressor genes—the genetic portion of the DNA that stops, inhibits, or suppresses cell division.
         (1) May also act to inhibit formation of cancers (Liotta & Liu, 2001) (Table 20-1).
         (2) Mutation and subsequent loss of tumor suppressor gene function may allow cells to proliferate beyond normal body needs.
         (3) A subtype of tumor suppressor gene, "DNA repair genes," repairs DNA damage caused by carcinogens (Ringer & Schnipper, 2001); mutations in these genes may also give rise to cancer.
         (4) *p53* is the most common mutated tumor suppressor gene currently found in human cancers (Rudin & Thompson, 2002).
            (a) Normally functions to stop cell proliferation and allows DNA damage to be repaired; can slow proliferation of cancer cells.
            (b) When mutated, *p53* restraint on cell proliferation is lost.
            (c) May also interfere with apoptosis, a genetically controlled process of programmed cell death that normally functions to eliminate aging or defective cells.
            (d) Failure of the apoptotic process may lead to malignancy.
            (e) *p53* mutations occur in bladder, breast, colorectal, esophageal, liver, lung, and ovarian carcinomas, and brain tumors, sarcomas, lymphomas and leukemias, and Li-Fraumeni cancer family syndrome.

TABLE 20-1
Selected Tumor Suppressor Genes Involved in Human Neoplasms

Subcellular Location	Gene	Function	Tumors Associated with Somatic Mutations	Tumors Associated with Inherited Mutations
Cell surface	TGF-ß receptor	Growth inhibition	Carcinomas of colon	Unknown
	E-cadherin	Cell adhesion	Carcinomas of stomach, breast	Familial gastric cancer
Under plasma membrane	NF-1	Inhibition of *ras* signal transduction	Schwannomas	Neurofibromatosis, type I; sarcomas
Cytoskeleton	NF-2	Unknown	Schwannomas, meningiomas	Neurofibromatosis, type II; acoustic schwannomas; meningiomas
Cytosol	APC	Inhibition of signal transduction	Carcinomas of stomach, colon, pancreas; melanomas	Familial adenomatous polyposis coli; colon cancers
Nucleus	Rb	Regulation of cell cycle	Retinoblastoma; osteosarcoma; carcinomas of breast, colon, lung	Retinoblastomas, osteosarcomas
	p53	Regulation of cell cycle and apoptosis in response to DNA damage	Most human cancers	Li-Fraumeni syndrome, multiple carcinomas and sarcomas
	WT-1	Nuclear transcription	Wilms' tumor	Wilms' tumor
	p16(INK4a)	Regulation of cell cycle by inhibiting cyclin-dependent kinases	Pancreatitis, esophageal cancers	Malignant melanomas
	BRCA1	DNA repair		Carcinomas of female breast and ovary
	BRCA2	DNA repair		Carcinomas of male and female breast

From Cotran RS, Kumar V, Robbins SL: *Robbins pathologic basis of disease,* ed 6, Philadelphia, 1999, WB Saunders, p. 287.
TGF, Transforming growth factor; *DNA,* deoxyribonucleic acid.

    c. Oncogenes: altered forms of normal proto-oncogenes; may give rise to cancers (Table 20-2).

       (1) Oncogenes can interfere with normal cell growth, differentiation, and apoptosis (Park, 2002).

       (2) Oncogenic mutations may produce abnormal growth factor receptors and other substances that alter the mechanisms of signal transduction. (Signal transduction is the process of transmitting information received on the cell membrane to the cell's nucleus.)

TABLE 20-2
Selected Oncogenes, Their Mode of Activation, and Associated Human Tumors

Category	Proto-oncogene	Mechanisms	Associated Human Tumor
GROWTH FACTORS			
PDGF-ß chain	*sis*	Overexpression	Astrocytoma
			Osteosarcoma
Fibroblast growth	*hst-1*	Overexpression	Stomach cancer
factors	*hst-2*	Amplification	Bladder cancer
			Breast cancer
			Melanoma
GROWTH FACTOR RECEPTORS			
EGF-receptor family	*erb-B1*	Overexpression	Squamous cell carcinomas of lung
	erb-B2	Amplification	Breast, ovarian, lung, stomach cancers
	erb-B3	Overexpression	Breast cancer
CSF-1 receptor	*fms*	Point mutation	Leukemia
	*ret**	Point mutation	Multiple endocrine neoplasia IIA and IIB
			Familial medullary thyroid carcinoma
		Rearrangement	Sporadic papillary carcinomas of thyroid
PROTEINS INVOLVED IN SIGNAL TRANSDUCTION			
GTP binding	*ras*	Point mutations	A variety of human cancers, including lung,
			colon, pancreas; many leukemias
Nonreceptor	*abl*	Translocation	Chronic myeloid leukemia
tyrosine kinase			Acute lymphoblastic leukemia
NUCLEAR REGULATORY PROTEINS			
Transcriptional	*myc*	Translocation	Burkitt's lymphoma
activators			
	N-myc	Amplification	Neuroblastoma
			Small cell carcinoma of lung
	L-myc	Amplification	Small cell carcinoma of lung
CELL CYCLE REGULATORS			
Cyclins	cyclin D	Translocation	Mantle cell lymphoma
		Amplification	Breast, liver, esophageal cancers
	CDK4	Amplification or	Glioblastoma, melanoma, sarcoma
		point mutation	

From Cotran RS, Kumar V, Robbins SL: *Robbins pathologic basis of disease,* ed 6, Philadelphia, 1999, WB Saunders, p. 279.
PDGF, Platelet-derived growth factor; *EGF,* epidermal growth factor; *CSF,* colony-stimulating factor; *GTP,* guanosine triphosphate.
ret proto-oncogene is a receptor for glial cell line–derived neurotrophic factor.

(3) The *ras* oncogenes are a frequently detected oncogene in human cancers.
(a) The *ras* family of proto-oncogenes normally functions to promote cellular growth.
(b) When mutated, *ras* oncogenes may allow cells to proliferate unrestrained.
(c) Overexpression of *ras* oncogenes has been identified in pancreatic, colorectal, lung, and thyroid cancers (Park, 2002).

    2. Clinical implications.
        a. Presence of certain mutated genes may have diagnostic and prognostic value.
        b. Presence of a genetic alteration may be associated with a favorable or poor prognosis. For example, mutant *p53* indicates a poor prognosis in breast cancer and a favorable prognosis in metastatic colon cancer (Pitot, 2002).
        c. Prevention of gene mutation is one focus of chemoprevention clinical trials.
        d. Understanding of genetic changes may result in new targets for treatment.
  C. Carcinogenesis: the process by which cancer arises (Figure 20-1).
    1. Likely involves a series of multiple steps and a number of genetic mutations that cause progressive alteration of normal cells into highly malignant derivatives (Hanahan & Weinberg, 2000).

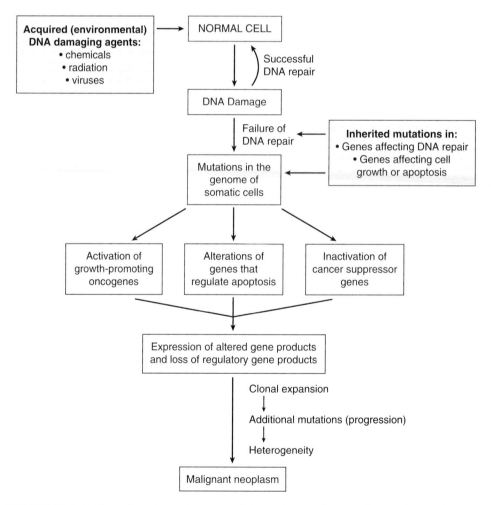

FIGURE 20-1 ■ Flow chart depicting a simplified scheme of the molecular basis of cancer. *DNA,* Deoxyribonucleic acid. (From Cotran RS, Kumar V, Robbins SL: *Robbins pathologic basis of disease,* ed 6, Philadelphia, 1999, WB Saunders, p. 278.)

2. The three-stage theory of causation (carcinogenesis) is a widely used explanation of the process by which a normal cell is transformed into a malignancy.
   a. Initiation—an initiating agent (a carcinogen or cancer-causing agent) may be chemical, physical, or biologic in nature (Pitot, 2002). The carcinogen damages the DNA by changing a specific gene; this gene may then do the following:
      (1) Undergo repair (thus no initiation occurs).
      (2) Become permanently changed (mutated) but not cause cancer unless subsequently exposed to threshold levels of cancer promoters.
      (3) Become mutated and produce a cancer cell line if the initiator is a complete carcinogen (acts as both an initiator and a promoter).
   b. Promotion—process by which carcinogens are subsequently introduced.
      (1) Promoters may alter the genetic structure of the cell or inhibit apoptosis of the cell (Pitot, 2002).
      (2) Results in one of the following changes:
         (a) Reversible damage to the proliferation mechanism of the cell; the effects of promoting factors may be inhibited by the following mechanisms:
            (i) Cancer-reversing or cancer-suppressing agents, such as vitamins (A, C, D, E, folic acid), minerals (calcium, selenium, iron, zinc), carotenoids, flavonoids, organosulfur compounds, isothiocyanates, and indoles, which may modify cancer risk (Milner et al., 2001).
            (ii) Host characteristics, such as immune function, age, hormonal factors.
            (iii) Time or dose limits on the exposure to the promoter.
            (iv) Growth-inhibiting peptides, such as transforming growth factor (Yuspa & Shields, 2001).
         (b) Irreversible damage to the proliferation mechanism, resulting in cancer cell transformation.
      (3) Characteristics of promoting factors.
         (a) Can induce tumors in initiated cells.
         (b) Will not cause tumors when applied *before* the initiating factor.
         (c) Have a threshold level—if a subthreshold dose or widely spaced doses are given, no effect occurs.
         (d) May also be initiators (e.g., cigarette smoke, asbestos, alcohol).
      (4) Time between exposure to initiators and promoters and development of cancer varies; may depend on dosage and length of exposure.
      (5) Clinical implications—understanding of the role of genetic changes in carcinogenesis may lead to new treatments.
   c. Progression—increasing genetic instability (mutations) occurs, which provides tumor cells with a growth advantage (Cahill & Lengauer, 2002).
      (1) Invasion—cells continue to divide; increased bulk, pressure, and secretion of enzymes result in local spread and invasion of surrounding structures (exception: carcinoma in situ—malignancy limited to the epithelium; has not yet invaded the basement membrane).
      (2) Angiogenesis—refers to a tumor's ability to stimulate the proliferation of new blood vessels from the host (Fidler et al., 2001) (Figure 20-2).

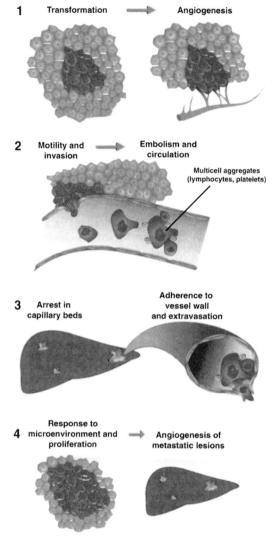

FIGURE 20-2 ▪ Angiogenesis is an essential process in primary and metastatic tumors. For a tumor mass to grow at a primary site, angiogenesis must occur, thereby allowing the tumor size to increase beyond the limits of oxygen diffusion (1 to 2 mm) *(1)*. Increases in vascular density increase the interactions among tumor cells and capillary channels, thereby increasing the chance of tumor cell embolization *(2)*. After a tumor cell has survived the circulation and invaded the organ of metastasis, angiogenesis is essential for tumor growth *(3, 4)*. (From Ellis LM: Tumor angiogenesis, *Horizons in cancer therapeutics: From bench to bedside* 3[1]:4-22, 2002.)

(a) Tumors larger than 0.5 mm require a vasculature in order to receive nutrients and oxygen.

(b) Permits growth of primary tumor cells and increases risk of metastases.

(c) Modulated by a number of factors, including vascular endothelial growth factor (VEGF), basic fibroblast growth factor, angiopoietins, and numerous other growth factors, genetic changes, and host factors.

(d) Clinical implication—antiangiogenesis factors may be useful in treating solid tumors and preventing metastases. Examples of agents under study include bevacizumab (Avastin), thalidomide (Thalomid), and semaxanib (SU5416).

(3) Metastasis—the spread of cancer cells for a primary tumor to distant sites in the patient's body (Figure 20-3). Additional genetic changes in the tumor cells may be associated with propensity to metastasize (Stetler-Stevenson & Kleiner, 2001).

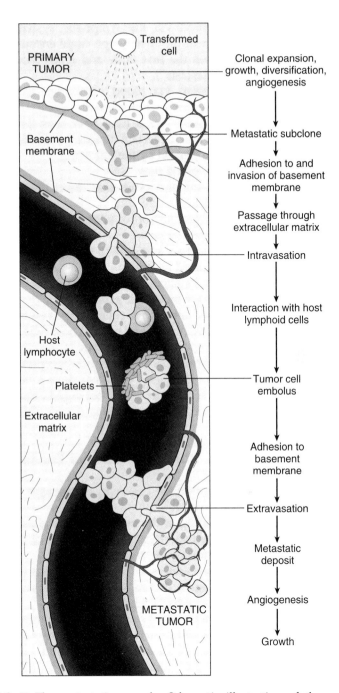

FIGURE 20-3 ■ The metastatic cascade. Schematic illustration of the sequential steps involved in the hematogenous spread of a tumor. (From Cotran RS, Kumar V, Robbins SL: *Robbins pathologic basis of disease,* ed 6, Philadelphia, 1999, WB Saunders, p. 30.)

(a) Routes of metastasis—cells may spread by the following routes:
  (i) Direct invasion into an adjoining organ.
  (ii) Seeding throughout a body cavity, such as the peritoneal cavity.

        (iii) Dissemination via the lymphatic system—entrapment may occur in the first lymph node encountered, or cells may bypass the first node and reach more distant sites ("skip metastasis").

        (iv) Dissemination via blood capillaries and veins; most metastases form by this method.

    (b) Sites: most common—bone, lung, liver, central nervous system (CNS). Predilection for certain tumors to metastasize to specific sites may be influenced by the following:

        (i) Patterns of blood flow.

        (ii) Cell receptors and genes that direct the cell to travel to specific sites.

        (iii) Tumor cell production of adhesion molecules that prefer certain distant organs.

        (iv) Chemical signals and growth factors, which can be found only in selected organs.

        (v) Inhibitor substances produced by organs that are not typically sites for metastatic growth.

        (vi) Collectively, items (ii) to (v) may be a result of "cross talk" between cancer cells and normal host cells. That is, cancer cells may release cytokines that induce the host cells to produce substances that recognize receptors on the cancer cells. Hence the cancer cells may have a "homing device" that attracts them to select host organs and may promote their growth in these distant tissues (Mareel & Leroy, 2003).

    (c) Clinical implications

        (i) Metastasis is the major cause of treatment failure and death.

        (ii) Most tumors have begun to metastasize at the time of detection.

        (iii) Understanding of the metastasis is leading to new therapies targeted specifically to the molecular changes associated with metastatic disease.

  (4) Tumor heterogeneity—refers to differences among individual cells within a tumor; degree of heterogeneity increases as the tumor grows (Stetler-Stevenson & Kleiner, 2001).

    (a) Differences include genetic composition, invasiveness, growth rate, production of hormones, growth factors and stimulators of angiogenesis, metastatic potential, and susceptibility to treatment and host immune response.

    (b) Caused by random mutations during tumor progression.

    (c) Clinical implications—can cause tumors to be highly resistant to any one specific therapy. Provides rationale for using combinations of chemotherapy instead of single-agent therapy.

II. What causes cancer (carcinogenesis)?

  A. Exposure to physical carcinogens (Ulrich, 2001).

    1. Radiation—cellular DNA is damaged by a physical release of energy.

      a. Ionizing radiation. Damage to the cell results in the following:

        (1) Is usually repaired and no mutation results.

        (2) May give rise to a malignancy when damage affects proto-oncogenes or tumor suppressor genes.

(3) Depends on numerous factors.
  (a) Level of tissue oxygenation—well-oxygenated cells are more radiosensitive.
  (b) Genetic composition—certain genetic disorders, particularly those associated with inefficient DNA repair mechanisms, increase risk.
  (c) Cell-cycle phase (Figure 20-4)—G_2 more sensitive than S or G_1.
  (d) Degree of differentiation—immature cells most vulnerable.
  (e) Cell proliferation rate—cells with high mitotic index most vulnerable.
  (f) Age—children and younger adults have greater susceptibility to radiation-induced cancers.
  (g) Tissue type—bone marrow, thyroid, lung, and breast are the most sensitive.
  (h) Total dose and rate of dose—the higher the cumulative dose and dose rate, the greater the likelihood of mutation.
(4) Most exposure is from natural, unavoidable sources; exposure may also come from diagnostic and therapeutic sources.
  (a) Examples of ionizing radiation from natural sources: cosmic rays, radioactive ground minerals, and gases—radon gas, radium, uranium.
  (b) Examples of ionizing radiation from diagnostic or therapeutic sources: diagnostic radiographs, radiation therapy (RT), radioisotopes used in diagnostic imaging.
(5) Cancers linked to exposure to ionizing radiation include skin, lung, thyroid, breast, and acute leukemias and chronic myelogenous leukemia.
b. Ultraviolet radiation (UVR) is a complete carcinogen; responsible for a large proportion of skin cancers.
  (1) Sources of UVR—sunlight, tanning salons, industrial sources (i.e., welding arcs, germicidal lights).
  (2) Risk of carcinogenesis by UVR is increased by the following:

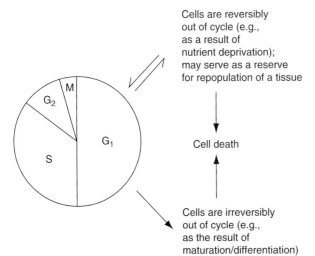

Cells are reversibly out of cycle (e.g., as a result of nutrient deprivation); may serve as a reserve for repopulation of a tissue

Cell death

Cells are irreversibly out of cycle (e.g., as the result of maturation/differentiation)

FIGURE 20-4 ■ Diagrammatic representation of the cell growth cycle, emphasizing the relationships between proliferating and nonproliferating cell populations. *M*, Mitosis; *S*, DNA synthesis phase; G_1, the time or "gap" between mitosis and S phase; G_2, the gap between the end of S phase and mitosis. (From Cooper MR, Cooper MR: Systemic therapy. In Lenhard RE, Osteen RT, Gansler T, editors: *Clinical oncology*, Atlanta, 2001, American Cancer Society, p. 176.)

(a) Prolonged exposure as a result of occupational or recreational activities.

(b) Hereditary diseases characterized by inefficient DNA repair mechanisms (e.g., xeroderma pigmentosum).

(c) Skin pigmentation—the greater the amount of melanin, the greater is the protection against UVR.

(d) Acuity of exposure—risk of melanoma is more associated with history of acute sunburn at an early age as opposed to chronic exposure over time.

(3) Skin cancers most commonly associated with UVR include melanoma, basal cell carcinoma, squamous cell carcinoma.

c. Asbestos—a group of fibers used for mining and industrial applications.

(1) Mechanism—asbestos fibers induce DNA damage and genetic mutation; inflammatory responses secondary to exposure may also enhance growth of mutated cells.

(2) Exposure results in increased risk for malignant mesothelioma; other cancers include bronchogenic, larynx, oropharynx, kidney, esophagus, and gallbladder.

(3) Exposure to asbestos and smoking interact to further increase risk for cancer.

B. Exposure to chemical carcinogens—chemical substances that alter DNA. Examples include tobacco smoke; arsenic; alcoholic beverages; aflatoxin; nickel compounds; crystalline silica; benzopyrene; beryllium; coal and tar pitch; soots; mustard gas; smoked, salted, and pickled foods; vinyl chloride; phenacetin; cadmium; cyclosporine A; benzene; antineoplastic agents; and others (Yuspa & Shields, 2001).

C. Exposure to viruses (Pitot, 2002) (Table 20-3).

1. Viruses infect DNA and ribonucleic acid (RNA); may result in oncogene formation, interference with apoptosis and cell-cycle regulation, and creation of immunosuppression and inflammation.

TABLE 20-3
Viruses That Play a Role in the Etiology of Human Cancers

Virus Types	Specific Viruses	Cancers
DNA	Epstein-Barr herpesvirus (EBV)	Burkitt's tumor, Hodgkin's disease (?), nasopharyngeal cancer
	Human papillomavirus (HPV)	Cervix uteri carcinoma, anal carcinoma
	Hepatitis B virus (HBV)	Hepatocellular carcinoma
RNA	Hepatitis C virus (HCV)	Hepatocellular carcinoma
	Human T-cell leukemia virus type 1 (HTLV-1)	Adult T-cell leukemia
	Human immunodeficiency virus (HIV)	Kaposi's sarcoma, non-Hodgkin's lymphoma, cervix uteri carcinoma, anal carcinoma

From Heath CW, Fontham ET: Cancer etiology. In Lenhard RE, Osteen RT, Gansler T, editors: *Clinical oncology*, Atlanta, 2001, American Cancer Society, p. 45.
DNA, Deoxyribonucleic acid; *RNA*, ribonucleic acid.

2. Effects modified by the following:
  a. Age—the very young and elderly are more susceptible.
  b. Immunocompetence—many viruses are oncogenic only if the host is immunocompromised.
D. Failure of immune surveillance.
  1. Immune surveillance against cancer—theory that proposes recognition and destruction of cancer cells by the immune system.
  2. Surveillance occurs via recognition of surface structures on tumor cells that mark some cancer cells as foreign.
    a. Components of the immune system may eliminate or inhibit the growth of tumors.
    b. Specifically, dendritic cells act as "sentries" and watch for foreign antigens and autoantigens.
      (i) Dendritic cells can quickly induce T-lymphocyte immune responses to cancer cells (Jefford et al., 2001).
    c. This process may eliminate some early-stage, transformed cancer cells but may not adequately activate T lymphocytes to curtail further cancer growth (Pardoll, 2003).
  3. The immune system also may fail to curtail cancers because of development of immune tolerance to cancer cells (Pardoll, 2003).
    a. Advanced tumors that invade and metastasize may develop mechanisms that allow them to spread without inducing an immune response sufficient to stop their activity.
    b. For example, some tumor cells may be able to activate systems that suppress the release of inflammatory "danger signals" that would otherwise activate a lethal immune reaction.
E. Genetic predisposition—predisposition to certain cancers may be inherited from one or both parents.
  1. Inherited cancers occur via carcinogenic mutations in germ cells (reproductive cells of the body).
  2. Cancers that arise because of inherited genetic mutations represent 0.1% to 10% of total cancers in the United States (Kinzler & Vogelstein, 2002).
  3. Examples of cancers linked to inherited genetic mutations include familial adenomatous polyposis (FAP), hereditary nonpolyposis colon cancer (HNPCC), familial breast cancer, von Hippel–Lindau syndrome, hereditary papillary renal cancer (HPRC), familial melanoma, retinoblastoma, neurofibromatosis, Wilms' tumor, Li-Fraumeni syndrome, and multiple endocrine neoplasia (MEN) (Middleton et al., 2002).
III. What are the characteristics of cancer cells?
  A. Microscopic studies show structural changes in cancer cells that are described in pathologic terms such as the following:
    1. Pleomorphism—cells are variable in size and shape.
    2. Hyperchromatism—nuclear chromatin more pronounced on staining.
    3. Polymorphism—nucleus enlarged and variable in shape.
    4. Abnormal chromosome arrangements (Kinzler & Vogelstein, 2002).
      a. Translocations—exchange of material between chromosomes.
      b. Deletions—loss of chromosome segments.
      c. Amplification—an increase in the number of copies of a DNA sequence.
      d. Aneuploidy—abnormal number of chromosomes.
  B. Biochemical studies show differences in cell metabolism and products such as the following:

1. Cell membrane changes (Cotran et al., 1999).
    a. Production of surface enzymes that may aid in invasion and metastasis.
    b. Loss of glycoproteins that normally aid in cell-to-cell adhesion and organization.
    c. Production of abnormal growth factor receptors that may independently "signal" the cell to grow and may cause the cell to be highly sensitive to presence of normal growth factors. Abnormal receptors can activate signal transduction without exposure to a growth factor and may persist in delivering growth signals to the cell (Gribbon & Loescher, 2000).
    d. Loss of antigens that otherwise label the cell as "self," and production of new tumor-associated antigens that mark the cell as "nonself."
        (1) Oncofetal antigens—antigens that are expressed by certain normal cells during fetal development but are subsequently suppressed; may reappear when cell becomes malignant; examples:
            (a) Carcinoembryonic antigen (CEA)—may be elevated in colorectal, breast, lung, liver, pancreatic, gynecologic cancers.
            (b) α-Fetoprotein (α-FP)—may be elevated in hepatocellular, testicular, lung, pancreatic, ovarian cancers.
        (2) Placental antigens—antigens normally produced by the placenta, such as human chorionic gonadotropin (HCG) and human placental lactogen (HPL), which usually are associated with gynecologic cancers.
        (3) Prostate-specific antigen (PSA)—protein produced by prostate gland cells. Elevation in PSA may indicate prostate cancer.
        (4) Differentiation antigens, which are found in normal differentiating tissue; associated with acute lymphocytic leukemia (ALL), chronic lymphocytic leukemia (CLL), and lymphoblastic lymphoma.
        (5) Lineage-associated determination antigens, such as CA 125, which is associated with ovarian cancer.
        (6) Viral antigens—appear in certain cancers associated with viral origins.
    e. Clinical usefulness—certain tumor antigens may be used as tumor markers (Table 20-4), which are biochemical substances synthesized and released by tumor cells.
        (1) May be used as indicators of tumor presence.
        (2) May also be present in a variety of benign conditions; many tumor markers lack specificity to cancer.
        (3) Most often not used for screening but as a tool to monitor response to therapy.
2. Abnormal glycolysis—higher rate of anaerobic glycolysis, making the cell less dependent on oxygen.
3. Abnormal production of substances that give rise to paraneoplastic syndromes (signs or symptoms that occur in a client with cancer but are not due directly to the local effects of the tumor) (Table 20-5).
C. Cell kinetic (growth and division) studies show the following (Ringer & Schnipper, 2001):
    1. Loss of contact inhibition (the normal inhibition of cell movement and division once in contact with other cells).
    2. Defect in cell-to-cell recognition and adhesion—cancer cells do not recognize and adhere to each other as well as normal cells do.

TABLE 20-4
Selected Tumor Markers and Applications to Diagnostic Medicine

Tumor Marker	Commonly Associated Malignant Neoplasms	Nonneoplastic Diseases
HORMONES		
Human chorionic gonadotropin (HCG)	Gestational trophoblastic disease, gonadal germ cell tumors	Pregnancy
Calcitonin	Medullary cancer of thyroid	—
Catecholamines and metabolites	Pheochromocytoma	—
ONCOFETAL ANTIGENS		
α-Fetoprotein	Hepatocellular carcinoma, gonadal germ cell tumors (especially endodermal sinus tumor)	Cirrhosis, toxic liver injury, hepatitis
Carcinoembryonic antigen	Adenocarcinomas of colon, pancreas, stomach, lung, breast, ovary	Pancreatitis, inflammatory bowel disease, hepatitis, cirrhosis, tobacco abuse
ISOENZYMES		
Prostatic acid phosphatase	Adenocarcinoma of prostate	Prostatitis; nodular prostatic hyperplasia
Neuron-specific enolase	Small cell carcinoma of lung; neuroblastoma	—
SPECIFIC PROTEINS		
Prostate-specific antigen	Adenocarcinoma of prostate	Nodular prostatic hyperplasia, prostatitis
Monclonal immunoglobulin	Multiple myeloma	Monoclonal gammopathy of unknown significance
CA 125	Epithelial ovarian neoplasms	Menstruation, pregnancy, peritonitis
CA 19-9	Adenocarcinoma of pancreas or colon	Pancreatitis; ulcerative colitis

From Pfeifer JD, Wick MR: Pathologic evaluation of neoplastic diseases. In Lenhard RE, Osteen RT, Gansler T, editors: *Clinical oncology,* Atlanta, 2001, American Cancer Society, p. 144.

3. Impaired control of proliferation.
   a. Most tumors have changes in signal transduction pathways (the communication "tree" within the cell that mediates cell proliferation, survival, energy utilization, cell death, and many other functions) (Livingston & Shivdasani, 2001). This allows cells to continue to replicate more times than normal cells.
   b. In a normal cell, cross talk (e.g., communication between various signaling pathways) is a normal process that occurs to maintain various cell functions. In cancer cells, cross talk between signal transduction pathways can enhance the disease progression, metastatic potential, and resistance to treatment. Conventio al chemotherapy or RT can contribute to cancer cells' resistance to treatment by creating cell signals that learn to avert normal apoptosis (Ding et al., 2001).

TABLE 20-5
Common Paraneoplastic Syndromes

Type of Syndrome	Proposed Mechanism	Associated Tumor Type
ENDOCRINOLOGIC		
SIADH	Production and release of anti-diuretic hormone by tumor cells	Small cell lung cancer, many others
Cushing's syndrome	Production and release of ACTH by tumor cells	Small cell lung cancer, bronchial carcinoid tumors
Hypercalcemia	Production and release of a polypeptide (possibly a growth factor with partial homology to parathormone) by tumor cells	Squamous cell lung cancer, squamous cell cancer of the head and neck, ovarian cancer
MUSCULOSKELETAL		
Dermatomyositis	Unknown (possibly an autoimmune reaction)	Visceral adenocarcinomas of lung, breast, colon, other sites
Hypertrophic pulmonary osteoarthropathy	Unknown	Lung carcinoma, particularly adenocarcinoma and large cell cancer
DERMATOLOGIC (VARIOUS)	Possibly caused by production of a growth factor (e.g., transforming growth factor–α, insulin-like growth factor, epidermal growth factor) by tumor cells	Gastric carcinoma, melanoma
NEUROLOGIC		
Eaton-Lambert syndrome	Autoimmune production of IgG reactive with motor end plate (possibly with calcium channels)	Small cell cancer
Subacute cerebellar degeneration	Possible autoimmune reaction to cerebellar Purkinje's cells	Small cell cancer, ovarian cancer, lymphoma

From Rosenthal PE: Paraneoplastic and endocrine syndromes. In Lenhard RE, Osteen RT, Gansler T, editors: *Clinical oncology,* Atlanta, 2001, American Cancer Society, p. 722.
SIADH, Syndrome of inappropriate antidiuretic hormone; *ACTH,* adrenocorticotropic hormone; *IgG,* immunoglobulin G.

4. Increased mitotic index (the proportion of cells in a tissue that are in mitosis at any given time).
   a. Large numbers of mitotic cells reflect the higher proliferative activity of the tumor.
   b. A high mitotic index is not unique to cancer; normal cells in the gastrointestinal (GI) system, bone marrow, and hair follicles have a rapid rate of cell turnover and thus a high mitotic index.
5. Abnormal longevity—cancer cells tend to live longer than normal cells and resist the process of apoptosis, a hallmark of cancer (Hanahan & Weinberg, 2000).
   a. May be because of the presence of telomerase, an enzyme that may allow cells to continue to replicate themselves beyond a normal life span (Kelland, 2001).
6. Abnormal cell differentiation.
   a. Differentiation—refers to the extent to which tumor cells resemble comparable normal cells, both morphologically and functionally.

    (1) Grade—an evaluation of the degree of differentiation of the malignant cells.

        (a) Grading criteria vary greatly for different tumors; based on degree to which tumor cells resemble their normal counterpart.

        (b) Often characterized as grade I, II, III, or IV.

            (i) Grade I—well differentiated; also termed low grade.

            (ii) Grade IV—poorly differentiated; also termed high grade.

    (2) Benign tumors composed of well-differentiated cells; tend to resemble the mature, functionally normal cells of the tissue of origin.

    (3) Malignant tumors may be composed of cells that range from well-differentiated to undifferentiated, primitive cells.

    (4) Anaplasia, or lack of differentiation, is a hallmark of malignancy and the result of proliferation of transformed cells that do not mature.

  b. Functional changes.

    (1) The greater the degree of differentiation of a cell, the more likely it will have some of the functional capabilities of its normal counterpart.

    (2) The more anaplastic the tumor, the less likely any specialized function will be present.

7. Growth characteristics—the length of time required for a tumor to become clinically detectable is influenced by the following (Cooper & Cooper, 2001):

  a. Growth fraction—the fraction of proliferating cells in the tumor.

    (1) Normal tissue—growth fraction varies depending on type of tissue. Example—intestinal epithelium contains approximately 16% actively proliferating cells; CNS cells are nonproliferating.

    (2) Type of malignancy—growth fraction also varies, depending on type of cancer. Example—in many solid tumors, 1% to 8% of cells are actively proliferating.

  b. Tumor volume–doubling time—time within which the total cancer cell population doubles; influenced by tumor type since most tumors have high proportion of nonproliferating cells, and tumor vascularity.

  c. Cell loss by continuous shedding from the primary tumor; death caused by toxic products released from other necrotic cells within the tumor.

  d. Hormone levels—certain cancers (that arise from hormone-dependent tissue) require hormones for growth.

    (1) Reduction in hormone levels reduces tumor growth.

    (2) Increased hormone levels promote growth.

  e. Gompertzian growth—refers to a hypothetical growth curve over the lifetime of an "average" tumor (Figure 20-5).

    (1) Growth increases exponentially at first (tumor growth doubles constantly over time).

    (2) Growth then slows owing to hypoxia, decreased availability of nutrients and growth factors, toxins, and faulty cell-to-cell communication.

  f. Clinical conclusions: tumor growth rates vary widely.

    (1) Smallest clinically detectable mass equals 1 g in weight, 1 cm^3 in diameter, 1 billion cells, or approximately 30 tumor volume–doubling times.

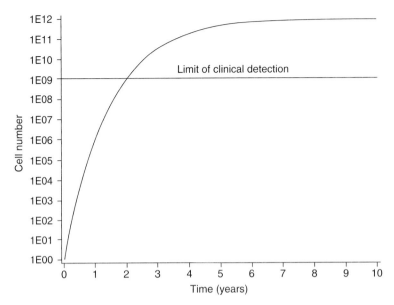

FIGURE 20-5 ▪ The gompertzian growth curve. During the early stage of development, growth is exponential. As a tumor enlarges, its growth slows. By the time a tumor becomes large enough to cause symptoms and is clinically detectable, most of its growth has already occurred, and the exponential phase is complete. (From Cooper MR, Cooper MR: Systemic therapy. In Lenhard RE, Osteen RT, Gansler T, editors: *Clinical oncology,* Atlanta, 2001, American Cancer Society, p. 179.)

        (2) Tumors increase in size because the rate of cell production exceeds rate of cell death.

    D. Tumor growth patterns.

        1. Noncancerous and precancerous growth changes.

            a. Hyperplasia—an increase in the number of cells in a tissue.

                (1) Can be a normal process (e.g., tissue hyperplasia that occurs in wound healing).

                (2) May occur in cancer but is not a unique or defining characteristic of cancer.

            b. Metaplasia—potentially reversible process involving replacement of one mature cell type by another mature cell type not usually found in the involved tissue (Pitot, 2002) (Figure 20-6).

                (1) Initiated by chronic irritation, inflammation, vitamin deficiency, or other pathologic process.

                (2) Example—replacement of columnar epithelial cells in respiratory passages of smokers with squamous cell epithelium.

FIGURE 20-6 ▪ Metaplasia. A schematic diagram of columnar to squamous metaplasia. (From Cotran RS, Kumar V, Robbins SL: *Robbins pathologic basis of disease,* ed 6, Philadelphia, 1999, WB Saunders, p. 37.)

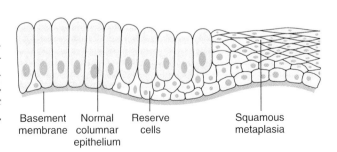

Basement membrane   Normal columnar epithelium   Reserve cells   Squamous metaplasia

      c. Dysplasia—alteration in normal adult epithelial cells (Pitot, 2002).
         (1) Loss of uniformity of cells; also characterized by variations in cell size, shape, organization (architecture).
         (2) May be reversible if stimulant is removed.
         (3) Although dysplasia does not always progress to cancer, it almost always appears before neoplastic changes.
   2. Cancerous conditions.
      a. Anaplasia—most often used to describe malignancy.
         (1) The cytologic and positional disorganization of cells.
         (2) Degree of anaplastic changes may vary.
            (a) Cells tend to be poorly differentiated and in varying sizes and shapes.
            (b) Cell nuclei are disproportionately large.
      b. *Neoplasm* versus *tumor*—interchangeable terms.
         (1) Refers to abnormal growth of tissue that serves no function and continues to grow unchecked once the stimulus is removed.
         (2) Can be benign or malignant.
      c. *Cancer*—common term for all malignancies.
 E. Tumor nomenclature (Table 20-6).
   1. Usually named according to tissue of origin (numerous exceptions exist).
   2. Benign tumors: labeled by adding the suffix *-oma* to the tissue of origin. Example—lipoma is benign tumor composed of lipid cells, and adenoma is benign tumor composed of glandular cells.
   3. Malignant tumors—classified according to tissue of origin, biologic behavior, anatomic site, degree of cell differentiation.
      a. Carcinomas arise in epithelial tissue. Prefixes describe specific type of epithelial tissue.
         (1) *Adeno-*: describes tumors arising from glandular epithelium (columnar). Organ of origin also included. Example—pancreatic adenocarcinoma (a malignant epithelial neoplasm located in the pancreas).
         (2) *Squamous*: describes tumors arising from squamous epithelium. Organ of origin is included. Example—squamous cell carcinoma of the skin.
      b. Sarcomas originate in connective tissue. Prefixes for specific connective tissue sarcomas include *osteo*—arising from bone, *chondro*—arising from cartilage, *lipo*—arising from fat, *rhabdo*—arising from skeletal muscle, and *leiomyo*—arising from smooth muscle.
      c. Hematologic malignancies.
         (1) Leukemias arise from hematopoietic cells: classified according to cell type and maturity. *Lympho-* denotes leukemia of lymphoid origin. *Myelo-* denotes leukemia of myeloid origin.
         (2) Lymphomas are malignancies of the lymphocytes. Subclassified as Hodgkin's disease and non-Hodgkin's lymphoma.
         (3) Multiple myeloma arises from the plasma cell line.
IV. What are the implications of diagnosis and staging on treatment goals and strategies?
 A. Decisions related to the treatment are made after review of the clinical, pathologic, laboratory, and diagnostic data by a multidisciplinary team of cancer specialists.
 B. Key factors to evaluate before making a treatment decision.
   1. Site of cancer: review of client history, physical examination, radiologic examination, laboratory data.

TABLE 20-6
Nomenclature of Tumors

Tissue of Origin	Benign	Malignant
COMPOSED OF ONE PARENCHYMAL CELL TYPE		
MESENCHYMAL TUMORS		
Connective tissue and derivatives	Fibroma	Fibrosarcoma
	Lipoma	Liposarcoma
	Chondroma	Chondrosarcoma
	Osteoma	Osteogenic sarcoma
Endothelial and related tissues		
Blood vessels	Hemangioma	Angiosarcoma
Lymph vessels	Lymphangioma	Lymphangiosarcoma
Synovium		Synovial sarcoma
Mesothelium		Mesothelioma
Brain coverings	Meningioma	Invasive meningioma
Blood cells and related cells		
Hematopoietic cells		Leukemias
Lymphoid tissue		Malignant lymphomas
Muscle		
Smooth	Leiomyoma	Leiomyosarcoma
Striated	Rhabdomyoma	Rhabdomyosarcoma
EPITHELIAL TUMORS		
Stratified squamous	Squamous cell papilloma	Squamous cell or epidermoid carcinoma
		Basal cell carcinoma
Basal cells of skin or adnexa		
Epithelial lining		
Glands or ducts	Adenoma	Adenocarcinoma
	Papilloma	Papillary carcinoma
	Cystadenoma	Cystadenocarcinoma
Respiratory passages		Bronchogenic carcinoma
		Bronchial adenoma (carcinoid)
Neuroectoderm	Nevus	Malignant melanoma
Renal epithelium	Renal tubular adenoma	Renal cell carcinoma
Liver cells	Liver cell adenoma	Hepatocellular carcinoma
Urinary tract epithelium (transitional)	Transitional cell papilloma	Transitional cell carcinoma
Placental epithelium (trophoblast)	Hydatidiform mole	Choriocarcinoma
Testicular epithelium (germ cells)		Seminoma
		Embryonal carcinoma
MORE THAN ONE NEOPLASTIC CELL TYPE—MIXED TUMORS, USUALLY DERIVED FROM ONE GERM LAYER		
Salivary glands	Pleomorphic adenoma (mixed tumor of salivary origin)	Malignant mixed tumor of salivary gland origin
Breast	Fibroadenoma	Malignant cystosarcoma phyllodes
Renal anlage		Wilms' tumor
MORE THAN ONE NEOPLASTIC CELL TYPE DERIVED FROM MORE THAN ONE GERM LAYER—TERATOGENOUS		
Totipotential cells in gonads or in embryonic rests	Mature teratoma, dermoid cyst	Immature teratoma, teratocarcinoma

From Cotran RS, Kumar V, Robbins SL: *Robbins pathologic basis of disease*, ed 6, Philadelphia, 1999, WB Saunders, p. 263.

2. Histologic type and grade of cancer.
   a. Diagnosis of cancer is determined by tissue biopsy.
      (1) Incisional biopsy—aspiration, fine-needle biopsy (removal of a core of tissue), or punch biopsy (removal of tissue tumor core).
      (2) Excisional biopsy—removal of tissue with client under general or local anesthesia. Provides an opportunity to remove the entire lesion. Serves as a mechanism for removal of an adequate sample of tissue for diagnosis.
      (3) Cytology—examination of fluid-containing cells that have been shed. A positive result from cytology examination may be adequate for diagnosis; a negative result is inconclusive, and additional attempts to obtain tissue for diagnosis are indicated.
   b. Tissue biopsy allows for histopathologic grading of tumor.
3. Extent of disease or stage of cancer.
   a. Knowledge of the usual pattern of spread of specific cancers provides guidelines for the staging workup.
   b. Obtaining an extensive history and physical examination is initial step of the staging procedure.
   c. Tests selected for the staging procedure are designed to evaluate the extent of local disease and potential sites of metastatic disease.
      (1) Noninvasive procedures, such as x-rays, computed tomographic (CT) scans, magnetic resonance imaging (MRI), ultrasound.
      (2) Invasive procedures, such as exploratory laparotomy.
   d. Staging systems: allow comparisons of treatment results across populations; serve as an aid to indicate appropriate and standard therapy.
      (1) TNM system—most widely accepted system for staging (Pitot, 2002). Includes determination of T—extent of primary tumor; N—absence or presence and extent of regional lymph node metastasis; and M—absence or presence of distant metastases.
      (2) Disease stage is typically divided into four classifications, with I, the earliest stage, and IV, the most extensive disease. Specific definitions and guidelines for staging each type of cancer have been developed.
4. Flow cytometry—may be used to determine cell size, surface marker expression, and DNA content. Results may assist with determination of treatment and prognosis (Pfeifer & Wick, 2001).
5. Diagnostic molecular genetics—procedures used to analyze genetic characteristics of the cancer cells (Pfeifer & Wick, 2001).
6. Tumor markers—procedures used to detect tumor markers (molecules in body fluids; see Table 20-6).
7. General health status of the client.
   a. Physical examination.
   b. Additional radiologic and laboratory tests are conducted to determine the ability of the client to withstand the demands of and potential consequences of the proposed therapies.
   c. Evaluation of pulmonary, renal, liver, GI, and cardiac function is often obtained.
   d. Performance status scales.
8. Types of therapy.
   a. Primary treatment—major modality used to treat the cancer.
   b. Adjuvant therapy—therapy given after the primary treatment to control potential or known sites of metastasis.

       c. Neoadjuvant treatment—adjuvant therapy given before the primary treatment to control potential or known sites of metastasis.

       d. Prophylactic treatment—treatment directed to a sanctuary site when the risk for developing cancer at the site is high.

   9. Goals of therapy.

       a. Cure—eradication of cancer cells in the body.

       b. Control—containment of the growth of cancer cells without complete eradication.

       c. Palliation—comfort and relief of symptoms when cure is no longer possible. Treatment may include any of the therapeutic modalities.

       d. Reconstruction—to return an individual to his/her optimum functional status.

  C. Treatment may include single and multimodal approaches.

   1. Single-modality approach for clients with small local disease and without evidence of predilection for metastasis.

   2. Multimodal approach.

       a. For clients with bulky tumors or a high likelihood of having or actually having metastatic disease.

       b. Surgery, RT, chemotherapy, and biotherapy may be combined sequentially or given concurrently.

  D. Evaluation of response to treatment: based on individual type of cancer.

V. How are these concepts related to nursing care?

  A. Form the basis for client teaching about prevention and health promotion.

   1. Avoidance of known carcinogens.

   2. Emphasis on health promotion and lifestyle choices.

   3. Investigative potential of reversing agents (e.g., chemoprevention trials).

   4. Emphasis on reversibility of cellular changes (as appropriate); behavior or lifestyle changes can make a difference.

   5. Clarification of misconceptions about carcinogenic potential of screening and diagnostic radiologic examinations: carcinogenic risk from diagnostic procedures is extremely small.

   6. Emphasis on risk of not undergoing screening radiography.

  B. Form the basis of client teaching about cancer diagnoses.

   1. Pathology examination necessary for cancer diagnosis.

   2. Cytologic examinations for detection before palpable lesion is present and promotion of chance for early cure.

   3. Tumor-associated antigens are used as tumor markers at time of diagnosis, during treatment, and after treatment to monitor recurrence or progression.

   4. Radiologic examinations are necessary for detection of micrometastases.

  C. Form the basis of client teaching about treatment.

   1. High mitotic index of certain cancer cells renders them more susceptible to cytotoxic effects of chemotherapeutic agents.

   2. Stable cells (bone, neural tissue) are less sensitive to effects of chemotherapy because of lower mitotic index.

   3. Use of hyperoxygenation procedures is based on principles of cell sensitivity to radiation effects.

   4. Tumor heterogeneity explains the necessity for the following:

       a. Intense initial treatment.

       b. Subsequent repeated treatments, with a variety of drugs.

       c. Novel treatment approaches targeted to the molecular basis of metastatic spread of disease.

    5. Adjuvant therapy is used for presumed micrometastases to kill the last remaining cancer cells.

    6. Use of hormonal manipulation for tumors is effective only in hormone-dependent tissues.

    7. Use of fractionated RT is to minimize damage to healthy tissue while achieving a lethal effect to malignant cells.

    8. Use of "targeted therapies" is designed to administer drugs that are targeted to cancer cells only and spare normal cells. This reduces toxicity while increasing the eradication of cancer (Johnson, 2003).

    9. Use of immune-modulated therapies is based on understanding of the immune surveillance theory.

    10. Carcinogenic potential of alkylating chemotherapeutic agents and RT necessitates long-term client follow-up to detect secondary malignancies.

  D. Form the basis for understanding treatment side effects.

  E. Account for paraneoplastic syndromes, which are caused by ectopic production of hormones and other substances by the malignant cells.

  F. Form the basis for client teaching and follow-up to detect metastasis.

    1. Likelihood of metastasis at time of diagnosis may necessitate extensive diagnostic workup, systemic approach to therapy, adjuvant therapy.

    2. Potential for disease recurrence via metastasis necessitates frequent and long-term follow-up.

VI. What are the implications for the professional development of the nurse?

  A. Promotes understanding of terminology and nomenclature necessary for client teaching and interdisciplinary communication or collaboration.

  B. Promotes understanding of cancer prevention and early detection.

  C. Forms basis for understanding the rationale for treatment protocols, timing of treatment, and diagnostic follow-up.

  D. Enhances understanding of reasons for intensity of initial treatment protocols.

  E. Forms basis for understanding current research and trends in care.

  F. Forms basis for understanding and initiating cancer nursing research.

  G. Promotes understanding of prognostic implications of disease.

  H. Enhances participation in identification and discussion of ethical issues related to disease and treatment.

REFERENCES

Cahill, D.P., & Lengauer, C. (2002). Tumor genome instability. In B. Vogelstein & K.W. Kinzler (Eds.). *The genetic basis of human cancer* (2nd ed.). New York: McGraw-Hill, pp. 129-130.

Cooper, M.R., & Cooper, M.R. (2001). Systemic therapy. In R.E. Lenhard, R.T. Osteen, & T. Gansler (Eds.). *Clinical oncology.* Atlanta: American Cancer Society, pp. 175-215.

Cotran, R.S., Kumar, V., & Robbins, S.L. (1999). *Robbins pathologic basis of disease* (6th ed.). Philadelphia: W.B. Saunders.

Ding, S., Chamberlain, M., McLaren, A., et al. (2001). Cross-talk between signaling pathways and the multi-drug resistant protein MDR-1. *British Journal of Cancer 85*(8), 1175-1184.

Fidler, I.J., Kerbel, R.S., & Ellis, L.M. (2001). Biology of cancer: Angiogenesis. In V.T. DeVita, S. Hellman, & S.A. Rosenberg (Eds.). *Cancer: Principles and practice of oncology* (6th ed.). Philadelphia: Lippincott Williams & Wilkins, pp. 137-147.

Gribbon, J., & Loescher, L. (2000). Biology of cancer. In C.H. Yarbro, M.H. Frogge, M. Goodman, & S.L. Groenwald (Eds.). *Cancer nursing: Principles and practice* (5th ed.). Sudbury, MA: Jones and Bartlett Publishers, pp. 17-34.

Hanahan, D., & Weinberg, R.A. (2000). The hallmarks of cancer. *Cell 100,* 57-70.

Jefford, M., Maralovsky, E., Cebon, J., & Davis, I. (2001). The use of dendritic cells in cancer therapy. *Lancet Oncology 2,* 343-353.

Johnson, D.H. (2003). Targeted therapy in non-small cell lung cancer: Myth or reality. *Lung Cancer 4*(Suppl. 1), S3-S8.

Kelland, L.R. (2001). Telomerase: Biology and phase I trials. *Lancet Oncology 2,* 95-102.

Kinzler, K.W., & Vogelstein, B. (2002). Introduction. In B. Vogelstein & K.W. Kinzler (Eds.). *The genetic basis of human cancer* (2nd ed.). New York: McGraw-Hill, pp. 3-6.

Liotta, L.A., & Liu, E.T. (2001). Essentials of molecular biology: Genomics and cancer. In V.T. DeVita, S. Hellman, & S.A. Rosenberg (Eds.). *Cancer: Principles and practice of oncology* (6th ed.). Philadelphia: Lippincott Williams & Wilkins, pp. 17-29.

Livingston, D.M., & Shivdasani, R. (2001). Toward mechanism-based cancer care. *Journal of the American Medical Association 285,* 588-593.

Mareel, M., & Leroy, A. (2003). Clinical, cellular, and molecular aspects of cancer invasion. *Physiological Reviews 83,* 337-376.

Middleton, L., Dimond, E., Calzone, K., et al. (2002). The role of the nurse in cancer genetics. *Cancer Nursing 25,* 196-206.

Milner, J.A., McDonald, S.S., Anderson, D.E., & Greenwald, P. (2001). Molecular targets for nutrients involved with cancer prevention. *Nutrition and Cancer 41*(1 & 2), 1-16.

Pardoll, D. (2003). Does the immune system see tumors as foreign or self? *Annual Review of Immunology 21,* 807-839.

Park, M. (2002). Oncogenes. In B. Vogelstein & K.W. Kinzler (Eds.). *The genetic basis of human cancer* (2nd ed.). New York: McGraw-Hill, pp. 177-196.

Pfeifer, J.D., & Wick, M.R. (2001). Pathologic evaluation of neoplastic diseases. In R.E. Lenhard, R.T. Osteen, & T. Gansler (Eds.). *Clinical oncology.* Atlanta: American Cancer Society, pp. 123-147.

Pitot, H.C. (2002). *Fundamentals of oncology* (4th ed.). New York: Marcel Dekker.

Ringer, D.P., & Schnipper, L.E. (2001). Principles of cancer biology. In R.E. Lenhard, R.T. Osteen, & T. Gansler (Eds.). *Clinical oncology.* Atlanta: American Cancer Society, pp. 21-35.

Rudin, C.M., & Thompson, C.B. (2002). Apoptosis and cancer. In B. Vogelstein & K.W. Kinzler (Eds.). *The genetic basis of human cancer* (2nd ed.). New York: McGraw-Hill, pp. 163-175.

Stetler-Stevenson, W.G., & Kleiner, D.E. (2001). Molecular biology of cancer: Invasion and metastases. In V.T. DeVita, S. Hellman, & S.A. Rosenberg (Eds.). *Cancer: Principles and practice of oncology* (6th ed.). Philadelphia: Lippincott Williams & Wilkins, pp. 123-136.

Ulrich, R.L. (2001). Etiology of cancer: Physical factors. In V.T. DeVita, S. Hellman, & S.A. Rosenberg (Eds.). *Cancer: Principles and practice of oncology* (6th ed.). Philadelphia: Lippincott Williams & Wilkins, pp. 123-136.

Yuspa, S.H., & Shields, P.G. (2001). Etiology of cancer: Chemical factors. In V.T. DeVita, S. Hellman, & S.A. Rosenberg (Eds.). *Cancer: Principles and practice of oncology* (6th ed.). Philadelphia: Lippincott Williams & Wilkins, pp. 179-193.

21 Immunology

KRISTI V. SCHMIDT

Theory

I. Definition.
   A. Study of the mechanisms with which the body defends itself against infectious agents and foreign substances.
   B. Includes innate and acquired defense mechanisms, such as physical barriers, chemical substances, physiologic reactions of tissues to injury or infection, and a network of specialized cells.
   C. Together, these components are able to initiate or inhibit specific immune responses, recognize "self versus nonself" of human histology, and identify and destroy malignant and/or altered cells (Lowell, 2001).
II. Core functions (U.S. Department of Health and Human Services, 2003).
   A. Hematopoiesis—regulation, production, and development of blood cells.
      1. Blood cell development begins with a single cell, the pluripotent stem cell.
      2. This cell divides to produce undifferentiated hematopoietic stem cells that are committed to one of two cell lineages or pathways, lymphoid or myeloid progenitor cells (Figure 21-1).
   B. Protection against infection by recognizing and destroying pathogens.
   C. Homeostasis—maintaining the balance of blood cell supply.
III. Anatomy and structure.
   A. Primary lymphoid organs.
      1. Allow for the maturation of lymphocytes, including the growth and expression of specific antigen receptors essential for future antigenic invasion. Includes the following (Male, 2001):
         a. Bone marrow—location of B-cell differentiation and maturation.
         b. Thymus—location of T-cell differentiation and maturation.
   B. Secondary lymphoid organs and tissues.
      1. Sites where foreign antigens encounter lymphocyte immune responses, which include the following (Abbas et al., 2000; Lydyard & Grossi, 2001):
         a. Waldeyer's ring (tonsils and adenoids)—mucosa-associated lymphoid tissue.
         b. Bronchus-associated lymphoid tissue—mucosa-associated lymphoid tissue.
         c. Lymph nodes—initiate immune responses to antigens circulating in the lymph, skin (subcutaneous lymph nodes), or mucosal surfaces.
         d. Spleen—responds to blood-borne antigens.
         e. Bone marrow—functions as both primary and secondary lymphoid organ.
         f. Peyer's patch—gastrointestinal (GI) mucosa–associated lymphoid tissue.
         g. Urogenital lymphoid tissue—mucosa-associated lymphoid tissue.

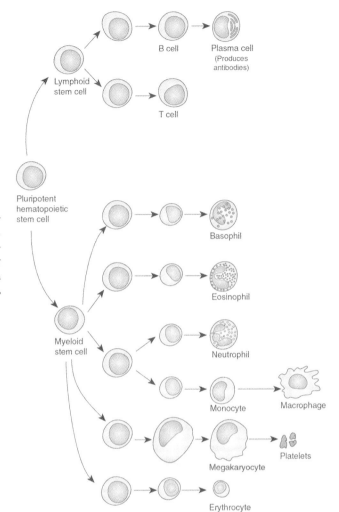

FIGURE 21-1 ■ Hematopoiesis—blood cell development. (From Genentech, Inc. *Biooncology masters curriculum: Introduction to oncology,* South San Francisco, 2003, The CELL Group.)

IV. Components of the immune system.
   A. Cells.
      1. Lymphocytes are derived from the lymphoid stem cell lineage and are key for all immune responses. The two types are as follows:
         a. B cells.
            (1) Develop in the bone marrow.
            (2) On recognition of a specific antigen, B cells multiply and further differentiate into plasma cells, which produce one of five types of immunoglobulins (IgG, IgA, IgM, IgE, IgD).
         b. T cells.
            (1) Migrate to the thymus gland for development.
            (2) Before antigen recognition by T cells, antigens are processed by antigen-presenting cells (APCs) displayed on the cell surface as peptides (Figure 21-2).
            (3) The different types of T cells include the following (Abbas et al., 2000; Roitt & Delves, 2001):
               (a) T helper cells (CD4+ cells): type 1 (Th1) secretes cytokines and interacts with mononuclear phagocytes to assist in their ability to destroy intracellular pathogens.

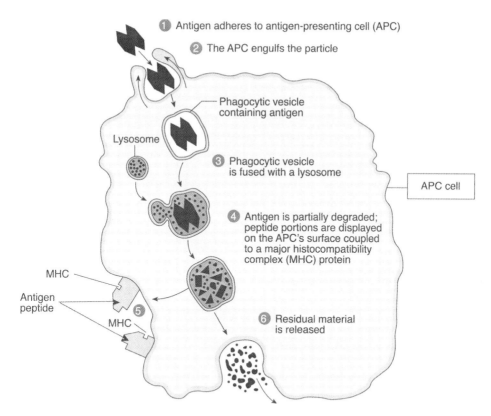

① Antigen adheres to antigen-presenting cell (APC)

② The APC engulfs the particle

Phagocytic vesicle containing antigen

Lysosome

③ Phagocytic vesicle is fused with a lysosome

APC cell

④ Antigen is partially degraded; peptide portions are displayed on the APC's surface coupled to a major histocompatibility complex (MHC) protein

MHC

Antigen peptide

MHC

⑤

⑥ Residual material is released

FIGURE 21-2 ■ Antigen-presenting cell (APC) process of antigen ingestion and presentation. (From Genentech, Inc. *Biooncology masters curriculum: Introduction to oncology,* South San Francisco, 2003, The CELL Group.)

    (b) T helper cells (CD4+ cells): type 2 (Th2) interacts with B cells, enhancing cell division, differentiation, and antibody production.

    (c) T cytotoxic cells (CD8+ cells): also referred to as Tc, destroy host cells with the direction of CD4+ cells.

2. Phagocytes—internalize (engulf) and consume pathogenic microorganisms and debris and function to engulf and destroy particles (Solomon & Komanduri, 2001).

  a. Mononuclear phagocytes—fixed and mobile phagocytic cells associated with blood monocytes and tissue macrophages (Roitt & Delves, 2001).

  b. Polymorphonuclear granulocytes (Roitt & Delves, 2001).

    (1) Polymorphonuclear neutrophils (PMNs).

      (a) Make up majority (60% to 70%) of the blood leukocytes (white cells).

      (b) Are short-lived cells that migrate into tissues (inflammatory response), where they engulf and destroy material (Male, 2001).

    (2) Eosinophil polymorphs—also known as eosinophils.

      (a) Make up 2% to 5% of blood leukocytes (Roitt & Delves, 2001).

      (b) Are attracted to large extracellular parasitic worms.

        (c) Cell kill is done by the release of the contents of their intracellular granules close to them.

        (d) Also release histamine and arylsulfatase to reduce an inflammatory response and granulocyte accumulation (Male, 2001; Roitt & Delves, 2001).

    (3) Basophils.

        (a) Make up less than 0.2% of leukocytes (Roitt & Delves, 2001).

        (b) Are circulating granulocytes that move to tissue sites where antigens are present and can create immediate hypersensitivity reactions.

        (c) Similar in function to mast cells, which are described below (Abbas et al., 2000).

3. Dendritic cells (DCs).

  a. Are derived from either lymphoid or mononuclear phagocyte cell lineages but most are related to the latter (Roitt & Delves, 2001).

  b. Function as APCs that initiate T-cell (CD4+, CD8+), as well as naive T-cell, dependent immune responses known as "priming" (Abbas et al., 2000).

  c. Are effective in stimulating both antiviral and antitumor immune responses in experimental animal and human models.

  d. Immature DCs are found in peripheral tissue and possess phagocytic and macropinocytotic functions that express multiple receptors that enhance antigen uptake with low surface expression of class I and II major histocompatibility complex (MHC) molecules.

  e. Mature DCs are influenced by inflammatory stimuli that lead to decreased phagocytosis and increased cell surface expression of class I and II molecules.

  f. Mature DCs are then able to migrate through the lymphatics to adjacent lymphoid tissue through specific molecular function to present antigen proteins to CD4+ and CD8+ T cells (Mullins et al., 2003).

4. Null cells.

  a. Are a separate lineage of lymphoid cells that express neither T-cell nor B-cell surface markers.

  b. Early in cell differentiation these cells display T-cell markers but with further maturation acquire markers found also on macrophages and neutrophils (Williams et al., 2001).

  c. Two types.

    (1) Natural killer (NK) cells.

        (a) Contain substances called *perforin*, serine proteases, and other enzymes that lyse targeted cells.

        (b) Activity is increased with the addition of cytokines such as IL-2, IL-12 (interleukins), and IFN-α (interferon).

        (c) Ultimate function is to identify and destroy virus-infected cells and certain tumor cells (Lydyard & Grossi, 2001).

    (2) Lymphokine-activated (LAK) cells.

        (a) Are produced when mononuclear cells (lymphocytes) are removed from a client's blood and cultured with IL-2 or alloantigens.

        (b) LAK subset of cells creates cytotoxicity in a wide spectrum of targeted cells.

        (c) Continued presence of IL-2 required and LAK cells must have direct contact with target cell for cytotoxic effect (Roitt & Delves, 2001).

   5. Mast cells.
      a. Granulocytes that have multiple mediators that produce inflammatory response within tissues.
      b. Are located close to blood vessels in all tissues and are often indistinguishable from basophils (Roitt & Delves, 2001).
      c. Two kinds of mast cells.
         (1) Mucosal mast cell (MMC).
         (2) Connective tissue mast cell (CTMC).
   6. Platelets.
      a. Aside from blood clotting, platelets have immunologic function that releases inflammatory mediators through the process of thrombogenesis or antigen-antibody complexes (Roitt & Delves, 2001).
B. Mediators of immune system function—specific molecules involved in the development and enhancement of the immune response.
   1. Complement system—an interactive network of approximately 20 unique serum and cell proteins present in plasma (Solomon & Komanduri, 2001).
      a. Complement proteins have the ability to leak out of the vascular spaces into tissue.
         (1) When an antibody adheres to an antigen, a portion of the antibody changes, making it possible for a preliminary complement protein to bind to the antibody.
      b. Once the first complement protein (C1) binds to the antibody, a cascade of reactions, which create enzymes, takes place, resulting in the following therapeutic effects.
         (1) Opsonization—phagocytosis is stimulated when products of the complement cascade interact with neutrophils and macrophages, enticing them to phagocytize antigen-antibody complexes.
         (2) Another product of the complement cascade, the lytic complex, is able to rupture the cell membranes of foreign cells.
         (3) Complement products make the outer coatings of invading cells sticky, resulting in agglutination, and can change the structures of some viruses, making them nonvirulent.
         (4) Complement products encourage basophils and mast cells to release histamines in the blood, which aids in the process of inflammation.
   2. Cytokines.
      a. A group of molecules produced by cells that enhance communication and induce growth and differentiation of lymphocytes and other cells within the immune and neuroendocrine system (Male, 2001). Includes the following:
         (1) Interferons (IFNs), which limit the spread of certain viral infections, are produced early in response to infection, and offer first line of viral resistance.
         (2) Interleukins (ILs), which are produced mainly by T cells; however, some production in mononuclear phagocytes or tissue cells.
         (3) Hematopoietic growth factors (referred to as colony-stimulating factors), which guide and direct cell division and differentiation of bone marrow stem cells and leukocytes.
         (4) Tumor necrosis factors (TNF-α or TNF-β) and transforming growth factor–β play key roles in mediating inflammation and cytotoxic reactions.
         (5) Chemokines are cytokines (proteins secreted by selected white blood cells [WBCs]) that guide leukocyte movement around the body between blood and tissues.

(a) May activate cells to perform specialized immunologic functions (Abbas et al., 2000).

C. Major histocompatibility complex (MHC) (Sompayrac, 2003; Williams et al., 2001).

1. MHC is the genetic region where immune surveillance is a key function (self-recognition).

2. MHC genes are coded on chromosome 6 in humans and chromosome 17 in mice and utilized for presentation of peptides.

3. MHC molecules expressed on the surface of human cells are also known as human leukocyte antigens (HLAs) (Abbas et al., 2000).

4. There are two main classes of membrane protein MHC molecules: class I (HLA-A, HLA-B, HLA-C) and class II (HLA-DR, HLA-DP, HLA-DQ).

   a. Class I MHC molecules are cell surface glycoproteins found on many cells and function by binding to and displaying a cell's peptides to specific immune cells, such as T cells.

      (1) Represents intercellular function of antigen presentation.

   b. Class II MHC molecules are membrane glycoproteins found only on specialized cells that have antigen presentation capabilities.

      (1) Represents extracellular function of antigen presentation.

V. Immune system response.

   A. Innate immunity.

   1. Is a cascade of mechanisms that occur before onset of infection, respond rapidly to microbes, and react in the same fashion to repeated infections (Abbas et al., 2000).

   2. Does not have the ability to target specific pathogens and includes the following:

      a. Mechanical barriers—intact skin and mucous membranes; cilia lining the respiratory tract.

      b. Chemical barriers—saliva, sweat, gastric acid, digestive enzymes.

      c. Fever, which results from the hypothalamus being stimulated by IL-1 when it is released by activated macrophages, lymphocytes, neutrophils, and NK cells during the inflammatory response, infection, or other exposure to antigen.

      d. Phagocytosis, a process found in both innate and acquired immunity (Figure 21-3).

         (1) Pseudopods extend around a microbe, surrounding it with a plasma membrane.

         (2) The surrounded microbe is then enclosed into a vacuole.

         (3) The microbe is subsequently destroyed within the vacuole (Roitt & Delves, 2001).

         (4) This process destroys the majority of bacteria, viruses, and other pathogens or foreign materials invading the body.

         (5) Performed by neutrophils, macrophages, and antigen-presenting cells, such as dendritic cells.

         (6) Can begin as a result of chemotaxis.

            (a) Chemotaxis occurs when tissue is invaded and becomes inflamed. Many different chemical and protein substances are produced in the area. These substances fall into three categories.

               (i) Bacterial toxins released before and after phagocytosis.

               (ii) Particles of destroyed inflamed tissue.

               (iii) Complement.

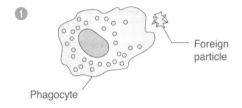

Foreign particle

Phagocyte

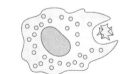

FIGURE 21-3 ▨ Phagocytosis. Genentech, Inc. *Biooncology masters curriculum: Introduction to oncology,* South San Francisco, 2003, The CELL Group.)

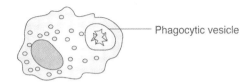

Phagocytic vesicle

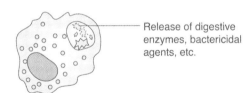

Release of digestive enzymes, bactericidal agents, etc.

e. Mononuclear phagocyte system (MPS) (Male, 2001).
   (1) Is a system of phagocytes composed of monocytes and macrophages.
   (2) Also referred to as reticuloendothelial system (RES), named when it was believed that macrophages were derived from endothelial cells.
   (3) Once an invading pathogen or other foreign substance is identified by the MPS, it is phagocytized.
      (a) If an invading pathogen is not destroyed in the tissues, it can move into the lymph system and travel to a lymph node to be destroyed by a tissue macrophage there.
      (b) Tissue macrophages are present in various blood- and lymph-filtering sites in the body and at points where pathogens frequently enter the body.
f. Inflammation—foreign invaders not destroyed by phagocytosis can cause tissue injury. Trauma, chemicals, burns, and many other events can also cause tissue injury. Specific chemicals and proteins are secreted in response to injury. This process is called *inflammation* (Roitt & Delves, 2001).

(1) Purpose of inflammation is to provide nonspecific defense against foreign invaders.

(2) Inflammation is a catalyst for destruction of invaders and repair of tissue.

    (a) Types of invaders that can stimulate inflammation include pathogens; allergens; another person's tissue (e.g., donated bone marrow, a kidney); and an artificial, foreign material (e.g., a Hickman catheter).

(3) Degree of inflammatory response is based on the following:

    (a) Degree of "foreignness" of the invader.

    (b) Intensity of exposure to foreign material.

    (c) Size and chemical makeup of the invader.

    (d) Complexity of the molecule: the more complex, the greater the immune response.

    (e) Severity of the invasion or injury.

    (f) Duration of exposure.

    (g) Size of exposure.

B. Acquired immunity.

  1. Begins with an antigen that is phagocytized by a macrophage and is presented to B or T lymphocytes and T helper cells (Male, 2001).

  2. Each antigen is unique because of its peculiar combination of proteins and polysaccharides.

  3. In order to be antigenic and recognized by a B or T lymphocyte as nonself, two characteristics must exist.

    a. The antigen must be of high molecular weight.

    b. On the surface of each antigen must be a pattern of recurring molecules called *epitopes.*

      (1) These serve as identifiers and are formed by genes within the organism.

      (2) The genes that pattern the epitope compose the major histocompatibility complex (MHC), also referred to as the human leukocyte antigen complex.

  4. B-cell, or humoral, immunity.

    a. B lymphocytes dwell in lymphoid tissue, waiting for macrophages to bring antigens to the unused B lymphocyte for processing (Male, 2001).

    b. Each B-cell lymphocyte develops to recognize only one type of antigen.

      (1) This characteristic is called *specificity.*

      (2) Once specificity develops, three processes occur.

        (a) Specific B-cell lymphocytes are produced at a fast pace.

        (b) Some specified B-cell lymphocytes differentiate to become plasma cells. Each specialized plasma cell produces one specific antibody; these committed, highly differentiated cells are not phagocytic.

        (c) Some specialized B-cell lymphocytes become memory cells and exist in the body capable of recognizing a particular antigen at future exposures and producing plasma cells to generate abundant antibody specific to the antigen.

    c. Some antibodies circulate in the bloodstream in addition to gathering at the site of invasion.

    d. Antibodies (immunoglobulins) protect the body from antigens and cells containing them by direct action via immune effector mechanisms, such as neutralization, antibody-dependent cell-mediated cytotoxicity

(ADCC), complement-dependent cytotoxicity (CDC), and apoptosis (Schmidt & Wood, 2003). Specifically the following events occur:

(1) Neutralization occurs when cell growth is stopped because of interference of the immunoglobulin with the antigen.

(2) ADCC occurs when the antibody binds to the antigen and forms a bridge to cause direct cell kill. In addition to the immunoglobulin, NK cells and macrophages participate in this process.

(3) Apoptosis (programmed cell death) occurs because of the attachment of the antibody to the antigen, sending a complex, multiple-step signal that causes breakage of the DNA within the cell nucleus.

(4) CDC is the interaction of serum and cell surface proteins along with other molecules via cascade mechanisms.

    (a) Complement is activated via the "classical pathway."

    (b) Is initiated when IgM binds to the antigen-antibody target and recruits two or more C1 molecules.

    (c) The end result is cell lysis and recruitment of other components of the immune system to enhance the effector cell response (Schmidt & Wood, 2003; Sompayrac, 2003).

5. T-cell immunity, or cell-mediated immunity.

  a. Occurs when antigens are exposed in the bloodstream and presented to T lymphocytes by macrophages via APCs (Male, 2001).

  b. T lymphocytes specific to the presented antigen are produced; they are referred to as activated T cells.

  c. Activated T cells are released into lymphatic fluid from the bloodstream. Then they move back and forth from the lymphatic ducts to the blood vessels.

  d. T-lymphocyte memory cells are also produced and are able to respond more quickly in producing more activated T lymphocytes when exposed to the same antigen in the future.

  e. Antigens can also attach to the membranes of T lymphocytes.

  f. There are three types of T lymphocytes that work within the immune system.

    (1) Helper T cells regulate immune system function through the secretion of lymphokines, which do the following:

      (a) Stimulate production and maturation of cytotoxic T cells.

      (b) Stimulate production and maturation of suppressor T cells.

      (c) Activate macrophages.

    (2) Cytotoxic T cells and NK cells are capable of directly attacking other cells and destroying them as part of cell-mediated immunity (Male, 2001).

      (a) CD8+ T cells use FasL (ligand for tumor necrosis factor molecule) and granules to kill targeted cells.

      (b) CD4+ T cells primarily use FasL to kill targeted cells.

      (c) NK cells use granules to kill targeted cells; specifically, NK cells bind to the antigens on the surface of cells that they recognize. After binding to the cells, the NK cell secretes enzymes as described earlier that create a hole in the membrane of the cell. Cytotoxic substances are released into the cell, resulting in swelling and disintegration of the cell.

      (d) Cytotoxic T cells and NK cells eliminate target cells through a process called ADCC by mechanisms described above.

         (3) Suppressor T cells are able to turn off the functioning of both cyto-
toxic and helper T cells.

    g. T lymphocytes are also able to recognize and bind to antigen.

       (1) T lymphocytes cannot read epitopes until the molecule is phago-
cytized and digested and its antigens are linked with the MHC
antigens on the surface of the NK T lymphocytes.

       (2) Some molecules resist digestion by phagocytes and therefore may
never be read by T lymphocytes.

    h. If T lymphocytes are reduced in number or are not functioning well,
invading cells and proteins may never be recognized.

VI. Tumor immunology.

    A. The science behind immune surveillance is that tumor cells express cellular
components recognized as nonself and are considered antigenic (recognized
as a foreign body). Therefore progression of tumors is related to an ineffective immune system (Williams et al., 2001).

    B. Tumor-associated antigens (TAAs)—changes can occur in cell surface mole-
cules when a cell transitions from normal to malignant; however, only a limited number of TAAs have been identified (e.g., HER2/neu, CEA, CA 125,
TAG-72, EGFR, PSA, ganglioside).

    C. Cell-mediated and humoral immune effector cell responses have been
demonstrated in vitro, leading to tumor cytotoxicity.

    D. Examples of how tumor cells do evade immune system effector functions
include the following (Abbas et al., 2000):

      1. Clients with T-cell immunodeficiencies are at higher risk of developing
malignancies because of oncogenic viral invasion, such as Epstein-Barr
virus (EBV). T cells play a critical role in immune surveillance.

      2. Class I MHC expression may be deregulated on tumor cells so that they
are not targeted by cytotoxic T cells.

      3. Tumor cells are created from host cells and resemble/function similar to
normal cells except tumor cells lose expression of antigens that do the following:

        a. Normally ignite an immune response.

        b. Secrete cytokines that suppress immune cell responses.

      4. Tumor cells fail to recruit cytotoxic T cells because the cells do not express
costimulators that normally induce cytotoxic T cells or class II MHC molecules.

      5. Cell turnover and rapid growth rates in malignant tumors may over-
power immune system effector cell functions intending to destroy and
eliminate the tumor cells.

REFERENCES

Abbas, A., Lichtman, A., & Pober, J. (2000). *Cellular and molecular immunology* (4th ed.).
Philadelphia: W.B. Saunders.

Genentech, Inc. (2003). *Biooncology masters curriculum: Introduction to oncology.* South San
Francisco: The CELL Group.

Lowell, C. (2001). Basic immunology. In T.G. Parslow, D.P. Stites, A.I. Terr, & J.B. Imboden
(Eds.). *Medical immunology* (10th ed.). Retrieved November 24, 2003 from the World Wide
Web: http://onlinestatref.com/document.

Lydyard, P., & Grossi, C. (2001). Cells, tissues and organs of the immune system. In I. Riott,
J. Brostoff, & D. Male (Eds.). *Immunology* (6th ed.). Edinburgh: Mosby, pp. 15-46.

Male, D. (2001). Introduction to the immune system. In I. Riott, J. Brostoff, & D. Male (Eds.).
Immunology (6th ed.). Edinburgh: Mosby, pp. 1-13, 164-170.

Mullins, D.W., Sheasley, S.L., Ream, R.M., et al. (2003). Route of immunization with peptide-pulsed dendritic cells controls the distribution of memory and effector T cells in lymphoid tissues and determines the pattern of regional tumor control. *Journal of Experimental Medicine 198*(7), 1023-1034.

Roitt, I., & Delves, P. (2001). *Essential immunology* (10th ed.). Malden, MA: Blackwell Science.

Schmidt, K., & Wood, B. (2003). Trends in cancer therapy: Role of monoclonal antibodies. In C. Yarbro & K. Schmidt (Eds.). *Seminars in Oncology Nursing (Emerging Therapies) 19*(3), 169-179.

Solomon, S., & Komanduri, K. (2001). The immune system. In P. Trahan Reiger (Ed.). *Biotherapy: A comprehensive nursing overview.* Sudbury, MA: Jones and Bartlett Publishers, pp. 39-64.

Sompayrac, L. (2003). *How the immune system works* (2nd ed.). Malden, MA: Blackwell Science.

U.S. Department of Health and Human Services. (2003). Understanding the immune system: How it works (electronic version). Retrieved January 22, 2004 from the World Wide Web: http://www.niaid.nih.gov-publications.

Williams, J., Lord, E., & Order, S. (2001). Basic concepts of tumor immunology and principles of immunotherapy. In P. Rubin & J. Williams (Eds.). *Clinical oncology: A multidisciplinary approach for physicians and students.* Philadelphia: W.B. Saunders, pp.185-198.

22 Genetics

KATHLEEN A. CALZONE

Theory

I. Organization and function of genetic material (Vogelstein & Kinzler, 2002).
   A. Most genetic information of a cell is organized, stored, and retrieved in structures called *chromosomes* that are made up of densely coiled deoxyribonucleic acid (DNA).
      1. Human body has 46 *chromosomes* consisting of 23 chromosome pairs, one copy from each parent.
         a. *Autosomes* represent the 22 chromosome pairs numbered 1 to 22, which do not determine gender.
         b. *Sex chromosomes* are the X and Y. Women have two X chromosomes, and men have one X chromosome and one Y chromosome.
   B. Nucleic acids form the building block for protein production, which controls cell function (Vogelstein & Kinzler, 2002).
      1. Consist of bases and a sugar and phosphate group.
      2. Two types of nucleic acids.
         a. DNA consists of two parallel nucleotide chains, running in opposite directions held together by hydrogen bonds. The parallel structure twists to form a double helix (Figure 22-1).
            (1) Two types of bases: purines and pyrimidines.
               (a) Two types of purines: adenine (A) and guanine (G).
               (b) Two types of pyrimidines: thymine (T) and cytosine (C).
            (2) DNA base pairs are complementary: A attaches to T, and G attaches to C.
         b. RNA (ribonucleic acid) consists of a single nucleotide chain that is a complementary copy of a strand of DNA.
            (1) Bases are the same as DNA except that the base uracil (U) replaces thymine (T).
            (2) Three primary types of RNA (Figure 22-2).
               (a) Messenger RNA (mRNA) contains information about the order of the amino acids in a protein.
                  (i) A codon is a chain of three mRNA nucleotides that specify the insertion of one of twenty different amino acids.
                  (ii) Some amino acids have more than one specific codon.
                  (iii) There are three stop codons, which stop the assembly of the amino acid chain.
               (b) Transfer RNA (tRNA) brings the amino acids to the site of protein synthesis.
               (c) Ribosomal RNA (rRNA) provides the structural support for the protein in addition to other functions.
            (3) *Transcription* refers to the process of making RNA from DNA.
            (4) *Translation* refers to the process of making proteins from RNA.

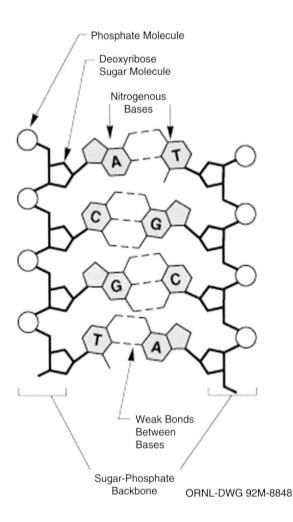

Phosphate Molecule

Deoxyribose
Sugar Molecule

Nitrogenous
Bases

A   T

C   G

G   C

T   A

Weak Bonds
Between
Bases

Sugar-Phosphate
Backbone   ORNL-DWG 92M-8848

FIGURE 22-1 ■ DNA structure. (Used with permission of U.S. Department of Energy Human Genome Program, http://www.ornl. gov/hgmis.)

ORNL-DWG B1M-17380

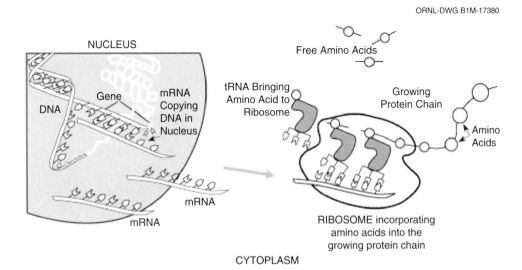

NUCLEUS

Free Amino Acids

Gene   mRNA
Copying
DNA in
Nucleus

DNA

tRNA Bringing
Amino Acid to
Ribosome

Growing
Protein Chain

Amino
Acids

mRNA

mRNA

RIBOSOME incorporating
amino acids into the
growing protein chain

CYTOPLASM

FIGURE 22-2 ■ Three types of RNA. (Used with permission of U.S. Department of Energy Human Genome Program, http://www.ornl.gov/hgmis.)

(a) *Proteins* consist of chains of amino acids. Sequence of the amino acids determines the function of the protein.

C. Genes are individual units of hereditary information located at a specific position on the chromosome (Figure 22-3) (Vogelstein & Kinzler, 2002).

  1. Consist of a sequence of DNA that codes for a specific protein.
  2. Consist primarily of exons and introns.
     a. *Exons* are protein-coding segments of a gene.
     b. *Introns* are nonprotein-coding segments of a gene.

II. Basic mechanisms of carcinogenesis, mutations, and heredity (Balmain et al., 2003; Tranin, 1997; Tranin et al., 2003; Vogelstein & Kinzler, 2002).

  A. Cancer has a multifactorial etiology with several genetic, environmental, and personal factors interacting to produce a malignancy.

  B. Genetic mutations and genetic instability are at the very core of cancer development.

  1. Most cancer is not the result of an inherited mutation.
  2. Most cancer is associated with genetic mutations that occur in single cells sometime during the life of an individual.
  3. A malignant tumor arises after a series of genetic mutations have accumulated.

  C. Genetic mutations that are acquired are associated with exogenous or indigenous factors. For example, carcinogens are thought to operate by causing genetic mutations.

  D. Malignant tumor is derived from genetic instability and genetic mutations in regulatory genes that control cell growth and proliferation.

  1. Types of regulatory genes.
     a. *Proto-oncogenes* are essential for normal cell development and growth regulation. Mutations of proto-oncogenes result in oncogene activation or dysregulation, which can result in uncontrolled cell growth.
     b. *Tumor suppressor genes* function as modulators of cell growth.
     c. *Mismatch repair genes* correct DNA replication errors.
     d. *Apoptosis* refers to the activation of a program that leads to programmed or normal cell death, which often occurs in response to DNA damage. Loss of response to apoptotic signals results in inappropriate maintenance of cell viability.

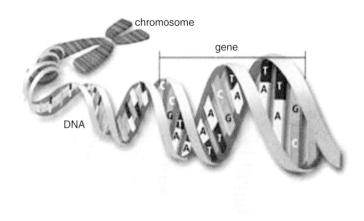

FIGURE 22-3 ■ Chromosomes to genes. (Used with permission of U.S. Department of Energy Human Genome Program, http://www.ornl.gov/hgmis.)

   e. *Telomerase* plays a role in cellular aging through the telomeres, which are the ends of the chromosome.
   (1) As cells age, telomerase is normally repressed and the telomeres progressively shorten.
   (2) In cancer, telomerase is reactivated, which keeps the telomeres intact, facilitating cell immortalization.
 2. *Knudson "two hit" hypothesis* refers to the inactivation of both copies of a given regulatory gene. Because all individuals are born with two copies of almost every gene, both functioning copies of the gene must be inactivated for cancer to occur.
 3. Mutations are variations in the sequence of DNA.
   a. Usually acquired; however, in someone with a genetic predisposition to cancer, a mutation has been inherited in the germline.
   (1) *Somatic* refers to acquired genetic mutations in single isolated cells.
   (2) *Germline* refers to inherited genetic mutations that are transmitted in the egg or sperm.
   (3) *De novo* refers to genetic mutations occurring in the egg or sperm.
   b. Types of mutations.
   (1) *Frameshift* mutations occur when one or more bases are added or deleted from the normal sequence, resulting in an altered form of the protein.
   (2) *Missense* mutations are single–base pair changes that result in the substitution of one amino acid for another in the protein being constructed. Some of the substituted amino acids may be critical to the function of the protein, others may not change protein function.
   (3) *Nonsense* mutations change an amino acid signal into a signal to stop adding amino acids to a growing protein. Nonsense mutations result in a truncated nonfunctional protein.
   (4) *RNA-negative* mutations result in the absence of RNA transcribed from a gene copy.
   (5) *Splicing* mutations occur when DNA that should be removed from the coding sequence is retained or DNA that should not be added is spliced in, resulting in frameshift mutations.
   (6) *Polymorphisms* are changes in the DNA sequence of a gene that often are not disease related and occur at variable frequency in the general population.
 4. Chromosomal abnormalities.
   a. *Translocations* refer to segments of one chromosome that break off and attach themselves to other chromosomes, potentially resulting in altered gene expression.
   b. *Aneuploidy* is an abnormal number of chromosomes.
   c. *Loss of heterozygosity* refers to the loss of a segment of both copies of a chromosome.
 E. Mendelian inheritance.
 1. *Dominant* inheritance requires only one altered copy of a gene to result in disease expression (Figure 22-4).
 2. *Recessive* inheritance requires two altered copies of a gene, one from each parent, to result in disease expression (Figure 22-5).
 3. *X-linked* inheritance is associated with the inheritance of genes located on the X chromosome. Men carry one X and one Y chromosome; genes on their X chromosome are hemizygous (having only one copy of a chromosome pair), and so a mutation in a gene on an X chromosome in a man can result in disease expression.

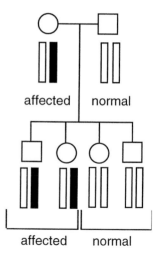

FIGURE 22-4 ■ Autosomal dominant inheritance.

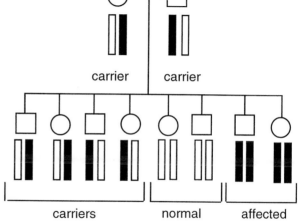

FIGURE 22-5 ■ Autosomal recessive inheritance.

III. Key technical characteristics of predisposition genetic testing (Vogelstein & Kinzler, 2002).
A. Techniques for identifying mutations.
1. *Direct sequencing* determines the sequence of the gene being tested and detects sequence changes in the regions being analyzed.
a. Detects sequence changes in the regions being analyzed but can miss mutations that are outside the coding region or mutations that are large genomic rearrangements or large deletions.
2. *Microarray* (Figure 22-6) (Ramaswamy & Golub, 2002).
a. Involves the attachment of large numbers (hundreds to thousands) of segments of DNA, RNA, protein, or tissue to slides at a precise location, which is followed by the application of a fluorescent label. The biosample under study is then processed so the genetic material of the sample binds to the genetic material on the slide. The slide is then scanned to measure the brightness of each fluorescent dot. The brighter the dot, the greater the activity.
b. Used for mutation detection as well as gene expression.

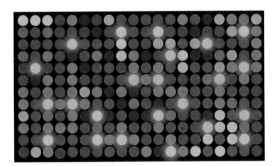

FIGURE 22-6 ■ Microarray. (Used with permission of U.S. Department of Energy Human Genome Program, http://www.ornl.gov/hgmis.)

    3. *Allele specific oligonucleotide (ASO).*
        a. Detects one single specific mutation that involves a short sequence of DNA.
    4. *Single-strand confirmation polymorphism analysis (SSCP).*
        a. Sequence change into DNA alters the size and/or shape of a DNA fragment, which can be detected by SSCP on a gel.
        b. Altered gene produces a band that is different from a normal gene.
        c. SSCP easily detects insertions or deletions of four or more bases of DNA; however, mutations that change one base for another without altering the length of the DNA fragment are difficult to detect.
    5. *Protein truncation assay* refers to an analysis of coding DNA, which is directly translated in the laboratory into protein.
        a. Shortened proteins can then be detected on a gel, based on the mobility differences between larger and smaller proteins.
        b. Sensitive for the detection of mutations in which the sequence change results in a shortened form of the protein but does not detect other types of mutations.
  B. Considerations in genetic testing laboratory selection (ASCO, 2003).
    1. Laboratories where genetic testing is performed should meet the following criteria:
        a. Clinical Laboratory Improvement Act (CLIA)–approved laboratory.
          (1) Does not evaluate proficiency of DNA testing.
        b. Laboratory director certified by the American Board of Medical Genetics.
    2. Resources for identifying laboratories performing testing include the following:
        a. Gene Tests website, http://www.geneclinics.org. Offers a clinic and laboratory directory as well as summaries on specific genetic syndromes.
IV. Common hereditary cancer syndromes and cancer susceptibility genes.
  A. The common hereditary cancer syndromes, clinical manifestations, inheritance patterns, and genes are outlined in Table 22-1 (Lindor & Greene, 1998).
  B. Features of hereditary cancer (Schneider, 2002; Tranin et al., 2003).
    1. Early age of cancer onset.
    2. Evidence of autosomal dominant inheritance pattern.
    3. Cancer in two or more close relatives.
    4. Bilaterality in paired organs.
    5. Multiple primary cancers in a single individual.
    6. Constellation of cancer in the family; part of a known hereditary cancer syndrome.

TABLE 22-1
Common Hereditary Cancer Syndromes and Cancer Susceptibility Genes

Syndrome	Clinical Manifestations	Gene	Testing Available	Mode of Inheritance
Ataxia-telangiectasia	Cerebral ataxia, oculocutaneous telangiectasias, radiation hypersensitivity, leukemia, lymphoma, breast cancer, other solid tumors	*ATM*	Available	Autosomal recessive
Breast/ovarian cancer syndrome	Breast cancer, ovarian cancer, fallopian tube, pancreas, melanoma, prostate cancer, colon cancer	*BRCA1* *BRCA2*	Available	Autosomal dominant
Cowden syndrome	Multiple mucocutaneous lesions, vitiligo, angiomas, benign proliferative disease of multiple organ systems, breast cancer, thyroid cancer, colon cancer, macrocephaly	*PTEN*	Available	Autosomal dominant
Familial adenomatous polyposis	Colon polyposis (adenomas), desmoid tumors, congenital hypertrophy of the retinal pigment, osteomas, thyroid cancer, small bowel cancer, hepatoblastoma	*APC*	Available	Autosomal dominant
Fanconi's anemia	Leukemia; squamous cell carcinomas of head/neck; esophageal cancer; hepatoma; hepatic adenoma; cancers of the cervix, vulva, anus; myelodysplastic syndrome	*FACC*	Available	Autosomal recessive
Gorlin's syndrome	Basal cell carcinoma, medulloblastoma, fibrosarcoma, ovarian cancer, odontogenic keratocyst, palmar/plantar pits, macrocephaly	*PTCH*	Available	Autosomal dominant
Hereditary non-polyposis colorectal cancer (Lynch syndromes)	Cancers of the colon, rectum, stomach, small intestine, liver and biliary tract, brain, endometrium, ovary; transitional cell carcinoma of the ureters and renal pelvis	*MSH2* *MLH1* *MSH6* *PMS1* *PMS2*	Available	Autosomal dominant
Li-Fraumeni syndrome	Breast cancer, sarcoma, brain tumors, leukemia, adrenocortical carcinoma	*p53*	Available	Autosomal dominant
Melanoma	Melanoma, astrocytoma, pancreatic cancer	*p16*	Available	Autosomal dominant
Muir-Torre syndrome	GI and GU cancers, sebaceous gland carcinomas, keratoacanthomas, breast cancer, benign breast tumors	*MSH2* *MLH1*	Available	Autosomal dominant
Multiple endocrine neoplasm, type I	Pancreatic islet cell tumors, parathyroid disease, adrenal cortical tumors, carcinoids, lipomas	*MEN1*	Available	Autosomal dominant
Multiple endocrine neoplasm, type II	Medullary thyroid cancer, pheochromocytoma, parathyroid disease	*RET*	Available	Autosomal dominant

(Continued)

TABLE 22-1
Common Hereditary Cancer Syndromes and Cancer Susceptibility Genes—cont'd

Syndrome	Clinical Manifestations	Gene	Testing Available	Mode of Inheritance
Neuro-fibromatosis	Neurofibromatosis, optic gliomas, meningioma, ependymomas, astrocytomas, schwannomas, café-au-lait macules	*NF1* *NF2*	Available	Autosomal dominant
Prostate cancer	Prostate, other cancer risks not fully defined	Several linkage sites and candidate genes are under study: *1q24-25, 1q42.2-43, Xq27-28, 1p36, 20q13, 17p*	Participation in research studies available	Varied: autosomal dominant, X linked
Retinoblastoma	Retinoblastoma, soft tissue sarcoma and osteosarcoma, lipomas	*RB1*	Available	Autosomal dominant
von Hippel–Lindau disease	Renal cell cancer; hemangioblastomas of brain, spinal cord, and retina; renal cysts; pheochromocytomas; endolymphatic tumors	*VHL*	Available	Autosomal dominant
Wilms' tumor	Wilms' tumor, aniridia, embryologic tumors	*WT1*	Available	Autosomal dominant
Xeroderma pigmentosum	Basal and squamous cell skin cancer; melanoma; brain, lung, and gastric cancers; leukemia; conjunctival papillomas; actinic keratosis; lid epitheliomas; keratoacanthomas; angiomas; fibromas	*RAD2*		Autosomal recessive

From Lindor NM, Greene MH: The concise handbook of family cancer syndromes, *J Natl Cancer Inst* 90:1039-1071, 1998.
GI, Gastrointestinal; *GU*, genitourinary.

C. Indications for cancer predisposition testing (ASCO, 2003).
 1. Criteria for predisposition genetic testing vary, depending on the gene tested.
  a. Universal criteria for predisposition genetic testing include the following:
   (1) Confirmed family history consistent with the hereditary cancer syndrome.
   (2) Informed consent by the client to be tested.
   (3) Test that can be interpreted once performed.
   (4) Test will be used to assist in medical decision making or will assist in diagnosis of a condition.

2. Not every client is appropriate for predisposition genetic testing for inherited cancer susceptibility.

D. Outcomes for cancer predisposition testing (Schneider, 2002; Tranin et al., 2003).

1. Predictive value of a negative test result varies depending on whether there is a known genetic mutation in the family.

a. Negative test result in the presence of a known genetic mutation indicates that the client is within the general population risk for the specific cancer or cancers associated with the mutation in that branch of the family.

(1) However, family history from the other parent and other personal risk factors still influence the risk of developing cancer.

b. A negative result with no known family genetic mutation can occur because of the following:

(1) Identifying a mutation in a cancer susceptibility gene may not be possible because of the limited sensitivity of the techniques used.

(2) Function of the gene can be affected by a mutation in a different gene.

(3) Cancer in the family may be associated with a cancer susceptibility gene other than the one tested.

(4) Cancer in the family is not the result of a germline genetic mutation.

2. Predictive value of a positive test result varies depending on the type of genetic mutation identified and the degree of certainty that the function of the gene has been affected.

a. *Penetrance* refers to the cancer risks associated with the specific genetic mutation. Penetrance may be different for different genetic mutations in the same cancer susceptibility gene.

b. A mutation of uncertain clinical significance is identified.

(1) Mutation is identified in which the association with cancer risk cannot be established.

V. Potential therapeutic interventions (Collins et al., 2003; Loud et al., 2002).

A. Pharmacogenetics (Innocenti & Ratain, 2002; Weinshilbourn, 2003).

1. The genetic basis for differences in treatment response that can be used to individualize treatment.

2. Individualized treatment based on the genetic characteristics of the tumor.

3. Drugs that are developed specifically aimed at the genetic change and/or altered protein product.

B. Proteomics (Patterson & Aebersold, 2003).

1. Analysis of the structure, composition, and function of proteins.

2. Aids in the diagnosis and enhances the understanding of the biologic basis of cancer.

C. Somatic gene therapy.

1. Introduction of a functioning gene into the somatic cells to replace missing or defective genes or to provide a new cellular function.

2. Investigational trials using somatic gene therapy for a variety of cancers are ongoing.

D. Germline gene therapy.

1. Introduction of a functioning gene into the egg or sperm to prevent transmission of a genetic mutation.

2. Germline gene therapy is not available. Germline gene therapy raises several ethical, legal, and social concerns.

VI. Medical management issues associated with the care of individuals harboring a cancer susceptibility gene (Schneider, 2002; Tranin et al., 2003).

   A. Management of cancer risk falls into four basic categories.

   1. Surveillance is monitoring to detect cancer as early as possible, when the chances for cure are greatest.

   2. Prophylactic surgery is the removal of as much of the tissue at risk as possible to reduce the risk of developing a cancer.

   3. Chemoprevention involves taking a medicine, vitamin, or other substance to reduce the risk of cancer.

   4. Risk avoidance is the avoidance of exposures that may increase the risk of certain cancers.

   B. Cancer risk management strategies available to individuals at high risk for cancer because of a mutation in a cancer susceptibility gene vary according to the gene and/or specific gene mutation identified.

   1. Each strategy has varying degrees of risks, benefits, and limitations as well as varying levels of evidence specific to the intervention.

VII. Ethical, legal, and social issues associated with genetic information.

   A. Predisposition genetic testing can have psychologic consequences, some of which could impact subsequent health behaviors and family communication (Scanlon & Fibison, 1995; Schneider, 2002; Tranin et al., 2003).

   1. Survivor guilt is often observed in clients who have not inherited the genetic mutation that is present in other close family members.

   2. Transmitter guilt is often observed when a family member passes on the genetic mutation to one of his/her offspring.

   3. Heightened anxiety can result when clients learn that they are at a substantially increased risk for developing cancer or another primary lesion.

   4. Depression and anger can occur regardless of genetic status.

   5. Personal identity issues result because genetic information involves the very essence of an individual.

   6. Regret of previous decisions can occur in clients who have made major decisions based on their perceived cancer risk and testing results are inconsistent with what they had previously thought.

   7. Uncertainty occurs because predisposition genetic testing does not provide information about if or when cancer develops. In many instances there is no proven risk-reducing strategy.

   8. Intrafamilial issues arise because predisposition genetic testing affects all family members. These issues include but are not limited to the following:

   a. Coercion regarding testing, disclosure of testing results to family members, and cancer risk management approaches.

   b. Effect of the genetic information on the partner who is not at risk physically but whose children may be impacted.

   9. Stigmatization can occur both within the family and within the individual's social network.

   B. Predisposition genetic testing also has social implications (Hall & Rich, 2000; Schneider, 2002; Tranin et al., 2003).

   1. Financial considerations.

   a. Predisposition genetic testing can be very expensive. Not all insurers will cover testing and counseling.

   b. Insurers may be reluctant to cover enhanced surveillance programs unless there is proven efficacy.

   c. Insurers may not be willing to cover the expense of prophylactic surgery unless it has proven benefit.

2. Quality assurance of laboratory testing is not certain because there is no regulation beyond CLIA approval for molecular laboratories performing testing (ASCO, 2003).
3. Availability and quality assurance of genetic counseling are of concern given the small number of trained providers in cancer genetics.

C. Legal issues for the client undergoing predisposition testing (Scanlon & Fibison, 1995; Schneider, 2002; Tranin et al., 2003).
   1. Insurance discrimination can occur for those harboring an altered cancer susceptibility gene because they may be considered as having a preexisting condition or may be too high a risk to insure (Rothenberg, 1995).
      a. Health insurance.
      b. Life insurance.
      c. Disability insurance.
      d. Long-term care insurance.
   2. State and federal legislative approaches have already been proposed or enacted, depending on the issue and state.
      a. Health Insurance Portability and Accountability Act (HIPAA) (1996) is a federal law that states that genetic information cannot be used as a preexisting condition nor to determine eligibility for insurance.
         (1) This protection only applies to group and self-funded plans.
         (2) This law does not protect against rate hikes, against access of insurers to an individual's genetic information, or from the insurer requiring genetic testing as a condition of insurance coverage.
   3. Self-insured employers are also exempt from state laws and regulations on health insurance because of the Employee Retirement Income Security Act of 1974 (ERISA), which governs employer pension plans as well as other benefits.
   4. Individuals may face discrimination from employers (Rothenberg et al., 1997).
      a. In March 1995, the U.S. Equal Employment Opportunity Commission released guidelines on the definition of "disability" under the Americans with Disabilities Act (ADA), which is now extended to include discrimination based on genetic information.
         (1) This set of guidelines is not law but simply is an interpretation of the language of the ADA and may be overturned in a court of law (U.S. Equal Employment Opportunity Commission, 1995).
   5. Risk of discrimination can also occur with education and housing.

D. Informed consent should precede genetic testing and consist of the following (ASHG, 1996; Geller et al., 1997; International Society of Nurses in Genetics, 2000; Rieger & Pentz, 1999; Schneider, 2002; Tranin et al., 2003):
   1. Purpose of the genetic test.
   2. Motivation for testing.
   3. Risks of genetic testing.
   4. Benefits of genetic testing.
   5. Limitations of genetic testing.
   6. Inheritance pattern of the gene being tested.
      a. Risk of misidentified paternity if applicable.
   7. Accuracy and sensitivity of genetic testing method.
   8. Outcomes of genetic testing.
   9. Confidentiality of genetic testing results.

       10. Possibility of discrimination.

       11. Alternatives to genetic testing.

       12. How testing will impact medical decision making.

       13. Cost of testing.

       14. Right to refuse.

       15. Testing in children (ASCO, 2003; Hoffman & Wulfsberg, 1995; Nelson et al., 2001).

    E. Genetic technology raises legal liability issues for the health care provider (ASCO, 2003; Schneider, 2002; Tranin et al., 2003).

       1. Privacy and confidentiality (International Society of Nurses in Genetics, 2001).

         a. Genetic information of all types should be handled in a confidential manner to prevent unauthorized access.

       2. Genetic testing and release of genetic information should be preceded by education, counseling, and informed consent.

       3. Health care providers may have a duty to inform clients regarding their potential for increased cancer risk because of an inherited susceptibility and the availability of predisposition genetic testing.

Assessment

  I. Assessment of a client with a family history of cancer.

    A. A pedigree is a graphic illustration of biologic relationships in a family as well as disease history (Figure 22-7) (Bennett et al., 1995; Schneider, 2002; Tranin et al., 2003).

       1. Components of a pedigree.

         a. Bilineal three-generation family history.

         b. Cancer history for each family member including the following:

           (1) Primary site.

           (2) Age at diagnosis.

           (3) Laterality in paired organs such as breasts, eyes.

         c. Previous prophylactic surgery to reduce cancer risk.

         d. Other health problems.

         e. Racial and ethnic background.

         f. Consanguinity.

         g. Pregnancy loss.

         h. Birth defects.

         i. Early infant death.

         j. Environmental and occupational exposures.

       2. Confirmation of the family history.

         a. Documentation of reported cancers by pathology records or the equivalent is suggested because evidence exists demonstrating that the further the relationship is from the affected family member, the more likely the primary site and age at diagnosis of cancer may not be accurate.

    B. Personal health history.

       1. Complete review of systems.

       2. Cancer history.

       3. Risk factor history, including exposures to environmental or occupational carcinogens.

       4. Current surveillance plan.

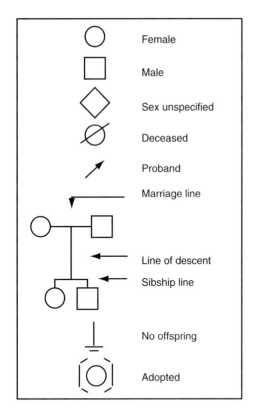

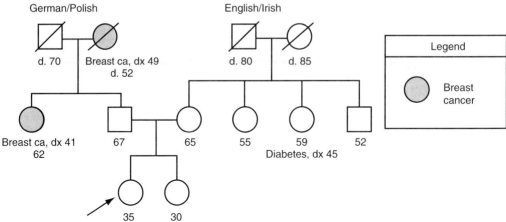

FIGURE 22-7 ■ Common pedigree symbols and sample pedigree. (From Bennett RL, Steinhaus KA, Uhrich SB, et al: Recommendations for standardized human pedigree nomenclature, *Am J Hum Genet* 56:745-752, 1995.)

    C. Psychosocial history.
        1. Perception of cancer risk.
        2. Beliefs about etiology of cancer in the family.
        3. Prior mental illness.
        4. Current support mechanisms.
        5. Previous patterns of stress management.
        6. Motivation for genetic testing.
        7. Insurance and employment status.

Nursing Diagnoses

  I. Deficient knowledge related to cancer genetics.
 II. Ineffective health maintenance.
III. Ineffective coping or altered family processes.

Outcome Identification

  I. Client and family, consistent with cultural, educational, and emotional status, describe the following:
  - **A.** Genetic basis of cancer.
  - **B.** Risks and benefits of predisposition genetic testing.
  - **C.** Alternatives for cancer risk management.
 II. Client identifies factors that may decrease or increase cancer risk.
  - **A.** Client describes cancer warning signals and the cancer risk management alternatives.
  - **B.** Client describes health promotion activities.
  - **C.** Client identifies the agencies in which cancer risk management services can be obtained.
  - **D.** Client describes and demonstrates self-examination procedures.
III. Client and family, consistent with cultural, physical, and psychosocial domain, do the following:
  - **A.** Identify personal and community resources that enhance coping.
  - **B.** Use identified coping strategies that lead to effective outcomes.
  - **C.** Participate in care and decision making.
  - **D.** Identify alternatives for coping when existing strategies are ineffective.
  - **E.** Establish contact with a member of the health care team as needed.
  - **F.** Communicate feelings about inherited cancer susceptibility.

Planning and Implementation

  I. Interventions to assist the client and family to understand cancer genetics and predisposition genetic testing.
  - **A.** Describe the organization and function of genetic material and the role of genetics in carcinogenesis.
  - **B.** Assess the client's beliefs about the etiology of cancer in the family and correct misconceptions.
  - **C.** Describe the process for cancer risk evaluation and predisposition genetic testing.
  - **D.** Discuss the risks and benefits of predisposition genetic testing.
 II. Interventions to decrease perceived and definite barriers to cancer risk management.
  - **A.** Educate and monitor the performance of self-examination techniques.
  - **B.** Provide education on the benefits of cancer risk management.
  - **C.** Facilitate the reimbursement for cancer risk management procedures.
  - **D.** Encourage communication regarding fears and concerns.
III. Interventions to enhance coping and adaptation.
  - **A.** Refer the client and/or family to community support services.
  - **B.** Refer the client and/or family to professional counseling services when indicated.
  - **C.** Encourage the use of coping strategies that have previously been effective.

Evaluation

The oncology nurse systematically and regularly evaluates the client's and/or family's responses to interventions in order to determine progress toward the achievement of expected outcomes. Relevant data are collected, and actual findings are compared with expected findings. Nursing diagnoses, outcomes, and plans of care are reviewed and revised as necessary.

REFERENCES

American Society of Clinical Oncology (ASCO). (2003). American Society of Clinical Oncology policy statement update: Genetic testing for cancer susceptibility. *Journal of Clinical Oncology 21*, 2397-2406.

American Society of Human Genetics (ASHG). (1996). American Society of Human Genetics Report: Statement on informed consent for genetic research. *American Journal of Human Genetics, 59*, 471-474.

Balmain, A., Gray, J., & Ponder, B. (2003). The genetics and genomics of cancer. *Nature Genetics 33*(Suppl.), 238-244.

Bennett, R.L., Steinhaus, K.A., Uhrich, S.B., et al. (1995). Recommendations for standardized human pedigree nomenclature. *American Journal of Human Genetics 56*, 745-752.

Collins, F.S., Green, E.D., Guttmacher, A.E., & Guyer, M.S. (2003). A vision for the future of genomics research: A blueprint for the genomic era. *Nature 422*, 835-847.

Geller, G., Botkin, J.R., Green, M.J., et al. (1997). Genetic testing for susceptibility to adult-onset cancer: The process and content of informed consent. *Journal of the American Medical Association 277*(18), 1467-1474.

Hall, M., & Rich, S. (2000). Genetic information and health insurance. *American Journal of Human Genetics 66*, 293-307.

Hoffman, D.E., & Wulfsberg, E.A. (1995). Testing children for genetic predispositions: Is it in their best interest? *Journal of Law Medicine and Ethics 23*, 331-344.

Innocenti, F., & Ratain, M.J. (2002). Update on pharmacogenetics in cancer chemotherapy. *European Journal of Cancer 38*, 639-644.

International Society of Nurses in Genetics. (2000). Informed decision-making and consent: The role of nursing. Retrieved March 1, 2003, 2003 from the World Wide Web: http://www.globalreferrals.com/consent.htm.

International Society of Nurses in Genetics. (2001). Privacy and confidentiality of genetic information: The role of the nurse. Retrieved March 1, 2003 from the World Wide Web: http://www.globalreferrals.com/privacy.htm.

Lindor, N.M., & Greene, M.H. (1998). The concise handbook of family cancer syndromes. *Journal of the National Cancer Institute 90*, 1039-1071.

Loud, J.T., Peters, J.A., Fraser, M., & Jenkins, J. (2002). Applications of advances in molecular biology and genomics to clinical cancer care. *Cancer Nursing 25*, 110-122.

Nelson, R.M., Botkin, J., Kodish, E.D., et al. (2001). Ethical issues with genetic testing in pediatrics. *Pediatrics 107*, 1451-1455.

Patterson, S.D., & Aebersold, R.H. (2003). Proteomics: The first decade and beyond. *Nature Genetics 33*(Suppl.), 311-323.

Ramaswamy, S., & Golub, T. (2002). DNA microarrays in clinical oncology. *Journal of Clinical Oncology 20*, 1932-1941.

Rieger, P., & Pentz, R. (1999). Genetic testing and informed consent. *Seminars in Oncology Nursing 15*, 104-115.

Rothenberg, K.H. (1995). Genetic information and health insurance: State legislative approaches. *Journal of Law Medicine and Ethics 23*, 312-319.

Rothenberg, K.H., Fuller, B., Rothstein, M., et al. (1997). Genetic information and the workplace. *Science 275*, 1755-1757.

Scanlon, C., & Fibison, W. (1995). *Managing genetic information: Implications for nursing education.* Washington, DC: American Nurses Association.

Schneider, K.A. (Ed.). (2002). *Counseling about cancer: Strategies for genetic counselors* (2nd ed.). Dennisport, MA: Graphic Illusions.

Tranin, A.S. (1997). Genetics and cancer. *Seminars in Oncology Nursing 12*, 67-144.

Tranin, A.S., Masny, A., & Jenkins, J. (Eds.). (2003). *Genetics in oncology practice: Cancer risk assessment.* Pittsburgh: Oncology Nursing Society.

U.S. Equal Employment Opportunity Commission. (1995). *Compliance manual section 902: Definition of the term "disability."* Washington, D.C. Retrieved July 29, 2004 from the World Wide Web: http://www.eeoc.gov/policy/docs/902cm.html.

Vogelstein, B., & Kinzler, K.W. (Eds.). (2002). *The genetic basis of human cancer* (2nd ed.). New York: McGraw-Hill.

Weinshilbourn, R. (2003). Inheritance and drug response. *New England Journal of Medicine 386,* 529-549.

23 Nursing Care of the Client with Breast Cancer

MARJORIE BERNICE

Theory

I. Physiology and pathophysiology.
  A. Anatomy of the breast.
    1. Adult female breast lies on the anterior chest wall between the sternum and midaxillary line from the second to sixth ribs.
    2. The stroma and subcutaneous tissue of the breast comprises connective tissue, nerves, blood vessels, lymphatic vessels, and fat (Osborne, 2000).
    3. The breast parenchyma consists of six to nine independent ductal systems, each converging at the nipple (Love, 2000).
    4. The terminal ductal-lobular unit (TDLU) is the hormonally sensitive lactational unit of the breast (Kuhns & Ackerman, 2002) and is the site from which the majority of malignant lesions arise (Bartow, 2002).
    5. Lymphatic fluid flows outward toward the lymph nodes, with the majority flowing to the axillary nodes.
  B. Histopathology.
    1. Breast cancer is a heterogeneous disease with 24 distinct histologic subtypes (Greene et al., 2002).
    2. Noninvasive breast cancer.
      a. Also called in-situ cancer or "precancer."
      b. Confined to the duct or lobule and has not spread into blood or lymphatic systems.
      c. Ductal carcinoma in situ (DCIS).
        (1) Also referred to as intraductal, stage 0, preinvasive.
        (2) Proliferation of cancerous cells within the mammary ductal-lobular system without invasion beyond the basement membrane.
        (3) Precursor lesion of invasive ductal carcinoma; woman with DCIS has a tenfold increased risk of developing invasive ductal carcinoma (Page et al., 2002).
        (4) Usually is not palpable and is often detected only by mammogram or as an incidental finding in biopsy of another lesion.
        (5) Categorized as micropapillary, papillary, solid, cribriform, or comedo; comedo lesions are more aggressive and carry a higher probability of recurrence and evolution to invasive carcinoma.
      d. Lobular carcinoma in situ (LCIS).
        (1) Also called lobular neoplasia.
        (2) Commonly multicentric.
        (3) Usually an incidental finding in biopsy, not detected by mammogram or clinical examination.

(4) Considered a marker for increased risk of invasive breast cancer in either breast rather than a premalignant lesion.

(5) Women with LCIS have a 1% per year risk of developing an invasive cancer in either breast (Morrow & Schnitt, 2000).

3. Invasive breast cancers.
   a. Also referred to as infiltrating.
   b. No longer completely contained within the basement membrane of the duct or lobule and has grown into surrounding tissue.
   c. Capable of spreading to other parts of the body.
   d. Subtypes.
      (1) Invasive ductal carcinoma—most common type, accounts for up to 70% to 80% of all breast cancers (National Cancer Institute [NCI], 2003).
      (2) Invasive lobular carcinoma—accounts for approximately 5% to 10% of all invasive breast cancers (Schnitt & Guidi, 2000).
      (3) Other less common types include tubular, papillary, mucinous, medullary, and cribriform.
      (4) Special manifestations.
         (a) Inflammatory.
            (i) Usually presents with sudden dramatic and diffuse inflammatory skin changes, often without a distinct mass.
            (ii) Classified as primary stage IIIB or greater.
            (iii) Most aggressive breast cancer; poor prognosis.
         (b) Paget's disease of the nipple.
            (i) Neoplastic eczematoid lesion of nipple-areolar complex.
            (ii) Usually associated with an underlying ductal carcinoma.

4. Factors affecting prognosis and treatment decisions (Clark, 2000).
   a. Lymph node status—lymph node positivity is associated with a poorer prognosis; prognosis progressively worsens as the number of positive lymph nodes increases.
   b. Tumor size—larger tumors are associated with an increased probability of nodal involvement and a poorer prognosis.
   c. Nuclear grade—high-grade, poorly differentiated tumors have a worse prognosis.
   d. Hormone receptor status—estrogen-receptor (ER) and progesterone receptor (PR) (ER/PR)–negative tumors are associated with a less favorable prognosis.
   e. Histologic type—inflammatory breast cancer carries the least favorable prognosis; noninvasive cancers have an excellent prognosis.
   f. Other histologic features—presence of tumor necrosis, peritumoral lymphatic or vascular invasion, and angiogenesis (tumor vascularity measured by microvessel count) are unfavorable prognostic factors.
   g. Deoxyribonucleic acid (DNA) ploidy—tumors with abnormal complement of DNA are termed *aneuploid* and are associated with a worse prognosis.
   h. Tumor proliferative indices associated with poor prognosis.
      (1) S-phase fraction (SPF).
      (2) Mitotic index (MI).
      (3) Thymidine labeling index (TLI).
      (4) Ki-67 monoclonal antibody antigen marker.
   i. Investigational factors associated with poor prognosis.

(1) Oncogenes (HER-2/neu, epidermal growth factor receptor gene).

(2) Tumor suppressor genes *(p53, nm23)*.

(3) Proteases (cathepsin D, urokinase plasminogen activator).

C. Metastatic patterns.

    1. Local spread within the breast occurs by direct infiltration into parenchyma, along mammary ducts, or via breast lymphatics.

    2. Principal site of regional node involvement is axillary; likelihood of involvement is directly related to tumor size.

    3. It takes approximately 5 years for a single cancer cell to multiply to 1 billion cells (1 cm); risk of systemic spread is believed to begin after tumor reaches size of 1 cm.

    4. Distant spread.

        a. Occurs via hematogenous or lymphatic pathways.

        b. Major sites of metastases are bone, lung, liver, and brain (Greene et al., 2002).

        c. Bone is the most frequent site of distant metastasis.

D. Trends in epidemiology.

    1. Most common cancer among women worldwide.

    2. Projected to account for 32% of all new cancer cases among American women in 2003 (Jemal et al., 2003).

    3. Projected to account for 15% of cancer deaths in American women in 2003; leading cause of cancer death for women between ages 20 and 59 years, second highest cancer killer of American women overall (Jemal et al., 2003).

    4. U.S. incidence rates increased by more than 40% between 1973 and 1998 (Howe et al., 2001).

    5. Increase in incidence may be largely, but not fully, attributable to increase in screening.

    6. U.S. age-adjusted incidence rates vary by ethnic group (Figure 23-1); highest among Caucasian, Hawaiian, and African American women and lowest among Korean, American Indian, and Vietnamese women (Clegg et al., 2002).

    7. Male breast cancer accounts for less than 1% of all breast cancers (Jemal et al., 2003).

II. Principles of medical management.

A. Screening procedures.

    1. Breast self-examination (BSE).

        a. American Cancer Society (ACS) recommends instruction and information about benefits and limitations of BSE be provided to all women beginning in their twenties (Smith et al., 2003).

        b. Effectiveness questionable since mortality reduction has not been demonstrated (Thomas et al., 2002).

        c. Sensitivity may be improved with use of various techniques and devices.

            (1) MammaCare is a systematic BSE skill training method.

            (2) The BSE Pad is a reusable pad approved by the U.S. Food and Drug Administration (FDA) and composed of ultrathin polyurethane with a small amount of lubricant sealed inside designed to reduce friction and therefore enhance tactile sensitivity during BSE.

    2. Clinical breast examination (CBE).

        a. ACS recommends CBE as part of a periodic health examination at least every 3 years between ages 20 and 39 years, then preferably annually from age 40 years (Smith et al., 2003).

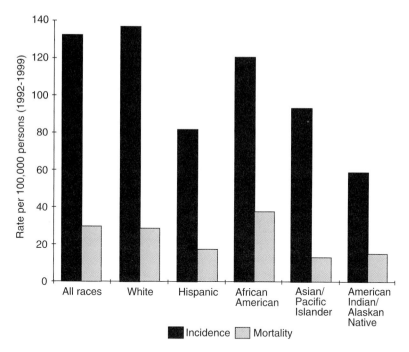

FIGURE 23-1 ■ U.S. breast cancer age-adjusted incidence and mortality rates 1992 to 1999. (Data from Ries L.A.G. et al: *SEER cancer statistics review, 1973-1999,* Bethesda, MD, 2002, National Cancer Institute. http://seer.cancer.gov/csr/1973_1999/.)

    b. Additive benefit when used in conjunction with mammography (Bobo et al., 2000).
  3. Mammography.
    a. There is a lack of consensus regarding optimal screening schedule.
      (1) ACS recommends annual mammograms for women age 40 years and over (Smith et al., 2003).
      (2) NCI recommends screening every 1 to 2 years for women age 40 years and over (NCI, 2002).
    b. Federal law (Mammography Quality Standards Act) mandates strict quality standards and certification of mammography facilities.
    c. BI-RADS system (American College of Radiology, 1998) provides a standardized lexicon for reporting results (Table 23-1).
    d. False negative rate is 10% to 15%.
    e. There are conflicting analyses regarding efficacy and cost-effectiveness.
      (1) Meta-analyses of mammogram screening trials have shown a large reduction in breast cancer mortality (Humphrey et al., 2002; Tabar et al., 2001).
      (2) Meta-analysis of Swedish and Canadian screening trials failed to find any evidence of reduced mortality (Olsen & Gotzsche, 2001; Miller et al., 2002).
  4. Mammography, BSE, and CBE are complementary screening modalities to be used in combination rather than singly.
  5. Screening decisions for older women should be individualized taking into account current health status and estimated life expectancy (Smith et al., 2003).

TABLE 23-1
Breast Imaging–Reporting and Data System (BI-RADS) Assessment Categories

Category	Assessment
0	Need additional imaging evaluation
1	Negative
2	Benign finding
3	Probably benign finding
4	Suspicious looking abnormality
5	Highly suggestive of malignancy

From American College of Radiology (ACR): *Breast Imaging Reporting and Data System (BI-RADS)*, Reston, VA, 1998: American College of Radiology, © 1998 by the American College of Radiology. Reprinted with permission of the American College of Radiology. No other representation of this material is authorized without expressed, written permission from the American College of Radiology.

6. New technology approved for general clinical use.
   a. Digital mammography—achieves higher resolution by computerizing, enhancing, and re-creating image.
   b. Computer-aided diagnosis (CAD)—computerized analysis of mammogram used by the radiologist as a "second opinion."
7. Ductal lavage is a promising new minimally invasive procedure to collect ductal cells for cytologic evaluation (Dooley et al., 2001; O'Shaughnessy et al., 2002).
   a. Presence of atypical cells indicates increased risk.
   b. Information useful for high-risk women.
8. Women at increased risk may benefit from screenings initiated earlier and done more frequently, as well as use of adjunctive imaging studies (Smith et al., 2003).
9. Adjunctive imaging studies.
   a. Ultrasonography.
      (1) Uses high-frequency sound waves to create an image.
      (2) Useful in distinguishing cystic from solid masses.
   b. Galactography (ductography).
      (1) Injection of contrast medium into the duct.
      (2) Useful in delineating the anatomy of the affected duct in cases of a spontaneous single-duct nipple discharge.
   c. Investigational imaging methods—may be useful in special circumstances but cost and technical limitations preclude routine use (Sumkin & Hardesty, 2001).
      (1) Magnetic resonance imaging (MRI).
      (2) Positron emission tomography (PET).
      (3) Scintimammography (technetium-99m sestamibi scanning).
B. Diagnostic procedures.
   1. Biopsy (Table 23-2).
      a. Microscopic evaluation is required to make the diagnosis of breast cancer.
      b. Considerations for method of biopsy include size and location of lesion, likelihood of malignancy, potential for follow-up, cost, and client preference.

TABLE 23-2
Breast Biopsy Techniques

Type of Biopsy	Method of Analysis	Palpable Lesion	Nonpalpable Lesion
Needle	Cytology	Fine-needle aspiration (FNA)	Stereotactic FNA
	Histology	Core biopsy	Stereotactic core biopsy (SCB)
Open	Histology	Incisional/excisional biopsy	Needle localization breast biopsy (NLBB)

    c. Two-step approach separates biopsy from definitive surgery and is preferred because it allows the client an opportunity to explore treatment alternatives after the diagnosis of cancer is made.

    d. Cytology evaluation.

        (1) Fine-needle aspiration (FNA)—insertion of 21- to 23-gauge needle into lesion for aspiration of cellular material.

        (2) Combination of mammography, physical examination, and FNA is referred to as "triple test" and is more reliable than each alone (Donegan, 2002).

    e. Histology evaluation.

        (1) Skin biopsy—punch biopsy may be diagnostic for Paget's disease or inflammatory carcinoma.

        (2) Needle core biopsy—needle with large lumen (usually 14 gauge) is used to remove a core of tissue.

        (3) Incisional biopsy—surgical removal of a portion of tumor through skin incision.

        (4) Excisional biopsy—surgical removal of entire tumor, generally with margin of normal tissue, through a skin incision.

    f. Core biopsy has higher sensitivity, higher specificity, and lower inadequate sample rate compared with FNA.

    g. Nonpalpable lesions require localization using ultrasound or mammographic guidance before biopsy.

        (1) Stereotactic localization involves use of specially designed computerized mammography equipment to triangulate the location of a nonpalpable abnormality for needle aspiration, core needle biopsy, or open biopsy.

        (2) Automated spring-loaded guns require separate needle insertions to obtain each sample.

        (3) Large-gauge directional vacuum suction probes facilitate removal of multiple contiguous cores of tissue from a targeted site via a single insertion (Dershaw, 2003).

C. Staging methods and procedures.

    1. Staging workup may include the following:

        a. Chest radiograph.

        b. Computed tomography (CT) of abdomen or liver ultrasound.

        c. Bone scan.

    2. Staging classification (Greene et al., 2002) (Figure 23-2).

        a. Stage 0—carcinoma in situ.

        b. Stage I—tumor diameter under 2 cm with negative nodes.

        c. Stage II—tumor diameter under 5 cm with positive axillary nodes or tumor over 5 cm with negative nodes.

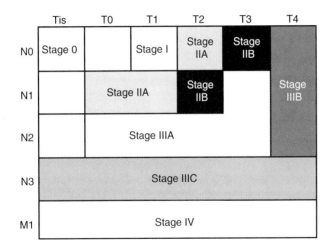

FIGURE 23-2 ■ Graphic for determining TNM stage based on T, N, and M components. *T*, Tumor; *N*, nodes; *M*, metastasis. (From Sugg SL, Donegan WL: Staging and prognosis. In Donegan WL, Spratt JS, editors: *Cancer of the breast*, ed 5, Philadelphia, 2002, WB Saunders, p. 484.)

    d. Stage III—tumor diameter over 5 cm with positive nodes or tumor of any size with direct extension to chest wall or skin; positive infraclavicular, supraclavicular, or internal mammary nodes; or axillary lymph nodes that are fixed or matted.

    e. Stage IV—any distant metastasis.

D. Treatment strategies.

    1. Individualized treatment is based on multiple factors, including stage, histologic type, prognostic indicators, hormone receptors, and client factors.

    2. Breast cancer management usually involves both local and systemic treatment.

    3. Multidisciplinary team approach provides comprehensive evaluation, treatment, education, support services, collaboration among treating disciplines, and coordination of care to optimize client outcomes and convenience (Link, 2000).

    4. Local treatments.

        a. Goal is to remove or destroy cancer cells in the breast area.

        b. Surgical treatments (Table 23-3).

            (1) Mastectomy—removes entire breast.

            (2) Breast conservation therapy (BCT)—preserves breast by removing only the tumor and surrounding tissue and, in cases of invasive cancer, is usually followed by radiation therapy (RT) to the breast (Table 23-4).

                (a) BCT with RT is considered standard treatment for women with early-stage breast cancer (Morrow et al., 2002).

                (b) Survival rates for BCT with RT are equivalent to modified radical mastectomy (Morrow et al., 2002).

                (c) Contraindications to BCT (Box 23-1).

            (3) Surgical management of axillary lymph nodes.

                (a) Axillary node dissection (AND) is current gold standard for staging invasive breast cancer (Spillane & Sacks, 2000).

                (b) Sentinel lymph node biopsy (SLNB) is an alternate axillary staging method for early breast cancer currently under investigation.

TABLE 23-3
Breast Cancer Surgical Procedures

BREAST-CONSERVING SURGERIES*

Lumpectomy	Excision of tumor with small margin of normal tissue around it
Segmental resection (tylectomy, quadrantectomy, partial mastectomy)	Excision of tumor with a wider margin of surrounding tissue

MASTECTOMIES

Subcutaneous mastectomy	Removes all breast tissue except overlying skin and nipple-areolar complex
Skin-sparing mastectomy	Removes above plus limited overlying "skin at risk" (biopsy scar, nipple-areolar complex)
Total (simple) mastectomy	Removes all breast tissue including skin, gland, nipple-areolar complex
Modified radical mastectomy	Removes above plus axillary lymph node dissection
Radical mastectomy	Removes above plus underlying pectoral muscles

*Usually done in conjunction with axillary node biopsy or dissection through a second incision.

TABLE 23-4
Comparison of Surgical Options for Early-Stage Invasive Breast Cancer

	Breast Conservation Therapy	Modified Radical Mastectomy
Removes only the malignant tumor and a small margin of surrounding normal tissue	X	
Removes the entire breast		X
Removes some lymph nodes from underarm	X	X
Includes radiation therapy following surgery	X	

Modified from V.M. Pressler, M.D., with permission of author.

      (i) Sentinel lymph node is the first lymph node to receive drainage from the cancer site.

     (ii) Lymphatic mapping technique uses blue dye and/or radiolabeled colloid injection to identify the sentinel node.

    (iii) SLNB spares cost and morbidity of AND in clients with clinically negative axillary nodes (Wong et al., 2002).

  (c) Local control following axillary node sampling with RT is equivalent to AND (Spillane & Sacks, 2000).

(4) Clinical trials underway to evaluate if timing of surgery during the luteal phase improves survival (NCI, 2003).

(5) Breast reconstruction.

BOX 23-1
CONTRAINDICATIONS TO BREAST CONSERVATION TREATMENT WITH RADIATION THERAPY

1. First- and second-trimester pregnancy*
2. Two or more gross malignancies in separate quadrants of the breast*
3. Prior therapeutic radiation to the breast*
4. Persistent positive margins*
5. History of collagen vascular disease†
6. Multiple gross tumors in same quadrant and indeterminate calcifications†
7. Large tumor in a small breast†
8. Large breast size†

Data from Morrow M et al: Standard for breast conservation therapy in the management of invasive breast carcinoma, *CA Cancer J Clin* 52:289, 2002.
*Absolute contraindication.
†Relative contraindication.

    (a) Surgically re-creates breast mound after mastectomy.
    (b) Has no adverse effect on survival or detection of local recurrence (Dixon, 2000).
    (c) May be immediate (at same time as mastectomy) or delayed (6 months or more following surgery).
    (d) Technique of skin-sparing mastectomy minimizes skin sacrifice and facilitates cosmesis following reconstruction (Robb, 2001).
    (e) Federal legislation passed in 1998 requires that insurers cover breast reconstruction as well as procedures necessary to restore symmetry with the opposite breast.
    (f) Methods using implants are simpler, are less costly, and require shorter recovery time compared with flap methods.
    (g) Tissue expander may be used to gradually stretch the skin to accommodate desired implant size.
    (h) Use of autologous tissue in flap methods results in a more natural texture and shape, but flap methods are more technically difficult and costly procedures.
        (i) Myocutaneous flaps (latissimus dorsi, transverse rectus abdominis myocutaneous [TRAM]) transfer skin and underlying muscle with blood supply intact.
        (ii) Free flap methods require microsurgical reconnection of blood vessels at distant site.
    (i) Techniques for nipple-areolar reconstruction include skin grafting from thigh crease or permanent tattooing.
  c. RT.
    (1) May be administered in conjunction with breast-conserving surgery to achieve local control and reduce risk of local recurrence.
    (2) May be administered before, sequentially with, or following chemotherapy.
    (3) May be administered as an adjunctive treatment for clients with tumor close to the chest wall, locally advanced tumors, or tumors from recurrent or inflammatory breast cancer (NCI, 2003).
    (4) May be administered to specific sites of bone metastasis for palliation of pain.

(5) Primary therapy is usually initiated 2 to 4 weeks after segmental resection when incisions have healed and shoulder range of motion is adequate.

(6) Total of 6000 cGy administered—4500 to 5000 cGy to entire breast, usually followed by 1000 to 1500 cGy to the tumor site by interstitial iridium-192 implants or electron beam "boost."

(7) Common immediate side effects are skin reactions and fatigue.

(8) Possible late effects include hyperpigmentation, soft tissue fibrosis, rib fractures, pneumonitis, cardiac events, brachial plexopathy, arm edema, and secondary malignancy.

(9) New operative approaches have been developed to deliver definitive RT targeted directly to the tumor bed (e.g., Mammosite, INTRABEAM) thereby decreasing length of treatment and minimizing radiation exposure to healthy tissue (Hogle et al., 2003).

5. Systemic treatments.
   a. Goal is to destroy or control overt or occult cancer cells anywhere in the body.
   b. May be given as adjuvant or metastatic treatment.
   c. Treatment recommendations are individualized based on factors such as age, nodal, menopausal, and hormone receptor status.
   d. Hormonal therapy.
      (1) ER and PR test results predict those clients likely to respond to hormonal therapy (Buzdar, 2001).
         (a) Response rate of 50% to 70% in women with ER/PR–positive tumors.
         (b) Less than 10% response rate in women with ER/PR–negative tumors.
      (2) Ablative therapies are directed at removing sources of estrogen.
         (a) Ovarian.
            (i) Major source of estrogen premenopausally.
            (ii) Ablation may be achieved by oophorectomy, ovarian radiation, or administration of luteinizing hormone–releasing hormone (LHRH) agonists/antagonists.
         (b) Adrenal.
            (i) Major source of postmenopausal estrogen.
            (ii) Ablation may be accomplished surgically by adrenalectomy or hypophysectomy or pharmacologically through administration of aromatase inhibitors.
      (3) Additive therapies block action of estrogen on the cancer cell (Table 23-5).
   e. Chemotherapy.
      (1) Commonly used agents are cyclophosphamide (Cytoxan) (C), doxorubicin (Adriamycin) (A), epirubicin (Ellence) (E), paclitaxel (Taxol) (P), docetaxel (Taxotere) (D), methotrexate (Mexate) (M), and fluorouracil (5-Fluorouracil) (F) (Dow, 2002).
      (2) Common adjuvant regimens include CAF, CEF, CMF, AC, EC, FAC-P, A-CMF.
      (3) Capecitabine (Xeloda), gemcitabine (Gemzar), vinorelbine (Navelbine), and etoposide (VP-16, Etopophos, VePesid) may be used in the treatment of recurrent and metastatic disease (Dow, 2002).
      (4) Neoadjuvant chemotherapy may be given to reduce size of tumor before surgery.

TABLE 23-5
Pharmacologic Endocrine Therapies for Breast Cancer Treatment

Category	Mechanism of Action	Agents
Estrogens	Bind to estrogen receptors, thereby inhibiting tumor growth	Diethylstilbestrol (Estratab)
Androgens	Have antiestrogenic effects and also block ovarian secretion of estrogen	Fluoxymesterone (Halotestin)
Progestins	May act by preventing estrogen from reaching tumor	Megestrol (Megace) Medroxyprogesterone (Depo-Provera)
LHRH agonists	Block release of LH and FSH, thereby preventing ovarian production of estrogen	Goserelin (Zoladex) Leuprolide (Lupron) Buserelin (Suprefact)
Selective estrogen receptor modulators (SERMs)	Bind to estrogen receptors; have both agonist and antagonist properties (selectively block action of estrogen in the breast but not in other organs)	Tamoxifen (Nolvadex) Toremifene (Fareston) Raloxifene (Evista) Arzoxifene (Arzox)
Aromatase inhibitors Nonselective	Prevent conversion of adrenal and ovarian androgens to estrogens by inhibiting the aromatase enzyme	Aminoglutethimide (Cytadren) Testolactone (Teslac)
Selective	Inhibit aromatase enzyme, thereby preventing the conversion of adrenal and ovarian androgens to estrogens	Formestane (Lentaron) Anastrozole (Arimidex) Letrozole (Femara) Exemestane (Aromasin) Fadrozole
Estrogen receptor down regulators	Bind to estrogen receptors and also induce degradation of estrogen receptor	Fulvestrant (Faslodex)

LHRH, Luteinizing hormone–releasing hormone; *LH*, luteinizing hormone; *FSH*, follicle-stimulating hormone.

(5) Conclusions from analyses of chemotherapy trials (National Institutes of Health [NIH], 2000).
  (a) Combination regimens have been demonstrated to be more effective than single-agent treatment.
  (b) Regimens that contain anthracyclines (such as doxorubicin, epirubicin appear to be more effective than regimens that do not include anthracyclines.
  (c) Four to six courses of treatment appear to provide optimal benefit; additional courses increase toxicity without substantially improving outcome.
  (d) Dose-intensified regimens have not been proven to be more effective than standard dose regimens.
  (e) Taxanes (docetaxel, paclitaxel) are among the most active agents for treatment of metastatic disease.
  f. Biologic therapies such as trastuzumab (Herceptin) (anti-HER-2/neu monoclonal antibody) selectively target critical steps in the processes required for tumor growth, viability, or invasion; may be added to chemotherapeutic regimens (Rosen et al., 2000).
  g. Immunotherapy vaccines are currently being developed to destroy breast cancer cells by stimulating immune response (Cheever & Disis, 2000).

    h. Use of complementary and alternative medicine (CAM) therapies, such as special diets, vitamins, minerals, herbs, acupuncture, homeopathy, naturopathy, biofeedback, reflexology, therapeutic touch, aromatherapy, prayer, meditation, and guided imagery, is increasing among women with breast cancer (Lengacher et al., 2002).

  6. Standard therapies by stage (NCI, 2003).

    a. Stage 0 (noninvasive cancers).

      (1) Goal of treatment is to prevent development of invasive disease.

      (2) Treatment options for DCIS.

        (a) Breast-conserving surgery and RT, with or without tamoxifen (Nolvadex).

        (b) Total mastectomy with or without tamoxifen.

        (c) Participation in clinical trial comparing breast-conserving surgery and tamoxifen with and without radiation.

      (3) Treatment options for LCIS.

        (a) Observation only.

        (b) Tamoxifen to decrease the incidence of subsequent breast cancer.

        (c) Participation in clinical trial for high-risk postmenopausal women that compares raloxifene (Evista) with tamoxifen in reducing incidence of breast cancer.

        (d) Bilateral prophylactic total mastectomy without axillary node dissection.

    b. Treatment for stages I, II, and IIIA.

      (1) Local-regional treatment options.

        (a) Breast-conserving therapy (lumpectomy, breast irradiation, surgical staging of the axilla).

        (b) Modified radical mastectomy (removal of the entire breast with level I or II axillary dissection) with or without breast reconstruction.

        (c) Role of sentinel node biopsy is under evaluation.

        (d) Adjuvant RT advised if more than four positive nodes; unclear role for regional RT if three or fewer positive nodes.

      (2) Adjuvant systemic treatment options with hormonal therapy and/or chemotherapy are individualized based on nodal status, ER/PR status, tumor grade, menopausal status, age.

    c. Treatment for stages IIIB, IV, recurrent and metastatic breast cancer.

      (1) Modified radical mastectomy or radical mastectomy with RT preoperatively or postoperatively, plus the following:

      (2) Systemic treatment with chemotherapy or hormone therapy (may be given preoperatively if very large tumor or fixed nodes).

    d. Stage IV.

      (1) Systemic chemotherapy or hormone therapy, plus the following:

      (2) Local treatments as needed for palliation.

E. Trends in survival.

  1. U.S. mortality rates for Caucasian women declined 1.6% per year from 1989 to 1995, then decreased by 3.5% per year from 1995 to 1998 (Howe et al., 2001).

  2. Five-year survival by stage at diagnosis (Ries et al., 2002).

    a. Localized—96.8%.

    b. Regional—78.4%.

    c. Distant—22.5%.

3. Survival rates vary by ethnic group (see Figure 23-1) and are poorer among African Americans, Hispanics, Hawaiians, and Filipinos compared with Caucasians (Clegg et al., 2002; Ries et. al., 2002), largely because of later stage at diagnosis and possibly because of disparity in care (Bradley et al., 2002; Brawley, 2002).

Assessment

I. Pertinent personal and family history.
  A. Gender—more than 99% of all breast cancer cases occur in women.
  B. Age—risk increases with age; majority of cases are in women over age 50 years.
  C. Personal history of breast cancer—threefold to fourfold increased risk of developing a new cancer in the same or opposite breast.
  D. Family history of breast cancer and genetics.
      a. Twofold to threefold increased risk in women with a first-degree relative (FDR) with breast cancer; risk increased further if bilateral, premenopausal, and with increased number of affected FDRs.
      b. Genetically determined breast cancers.
          (1) Account for only 5% to 10% of all cases (Mills & Rieger, 2001).
          (2) Are more likely to be bilateral, occur at younger ages, and appear in multiple family members over three or more generations.
          (3) Mutations of *BRCA1* and *BRCA2* genes are linked to a high risk of breast and ovarian cancers.
          (4) Family history characteristics suggestive of increased breast cancer risk (Smith et al., 2003).
              (a) Two or more relatives with breast or ovarian cancer.
              (b) Breast cancer onset before age 50 years in affected relative.
              (c) Relatives with bilateral breast cancer or both breast and ovarian cancers.
              (d) Male relatives with breast cancer.
              (e) Family history of breast or ovarian cancer and Ashkenazi Jewish heritage.
  E. Hormonal factors.
      1. Reproductive.
          a. Increased risk in women who have never had children.
          b. Risk is highest in women who had their first full-term pregnancy after age 30 years.
          c. Prolonged breastfeeding may be protective (Lipworth et al., 2000).
      2. Menstrual.
          a. Early menarche (before age 12 years) increases risk.
          b. Late menopause (after age 55 years) increases risk.
          c. Oophorectomy before age 40 years is protective.
      3. Exogenous hormones.
          a. Postmenopausal hormone replacement therapy with estrogen plus progestin is associated with increased risk (Women's Health Initiative Investigators Writing Group, 2002).
          b. Possible slightly increased risk associated with current or recent use of oral contraceptives (Brinton et al., 2002).
          c. Tamoxifen has been demonstrated to decrease breast cancer incidence in high-risk women by 49%; efficacy of other selective estrogen receptor modulators (SERMs) and aromatase inhibitors in prevention is under investigation (Goss, 2002; Powles, 2002).

F. Proliferative breast disease (Page et al., 2002).
  1. Proliferative lesions without atypia are associated with slightly increased risk.
  2. Atypical hyperplasia is associated with fourfold to fivefold increased risk.
G. Radiation exposure.
H. Personal history of endometrial, ovarian, or colon cancer doubles relative risk.
I. Role of lifestyle, dietary, and environmental factors is currently under investigation.

II. Physical examination.
A. Early signs and symptoms.
  1. Usually asymptomatic.
  2. Most cancers less than 1 cm are nonpalpable and are detected only by mammogram (Donegan, 2002).
  3. Suspicious mammogram findings may include mass, microcalcifications, or architectural distortion.
  4. Palpable cancers.
    a. Majority are discovered by the client rather than her health provider.
    b. Half of all breast cancers occur in the upper outer quadrant of the breast (Greene et al., 2002).
    c. Most commonly present as a painless lump or thickening, but about 11% are associated with some discomfort (Donegan, 2002).
  5. Spontaneous unilateral nipple discharge may be present early or late; increased suspicion for cancer if discharge is from a single duct and/or Hemoccult positive.
B. Later signs and symptoms.
  1. Primary tumor changes.
    a. Dimpling of the skin.
    b. Nipple retraction or deviation.
    c. Asymmetry of breasts.
    d. Peau d'orange skin changes—skin edema with prominent pores (appearance similar to the peel of an orange) resulting from obstructed lymphatic drainage.
    e. Grossly bloody discharge from the nipple.
    f. Ulceration of the breast.
  2. Nodal involvement.
    a. Firm, enlarged axillary lymph nodes.
    b. Palpable supraclavicular nodes.
  3. Distant metastasis.
    a. Pain in shoulder, hip, lower back, or pelvis.
    b. Persistent cough.
    c. Anorexia or unexplained weight loss.
    d. Digestive disturbances.
    e. Persistent dizziness, blurred vision, or headache.

III. Laboratory data specific to breast cancer.
A. Pathology report of breast lesion (including HER-2/neu and hormone receptor status).
B. Baseline serum tumor markers may be obtained in some settings.
  1. Carcinoembryonic antigen (CEA).
  2. CA 15-3 and CA 27-29.
  3. HER-2/neu.
C. Complete blood count with platelet count.
D. Liver function tests.

Nursing Diagnoses

    I. Deficient knowledge related to disease process, treatment options, side effects, self-care.

    II. Decisional conflict related to treatment options.

    III. Disturbed body image related to surgical changes, chemotherapy-induced alopecia, possible treatment-related weight gain.

    IV. Ineffective sexuality patterns related to altered body image, pain, premature menopause.

    V. Impaired physical mobility related to surgical drains, pain, scar tissue.

    VI. Risk for infection related to surgical wound, lymph node removal, chemotherapy-induced neutropenia.

    VII. Fatigue.

    VIII. Ineffective coping.

    IX. Compromised family coping.

    X. Interrupted family processes related to role changes, treatment-related physical limitations.

Outcome Identification

    I. Client describes the state of the disease and therapy at a level consistent with her educational background and emotional status.

    II. Client participates in the decision-making process pertaining to the plan of care to the extent desired or possible.

    III. Client describes the schedule for ongoing therapy and long-term follow-up care.

    IV. Client identifies appropriate community and personal resources that provide information, facilitate coping, and assist with changes in body image and sexuality (e.g., Reach to Recovery, Look Good Feel Better, local support groups).

    V. Client engages in open communication with significant other regarding changes in sexuality.

    VI. Client adopts behaviors to prevent infection and lymphedema in the affected arm.

    VII. Client identifies the early signs and symptoms of infection.

    VIII. Client performs exercises to regain full mobility of the affected shoulder and arm.

    IX. Client modifies her activities as necessary and desired.

    X. Client communicates feelings about living with cancer and body image changes.

    XI. Client and her significant others adapt to changes in family roles.

Planning and Implementation

    I. Interventions to increase knowledge and facilitate treatment decision making (Davison & Degner, 2002).

        A. Explain treatment options in a nonjudgmental way and at the client's level of understanding.

        B. Encourage discussion regarding potential physical and emotional changes resulting from treatment and exploration of her personal values and beliefs as they relate to treatment options.

        C. Facilitate client's involvement in treatment decision making to the extent desired.

II. Interventions to maximize safety for the client.
  A. Prevent fluid accumulation under the chest wall incision by maintaining patency of surgical drains.
    1. Drains are usually left in for approximately 1 week or until output is less than 30 ml/24 hr.
    2. Teach client and significant other how to care for drain before discharge from hospital.
  B. Promote venous lymphatic drainage.
    1. Elevate affected arm with the hand higher than the elbow and the elbow higher than the shoulder to facilitate venous drainage.
    2. Place a sign on the bed advising that no blood pressure readings, injections, or blood testing should be done on the affected arm.
  C. Adduct arm in the first 24 hours to minimize tension on suture lines.
  D. Promote functional recovery of arm and shoulder.
    1. Perform limited exercise for the first 24 hours (squeezing ball, wrist and elbow flexion and extension).
    2. Encourage the client to use the affected arm for activities of daily living (e.g., eating, hair brushing).
    3. Begin active range of motion exercises, usually on the second to third day or as ordered by the physician.
    4. Refer for physical therapy if full range of motion not regained within 4 to 8 weeks postoperatively.
III. Interventions to monitor for unique side effects of treatment for breast cancer.
  A. Teach the client to measure the circumference of the affected arm and to notify the physician if it increases.
  B. Inform the client about altered arm and breast sensations (numbness and tingling of arm, lack of sensation on chest wall, phantom breast sensation after mastectomy) that may persist indefinitely following surgery.
  C. Assess for menopausal symptoms (hot flashes, vaginal dryness) that may be associated with adjuvant endocrine therapy or chemotherapy-induced ovarian failure.
  D. Monitor for and manage side effects of surgery, radiation, biotherapy, and chemotherapy (see Chapters 35 to 38).
IV. Interventions to enhance adaptation and rehabilitation.
  A. Facilitate communication between client and her health care providers; alert the health care team to the client's concerns about breast cancer and its treatment.
  B. Assess coping skills, support system, feelings about body image, sexual identity, role relationships; see Chapter 6 discussion on sexual dysfunction for interventions to manage problems with sexuality.
  C. Provide client with information regarding community resources available for support, rehabilitation, and breast prostheses.
  D. Prepare client for long-term follow-up: office visits every 3 months for the first 2 to 3 years, every 6 months for the next 2 to 3 years, and then at least annually thereafter.
  E. Teach the client with a mastectomy the importance of examining the mastectomy incision and chest wall as well as practicing BSE of the remaining breast; teach the client with BCT how to recognize changes in BSE (breast will look and feel different following radiation).
  F. Teach the client and family precautions to take with the affected arm to prevent trauma and infection, which can lead to lymphedema (Box 23-2; see also Chapter 17).

BOX 23-2
EIGHTEEN STEPS TO PREVENTION OF LYMPHEDEMA

1. Never ignore any swelling in the arm, hand, fingers, or chest wall; consult with physician immediately if present.
2. Never allow an injection or a blood draw in the affected arm or arms; wear a LYMPHEDEMA ALERT bracelet.
3. Never have blood pressure checked on the affected arm; use thigh if bilateral lymphedema at-risk arms.
4. Keep the at-risk arm or arms clean. Use lotion after bathing. Dry gently, making sure to thoroughly dry in any creases and between the fingers.
5. Avoid vigorous, repetitive movements against resistance (scrubbing, pushing, pulling) with the affected arm.
6. Avoid heavy lifting with the affected arm. Never carry heavy handbags or bags with over-the-shoulder straps on your affected side.
7. Do not wear tight jewelry or elastic bands around affected fingers, arm, or arms.
8. Avoid exposing arm to extreme temperatures, such as saunas, hot tubs, hot bath water or dishwater. Protect the arm from the sun at all times.
9. Try to avoid any type of trauma (bruising, cuts, sunburn or other burns, sports injuries, insect bites, cat scratches) to the arm or arms. If injury occurs, watch carefully for subsequent signs of infection.
10. Wear gloves while doing housework, gardening, or any type of work that could result in even a minor injury.
11. Avoid cutting your cuticles.
12. Exercises such as walking, swimming, light aerobics, bike riding, ballet, or yoga are recommended. Avoid lifting more than 15 pounds. Be careful not to overtire at-risk arm; if it starts to ache, lie down and elevate it.
13. When traveling by air, wear a well-fitted compression sleeve. Additional bandages may be required on a long flight. Increase fluid intake while in the air.
14. Wear a well-fitted bra and prosthesis. Avoid heavy prostheses, under wire, and binding shoulder straps.
15. Use an electric razor to shave underarm.
16. Clients with lymphedema should wear a well-fitted compression sleeve during all waking hours. Have sleeve refitted at least every 4 to 6 months.
17. Watch for any signs of infection, such as rash, itching, redness, warmth, pain, or fever. See your physician immediately if present.
18. Maintain your ideal weight through a well-balanced, low-sodium, high-fiber diet. Avoid smoking and alcohol. Do not limit protein since it will not reduce lymphedema.

© January 2003 by the National Lymphedema Network, 1-800-541-3259, www.lymphnet.org. Modified with permission.

V. Interventions to incorporate the client and family in care.
   A. Assess psychologic status and concerns of spouse or significant other—level of distress, ability to serve as support system.
   B. Include significant others in teaching and care to the extent desired by client.
   C. Teach female first-degree relatives of client regarding their increased risk and the importance of regular breast cancer screening.
   D. Facilitate mother-child discussion about the breast cancer that is developmentally appropriate and facilitates the child's expression of questions and feelings (Shands et al., 2000).
   E. Facilitate communication and problem solving between client and significant others about issues related to the breast cancer.

Evaluation

The oncology nurse systematically and regularly evaluates the client's and/or family's responses to interventions in order to determine progress toward the achievement of expected outcomes. Relevant data are collected, and actual findings are compared with expected findings. Nursing diagnoses, outcomes, and plans of care are reviewed and revised as necessary.

REFERENCES

American College of Radiology. (1998). *Breast Imaging Reporting and Data System (BI-RADS)* (3rd ed.). Reston, VA: American College of Radiology. Retrieved July 1, 2003 from the World Wide Web: http://www.acr.org/mammography.

Bartow, S.A. (2002). Normal anatomy and physiologic changes. In S.G. Silverberg (Ed.). *Atlas of breast pathology*. Philadelphia: W.B. Saunders, pp. 19-25.

Bobo, J.K., Lee, N.C., & Thames, S.F. (2000). Findings from 752,081 clinical breast examinations reported to a national screening program from 1995-1998. *Journal of the National Cancer Institute 92*, 971-976.

Bradley, C.J., Given, C.W., & Roberts, C. (2002). Race, socioeconomic status, and breast cancer treatment and survival. *Journal of the National Cancer Institute 94*, 90-96.

Brawley, O.W. (2002). Disaggregating the effects of race and poverty on breast cancer outcomes [editorial]. *Journal of the National Cancer Institute 94*, 471-473.

Brinton, L., Lacey, J., & Devesa, S.S. (2002). Epidemiology of breast cancer. In W.L. Donegan & J.S. Spratt (Eds.). *Cancer of the breast* (5th ed.). Philadelphia: W.B. Saunders, pp. 111-132.

Buzdar, A.U. (2001). Endocrine therapy for breast cancer. In K.K. Hunt, G.L. Robb, E.A. Strom, & N.T. Ueno (Eds.). *Breast cancer*. New York: Springer-Verlag, pp.366-381.

Cheever, M.A., & Disis, M.L. (2000). Immunology and immunotherapy. In J.R. Harris, M.E. Lippman, M. Morrow, & C.K. Osborne (Eds.). *Diseases of the breast* (2nd ed.). Philadelphia: Lippincott Williams & Wilkins, pp. 811-824.

Clark, G.M. (2000). Prognostic and predictive factors. In J.R. Harris, M.E. Lippman, M. Morrow, & C.K. Osborne (Eds.). *Diseases of the breast* (2nd ed.). Philadelphia: Lippincott Williams & Wilkins, pp. 489-514.

Clegg, L.Y., Li, F.P., Hankey, B.F., et al. (2002). Cancer survival among U.S. whites and minorities: A SEER program population-based study. *Archives in Internal Medicine 162*, 1985-1993.

Davison, B.J., & Degner, L.F. (2002). Feasibility of using a computer-assisted intervention to enhance the way women with breast cancer communicate with their physicians. *Cancer Nursing 25*, 417-424.

Dershaw, D.D. (2003). Needles and biopsy probes. In D.D. Dershaw (Ed.). *Imaging—guided interventional breast techniques*. New York: Springer-Verlag, pp. 69-86.

Dixon, J.M. (2000). Breast reconstruction after mastectomy. In J.M. Dixon (Ed.). *Breast cancer: Diagnosis and management*. Amsterdam: Elsevier, pp. 207-213.

Donegan, W. (2002). Diagnosis of breast cancer. In W.L. Donegan & J.S. Spratt (Eds.). *Cancer of the breast* (5th ed.). Philadelphia: W.B. Saunders, pp. 329-220.

Dooley, W.C., Ljung, B.M., Veronesi, U., et al. (2001). Ductal lavage for detection of cellular atypia in women at high risk for breast cancer. *Journal of the National Cancer Institute 93*, 1624-1632.

Dow, K.H. (2002). *Pocket guide to breast cancer* (2nd ed.). Sudbury, MA: Jones and Bartlett Publishers, pp. 116-124.

Goss, P.E. (2002). Aromatase inhibitors and chemoprevention of breast cancer. In W.R. Miller & J.N. Ingle (Eds.). *Endocrine therapy in breast cancer*. New York: Marcel Dekker, pp. 309-317.

Greene, F.L., Page, D.L., Fleming, I.D., et al. (Eds). (2002). *American Joint Committee on cancer (AJCC) cancer staging handbook* (6th ed.). New York: Springer-Verlag, pp. 223-229.

Hogle, W.P., Quinn, A.E., & Heron, D.E. (2003). Advances in brachytherapy: New approaches to target breast cancer. *Clinical Journal of Oncology Nursing 7*, 324-328.

Howe, H.L., Wingo, P.A., Thun, J.J., et al. (2001). Annual report to the nation on the status of cancer (1973-1998), featuring cancers with recent increasing trends. *Journal of the National Cancer Institute 93*, 824-842.

Humphrey, L.L., Helfand, M., Chan, B.K., & Woolf, S.H. (2002). Breast cancer screening: A summary of the evidence for the U.S. Preventive Services Task Force. *Annals of Internal Medicine 137*, 347-360.

Jemal, A., Murray, T., Samuels, A., et al. (2003). Cancer statistics, 2003. *CA: A Cancer Journal for Clinicians 53*, 5-26.

Kuhns, J.G., & Ackerman, D.M. (2002). Microscopic anatomy of the breast. In W.L. Donegan & J.S. Spratt (Eds.). *Cancer of the breast* (5th ed.). Philadelphia: W.B. Saunders, pp. 21-27.

Lengacher, C.A., Bennet, M.P., Kip, K.E., et al. (2002). Frequency of use of complementary and alternative medicine in women with breast cancer. *Oncology Nursing Forum 29*, 1445-1452.

Link, J.S. (2000). History and overview of comprehensive interdisciplinary breast centers. *Surgical Oncology Clinics of North America 9*, 147-157.

Lipworth, L., Bailey, L.R., & Trichopoulos, D. (2000). History of breast-feeding in relation to breast cancer risk: A review of the epidemiologic literature. *Journal of the National Cancer Institute 92*, 302-312.

Love, S. (2000). *Dr. Susan Love's breast book* (3rd ed.). Cambridge, MA: Perseus Publishing, pp. 10-11.

Miller, A.B., To, T., Baines, C.J., & Wall, C. (2002). The Canadian National Breast Screening Study–1: Breast cancer mortality after 11-16 years of follow-up. *Annals of Internal Medicine 137*, 305-312.

Mills, G.B., & Rieger, P.T. (2001) Genetic predisposition to breast cancer. In K.K. Hunt, G.L. Robb, E.A. Strom, & N.T. Ueno (Eds.). *Breast cancer*. New York: Springer-Verlag, pp. 55-81.

Morrow, M., & Schnitt, S.J. (2000). Lobular carcinoma in situ. In J.R. Harris, M.E. Lippman, M. Morrow, & C.K. Osborne (Eds.). *Diseases of the breast* (2nd ed.). Philadelphia: Lippincott Williams & Wilkins, pp. 377-381.

Morrow, M. Strom, E.A., Bassett, L.W., et al. (2002). Standard for breast conservation therapy in the management of invasive breast carcinoma. *CA: A Cancer Journal for Clinicians 52*, 277-300.

National Cancer Institute (NCI). (2003). Breast cancer physician's data query (PDQ): Treatment health professional version (modified 6/19/03). Retrieved July 1, 2003 from the World Wide Web: http://cancer.gov/cancerinfo/pdq/treatment/breast/healthprofessional/.

National Cancer Institute (NCI). (2002). NCI statement on mammography screening (posted 1/31/02). Retrieved July 1, 2003 from the World Wide Web: http://www.nci.nih.gov/news-center/mammstatement 31 Jan 02.

National Institutes of Health (NIH). (2000). Adjuvant therapy for breast cancer. NIH consensus statement online 2000 November 1-3, 17, 1-23. Retrieved July 1, 2003 from the World Wide Web: http://odp.od.nih.gov/consensus/cons/114/114_statement.htm.

National Lymphedema Network. (2003). *Eighteen steps to prevention of lymphedema: Fact sheet*. National Lymphedema Network.

Olsen, O., & Gotzsche, P.C. (2001). Cochrane review on screening for breast cancer with mammography. *Lancet 358*, 1340-1342.

Osborne, M.P. (2000). Breast anatomy and development. In J.R. Harris, M.E. Lippman, M. Morrow, & C.K. Osborne (Eds.). *Diseases of the breast* (2nd ed.). Philadelphia: Lippincott Williams & Wilkins, pp. 1-13.

O'Shaughnessy, J.A., Ljung, B.M., Dooley, W.C., et al. (2002). Ductal lavage and the clinical management of women at high risk for breast carcinoma. *Cancer 94*, 292-298.

Page, D.L., Rogers, L.W., Schuyler, P.A., et al. (2002). The natural history of ductal carcinoma in situ of the breast. In M.J. Silverstein (Ed.). *Ductal carcinoma in situ of the breast* (2nd ed.). Philadelphia: Lippincott Williams & Wilkins, pp. 17-21.

Powles, T.J. (2002). Use of selective antiestrogens for the chemoprevention of breast cancer. In W.R. Miller & J.N. Ingle (Eds.). *Endocrine therapy in breast cancer*. New York: Marcel Dekker, pp. 303-308.

Ries, L.A.G., Eisner, M.P., Kosary, C.L., et al. (Eds). (2002). *SEER cancer statistics review, 1973-1999*. Bethesda, MD: National Cancer Institute. Retrieved July 1, 2003 from the World Wide Web: http://seer.cancer.gov/csr/1973_1999/.

Robb, G.L. (2001). Reconstructive surgery. In K.K. Hunt, G.L. Robb, E.A. Strom, & N.T. Ueno (Eds.). *Breast cancer*. New York: Springer-Verlag, pp. 223-253.

Rosen, N., Sepp-Lorenzino, L., & Lippman, M.E. (2000). Biologic therapy. In J.R. Harris, M.E. Lippman, M. Morrow, & C.K. Osborne (Eds.). *Diseases of the breast* (2nd ed.). Philadelphia: Lippincott Williams & Wilkins, pp. 825-839.

Schnitt, S.J,. & Guidi, A.J. (2000). Pathology and biological markers of invasive breast cancer. In J.R. Harris, M.E. Lippman, M. Morrow, & C.K. Osborne (Eds.). *Diseases of the breast* (2nd ed.). Philadelphia: Lippincott Williams & Wilkins, pp. 425-470.

Shands, M.E., Lewis, F.M., & Zahlis, E.H. (2000). Mother and child interactions about the mother's breast cancer: An interview study. *Oncology Nursing Forum 27,* 77-85.

Smith, R.A., Saslow, D., Sawyer, K.A., et al. (2003). American Cancer Society guidelines for breast cancer screening: Update 2003. *CA: A Cancer Journal for Clinicians 53,* 141-169.

Spillane, A.J., & Sacks, N.P.M. (2000). Axillary surgery in breast cancer: An overview. In J.M. Dixon (Ed.). *Breast cancer: Diagnosis and management.* Amsterdam: Elsevier Science B.V., pp. 247-259.

Sumkin, J., & Hardesty, L.A. (2001). New horizons in breast imaging. In V. Vogel (Ed.). *Management of patients at high risk for breast cancer.* Malden, MA: Blackwell Science, pp. 148-165.

Tabar, L., Vitak, B., Chen, H.H.T., et al. (2001). Beyond randomized controlled trials: Organized mammographic screening substantially reduces breast carcinoma mortality. *Cancer 91,* 1724-1731.

Thomas, D.B., Gao, D.L., Ray, R.M., et al. (2002). Randomized trial of breast self-examination in Shanghai: Final results. *Journal of the National Cancer Institute 94,* 1445-1457.

Women's Health Initiative Investigators Writing Group. (2002). Risks and benefits of estrogen plus progestin in healthy postmenopausal women: Principal results from the Women's Health Initiative randomized controlled trial. *Journal of the American Medical Association 288,* 321-333.

Wong, S.L., Chao, C., Edwards, M.J., & McMasters, K.M. (2002). Lymphatic mapping and sentinel node biopsy. In W.L. Donegan & J.S. Spratt (Eds.). *Cancer of the breast* (5th ed.). Philadelphia: W.B. Saunders, pp. 567-578.

24 Nursing Care of the Client with Lung Cancer

MARIE FLANNERY

Theory

I. Physiology and pathophysiology associated with lung cancer (Lind, 1998; Rhoades & Tanner, 2003; Sekido et al., 2001).
  A. Anatomy—see Figure 24-1 for schematic representation of the lungs, locations, and presenting symptoms of various types of tumors.
  B. Primary functions of the lungs are air exchange and filtering of microparticles from the air.
    1. Normal bronchial epithelial cells serve as a lining and have a protective function.
    2. Columnar epithelial cells line the tracheobronchial tree from the trachea to the terminal bronchioles.
    3. Columnar cells consist of ciliated cells that filter particles from the air and mucus-secreting cells that facilitate clearance of particles from the lungs.
  C. Cellular changes associated with cancer.
    1. Long-term exposures to cigarette smoke or irritants such as coal dust damage the ciliated cells and mucus-producing cells and result in replacement by dysplastic cells.
    2. Chromosomal and structural abnormalities and gene abnormalities of lung cancer cells are currently being identified (Sekido et al., 2001).
      a. Genetic alterations associated with lung cancer, in particular adenocarcinoma, provide additional opportunities for diagnosis, prognosis, monitoring of disease status with tumor markers, and targeted treatment options.
      b. The gene expression patterns of individuals with lung cancer have already been identified (Meyerson et al., 2004).
  D. Classification by histologic types is the most commonly accepted system (Franklin, 2000; Laskin et al., 2003).
    1. Non–small cell lung cancer (NSCLC).
      a. Squamous carcinoma—includes well or poorly differentiated.
      b. Adenocarcinoma—is the most common type and its incidence is increasing. Also includes acinar, papillary, bronchoalveolar.
      c. Large cell—includes undifferentiated and neuroendocrine.
      d. Spindle cell—includes pleomorphic, giant cell, carcinosarcoma.
    2. Small cell lung cancer (SCLC)—only 15% of cases and is a more aggressive subtype. Includes the following:
      a. Small cell carcinoma.
      b. Combined.
    3. Mesothelioma—usually associated with asbestos exposure.

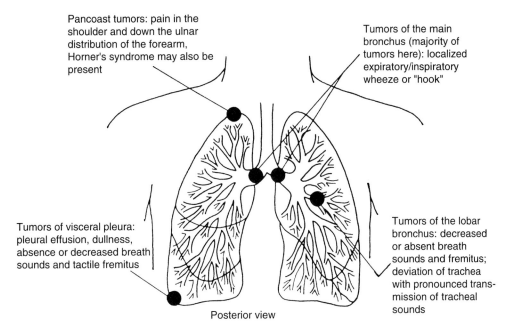

Pancoast tumors: pain in the shoulder and down the ulnar distribution of the forearm, Horner's syndrome may also be present

Tumors of the main bronchus (majority of tumors here): localized expiratory/inspiratory wheeze or "hook"

Tumors of visceral pleura: pleural effusion, dullness, absence or decreased breath sounds and tactile fremitus

Tumors of the lobar bronchus: decreased or absent breath sounds and fremitus; deviation of trachea with pronounced transmission of tracheal sounds

Posterior view

FIGURE 24-1 ■ Anatomic relationships and tumor locations in the lung. (From Frank-Stromborg M, Cohen R: Assessment and interventions for cancer prevention and detection. In Groenwald S, Frogge MH, Goodman M, et al, editors: *Cancer nursing principles and practice,* Sudbury, MA, 1990, Jones and Bartlett Publishers, p. 128.)

E. Presentation and metastatic patterns (see Figure 24-1).
   1. Early signs and symptoms may be absent.
      a. Disease may be detected when chest x-ray completed for some other reason.
   2. Late signs and symptoms may include respiratory changes, cough, hemoptysis, pneumonia, weight loss, pain, or fatigue.
      a. Symptoms of metastatic spread may be present, such as changes from brain metastasis or a pathologic fracture.
   3. Metastatic patterns.
      a. Local recurrence in the lung that may cause obstruction, pleural effusion, and lymph node involvement.
      b. Systemic spread to the brain, liver, adrenal glands, and bone is common.
      c. Individuals with lung cancer are at risk for oncologic emergencies, such as hypercalcemia, syndrome of inappropriate antidiuretic hormone (SIADH), spinal cord compression (SCC), and uncontrolled pain (see Chapters 1, 18, and 19).
F. Trends in epidemiology (American Cancer Society [ACS], 2004; Jemal et al., 2003).
   1. Lung cancer is the leading cause of deaths from cancer for both men and women in the United States. Accounts for the following:
      a. In men, 14% of new cases and 32% of cancer deaths.
      b. In women, 12% of new cases and 25% of cancer deaths.
      c. Projections for 2004 are 173,770 new cases and 160,440 deaths from lung cancer in the United States.

2. Probability of developing lung cancer is 1 in 13 for men and 1 in 17 for women.
3. Lung cancer rates have declined or stabilized in Caucasian men.
   a. Incidence and mortality are increasing in all other non-Caucasian ethnic groups.
4. Increase in lung cancer deaths in women is attributed to the increase in the number of women smoking.
5. Tobacco smoking accounts for approximately 90% of lung cancers and is closely associated with all histologic types.
   a. Smoking is the greatest risk factor for developing lung cancer.
   b. Compared with nonsmokers, lung cancer rates are 22 times higher for current male smokers and 12 times higher for female smokers.
   c. Secondary smoking risks are well established.
   d. Tobacco smoke also promotes the carcinogenic effect of other carcinogens.
6. Never smoking greatly decreases the risk for lung cancer.
   a. Current smokers should stop smoking.
      (1) Smoking cessation is associated with a gradual decrease in the risk of lung cancer (see Chapter 42).
      (2) Five or more years must elapse before an appreciable decrease in risk occurs.
      (3) Symptomatic improvements may be noted immediately on smoking cessation.
7. Environmental and occupational factors.
   a. Asbestos exposure has been linked to the incidence of lung cancer (especially mesothelioma) in shipyard workers, miners, and pipe fitters.
   b. Uranium miners appear to have a particularly high incidence of SCLC (probably caused by radon, which is a radioactive gas that exists in the atmosphere).
   c. Indoor exposure to radon seems to present a risk for lung cancer, but current epidemiologic studies are inconclusive in estimating risks of exposure to radon gas.
8. Trends in survival.
   a. Overall survival rate for lung cancer at 5 years is only 15% in all clients.
   b. Survival depends on the size, location, and extent of metastases at the time of diagnosis.
   c. Survival rates have improved only slightly over the past 10 years.

II. Principles of medical management.
   A. Screening tests (Bach et al., 2003).
      1. No reliable screening or early detection methods exist.
      2. Chest x-ray examinations, lung health questionnaires, and sputum cytology at regular intervals are ineffective in screening.
         a. Spiral computed tomography (CT) and positron emission tomography (PET) scans detect earlier cancers but are not established for screening.
      3. Screening for high-risk individuals may be done in clinical trials.
         a. Continued research explores efficacy of spiral CT based on more positive outcomes for detecting early-stage, resectable, limited lesions.
         b. National Lung Cancer Screening Trial has completed enrollment (nearly 50,000) of high-risk individuals, current or former smokers, randomizing to standard chest x-ray or spiral computed tomography.
            (1) Data will be collected and analyzed for 8 years.
            (2) Study completion may result in change to screening guideline recommendations.

B. Diagnostic tests (Patz, 2000).
   1. Tests to determine the size, histology, location of the primary tumor, and lymph node involvement.
      a. Chest x-ray examination.
      b. CT scan or magnetic resonance imaging (MRI) of chest.
      c. Bronchoscopy (with brush or needle biopsy).
      d. Transthoracic fine-needle aspiration biopsy.
      e. Mediastinoscopy.
      f. Scalene node biopsy.
   2. Tests that aid in detecting distant metastases.
      a. Liver, spleen, and adrenal imaging.
      b. Bone scan.
      c. Brain imaging.
      d. Thoracentesis (to detect tumor cells in pleural fluid).
C. Staging methods and procedures (Mountain, 1997).
   1. Staging system (Table 24-1).
   2. TNM system (Table 24-2).
   3. Performance scales that measure physical status.
   4. Procedures as outlined above under diagnostic tests section.
D. Types of treatment.
   1. Clinical trials (National Cancer Institute [NCI], 2004).
      a. Given the poor prognosis of lung cancer, participation in a clinical trial is recommended.
      b. Review of the NCI clinical trials database reveals multiple active trials at any time (http://www.cancer.gov/clinicaltrials).
         (1) For example, 153 trials for NSCLC and 53 active trials for SCLC (retrieved March 20, 2004).
   2. Surgery—treatment of choice for cure of NSCLC.
      a. Lobectomy—removal of a lobe of the lung.
         (1) Associated with lower morbidity and mortality rates than pneumonectomy.
         (2) Generally the preferred treatment for small tumors.

TABLE 24-1
Lung Cancer Stage Grouping with TNM Subsets

Stage	TNM Subset
0	T is (carcinoma in situ)
IA	T1N0M0
IB	T2N0M0
IIA	T1N1M0
IIB	T2N1M0
	T3N0M0
IIIA	T3N1M0
	T1N2M0
	T2N2M0
	T3N2M0
IIIB	Any T, N3M0
	T4, Any N, M0
IV	Any T, any N, M1

From Mountain C: Revisions in the international system for staging lung cancer, *Chest* 111:1710-1717, 1997.

TABLE 24-2
TNM Classification of Carcinoma of the Lung

Stage	Description
PRIMARY TUMOR = T	
TX	Primary tumor cannot be assessed, or tumor proven by the presence of malignant cells in septum or bronchial washings but not visualized by imaging or bronchoscopy
T0	No evidence of primary tumor
Tis	Carcinoma in situ
T1	Tumor ≤3 cm in greatest dimension, surrounded by lung or visceral pleura, without bronchoscopic evidence of invasion more proximal that the lobar bronchus* (i.e., not in the main bronchus)
T2	Tumor with any of the following features in size or extent: ■ >3 cm in greatest dimension ■ Involves main bronchus, ≥2 cm distal to the carina ■ Invades the visceral pleura ■ Associated with atelectasis or obstructive pneumonitis that extends to the hilar region but does not involve the entire lung
T3	Tumor of any size that directly invades any of the following: chest wall (including superior sulcus tumors), diaphragm, mediastinal pleura, parietal pericardium; or tumor is in the main bronchus <2 cm distal to the carina, but without involvement of the carina; or associated atelectasis or obstructive pneumonitis of the whole lung
T4	Tumor of any size that invades any of the following: mediastinum, heart, great vessels, trachea, esophagus, vertebral body, carina; or tumor with a malignant pleural or pericardial effusion,[†] or with satellite tumor nodule(s) within the ipsilateral primary-tumor lobe of the lung
REGIONAL LYMPH NODES = N	
NX	Regional lymph node cannot be assessed
N0	No regional lymph node metastasis
N1	Metastasis to ipsilateral peribronchial and/or ipsilateral bilar lymph node, and intrapulmonary nodes involved by direct extension of the primary tumor
N2	Metastasis to ipsilateral mediastinal and/or subcarinal lymph node(s)
N3	Metastasis to contralateral mediastinal, contralateral hilar, ipsilateral or contralateral scalene, or supraclavicular lymph node(s)
DISTANT METASTASIS = M	
MX	Presence of distant metastasis cannot be assessed
M0	No distant metastasis
M1	Distant metastasis present[‡]

From Mountain C: Revisions in the international system for staging lung cancer, *Chest* 111:1710-1717, 1997.
*The uncommon superficial tumor of any site with its invasive component limited to the bronchial wall, which may extend proximal to the main bronchus, is also classified T1.
†Most pleural effusions associated with lung cancer are due to tumor. However, there are a few clients in whom multiple cytopathologic examinations of pleural fluid show no tumor. In these cases, the fluid is nonbloody and is not an exudate. When these elements and clinical judgment dictate that the effusion is not related to the tumor, the effusion should be excluded as a staging element and the client's disease should be staged T1, T2, or T3. Pericardial effusion is classified according to the same rules.
‡Separate metastatic tumor nodule(s) in the ipsilateral nonprimary tumor lobe(s)of the lung also are classified M1.

    b. Pneumonectomy—removal of one lung.
        (1) Higher incidence of perfusion and ventilation problems, circulatory overload, pulmonary hypertension.
    c. Contraindications.
        (1) Metastasis outside the lung to contralateral lung, or scalene nodes.
        (2) Inadequate pulmonary function or extensive comorbidities.

    d. Approximately 50% of lung cancer clients are candidates for surgery; but about one half of those people do not have a resection after the opening of the chest because metastases are found during surgery.

3. Radiation therapy (RT)—external beam radiotherapy.

    a. Alone with curative intent for stage I or II NSCLC if lung function is impaired or other conditions preclude surgery (commonly 60 Gy).

    b. As adjuvant to surgery, either preoperatively or postoperatively; the impact on overall survival is minimal, but local response may be improved (Wagner, 2000).

    c. In combination or sequentially with chemotherapy, especially for stage IIIB disease (Belani, 2000a).

    d. Prophylactic cranial irradiation (PCI) to prevent or delay the incidence of brain metastases in SCLC.

    e. As palliation for control of symptoms associated with lung cancer (severe cough, hemoptysis, pain, obstructive pneumonitis, superior vena cava syndrome).

    f. Newer techniques such as 3-D imaging have improved fields and minimized toxicities.

4. Chemotherapy (Bunn & Kelly, 2000; Simon & Wagner, 2003).

    a. Treatment of choice for SCLC.

        (1) Improves survival rates.

            (a) About a 20% cure rate for limited-stage disease.

            (b) Survival for limited-stage disease approaching 2 years.

            (c) For extensive-stage disease, median survival is about 9 months.

            (d) Overall response rates high (50% to 78%) but duration of response is limited.

            (e) Recommended duration is 4 to 6 cycles.

        (2) The following combinations produce similar response rates.

            (a) Etoposide (VP-16) plus either cisplatin (Platinol) or carboplatin (Paraplatin).

            (b) Cyclophosphamide (Cytoxan)-doxorubicin (Adriamycin)-vincristine (Oncovin).

            (c) Cyclophosphamide-doxorubicin–etoposide.

            (d) Ifosfamide (Ifex)-carboplatin-etoposide.

    b. May be used as adjuvant therapy in NSCLC (Johnson, 2000).

        (1) Improved quality of life outcomes versus best supportive care.

            (a) Improved symptom control for limited number of cycles and individuals with good performance status (PS).

        (2) Response rates as high as 40%.

            (a) Modest improvements in survival, about a 10% improvement in 1-year survival (Schiller, 2001).

        (3) May be combined with RT, concurrently or sequentially.

        (4) Platinum-based combinations are the standard of care for NSCLC, inoperable Stage III, and Stage IV (ASCO, 1997; Belani, 2000b). Examples of regimens include:

            (a) Cisplatin and etoposide (VP-16).

            (b) Carboplatin and paclitaxel (Taxol).

        (5) Additional regimens include cyclophosphamide and doxorubicin-cisplatin, gemcitabine (Gemzar), vinorelbine (Navelbine), and taxanes (docetaxel and paclitaxel), topotecan (Hycamtin), irinotecan (Camptosar).

    c. Commonly used for recurrent advanced disease.

       (1) Second-line therapies generally yield frequent but brief response rates (up to 40% in some studies).

       (2) Docetaxel (Taxotere) as a single agent is recommended for second-line therapy of nonresectable and metastatic disease (ASCO, 2003).

       (3) Cisplatin-based combinations or single agents such as gemcitabine and topoisomerase inhibitors (topotecan [Hycamtin]; irinotecan) are also used.

    d. Newer agents.

       (1) Gefitinib (Iressa) has been approved as single-agent therapy for NSCLC clients with advanced disease who have failed platinum-based chemotherapy (Treat et al., 2002).

       (2) Cyclooxygenase-2 inhibitors have demonstrated benefit when combined with chest RT (Saha & Choy, 2003).

       (3) Agents with novel mechanisms, such as angiogenesis agents, receptor protein kinases, matrix metalloproteinase (MMP) inhibitors, monoclonal antibodies, growth factors, and other biologic response modifiers, are under investigation.

          (a) Review of the literature for ongoing clinical trial findings is recommended since new therapies with novel mechanisms of action may be approved (Bunn et al., 2000).

  5. Treatment options by stage (Alberts, 2003; Ettinger et al., 1996; Demetri et al., 1996).

    a. NSCLC.

       (1) Stage I (Smythe, 2003).

          (a) Lobectomy or pneumonectomy preferred over wedge resection.

          (b) RT with curative intent for potentially resectable clients who have medical contraindications to surgery.

          (c) Clinical trials of adjuvant chemotherapy following resection.

       (2) Stage II (Scott et al., 2003).

          (a) Lobectomy, pneumonectomy, or segmental resection.

          (b) RT with curative intent for potentially operable tumors in clients who have medical contraindications to surgery.

          (c) Adjuvant RT for improved local control or on clinical trial.

          (d) Adjuvant chemotherapy in the clinical trial setting.

       (3) Stage IIIA (Robinson et al., 2003).

          (a) Surgery alone in highly selected cases.

          (b) Chemotherapy with concurrent or sequential RT for unresectable disease or in a clinical trial as adjuvant.

          (c) RT alone.

       (4) Stage IIIB (Jett et al., 2003).

          (a) Chemotherapy with concurrent RT for individuals with good performance status.

          (b) Chemotherapy and sequential RT for those with poor performance status.

          (c) RT alone or chemotherapy alone for selected cases.

       (5) Stage IV.

          (a) Chemotherapy or palliative-focused care.

    b. SCLC.

       (1) Limited stage.

          (a) Combination chemotherapy and chest RT (with or without PCI given to clients with complete responses).

(b) Combination chemotherapy and RT sequentially, especially for clients with impaired pulmonary function or poor performance status.

(c) Surgical resection of pulmonary tumor in highly selected cases, followed by combination chemotherapy with or without PCI.

(2) Extensive stage.

(a) Initial treatment may depend on presenting problem (e.g., RT to the brain).

(i) Performance status and client/family preference may influence choice.

(ii) For individuals with PS of 2 or less, may select single-agent chemotherapy or palliative care.

(b) Platinum-based chemotherapy for 4 to 6 cycles.

(c) Selected cases may be treated with chemotherapy and RT in combination or sequentially (localized, symptomatic lung disease).

(d) Palliative RT to sites of metastatic disease (bone, brain, airway obstruction).

c. Recurrent disease.

(1) Salvage therapy for relapsed disease includes palliative-focused chemotherapy or choice of palliative symptom management.

Assessment (Ingle, 2000; Lind, 1998)

I. Pertinent personal and environmental history (risk factors) (Otto, 2001).

A. Tobacco use (number of packs per day multiplied by number of years smoked).

1. At highest risk are people over 45 years who have smoked two or more packs per day for 10 years or more (20 pack years).

2. Mortality rates for 20–pack year persons are 15 to 25 times higher than for nonsmokers.

B. Occupational and environmental exposures (i.e., asbestos, uranium, radon).

C. Onset and duration of symptoms, including client's understanding of disease and treatment.

II. Physical examination (client may be asymptomatic).

A. Pulmonary manifestations.

1. Cough.

2. Hemoptysis.

3. Dyspnea.

4. Pneumonia.

B. Local manifestations (related to the growth of tumor and compression of adjacent structures).

1. Shoulder pain.

2. Arm pain.

3. Superior vena cava syndrome (distention of arm and neck veins; facial, neck, arm edema).

III. Evaluation of laboratory data.

A. Metabolic complications (especially small cell).

1. Elevated antidiuretic hormone (ADH) level because ADH mimic may be produced by the tumor.

2. Elevated adrenocorticotropic hormone (ACTH) level because ACTH mimic may be produced by the tumor.

    B. Blood gas values.

    C. Pulmonary functions test results.

        1. FEV_1 greater than 70%, lung function normal.

        2. FEV_1 35% to 70%, mild to moderate ventilatory impairment.

        3. FEV_1 less than 35%, severe ventilatory impairment.

Nursing Diagnoses

   I. Acute or chronic pain.

  II. Impaired gas exchange.

 III. Imbalanced nutrition: less than body requirements.

 IV. Deficient knowledge related to diagnosis and treatment of lung cancer.

  V. Anxiety.

Outcome Identification

   I. Client states adequate pain relief.

  II. Client maintains optimal gas exchange with oxygen saturation within normal range and remains alert and oriented.

 III. Client weighs within 10% of ideal body weight.

 IV. Client discusses rationale, schedule, and personal demands of treatment and follow-up plan.

    A. Client lists potential side effects of disease and treatment.

    B. Client describes and uses self-care measures to manage the effects of the disease and treatment.

    C. Client and family specify symptoms to report immediately to the health care team.

        1. Signs and symptoms of upper respiratory infection (i.e., fever, cough, yellow or green expectoration).

        2. Signs and symptoms of decreased oxygenation (i.e., fatigue, dyspnea, change in level of consciousness).

        3. Signs and symptoms of SIADH (see Chapter 18).

        4. Pain.

        5. Changes in affect or personality, mental status, seizure activity, or gait imbalance.

        6. Jaundice.

  V. Client describes a reduction in level of anxiety experienced.

    A. Client demonstrates positive coping behaviors.

    B. Client identifies sources of emotional and psychologic support.

Planning and Implementation (Ingle, 2000; Lind, 1998)

   I. Interventions to decrease severity of symptoms associated with the disease and/or treatment.

    A. Interventions related to surgical treatment (Otto, 2001).

        1. Postoperative interventions to maximize client safety by prevention and detection of hemorrhage, pneumothorax, and/or mediastinal shift.

            a. Check the chest tube drainage system for obstruction every 1 to 2 hours; observe and document the following:

                (1) Absence of fluctuations in the water-seal chamber.

                (2) Lack of drainage fluid in the drainage tubing or collection chamber.

      (3) Excessive drainage.

    b. Reposition the chest tube drainage tubing as frequently as necessary.

      (1) Secure chest tubes with a tight dressing.

      (2) Minimize chest tube movement by securing tubes to body.

      (3) Avoid kinks or dependent loops in drainage tubes.

    c. Examine the drainage tubing and connections for clots and/or debris.

    d. Assess the drainage system for breaks in the system every 8 hours and as needed; document findings; immediately report:

      (1) Continuous large amount of bubbling in the water-seal chamber.

      (2) "Air leak" noises in the system.

    e. Assess for cause of air leak by checking the following:

      (1) For occlusive seal at the insertion site.

      (2) To determine if the chest tube has moved; if so, notify physician.

      (3) For an improper fit at the connector site.

      (4) For a defect in the equipment.

    f. Auscultate and document breath sounds every 2 to 4 hours.

    g. Monitor and document early signs of respiratory distress—increased respiratory rate, nasal flaring, use of accessory muscles.

    h. Instruct the client to report increase in shortness of breath.

    i. Document client teaching.

    j. Assess and document signs of pneumothorax every 2 to 4 hours—absent breath sounds unilaterally, tracheal deviation, increased shortness of breath.

    k. Obtain chest x-ray examination and blood gas values as ordered and monitor reports.

    l. Monitor position of trachea, and report shift from midline.

    m. Avoid deep suctioning that may cause trauma to suture line.

  2. Teach the client and family preoperatively about equipment (may receive mechanical ventilation or supplemental oxygen immediately postoperatively), breathing exercises, and postoperative recovery.

  3. Apply elastic stockings, and teach leg exercises to prevent postoperative emboli.

  4. Provide pain relief to promote comfort, early ambulation, and coughing and deep breathing.

  5. Position the client to protect remaining lung tissue.

    a. After lobectomy—promote expansion to fill lung space by avoiding prolonged lying on operative side.

    b. After pneumonectomy—client may lie on back or operated side only.

  6. Promote optimal pulmonary function—coughing and deep breathing, hydrating, changing positions, ambulating.

  7. Teach breathing exercises and the need for cessation of smoking.

 B. Interventions related to RT of pulmonary and/or cranial fields (see Chapter 36).

 C. Nursing interventions related to chemotherapy (see Chapter 38).

 D. Interventions for clients with advanced disease.

  1. Individuals with lung cancer often have greater symptom distress and a higher incidence and severity of symptoms.

    a. Systematic nursing assessment with a comprehensive review of systems has been shown to improve outcomes (Cooley, 2000; Sarna, 1998).

    b. Evaluate for weight loss, fatigue, pain, dyspnea, sleep disturbance, coping deficits, anticipatory grieving.

II. Interventions to monitor disease progression.

 A. Schedule follow-up care.

     B. Discuss purpose of scans or other surveillance procedures for metastatic disease.

     C. Teach the client and family signs and symptoms of metastatic disease.

       1. Changes in affect or personality.

       2. Bone pain.

       3. Changes in respiratory status.

       4. Jaundice.

       5. Headache.

       6. New-onset seizures.

III. Interventions to enhance adaptation and rehabilitation.

     A. Pulmonary rehabilitation.

     B. Range of motion exercises on side of the thoracotomy.

IV. Interventions to incorporate the client and family in care.

     A. Help family to allow the client to maintain roles and activities most important to him/her.

       1. Place emphasis on short-term goals in daily care and priority setting.

       2. Refer to local community resources as appropriate and available (see Chapter 8).

     B. Teach supportive care skills.

       1. Instruct the client and family in the use of oxygen equipment, postural drainage, and how to self-pace to conserve energy, as appropriate.

       2. Teach general strengthening exercises.

       3. Instruct in relaxation techniques.

       4. Assist to maintain realistic hope, yet prepare for changes in lifestyle if prognosis is poor.

       5. Assist to resume previous roles and responsibilities if prognostic factors are favorable (small, solitary, isolated lesion).

Evaluation

The oncology nurse systematically and regularly evaluates the client's and/or family's responses to interventions to determine progress toward the achievement of expected outcomes. Relevant data are collected, and actual findings are compared with expected findings. Nursing diagnoses, outcomes, and plans of care are reviewed and revised as necessary.

REFERENCES

Alberts, M. (2003). Lung cancer guidelines: Introduction. *Chest 123*, 1S-23S.

American Cancer Society (ACS). (2004). *Cancer facts & figures 2004.* Atlanta: American Cancer Society.

American Society of Clinical Oncology (ASCO). (2003). American Society of Clinical Oncology treatment of unresectable non-small cell lung cancer guideline: Update 2003. *Journal of Clinical Oncology 22*, 330-353.

American Society of Clinical Oncology (ASCO). (1997). Clinical practice guidelines for the treatment of unresectable non-small-cell lung cancer. *Journal of Clinical Oncology 8*, 2996-3018.

Bach, P.B., Niewoehner, D.E., & Black, W.C. American College of Chest Physicians. (2003). Screening for lung cancer: The guidelines. *Chest 123*, 83S-88S.

Belani, C. (2000a). Combined modality therapy for unresectable Stage III non-small cell lung cancer: New chemotherapy combinations. *Chest 117*, 127S-132S.

Belani, C. (2000b). Paclitaxel and docetaxel combinations in non-small cell lung cancer. *Chest 117*, 144S-151S.

Bunn, P., & Kelly, K. (2000). New combinations in the treatment of lung cancer: A time for optimism. *Chest 117*, 138S-143S.

Bunn, P., Soriano, A., Johnson, G., & Heasley, L. (2000). New therapeutic strategies for lung cancer: Biology and molecular biology come of age. *Chest 114*, 163S-168S.

Cooley, M. (2000). Symptoms in adults with lung cancer: A systematic research review. *Journal of Pain and Symptom Management 19*, 137-153.

Demetri G., Elias A., Gershenson D., et al. (1996). NCCN small-cell lung cancer practice guidelines. The National Comprehensive Cancer Network. *Oncology 10* (Suppl. 11), 179-194.

Ettinger D.S., Cox J.D., Ginsberg R.J., et al. (1996). NCCN non-small cell lung cancer practice guidelines. The National Comprehensive Cancer Network. *Oncology 10* (Suppl. 11), 81-111.

Franklin, W. (2000). Diagnosis of lung cancer: Pathology of invasive and preinvasive neoplasia. *Chest 117*, 80S-89S.

Ingle, R. (2000). Lung cancer. In C.H. Yarbro, M.H. Frogge, M. Goodman, & S.L. Groenwald (Eds.). *Cancer nursing: Principles and practice* (5th ed.). Sudbury, MA: Jones and Bartlett Publishers.

Jemal, A., Murray, T., Samuela, A., et al. (2003). Cancer statistics, 2003. *CA: A Journal for Clinicians 53*, 5-26.

Jett, J., Scott, W., Rivera, M., & Sause, W. (2003). Guidelines on treatment of Stage IIIB non-small cell lung cancer. *Chest 123*, 221S-225S.

Johnson, D. (2000). Evolution of cisplatin-based chemotherapy in non-small cell lung cancer: A historical perspective and the eastern cooperative group experience. *Chest 117*, 133S-137S.

Laskin, J., Sandler, A., & Johnson, D. (2003). An advance in small-cell lung cancer treatment—more or less (editorial). *Journal of the National Cancer Institute 95*, 1099-1101.

Lind, J. (1998). Nursing care of the client with lung cancer. In J. Itano & K. Taoka (Eds.). *Core curriculum for oncology nursing* (3rd ed.). Philadelphia: W.B. Saunders.

Meyerson, M., Franklin, W., & Kelley, M. (2004). Molecular classification and molecular genetics of human lung cancers. *Seminars in Oncology 31* (Suppl. 1), 4-19.

Mountain, C. (1997). Revisions in the international system for staging lung cancer. *Chest 111*, 1710-1717.

National Cancer Institute (NCI). (2004). Clinical trials. Retrieved March 26, 2004 from the World Wide Web: http://www.cancer.gov/.

National Comprehensive Cancer Network (NCCN). (1996b). NCCN small-cell lung cancer practice guidelines. *Oncology 10* (Suppl.), 179-194.

Otto, S. (2001). *Oncology nursing* (4th ed.). St. Louis: Mosby.

Patz, E. (2000). Imaging bronchogenic carcinoma. *Chest 117*, 90S-95S.

Rhoades, R., & Tanner, G. (2003). *Medical physiology* (2nd ed.). Philadelphia: Lippincott Williams & Wilkins.

Robinson, L., Wagner, H., & Ruckdeschel, J. (2003). Treatment of Stage IIIA lung cancer. *Chest 123*, 202S-220S.

Saha, D., & Choy, H. (2003). Potential for combined modality therapy of cyclooxygenase inhibitors and radiation. *Progress in Experimental Tumor Research 37*, 193-209.

Sarna, L. (1998). Effectiveness of structured nursing assessment of symptom distress in advanced lung cancer. *Oncology Nursing Forum 25*(6), 1041-1048.

Schiller, S. (2001). Current standards of care in small-cell and non-small cell lung cancer. *Oncology 61*(Suppl.), 3-13.

Scott, W., Howington, J., & Movsas, B. (2003). Treatment of Stage II non-small cell lung cancer. *Chest 123*, 188S-201S.

Sekido, Y., Fong, K., & Minna, J. (2001). Cancer of the lung. In V. DeVita, S. Hellman, & S. Rosenberg (Eds.). *Cancer: Principles & practice of oncology* (6th ed.). Philadelphia: Lippincott Williams & Wilkins.

Simon, G., & Wagner, H. (2003). Small cell lung cancer. *Chest 123*, 259S-271S.

Smythe, W. (2003). Treatment of stage I non-small cell lung carcinoma. *Chest 123*, 181S-187S.

Treat, J., Schiller, J., Quoix, E., et al. (2002). ZD0473 treatment in lung cancer: An overview of the clinical trial results. *European Journal of Cancer 38*(Suppl.), S13-S18.

Wagner, H. (2000). Postoperative adjuvant therapy for patients with resected non-small cell lung cancer: Still controversial after all these years. *Chest 117*, 110S-118S.

25 Nursing Care of the Client with Cancers of the Gastrointestinal Tract

ROBERTA ANNE STROHL

ESOPHAGEAL CANCER

Theory

I. Anatomy/physiology and pathophysiology associated with esophageal cancer.
   A. Anatomy.
      1. Located behind the trachea and between hypopharynx and stomach.
      2. Originates at cricoid cartilage at the sixth cervical vertebra.
      3. Sections.
         a. Cervical esophagus is about 5 cm long.
         b. Thoracic esophagus is 20 to 25 cm long.
            (1) Begins at the thoracic inlet and ends at the gastroesophageal junction (Odze & Antonioli, 2003).
      4. Is a distensible structure (2 cm in diameter).
         a. Upper one third is striated muscle.
         b. Lower two thirds is smooth muscle.
      5. Critical adjacent structures.
         a. Trachea.
         b. Aorta.
         c. Lung.
   B. Normal functions.
      1. Conducts food and fluids from pharynx to stomach.
      2. Facilitates swallowing through primary and secondary peristalsis.
      3. Prevents reflux of stomach contents by contraction of lower esophageal sphincter (Odze & Antonioli, 2003).
   C. Changes in function because of cancer.
      1. Symptoms occur late when circumference is less than 13 mm.
         a. Achalasia is a benign spasm of lower esophageal sphincter with marked dilation of the esophagus.
         b. Difficulty swallowing that is progressive, unremitting, and of short duration.
         c. Painful swallowing of food (odynophagia).
         d. Regurgitation.
         e. Retrosternal or epigastric pain.
         f. Hematemesis.
         g. Melena (Schmitt & Brazer, 2003).

D. Metastatic patterns.
  1. Local spread.
  2. Visceral metastases.
   a. Liver.
   b. Lung.
   c. Pleura.
   d. Stomach.
   e. Peritoneum.
   f. Kidney.
   g. Adrenal gland.
   h. Bone.
   i. Brain (Schmitt & Brazer, 2003).
 II. Trends in epidemiology.
  A. United States (U.S.).
   1. Uncommon cancer, accounts for about 2% of U.S. cancer deaths; 12,000 new cases annually.
   2. Sixth most common cause of death.
   3. One of top five causes of death in men.
   4. Ninety percent of esophageal cancers are squamous cell carcinomas.
   5. Squamous cell cancer of esophagus has a higher incidence in African Americans.
   6. Adenocarcinoma of esophagus has a higher incidence in Caucasians; incidence appears to be increasing (Schmitt & Brazer, 2003).
  B. Worldwide.
   1. Eighth most common cancer worldwide.
   2. Highest in southern and eastern Africa and China.
   3. Squamous cell cancer most common worldwide.
   4. Adenocarcinoma increasing in United States, Europe, Scandinavia, New Zealand, and Australia (Schmitt & Brazer, 2003).
III. Principles of medical management.
  A. Screening.
   1. Routine screening has not been reported.
  B. Diagnostic procedures.
   2. Esophagoscopy and biopsy.
   3. Esophagogram.
   4. Computed tomography (CT) of the chest.
   5. Endoscopic ultrasound.
   6. Chest radiography.
   7. Assessment of the head and neck because 20% of clients may present with a second primary lesion.
   8. Positron emission tomography (PET) scan to detect distant metastases (Schmitt & Brazer, 2003).
  C. Staging.
   1. Tumor-node-metastasis (TNM) system used (Table 25-1).
   2. CT of the chest, bone scan, bronchoscopy, pulmonary function studies may add to staging.
   3. Surgical staging with lymph node sampling.
  D. Treatment strategies.
   1. Surgery.
    a. Surgical approaches (Table 25-2).
     (1) Endoscopic mucosal resection in T1 disease.
    b. Surgery may be curative or palliative.

TABLE 25-1
Staging of Esophageal Cancer

Stage	Description
T = PRIMARY TUMOR	
TX	Minimum requirements to assess the primary tumor cannot be seen
T0	No evidence of primary tumor
Tis	Preinvasive carcinoma (carcinoma in situ)
T1	Tumor invades into but not beyond the submucosa
T2	Tumor invades but not beyond the muscularis propria
T3	Tumor invades into the adventitia
T4	Tumor invades contiguous structures
N = REGIONAL LYMPH NODES	
Cervical esophagus (cervical and supraclavicular lymph nodes)	
NX	Lymph nodes cannot be assessed
N0	No demonstrable metastasis to regional lymph nodes
N1	Regional lymph nodes contain metastatic tumor
Thoracic esophagus (nodes in the thorax, not those of cervical, supraclavicular, or abdominal area)	
N0	No nodal involvement
N1	Nodal involvement
M = DISTANT METASTASIS	
MX	Distant metastasis cannot be assessed
M0	No evidence of distant metastasis
M1	Distant metastasis present

From Greene FL, Page DL, Fleming ID, et al., editors. *American Joint Committee on Cancer (AJCC). Cancer staging handbook*, ed 6, New York, 2002, Springer-Verlag.

        (1) Disease is often systemic at diagnosis with lymph node involvement and distant metastases.

    c. Preoperative considerations.

        (1) Preoperative pulmonary function values are obtained; forced expiratory volume (FEV) should be at least 70%.

        (2) Cardiac assessment.

        (3) Nutritional status.

        (4) Oral sepsis increases risk of intrathoracic infection, indicating the need for preoperative dental evaluation (Marshall & Kaiser, 2003).

  2. Radiation therapy (RT).

    a. Palliative radiation as single modality for client in poor condition or with metastatic disease.

    b. To alleviate obstruction, control pain, or restore swallowing.

    c. Combined with surgery preoperatively or postoperatively.

    d. Combined with chemotherapy and surgery (Marshall & Kaiser, 2003).

  3. Chemotherapy.

    a. Combined with RT; simultaneously administered external beam with fluorouracil (5-FU), cisplatin (Platinol), or mitomycin C (Mutamycin) (chemoradiation).

    b. Trials ongoing with radiosensitizers.

    c. Other agents used include bleomycin (Blenoxane), vinblastine (Velban), etoposide (VP-16), doxorubicin (Adriamycin), or paclitaxel (Taxol) (Marshall & Kaiser, 2003).

  4. Photodynamic therapy.

TABLE 25-2
Surgical Approaches in Esophageal Cancer

Location of Lesion	Procedure	Technique	Morbidity Related to *All* Techniques of Esophageal Resection
Lower third of esophagus and cardia	Transthoracoscopy Esophagectomy	Removes distal esophagus and proximal stomach with clear margins of 5-10 cm Resection includes paraesophageal, pericardial, left gastric, and celiac nodes Stomach is mobilized with vascular pedicle, advanced into thorax with end-to-side anastomosis	Atelectasis Pneumonia Postoperative hypoxia (secondary to atelectasis and increased intrapulmonary shunting) Dehiscence of esophageal anastomosis (7-10 days postoperative) Early symptoms of leak Low-grade fever, chest pain Late signs: dyspnea, tachycardia, cervical crepitus, pneumothoraces, pleural effusion (on operative side with brown fluid) Postoperative bleeding Recurrent laryngeal nerve paralysis (cervical sites)
	En bloc esophagectomy	Dissection includes esophagus surrounding pleura, thoracic duct, lymphatics, and adjacent portions of pericardium and diaphragm	
Upper and middle thirds	Combined right thoracotomy and abdominal approach	Requires anastomosis at or above aortic arch Resection of whole intrathoracic esophagus and dissection of lymph nodes Mobilization of gastric or intestinal conduit for bypass	
Cervical esophagus		Dissection includes head and neck as well as thorax; surgery may require resection of larynx and hypopharynx	

    a. Intravenous (IV) administration of an agent that sensitizes tumors to light at certain wavelengths.

    b. Used in superficial and mucosal lesions.

IV. Trends in survival.

    A. Prognosis remains poor because most cancers are diagnosed late.

    B. Five-year survival is 15% in Caucasians and 9% in African Americans.

    C. Survival rates have doubled in last 40 years but remain poor (Schmitt & Brazer, 2003).

Assessment

I. Pertinent client and family history.

    A. Risk factors.

        1. Predisposing conditions.

    a. Tylosis.
       (1) Hyperkeratosis of the skin of palms and soles.
       (2) Papillomata of the esophagus.
       (3) Inherited in an autosomal dominant fashion.
       (4) Squamous cell cancer of the esophagus in affected families.
    b. Achalasia.
       (1) Benign spasm of lower esophageal sphincter; a neuromuscular disorder resulting from absent or defective nerves of the myenteric plexus.
       (2) Risk of esophageal cancer is 20%.
       (3) Most common in middle third of the esophagus.
       (4) Seventeen years from diagnosis of achalasia to cancer.
    c. Barrett's esophagus.
       (1) Mechanism unclear, may be related to esophageal damage from gastroesophageal reflux disease (GERD).
       (2) Failure of normal developmental progression from columnar to epithelial cells in utero. Environmental factors contribute to progression over time.
       (3) May be related to congenitally short esophagus.
       (4) Acquired condition related to cephalad migration of gastric columnar epithelium in response to reflux injury of squamous epithelium.
       (5) Premalignant in cases when Barrett's lesion extends from proximal to distal 10 cm of the esophagus.
       (6) Results in adenocarcinoma.
    d. Caustic injury.
       (1) Cancer develops in 1% to 45% of clients with lye strictures.
       (2) May occur as late as 40 years after injury.
    e. Esophageal webs.
       (1) Plummer-Vinson iron deficiency anemia, glossitis, cheilosis, koilonychia, brittle fingernails, splenomegaly.
       (2) More common in females.
    f. Secondary primary with lung and head and neck tumors
       (1) Other cancers associated with risk factors (tobacco, alcohol).
       (2) Most arise in upper aerodigestive epithelium.
    g. Age and gender.
       (1) Most common in those 55 to 65 years old.
       (2) More common in males.
2. Dietary factors and lifestyle risk factors.
    a. Tobacco abuse.
    b. Alcohol abuse.
       (1) Synergistic effect when combined with tobacco.
    c. Low-calorie diet.
    d. Low-protein diet.
    e. Pickled vegetables.
    f. Exposure to carbon black, nitrosamines (rubber workers), and sulfuric acid (food industry).
    g. Deficiencies in vitamins A, C, E, B_{12}, folic acid, and riboflavin (Nakagawa et al., 2003).
    h. Obesity.
       (2) Excessive adipose tissue may predispose to reflux. May be related to increase in intraabdominal pressure.

   3. Genetic factors.
      a. Human papillomavirus leads to oncogene activation and tumor suppressor gene inactivation.
      b. Epidermal growth factor receptors contribute to abnormal cell growth (Waxman & Herbst, 2000).
      c. Gene *c-myc* implicated in cell proliferation, differentiation seen amplified in 15% of esophageal cancers.
      d. Gene *p53* seen frequently as early indicator of dysplasia (Nakagawa et al., 2003).
II. Physical examination.
   A. Weight loss.
   B. Dysphagia.
   C. Odynophagia.
   D. "Food sticking."
   E. Melena.
   F. Cough (with tracheoesophageal fistula).
   G. Hematemesis.
   H. Horner's syndrome.
      1. Miotic pupils and ptosis of the eyelid.
      2. Loss of sweating over affected side.
      3. Enophthalmos (recession of the eyeball into the orbit) caused by paralysis of the cervical sympathetic trunk.
      4. Exsanguinating hemorrhage with aortic erosion.
III. Laboratory data.
   A. Hemoglobin, hematocrit levels.
   B. Liver enzyme studies.
   C. Electrolyte levels (Schmitt & Brazer, 2003).

Nursing Diagnoses

   I. Acute or chronic pain.
  II. Anxiety.
 III. Imbalanced nutrition: less than body requirements.
  IV. Risk for aspiration.
   V. Deficient knowledge related to diagnosis and treatment of esophageal cancer.
  VI. Impaired swallowing.

Outcome Identification

   I. Client states adequate pain relief or ability to cope with current level of pain.
  II. Client describes a reduction in level of anxiety experienced.
      A. Client demonstrates positive coping behaviors.
 III. Client weighs within 10% of ideal body weight.
  IV. Client maintains patent airway and does not aspirate fluids or foods.
   V. Client discusses rationale, schedule, and personal demands of treatment and follow-up plan.
      A. Client lists potential side effects of disease and treatment.
      B. Client describes and uses self-care measures to manage the effects of the disease and treatment.
      C. Client and family specify symptoms to report immediately to the health care team.

    1. Bleeding.
    2. Aspiration.
    3. Shortness of breath.
    4. Fever.
    5. Intractable nausea and vomiting.
    6. Dizziness and syncope.
VI. Client does not aspirate foods or fluids.

Planning and Implementation

  I. Interventions to decrease incidence and severity of complications of treatment unique to esophageal cancer.
    A. Monitor for postoperative complications.
      1. Wound healing.
    B. Management of multiple incision and drains.
      1. Anastomotic leak.
      2. Aspiration.
      3. Respiratory complications.
        a. Severe atelectasis.
        b. Pulmonary edema.
        c. Adult respiratory distress syndrome (ARDS).
      4. Assess need for jejunostomy tube for initial postoperative enteral feeding.
    C. Monitor for side effects of radiation.
      1. Nausea and vomiting.
      2. Dysphagia.
      3. Fatigue.
      4. Myelosuppression in combined radiation/chemotherapy regimen.
      5. Fistula (in advanced lesions, a tracheoesophageal fistula may occur as the tumor regresses).
    D. Monitor for side effects of chemotherapy.
      1. Mucositis.
      2. Nausea and vomiting.
      3. Diarrhea.
      4. Myelosuppression.
      5. Neurotoxicity.
    E. Pharmacologic interventions.
      1. Administer antiemetics, antimicrobials, antidiarrhea drugs, and human growth factors, as needed.
      2. Assess pain, and administer pain medications as needed.
    F. Nonpharmacologic intervention.
      1. Refer for swallowing therapy.
      2. Provide outlet for discussions of fear and anxiety since many individuals present with advanced disease.
      3. Consider relaxation, meditation, and other techniques to manage anxiety and pain.
    G. Monitor for imbalanced nutrition.
      1. Refer to dietitian for nutritional support assessment.
      2. Swallowing therapy.
      3. Weigh at least weekly.
  II. Interventions to incorporate the client and family in care.
    A. Prevention and early detection.

1. Instruct family members about predisposing conditions and risk factors for esophageal cancer.
        2. Refer the client and family to substance abuse programs, if indicated.
        3. Teach the family to recognize signs and symptoms of esophageal cancer.
    B. Treatment and follow-up demands.
        1. Educate the client and family about self-care measures to reduce complications of disease and treatment.
        2. Inform them about written and service resources (see Chapter 8).
        3. Refer to Alcoholics Anonymous or other substance abuse programs.
        4. Encourage participation in smoking cessation programs.
        5. Teach the client and family signs and symptoms to report immediately to the health care team, including fever, bleeding, intractable nausea and vomiting, dizziness and syncope, aspiration, and shortness of breath.

Evaluation

The oncology nurse systematically and regularly evaluates the client's and/or family's responses to interventions to determine progress toward the achievement of expected outcomes. Relevant data are collected, and actual findings are compared with expected findings. Nursing diagnoses, outcomes, and plans of care are reviewed and revised as necessary.

GASTRIC CANCER

Theory

I. Anatomy/physiology and pathophysiology associated with gastric cancer.
    A. Anatomy.
        1. Begins at the gastroesophageal junction, ends at the pylorus.
        2. Divided into three major parts.
            a. Fundus.
            b. Corpus or body.
            c. Antrum.
        3. Critical adjacent structures.
            a. Diaphragm.
            b. Liver.
            c. Abdominal wall.
            d. Colon.
            e. Greater omentum.
            f. Spleen.
            g. Pancreas.
            h. Left adrenal gland and kidney.
            i. Duodenum (Farrell & Wang, 2003).
    B. Normal functions.
        1. Storage of food until it can enter the lower portion of gastrointestinal (GI) tract.
        2. Mixing of food with gastric secretions until chyme, a semifluid mixture, is formed.
        3. Slow emptying of food into small intestine at rate that accommodates absorption and digestion.
    C. Changes in function because of cancer.
        1. Early gastric cancer is often asymptomatic.

      2. If symptoms reported, often are nonspecific and may include the following:

        a. Epigastric discomfort.

        b. Dysphagia.

        c. Early satiety.

        d. Persistent vomiting.

        e. Weight loss.

        f. Pain (Goldberg, 2000).

      3. Late symptoms are due to metastatic spread.

    D. Metastatic patterns.

      1. Penetration of gastric wall.

      2. Invasion of intramural lymphatics.

      3. Local spread to esophagus or duodenum.

      4. Through the serosa to the omentum, spleen, liver, kidney, pancreas, bowel, and lung (Goldberg, 2000).

II. Trends in epidemiology.

  A. United States.

    1. Tenth most common cancer in men, fourteenth in women.

    2. Incidence declining in last 60 years.

    3. Ninety percent of cancers are adenocarcinomas.

      a. Other lesions with greater than 1% incidence are gastric lymphoma and leiomyosarcoma (Kurtz, 2003).

  B. Worldwide.

    1. Leading cause of cancer death in Japan.

    2. High incidence in Thailand, Finland, and mountainous regions of Colombia (Kurtz, 2003).

III. Principles of medical management.

  A. Screening and diagnostic procedures.

    1. High-risk areas (Japan) screen with double-contrast upper GI barium studies and upper GI endoscopy.

  B. Diagnostic procedures.

    1. Results of barium study with biopsy yield diagnosis.

    2. Abdominal and chest radiographs.

    3. Endoscopic ultrasonography (EUS) (Kurtz, 2003).

  C. Staging methods and procedures.

    1. TNM system used (Table 25-3).

    2. Surgical staging with lymph node sampling.

  D. Treatment strategies.

    1. Surgery.

      a. Surgical approaches (Table 25-4).

      b. Curative modality in local disease.

      c. Nutritional assessment is critical preoperatively.

      d. Feeding jejunostomy may be needed in those who are nutritionally compromised (Osteen, 2003).

    2. Chemotherapy.

      a. Postoperative in high-risk clients.

      b. Combination regimens include the following:

        (1) FAM—Fluorouracil (5-FU), Adriamycin (doxorubicin), mitomycin C (Mutamycin).

        (2) FAP—5-FU, Adriamycin, Platinol (cisplatin).

        (3) FAMTX—5-FU, Adriamycin, methotrexate (Folex, Mexate) (with rescue leucovorin [Wellcovorin]).

        (4) EAP—Etoposide (VP-16), Adriamycin, Platinol.

TABLE 25-3
Staging of Gastric Cancer

Stage	Description
T = PRIMARY TUMOR	
TX	Primary tumor cannot be assessed
T0	No evidence of primary tumor
Tis	Carcinoma in situ
T1	Tumor invades lamina propria or submucosa
T2	Tumor invades muscularis propria
T3	Tumor invades adventitia
T4	Tumor invades adjacent structures
N = REGIONAL LYMPH NODES	
NX	Regional lymph node(s) cannot be assessed
N0	No regional lymph node metastasis
N1	Metastasis in perigastric lymph node(s) within 3 cm of primary tumor
N2	Metastasis in perigastric lymph node(s) more than 3 cm from edge of primary tumor or in lymph nodes along left gastric, common hepatic, splenic, or celiac arteries
M = DISTANT METASTASIS	
MX	Presence of distant metastasis cannot be assessed
M0	No distant metastasis
M1	Distant metastasis

Stage Grouping

Stage 0	Tis	N0	M0
Stage IA	T1	N0	M0
Stage IB	T1	N1	M0
	T2	N0	M0
Stage II	T1	N2	M0
	T2	N1	M0
	T3	N0	M0
Stage IIIA	T2	N2	M0
	T3	N1	M0
	T4	N0	M0
Stage IIIB	T3	N2	M0
	T4	N1	M0
Stage IV	T4	N2	M0
	Any T	Any N	M1

From Greene FL, Page DL, Fleming ID, et al., editors. *American Joint Committee on Cancer (AJCC). Cancer staging handbook,* ed 6, New York, 2002, Springer-Verlag.

    c. Single agents include the following:
        (1) 5-FU.
        (2) Doxorubicin.
        (3) Cisplatin.
        (4) Etoposide.
        (5) Mitomycin C.
        (6) Nitrosoureas—bischloroethylnitrosourea (BCNU) (Carmustine), methyl-CCNU (Semustine)
    d. Delivery systems.

TABLE 25-4
Surgical Approaches to Gastric Cancer

Procedure	Anatomic Site of Lesion	Technique	Advantages/Disadvantages	Continuity of GI Tract
Radical distal subtotal resection	Body or antrum of stomach	Billroth I—removes first portion of duodenum, distal stomach, pylorus	Procedure of choice for elderly or debilitated clients because surgical time is limited; however, scope of resection is also limited	Gastroduodenostomy
		Billroth II—removes 80% of stomach, first portion of duodenum, gastrohepatic and gastrocolic omentum, and nodal tissue adjacent to celiac axis	Preserves a small part of the stomach, which is a better material for anastomosis than esophagus; limited by tumor extent; if clear margins cannot be obtained, total gastrectomy is needed	Gastrojejunostomy
Total gastrectomy	Extensive or proximal lesions	Entire stomach is removed along with lymph nodes and structures as indicated above; in addition, spleen and distal pancreas may be removed	Increased morbidity/mortality related to anastomotic leaks; extensive lesions can be treated	Esophagoduodenostomy Esophagojejunostomy

GI, Gastrointestinal.

(1) Intraperitoneal, intraoperative, intraarterial administration.
(2) Systemic (Minsky, 2003).
      3. RT.
         a. As adjuvant with chemotherapy and/or surgery.
         b. Palliatively to alleviate bleeding, obstruction, and pain (Minsky, 2003).
IV. Trends in survival.
   A. Most gastric cancer in the United States diagnosed at an advanced stage.
   B. Five-year survival is 60% without serosal or nodal involvement and tumor at line of resection; it is less than 5% with these factors present (Goldberg, 2000).

Assessment

   I. Pertinent client and family history.
      A. Risk factors.
         1. Two variants of gastric cancer have different etiologic factors.
            a. Intestinal.
               (1) More common in men.
               (2) More common in older individuals.
               (3) More common in areas where gastric cancer is epidemic, suggesting environmental etiology.
               (4) Preexisting disease—arises from precancerous areas, such as gastric atrophy or intestinal metaplasia.
            b. Diffuse.
               (1) More frequent in women.
               (2) More frequent in younger individuals.
               (3) Preexisting disease not a factor.
               (4) Familial pattern suggesting genetic predisposition (Kurtz, 2003).
         2. Dietary and lifestyle factors.
            a. Low fat and protein.
            b. Salted meat and fish.
            c. High nitrate.
            d. Low vitamin A and vitamin C.
            e. Smoked and pickled foods.
            f. Smoking.
         3. Environmental factors.
            a. Lack of refrigeration.
            b. Poor-quality drinking water.
            c. Occupational exposure (rubber and coal workers) (Farrell & Wang, 2003).
         4. Medical factors.
            a. Prior gastric surgery (i.e., Billroth II with resulting atrophic gastritis).
            b. *Helicobacter pylori* infection.
         5. Gastric atrophy and gastritis.
         6. Barrett's esophagus with increased risk of adenocarcinoma of gastric cardia.
            a. Genetic factor.
               (1) Familial clustering of *H. pylori.*
               (2) Familial diffuse gastric cancer.
               (3) Hereditary nonpolyposis colorectal cancer (Farrell & Wang, 2003).
  II. Physical examination.
      A. Epigastric discomfort.
      B. Dysphagia.
      C. Weight loss.

    D. Fatigue.

    E. Epigastric mass.

    F. Vomiting.

    G. Vague symptoms often present; retrosternal or back pain.

    H. Jaundice in advanced disease.

III. Laboratory data.

    A. Decreased hemoglobin and hematocrit levels since 50% present with anemia.

    B. Elevated liver enzyme levels from liver metastasis (Kurtz, 2003).

Nursing Diagnoses

   I. Acute or chronic pain.

  II. Anxiety.

 III. Imbalanced nutrition: less than body requirements.

  IV. Risk for deficit fluid volume.

   V. Deficient knowledge related to diagnosis and treatment of gastric cancer.

Outcome Identification

   I. Client states adequate pain relief or ability to cope with current level of pain.

  II. Client describes a reduction in level of anxiety experienced.

    A. Client demonstrates positive coping behaviors.

 III. Client weighs within 10% of ideal body weight.

  IV. Client does not experience symptoms related to postgastrectomy dumping syndrome.

   V. Client discusses rationale, schedule, and personal demands of the treatment and follow-up plans.

    A. Client lists potential side effects of the disease and treatment.

    B. Client describes and uses self-care measures to manage the effects of the disease and treatment.

    C. Client and family/significant other specify symptoms to report immediately to the health care team.

        1. Intractable vomiting.

        2. Symptoms of bowel obstruction.

        3. Bleeding.

        4. Fever.

        5. Pain.

Planning and Implementation

   I. Interventions to decrease the incidence and severity of complications of treatment unique to gastric cancer.

    A. Monitor for side effects of surgery.

        1. Dumping syndrome.

        2. Poor wound healing.

        3. Infection.

        4. Anastomotic leak.

        5. Reflux aspiration.

        6. Bezoar formation (food at gastric outlet).

    B. Monitor for side effects of chemotherapy.

        1. Mucositis.

        2. Diarrhea.

  3. Nausea and vomiting.

  4. Myelosuppression.

 C. Monitor for side effects of radiation.

  1. Nausea.

  2. Vomiting.

  3. Fatigue.

II. Interventions to incorporate the client and family in care.

 A. Prevention and early detection.

  1. Instruct family members about familial and dietary risks for gastric cancers.

  2. Discuss recommended screening if at high risk.

  3. Teach the family to recognize signs and symptoms of gastric cancer.

 B. Treatment and follow-up demands.

  1. Educate client and family about self-care measures to reduce complications of disease and treatment.

  2. Inform about written and service resources (see Chapter 8).

  3. Signs and symptoms to report immediately to health care team, such as intractable vomiting, fever, pain, signs of bowel obstruction and bleeding.

Evaluation

The oncology nurse systematically and regularly evaluates the client's and/or family's responses to interventions to determine progress toward the achievement of expected outcomes. Relevant data are collected, and actual findings are compared with expected findings. Nursing diagnoses, outcomes, and plans of care are reviewed and revised as necessary.

COLORECTAL CANCER

Theory

 I. Anatomy/physiology and pathophysiology associated with colorectal cancer.

  A. Anatomy.

   1. Colon (Figure 25-1).

    a. Extends from the terminal ileum to the anal canal.

    b. Consists of four parts—ascending or right colon, transverse or middle colon, descending or left colon, sigmoid colon.

   2. Rectum (see Figure 25-1).

    a. Is continuous with the sigmoid colon and terminates at the distal anal canal.

    b. Contains a transitional zone between keratinized and nonkeratinized stratified squamous epithelium at the anal verge.

    c. Is covered with peritoneum.

   3. Anus.

    a. Terminal 4 to 6 cm of GI tract.

    b. Area between anal verge and anorectal ring where there is a transition in epithelium from squamous to columnar epithelium.

   4. Critical adjacent structures.

    a. Venous drainage from the colon and upper to middle third of the rectum enters the portal system to the liver.

    b. Lower third of the rectum drains to the portal vein and inferior vena cava.

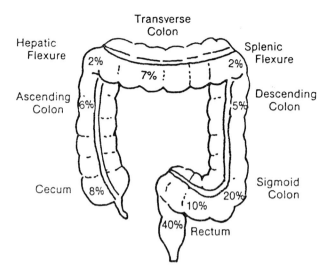

FIGURE 25-1 ■ Anatomic regions of the colon and associated cancer incidence. Two thirds of all colorectal cancers occur in the rectosigmoid and rectum. Many of these cancers are within reach of the examining finger, and 50% are within the reach of a sigmoidoscope. (From Otte DM: Nursing management of the patient with colon and rectal cancer, *Semin Oncol Nurs* 4[4]:286, 1988.)

      c. Colon, rectum, and anus lie in proximity to the vagina in females and to the bladder, seminal vesicles, prostate, and urethra in males.

  B. Normal functions.

    1. Processing of ileal contents.

      a. Colon receives 800 to 1000 ml of ileal contents per day.

      b. Absorption of water and electrolytes occurs primarily in the proximal or right colon.

      c. Feces in the right colon are more fluid than in the sigmoid colon.

    2. Movement of ileal contents through bowel.

      a. Innervation of gut responds to both parasympathetic and sympathetic signals.

      b. Secretion, blood flow, and sensory perception are controlled by submucosal structures.

      c. Ileal contents are moved through the colon by a mixture of circular constrictions and longitudinal contractions.

      d. Fecal material is exposed to the bowel wall for absorption of nutritional elements.

      e. Feces are pushed into the rectum.

    3. Storage of feces in the left colon until defecation.

    4. Defecation.

      a. Rectal wall is distended by feces.

      b. Peristalsis is initiated; the anal sphincter relaxes, and defecation occurs.

      c. External anal sphincter is controlled by the conscious mind and can inhibit defecation.

      d. If the impulse for defecation is ignored, the reflex fades.

  C. Changes in function because of cancer.

    1. Increase or decrease in consistency of stool.

    2. Changes in color of stool.

      3. Inability to move stool through bowel (obstruction) or pencil-shaped stool because of partial obstruction of bowel (Alquist & Pasha, 2003).

      4. Symptoms vary by location of cancer (see Table 25-8).

   D. Metastatic patterns.

      1. Colorectal cancers.

         a. Local extension through penetration of layers of bowel.

         b. Deeper penetration increases chance of spread.

         c. Tumors that have invaded beyond submucosal layer have direct access to vascular and lymphatic systems.

         d. Distant metastases most frequently occur in the liver and lungs and less frequently occur in the brain, bone, and adrenal glands.

      2. Anal cancers.

         a. Local extension to sphincter ani muscles, prostate, urethra, and bladder in males and vagina in females.

         b. Distant metastases occur in lung and liver (Goldberg, 2000).

II. Trends in epidemiology.

   A. United States.

      1. Third in incidence in men and women; 148,300 new cases each year.

      2. Incidence increases with age, but 3% occur in individuals under 40 years (Goldberg, 2003).

      3. Accounts for 11% of cancer mortality.

      4. Second to lung cancer in mortality; 57,000 deaths annually.

   B. Worldwide.

      1. Colorectal cancer is a common tumor, second only to lung cancer in the number of new cases.

      2. Worldwide, 600,000 cases annually.

III. Principles of medical management.

   A. Screening.

      1. Digital examination detects 10% of anorectal lesions.

      2. Checking stool for occult blood is controversial with respect to cost-effectiveness as a screening test.

      3. Flexible fiberoptic colonoscopy allows examination of up to 60 cm of colon.

      4. Screening guidelines: over age 50 years, annual fecal occult blood and rectal exam, sigmoidoscopy, or colonoscopy every 3 to 5 years.

   B. Diagnostic procedures (Table 25-5).

   C. Staging.

      1. TNM system is used (Table 25-6).

         a. TNM has replaced Duke's staging system.

      2. Staging based on clinical data or surgical data.

   D. Treatment strategies.

      1. Surgery.

         a. Surgical resection is the primary treatment for 75% of clients with colorectal cancer.

         b. Surgical approaches may or may not require ostomy (Table 25-7) (Owens & Bleday, 2003).

      2. RT.

         a. Preoperative RT used to do the following:

            (1) Decrease tumor size and render the tumor resectable.

            (2) Eradicate microscopic disease.

            (3) Decrease the incidence of local recurrence.

TABLE 25-5
Diagnostic Tests for Colorectal Cancer

Description/Purpose	Time Required for Test	Sensations Experienced	Potential Side Effects/ Complications	Self-Care Measures	Critical Symptoms to Report to Health Care Team
BARIUM ENEMA					
Identify extent of lesion in colon Identify obstruction	30-45 min	Fullness, abdominal pain, discomfort, urge to defecate	Perforation Bowel obstruction	Preparation includes liquid diet day before and low-residue diet 1-3 days before test Bowel preparation—laxatives or enema before and after examination. Client must hold anal sphincter against tube and breathe slowly to minimize discomfort	Failure to pass barium Signs of GI obstruction
COMPUTED AXIAL TOMOGRAPHIC (CAT) SCAN					
Identify lymph node involvement, liver metastases	45-60 min	May be claustrophobic when in scanner Sound of machine going on and off Warm feeling with injection of dye	Allergic reaction to dye Nausea from dye Blood samples for determining BUN and creatinine levels are drawn first to assess renal function	May receive nothing by mouth or be instructed to eat lightly before examination because of potential nausea from dye	With contrast, immediately report any discomfort, breathing difficulty, itching

STOOL FOR OCCULT BLOOD

Preparation—48-72 hr

False positive results: meat in diet, hemorrhoids, fissures, peroxidases in skin of vegetables and fruits (cherries, tomatoes), gastritis from aspirin

False negative results: failure to use high-residue, high-fiber diet

72 hr before test
Vitamin C in diet
Delay between collection and examination
Failure to prepare slide properly
Lesion not bleeding at time of examination

No red meat, poultry, fish, turnips, horseradish for 72 hr before test
Withhold iron and aspirin

Collect three specimens

Client urinates first into toilet, uses bedpan to collect stool
Send specimen to laboratory or return as instructed

COLONOSCOPY, SIGMOIDOSCOPY, PROCTOSCOPY

Visualize GI tract   15-30 min

Pressure discomfort
IV infusion with sedation
Lying on left side
Scope feels cool
Sensation of need to defecate

If tissue removed, bleeding
Adverse effects from sedatives

Clear liquid diet for 24 hr, laxative evening before, cleansing enema 3-4 hr before test
Deep breathing during examination
Expect a large amount of flatus after examination

Pain
Bleeding

GI, Gastrointestinal; *BUN,* blood urea nitrogen; *IV,* intravenous.

TABLE 25-6
Staging of Colorectal Cancer

Stage	Description
T = PRIMARY TUMOR	
TX	Primary tumor cannot be assessed
T0	No evidence of primary tumor
Tis	Carcinoma in situ
T1	Tumor invades submucosa
T2	Tumor invades muscularis propria
T3	Tumor invades through muscularis propria into subserosa or into nonperitonealized pericolic or perirectal tissues
T4	Tumor perforates visceral peritoneum or directly invades other organs or structures
N = LYMPH NODES	
NX	Regional lymph nodes cannot be assessed
N0	No regional lymph node metastasis
N1	Metastasis in one to three pericolic or perirectal lymph nodes
N2	Metastasis in four or more pericolic or perirectal lymph nodes
N3	Metastasis in any lymph node along course of a major named vascular trunk
M = DISTANT METASTASIS	
MX	Presence of distant metastasis cannot be assessed
M0	No distant metastasis
M1	Distant metastasis

Stage Grouping

0	Tis	N0	M0
I	T1	N0	M0
	T2	N0	M0
II	T3	N0	M0
	T4	N0	M0
III	Any T	N1	M0
	Any T	N2	M0
	Any T	N3	M0
IV	Any T	Any N	M1

Histopathologic Grade

GX	Grade cannot be assessed
G1	Well differentiated
G2	Moderately well differentiated
G3	Poorly differentiated
G4	Undifferentiated

From Greene FL, Page DL, Fleming ID, et al., editors: *American Joint Committee on Cancer (AJCC). Cancer staging handbook,* ed 6, New York, 2002, Springer-Verlag.

    b. Postoperative RT used to eradicate remaining disease if the following are true:

        (1) Surgical margins are positive for cancer.

        (2) Residual tumor is present.

        (3) Sphincter preservation is possible.

    c. Combined preoperative and postoperative RT may be used.

TABLE 25-7
Surgical Management of Colorectal Cancer

Site	Procedure	Technique	Physical Alterations	Possible Complications
Rectum	Low anterior resection—for lesions >10 cm from anal verge	Resect tumor and 2- to 5-cm margins; staple or suture bowel, conserving sphincter	Sphincter preserved	Anastomotic leak Abscess, infection, irregular bowel function
	Abdominal incision—remove tumor and adjacent involved or potentially involved structures	Performed through abdomen and perineum; perineal wound closed with drain or open to heal by granulation	Colostomy Perineal wound Foley catheter postoperatively Nasogastric tube postoperatively until peristalsis returns	Urinary dysfunction Wound infection Stomal complications Impotence in males Sexual dysfunction related to scarring in females
Anus	Removal of perianal skin, anal canal	Wide excision; antero-posterior resection may include total pelvic exenteration if lesions involve bladder or urethra	Colostomy Urinary diversion if total pelvic exenteration	As above
Colorectum	Hemicolectomy	Small tumors may be resected with enough margin so that permanent colostomy not needed; may have temporary colostomy	Temporary colostomy possible	Anastomotic leak
	Single-barreled colostomy	Proximal colon brought out and sutured to abdominal wall Defunctionalized colon removed or placed into abdomen (Hartmann's pouch)	Permanent colostomy Type of stool depends on location of stoma— *ascending*, fluid, semifluid; *transverse,* mush, semi-mush; *descend-ing*, solid; *rectum*, solid; *anus*, hard solid	Stomal complications Herniation Prolapse Hemorrhage
	Double-barreled colostomy	Two stomas Defunctionalized colon not removed Proximal portion sutured to abdominal wall end Stoma Distal mucous fistula		
All sites	Relief of obstruction May be done for palliation of symptoms	Debulking	May have tempo-rary colostomy, nasogastric tube	

    d. Early rectal cancers in the low-rectal and midrectal regions and anal cancer have been treated with endocavitary radiation (three treatments to a total dose of 8000 to 15,000 cGy).

    e. High complication rate resulting from superficial effect of high doses of radiation, although they are delivered with low-energy sources, including the following:

        (1) Radionecrosis.

        (2) Anal canal ulcers.

        (3) Strictures.

        (4) Bleeding (Clark & Willett, 2003).

3. Chemotherapy.

    a. Used in combination with surgery and RT.

    b. Fluorouracil (5-FU) remains mainstay.

    c. Other agents include irinotecan (Camptosar), oxaliplatin (Eloxatin), and capecitabine (Xeloda) (Clark & Willett, 2003).

    d. Oxaliplatin in combination with 5-FU and leucovorin (Wellcovorin) being studied in advanced colorectal tumors (Berg, 2003).

4. Biotherapy.

    a. Monoclonal antibodies as antiepidermal growth factors.

    b. Clinical trials are ongoing.

    c. Targeted therapy; such as bevacizumab (Avastin) approved for metastatic disease.

IV. Trends in survival.

    A. Survival is determined by the stage of disease, grade of tumor, histologic type of tumor, and general health status of the client.

    B. Colon cancer—general 5-year survival rate by stage.

        1. Stage I, 90% to 95%.

        2. Stage II, 75% to 80%.

        3. Stage III, 40% to 70%.

        4. Stage IV, 5%.

    C. Anal cancer overall 5-year survival rate is 48% to 66% (Goldberg, 2000).

Assessment

I. Pertinent client and family history.

    A. Risk factors.

        1. Age.

            a. Incidence increases slightly at 40 years; increases sharply at 50 years; doubles each decade thereafter.

        2. Medical factors.

            a. Villous adenoma.

                (1) Polyps most likely to become malignant.

                (2) Excision of polyps recommended, with annual colonoscopy follow-up examinations.

            b. Ulcerative colitis.

                (1) Increased duration of colitis increases risk for malignant change.

                (2) The longer the length of involved bowel, the greater the risk for malignancy.

            c. Crohn's disease—risk of malignancy is related to duration and extent of disease.

            d. Irritation of anal canal related to condylomata, fistula, fissures, abscesses, hemorrhoids.

  e. History of other cancers, such as breast and gynecologic cancers.
 3. Dietary factors.
  a. High-fat intake is proposed as an increased risk for colorectal cancer.
  b. Low-fiber diet increases transit time in the colon; therefore fecal bile acids and carcinogens in stool have a longer time to interact with mucosa.
 4. Environmental factors.
  a. Petroleum workers.
  b. Synthetic fabric manufacturers.
  c. Inhalation of wood or metal dust in rectal cancer (Alquist & Pasha, 2003).
 5. Genetic factors. Colorectal cancer is a genetic disease with important environmental influences.
  a. Familial polyposis, gene leads to successive chromosomal loss.
  b. Gardner's syndrome.
  c. Turcot's syndrome.
  d. Peutz-Jeghers syndrome.
  e. Juvenile polyposis.
  f. Family cancer syndrome.
  g. Changes in 5q chromosome and *ras* oncogene lead to deletion in region of chromosome.
  h. Diethyldithiocarbamic acid (DCC) deleted in colon cancer gene.
   (1) Role in cell-to-cell contact.
   (2) Loss of contact inhibition.
  i. Allelic loss of tumor suppressor gene such as *p53*, or adenomatous polyposis gene (APC) (Carethers, 2003).
 6. Physical examination.
  a. Early signs and symptoms.
   (1) Malaise and fatigue.
   (2) Signs and symptoms depend on location of cancer (Table 25-8).
   (3) Palpation of a mass in the transverse or right colon.
   (4) Occult or frank blood in stool.
  b. Late signs and symptoms.
   (1) Pain.
   (2) Weight loss.
   (3) Presence of symptoms of metastatic disease.
 7. Pulmonary—cough, chest pain, dyspnea, hemoptysis, wheezing, or dysphagia.
 8. Hepatic—ascites, abdominal distention, nausea, anorexia, increasing abdominal girth, jaundice, changes in color of urine and stool, or pruritus.
II. Laboratory data.
 A. Hemoglobin and hematocrit levels.
  1. Anemia commonly found with lesions on the right side.
 B. Liver function tests.
  1. Elevated lactate dehydrogenase (LDH), serum glutamate pyruvate transaminase (SGPT), or serum glutamic oxaloacetic transaminase (SGOT) caused by liver metastasis.
 C. Carcinoembryonic antigen (CEA).
  1. Although not valuable as a diagnostic or screening test, CEA has been used to monitor the response to therapy and follow-up care (Alquist & Pasha, 2003).
 D. Fecal occult blood testing.

TABLE 25-8
Characteristics of Colorectal Cancer

Site	Pathology	Characteristics	Presentation
Colon	Adenocarcinoma	Most are relatively slow growing, poorly differentiated, more aggressive; lymph node involvement common with progression	
Ascending			Anemia, nausea, weight loss, pain (vague, dull); palpable mass uncommon Late symptoms—diarrhea, constipation, anorexia
Transverse			Palpable mass, blood in stool, change in bowel habits, obstruction
Descending			Obstruction, pain (cramps), change in bowel habits
Sigmoid			Blood in stool, constipation, pencil-like stool, obstruction
Rectum	Adenocarcinoma	Same as above	Mucous discharge, bright red rectal bleeding (most common), tenesmus, sense of incomplete evacuation, mucous diarrhea, pain Late symptoms—feeling of rectal fullness, constant ache
Anus	Adenocarcinoma	Higher incidence in fifth through seventh decades; tend to be highly malignant; increasing incidence in male homosexuals	Rectal bleeding, pruritus, mucous discharge, tenesmus, pain or pressure in rectal region
	Squamous cell	May be multifocal; generally well differentiated and slow growing	
	Basal cell	Local spread only but may be highly malignant; does not behave like basal cell in skin—may metastasize	Sensation of lump, bleeding, pruritus, mucous discharge
	Kaposi's sarcoma (see Chapter 34)		

Nursing Diagnoses

I. Acute or chronic pain.
II. Anxiety.
III. Imbalanced nutrition: less than body requirements.
IV. Disturbed body image.
V. Sexual dysfunction.
VI. Deficient knowledge related to diagnosis and treatment of colorectal cancer.

Outcome Identification

I. Client states adequate pain relief or ability to cope with current level of pain.
II. Client describes a reduction in level of anxiety experienced.
   A. Client demonstrates positive coping behaviors.
III. Client weighs within 10% of ideal body weight.
IV. Client expresses feelings about ostomy.
V. Client describes strategies he/she can use in response to actual or potential sexual changes.
   A. Client identifies satisfactory alternative methods for expressing sexuality.
VI. Client discusses rationale, schedule, and personal demands of the treatment and follow-up plans.
   A. Client lists potential side effects of the disease and treatment.
   B. Client describes and uses self-care measures to manage the effects of the disease and treatment.
   C. Client and family specify symptoms to report immediately to the health care team.
      1. Changes in structure or function of ostomy.
      2. Symptoms of obstruction.
      3. Blood in stool.
      4. Symptoms of metastatic disease to lung or liver.

Planning and Implementation

I. Interventions to decrease the incidence and severity of complications of treatment unique to colorectal cancer.
   A. Stoma placement to decrease the incidence of skin reactions.
      1. Mark site at least 2 inches below the waist and away from leg creases.
         a. Avoid stoma placement near scars, bony prominence, skin folds, fistulas, pendulous breasts, or belt line.
         b. Allow for 2 inches of smooth skin around stoma for appliance adherence.
      2. Mark the site while client is lying flat, sitting, standing, and bending.
      3. Mark the site within borders of rectus muscles to minimize risk of herniation and prolapse.
   B. Appliance selection is based on character of stool, contour of skin surrounding stoma, client's manual dexterity, and cost.
   C. Stoma care.
      1. Change appliance every week.
      2. Use skin barriers cut to fit the stoma exactly.
      3. Avoid use of skin products and appliances that contain materials that cause allergic reactions.
      4. Assess the stoma and skin around stoma for complications with each appliance change—erythema; edema; erosion; bleeding; stomal protrusion, retraction, herniation, or narrowing.
   D. Management of common problems associated with an ostomy.
      1. Physiologic problems (see Table 25-9).
      2. Adjusting to body image change (see Chapter 3).
II. Interventions to monitor for side effects of treatment.
   A. Monitor for postoperative complications related to bowel surgery.
      1. Obstruction or paralytic ileus—pain, diarrhea, nausea, vomiting, or abdominal distention.

TABLE 25-9
Nursing Management of Common Problems Associated with an Ostomy

Problem	Nursing Management
Fecal odor due to normal intestinal flora or food	Good hygiene, odor proof pouch with charcoal filter, pouch deodorant, air freshener. Dietary experimentation (i.e., yogurt, parsley, and orange juice). Use of medications (chlorophyllin copper complex (Derifil), Bismuth subgallate, or Bismuth subcarbonate).
Urinary odor due to poor hygiene, infection, or concentrated urine.	Pouch deodorant; soak appliance in vinegar-water solution (1:4). Reassess client/family technique in care of the ostomy. Treat infection and increase fluid intake.
Peristomal skin irritation due to improper stoma size/placement, leakage, poor technique, or allergy.	Revise stoma. Alter pouch/skin barrier aperture, change/add convex skin barrier wafer, wafer strips, or powder/paste. Reassess client/family technique. Identify/remove allergen, avoid related products, dust with skin barrier power/apply topical corticosteriod agent.
Pressure, friction, or shear injuries due to abrasive cleaning technique or poor fitting appliance.	Reassess client/family technique. Alter pouch aperture and type of system as indicated.
Pseudooverrucous lesions due to prolonged exposure to moisture (seen in urostomies and high output stomas).	Alter pouch/skin barrier aperture and type of system. Change/add convexity. Refer to WOCN.
Candidiasis due to warm, moist peristomal region and antibiotic therapy.	Apply topical antifungal powder and skin barrier powder with pouch change. Reassess pouching system, wearing time, and barrier type.

WOCN, Wound ostomy and continent nurse.
Data from Erwin-Toth, P: Caring for a stoma, *Nursing* 31:36-40, 2001; Hampton BG, Bryant RA: *Ostomies and Continent Diversions: Nursing Management*, St Louis, 1992, Mosby; Rowbotham JL: *Managing colostomies*, Pub. No. 3422-PE, Atlanta, 1982, American Cancer Society.

   2. Bleeding—pulse rate, respiratory rate, blood pressure, amount and color of drainage from wound and/or stoma.
   3. Infection—fever, pain, redness at incision site, edema, or changes in amount or color of wound drainage.
   4. Stomal complications—retraction, changes in color of stoma, protrusion of stoma onto abdomen, narrowing of stomal opening, herniation, or drainage from fistulous tracts around the stoma.
   5. Changes in sexual function (see also Chapter 6).
      a. Males—may have erectile and ejaculatory problems with severing of nerves (vertebral segments S2 to S4 and L2 to L4).
      b. Females—enervation not a problem but they may have a decrease in length of the vagina, lack of lubrication, or discomfort with intercourse because of surgical dissection in which the vagina is separated from the rectum.
   B. Monitor for return of bowel function.
      1. Presence of bowel sounds, passage of flatus, passage of stool.
      2. Tolerance of progressive oral diet.

C. Monitor for complications of RT to the GI tract.
 1. Inflammation of the bowel or bladder.
 2. Blood in stool or urine.
 3. Ulceration of GI mucosa—pain.
 4. Necrosis.
 5. Changes in sexual activity related to inflammation of perineal skin.
 D. Monitor for complications of chemotherapy for colorectal cancers—fluorouracil, leucovorin, cisplatin, methotrexate, semustine.
 1. Mucositis.
 2. Diarrhea.
 3. Nausea and vomiting.
 4. Myelosuppression.
 5. Decreased libido.
III. Interventions to incorporate the client and family in care.
 A. Prevention and early detection.
 1. Instruct family members about familial risks for colorectal cancers.
 2. Discuss recommended screening guidelines for high-risk individuals.
 3. Suggest dietary modifications to reduce risks of colorectal cancers.
 4. Teach the family to recognize early signs and symptoms of colorectal cancers.
 B. Treatment and follow-up demands.
 1. Educate the client and family about self-care measures to reduce complications of the disease and treatment.
 2. Inform them about written and service resources available for client and family facing a diagnosis of colorectal cancer (see Chapter 8).
 3. Teach the client and family signs and symptoms to report immediately to health care team (e.g., changes in structure or function of ostomy, symptoms of obstruction, blood in stool, symptoms of metastatic disease to lung or liver).

Evaluation

The oncology nurse systematically and regularly evaluates the client's and/or family's responses to interventions to determine progress toward the achievement of expected outcomes. Relevant data are collected, and actual findings are compared with expected findings. Nursing diagnoses, outcomes, and plans of care are reviewed and revised as necessary.

PANCREATIC CANCER

Theory

 I. Anatomy/physiology and pathophysiology associated with pancreatic cancer.
 A. Anatomy.
 1. Lies obliquely in upper retroperitoneal area.
 a. Head tucked behind the stomach into the curve of the duodenum.
 b. Body anterior to first and second lumbar vertebrae.
 c. Tail touching the spleen, anterior to the superior pole of the left kidney.
 2. Composed of soft lobules of glandular tissue mixed with adipose tissue.

     3. Critical adjacent structures.
        a. Aorta.
        b. Celiac axis.
        c. Superior mesenteric artery.
        d. Inferior vena cava.
        e. Splenic artery and vein.
  B. Normal functions.
     1. Digestion of proteins, carbohydrates, and fats by pancreatic enzymes.
     2. Secretion of insulin and glucagon.
  C. Changes in function.
     1. Early symptoms are vague and nonspecific.
        a. Indigestion.
        b. Weight loss.
        c. Abdominal pain.
     2. Specific systems develop late and are due to loss of pancreatic function or invasion or obstruction of nearby structures.
        a. Increased abdominal pain.
        b. Jaundice.
        c. Nausea, diarrhea, obstipation.
        d. Diabetes mellitus.
  D. Metastatic patterns.
     1. Liver.
     2. Peritoneum (Goldberg, 2000; Reiser & Schmiegel, 2003).
II. Trends in epidemiology.
  A. United States.
     1. 28,000 new cases annually and 25,000 deaths.
     2. Fifth leading cause of cancer deaths.
  B. Worldwide.
     1. Incidence highest in North America and New Zealand (Reiser & Schmiegel, 2003).
III. Principles of medical management.
  A. Screening.
     1. Routine screening has not been reported.
  B. Tumor markers.
     1. Lack sensitivity and tumor specificity.
     2. CA 19-9 suggested but is not sensitive enough for screening.
  C. Diagnostic procedures.
     1. Abdominal ultrasound.
     2. CT.
     3. Magnetic resonance imaging (MRI).
     4. Endoscopic retrograde cholangiopancreatography (ERCP).
     5. Endoscopic ultrasound.
     6. PET scan.
  D. Staging.
     1. TNM staging (Table 25-10).
     2. Most clients present with advanced disease (Goldberg, 2000).
  E. Treatment strategies.
     1. Surgery.
        a. Pancreaticoduodenectomy (Whipple's procedure) is the removal of distal third of stomach; gallbladder; cystic and common bile duct; head of pancreas; parts of tail and body; duodenum; proximal 10 cm of

TABLE 25-10
Staging of Pancreatic Cancer

Stage	Description
T = PRIMARY TUMOR	
TX	Primary tumor indeterminate
T0	No primary tumor detected
Tis	Carcinoma in situ
T1	Tumor confined to the pancreas, 2 cm or less
T2	Tumor confined to the pancreas, >2 cm
T3	Infiltration of the duodenum, bile duct, or peripancreatic tissue
T4	Infiltration of stomach, colon, spleen, or large vessels
N = LYMPH NODE	
NX	Regional lymph node indeterminate
N0	No regional lymph node metastases
N1	Regional lymph node metastases
M = DISTANT METASTASIS	
MX	Distant metastases indeterminate
M0	No distant metastases
M1	Distant metastases

From Reiser M, Schmiegel W: Clinical aspects of pancreatic and ampullary cancers. In Rustgi A, editor: *Gastrointestinal cancer*, New York, 2003, WB Saunders, pp. 507-519.

jejunum; and superior mesenteric, peripancreatic, and hepatoduodenal lymph nodes.
   b. Total pancreatectomy.
   c. Pylorus-preserving pancreatectomy-antrectomy not included.
   d. Limited surgery for palliation of obstructive symptoms (i.e., biliary bypass or bowel resection/bypass) (Gibbs et al., 2003).
  2. Chemotherapy.
   a. Response rate in recent trials is under 15%.
   b. Gemcitabine (Gemzar) as single agent or gemcitabine plus fluorouracil.
   c. Other agents being studied include camptothecin, topotecan (Hycamtin), taxanes, doxorubicin (Adriamycin), and ifosfamide (IFEX).
  3. Radiation.
   a. Limited role as single agent.
   b. Used in trials with 5-FU in unresectable tumors (Gibbs et al., 2003).
IV. Trends in survival.
  A. Lowest 5-year survival of all GI cancers (<5%) because of the following:
   1. Lack of early symptoms.
   2. Lack of sensitive and specific screening tools.
   3. Majority present with stage IV disease.
  B. Fewer than 20% of clients survive the first year.

    C. Even with resection and all negative nodes, 5-year survival rate is 55%.

    D. Median survival in nonresectable or metastatic disease is 2 to 6 months (Goldberg, 2000).

Assessment

  I. Pertinent client and family history.

    A. Risk factors.

      1. Age over 50 years.

      2. Lifestyle factors.

        a. Alcohol consumption.

        b. Cigarette smoking.

      3. Environmental factors.

        a. Exposure to aromatic amines (chemical industry).

      4. Medical factors.

        a. Diabetes mellitus.

        b. Hereditary metabolic disease.

    B. Hereditary pancreatitis.

    C. Cystic fibrosis (Reiser & Schmiegel, 2003).

      1. Genetic factors.

        a. Activation of *Kras* oncogene.

        b. Inactivation of *p53, p16,* and *BRCA-2* tumor suppressor genes.

        c. Two or more first-degree relatives.

        d. Cancer syndromes, such as familial polyposis, familial breast cancer, or familial atypical multiple mole melanoma.

 II. Physical examination.

    A. Early signs and symptoms.

      1. Most signs and symptoms are late.

      2. Painless jaundice most common presentation in individuals with a potentially curable lesion.

    B. Late signs and symptoms.

      1. Pain most common; 80% present with pain associated with advanced disease.

      2. Weight loss.

      3. Diabetes mellitus.

      4. Palpable gallbladder.

      5. Nausea, vomiting, obstipation.

      6. Upper GI hemorrhage.

      7. Splenomegaly.

Nursing Diagnoses

  I. Acute or chronic pain.

 II. Anticipatory grieving.

III. Deficient knowledge related to diagnosis and treatment.

IV. Impaired nutrition: less than body requirements.

Outcome Identification

  I. Client states adequate pain relief or ability to cope with current level of pain.

 II. Client verbalizes feelings about pending death.

    A. Client establishes and maintains functional support systems.

III. Client discusses rationale, schedule, and personal demands of the treatment and management of symptoms.
  A. Client lists potential effects of the disease and treatment.
  B. Client describes and uses self-care measures to manage the effects of the disease and treatment.
  C. Client and family/significant other specify symptoms to report immediately to the health care team.
    1. Intractable pain.
    2. Intractable vomiting.
    3. Symptoms of bowel obstruction.
    4. Bleeding (Reiser & Schmiegel, 2003).
IV. Client weighs within 10% of ideal body weight.

Planning and Implementation

  I. Interventions to decrease the incidence and severity of complications unique to pancreatic cancer.
  A. Monitor for surgical complications.
    1. Sepsis.
    2. Abscess formation.
    3. Hemorrhage.
    4. Pancreatic and biliary fistulas.
  B. Monitor for side effects of radiation.
    1. Nausea and vomiting.
    2. Fatigue.
  C. Monitor for side effects of chemotherapy.
    1. Mucositis.
    2. Nausea and vomiting.
    3. Diarrhea.
    4. Myelosuppression.
 II. Interventions to include client and family in care.
  A. Provide information about symptom management.
  B. Provide support during decision-making process.
  C. Work with health care providers to determine palliative care needs (Goldberg, 2000).

Evaluation

The oncology nurse systematically and regularly evaluates the client's and/or family's responses to interventions in order to determine progress toward the achievement of expected outcomes. Relevant data are collected, and actual findings are compared with expected findings. Nursing diagnoses, outcomes, and plans of care are reviewed and evaluated as necessary.

REFERENCES

Alquist, D., & Pasha,T. (2003).Clinical aspects of sporadic colorectal cancer. In A. Rustgi (Ed.). *Gastrointestinal cancers.* New York: W.B. Saunders, pp. 379-407.

Berg, D. (2003). Oxaliplatin: A novel platinum analog with activity in colorectal cancer. *Oncology Nursing Forum* 30(6), 957-966.

Carethers, J. (2003). Biology and genetics of colorectal cancer. In A. Rustgi (Ed.). *Gastrointestinal cancer.* New York: W.B. Saunders, pp. 407-421.

Clark, J., & Willett, C. (2003). Chemotherapy and radiation therapy of colorectal cancer. In A. Rustgi (Ed.). *Gastrointestinal cancer.* New York: W.B. Saunders, pp. 453-473.

Farrell, J., & Wang, T. (2003). Biology of gastric cancer. In A. Rustgi (Ed.). *Gastrointestinal cancer.* New York: W.B. Saunders, pp. 299-329.

Gibbs, J., Smith, J., & Douglass, H. (2003). Surgery of pancreatic cancer. In A. Rustgi (Ed.). *Gastrointestinal cancers.* New York: W.B. Saunders, pp. 541-549.

Goldberg, R. (2000). Gastrointestinal tract cancers. In D. Casciato & B. Lowitz (Eds.). *Manual of clinical oncology.* New York: Lippincott Williams & Wilkins, pp. 172-218.

Greene, F.L., Page, D.L., Fleming, I.D., et al. (Eds.). (2002). *American Joint Committee on Cancer (AJCC) cancer staging handbook* (6th ed.). New York: Springer-Verlag.

Kurtz, R. (2003). Clinical aspects of gastric cancer. In A. Rustgi (Ed.). *Gastrointestinal cancers.* New York: W.B. Saunders, pp. 291-299.

Marshall, M., & Kaiser, I. (2003). Surgery of esophageal cancer. In A. Rustgi (Ed.). *Gastrointestinal cancers.* New York: W.B. Saunders, pp. 271-283.

Minsky, B. (2003). Chemotherapy and radiation therapy of gastric cancer. In A. Rustgi (Ed.). *Gastrointestinal cancers.* New York: W.B. Saunders, pp. 345-355.

Nakagawa, H., Katzka, D., & Rustgi, A. (2003). Biology of esophageal cancer. In A. Rustgi (Ed.). *Gastrointestinal cancers.* New York: W.B. Saunders, pp. 241-253.

Odze, R., & Antonioli, D. (2003). Pathology of esophageal cancer. In A. Rustgi (Ed.). *Gastrointestinal cancers.* New York: W.B. Saunders, pp. 253-271.

Osteen, R. (2003). Surgery of gastric cancer. In A. Rustgi (Ed.). *Gastrointestinal cancers.* New York: W.B. Saunders, pp. 331-345.

Owens, C., & Bleday, R. (2003). Surgery of colorectal cancer. In A. Ristgi (Ed.). *Gastrointestinal cancers.* New York: W.B. Saunders, pp. 473-491.

Reiser, M., & Schmiegel, W. (2003). Clinical aspects of pancreatic and ampullary cancers. In A. Rustgi (Ed.). *Gastrointestinal cancer.* New York: W.B. Saunders, pp. 507-519.

Schmitt, C., & Brazer, S. (2003). Clinical aspects of esophageal cancer. In A. Rustgi (Ed.). *Gastrointestinal cancers.* New York: W.B. Saunders, pp. 215-241.

Waxman, E., & Herbst, R. (2000). The role of the epidermal growth factor receptor in the treatment of colorectal cancer. *Seminars in Oncology Nursing* (Suppl.) *18*(2):20-29.

Nursing Care of the Client with Cancers of the Reproductive System

SUSAN VOGT TEMPLE AND CYNTHIA H. UMSTEAD*

CERVICAL CANCER

Theory

I. Physiology and pathophysiology associated with cervical cancer (DiSaia & Creasman, 2002e; Solomon et al., 2002; Stehman et al., 2000).
   A. Anatomy of the cervix.
      1. Consists of the lower portion of the uterus, which is contiguous with the upper portion of the vagina.
      2. Composed of the exocervix and the endocervix.
      3. Surrounded by paracervical tissues rich in lymph nodes.
   B. Changes associated with cancer of the cervix.
      1. Cellular changes exist on a continuum from premalignant changes (mild to moderate to severe cervical intraepithelial neoplasia [CIN]) to carcinoma in situ (CIS) to invasive disease.
      2. The causative agents and risk factors associated with invasive cervical carcinoma have been a major focus of research. Certain subtypes of the human papillomavirus (HPV) are known to be oncogenic; multiple cofactors have been identified.
      3. Most cases of invasive cervical cancer arise in the transformation zone at the squamocolumnar junction (Figure 26-1).
         a. Exophytic, fungating, or cauliflower-like lesions protrude from the cervix.
         b. Excavating or ulcerative necrotic lesions replace the cervix or upper vagina.
         c. Endophytic lesions extend within the cervical canal.
      4. The two main histologic types of cervical cancer are squamous carcinoma and adenocarcinoma.
         a. Squamous carcinoma is most common (85% to 90%).
         b. Adenocarcinoma occurs in younger women and carries a poorer prognosis; bulky endocervical tumors are aggressive in nature and less responsive to treatment.

---

*Susan Vogt Temple and Cynthia H. Umstead are full-time employees of GlaxoSmithKline (GSK). The views and opinions expressed herein are those of the authors/editors and do not necessarily reflect those of GSK.

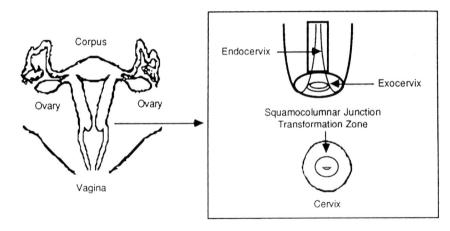

FIGURE 26-1 ■ Female reproductive organs with anatomy of the cervix.

C. Metastatic patterns.
1. Direct extension into the parametrium, vagina, lower uterine segment, the abdomen and other pelvic structures.
2. Lymph node metastases.
3. Metastasis to lung, liver, and bone through the hematologic route.
D. Trends in epidemiology.
1. Worldwide, invasive cervical cancer is one of the leading causes of morbidity and mortality in women.
2. Incidence of invasive cervical cancer in the United States (U.S.) has decreased significantly since 1945 because of successful screening programs (Papanicolaou [Pap] smear/test) with an increase in the diagnosis of preinvasive disease.
II. Principles of medical management.
A. Screening and diagnostic procedures.
1. Screening procedures.
a. Pap smear/test with bimanual pelvic examination is recommended as the screening test for premalignant and malignant cervical disease (American Cancer Society [ACS], 2003).
(1) ACS recommendations: initial Pap smear 3 years following initiation of vaginal intercourse but no later than 21 years of age, then
(2) Screening every year with Pap smear or every 2 years when using liquid-based Pap test, and
(3) Beginning at age 30 years, after three consecutive normal Pap smear/test results, repeat screening every 2 to 3 years at discretion of physician. If abnormal Pap test after age 30 years, consider hybrid capture for HPV subtyping for high-risk strains.
2. Diagnostic procedures (ACS, 2003; DiSaia & Creasman, 2002g; Stehman et al., 2000).
a. Colposcopy (examination of the cervix under magnification after application of acetic acid) is recommended as a component of evaluation of the cervix after obtaining an abnormal result from a Pap smear/test.
b. HPV deoxyribonucleic acid (DNA) testing for high-risk types of HPV for Pap tests revealing abnormal squamous cells (Solomon et al., 2002; Wright et al., 2002).

   c. Cervical biopsy is recommended when abnormalities are identified on the cervix by colposcopy.
   d. Endocervical curettage is recommended when the upper limits of cervical abnormalities are not visualized or the transformation zone within the endocervical canal is not visualized completely.
   e. Cone biopsy (Figure 26-2) or loop electrosurgical excision procedure (LEEP) may be recommended to obtain a larger wedge of tissue and to rule out invasive cancer.
B. Staging methods and procedures (DiSaia & Creasman, 2002e; Stehman et al., 2000).
   1. The Bethesda System describing Pap results was revised in 2001 (Solomon et al., 2002). General categories include the following:
      a. Negative for intraepithelial lesion or malignancy.
      b. Epithelial cell abnormalities (includes atypical squamous cells, squamous intraepithelial lesions, squamous cell carcinoma, atypical glandular cells).
      c. Other malignant neoplasms (to include melanoma, sarcomas, lymphoma).
   2. Biopsy reports cervical intraepithelial neoplasia including the following (DiSaia & Creasman, 2002g; Solomon et al., 2002; Stehman et al., 2000; Wright et al., 2002):
      a. CIN 1 (mild dysplasia).
      b. CIN 2 (moderate dysplasia).
      c. CIN 3 (severe dysplasia and carcinoma in situ).
      d. Squamous cell cancer of the cervix.
   3. For invasive cervical cancer, examination with the client under anesthesia is done to evaluate extent of disease. Extension of disease to the bladder or rectum is determined by cystoscopy, intravenous pyelogram (IVP), sigmoidoscopy, proctoscopy, or barium enema.
   4. Abdominal or pelvic computed tomographic (CT) scan, ultrasound, magnetic resonance imaging (MRI), or positron emission tomography (PET) scanning may be done to evaluate the extent of the local lesion and metastasis to regional lymph nodes.
   5. Chest x-ray examination is used to rule out lung metastasis.
   6. Invasive cervical cancer is clinically staged and is not altered by subsequent surgical findings (Table 26-1).

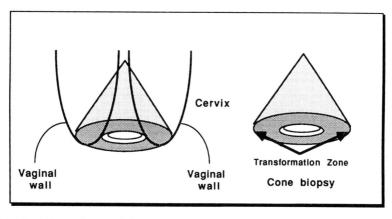

FIGURE 26-2 ■ Cone biopsy of the cervix.

TABLE 26-1
FIGO Staging for Cervical Cancer

Stage	Description
I	The carcinoma is strictly confined to the cervix.
IA	Invasive cancer identified only microscopically. All gross lesions even with superficial invasion are stage IB cancers. Invasion is limited to measured stromal invasion with maximum depth of 5 mm and no wider than 7 mm.
IA1	Measured invasion of stroma no greater than 3 mm in depth and no wider than 7 mm.
IA2	Measured invasion of stroma greater than 3 mm and no greater than 5 mm and no wider than 7 mm. The depth of invasion should not be more than 5 mm taken from the base of the epithelium, either surface or glandular, from which it originates. Preformed space involvement (vascular or lymphatic) should not alter the staging but should be specifically recorded so as to determine whether it should affect treatment decisions in the future.
IB	Clinical lesions confined to the cervix or preclinical lesions greater than 1A.
IB1	Clinical lesions no greater than 4 cm in size.
IB2	Clinical lesions greater than 4 cm in size.
II	The carcinoma extends beyond the cervix but has not extended to the pelvic wall. The carcinoma involves the vagina but not as far as the lower one third.
IIA	No obvious parametrial involvement.
IIB	Obvious parametrial involvement.
III	The carcinoma has extended to the pelvic wall. On rectal examination, there is no cancer-free space between the tumor and the pelvic wall. The tumor involves the lower one third of the vagina. All cases with hydronephrosis or nonfunctioning kidney are included unless they are known to be due to other causes.
IIIA	No extension to the pelvic wall.
IIIB	Extension to the pelvic wall and/or hydronephrosis or nonfunctioning kidney.
IV	The carcinoma has extended beyond the true pelvis or has clinically involved the mucosa of the bladder or rectum. A bullous edema as such does not permit a case to be allotted to stage IV.
IVA	Spread of the growth to adjacent organs.
IVB	Spread to distant organs.

Derived from AJCC Cancer Staging Manual, Sixth Edition. For a complete, official description of TNM, Stage Grouping and Histologic Grade for this site, please consult Greene F.L., Page D.L., Fleming, I.D., et al. *AJCC Cancer Staging Manual*, Sixth Edition. New York: Springer-Verlag, 2002.
FIGO, International Federation of Gynecology and Obstetrics.

    C. Treatment strategies (DiSaia & Creasman, 2002e, 2002g; Stehman et al., 2000).
        1. Preinvasive disease—biopsy, cautery, cryotherapy, laser therapy, conization, LEEP, or hysterectomy. Treatment depends on the following:
            a. Size and location of CIN visualized.
            b. Client's desire for preservation of childbearing capacity.
            c. Physician's skills and preference.
        2. Invasive disease—surgery and/or radiation.
            a. Treatment choice depends on client's age, physical condition, body habitus, tumor volume, and desire to maintain ovarian function.
            b. Primary surgical treatment—early-stage disease.
                (1) Radical trachelectomy (amputation of the cervix) in very select client populations desiring to preserve fertility (Shepherd et al., 2001).
                (2) Radical hysterectomy with pelvic lymphadenectomy and paraaortic lymph node dissection is the standard of care.
                (3) Bilateral salpingo-oophorectomy included in postmenopausal women or those over age 40 years/no longer desirous of childbearing.

    c. Primary radiation therapy (RT) treatment—early- or advanced-stage disease.
      (1) Combination of external and either high-dose outpatient or conventional inpatient intracavitary brachytherapy implants.
      (2) Intracavitary implants may be given before or after external RT is completed.
      (3) Radiosensitization with cisplatin (Platinol), 40 mg/m^2 weekly during radiation.
    d. Combination of surgery and radiation/chemotherapy for advanced-stage disease or early-stage disease with positive lymph nodes or positive surgical margins.

  3. Recurrent disease (DiSaia & Creasman, 2002e; Fischer, 2002; Stehman et al., 2000).
    a. Central recurrence only—anterior, posterior, or total pelvic exenteration.
      (1) Triad of unilateral leg edema, sciatic pain, and ureteral obstruction is indicative of recurrent and unresectable disease.
      (2) Extensive preoperative workup is done to rule out extrapelvic disease.
      (3) Initial pelvic sidewall biopsies/lymph node evaluation/frozen sections to rule out metastatic disease (intraoperatively).
      (4) Total pelvic exenteration includes removal of all pelvic viscera and creation of urinary conduit/colostomy.
    b. Unresectable or disseminated disease.
      (1) Chemotherapy is palliative with single agents. Agents with known activity include cisplatin, paclitaxel (Taxol), fluorouracil (5-Fluorouracil, 5-FU), methotrexate (Mexate), ifosfamide (Ifex), cyclophosphamide (Cytoxan), gemcitabine (Gemzar), topotecan (Hycamtin), and vinorelbine (Navelbine); response rates are low.

D. Trends in survival.
  1. No overall change in survival rate has occurred for clients with invasive cervical cancer, although mortality rate has decreased because of decreased incidence.
  2. Prognosis is related to stage of disease.
  3. Thirty-five percent of women have recurrent disease within 3 years of initial therapy.
  4. Cause of death associated most often with uremia, infection, or hemorrhage.

Assessment (DiSaia & Creasman, 2002e; Fischer, 2002; Stehman et al., 2000)

I. Pertinent personal and family history.
  A. Average age is between 45 and 55 years.
  B. Presence of HPV oncogenic subtypes, including HPV 16, 18, 33, 35, and 45.
  C. Initiation of sexual intercourse during teenage years.
  D. Multiple sexual partners and sexual partners who have had multiple sexual partners.
  E. History of CIN.
  F. Cigarette smoking.
  G. Immunosuppression (e.g., with acquired immunodeficiency disease [AIDS] or after transplantation).

II. Physical examination.
- **A.** Early signs and symptoms—most women are asymptomatic until disease is advanced.
  - **1.** May have a thin, watery vaginal discharge or painless, intermittent, postcoital, intramenstrual, or postmenopausal vaginal bleeding or an increase in the length and amount of menstrual flow.
- **B.** Late signs and symptoms—pain referred to the flank or leg, lower extremity edema.
  - **1.** Urinary symptoms include dysuria, urinary retention, urinary frequency, or hematuria.
  - **2.** Bowel symptoms may include rectal bleeding, constipation, or bowel obstruction.

III. Evaluation of laboratory data.
- **A.** Elevated blood urea nitrogen (BUN) and/or creatinine levels.
- **B.** Decreased hemoglobin or hematocrit levels.
- **C.** Increased white blood cell count.

Nursing Diagnoses

- **I.** Disturbed body image.
- **II.** Sexual dysfunction.
- **III.** Anticipatory or dysfunctional grieving.
- **IV.** Constipation.
- **V.** Impaired urinary elimination.
- **VI.** Ineffective coping.
- **VII.** Compromised family coping.
- **VIII.** Deficient knowledge related to personal risk factors, treatment, side effect management, and so on.

Outcome Identification

- **I.** Client describes personal risk factors for cervical cancer, methods to minimize risks, and plan for screening with Pap smear/test and pelvic examination.
- **II.** Client discusses rationale, schedule, and personal demands of treatment and follow-up care. Maintains vaginal vault access through regular intercourse or dilation.
- **III.** Client lists potential side effects of disease and treatment.
- **IV.** Client describes self-care measures to decrease the incidence and severity of complications of treatment.
- **V.** Client and family list signs and symptoms of recurrent disease to report to the health care team—pain in hips or lower back, vaginal bleeding, swelling of lower extremities, or unexplained weight loss.
- **VI.** Client and family describe community resources to potentially meet demands of treatment and survivorship (e.g., American Cancer Society, National Cervical Cancer Coalition, National Coalition for Cancer Survivorship).

Planning and Implementation (Fischer, 2002; Spinelli, 2002)

- **I.** Interventions to maximize safety for the client.
  - **A.** Teach changes in lifestyle that can modify risks of cervical cancer.
    - **1.** Limit number of sexual partners.

2. Use of barrier-type contraceptives—diaphragm or condom, although not protective for HPV exposure, protective for other sexually transmitted diseases (STDs).
3. Discontinuation of cigarette smoking.
4. Screening with a Pap smear/test as recommended to detect premalignant changes.

B. See Chapters 35 and 36 for safety concerns with surgery and radiation therapy (RT).

II. Interventions to decrease the severity of symptoms associated with disease and treatment.

A. Teach the client about possible symptoms associated with treatment modality options.

B. Primary symptoms related to surgery.
1. Inability to void—innervation to the bladder is disrupted during radical hysterectomy, resulting in an inability to sense the need to void and an inability to empty the bladder completely; a suprapubic catheter is placed postoperatively. Initiate bladder training by clamping the catheter for 2 to 3 hours. Encourage the client to drink fluids unless contraindicated by physiologic status. Remove the catheter after less than 50 ml of residual urine remains after voiding as ordered. *Alternatively,* client can be taught intermittent self-catheterization before discharge from the hospital.
2. Constipation—bowel is manipulated during radical surgery; peristalsis may not return for several days (see Chapter 15).
3. Shortened vagina—approximately one third of the upper vagina may be excised with hysterectomy; remaining margins are sutured to form a vaginal cuff.
4. Urinary and stool diversions with pelvic exenteration (see Chapter 15).

C. Primary symptoms related to RT (see Chapter 36 for nursing implications of RT to the ovary, urinary bladder, gastrointestinal [GI] tract, and skin).

III. Interventions to monitor for sequelae of disease or treatment.

A. Surgery.
1. Assess changes in bowel pattern—constipation, bowel obstruction, rare fistula formation.
2. Evaluate changes in bladder pattern—recurrent urinary tract infection, fistula formation.

B. RT.
1. Assess changes in bowel pattern—diarrhea, bowel obstruction, rectal ulcers, rectovaginal fistulas.
2. Assess changes in bladder pattern—urinary retention, cystitis, vesicovaginal fistulas.
3. Evaluate changes in vaginal tissues—atrophy, stenosis, dryness.

C. Recurrent disease.
1. Assess for history of vaginal bleeding.
2. Evaluate occurrence of new pain, particularly in hips or lower back.
3. Evaluate lower extremities for edema.
4. Assess for changes in appetite with weight loss.

IV. Interventions to incorporate the client and family in care.

A. Encourage open communication about the impact of disease and treatment on the client and significant others.

B. Teach the client and significant other new self-care skills required during or after treatment.

C. Identify concerns the client and sexual partner may have about resuming intercourse after treatment.

Evaluation

The oncology nurse systematically and regularly evaluates the client's and/or family's responses to interventions to determine progress toward the achievement of expected outcomes. Relevant data are collected, and actual findings are compared with expected findings. Nursing diagnoses, outcomes, and plans of care are reviewed and revised as necessary.

ENDOMETRIAL CANCER

Theory

I. Physiology and pathophysiology associated with endometrial cancer (Barakat et al., 2000; DiSaia & Creasman, 2002a).
   A. Anatomy of the endometrium.
      1. Inner layer of three layers of the uterus (endometrium, myometrium, parietal peritoneum).
      2. Highly vascular mucous membrane lining.
   B. Primary functions of the endometrium—provides vascular and nutrient supply for developing fetus and responds to variations in estrogen and progesterone levels in a cyclic fashion.
   C. Changes associated with cancer of the endometrium.
      1. Underlying cause of endometrial cancer is believed to be abnormal production and metabolism of endogenous estrogen.
      2. Atypical hyperplasia that may progress to invasive cancer.
      3. Histology is 90% adenocarcinoma (type 1); rarer types include clear cell, uterine papillary serous (type 2), adenosquamous, and sarcoma histology.
   D. Metastatic patterns.
      1. Invades inner one third of the endometrium and progresses to the full thickness of the endometrium.
      2. Metastasis occurs through local extension to adjacent structures, such as the cervix and vagina, and distantly to intraabdominal sites and lung.
      3. Metastasis occurs in femoral, iliac, hypogastric, paraaortic, and obturator lymph nodes.
      4. Hematologic metastasis is uncommon except in rarely occurring sarcoma.
   E. Trends in epidemiology.
      1. Most common gynecologic malignancy among women in the United States.
      2. Fourth most common cancer in women in the United States.
      3. Incidence has increased over the past several decades and has been associated with increased use of estrogen replacement therapy (without progestins).
II. Principles of medical management (Barakat et al., 2000; DiSaia & Creasman, 2002a; Kim et al., 2002; Levine & Hoskins, 2002).
   A. Screening procedures.
      1. Ultrasound has not been found to be cost effective as a screening modality for endometrial cancer.
      2. Bimanual pelvic examination to palpate the size and shape of the uterus.

B. Diagnostic procedures.
   1. Endometrial aspiration or biopsy.
   2. Endocervical curettage to rule out cervical cancer.
   3. Fractional dilation and curettage (D and C) if previous endometrial biopsy results have been negative, stenosis makes endometrial biopsy impossible, and/or abnormal bleeding persists.
C. Staging methods and procedures.
   1. Procedures.
      a. Suspected bladder or bowel involvement—cystoscopy, barium enema, proctoscopy, or sigmoidoscopy.
      b. Chest x-ray examination to rule out metastasis.
   2. Surgical staging based on findings from exploratory laparotomy, total abdominal hysterectomy–bilateral salpingo-oophorectomy (TAH-BSO), and peritoneal washings.
   3. Results of staging reported as anatomic stage, histopathologic grade, depth of myometrial invasion, and evaluation of peritoneal cytology (Table 26-2).
D. Treatment strategies (Barakat et al., 2000; DiSaia & Creasman, 2002a; Kim et al., 2002; Levine & Hoskins, 2002).
   1. Treatment decisions are based on stage of disease, grade, depth of myometrial invasion, presence or absence of prognostic features within the tumor specimen, and client characteristics.
   2. Preinvasive disease—administration of progesterone or simple hysterectomy.
   3. Invasive disease—surgery and/or RT.
      a. Surgery.
         (1) Surgical staging procedure (TAH-BSO with peritoneal cytologic examination) serves as primary treatment for early-stage disease.
         (2) Pelvic and paraaortic lymphadenectomy and omental biopsy included for grade 2 and 3 lesions.
      b. RT is the primary treatment for high-risk surgical candidates (Grigsby, 2002).

TABLE 26-2
FIGO Staging for Endometrial Cancer

Stage	Description
IA	Tumor limited to the endometrium
IB	Invasion to less than one half of the myometrium
IC	Invasion of more than one half of the myometrium
IIA	Endocervical gland involvement only
IIB	Cervical stromal invasion
IIIA	Invasion of uterine serosa and/or adnexa and/or positive peritoneal cytology
IIIB	Vaginal metastases
IIIC	Metastases to pelvic and/or paraaortic nodes
IVA	Invasion of bladder and/or bowel mucosa
IVB	Distant metastases, including intraabdominal metastases and/or inguinal lymph nodes

Derived from AJCC Cancer Staging Manual, Sixth Edition. For a complete, official description of TNM, Stage Grouping and Histologic Grade for this site, please consult Greene F.L., Page D.L., Fleming, I.D., et al. *AJCC Cancer Staging Manual*, Sixth Edition. New York: Springer-Verlag, 2002.
FIGO, International Federation of Gynecology and Obstetrics.

      c. Adjuvant RT.
- (1) Preoperative therapy for clients with extensive lesions involving the cervix or high-grade lesions.
- (2) Postoperative therapy for clients with risk factors for recurrent disease; high-grade lesions, deep myometrial invasion; or lower uterine segment/cervical involvement.
- (3) Techniques include intracavitary brachytherapy and teletherapy.

      d. Disseminated disease (Barakat et al., 2000; DiSaia & Creasman, 2002a; Kim et al., 2002; Levine & Hoskins, 2002).
- (1) Hormonal agents include synthetic progestational agents—megestrol acetate (Megace), medroxyprogesterone acetate (Depo-Provera), tamoxifen (Nolvadex), and numerous other agents have been investigated for activity.
- (2) Single-agent and combination chemotherapy—agents with known activity include cyclophosphamide (Cytoxan), doxorubicin (Adriamycin), paclitaxel (Taxol), carboplatin (Paraplatin), and cisplatin (Platinol).

      e. Recurrent disease—surgery or RT to previously untreated areas, chemotherapy, or hormonal therapy.

  E. Trends in survival.
1. Most curable gynecologic malignancy.
2. Prognostic factors include stage, grade, and depth of myometrial invasion, peritoneal cytology, and hormone receptor status.
3. Twenty-five to thirty-five percent of clients have recurrent disease.

Assessment

  I. Pertinent personal and family history (Barakat et al., 2000; DiSaia & Creasman, 2002a; Levine & Hoskins, 2002; Porter, 2002).
- **A.** Age—peak incidence, 50 to 59 years.
- **B.** Menopausal status—80% of clients are postmenopausal.
- **C.** Socioeconomic status—higher status places women at increased risk.
- **D.** History of changes in hormone levels—obesity, nulliparity, late menopause, infertility, anovulation, irregular menstrual history, Stein-Leventhal syndrome, and estrogen replacement therapy without progestational agents.
- **E.** Personal history of endometrial hyperplasia; breast, ovarian, or colorectal cancers.
- **F.** Family history of hereditary nonpolyposis colorectal cancer, multiple endocrine-related cancers.
- **G.** Triad of obesity, diabetes, and hypertension greatly increases risk.
- **H.** Exposure to external carcinogens.

  II. Physical examination.
- **A.** Early signs and symptoms—bleeding in postmenopausal women, irregular or heavy menstrual flow in premenopausal women, intermenstrual spotting, vaginal discharge, lumbosacral pain.
- **B.** Late signs and symptoms—hemorrhage, ascites, jaundice, bowel obstruction, respiratory distress.

  III. Evaluation of laboratory data.
- **A.** Decreased hemoglobin or hematocrit level.
- **B.** Abnormal liver enzyme levels.
- **C.** Abnormal chemistry profile results.

Nursing Diagnoses

  I. Disturbed body image.
  II. Sexual dysfunction.
  III. Ineffective coping.
  IV. Compromised family coping.
  V. Fear.
  VI. Deficient knowledge related to personal risk factors, treatment, side effects, and so on.

Outcome Identification

  I. Client describes personal risk factors for endometrial cancer.
  II. Client discusses rationale, schedule, and personal demands of treatment and follow-up care.
  III. Client and family list potential side effects of disease and treatment.
  IV. Client describes self-care measures to decrease the incidence and severity of complications of treatment.
  V. Client and family list signs and symptoms of recurrent disease to report to the health care team, such as vaginal bleeding, constipation, and pelvic pain.
  VI. Client and family describe potential community resources to meet demands of treatment and survivorship.

Planning and Implementation

  I. Interventions to maximize safety for the client (Barakat et al., 2000; DiSaia & Creasman, 2002a; Porter, 2002).
    A. Teach changes in lifestyle that can modify risks of endometrial cancer.
      1. Encourage the client to maintain ideal body weight.
      2. Encourage the client to report any unexpected bleeding or spotting to physician.
      3. If client requests, estrogen and progesterone hormone replacement postmenopausally if the uterus is present.
    B. See Chapters 35 and 36 for safety concerns about surgery and RT.
  II. Interventions to decrease the severity of symptoms associated with disease and treatment from surgery and RT, such as altered urinary and bowel function and pain.
    A. Venous stasis.
      1. Encourage turning in bed and ambulating as soon as possible.
      2. Teach isometric leg exercises to do while in bed.
      3. Apply antiembolic stockings.
      4. Monitor for discomfort in legs and thighs.
      5. Avoid use of a knee gatch in the bed.
    B. Urinary retention.
      1. Monitor urinary output.
      2. Assess for bladder distention above the symphysis pubis.
      3. Assess for lower abdominal discomfort.
  III. Interventions to monitor for sequelae of disease and treatment.
    A. See Chapters 14 and 15 for issues related to nutrition and elimination and Chapter 1 for comfort issues.
    B. See Chapters 2, 3, and 6 for coping, body image, and sexuality issues.

    C. Assess for signs of recurrent disease.
        1. Vaginal bleeding.
        2. Change in bowel habits—constipation.
        3. Pelvic pain.

Evaluation

The oncology nurse systematically and regularly evaluates the client's and/or family's responses to interventions to determine progress toward the achievement of expected outcomes. Relevant data are collected, and actual findings are compared with expected findings. Nursing diagnoses, outcomes, and plans of care are reviewed and revised as necessary.

OVARIAN CANCER

Theory

  I. Physiology and pathophysiology of ovarian cancer (DiSaia & Creasman, 2002b; Ozols et al., 2000).
    A. Anatomy of the ovary.
        1. Ovaries are located on each side of the uterus behind the fallopian tubes.
        2. Ovarian lymphatics drain into the iliac and periaortic lymph nodes.
    B. Primary functions of the ovary—production and release of ova and production of hormones to meet needs of female for development, growth, and function (estrogen, progesterone, testosterone).
    C. Metastatic patterns.
        1. Local extension to adjacent organs.
        2. Exfoliation of the ovarian capsule.
        3. Serosal seeding by tumor nests throughout the peritoneal cavity.
        4. Lymphatic spread.
        5. Hematologic spread is rare.
    D. Trends in epidemiology—steady increase in the incidence of ovarian cancer.
  II. Principles of medical management.
    A. Screening procedures (Cherry & Vacchiano, 2002; DiSaia & Creasman, 2002b; O'Rourke & Mahon, 2002; Ozols et al., 2000).
        1. Bimanual pelvic examination.
           a. Increase in size or irregularity of the ovary.
           b. Palpable ovary in a postmenopausal woman.
        2. Serial CA 125 determinations in high-risk women supplemented by transvaginal ultrasound remain controversial but are often used for high-risk women.
    B. Diagnostic procedures (DiSaia & Creasman, 2002b; Martin, 2002; Ozols et al., 2000).
        1. Laparoscopy or exploratory laparotomy to obtain tissue for diagnosis.
        2. Paracentesis of ascitic fluid.
    C. Staging (Table 26-3) procedures and methods.
        1. CT scan of the abdomen and pelvis.
        2. Barium enema/colonoscopy.
        3. Pulmonary involvement—chest x-ray examination, cytologic evaluation of pleural fluid.
        4. Surgical staging laparotomy is mandatory to evaluate pelvic and abdominal contents—TAH-BSO; peritoneal cytology; omentectomy; lymph node

TABLE 26-3
FIGO Staging for Ovarian Cancer

Stage	Description
I	Growth limited to the ovaries
IA	Growth limited to one ovary, no ascites, no tumor on the external surface, capsule intact
IB	Growth limited to both ovaries, no ascites, no tumor on the external surface, capsules intact
IC	Tumor stage IA or IB, but with tumor on the surface of one or both ovaries, with capsule ruptured, with ascites present containing malignant cells, or with positive peritoneal washings
II	Growth involving one or both ovaries with pelvic extension
IIA	Extension or metastases to the uterus or tubes
IIB	Growth involving one or both ovaries with pelvic extension
IIC	Tumor either stage IIA or IIB with tumor on the surface of one or both ovaries, with capsules ruptured, with ascites present containing malignant cells, or with positive peritoneal washings
III	Tumor involving one or both ovaries with peritoneal implants outside the pelvis or positive retroperitoneal or inguinal nodes, superficial liver metastases equal stage III, tumor limited to the true pelvis but with histologically verified malignant extension to small bowel or omentum
IIIA	Tumor grossly limited to the true pelvis with negative nodes but with histologically confirmed microscopic seeding of abdominal peritoneal surfaces
IIIB	Tumor of one or both ovaries with histologically confirmed implants of abdominal peritoneal surfaces, none exceeding 2 cm in diameter, nodes negative
IIIC	Abdominal implants greater than 2 cm in diameter, or positive retroperitoneal or inguinal nodes
IV	Growth involving one or both ovaries with distant metastases: if pleural effusion is present, there must be positive cytologic test results to allot a case to stage IV; parenchymal liver metastases equal stage IV

Derived from AJCC Cancer Staging Manual, Sixth Edition. For a complete, official description of TNM, Stage Grouping and Histologic Grade for this site, please consult Greene F.L., Page D.L., Fleming, I.D., et al. *AJCC Cancer Staging Manual*, Sixth Edition. New York: Springer-Verlag, 2002.
FIGO, International Federation of Gynecology and Obstetrics.

biopsies or removal; multiple biopsies of bladder, bowel, liver, and diaphragm surfaces; appendectomy; and debulking cytoreduction of all visible tumor.

5. Majority of clients with ovarian cancer are diagnosed with late-stage disease.
6. CA 125; other proteins are under evaluation as markers.

D. Treatment strategies (DiSaia & Creasman, 2002b; Kim et al., 2002; Martin, 2002; Ozols, 2002; Ozols et al., 2000).

1. Primary surgical treatment.
   a. Cytoreduction, with removal of all tumor or tumors greater than 1 to 2 cm in size so that minimal residual disease remains (optimal debulking).
   b. Surgery may be used alone to treat early-stage disease or borderline tumors with "low malignant potential."
   c. Surgery may be used to evaluate the response to chemotherapy treatment ("second-look" procedures), for secondary cytoreduction, and for palliation of recurrent bowel obstruction.
      (1) Goals are to detect residual tumor, debulk remaining tumor, and determine further treatment.
      (2) Second-look procedures are done only in the presence of a complete response clinically.
      (3) One fourth to one third of clients with a complete response clinically have evidence of disease on second look.

2. Adjuvant chemotherapy.
   a. For clients with early-stage or poorly differentiated disease or more advanced disease.
   b. Combination chemotherapy with paclitaxel (Taxol) and cisplatin (Platinol)/carboplatin (Paraplatin) is now first-line therapy. Recurrent progressive disease may be treated with a number of agents, including cisplatin, cyclophosphamide (Cytoxan), liposomal doxorubicin (Doxil), paclitaxel, docetaxel (Taxotere), hexamethylmelamine (Hexalen), topotecan (Hycamtin), etoposide (VP-16, Etopophos, VePesid), gemcitabine (Gemzar), oxaliplatin (Eloxatin), melphalan (Alkeran), and/or vinorelbine (Navelbine).
   c. Chemotherapy may be administered orally, intravenously, or intraperitoneally; advantages of the intraperitoneal method include the following:
      (1) Higher concentrations of drug to the surface of the tumor.
      (2) Decreased systemic side effects.
      (3) Systemic tolerance of higher doses of drug.
   d. Hormonal therapy may be used (e.g., megestrol acetate [Megace], tamoxifen [Nolvadex]) for consolidation therapy or for clients unable to tolerate more aggressive regimens.
   e. Adjuvant RT.
      (1) Pelvic or whole abdominal extended fields may be used for treatment of metastatic disease to the pelvis or abdomen.
      (2) Acute and chronic GI complications are common.
      (3) Radioactive isotopes, such as phosphorus-32, may also be given intraperitoneally to treat abdominal metastases.
   f. Biologic response modifiers are used as single agents and in combination with chemotherapy as adjuvant therapy.
      (1) Biologic response modifiers can be administered intravenously or intraperitoneally.
      (2) Interferon, interleukin-2, and monoclonal antibodies are under investigation.
E. Trends in survival.
   1. Overall 5-year survival rate is 53%.
   2. Stage, grade, and amount of residual disease following initial surgery (optimal versus suboptimal debulking) are important prognostic factors.
   3. Abdominal carcinomatosis commonly occurs and results in intestinal obstruction, malabsorption, and fluid and electrolyte imbalances.

Assessment (DiSaia & Creasman, 2002b; Martin, 2002; O'Rourke & Mahon, 2002; Ozols et al., 2000)

I. Pertinent personal and family history.
   A. Age—occurs commonly in premenopausal women ages 40 to 65 years old. Peak incidence is at age 60 to 64 years.
   B. Germ cell tumors are more common in children and adolescents.
   C. Infertility.
   D. Nulliparity.
   E. Personal history of breast, endometrial, or colon cancer.
   F. Family history of breast, endometrial, or colon cancer.
   G. Ten percent of epithelial ovarian cancers are familial, receiving great investigative attention including genetic investigation.
   H. Environmental factors.

II. Physical examination.
   A. Early signs and symptoms are vague and diffuse—GI distress, dyspepsia, abdominal discomfort, bloating, flatulence, eructation, increased pelvic pressure, vaginal bleeding.
   B. Late signs and symptoms—palpable abdominal or pelvic mass, increased abdominal girth, ascites, pleural effusions, intestinal obstruction, weight loss, vaginal bleeding.
III. Evaluation of laboratory data.
   A. CA 125 may be used to monitor treatment response or disease recurrence.
   B. Beta–human chorionic gonadotropin (β-HCG) and alpha-fetoprotein (α-FP) levels may be used to detect and monitor germ cell tumors.

Nursing Diagnoses

   I. Disturbed body image.
   II. Constipation.
   III. Imbalanced nutrition: less than body requirements.
   IV. Ineffective coping.
   V. Compromised family coping.
   VI. Anticipatory grieving.
   VII. Sexual dysfunction.
   VIII. Deficient knowledge related to personal risk factors, treatment, side effects, and so on.

Outcome Identification

   I. Client describes personal risk factors for ovarian cancer.
   II. Client and family discuss rationale, schedule, and personal demands of treatment and follow-up care.
   III. Client lists potential side effects of disease and treatment.
   IV. Client describes self-care measures to decrease the incidence and severity of complications of treatment.
   V. Client and family identify signs and symptoms of recurrent disease to report to the health care team.
   VI. Client and family describe community resources to meet potential demands of treatment and survivorship (e.g., the Wellness Community, National Ovarian Cancer Coalition, Ovarian Cancer National Alliance, CONVERSATIONS! The International Newsletter for Those Fighting Ovarian Cancer).

Planning and Implementation

   I. Interventions for management of symptoms related to disease and treatment modalities, that is, surgery and chemotherapy.
      A. See Chapters 14 and 15 for issues related to nutrition and elimination and Chapter 1 for comfort issues.
      B. See Chapters 2, 3, 6, and 7 for coping, body image, sexuality, and death and dying issues.
   II. Aggressive symptom management is necessary while women receive complex chemotherapy regimens (e.g., antiemetic control, prevention of neuropathies, maintenance of fluid and electrolyte balance).
   III. Coping issues need to be addressed because diagnosis is often delayed, therapy may be prolonged, and prognosis is poor.

Evaluation

The oncology nurse systematically and regularly evaluates the client's and/or family's responses to interventions to determine progress toward the achievement of expected outcomes. Relevant data are collected, and actual findings are compared with expected findings. Nursing diagnoses, outcomes, and plans of care are reviewed and revised as necessary.

GESTATIONAL TROPHOBLASTIC NEOPLASIA

Theory

I. Physiology and pathophysiology associated with gestational trophoblastic neoplasia (GTN) (Berkowitz & Goldstein, 2000; Burger & Creasman, 2002; Door, 2002a, 2002b).
   A. A spectrum of neoplasia associated with the products of conception.
   B. Chromosomal abnormalities involved in fertilization, differentiation and pronuclear cleavage, decidual implantation, and invasion under investigation.
   C. Metastatic patterns—most common sites of metastases are the lung, vagina, liver, and brain.
II. Principles of medical management.
   A. Diagnostic evaluation—history and physical examination including pelvic examination, ultrasound to evaluate suspected pregnancy if fetal abnormality or absence, quantitative serum β-HCG, and metastatic workup if necessary (complete blood count [CBC]; chemistries; CT or MRI of head, chest, abdomen).
   B. Staging methods and procedures include ultrasound; D and C with suction evacuation; metastatic evaluation of chest, abdomen, and brain if appropriate (Table 26-4).
   C. Treatment strategies.
      1. Depend on classification and desired fertility.
         a. Suction evacuation of uterine contents eliminates mole and preserves childbearing.
         b. Hysterectomy may be done if childbearing is not desired.
      2. Invasive disease—removal of uterine contents with suction.
      3. Chemotherapy is extremely effective in management of GTN.
         a. Single-agent therapy with methotrexate (Mexate) or actinomycin-D (Cosmegen) for nonmetastatic or good prognosis disease.
         b. Multiagent chemotherapy for clients with poor prognosis metastatic GTN (Box 26-1).
      4. Surgical removal of isolated chemotherapy-resistant metastasis.
      5. RT of resistant metastatic sites.
   D. Trends in survival—90% of clients with metastatic disease are cured.

Assessment

I. Pertinent personal and family history.
   A. Age—highest risk for women over 40 years of age becoming pregnant. Some increased risk for women under 20 years.
   B. Previous molar pregnancy greatest risk factor.
II. Physical examination: early signs and symptoms include delayed menses (presumed pregnant), abnormal uterine bleeding while presumed pregnant; abdominal pain; absence of fetal heartbeat; uterine size large for gestational dates.
III. Evaluation of laboratory data: quantitative β-HCG extremely sensitive. Weekly serial tests until results are normal for 3 weeks, then monthly until normal for

TABLE 26-4
FIGO Staging for Gestational Trophoblastic Tumors*

Stage	Description
I	Tumor confined to the uterus
II	Tumor extends to other genital structures (ovary, tube, vagina, broad ligaments) by metastasis or direct extension
III	Lung metastasis
IV	All other distant metastases

Risk factors	Score 0	Score 1	Score 2	Score 4
Age (yr)	<40	>40		
Antecedent pregnancy	Hydatidiform mole	Abortion	Term pregnancy	
Interval (mo) from index pregnancy	<4	4-<7	7-12	>12
Pretreatment HCG	$<10^3$	$\geq 10^3 - <10^4$	$10^4 - <10^5$	$\geq 10^5$
Largest tumor size (cm) including uterus	<3	3-<5	≥ 5	
Site of metastases	Lung	Spleen, kidney	GI tract	Brain, liver
Number of metastases		1-4	5-8	>8
Previous failed chemotherapy			Single drug	Two or more drugs
Total Score				

Derived from AJCC Cancer Staging Manual, Sixth Edition. For a complete, official description of TNM, Stage Grouping and Histologic Grade for this site, please consult Greene F.L., Page D.L., Fleming, I.D., et al. *AJCC Cancer Staging Manual,* Sixth Edition. New York: Springer-Verlag, 2002.
FIGO, International Federation of Gynecology and Obstetrics; *HCG,* human chorionic gonadotropin; *GI,* gastrointestinal.
*The score on the Prognostic Scoring Index is used to substage patients. Each stage is defined as substage A (low risk—prognostic score of 7 or less) or B (high risk—prognostic score of 8 or more).

BOX 26-1
POOR PROGNOSIS METASTATIC GTN

Tumor volume (size and number of metastases)
Sites of involvement
Urinary β-HCG >100,000 milli international units/24 hr or serum β-HCG >40,000 milli international units/ml
Failed prior therapy
Symptoms >4-mo duration
Antecedent term pregnancy (?)

From Berkowitz R, Goldstein D: Gestational trophoblastic diseases. In Hoskins WJ, Perez CA, Young RC, editors: *Principles and practice of gynecologic oncology,* ed 3, Philadelphia, 2000, Lippincott Williams & Wilkins, pp 1117-1137; and DiSaia, PJ, Creasman, WT. Gestational trophoblastic neoplasia. In DiSaia PJ, Creasman WT, editors. *Clinical gynecologic oncology,* ed 6, St. Louis, 2002, Mosby, pp 185-210.
GTN, Gestational trophoblastic neoplasia; *β-HCG,* beta human gonadotropic hormone.

1 year and up to 2 years in clients with poor prognosis. Used to monitor presence of disease, response to treatment, and recurrence.

Nursing Diagnoses

I. Disturbed body image.
II. Sexual dysfunction.

  III. Anticipatory or dysfunctional grieving.

  IV. Ineffective coping.

   V. Compromised family coping.

  VI. Deficient knowledge related to personal risk factors, treatment, side effects, fertility, and so on.

Outcome Identification

   I. Client describes personal risk factors for GTN; methods for screening.

  II. Client discusses rationale, schedule, and personal demands of treatment and follow-up care, especially obtaining routine β-HCG.

 III. Client and family list potential side effects of disease and treatment.

  IV. Client identifies self-care measures to decrease the incidence and severity of complications of treatment.

   V. Client and family address issues of loss related to pregnancy and/or future fertility.

  VI. Client and family describe community resources to meet potential demands of treatment and survivorship, such as the American Cancer Society and National Coalition for Cancer Survivorship.

Planning and Implementation

   I. Interventions to decrease the severity of symptoms associated with disease and treatment.

     A. See Chapters 14 and 15 for issues related to nutrition and elimination and Chapter 1 for comfort issues.

     B. See Chapters 2, 3, and 6 for coping, body image, and sexuality issues.

  II. Interventions to incorporate the client and family in care.

     A. Encourage open communication about the impact of disease and treatment on the client and significant others.

     B. Teach the client and significant other new self-care skills required during or after treatment.

     C. Instruct client to use oral contraceptives during treatment and follow-up. Time frame variable; dependent upon clinical situation.

     D. Identify concerns the client and her sexual partner may have about future fertility.

Evaluation

The oncology nurse systematically and regularly evaluates the client's and/or family's responses to interventions to determine progress toward the achievement of expected outcomes. Relevant data are collected, and actual findings are compared with expected findings. Nursing diagnoses, outcomes, and plans of care are reviewed and revised as necessary.

VULVAR CANCER

Theory

   I. Physiology and pathophysiology associated with vulvar cancer (Burke et al., 2000; DiSaia & Creasman, 2002d; Door, 2002b; Eifel et al., 2001).

     A. Anatomy of the vulva—comprises the external genital organs: mons pubis, labia majora and minora, clitoris, vaginal vestibule, perineal body, supporting subcutaneous tissue.

    B. Changes associated with cancer of the vulva.

        1. Cellular changes exist on a continuum from premalignant changes to invasive carcinoma.

            a. HPV-related changes.

            b. Other/granulomatous.

        2. Histology—85% squamous; rare—melanoma, sarcoma, basal cell.

    C. Metastatic patterns.

        1. Direct extension to adjacent structures.

        2. Lymph node metastases (femoral and inguinal, iliac nodes).

        3. Hematogenous spread to distant sites including lung.

    D. Trends in epidemiology—very rare cancer, comprises only 8% of all female cancers.

II. Principles of medical management (Burke et al., 2000; DiSaia & Creasman, 2002d; Door, 2002b; Eifel et al., 2001).

    A. Screening and diagnostic procedures.

        1. Screening procedures—careful visual and pelvic inspection and examination; acetic acid staining and colposcopy may be used to evaluate any suspicious lesions. Cystoscopy and proctoscopy for advanced disease.

        2. Diagnostic procedure—biopsy.

    B. Staging methods and procedures include biopsy of suspected area and evaluation of lymph node involvement with CT, cystoscopy, and proctoscopy. The International Federation of Gynecology and Obstetrics (FIGO) system is used (Table 26-5).

    C. Treatment strategies.

        1. Stage 1A—surgical management with wide local excision.

        2. Stages 1B and 2—surgery has been the major modality (i.e., radical excision/vulvectomy and nodal evaluation/dissection).

        3. Advanced disease—chemotherapy/RT as an adjunct preoperatively or postoperatively.

    D. Five-year survival rates of 80% to 90% reported for stages I and II disease; survival rates for clients with advanced disease are poor: 60% for stage III

TABLE 26-5
FIGO Staging for Invasive Cancer of the Vulva

Stage	Description
0	Carcinoma in situ; intraepithelial carcinoma
IA	Lesions 2 cm or less in size confined to the vulva or perineum and with stromal invasion no greater than 1 mm (no nodal metastases)
IB	Lesions 2 cm or less confined to the vulva or perineum and with stromal invasion greater than 1 mm (no nodal metastases)
II	Tumor confined to the vulva and/or perineum—more than 2 cm in greatest dimension (no nodal metastases)
III	Tumor any size with adjacent spread to the urethra, vagina, or anus with unilateral regional lymph node metastasis
IVA	Tumor invades the upper urethra, bladder mucosa, rectal mucosa, pelvic bone, or bilateral regional lymph node metastases
IVB	Any distant metastasis, including pelvic lymph nodes

Derived from AJCC Cancer Staging Manual, Sixth Edition. For a complete, official description of TNM, Stage Grouping and Histologic Grade for this site, please consult Greene F.L., Page D.L., Fleming, I.D., et al. *AJCC Cancer Staging Manual,* Sixth Edition. New York: Springer-Verlag, 2002.
FIGO, International Federation of Gynecology and Obstetrics.

and 15% for stage IV. Prognosis is related to inguinal nodal metastasis, tumor size, depth of invasion, and tumor thickness.

Assessment

I. Pertinent personal and family history.
  A. Age—postmenopausal women at ages ranging from 65 to 75 years have peak incidence; 15% of cases occur in women younger than 40 years.
  B. History of HPV infections, vulvar inflammation, and other genitourinary (GU) cancers increases risk.
II. Physical examination.
  A. Early signs and symptoms—vaginal lump, itching, pain.
  B. Late signs and symptoms—bleeding, discharge, dysuria.

Nursing Diagnoses

I. Disturbed body image.
II. Sexual dysfunction.
III. Ineffective coping.
IV. Compromised family coping.
V. Deficient knowledge related to personal risk factors, treatment, side effects, and so on.

Outcome Identification

I. Client describes personal risk factors to minimize risks and plan for screening.
II. Client discusses rationale, schedule, and personal demands of treatment and follow-up care.
III. Client and family list potential side effects of disease and treatment.
IV. Client and family address concerns of altered sexual functioning and perception.
V. Client and family describe community resources to meet potential demands of treatment and survivorship.

Planning and Implementation (Door, 2002b)

I. Interventions to decrease the severity of symptoms associated with disease and treatment.
  A. Teach client about possible symptoms associated with treatment modality options (e.g., attention to skin care and promotion of healing without infection or pain are important after surgery). (See Chapter 35.)
II. Monitor for the development of leg edema if lymph node dissection completed.
III. Identify concerns the client and her sexual partner may have about resuming sexual functioning after treatment.

Evaluation

The oncology nurse systematically and regularly evaluates the client's and/or family's responses to interventions to determine progress toward the achievement of expected outcomes. Relevant data are collected, and actual findings are compared with expected findings. Nursing diagnoses, outcomes, and plans of care are reviewed and revised as necessary.

VAGINAL CANCER

Theory

I. Physiology and pathophysiology associated with vaginal cancer (DiSaia & Creasman, 2002c; Door, 2002b; Perez et al., 2000).
   A. Anatomy of the vagina—the mucous membrane tube forming the passageway between the uterus and the vulva.
   B. Associated changes can be premalignant to invasive.
   C. Role of HPV under investigation as causative agent.
   D. Pathology—squamous cell carcinoma 85%; rarely melanoma, adenocarcinoma, clear cell cancers.
   E. Metastatic patterns.
      1. Local extension and lymph node involvement.
      2. More commonly a metastatic site for cervical cancer.
   F. Incidence—extremely rare cancer; comprises 1% to 2% of female GU cancers.
II. Principles of medical management (DiSaia & Creasman, 2002c; Door, 2002b; Perez et al., 2001).
   A. Screening procedures.
      1. Careful pelvic inspection and examination.
      2. Cytologic washings, even after hysterectomy.
   B. Diagnostic procedures.
      1. Biopsy of lesion, usually an outpatient procedure.
      2. Examination with client under anesthesia—cystoscopy, proctoscopy.
      3. Chest x-ray examination, CT of abdomen and pelvis.
   C. The FIGO staging system is used.
   D. Treatment strategies.
      1. Preinvasive disease—vaginal intraepithelial neoplasia: fluorouracil (5-Fluorouracil, 5-FU) local application, laser vaporization, brachytherapy, or surgical excision.
      2. Invasive disease—surgery and/or RT.
         a. Surgery—vaginectomy and hysterectomy for early-stage disease.
         b. RT—main treatment for all stages, implant may be added to teletherapy, lymph node fields depend on staging.
      3. Recurrent disease—surgery or RT to previously untreated areas.

Assessment

I. Pertinent personal and family history.
   A. Age—primarily a disease of the elderly, over age 60 years.
   B. Personal history of maternal diethylstilbestrol use during pregnancy; should be screened for rare clear cell pathology.
   C. Prior history of invasive cervical carcinoma (ICC) increases risk.
II. Physical examination.
   A. Early signs and symptoms—vaginal bleeding or discharge.
   B. Late signs and symptoms—GI or GU changes.

Nursing Diagnoses

I. Disturbed body image.
II. Sexual dysfunction.
III. Ineffective coping.

    IV. Compromised family coping.
    V. Deficient knowledge related to risk factors, treatment, side effects, and so on.

Outcome Identification

    I. Client describes personal risk factors for vaginal cancer.
    II. Client discusses rationale, schedule, and personal demands of treatment and follow-up care.
    III. Client and family list potential side effects of disease and treatment.
    IV. Client identifies self-care measures to decrease the incidence and severity of complications of treatment.
    V. Client lists signs and symptoms of recurrent disease to report to the health care team.
    VI. Client and family describe community resources to meet potential demands of treatment and survivorship.

Planning and Implementation

    I. Interventions to monitor for sequelae of disease and treatment.
       A. See Chapters 14 and 15 for issues related to nutrition and elimination and Chapter 1 for comfort issues.
       B. See Chapters 2, 3, and 6 for coping, body image, and sexuality issues.
    II. Interventions to incorporate the client and family in care.
       A. Identify concerns the client and her sexual partner may have about resuming sexual functioning after treatment.

Evaluation

The oncology nurse systematically and regularly evaluates the client's and/or family's responses to interventions to determine progress toward the achievement of expected outcomes. Relevant data are collected, and actual findings are compared with expected findings. Nursing diagnoses, outcomes, and plans of care are reviewed and revised as necessary.

TESTICULAR CANCER

Theory

    I. Physiology and pathophysiology associated with testicular cancer (Bosl et al., 2001; Poirier & Rawl, 2000).
       A. Anatomy of the testes—testes are ovoid glands located in the scrotal sac that descend from the abdomen through the inguinal canal during the seventh month of fetal life.
       B. Primary functions of the testes include spermatogenesis and production of a hormone (testosterone) for male development, growth, and function.
       C. Changes associated with cancer of the testes.
          1. Testicular cancers arise from germinal epithelium.
          2. Usually occurs in only one testis.
          3. Etiology is unknown. Risk factors include cryptorchidism, chromosomal abnormalities (e.g., Klinefelter's syndrome), and abnormalities in reproductive tract development in utero (ACS, 2003).

4. Behavior of testicular cancer varies with histologic subtype (Bosl et al., 2001).
   a. Seminomas.
      (1) Occur in approximately 50% of cases.
      (2) Spread slowly, primarily through the lymphatics.
      (3) Are responsive to RT.
   b. Nonseminoma germ cell testicular tumors (NSGCTTs)—embryonal tumor (20%), teratoma, choriocarcinoma; yolk sac, interstitial cell, and gonadal stromal tumors.
      (1) More aggressive than pure seminomas; 60% to 70% have lymph node spread at diagnosis.
      (2) Embryonal tumors invade the spermatic cord and metastasize to lung.
      (3) Embryonal tumors are not responsive to RT.
   c. Mixed cell types are fairly common.
   D. Metastatic patterns.
      1. Direct extension to adjacent structures.
      2. Lymphatic spread.
      3. Hematologic metastasis to the lung, brain, bone, and liver.
   E. Trends in epidemiology.
      1. Very rare cancer, incidence approximately 1% in American males.
      2. Most commonly occurring cancer among men ages 15 to 35 years.
      3. Incidence is higher and is increasing among Caucasian males.
II. Principles of medical management (Bosl et al., 2001).
   A. Screening and diagnostic procedures.
      1. Screening procedures.
         a. Monthly testicular self-examination.
         b. Annual bimanual palpation and examination of the testes by the health care provider.
      2. Diagnostic procedure—ultrasound to diagnose mass; tissue biopsy by radical inguinal orchiectomy.
   B. Staging methods and procedures.
      1. Chest x-ray, CT scan of chest and abdomen.
      2. CT/MRI of brain if symptomatic.
      3. IVP to evaluate displacement of the ureter or kidney.
      4. Clinical evaluation and histologic determination are required for clinical staging.
      5. Pathologic staging dependent upon surgical findings.
      6. Alpha-fetoprotein (α-FP), lactate dehydrogenase (LDH), and beta–human chorionic gonadotropin (β-HCG) testing.
   C. Treatment strategies (vary by histology).
      1. Surgery.
         a. Transinguinal orchiectomy is the primary treatment for seminomas and nonseminomas.
         b. Retroperitoneal lymph node dissection (RPLND).
         c. Surgery may be used to resect residual disease and isolated metastatic lesions of lung, liver, and retroperitoneum.
      2. RT.
         a. Primary or adjuvant treatment for early-stage seminomas.
         b. Fields may include iliac, retroperitoneal, and paraaortic lymph nodes or whole abdomen.
         c. Use of RT to lung fields limits use of bleomycin (Blenoxane) for recurrent disease because the risk of pulmonary fibrosis increases.

    3. Chemotherapy.
       a. Treatment for NSGCTT and high-risk seminoma; clients with elevated tumor markers, advanced-stage disease, or recurrent disease.
       b. Aggressive combination chemotherapy regimens (agents commonly used include cisplatin [Platinol], vinblastine [Velban], bleomycin [Blenoxane], etoposide [VP-16, Etopophos, VePesid], ifosfamide [Ifex], vincristine [Oncovin], and paclitaxel [Taxol]). Response rates are high—complete response (70%) and partial response (30%).
    4. Recurrent disease also responds to chemotherapy. Surgical resection of recurrent disease or isolated resistant metastasis may be done.
  D. Trends in survival.
    1. Survival from testicular cancer has increased dramatically.
    2. Testicular cancer is almost always considered curable, and the prognosis for clients is excellent.
    3. Prognosis depends on bulk of disease at diagnosis (Table 26-6).
    4. Recurrences usually occur within 2 years; however, recurrences beyond 5 years have been reported, and recurrent disease is also responsive to treatment.

Assessment

  I. Pertinent personal and family history.
    A. Age.
      1. Most commonly occurs in men age 20 to 35 years.
      2. Incidence decreases for men age 40 to 60 years and increases again after age 60 years.

TABLE 26-6
Germ Cell Tumor Risk Classification: International Consensus

Risk	Seminoma	Nonseminoma
Good risk	Any HCG	α-FP <1000 ng/ml
	Any LDH	HCG <5000 milli international units/ml
	Nonpulmonary visceral metastases (mets) absent	LDH <1.5 × ULN
		Nonpulmonary visceral mets absent
	Any primary site	Gonadal or retroperitoneal primary tumor
Intermediate risk	Nonpulmonary visceral metastases present	α-FP 1000-10,000 ng/ml
	Any HCG	HCG 5000-50,000 milli international units/ml
	Any LDH	LDH 1.5-10 × ULN
	Any primary site	ULN
		Nonpulmonary visceral mets absent
		Gonadal or retroperitoneal primary site
Poor risk		Mediastinal primary site
		Nonpulmonary visceral mets present (e.g., bone, liver, brain)
		α-FP ≥10,000 ng/ml
		HCG ≥50,000 milli international units/ml
		LDH ≥10 × ULN

From Bosl G, Bajorin D, Sheinfeld J, et al: Cancer of the testis. In DeVita VT Jr, Hellman S, Rosenberg SA, editors: *Cancer: principles and practice of oncology*, ed 6, Philadelphia, 2001, Lippincott Williams & Wilkins, pp. 1491-1518. *HCG*, Human chorionic gonadotropin; *LDH*, lactate dehydrogenase; *α-FP*, alpha-fetoprotein; *ULN*, upper limit of normal.

    B. Cryptorchidism (undescended testis) increases risk twentyfold to fortyfold; if orchipexy is done after 6 years of age, protection is lost.

    C. Polythelia (multiple nipples) is associated with increased risk.

II. Physical examination.

    A. Early signs and symptoms are usually absent. Clients may have an asymptomatic mass; gynecomastia; infertility; or testicular fullness, heaviness, swelling, or pain.

    B. Late signs and symptoms are back pain, bone pain, or respiratory distress.

III. Evaluation of laboratory data.

    A. Serum tumor markers—α-FP and β-HCG to establish a differential diagnosis, assess response to treatment, and monitor long-term responses.

    B. NSGCTT more commonly has elevated levels of markers—α-FP (70%) and β-HCG (50%). α-FP is not elevated in pure seminomas.

    C. LDH reflects tumor burden, growth rate, and cellular proliferation. Elevated in approximately 60% of NSGCTT cases and in 80% of clients with advanced seminoma.

Nursing Diagnoses

   I. Disturbed body image.

  II. Sexual dysfunction.

 III. Ineffective coping.

  IV. Compromised family coping.

   V. Deficient knowledge related to risk factors, treatment, side effects, fertility, and so on.

  VI. Anticipatory grieving.

Outcome Identification

   I. Client describes personal risk factors for testicular cancer and a plan for testicular self-examination.

  II. Client discusses rationale, schedule, and personal demands of treatment and follow-up care.

 III. Client and family list potential side effects of disease and treatment.

  IV. Client identifies self-care measures to decrease the incidence and severity of complications of treatment.

   V. Client and family list signs and symptoms of recurrent disease to report.

  VI. Client and family describe community resources to meet potential demands of treatment and survivorship.

Planning and Implementation (Bosl et al., 2001; Poirier & Rawl, 2000)

   I. Teach adolescent men to perform monthly testicular self-examination (TSE).

  II. See Chapters 35 and 38 for interventions related to surgical needs and chemotherapy. Chemotherapy regimens are aggressive and require intensive nursing support and symptom management for fluid and electrolyte maintenance, monitoring renal function, antiemetic control, and prevention of constipation and neuropathies.

 III. Interventions to decrease the severity of symptoms associated with disease and treatment.

    A. Inguinal orchiectomy is performed as an outpatient procedure for both diagnostic and therapeutic purposes. Client education specific for pain management, activity, and incisional wound care.

    B. Other considerations include pulmonary, GI, and fertility concerns.

    C. Psychosexual issues.

       1. Discuss the potential of sperm banking as an option before treatment begins.

       2. Encourage open discussion about changes in body image between the client and his sexual partner; long-term sexual dysfunction has been reported in approximately 25% of testicular cancer survivors.

IV. Interventions to incorporate the client and family in care. Identify concerns the client and his sexual partner may have about resuming sexual functioning after treatment.

Evaluation

The oncology nurse systematically and regularly evaluates the client's and/or family's responses to interventions to determine progress toward the achievement of expected outcomes. Relevant data are collected, and actual findings are compared with expected findings. Nursing diagnoses, outcomes, and plans of care are reviewed and revised as necessary.

PENILE CANCER

Theory

  I. Physiology and pathophysiology associated with penile cancer (Herr et al., 2001).

    A. Anatomy of the penis.

       1. Composed of the shaft and the glans.

       2. Shaft has three cylindric layers—bilateral corpus spongiosum, corpora cavernosa, and erectile tissues.

    B. Primary functions of the penis are urination and copulation.

    C. Causative factors unknown; HPV investigated; poor penile hygiene and no circumcision increase risk.

    D. Metastatic patterns.

       1. Direct extension to adjacent tissues.

       2. Metastasis to regional lymphatics—inguinal and iliac nodes.

  II. Principles of medical management (Herr et al., 2001).

    A. Diagnostic procedures include incisional or excisional biopsy of the penile lesion.

    B. Staging methods and procedures.

       1. Abdominal CT scan and MRI examination to evaluate regional lymph nodes; intravenous (IV) urography, lymphangiography, chest x-ray examination, liver and bone scans.

       2. Nodal status is most significant prognostic variable predicting survival.

    C. Treatment strategies.

       1. Premalignant lesions—local excision, topical fluorouracil, or laser therapy.

       2. Invasive cancer.

          a. Surgery.

             (1) Wide excision or partial penectomy with or without inguinal lymph node dissection for small and localized tumors.

             (2) Partial or total penectomy with groin node dissection is controversial.

(3) Total penectomy requires creation of a perineal urostomy for urination.

(4) Radical lymphadenectomy or lymph node sampling may be done, depending on the stage of disease.

b. RT.

(1) Interstitial, surface mold, or external beam therapy may be used for small penile lesions.

(2) RT may also be used for palliative treatment.

c. Chemotherapy.

(1) May be used as palliative treatment for clients with stage III or IV disease.

(2) Chemotherapy agents—cisplatin (Platinol), methotrexate (Mexate), and bleomycin (Blenoxane) are used.

(3) Other agents with known activity in squamous cell cancers of the cervix and head and neck may be useful.

D. Trends in survival—because the disease is extremely rare in the United States, accurate trends in survival are not available.

Assessment

I. Pertinent personal and family history.

A. Age—60 years or older.

B. Penile hygiene practices—poor hygiene increases risk.

C. Circumcision status—no circumcision increases risk.

II. Physical examination.

A. Early signs and symptoms—mass, nodule, or ulceration of the penis; foul-smelling penile discharge; inguinal lymphadenopathy; bleeding on the surface of the penis.

B. Late signs and symptoms—fungating lesion of the penis, bone pain, respiratory distress.

III. Evaluation of laboratory data—none specific to penile cancer.

Nursing Diagnoses

I. Disturbed body image.

II. Sexual dysfunction.

III. Ineffective coping.

IV. Compromised family coping.

V. Deficient knowledge related to personal risk factors, treatment, side effects, and so on.

Outcome Identification

I. Client describes personal risk factors for penile cancer.

II. Client discusses rationale, schedule, and personal demands of treatment and follow-up care.

III. Client and family list potential side effects of disease and treatment.

IV. Client identifies self-care measures to decrease the incidence and severity of complications of treatment.

V. Client and family list signs and symptoms of recurrent disease to report.

VI. Client and family describe community resources to meet potential demands of treatment and survivorship.

Planning and Implementation

I. Interventions to maximize safety for the client.
- **A.** Discuss the option of circumcision before puberty for protective effect.
- **B.** Instruct high-risk clients in penile self-examination.
- **C.** Teach penile hygiene practices.
  - **1.** Retraction of foreskin for cleansing.
  - **2.** Washing penis with mild soap and water.

II. For clients requiring assistance with urinary continence and maintenance, see Chapter 15.

III. Interventions to enhance adaptation and rehabilitation.
- **A.** Encourage open discussion of sexual concerns.
  - **1.** Reinforce information that clients with partial penectomy maintain sexual desire and the ability to penetrate, reach orgasm, and ejaculate.
  - **2.** Discuss prosthetic options with clients who have had a total penectomy.
- **B.** Discuss alternate forms of sexual expression with the client and his sexual partner.

Evaluation

The oncology nurse systematically and regularly evaluates the client's and/or family's responses to interventions to determine progress toward the achievement of expected outcomes. Relevant data are collected, and actual findings are compared with expected findings. Nursing diagnoses, outcomes, and plans of care are reviewed and revised as necessary.

REFERENCES

American Cancer Society (ACS). (2003). *What are the risk factors for cervical cancer? What are the risk factors for testicular cancer?* Retrieved February 16, 2003 from the World Wide Web: www.cancer.org.

Barakat, R., Grigsby, P., Sabbatini, P., & Zaino, R. (2000). Corpus: Epithelial tumors. In W.J. Hoskins, C.A. Perez, & R.C. Young (Eds.). *Principles and practice of gynecologic oncology* (3rd ed.). Philadelphia: Lippincott Williams & Wilkins, pp. 919-960.

Berkowitz, R., & Goldstein, D, (2000). Gestational trophoblastic diseases. In W.J. Hoskins, C.A. Perez, & R.C. Young (Eds.). *Principles and practice of gynecologic oncology* (3rd ed.). Philadelphia: Lippincott Williams & Wilkins, pp. 1117-1137.

Bosl, G., Bajorin, D., Sheinfeld, J., et al. (2001). Cancer of the testis. In V.T. DeVita, Jr., S. Hellman, & S.A. Rosenberg (Eds.). *Cancer: Principles and practice of oncology* (6th ed.). Philadelphia: Lippincott Williams & Wilkins, pp. 1491-1518.

Burger, R.A., & Creasman, W.T. (2002). Gestational trophoblastic neoplasia. In P.J. DiSaia & W.T. Creasman (Eds.). *Clinical gynecologic oncology* (6th ed.). St. Louis: Mosby, pp. 185-210.

Burke, T.W., Eifel, P.J., McGuire, W.P., & Wilkinson, E.J. (2000). Vulva. In W.J. Hoskins, C.A. Perez, & R.C. Young (Eds.). *Principles and practice of gynecologic oncology* (3rd ed.). Philadelphia: Lippincott Williams & Wilkins, pp. 775-810.

Cherry, C., & Vacchiano, S. (2002). Ovarian cancer screening and prevention. *Seminars in Oncology Nursing 18*(3), 167-173.

DiSaia, P.J., & Creasman, W.T. (2002a). Adenocarcinoma of the uterus. In P.J. DiSaia & W.T. Creasman (Eds.). *Clinical gynecologic oncology* (6th ed.). St. Louis: Mosby, pp. 137-172.

DiSaia, P.J., & Creasman, W.T. (2002b). Epithelial ovarian cancer. In P.J. DiSaia & W.T. Creasman (Eds.). *Clinical gynecologic oncology* (6th ed.). St. Louis: Mosby, pp. 289-350.

DiSaia, P.J., & Creasman, W.T. (2002c). Invasive cancer of the vagina and urethra. In P.J. DiSaia & W.T. Creasman (Eds.). *Clinical gynecologic oncology* (6th ed.). St. Louis: Mosby, pp. 241-258.

DiSaia, P.J., & Creasman, W.T. (2002d). Invasive cancer of the vulva. In P.J. DiSaia & W.T. Creasman (Eds.). *Clinical gynecologic oncology* (6th ed.). St. Louis: Mosby, pp. 211-239.

DiSaia, P.J., & Creasman, W.T. (2002e). Invasive cervical cancer. In P.J. DiSaia & W.T. Creasman (Eds.). *Clinical gynecologic oncology* (6th ed.). St. Louis: Mosby, pp. 53-112.

DiSaia, P.J., & Creasman, W.T. (2002f). Gestational trophoblastic neoplasia. In P.J. DiSaia & W.T. Creasman (Eds.). *Clinical gynecologic oncology* (6th ed.). St. Louis: Mosby, pp. 185-210.

DiSaia, P.J., & Creasman, W.T. (2002g). Preinvasive disease of the cervix. In P.J. DiSaia & W.T. Creasman (Eds.). *Clinical gynecologic oncology* (6th ed.). St. Louis: Mosby, pp. 1-33.

Door, A. (2002a). Gestational trophoblastic disease. *Journal of Gynecologic Oncology Nursing* 12(2), 19-21.

Door, A. (2002b). Less common gynecologic malignancies. *Seminars in Oncology Nursing* 18(3), 207-222.

Eifel, P.J., Berek, J.S., & Thigpen, J.T. (2001). Cancer of the cervix, vagina, and vulva. In V.T. DeVita, Jr., S. Hellman, & S.A. Rosenberg (Eds.). *Cancer: Principles and practice of oncology* (6th ed.). Philadelphia: Lippincott Williams & Wilkins, pp. 1526-1573.

Fischer, M. (2002). Cancer of the cervix. *Seminars in Oncology Nursing* 18(3), 193-199.

Greene, F.L., Page, D.L., Fleming, I.D., et al. (Eds.). (2002). *AJCC cancer staging manual* (6th ed.). New York: Springer-Verlag.

Grigsby, P. (2002). Update on radiation therapy for endometrial cancer. *Oncology* 16(6), 777-790.

Herr, H.W., Dalbagni, G., Bajorin, D., & Shipley, W. (2001). Cancer of the urethra and penis. In V.T. DeVita, Jr., S. Hellman, & S.A. Rosenberg (Eds.). *Cancer: Principles and practice of oncology* (6th ed.). Philadelphia: Lippincott Williams & Wilkins, pp. 1480-1489.

Kim, R., Omura, G., & Alvarez, R. (2002). Advances in the treatment of gynecologic malignancies. II. Cancers of the uterine corpus and ovary. *Oncology* 16(12), 1669-1678.

Levine, D., & Hoskins, W. (2002). Update in the management of endometrial cancer. *Cancer Journal* 8(3, Suppl. 1), S31-S40.

Martin, V. (2002). Ovarian cancer. *Seminars in Oncology Nursing* 18(3), 174-183.

O'Rourke, J., & Mahon, S. (2002). A comprehensive look at the early detection of ovarian cancer. *Clinical Journal of Oncology Nursing* 7(1), 41-47.

Ozols, R. (2002). Update in the management of ovarian cancer. *Cancer Journal* 8(3, Suppl. 1), S22-S30.

Ozols, R., Rubin, S., Thomas, G., & Robboy, S. (2000). Epithelial ovarian cancer. In W.J. Hoskins, C.A. Perez, & R.C. Young (Eds.). *Principles and practice of gynecologic oncology* (3rd ed.). Philadelphia: Lippincott Williams & Wilkins, pp. 981-1058.

Perez, C., Gersell, D., McGuire, W., & Morris, M. (2000). Vagina. In W.J. Hoskins, C.A. Perez, & R.C. Young (Eds.). *Principles and practice of gynecologic oncology* (3rd ed.). Philadelphia: Lippincott Williams & Wilkins, pp. 811-840.

Poirier, S., & Rawl, S. (2000). Testicular germ cell cancer. In C.H. Yarbro, M.H. Frogge, M. Goodman, & S.L. Groenwald (Eds.). *Cancer nursing: Principles and practice* (5th ed.). Sudbury, MA: Jones & Bartlett Publishers, pp. 1494-1510.

Porter, S. (2002). Endometrial cancer. *Seminars in Oncology Nursing* 18(3), 200-206.

Shepherd, J., Mould, T., & Oram, D. (2001). Radical trachelectomy in early stage carcinoma of the cervix: Outcome as judged by recurrence and fertility rates. *British Journal of Obstetrics and Gynaecology* 108(8), 882-885.

Solomon, D., Davey, D., Kurman, R., et al. (2002). The 2001 Bethesda System. Terminology for reporting results of cervical cytology. *Journal of the American Medical Association* 287(16), 2114-2119.

Spinelli, A. (2002). Preinvasive disease of the cervix, vulva, and vagina. *Seminars in Oncology Nursing* 18(3), 184-192.

Stehman, F., Perez, C., Kurman, R., & Thigpen, J. (2000). Uterine cervix. In W.J. Hoskins, C.A. Perez, & R.C. Young (Eds.). *Principles and practice of gynecologic oncology* (3rd ed.). Philadelphia: Lippincott Williams & Wilkins, pp. 841-918.

Wright, Jr., T.C., Cox, J., Massad, L., et al. (2002). 2001 Consensus guidelines for the management of women with cervical cytological abnormalities. *Journal of the American Medical Association* 287(16), 2120-2129.

27 Nursing Care of the Client with Cancers of the Urinary System

MAUREEN E. O'ROURKE

KIDNEY CANCER

Theory

I. Physiology and pathophysiology.
  A. Anatomic placement of a kidney (Figures 27-1 and 27-2).
  B. Primary function.
    1. Pair of organs, each measuring approximately 10 cm in length by 5.5 cm in width, positioned behind the peritoneum in a mass of fatty tissue.
    2. Urine production occurs in the renal lobes. Ducts within papillae drain urine into renal calyces, into renal pelvis, and ultimately to the renal sinus, which is connected to the ureter. Urine drains from the ureter into the bladder.
    3. The nephron is the basic structural and functional unit of the kidney (Martini et al., 2000).
  C. Changes associated with cancer: excessive cell production results in growth into adjacent organs and gradual loss of function in the affected kidney.
  D. Major types of kidney cancer (Pantuck et al., 2001).
    1. Clear cell carcinoma: also known as conventional or nonpapillary.
      a. Seventy to eighty percent of cases.
      b. Thought to arise from proximal renal tubule.
      c. Hereditary and sporadic forms.
    2. Papillary renal cell carcinoma.
      a. Ten percent of cases.
      b. Thought to arise from proximal renal tubular epithelium.
      c. Hereditary and sporadic forms.
    3. Chromophobe renal cell carcinoma.
      a. Five percent of cases.
      b. Arises from renal tubular epithelium, proposed to originate in collecting ducts.
      c. Excellent prognosis—better than papillary or clear cell.
    4. Collecting duct carcinoma, or Bellini's duct carcinoma of the kidney.
      a. Fewer than 1% of all cases.
      b. Arises in medullary collecting ducts.
      c. Aggressive with rapid metastasis.

The author acknowledges prior authors of this chapter for their contributions, most recently Julena Lind, RN, MN.

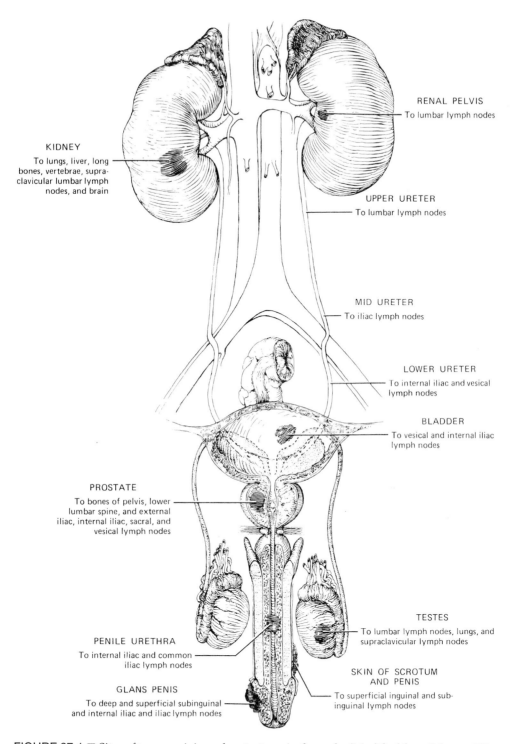

FIGURE 27-1 ■ Sites of tumor origin and metastases in the male. (Modified from Johnson DE, Swanson DA, von Eschenbach AC: Tumors of the genitourinary tract. In Tanagho EA, McAninch JW, editors: *Smith's general urology*, ed 12, San Mateo, Calif, 1987, Appleton & Lange, p. 332.)

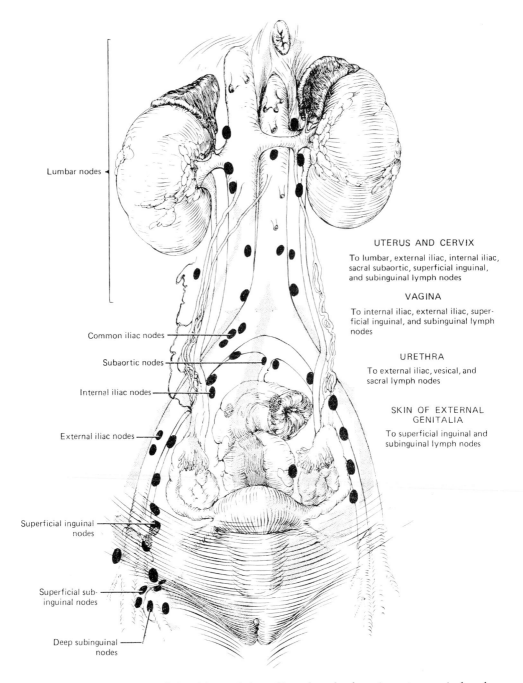

FIGURE 27-2 ■ Anatomic relationships and sites of lymph nodes for urinary tumors in females. (Modified from Johnson DE, Swanson DA, von Eschenbach AC: Tumors of the genitourinary tract. In Tanagho EA, McAninch JW, editors: *Smith's general urology*, ed 12, San Mateo, Calif, 1987, Appleton & Lange, p. 333.)

   d. Subtype of collecting duct carcinoma.
      (1) Renal medullary carcinoma (RMC).
      (2) Occurs almost exclusively in African American men with sickle cell disease (Pantuck et al., 2001; Yip et al., 2001).
   5. Unclassified renal cell carcinoma.
      a. Remains as diagnostic category for tumors that do not fit other categories.

    b. Sarcomatoid is no longer considered a distinct category but is viewed as a manifestation of high-grade carcinoma.

  6. Tumors of the renal pelvis (American Joint Commission on Cancer [AJCC], 2002).

    a. Very rare, 5% or less of all cases.

    b. Urothelial or transitional cell carcinomas.

    c. May occur at any site within the upper urinary collecting system.

    d. Generally multifocal.

    e. Incidence has decreased over past decades (Moyad, 2001).

  7. Renal cell cancers tend to grow toward the medullary portion of the kidney and spread in direct extrusion to the renal vein or the vena cava.

  8. Thirty percent of clients have metastasis at diagnosis. Even among those with early-stage disease, 40% will develop recurrence (Zweizig, 2002).

 E. Trends in epidemiology.

  1. Kidney cancer is relatively rare in the United States (U.S.), accounting for only 3% of all cancers (Jemal et al., 2003).

    a. Both incidence and death rates have been rising since 1973 (Vogelzang & Stadler, 1998).

    b. Rising incidence may be related to common use of high-resolution imaging and incidental finding of tumors among asymptomatic persons.

    c. Two thirds of renal carcinomas are now discovered incidentally during pelvic and abdominal scanning (Zweizig, 2002).

  2. Male predominance, 1.5:1 (Zweizig, 2002).

  3. Risk factors include the following:

    a. Cigarette smoking, obesity, hypertension, unopposed estrogen use, diuretic treatment, prior radiation therapy (RT), occupational exposure to petroleum products or heavy metals, asbestos exposure, and dialysis-acquired cystic kidney disease.

    b. Dietary factors have also been implicated: high-fat diets, high-protein diets, diets low in antioxidants.

    c. Genetic predisposition, von Hippel–Lindau (VHL) disease, non-Hodgkin's lymphoma, and sickle cell disease are also linked with an increased risk of kidney cancer (Lindblad et al., 1995; Mandel et al., 1995; Mellemgaard et al., 1995; Moyad, 2001).

  4. Clear cell carcinomas are strongly associated with loss or inactivation of the short arm of chromosome 3p.

    a. Alterations found in 80% of clients (Zhou & Rubin, 2001).

    b. This association is also found with von Hippel–Lindau disease.

  5. Papillary renal cell carcinoma.

    a. Normal 3p but often trisomies 3q, 8, 12, 17, and 20 are noted.

    b. Trisomies 7 and 17 and the loss of the Y chromosome are also reported (Zhou & Rubin, 2001).

  6. Chromophobe renal cell carcinoma is associated with loss of chromosomes 1, 2, 6, 10, 23, and 21 and alterations of chromosome 17 (Zhou & Rubin, 2001).

II. Principles of medical management.

 A. Screening and diagnostic tests—no screening tests are available for kidney cancer.

  1. Screening with ultrasound would not be cost effective because of the low prevalence of the disease.

  2. Clients with multiple affected relatives should be referred for genetic counseling and possible surveillance.

    B. Diagnostic tests.

        1. Kidney, ureter, and bladder (KUB) radiography (Table 27-1).

        2. Intravenous pyelography (IVP; also referred to as excretory urography): commonly used to evaluate clients presenting with hematuria (see Table 27-1).

        3. Renal ultrasound.

        4. Pelvic/abdominal computerized tomography (CT) scan—diagnostic test of choice.

        5. Renal angiography—less commonly performed, may be necessary because of large vascular mass if renal artery embolization is planned.

        6. Magnetic resonance imaging (MRI)—especially important if vena caval involvement.

        7. Retrograde urography (see Table 27-1).

    C. Staging methods and procedures.

        1. There is no known tumor or molecular marker to confirm diagnosis, remission, progression, or relapse (Mejean et al., 2002).

        2. Based on factors that influence survival—regional lymph node involvement, invasion through the renal capsule, extension to contiguous organs, vena cava or renal vein involvement, and distant metastases (AJCC, 2002).

        3. TNM staging was revised in 2002. Changes include the subdivision of T1 lesions into T1a (tumors of 4 cm or less) and T1b (tumors greater than 4 cm but less than 7 cm) (see revised TNM system, Table 27-2; AJCC, 2002).

TABLE 27-1
Urologic Diagnostic Tests and Nursing Interventions

Test	Preparation	Nursing Interventions
X-ray examination of kidneys, ureter, bladder (KUB)	None—plain film of abdomen	Explain client will lie flat on x-ray examination table. Do not schedule after barium studies (will obscure kidneys).
Excretory urography	Dye excreted unchanged by kidneys; therefore hydration is important, followed by nothing by mouth 6-8 hr before test Dye injected intravenously; anaphylactic or allergic reaction to dye may occur; may premedicate with antihistamines	Assess history of allergy to iodine dyes or contrast media before test; pretesting may be indicated. Use of iodine dyes may be contraindicated in clients with severe renal or hepatic disease or clinical hypersensitivity (severe allergies, asthma). Have emergency equipment and personnel available before injection (anaphylaxis and cardiovascular reactions may occur) and 30-60 min after test (delayed reactions). Observe for adverse reactions to dye—angina, chest pain, arrhythmias, hypotension, dizziness, blurred vision, headache, fever, convulsions, dyspnea, rhinitis, laryngitis, nausea.
Retrograde urography	General anesthesia or narcotic analgesia may be used; cystoscope is inserted; iodinated dye is injected via the urethral catheter Laxatives at bedtime before test may be used to cleanse bowel	Observe for reaction to anesthetic or analgesic. Monitor for bleeding, symptoms of urinary tract infections, dysuria, or difficulty voiding after test.

TABLE 27-2
TNM Staging—Kidney Cancer

PRIMARY TUMOR (T)

TX	Primary tumor cannot be assessed
T0	No evidence of primary tumor
T1	Tumor 7 cm or less in greatest dimension, limited to kidney
T1a	Tumor 4 cm or less in greatest dimension, limited to kidney
T1b	Tumor more than 4 cm but not more than 7 cm in greatest dimension, limited to kidney
T2	Tumor more than 7 cm in greatest dimension, limited to kidney
T3	Tumor extends into major veins or invades adrenal gland or perinephric tissues but not beyond Gerota's fascia
T3a	Tumor directly invades adrenal gland or perirenal and/or renal sinus fat but not beyond Gerota's fascia
T3b	Tumor grossly extends into the renal vein or its segmental (muscle-containing) branches, or vena cava below the diaphragm
T3c	Tumor grossly extends into vena cava above diaphragm or invades wall of vena cava
T4	Tumor invades beyond Gerota's fascia

REGIONAL LYMPH NODES (N)*

NX	Regional lymph nodes cannot be assessed
N0	No regional lymph node metastases
N1	Metastases in a single regional lymph node
N2	Metastasis in more than one regional lymph node

DISTANT METASTASIS (M)

MX	Distant metastasis cannot be assessed
M0	No distant metastasis
M1	Distant metastasis

STAGE GROUPING

Stage I	T1	N0	M0
Stage II	T2	N0	M0
Stage III	T1	N1	M0
	T2	N1	M0
	T3	N0	M0
	T3	N1	M0
	T3a	N0	M0
	T3a	N1	M0
	T3b	N0	M0
	T3b	N1	M0
	T3c	N0	M0
	T3c	N1	M0
Stage IV	T4	N0	M0
	T4	N1	M0
	Any T	N2	M0
	Any T	Any N	M1

Derived from AJCC Cancer Staging Manual, Sixth Edition. For a complete, official description of TNM, Stage Grouping and Histologic Grade for this site, please consult Greene F.L., Page D.L., Fleming, I.D., et al. *AJCC Cancer Staging Manual,* Sixth Edition. New York: Springer-Verlag, 2002.
*Laterality does not affect the N classification.
Note: If a lymph node dissection is performed, then pathologic evaluation would ordinarily include at least eight nodes.

4. Prognostic factors include histologic grade and type, performance status, client age, number and location of metastatic sites, time to appearance of metastasis, and prior nephrectomy (Mejean et al., 2002).

5. The production of antithyroid antibodies stimulated by interleukin-2 (IL-2) immunotherapy may be associated with improved survival (Franzke et al., 1999).

D. Treatment strategies.

1. Radical nephrectomy, which includes excision of the kidney, surrounding lymph nodes, fat, and fascia, as well as the adrenal gland on the affected side, has been the primary treatment since 1960 (Zweizig, 2002).

a. Nephron-sparing surgery now more commonly practiced; reviews suggest partial nephrectomy may be equieffective in selected clients (Novick et al., 2002).

b. Laparoscopic partial nephrectomy widely accepted for clients with solitary tumors and clients with poorly functioning contralateral kidneys (Bernado & Gill, 2002).

2. The utility of regional lymphadenectomy and ipsilateral adrenalectomy has been challenged. These do not appear to provide a therapeutic advantage but may provide important prognostic information (Pantuck et al., 2001).

3. Radiotherapy and chemotherapy.

a. Renal cell cancers are unresponsive to radiotherapy. Radiotherapy is indicated for palliative management of skeletal metastasis, however.

b. Adjuvant chemotherapy has not improved survival.

4. Biotherapy: based on rationale that cytokines bind to specific receptors responsible for intracellular and intercellular signaling with indirect effects on cancer cells.

a. IL-2: most effective immunotherapy available to date, but highly toxic. No direct antitumor effects. Overall response rates vary greatly.

b. Interferon-alpha (IFN-α): also reported to have some efficacy either as a solo agent or in combination with other agents such as 5-fluorouracil (5-FU) (Fishman & Seigne, 2002).

E. Five-year survival rate (Tsui et al., 2000).

1. Stages I and II—91% to 74%, respectively.

2. Stage III—67%.

3. Stage IV—32%; 5-year survival rates of 5% to 10%, however, are widely reported in the literature.

Assessment

I. Pertinent client and family history.

A. Assessment of risk factors associated with kidney cancer (see Section I.E.3. of Theory).

II. Physical examination.

A. Renal cell carcinomas generally remain clinically occult until signs of metastasis prompt diagnostic evaluation.

B. The classic triad of pain, hematuria, and a flank mass is noted in fewer than 10% of clients with kidney cancer and signals advanced disease (Zweizig, 2002).

C. Most common presenting signs: hematuria—60% of clients; abdominal pain—40% of clients; palpable mass—30% to 40% of clients (Zweizig, 2002).

III. Evaluation of diagnostic data.
   A. Gross hematuria found on urinalysis.
   B. CT scan demonstrates renal mass.
   C. Obstruction or blockage related to tumor presence as demonstrated in IVP/excretory urogram.
   D. Differential diagnosis of renal cysts versus neoplasms demonstrated by CT and/or renal ultrasound.
   E. MRI shows vena cava involvement.

Nursing Diagnoses

   I. Risk for altered respiratory function.
   II. Risk for imbalanced fluid volume.
   III. Acute pain.
   IV. Impaired tissue integrity.
   V. Risk for infection.
   VI. Anxiety.
   VII. Fear.
   VIII. Risk for spiritual distress.
   IX. Risk for caregiver role strain.
   X. Deficient knowledge related to diagnosis, treatment, impact on quality of life.

Outcome Identification

   I. Client will demonstrate the ability to turn, cough, and deep breathe and will use incentive spirometer as prescribed.
   II. Client's urine volume and quality are within normal limits. Client verbalizes understanding of need to maintain a liberal oral intake after discharge.
   III. Client verbalizes pain relief or demonstrates through nonverbal cues.
   IV. Client's wound healing progresses without signs of exudate or erythema.
   V. Client exhibits no signs of infection: white blood cell count (WBC) and temperature within normal limits.
   VI. Client and family members verbalize fears and concerns with trusted others.
   VII. Client and family use available resources.
   A. Identify local support groups and American Cancer Society as potential resources.
   VIII. With assistance, caregiver and client will identify activities for which assistance is needed. Caregiver will share frustrations and identify at least one source of support.
   IX. Client and family explain their understanding of diagnosis and treatment plan.
   A. Demonstrate the ability to perform dressing changes and/or management of any necessary medical equipment.
   X. Client participates in follow-up care.
   A. Verbalizes the schedule for follow-up appointments and the rationale for blood pressure monitoring, chest x-rays, CT scans, and other diagnostic tests, as well as scheduled physician's appointments
   B. Reports signs and symptoms of recurrence—for example, abdominal or flank pain, hematuria, bone pain, respiratory changes.
   C. Reports signs and symptoms of renal dysfunction—for example, decreased urine output, fluid retention, hypertension.

Planning and Implementation

I. Interventions to maximize safety.
   A. Prevention of atelectasis and pneumonia.
      1. Because of the close proximity of the nephrectomy incision to the diaphragm, deep breathing and coughing cause pain.
      2. Medicate client based on assessment findings to facilitate ability to move and perform coughing and deep breathing.
      3. Teach proper splinting, and instruct to take at least 10 deep breaths every hour while awake.
      4. Incentive spirometry.
   B. Observation for signs of hemorrhage.
      1. Bleeding is a postoperative risk because of the kidney's highly vascular nature.
         a. Acute massive hemorrhage is manifested by profuse drainage and distention at the suture line.
         b. Examine the nephrectomy dressing and underlying sheets frequently for any signs of bleeding.
         c. Closely monitor vital signs for signs of hemorrhage, for example, falling blood pressure (BP), rapid pulse rate.
   C. Monitor urine output postoperatively for volume of at least 30 ml/hr.
   D. Maintenance of water-seal drainage for chest tubes if thoracic-abdominal incision is used.
      1. Auscultate lung for reinflation.
      2. Auscultate unaffected lung for signs of respiratory compromise, for example, diminished breath sounds, crackles.
II. Interventions to decrease severity of symptoms associated with treatment.
   A. Pain relief measures.
      1. Postnephrectomy pain may be severe and related to both surgical positioning and extensive tissue trauma.
      2. Pain assessment using available reliable and valid scales must be implemented immediately in the postoperative period.
      3. Pain medication should be given on a scheduled basis, titrated to the individual needs of the client (see Chapter 1).
   B. Prevention and observation for paralytic ileus.
      1. Clients are at risk for paralytic ileus following nephrectomy related to bowel manipulation during the surgical procedure and later related to the need for narcotic analgesia.
      2. Ambulation and side-to-side positioning will promote peristalsis.
      3. Observe for abdominal distention, and auscultate bowel sounds every 2 to 4 hours.
      4. A bowel regimen should be instituted as soon as possible to accompany narcotic use.
   C. Prevention of loss of function of remaining kidney.
      1. Teach the client and family the importance of continuing liberal oral intake.
      2. Teach the client and family to avoid potentially nephrotoxic drugs (e.g., nonsteroidal antiinflammatory drugs [NSAIDs]) without first checking with the physician or nurse.
      3. Teach the client and family about risk of injury to the remaining kidney. Resumption of normal activities is the ultimate goal, but clients should be cautioned about participation in contact sports.

4. Teach the client and family signs and symptoms of urinary tract infection.
5. Teach clients to check with physician before taking any complementary therapies or over-the-counter medications. All caregivers must be aware of nephrectomy history.
III. Interventions to promote well-being at home.
    A. Teach the client and family follow-up monitoring.
        1. Frequent BP and renal function tests to monitor function of remaining kidney.
        2. Explain possible follow-up tests.
            a. CT scans to rule out metastases.
            b. Chest x-rays to rule out lung metastases.
            c. Bone scans to detect bony metastases.
    B. Teach the client and family to report signs of respiratory distress, hemoptysis, pain, or fractures.
    C. If appropriate, teach client and family about biologic agents and the management of potential common side effects (see Chapter 37).

Evaluation

The oncology nurse systematically and regularly evaluates the client's and/or family's responses to interventions to determine progress toward the achievement of expected outcomes. Relevant data are collected, and actual findings are compared with expected findings. Nursing diagnoses, outcomes, and plans of care are reviewed and revised as necessary.

BLADDER CANCER

Theory

I. Physiology and pathophysiology.
    A. Anatomy of the bladder.
        1. Hollow muscular organ that serves as temporary reservoir for urine, which is then discharged through the urethra (Martini et al., 2000).
        2. In men, critical adjacent structures include the prostate, seminal vesicles, urethra, nerves at the base of the penis, and local lymph nodes (see Figure 27-1).
        3. In women, critical adjacent structures include the uterus, ovaries, fallopian tubes, urethra, and local lymph nodes (see Figure 27-2).
    B. Changes associated with cancer.
        1. Proliferation of abnormal tissue in one or more places within the bladder.
        2. Clinical changes—bleeding, if the tumor has produced a bladder wall lesion; and, occasionally, urethral obstruction.
    C. Major types of bladder cancer.
        1. Reclassification by World Health Organization (WHO) and International Society of Urologic Pathology to standardize terminology for worldwide comparison and communication (Bostwick et al., 1999).
        2. In the United States, 90% of bladder tumors are urothelial carcinomas, formerly called transitional cell carcinomas; these are often multifocal.
            a. These tumors arise from the epithelial layer of the bladder, which rests on the basement membrane.
            b. If the basement membrane remains intact, metastasis to the vascular or lymphatic system is unlikely.

       c. Remaining bladder cancers include squamous cell carcinomas, approximately 5%, and adenocarcinomas, approximately 1%.

       d. Within the urothelial classification, the tumors are further subdivided—carcinoma in situ (confined to urothelial lining), papillary infiltrating, papillary noninfiltrating, and solid tumors (Bostwick et al., 1999).

          (1) Seventy to eighty percent are considered "superficial" disease (Pashos et al., 2002), although the WHO has recommended that this term be abandoned.

          (2) Papillary tumors are confined to the first two layers of the bladder, but they project toward the lumen (Pashos et al., 2002).

             (a) These tumors demonstrate changes to chromosome 9 and an overexpression of vascular endothelial growth factor leading to angiogenesis (Pashos et al., 2002).

   3. Tumors can involve one or both ureteral orifices.

   4. Tumor depth is an important prognostic indicator.

   5. Metastasis takes place via direct extension.

      a. Can spread by direct extension to adjacent structures, such as the colon, rectum, prostate, uterus, or vagina.

      b. Tumor can obstruct ureters or bladder neck.

   6. Tumor grade, size, location, biomarkers such as the *p21* gene and ki67 antigen, cellular adhesion models, and response to therapy are important prognostic indicators (Pashos et al., 2002).

  D. Trends in epidemiology.

   1. Incidence rates are high in the United States and Africa, especially Egypt where schistosomiasis is endemic (el-Mawla et al., 2001).

   2. Incidence has been gradually increasing over the past 30 years in most industrialized countries.

   3. Some increases may be related to reporting using the new classification system, for example, papillomas that were formerly classified as benign.

   4. Estimated new cases in the United States for 2003: 57,400 (Jemal et al., 2003).

   5. Male/female ratio: nearly 4:1.

   6. Median age at diagnosis is 65 years; rarely diagnosed before age 40 years (National Comprehensive Cancer Network [NCCN], 2002).

   7. Estimated deaths from bladder cancer in 2004 in the United States: 12,710 (American Cancer Society [ACS], 2004.

   8. African Americans continue to lag behind Caucasians in 5-year survival rates for all stages of urinary bladder cancer (Jemal et al., 2003).

   9. Most significant risk factor: cigarette smoking, accounting for 50% to 66% of all bladder tumors in men, 25% in women (Marcus et al., 2000).

  10. Other important risk factors include work-related contact with cyclic chemicals, especially benzenes and arylamines; heavy exposure to chemicals used in dyes, rubbers, textiles, paints, and leathers (Pashos et al., 2002).

  11. Diets high in consumption of fried meats and fats are associated with increased risk (Kamat & Lamm, 1999).

  12. Diets high in consumption of vitamins A, E, and zinc have been suggested to be highly protective (Kamat & Lamm, 1999).

II. Principles of medical management.

  A. Screening and diagnostic tests.

   1. Screening is not currently recommended by any major preventive group in the United States.

2. High-risk groups may benefit from screening as technology evolves.
3. A variety of assays are now available, at least one with U.S. Food and Drug Administration (FDA) approval (the NMP22 assay), for the surveillance and monitoring of clients with noninvasive disease (Schoenberg, 2000).
4. The most common presenting symptom is hematuria, leading to a full diagnostic workup (Pashos et al., 2002).
5. Physical examination is generally normal; only rarely is a mass palpated on rectal examination.
6. Diagnostic tests include the following (O'Rourke, 2001b):
    a. Intravenous pyelogram (IVP), also referred to as excretory urogram, allows visualization of upper tracts to determine whether the source is intravesicular—within the bladder—or located elsewhere (see Table 27-1).
    b. Cystoscopy with bladder washings and biopsies.
    c. Urinary cytology—for best results, specimens are obtained from late-morning or early-afternoon urine.
    d. Flow cytometry—technique used to examine the deoxyribonucleic acid content of urinary cells; provides information for staging purposes.
    e. CT—aids in defining the extent of local tumor and in identifying pelvic lymph node metastasis.
    f. MRI—to distinguish the tumor from the normal bladder wall and to identify the presence of pelvic lymph node involvement.
B. Staging methods and procedures.
    1. Staging: revised TNM system (AJCC, 2002) (Table 27-3).
    2. Tumor grade (grades X, 1, 2, 3, 4): refers to the degree of tumor cell differentiation and aggressive nature of the tumor cells.
C. Treatment strategies.
    1. Noninvasive cancer.
        a. Goal: to prevent disease progression and invasion, avoid loss of bladder, and increase survival (Pashos et al., 2002).
        b. Primary mode of treatment: cystoscopy to confirm tumor presence followed by transurethral resection (TUR). Tumor removal is achieved by fulguration (burning with electrical current) or laser therapy (Pashos et al., 2002).
            (1) Most common side effects include bleeding and infection.
            (2) Perforation of surrounding tissues is also risk of treatment.
        c. Intravesicular chemotherapy has been found to be more effective than TUR alone in preventing tumor recurrence (Duque & Loughlin, 2000).
        d. Most common drugs are mitomycin C (Mutamycin) (generally first line); or a combination of mitomycin C and bacillus Calmette-Guerin (BCG) (TheraCys, TICE BCG), thiotepa (Thioplex), and doxorubicin (Adriamycin) has also been used.
        e. Nursing considerations.
            (1) BCG contraindicated in clients with immune system compromise because of human immunodeficiency virus (HIV) or steroid use, urinary tract infections, or past reactions to tuberculosis strains. Clients can develop systemic tuberculosis.
            (2) Thiotepa: low molecular weight leads to high rates of systemic absorption, leading to severe myelosuppression.
            (3) Mitomycin C: higher molecular weight, lower risk of systemic side effects.

TABLE 27-3
TNM Staging—Bladder Cancer

PRIMARY TUMOR (T)
TX   Primary tumor cannot be assessed
T0   No evidence of primary tumor
Ta   Noninvasive papillary tumor
Tis   Carcinoma in situ: "flat tumors"
T1   Tumor invades subepithelial connective tissue
T2   Tumor invades muscle
pT2a   Tumor invades superficial muscle (inner half)
pT2b   Tumor invades deep muscle (outer half)
T3   Tumor invades perivesicular tissue
pT3a   Microscopically
pT3b   Macroscopically (extravesicular mass)
T4   Tumor invades any of the following: prostate, uterus, vagina, pelvic wall, abdominal wall
T4a   Tumor invades prostate, uterus, vagina
T4b   Tumor invades pelvic wall, abdominal wall

REGIONAL NODES (N)*
NX   Regional lymph nodes cannot be assessed
N0   No regional lymph node metastasis
N1   Metastasis in a single lymph node, 2 cm or less in greatest dimension
N2   Metastasis in a single node, more than 2 cm, but not more than 5 cm in greatest dimension
N3   Metastasis in a lymph node, more than 5 cm in dimension

DISTANT METASTASIS (M)
MX   Distant metastasis cannot be assessed
M0   No distant metastasis
M1   Distant metastasis

STAGE GROUPING

Stage 0a	Ta	N0	M0
Stage 0is	Tis	N0	M0
Stage I	T1	N0	M0
Stage II	T2a	N0	M0
	T2b	N0	M0
Stage III	T3a	N0	M0
	T3b	N0	M0
	T4a	N0	M0
Stage IV	T4b	N0	M0
	Any T	N1	M0
	Any T	N2	M0
	Any T	N3	M0
	Any T	Any N	M1

Derived from AJCC Cancer Staging Manual, Sixth Edition. For a complete, official description of TNM, Stage Grouping and Histologic Grade for this site, please consult Greene F.L., Page D.L., Fleming, I.D., et al. *AJCC Cancer Staging Manual*, Sixth Edition. New York: Springer-Verlag, 2002.
*Regional nodes are those within the true pelvis; all other nodes are distant lymph nodes.

    (a) Generally a first-line agent.
    (b) May cause dysuria, frequency, and less commonly, allergic reactions and myelosuppression (Duque & Loughlin, 2000).
  2. Treatment of invasive disease.
    a. Radical cystectomy with urinary diversion.
      (1) In men, the procedure involves removal of the bladder and prostate.

(2) In women, the procedure also involves a hysterectomy.
(3) For both men and women, the procedure is associated with high risk of infection, bleeding, and subsequent sexual dysfunction.
(4) Presurgical chemotherapy using MVAC (methotrexate [Mexate], vinblastine [Velban], Adriamycin [doxorubicin], cisplatin [Platinol]) has been demonstrated to double survival rates for clients with advanced bladder cancer as compared with surgery alone (Natale, 2001).
(5) Types of urinary diversions (see Chapter 15).
    (a) Ileal conduit (Figure 27-3)—well-known urinary diversion performed with cystectomy.
        (i) Portion of the terminal end of the ileum is isolated, the proximal end is closed, and the distal end is brought out through an opening in the abdominal wall and is sutured to the skin, creating a stoma.
        (ii) Ureters are implanted into the ileal segment, urine flows into the conduit, and peristalsis propels urine out through the stoma.

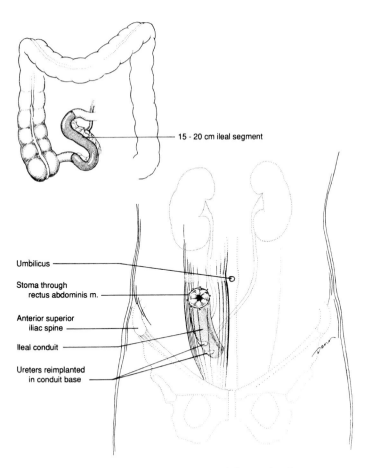

15 - 20 cm ileal segment

Umbilicus

Stoma through rectus abdominis m.

Anterior superior iliac spine

Ileal conduit

Ureters reimplanted in conduit base

FIGURE 27-3 ■ Urinary diversion using a segment of ileum. As short a segment as possible is used, and it is usually positioned in the right lower quadrant of the abdomen in an isoperistaltic direction. (From Carroll PR, Barbour S: Urinary diversion and bladder substitution. In Tanagho EA, McAninch JW, editors: *Smith's general urology*, ed 13, San Mateo, Calif, 1992, Appleton & Lange, p. 427.)

(b) Continent ileal reservoir (Figure 27-4)—technique that provides an intraabdominal pouch for storage of urine.
  (i) Typically has a nipple valve stoma to prevent ureteral reflux. Stoma is generally placed below undergarment line.
  (ii) No external collecting device is needed; urine remains in the reservoir until client self-catheterizes through stoma, approximately every 6 hours (O'Rourke, 2001b).

  b. Bladder preservation therapy.
   (1) Although radical cystectomy is the current primary treatment modality, some clients cannot tolerate cystectomy or are unwilling to undergo the procedure.
   (2) Bladder preservation strategies include the following:
     (a) External beam radiation therapy (XRT).
     (b) Trimodality therapy: TUR, XRT, and systemic chemotherapy (Zietman et al., 2000).

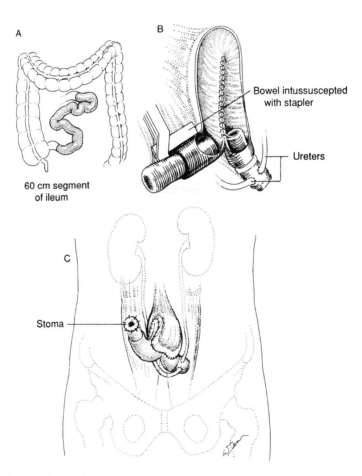

FIGURE 27-4 ■ Kock pouch urinary reservoir. **A,** Shaded area indicates section of small intestine selected for reservoir construction. **B,** Afferent (nonrefluxing) limb for ureteral implantation and efferent limb (with nipple valve) for stoma created by using stapling devices. **C,** Completed reservoir with the efferent limb drawn through the abdominal wall and stoma created. (From Carroll PR, Barbour S: Urinary diversion and bladder substitution. In Tanagho EA, McAninch JW, editors: *Smith's general urology*, ed 13, San Mateo, Calif, 1992, Appleton & Lange, p. 432.)

3. Advanced bladder cancer is often treated with single-agent or combination systemic chemotherapy.
   a. Single-agent therapy has demonstrated limited success, with cisplatin, proving to be the most effective agent.
   b. Combination chemotherapy—MVAC (methotrexate, vinblastine, Adriamycin [doxorubicin], cisplatin); other combinations include cisplatin, methotrexate, and vinblastine; and cisplatin, cyclophosphamide (Cytoxan), and doxorubicin (Pashos et al., 2002).
   c. Other clinical trials are underway examining the efficacy of combinations such as gemcitabine (Gemzar), paclitaxel (Taxol), and cisplatin; and cisplatin, gemcitabine, and gefitinib (Iressa) (http://www.cancer.gov/search/clinical_trials/results_clinicaltrials.aspx?version=patient&cdrid=694439&clickite accessed April 7, 2003).
   d. Protocols for relapse or incomplete responses include the use of ifosfamide, gemcitabine, and paclitaxel (if this agent has not already been used) (NCCN, 2002).
4. RT.
   a. Useful in the management of invasive disease.
   b. Linear accelerator with multiple fields, daily or twice daily.
   c. Clients must have an empty bladder for both simulation and treatment.
   d. Radiation is usually preceded by TUR.
   e. Often used as combined modality therapy with chemotherapy.
   f. Dose range to whole bladder: 40 to 55 Gy with an additional boost of 9 to 11 Gy for total of 49 to 66 Gy (NCCN, 2002).
5. Phototherapy.
   a. Has shown promise for carcinoma in situ.
   b. Use of light-sensitive chemical followed by exposure of bladder to light. Chemical converts oxygen into free radicals, which are cytotoxic.
   c. Clients experience irritable bladder symptoms, such as frequency, dysuria, and microscopic hematuria. They may also experience sunburn from the residual chemicals in the body (Walther, 2000).

Assessment

I. Assess major risk factors associated with increased risk of bladder cancer.
   A. Race—age-adjusted bladder cancer rate in Caucasian men in the United States is twice the rate of African American men.
   B. Gender—male/female ratio is 4:1.
   C. Age—most tumors occur in men over 65 years old.
   D. Geographic location.
      1. Africa and Egypt: high rates secondary to parasitic infection with schistosomiasis infection (el-Mawla et al., 2001).
   E. Occupational risks—dyes, cyclic chemicals, benzene derivative, arylamines.
   F. Cigarette smoking.
II. Physical examination.
   A. Client presentation.
      1. Eighty to ninety percent of clients present with gross or microscopic hematuria that is sporadic and often painless (Metts et al., 2000).
      2. May present with symptoms of bladder irritability: frequency, urgency, dysuria.

3. Clients may present with urinary obstructive symptoms: urinary hesitancy, diminished stream force, and flank pain if urethral obstruction occurs causing hydronephrosis (O'Rourke, 2001b).
4. Back pain, rectal pain, and suprapubic pain are late signs and may indicate metastasis (O'Rourke, 2001b).

III. Evaluation of diagnostic data.
   A. Gross or microscopic hematuria on urinalysis.
   B. CT demonstrates mass/masses, lymph node involvement.
   C. Urine cytology indicates presence of malignant cells.
   D. Bladder washings indicate presence of malignant cells.
   E. Bimanual examination (with client under anesthesia) indicates mass.
   F. Cystoscopy reveals mass/masses.
   G. Biopsy specimens taken at cystoscopy reveal malignancy.
   H. MRI and CT scans of pelvis and abdomen are used when there is a large mass or suspicion of metastatic disease.
   I. Chest x-ray and bone scan may be performed to evaluate metastatic disease.

Nursing Diagnoses

   I. Impaired urinary elimination.
   II. Risk for infection (e.g., pyelonephritis, surgical wound, peritonitis).
   III. Acute pain.
   IV. Risk for impaired skin integrity.
   V. Disturbed body image.
   VI. Risk for sexual dysfunction.
   VII. Deficient knowledge related to diagnosis, treatment, and impact on quality of life.

Outcome Identification

   I. Client's urine volume and quality are within normal limits.
   II. Client does not develop urinary tract infection.
   III. Client's stoma healing progresses without signs of infection: elevated temperature, leukocytosis, exudate at stoma site.
   IV. Client verbalizes pain relief or demonstrates it through nonverbal cues.
   V. Client participates actively in ostomy care and demonstrates an ability to perform skin and pouch changes if necessary.
   VI. Client will demonstrate willingness and ability to resume self-care role and responsibilities.
   VII. Client will be able to identify potential sexual limitations imposed by treatment and modifications/interventions in response to these limitations.
   VIII. Client verbalizes an understanding of disease and rationale and outcomes of treatment.
   IX. Client explains care at home following discharge, including the following:
      A. Describes a viable stoma (i.e., pink, moist).
      B. Describes desired urinary output (>30 ml/hr).
      C. Lists the signs and symptoms of urinary tract infection and measures to prevent it.
      D. Describes strategies to prevent ammonia salt encrustation.
      E. Demonstrates pouch change.
      F. Describes the use of skin barriers.

G. Demonstrates the steps of peristomal skin care.

H. Describes potential changes in sexual functioning.

I. Verbalizes understanding of the schedule for follow-up care and monitoring, including physician appointments, scans, and so on.

J. Client identifies selected resources—enterostomal therapy, home care, support services (e.g., American Cancer Society).

Planning and Implementation

I. Interventions to maximize safety of the client preoperatively.

A. Teach the client and family the importance of a low-residue diet 2 days before surgery, followed by clear liquid diet on the day before surgery.

B. Teach the client and family the importance of using the prescribed antibiotics and cathartics before surgery since incomplete adherence to the preoperative regimen increases the risk of infection.

C. Initiate referral to enterostomal therapist for preoperative marking and optimal positioning of stoma, avoiding skinfolds, scars, bony prominences, and belt lines that interfere with adherence of appliance and client comfort.

II. Interventions to maintain adequate urinary elimination.

A. Monitor urinary output—at least 30 ml/hr.

B. Monitor hematuria—should be clear within 2 days postoperatively.

1. Decreased urine output may be a sign of obstruction of urinary drainage or renal failure.

2. Maintain current input and output records; the urinary flow should be generally continuous.

3. Teach client and family the importance of maintaining adequate hydration.

III. Interventions to minimize risk of infection.

A. Assess the client for signs of peritonitis related to anastomotic leak.

1. Abdominal distention or tenderness, elevated temperature, leukocytosis.

2. Sudden decrease in urinary output or presence of malodorous abdominal wound drainage.

B. Monitor signs of urinary tract infection—elevated temperature, flank pain, malodorous urine, and/or hematuria.

1. Administer antibiotics.

2. Maintain hydration status.

C. Monitor abdominal wound/surgical incision site.

1. Change dressings as prescribed.

2. Monitor for signs of infection: erythema, exudate, leukocytosis, elevated temperature.

IV. Interventions to decrease pain.

A. Assess client's pain status using a 1 to 10 scale, a pictorial scale, or a visual analogue scale.

B. Medicate client on a routine schedule for pain as opposed to as-needed (prn) dosing.

C. Splint abdomen with pillow when the client is coughing or doing deep-breathing exercises.

D. Position with pillows when turning the client.

E. Teach client relaxation exercises to augment pharmacologic pain management.

V. Interventions to prevent impairment of the integumentary system.

A. Monitor and document color and condition of stoma.

      1. Color of the intestinal stomal tissue can be compared with the mucosal lining of the mouth.

      2. Stoma may bleed when rubbed because of the capillaries in the area.

      3. Normal color of the stoma is a deep pink to dark red; a dusky appearance ranging from purple to black may develop if circulation is seriously impaired.

      4. Stomal edema is normal in the early postoperative period.

      5. Edema should resolve during the first 1 or 2 weeks after surgery.

      6. Attach straight drainage bag to pouch when the client is in bed or at bedtime to prevent infections and damage to stomal tissue.

  B. In consultation with enterostomal therapist, teach client and family members proper care of the stoma and peristomal skin areas.

      1. Use of skin barriers.

      2. Proper cleansing of stoma.

      3. Selection of proper sizing of opening of pouch.

      4. Avoidance of topical irritants (e.g., solutions containing alcohol).

  C. Assess abdominal wound/surgical incision site for proper healing.

      1. Monitor for signs of infection: erythema, exudate, leukocytosis, elevated temperature.

      2. Assess incision for approximation and integrity of sutures or staples.

      3. Teach client and family members care of incision site.

VI. Interventions to enhance adaptation and rehabilitation related to alterations in body image and sexuality.

  A. Assess the client and family for signs of readiness to learn self-care of the stoma.

      1. Provide written instructions at low readability level with diagrams and photos.

      2. Encourage the client to observe pouch change and gradually to participate in self-care.

      3. Encourage the client and family to participate in ostomy care: pouch changes, skin care.

      4. Refer to the home health nursing agency if indicated for continued teaching and monitoring.

  B. Assess client and significant other's readiness to discuss sexuality issues.

      1. PLISSIT model guides care: give *p*ermission, *l*imited *i*nformation, *s*pecific *s*uggestions, or refer for *i*ntensive *t*herapy (Annon, 1976).

      2. Give permission for discussion by initiating topic in private setting.

      3. Provide limited information regarding potential sexual changes as related to treatment (Sprunk & Alteneder, 2000).

      4. Encourage openness between partners.

      5. Provide reassurance that treatment is available.

      6. Encourage clients to discuss specific interventions as they relate to their specific treatment with their physicians.

VII. Interventions for deficient knowledge regarding diagnosis, treatment, and impact on quality of life.

  A. Encourage client and family members to ask questions.

  B. Teach the client and family care of the stoma, and schedule return demonstrations until proper technique is achieved.

  C. Teach the client and family preventive elements of care (Table 27-4).

      1. Prevention of malodorous urine.

TABLE 27-4
Management of Common Ileal Conduit Problems

Problem	Interventions
Urinary odor	Avoid rubber pouch
	Soak appliance in vinegar/water, 1:4
Rash around stoma or under pouch	Dry and powder skin except under adhesive
	Use a skin barrier (e.g., Stomahesive)
Macerated skin around stoma	Dry skin, and apply a hydroponic skin barrier
	Decrease size of pouch opening
Crystals on or around stoma	Apply vinegar compresses on stoma and inside pouch
Ulcerated stoma	Enlarge pouch opening
	Consult enterostomal therapist if not partially healed in 1 wk
Monilial infection following antibiotic therapy	Dry skin, and apply nystatin (Mycostatin) powder
	Encourage oral fluids
Hyperplasia of skin around stoma	Decrease pouch opening size
Fistula	Revision of stoma at new site

    a. Avoid ingestion of large quantities of alkaline liquids, such as carbonated beverages.
    b. Drink fluids with high vitamin C content.
    c. Clean reusable pouch regularly with soap and water, rinsing with vinegar if desired.
    d. Avoid foods (e.g., fish, asparagus) that cause urinary odors.
  2. Prevention of urinary tract infection.
    a. Drink at least 2 L of fluid per day.
    b. Use straight drainage bag at bedtime, and clean the system each morning.
  3. Prevention of ammonia salt encrustation—ingest food and fluid (cranberry juice) that keep the urine acid.
  4. Prevention of peristomal skin breakdown.
    a. Use a skin barrier if irritation is present.
    b. Use appropriate stoma opening in the barrier and the pouch.
    c. Remove pouch if burning or itching occurs.
    d. Change pouch on a regular basis (e.g., every 3 to 7 days).
    e. Do not use preparations that are greasy or that contain benzoin or alcohol on irritated skin.
    f. Contact nurse, physician, or enterostomal therapist for assistance if problems occur.
D. Arrange preoperative and/or postoperative visit by rehabilitated client with similar diversion.

Evaluation

The oncology nurse systematically and regularly evaluates the client's and/or family's responses to interventions to determine progress toward the achievement of expected outcomes. Relevant data are collected, and actual findings are compared with expected findings. Nursing diagnoses, outcomes, and plans of care are reviewed and revised as necessary.

PROSTATE CANCER

Theory

I. Physiology and pathophysiology.
   A. Anatomy.
      1. Small, muscular organ, roughly the size of a walnut—4 cm in diameter (Martini et al., 2000).
      2. Located posterior to the symphysis pubis, inferior to the bladder, and in front of the rectum (see Figure 27-1).
      3. Prostate gland encircles the urethra as it leaves the bladder.
      4. Prostate gland comprises three zones: the transitional zone, central zone, and peripheral zone.
   B. Primary function.
      1. A secondary sex organ that secretes a component of seminal fluid.
   C. Changes associated with cancer.
      1. Most cancers develop in the peripheral zone (Scher et al., 2000).
      2. Malignant cell growth spreads locally to the seminal vesicles, bladder, and peritoneum (see Figure 27-1).
      3. Lymphatic and hematogenous spread is also common.
         a. Pelvic lymph node invasion.
         b. Hematogenous spread of prostatic cancer typically involves the lung, liver, kidneys, and bones.
   D. Types of prostate cancer.
      1. Ninety-five percent of all prostate cancers are adenocarcinomas.
      2. Sarcomas, ductal carcinomas, and transitional cell carcinomas comprise the remaining 5% (Frank et al., 1991).
   E. Trends in epidemiology.
      1. National trend in prostate cancer incidence: increased rates from 1988 to 1992 coinciding with the advent of widespread prostate specific antigen (PSA) testing; sharp declines from 1992 to 1995, followed by a leveling off from 1995 to 1999.
      2. Projections for 2004: 230,110 new cases and 29,900 deaths within the United States (ACS, 2004).
      3. Accounts for one third of all male cancers.
      4. Five-year survival rates have continued to improve steadily since 1974 for both Caucasians and African Americans; however, African Americans continue to have lower 5-year survival rates for all stages of prostate cancer (Jemal et al., 2003).
      5. Risk factors.
         a. Age.
            (1) More than 75% of prostate cancers are diagnosed in men 65 years or older.
            (2) Autopsy studies have shown that 30% of men aged 50 years have evidence of adenocarcinoma of the prostate, and by age 90 years that percentage rises to 57% (Scott et al., 1969).
         b. Ethnicity.
            (1) Higher mortality in Western versus non-Western countries (e.g., developing countries such as in Asia and the Middle East) (Brawley & Barnes, 2001).
            (2) Highest incidence and mortality rates in the world are among African Americans (Brawley & Barnes, 2001).

        (3) High mortality rates also noted among men of African heritage in Jamaica and Brazil (Glover et al., 1998).

    c. Dietary factors (Brawley & Barnes, 2001).

        (1) Possible role of high-fat diets in promotion of prostate cancer.

        (2) Diets high in vitamins E, D, and selenium may inhibit or prevent prostate cancer.

        (3) Diets high in lycopene have been linked with a low incidence of prostate cancer (Gann et al., 1999).

    d. Occupational exposures.

        (1) Farming and cadmium exposure through welding and battery manufacturing have also been associated with increased risk (Brawley & Barnes, 2001).

    e. Genetic factors.

        (1) Prostate cancer susceptibility locus called *HPC1* located on chromosome 1—thought to be responsible for 33% of all hereditary prostate cancer and 3% of cases overall (Cooney et al., 1997).

        (2) Gene mutations implicated in breast cancer, *BRCA1* and *BRCA2*, have also been implicated in prostate cancer (Ekman, 1999).

        (3) Having a single first-degree relative with prostate cancer increases risk twofold to threefold; having a first- and second-degree relative affected increases risk sixfold (Zlotta & Schulman, 1998).

II. Principles of medical management.

  A. Screening tests.

    1. There continues to be a high level of controversy at the national level surrounding routine screening for prostate cancer using PSA testing.

      a. Central issue: PSA testing may reveal clinically insignificant tumors that are treated with significant side effects, resulting in diminished quality of life.

    2. The American Cancer Society (ACS) recommends digital rectal examination (DRE) and PSA testing annually for men beginning at age 50 years who have a life expectancy of at least 10 years.

      a. For high-risk men, including African American men and those with a first-degree relative affected with prostate cancer, testing should begin at age 45 years (Smith et al., 2001).

    3. Other major health groups disagree: the U.S. Preventive Services Task Force (2002) concluded that there is insufficient evidence to determine if the benefits of PSA testing outweigh the harms.

    4. Normal range for PSA varies by age, race, and prostate size—0 to 4 ng/ml is considered the standard norm. Other important markers include PSA density and PSA velocity (Mettlin et al., 1994).

  B. Diagnostic tests.

    1. DRE: assess for size, lesions, symmetry, texture.

      a. Simple/inexpensive, but only the posterior and lateral areas can be palpated.

    2. Transrectal ultrasound (TRUS): evaluation of the prostate volume.

    3. Biopsy.

      a. Performed with TRUS for guidance.

      b. Transrectal route preferred, six specimens from both sides of the prostate.

    4. Pelvic MRI to evaluate capsular penetration and lymph node metastasis, seminal vesicles.

5. Bone scans: to evaluate possible bone metastasis. Generally not performed unless PSA level is above 10 or client complains of skeletal symptoms (Lee, 2002; National Comprehensive Cancer Network [NCCN], 2003).
6. Laboratory studies.
   a. PSA—increased levels may be significant as an adjunct in differential diagnosis or as a marker for disease progression.
      (1) Men should abstain from ejaculation for 48 hours before test.
      (2) Finasteride (Propecia), androgen receptor blockers, PC SPES may also affect PSA levels (NCCN, 2003).
C. Staging methods and procedures.
   1. TNM staging (Table 27-5).
   2. Gleason score: optimal method of grading based on assessment of tumor histology (Stoller & Carroll, 2003).
      a. Primary grade is based on evaluation of architecture of malignant glands in the largest portion of the specimen.
      b. Secondary grade is assigned to the next largest area of malignant growth.
      c. Score is computed by adding the primary and secondary grades together.

TABLE 27-5
TNM Staging—Prostate Cancer

PRIMARY TUMOR (T)
CLINICAL

TX	Primary tumor cannot be assessed
T0	No evidence of primary tumor
T1	Clinically inapparent tumor neither palpable nor visible by imaging
T1a	Tumor incidental histologic finding in 5% or less of tissue resected
T1b	Tumor incidental finding in more than 5% of tissue resected
T1c	Tumor identified by needle biopsy (e.g., because of elevated PSA)
T2	Tumor confined within prostate*
T2a	Tumor involves one half of one lobe or less
T2b	Tumor involves more than one half of one lobe but not both lobes
T2c	Tumor involves both lobes
T3	Tumor extends though the prostate capsule†
T3a	Extracapsular extension (unilateral or bilateral)
T3b	Tumor invades seminal vesicle(s)
T4	Tumor is fixed or invades adjacent structures other than seminal vesicles: bladder neck, external sphincter, levator muscles, and/or pelvic wall

PATHOLOGIC

pT2‡	Organ confined
pT2a	Unilateral, involving one half of one lobe or less
pT2b	Unilateral, involving more than one half of one lobe but not both lobes
pT2c	Bilateral disease
pT3	Extraprostatic extension
pT3a	Extraprostatic extension¶
pT3b	Seminal vesicle invasion
pT4	Invasion of bladder, rectum

REGIONAL LYMPH NODES (N)

NX	Regional nodes not sampled
N0	No regional node metastasis
N1	Metastasis in regional node(s)

TABLE 27-5
TNM Staging—Prostate Cancer—cont'd

DISTANT METASTASIS (M)

MX	Distant metastasis cannot be assessed (not evaluated by any modality)
M0	No distant metastasis
M1	Distant metastasis
M1a	Nonregional lymph node(s)
M1b	Bone(s)
M1c	Other site(s) with or without bone disease

HISTOLOGIC GRADE

GX	Grade cannot be assessed
G1	Well differentiated (slight anaplasia) (Gleason 2-4)
G2	Moderately differentiated (moderate anaplasia) (Gleason 5-6)
G3-4	Poorly differentiated/undifferentiated (marked anaplasia) (Gleason 7-10)

STAGE GROUPING

Stage I	T1a	N0	M0	G1
Stage II	T1a	N0	M0	G2, 3-4
	T1b	N0	M0	Any G
	T1c	N0	M0	Any G
	T1	N0	M0	Any G
	T2	N0	M0	Any G
Stage III	T3	N0	M0	Any G
Stage IV	T4	N0	M0	Any G
	Any T	N1	M0	Any G
	Any T	Any N	M1	Any G

Derived from AJCC Cancer Staging Manual, Sixth Edition. For a complete, official description of TNM, Stage Grouping and Histologic Grade for this site, please consult Greene F.L., Page D.L., Fleming, I.D., et al. *AJCC Cancer Staging Manual*, Sixth Edition. New York: Springer-Verlag, 2002.
PSA, Prostate specific antigen.
*Note: Tumor found in one or both lobes by needle biopsy but not palpable or reliably visible by imaging is classified as T1c.
†Note: Invasion into the prostatic apex or into (but not beyond) the prostatic capsule is classified not as T3 but as T2.
‡Note: There is no pathologic T1 classification.
¶Note: Postsurgical margin should be indicated by an R1 descriptor (residual microscopic disease).

      d. Scores of 2 to 10 are possible; higher scores indicate aggressive disease with a poor prognosis.
    3. Other diagnostic tests (discussed above) may be performed to evaluate possible metastasis.
  D. Treatment strategies.
    1. Early-stage disease.
      a. Treatment options: observation or expectant management, radical prostatectomy + lymph node dissection, three-dimensional conformal radiotherapy (3D-CRT), or brachytherapy.
        (1) Radical prostatectomy: complete removal of prostate, lymph node sampling. Walsh nerve-sparing technique is linked with less impotence postoperatively (Walsh, 1998).
          (a) Laparoscopic prostatectomy: newer option available at some major cancer centers, minimally invasive and associated with less blood loss than open surgery (Guillonneau et al., 2003), although rectal injury and urinary leakage rates are higher in this group (Rassweiler et al., 2003).

   (b) Robotic laparoscopic prostatectomy is now being performed at some centers (Antiphon et al., 2003).
   (2) 3D-CRT: radiation doses to prostate greater than 81 Gy (Iwamoto & Maher, 2001). Intensity modulated radiation therapy (IMRT) replacing 3D in major cancer centers.
   (3) Brachytherapy: guided by transrectal ultrasound, radioactive seed placement into the prostate gland via the perineum through a grid template (Iwamoto & Maher, 2001).
   (a) Isotopes used: iodine-125 or palladium-103.
   (4) Expectant management: careful follow-up monitoring with PSA testing, ultrasound, and DRE, followed by active treatment if disease progression is noted (Griffin & O'Rourke, 2001).
   (5) Cryosurgery: direct application of freezing temperatures to the prostate via percutaneously inserted cryogenic probes (O'Rourke, 2001a).

2. Complications of treatment.
   a. Incontinence: conflicting data because of imprecise measurement; estimates range from 3% to 87% after radical prostatectomy, 3% to 7% for external beam radiotherapy, and 6% for brachytherapy. Other complications include urethral stricture, urethral sloughing, and bladder outlet obstruction (O'Rourke, 2001a).
   b. Impotence: nerve-sparing prostatectomy techniques lessen incidence; imprecise definitions and measurement make comparisons difficult. High rates reported after surgery, and 6% to 61% of cases after brachytherapy have some form of impotence (Abel et al., 2003; Merrick et al., 2001).
   c. Gastrointestinal (GI) dysfunction: diarrhea, proctitis, and rectal bleeding have been associated with both RT and brachytherapy.
   (1) High correlations reported between bowel dysfunction and poor quality of life (Krupski et al., 2000).

3. Treatment for advanced prostate cancer.
   a. Hormonal manipulation—accepted standard for management of metastatic prostate cancer and also used in management of clients at high risk for relapse.
   (1) Orchiectomy—surgical removal of testicles; produces rapid response. Indicated for clients who are unreliable in taking medication or for whom estrogen is contraindicated.
   (a) Not acceptable as an option for many men.
   (b) Psychologic trauma as a result of surgical castration.
   (2) Luteinizing hormone–releasing hormones (LHRH analogues; e.g., leuprolide [Lupron], goserelin [Zoladex])—decrease production of testosterone; may produce fewer side effects than estrogens, used with flutamide (Eulexin) to reduce "flare," which is the sudden exacerbation of symptoms (Held-Warmkesel, 2001).
   (a) Flare can be life threatening with spinal cord compression and ureteral obstruction (Held-Warmkessel, 2001).
   (b) Other side effects include hot flashes, loss of libido, impotence, and gynecomastia.
   (3) Antiandrogens (flutamide, megestrol acetate [Megace])—interfere with intracellular androgen activity; effects may be delayed 1 to 2 months.

(4) Estrogen therapy—generally diethylstilbestrol (DES); results in decreased pain, weight gain, decreased tumor size, decreased urinary symptoms (Held-Warmkessel, 2001).

    (a) Associated with gynecomastia, sodium retention, and severe cardiovascular and thrombotic complications. In addition, this therapy is associated with relapse within 2 to 3 years, and at the time of relapse, disease often becomes resistant to further hormonal treatment.

(5) Ketoconazole (Nizoral): suppresses adrenal testosterone production.

    (a) Administered with hydrocortisone to reduce risk of adrenal insufficiency (O'Rourke, 2003).

  b. RT—for local extension and distant metastases.

    (1) May be primary treatment for stage D lesions if hormonal manipulation is ineffective or contraindicated and may be used as a component of combined-modality therapy.

    (2) Used for palliation of pain from bone metastasis.

    (3) Emergency treatment for spinal cord compression.

  E. Trends in survival in the United States (Jemal et al., 2003).

    1. Localized—5-year survival rate: 96.9% for Caucasians, 85.9% for African Americans.

    2. Five-year survival for all stages combined: 89.9% for Caucasians, 65.5% for African Americans.

Assessment

  I. Assess risk factors listed above: age, ethnicity, occupational exposures, and genetic/familial links.

  II. Physical examination.

    A. Early disease.

      1. Client may be asymptomatic or may present with complaints of dysuria, hesitancy, straining to start stream; weak urinary stream, nocturia, dribbling, urgency, sensation of incomplete voiding.

      2. Findings on physical examination.

        a. DRE: prostate nodule.

        b. Distended/palpable bladder: urinary retention.

    B. Advanced disease—client may present with lumbosacral back pain, migratory back pain, hip pain, lethargy.

      1. Findings on physical examination.

        a. DRE: hard and stonelike nodule, may be induration; hematuria.

        b. Weight loss.

        c. Lymphedema: caused by lymph node metastasis.

  III. Evaluation of laboratory data (Sacher & McPherson, 2000).

    A. Elevated serum alkaline phosphatase level: may be elevated if bone metastasis present.

      1. Largely replaced by the PSA.

    B. Serum calcium: may be elevated in the presence of bone metastases.

    C. Elevated serum acid phosphatase level: may be elevated in the presence of prostate cancer outside the confines of the prostate gland.

    D. Elevated PSA level: indicative of benign prostatic hypertrophy (BPH) or inflammation or malignancy of the prostate.

Nursing Diagnoses

 I. Impaired urinary elimination.
 II. Acute pain.
 III. Risk for infection.
 IV. Sexual dysfunction.
 V. Deficient knowledge related to diagnosis, treatment, and self-care management.

Outcome Identification

 I. Client maintains adequate urinary output: 30 ml/hr.
 II. Client demonstrates relief from pain: verbal or nonverbal communication, comparative scoring on pain assessment tools.
 III. Client exhibits no signs of infection: surgical wound is without exudates, normal WBC, temperature within normal limits, urine clear and free of bacteria on culture.
 IV. Client and partner verbalize their understanding of sexual implications of treatment plan.
    A. Client and partner can identify resources for dealing with impotence.
 V. Client and partner explain their understanding of diagnosis and treatment plan.
    A. Identify a follow-up schedule of every 6 to 12 months (or as prescribed).
    B. Demonstrate proper care of urinary catheter.

Planning and Implementation

 I. Interventions to maintain urinary output above 30 ml/hr.
    A. Maintain closed urinary catheter drainage system and aseptic technique during irrigation to prevent infection.
    B. Maintain patency of urinary and/or bladder irrigation systems; risk of blockage greatest in first 3 hours after surgery.
       1. Maintain continuous or intermittent bladder irrigation to remove blood clots and/or mucous plugs for clients after transurethral resection of prostate (TURP).
       2. Avoid kinked tubing by positioning of client and securing of tubes.
       3. Intravenous (IV) fluids; oral (PO) fluids when tolerated.
       4. Maintain positioning and patency of urethral catheter (serves as splint for urethral anastomosis and for bladder drainage after radical prostatectomy); usually left in place for 2 to 3 weeks.
 II. Interventions to promote comfort.
    A. Administer antispasmodics and/or analgesics for bladder spasms; initiate use of stool softeners with antispasmodics to avoid constipation.
    B. Consult with enterostomal therapist as indicated for perineal wound care, radiation reactions, or management of incontinence.
    C. Administer antidiarrheal medications as ordered for proctitis, and teach client to avoid a high-residue diet.
    D. Topical analgesics for rectal irritation.
 III. Interventions to prevent infection and promote healing.
    A. Assess wound for exudates.
    B. Irrigate wound.
    C. Provide sitz baths for comfort and cleanliness.
    D. Maintenance of closed urinary drainage system, aseptic technique.
 IV. Interventions to promote optimal sexual functioning—based on the PLISSIT model (Annon, 1976).

A. Facilitate physician/nurse/client discussion of potential impact of treatment on sexual functioning and interventions to minimize effects.
   1. Give permission before and after treatment to discuss functional and anatomic changes with treatment and resultant sexual concerns.
      a. Respect reticence in discussing sexual concerns.
      b. Use terminology appropriate to social and cultural level.
   2. Provide written information and anatomic drawings as indicated for clarity and to reinforce teaching.
   3. Provide specific suggestions related to treatment used and alternatives.
      a. Teach client and partner about available options for the treatment of impotence—pharmacologic, mechanical, surgical.
   4. Initiate referral for sexual counseling if indicated (Dest & Wallace, 2001).

V. Interventions to promote knowledge and self-care.
   A. Teach client and partner care of urinary catheter.
   B. Teach perineal exercises to manage dribbling, urgency, or urinary incontinence (in most cases, problem gradually diminishes).
   C. Teach client to report symptoms of urinary obstruction promptly—diminished stream, abdominal pain and distention, dysuria, retention with dribbling, bladder spasms.
   D. Teach client to report early symptoms of urinary tract infection—fever, dysuria, urgency, hematuria.
   E. Inform clients to report lymphedema of legs, scrotum, or penis after lymph node dissection.
   F. Teach client to report symptoms of recurrence—hematuria, urinary obstruction, bone pain, abdominal pain, neuritic pain, weight loss, debilitation, back pain.
   G. Teach client and partner side effects relative to each treatment: impotence, incontinence, bowel dysfunction, proctitis. For clients receiving hormonal therapy: fluid retention, edema, mood changes, gynecomastia, hot flashes.
   H. Describe follow-up schedule.
   I. Identify resources, as needed, for home care, follow-up, reconstructive treatment, or palliation.

Evaluation

The oncology nurse systematically and regularly evaluates the client's and/or family's responses to interventions to determine progress toward the achievement of expected outcomes. Relevant data are collected, and actual findings are compared with expected findings. Nursing diagnoses, outcomes, and plans of care are reviewed and revised as necessary.

REFERENCES

Abel, L., Dafoe-Lambie, J., Butler, W.M., & Merrick, G.S. (2003). Treatment outcomes and quality of life issues for patients treated with prostate brachytherapy. *Clinical Journal of Oncology Nursing 7*(1), 48-54.

American Cancer Society (ACS). (2004). *Cancer facts and figures 2004.* Atlanta: Author.

Annon, J.S. (1976). *Behavioral treatment of sexual problems: Brief therapy.* Hagerstown, PA: Harper & Row.

Antiphon, P., Hoznek, A., Benyoussef, A., et al. (2003). Complete solo laparoscopic radical prostatectomy: Initial experience. *Urology 61*(4), 724-728.

Bernado, N.O., & Gill, I.S. (2002). Laparoscopic partial nephrectomy: Current status. *Archivos Espanoles de Urologia 55*(7):868-880.

Bostwick, D.G., Ramnani, D., & Cheng, L. (1999). Diagnosis and grading of bladder cancer and associated lesions. *Urologic Clinics of North America 26,* 493-507.

Brawley, O.W., & Barnes, S. (2001). The epidemiology of prostate cancer in the United States. *Seminars in Oncology Nursing 17*(2), 72-77.

Cooney, K.A., McCarthy, J.D., Lange, E., et al. (1997). Prostate cancer susceptibility locus on chromosome 1q: A confirmatory study. *Journal of the National Cancer Institute 89,* 955-959.

Dest, V.M., & Wallace, M. (2001). Prevalent issues in patient education. In M. Wallace & L.L. Powell (Eds.). *Prostate cancer: Nursing assessment, management, and care.* New York: Springer Publishing, pp. 140-152.

Duque, J.L., & Loughlin, K.R. (2000). An overview of the treatment of superficial bladder cancer: Intravesicular chemotherapy. *Urologic Clinics of North America 27,* 125-135.

Ekman, P. (1999). Genetic and environmental factors in prostate cancer genesis: Identifying high-risk cohorts. *European Urology 35,* 362-369.

el-Mawla, N.G., el-Bolkainy, M.N., & Khaled, H.M. (2001). Bladder cancer in Africa: Update. *Seminars in Oncology 28*(2), 174-178.

Fishman, M., & Seigne, M.B. (2002). Immunotherapy of metastatic renal cell cancer. *Cancer Control 9*(4), 293-304.

Frank, I., Granham, S., & Neighbors, W. (1991). Urologic and male genital cancers. In A. Holleb, D. Fink, & G. Murphy (Eds.). *American Cancer Society textbook of clinical oncology.* Atlanta: American Cancer Society, pp. 271-289.

Franzke, A., Peest, D., Probst-Kepper, M., et al. (1999). Autoimmunity resulting from cytokine treatment predicts long term survival in patients with metastatic renal cell cancer. *Journal of Clinical Oncology 17,* 529-533.

Gann, P.H., Ma, J., & Giovannucci, E., et al. (1999). Lower prostate cancer risk in men with elevated plasma lycopene levels: Results of a prospective analysis. *Cancer Research 59,* 1225-1230.

Glover, F.E., Jr., Coffey, D.S., Douglas, L.L., et al. (1998). The epidemiology of prostate cancer in Jamaica. *Journal of Urology 159*(6), 1984-1986.

Greene, F.L., Page, D.L., Fleming, I.D., et al. (Eds.). (2002). *AJCC cancer staging manual* (6th ed.). New York: Springer-Verlag.

Griffin, A.S., & O'Rourke, M.E. (2001). Expectant management of prostate cancer. *Seminars in Oncology Nursing 17*(2), 101-107.

Guillonneau, B., el-Fettouh, H., Baumert, H., et al. (2003). Laparoscopic radical prostatectomy: Oncological evaluation after 1,000 cases at Montsouris Institute. *Journal of Urology 169*(4), 1261-1266.

Held-Warmkessel, J. (2001). Treatment of advanced prostate cancer. *Seminars in Oncology Nursing 17*(2), 118-128. Retrieved April 7, 2003 from the World Wide Web. http://www.cancer.gov/search/clinical_trials/results_clinicaltrials.aspx—version=patient&cdrid=64439&clickitem=ClinicalTrialsSearchResults.

Iwamoto, R., & Maher, K.E. (2001). Radiation therapy for prostate cancer. *Seminars in Oncology Nursing 17*(2), 90-100.

Jemal, J., Murray, T., Samuels, A., et al. (2003). Cancer statistics 2003. *CA: A Cancer Journal for Clinicians 53,* 5-26.

Kamat, A.M., & Lamm, D.L. (1999). Chemoprevention of urological cancer. *Journal of Urology 161,* 1748-1760.

Krupski, T., Petroni, G.R., Bissonette, E.A., & Theodorescu, D. (2000). Quality-of-life comparison of radical prostatectomy and interstitial brachytherapy in the treatment of clinically localized prostate cancer. *Urology 55*(5), 736-742.

Lee, U.H. (2002). Assessment, screening and diagnosis of prostate cancer. In M. Wallace & L. Powell. *Prostate cancer: Nursing assessment, management, and care.* New York: Springer, pp. 33-45.

Lindblad, P., Mellemgaard, A., Schlehofer, B., et al. (1995). International renal cell cancer study. V. Reproductive factors, gynecologic operations and exogenous hormones. *International Journal of Cancer 61,* 192-198.

Mandel, J.S., McLaughlin, J.K., Schlehofer, B., et al. (1995). International renal cell cancer study IV. Occupation. *International Journal of Cancer 61,* 601-605.

Marcus, P.M., Hayes, R.B., Vineis, P., et al. (2000). Cigarette smoking, N-acetyltransferase 2 acetylation status, and bladder cancer risk: A case-series meta-analysis of a gene-environment interaction. *Cancer Epidemiology, Biomarkers, and Prevention 9*(5), 461-467.

Martini, F.H., Timmons, M.J., & McKinley, M.P. (Eds.). (2000). *Human anatomy* (3rd ed.). Englewood Cliffs, NJ: Prentice-Hall, pp. 686-707.

Mejean, A., Oudard, S., & Thiounn, N. (2002). Prognostic factors of renal cell carcinoma. *Journal of Urology 169*(3), 821-827.

Mellemgaard, A., Lindblad, P., Schlehofer, B., et al. (1995). International renal cancer cell study. III. Role of weight, height, physical activity and use of amphetamines. *International Journal of Cancer 60*, 350-354.

Merrick, G.S., Butler, W.M., Lief, J.H., & Galbreath, R.W. (2001). Permanent prostate brachytherapy: Acute and late toxicity. *Journal of Brachytherapy International 17*, 229-236.

Mettlin, C., Littrup, P.J., Kane, R.A., et al. (1994). Relative sensitivity and specificity of serum prostate specific antigen (PSA) level compared with age-referenced PSA, PSA density, and PSA change. Data from the American Cancer Society National Prostate Cancer Detection Project. *Cancer 74*, 1615-1620.

Metts, M.C., Metts, J.C., Militio, S.J., & Thomas, C.T. (2000). Bladder cancer: A review of diagnosis and management. *Journal of the National Medical Association 92*, 285-294.

Moyad, M.A. (2001). Obesity, interrelated mechanisms, and exposures in kidney cancer. *Seminars in Urologic Oncology 19*(4), 270-279.

Natale, R. (2001). *ASCO 2001 highlights: Pre-surgical chemotherapy may improve survival in bladder cancer.* Retrieved April 7, 2003 from the World Wide Web: http://www.cancer.gov/clinicaltrials/results/pre-surgical-chemo0501.

National Comprehensive Cancer Network (NCCN). (2003). *Clinical guidelines version 1, 2003: Prostate cancer early detection.* Retrieved April 7, 2003 from the World Wide Web: http://www.nccn.org/physician_gls/f_guidelines.html.

National Comprehensive Cancer Network (NCCN). (2002). *Clinical practice guidelines in oncology-v.1.2002. Bladder cancer.* Retrieved April 7, 2003 from the World Wide Web: http://www.nccn.org/physician_gls/f_guidelines.html.

Novick, A.C., Streem, S., Montie, J.E., et al. (2002). Conservative surgery for renal cell carcinoma: A single-center experience with 100 patients. *Journal of Urology 167*(2), 878-883.

O'Rourke, M.E. (2001a). Decision making and prostate cancer treatment selection: A review. *Seminars in Oncology Nursing 17*(2), 108-117.

O'Rourke, M.E. (2001b). Genitourinary cancers. In S. Otto (Ed.). *Oncology nursing.* St. Louis: Mosby, pp. 213-247.

O'Rourke, M.E. (2003). Ketoconazole in the treatment of prostate cancer. *Clinical Journal of Oncology Nursing 7*(2), 235.

Pantuck, A.J., Zisman, A., & Belldegrun, A. (2001). Biology of renal cell carcinoma: Changing concepts in classification and staging. *Seminars in Urologic Oncology 19*(2), 72-79.

Pashos, C.L., Botteman, M.F., Laskin, B.L., & Redaelli, A. (2002). Bladder cancer: Epidemiology, diagnosis, and management. *Cancer Practice 10*(2), 311-322.

Rassweiler, J., Seemann, O., Schulze, M., et al. (2003). Laparoscopic versus open radical prostatectomy: A comparative study at a single institution. *Journal of Urology 169*(5), 1689-1693.

Sacher, R.A., & McPherson, R.A. (2000). *Widmann's clinical interpretation of laboratory tests* (11th ed.). Philadelphia: F.A. Davis.

Scher, H.I., Isaacs, J.T., Zelefsky, M.J., & Scardino, P.T. (2000). Prostate cancer. In M.D. Abeloff, J.O. Armitage, A.S. Lichter, & J.E. Niederhuber (Eds.). *Clinical oncology* (2nd ed.). New York: Churchill Livingstone, pp. 1823-1884.

Schoenberg, M. (2000). *State of the science: Genitourinary cancer. Diagnosis, surveillance, and in vitro diagnostics for bladder cancer.* Retrieved April 7, 2003 from the World Wide Web: http://www.webtie.org/sots/Meetings/Genitourinary/gu2/transcripts/03/transcripts.htm.

Scott, R., Mutchnik, D.L., Laskowski, T.Z., & Schmalhorst, W.R. (1969). Carcinoma of the prostate in elderly men: Incidence, growth characteristics and clinical significance. *Journal of Urology 101*, 602-607.

Smith, R.A., von Eschenbach, A.C., Wender, R., et al. (2001). American Cancer Society guidelines for the early detection of cancer: Update of early detection guidelines for prostate, colorectal and endometrial cancers. *CA: A Cancer Journal for Clinicians 51*, 31-75.

Sprunk, E., & Alteneder,, R.R. (2000). The impact of an ostomy on sexuality. *Clinical Journal of Oncology Nursing 4*(2), 85-88.

Stoller, M.L., & Carroll, P.R. (2003). Urology. In L.M. Tierney, S.J. McPhee, & M.A. Papadakis (Eds.). *CMDT: Current medical diagnosis and treatment.* (42nd ed.). New York: Lange Medical Books/McGraw-Hill, pp. 903-945.

Tsui, K.H., Shuarts, O., Smith, R.B., et al. (2000). Prognostic indicators for renal cell carcinoma: A multivariate analysis of 643 patients using the revised 1997 TNM staging criteria. *Journal of Urology 163*(4), 1090-1095.

United States Preventive Services Task Force. (2002). Screening for prostate cancer: Recommendations and rationale. *Annals of Internal Medicine 137,* 915-916.

Vogelzang, N.J., & Stadler, W.M. (1998). Kidney cancer. *Lancet 352*(9141), 1691-1696.

Walsh, P.C. (1998). Anatomic radical retropubic prostatectomy. In P.C. Walsh, A.B. Retick, E.D. Vaughan, & A.J. Wein (Eds.). *Campbell's urology* (7th ed.). Philadelphia: W.B. Saunders, pp. 2565-2587.

Walther, M.M. (2000). The role of photodynamic therapy in the treatment of recurrent superficial cancer. *Urologic Clinics of North America 27,* 163-170.

Yip, D., Steer, C., al-Nawab, M., et al. (2001). Collecting duct carcinoma of the kidney associated with the sickle cell trait. *International Journal of Clinical Practice 55*(6), 415-417.

Zhou, M., & Rubin, M.A. (2001). Molecular markers for renal cell carcinoma: Impact on diagnosis and treatment. *Seminars in Urologic Oncology 19*(2), 80-87.

Zietman, A.L., Shipley, W.U., & Kaufman, D.S. (2000). Organ conserving approaches to muscle invasive bladder cancer: Future alternatives to radical cystectomy. *Annals of Medicine 32,* 34-42.

Zlotta, A.R., & Schulman, C.C. (1998). Etiology & diagnosis of prostate cancer: What's new? *European Urology 33,* 351-358.

Zweizig, S.L. (2002). Cancer of the kidney. *Clinical Obstetrics and Gynecology 45*(3), 884-891.

28 Nursing Care of the Client with Skin Cancer

ALICE J. LONGMAN

Theory

I. Physiology and pathophysiology associated with skin cancer (Longman, 1998).
  A. Anatomy of the skin.
    1. Epidermis is the uppermost layer—composed of keratinocytes: flat, scale-like, stratified squamous epithelial cells and spherical-shaped basal cells.
    2. Dermis, or corium, is the underlying layer—contains collagen-producing fibroblasts, giving skin strength.
    3. Melanocytes, cells that produce melanin, are in the epidermis among the basal cells.
  B. Primary organ functions.
    1. Protects the body from mechanical, thermal, and chemical injuries and from infection-causing microorganisms.
    2. Helps maintain homeostasis and temperature regulatory functions.
    3. Carries the cutaneous and autonomic nerves, produces vitamin D, and stores water and fat.
  C. Changes in function associated with skin cancer (Jerant et al., 2000).
    1. Ultraviolet portion of the solar spectrum affects the incidence of skin cancer.
    2. Aging skin.
      a. Epidermis flattens and thins with age—wrinkling and sagging skin may result.
      b. Melanin production decreases with changes in skin and hair color.
  D. Metastatic pattern.
    1. Basal cell carcinoma.
      a. Recurrence rates vary, depending on the size of the tumor and length of follow-up.
      b. Rarely metastasizes but has the possibility of creating extensive local spread.
    2. Squamous cell carcinoma.
      a. Recurrence rates vary, but most develop within 2 years of diagnosis.
      b. Metastasizes to regional lymph nodes, lungs, and liver.
      c. Degree of metastasis varies according to causative factors, morphologic characteristics, and size and depth of the tumor.
    3. Malignant melanoma (Rigel & Carucci, 2000).
      a. Most important prognostic features are the depth of the primary lesion and stage at the time of removal.
      b. Metastasizes to regional lymph nodes, lungs, and brain.
      c. Difficult and unpredictable problem of hematogenous dissemination has not been solved.

E. Trends in epidemiology (American Cancer Society [ACS], 2003).
  1. Nonmelanoma skin cancers (basal cell and squamous cell carcinoma).
     a. Most common malignant neoplasms in the United States (U.S.) Caucasian population.
     b. Estimated 1,000,000 new cases in 2003 in the United States.
  2. Cutaneous malignant melanoma.
     a. Accounts for 3% of all skin cancer.
     b. Estimated 54,200 cases in 2003 in the United States.
     c. Accounts for an estimated 7600 deaths annually.
     d. Highest rates are found in southern Arizona.
F. Characteristics of skin cancer.
  1. Nonmelanoma skin cancers (basal cell and squamous cell carcinoma) (Albert & Weinstock, 2003; Jerant et al., 2000) (Table 28-1).
     a. Nodular basal cell carcinoma.
        (1) Bulky nodular growth caused by lack of keratinization in the epidermis.
        (2) Semitransparent surface producing a shiny, translucent, pearly hue.
        (3) Ulcerated center with elevated margins.
     b. Pigmented basal cell carcinoma.
        (1) Melanin in the epidermis and dermis and in the lesion itself.
        (2) Blue, black, or brown appearance.
        (3) Contains telangiectases and has a raised, pearly border.
     c. Morpheaform or sclerotic basal cell carcinoma.
        (1) Flat or depressed scarlike plaque that is pale yellow or white.
        (2) Nodularity, ulceration, and bleeding may occur.
        (3) Fingerlike projections of fibroepitheliomatous strands of tumor.
     d. Superficial basal cell carcinoma.
        (1) Develops in multiple sites growing peripherally across the skin surface.
        (2) Well-demarcated, erythematous, scaly patch.
        (3) Raised, pearly border.
     e. Squamous cell carcinoma.
        (1) Arises from the keratinizing cells of the epidermis.
        (2) Round to irregular shape with a plaquelike or nodular character.
        (3) Varies from an ulcerated infiltrating mass to an elevated, erythematous, nodular mass.
        (4) Potential for metastasis to regional and distant sites.

TABLE 28-1
Common Sites of Nonmelanoma Skin Cancers

Type of Skin Cancer	Common Sites
Nodular basal cell carcinoma	Face, head, neck
Pigmented basal cell carcinoma	Face, head, neck
Morpheaform basal cell carcinoma	Head, neck
Superficial basal cell carcinoma	Trunk, extremities
Squamous cell carcinoma	Head, neck, border of lips, hands, forearms, upper trunk, lower legs

TABLE 28-2
Common Sites of Malignant Melanoma

Type of Melanoma	Common Sites
Superficial spreading melanoma	Backs of men and women, legs of women
Nodular melanoma	Trunk, head, neck
Lentigo maligna melanoma	Face, neck, trunk, dorsum of hands
Acral-lentiginous melanoma	Palms of hands, soles of feet, nail beds, mucous membranes

2. Malignant melanoma (Rigel & Carucci, 2000) (Table 28-2).
   a. Major features.
      (1) Arises from melanocytes, cells specializing in the biosynthesis and transport of melanin.
      (2) Characterized by radial and vertical growth.
      (3) Precursor lesions.
         (a) Dysplastic nevi that may be familial (B-K moles) or nonfamilial (sporadic dysplastic nevi).
         (b) Congenital melanocytic nevi covering large areas of the body.
   b. Classification of malignant melanoma.
      (1) Superficial spreading melanoma (SSM).
         (a) Commonly arises in preexisting nevus.
         (b) Variety of colors, ranging from tan, brown, or black to a characteristic red, white, blue, and gray.
         (c) Irregular plaque, scaly, crusty, surface-notched border.
      (2) Nodular melanoma (NM).
         (a) Raised, dome-shaped, blue-black lesion.
         (b) Elevated lesion with well-demarcated borders.
         (c) Rapid vertical growth phase.
      (3) Lentigo maligna melanoma (LMM).
         (a) Found in chronically sun-exposed skin.
         (b) Large, frecklelike lesion, tan to black in color.
         (c) Raised nodule with notched border.
      (4) Acral-lentiginous melanoma (ALM).
         (a) Flat and irregular in shape.
         (b) Variegated colors in shades of tan, blue, and black.
         (c) Smooth or ulcerated lesion that may be raised or flat.
   c. Features of early malignant melanoma (Rigel & Carucci, 2000).
      (1) Asymmetry—uneven rate of growth resulting in an asymmetric pattern.
      (2) Border irregularity—uneven rate of growth resulting in an irregular border.
      (3) Color variegation—irregular growth causes new shades of black and light and dark brown.
      (4) Diameter greater than 6 mm—considered suspicious of melanoma.
II. Principles of medical management.
   A. Diagnostic procedures.
      1. General procedures.
         a. Nonmelanoma skin cancers (Albert & Weinstock, 2003).
            (1) Electrosurgery and histology with 0.5- to 1-cm margins are recommended if the lesion is small.

(2) Incisional biopsy, including a 1-cm margin, is justified for larger lesions.
    b. Malignant melanoma.
        (1) Most important characteristic is the vertical depth of melanotic penetration through the skin.
        (2) Refinement of classification relates the prognosis of melanoma to the actual measured depth or thickness of invasion.
    2. Specific procedures.
        a. Accurate histologic diagnosis.
            (1) Excisional biopsy, yielding a specimen with a few millimeters of normal tissue.
            (2) Step sections of biopsy specimen at 3 mm or closer.
        b. Microstaging describes the level of invasion of malignant melanoma and maximal tumor thickness.
B. Staging methods and procedures—parameters assessing the depth of invasion of malignant melanoma (Brenner & Tamir, 2002).
    1. Level of invasion in relation to the anatomic structures of the skin (Clark's five histologic levels).
    2. Measure of vertical thickness of the tumor in millimeters (Breslow's index—five measures in millimeters).
    3. Staging system for melanoma (Greene et al., 2002).
C. Treatment strategies.
    1. Nonmelanoma skin cancers—definitive treatment depends on location and size of the lesion, exact histologic type, possible extension into nearby structures, metastases, previous treatment, anticipated cosmetic results, age, and general condition of the client (Albert & Weinstock, 2003).
        a. Surgery.
            (1) Excision of the lesion.
            (2) Curettage and electrodesiccation for small, superficial, or recurrent lesions.
            (3) Mohs' micrographic surgery—surgically removes tissue in multiple, progressively thin layers.
        b. Radiotherapy.
            (1) Recommended for lesions that are inoperable and greater than 1 mm but smaller than 10 cm.
            (2) Administered in fractional doses.
        c. Cryotherapy.
            (1) Tumor destruction by use of liquid nitrogen to freeze and thaw tumor tissue.
            (2) Lesions with well-defined margins benefit from treatment.
        d. Chemotherapy.
            (1) Topical fluorouracil (5-Fluorouracil, 5-FU) for premalignant keratosis.
            (2) For recurrent skin cancers, particularly squamous cell carcinoma, no longer manageable by surgery or radiotherapy, cisplatin (Platinol) and doxorubicin (Adriamycin) have been used.
    2. Malignant melanoma.
        a. Surgery.
            (1) Local excision, leaving a 2- to 3-cm margin if anatomically possible.
            (2) Split-thickness skin grafting may be required for cosmetic reasons.
            (3) Regional lymph node dissection may be indicated but is controversial.

        (4) Sentinel lymph node dissection may be indicated but is controversial.

        (5) Used for palliative management in relief of symptoms or solitary lesions.

    b. Radiotherapy.

        (1) Most effective when tumor volume is low.

        (2) Used for palliative management when subcutaneous, cutaneous, and nodal metastases are inaccessible for surgical removal.

    c. Chemotherapy—agents with consistent activity include dacarbazine (DTIC), the nitrosoureas (carmustine [BCNU], lomustine [CCNU], semustine [MeCCNU], chlorozotocin), and an imidazotetrazine oral agent, temozolamide (Temodar).

    d. Biologic response modifiers—advances have been made with interferon-alpha (IFN-α), interferon-gamma (IFN-γ), and interleukin-2 (IL-2).

    e. Biochemotherapy—combination of cytokines with chemotherapy, specifically cisplatin-based chemotherapy, has been used (Fu et al., 2002).

    f. Promising modalities include novel chemotherapeutic agents, immunotherapy, and gene therapy (Rigel & Carucci, 2000).

  3. Special considerations.

    a. Primary melanoma of the eye.

        (1) Melanoma primarily in the iris responds well to local resection.

        (2) Ciliary body and choroidal melanoma require enucleation.

        (3) Success of treatment for metastatic disease from eye melanoma is uniformly poor.

    b. Local advanced disease.

        (1) Massive, local disease, frequently in the neck and in axillary or inguinal nodal areas, may develop.

        (2) Combination of radiotherapy and hyperthermia offers palliation.

Assessment

  I. Pertinent personal and family history.

    A. Risk factors (basal cell and squamous cell carcinoma) (Table 28-3).

TABLE 28-3
Risk Factors in the Development of Basal Cell and Squamous Cell Carcinoma

Risk Factor	Skin Cancer Risk
Personal factors	Excessive exposure to sunlight
	Easily burned
	Increasing age
	Premalignant states
Lifestyle	Outdoor work
	Outdoor recreational activities
	Chronic exposure to chemical agents
Drugs	Treatment for psoriasis (psoralen ultraviolet A [PUVA])
Immunologic factor	Organ transplant recipients

      1. Exogenous factors.
          a. Ultraviolet radiation from sunlight over a long period of time.
          b. Exposure to ionizing radiation, arsenic, or petroleum.
          c. Scars following injury.
      2. Endogenous factors.
          a. Fair or freckled complexion.
          b. Red, blond, or light brown hair.
          c. Light-colored eyes.
          d. Xeroderma pigmentosum, basal cell nevus syndrome, albinism, and epidermodysplasia verruciformis.
      3. Premalignant states or lesions.
          a. Actinic, or senile, keratoses.
          b. Seborrheic keratoses.
          c. Bowen's disease.
   B. Risk factors (malignant melanoma) (Rigel & Carucci, 2000) (Box 28-1).
      1. Exogenous factors.
          a. Poor tolerance of ultraviolet radiation from sunlight.
          b. Intense, intermittent exposure to sunlight.
   C. Pertinent history (Saraiya et al., 2002).
      1. Skin exposure to sunlight.
          a. Time of day during exposure.
          b. Geographic area of residence or recreation.
          c. Altitude or overcast weather conditions.
          d. Time of year exposed to the sun.
          e. Length of exposure or exposures.

BOX 28-1
RISK FACTORS IN THE DEVELOPMENT OF MALIGNANT MELANOMA

Family history of malignant melanoma
Presence of blond or red hair
Presence of marked freckling on the upper back
History of three or more blistering sunburns before age 20 years
History of 3 or more years of an outdoor job as a teenager
Presence of actinic keratoses

From Rigel DS, Carucci JA: Malignant melanoma: Prevention, early detection, and treatment in the 21st century, *CA: Cancer J Clin* 50:218, 2000.

TABLE 28-4
Skin Types and Skin Reactions

Skin Type	Skin Reactions
1	Burns easily and severely; tans minimally or not at all
2	Burns easily and severely; tans minimally or lightly
3	Burns moderately; tans approximately average
4	Burns minimally; tans easily
5	Burns rarely; tans easily and substantially
6	Never burns; tans profusely

      2. Skin type (Table 28-4).
         a. Pigmentation or erythema type.
         b. Genetic history.
 II. Physical examination.
    A. Skin assessment.
      1. Inspection and palpation of all accessible skin surfaces.
      2. Assessment of preexisting lesions.
      3. Inspection of the scalp and entire hairline.
      4. Inspection of the face, lips, and neck.
      5. Inspection and palpation of all surfaces of upper extremities.
      6. Inspection and palpation of the skin of the back, buttocks, and back of the legs.
    B. Signs and symptom—changes in existing moles.
      1. Size.
      2. Shape.
      3. Color.
      4. History of itching in existing moles.
      5. History of burning in existing moles.

Nursing Diagnoses

  I. Deficient knowledge (e.g., individual risk factors for skin cancer).
 II. Ineffective coping.
III. Compromised family coping.

Outcome Identification

   I. Prevention and early detection of skin cancer.
    A. Client identifies factors that place an individual at risk for skin cancer.
    B. Client describes specific health-promoting activities, such as minimal skin exposure to ultraviolet radiation during specific hours of the day.
  II. Skin self-assessment.
    A. Client describes systematic assessment of the skin for suspicious lesions.
    B. Client identifies resources that provide information.
 III. Warning signs of early malignant melanoma.
    A. Client describes importance of assessing for early signs of changes in nevi.
    B. Client and/or nurse conducts a family pedigree to determine family history of skin cancer.
  IV. Coping related to diagnosis of malignant melanoma (Thompson et al., 2001).
    A. Client participates in care and ongoing decision making.
    B. Client sets realistic goals.
   V. Changes in recreational activities or work because of skin cancer.
    A. Client uses appropriate personal and community resources in managing changes.
    B. Client identifies alternative resources when present strategies do not meet needs.
  VI. Changes in lifestyle as a result of the diagnosis of malignant melanoma.
    A. Client and family participate in the decision-making process pertaining to the plan of care and life activities.
    B. Client and family identify community resources that assist coping.

Planning and Implementation

I. Nonmelanoma skin cancers (basal cell and squamous cell carcinoma).
   A. Preventive measures.
      1. Minimize exposure to sunlight between the hours of 10 AM and 3 PM.
      2. Use protective clothing, such as a long-sleeved shirt, long pants, and a hat, during prolonged exposure to the sun.
      3. Use sunscreens (absorbers) and sun blocks (reflectors).
         a. Use commercial sunscreens with a sun protection factor (SPF) of 15 or more.
         b. Reapply sunscreen every 2 to 3 hours during prolonged exposure to the sun; reapply sunscreen after swimming.
      4. Use sunglasses that meet ultraviolet requirements.
      5. Use sunscreen with benzophenones because of photosensitivity if taking thiazides, sulfonamides, and antineoplastic agents.
      6. Avoid tanning salons and sun beds.
      7. Keep infants out of the sun.
   B. Screening and early detection measures.
      1. Obtain a history of any recent changes in lesions.
      2. Teach systematic assessment of skin lesions for changes.
      3. Use educational resources.
         a. American Academy of Dermatology—*The Sun and Your Skin.*
         b. American Cancer Society—*Cancer of the Skin.*
         c. Skin Cancer Foundation—*Sun and Skin News.*
         d. American Academy of Family Physicians—*How to Prevent Skin Cancer.*
   C. Therapeutic measures.
      1. Prepare the client and family for surgical intervention and other treatment.
      2. Stress importance of early treatment.
   D. Rehabilitative measures.
      1. Assess impact of treatment for skin cancer.
      2. Stress importance of evaluation at regular intervals for potential recurrence.
II. Malignant melanoma.
   A. Preventive measures.
      1. Teach high-risk clients to do monthly skin self-examination.
      2. Stress importance of monthly skin self-examination.
   B. Screening and early detection.
      1. Do a family pedigree to determine family history of malignant melanoma.
      2. Use educational resources.
         a. American Academy of Dermatology—*Melanoma Skin Cancer.*
         b. National Cancer Institute—*What You Need to Know About Melanoma.*
         c. Skin Cancer Foundation—*The Melanoma Letter.*
         d. American Academy of Family Physicians—*How to Prevent Skin Cancer.*
   C. Therapeutic measures (Thompson et al., 2001).
      1. Prepare the client and family for extensive intervention and treatment.
      2. Use an open, optimistic approach in discussing feelings and attitudes about the diagnosis and treatment.
   D. Rehabilitative measures.
      1. Stress importance of evaluation at regular intervals for potential recurrence.

2. Stress importance of changes in lifestyle in relation to sun exposure for high-risk individuals and families to decrease chances of further development of malignant melanoma.

Evaluation

The oncology nurse systematically and regularly evaluates the client's and/or family's responses to interventions to determine progress toward the achievement of expected outcomes. Relevant data are collected, and actual findings are compared with expected findings. Nursing diagnoses, outcomes, and plans of care are reviewed and revised as necessary.

REFERENCES

Albert, M.R., & Weinstock, M.A. (2003). Keratinocyte carcinoma. *CA: A Cancer Journal for Clinicians 53,* 292-302.

American Cancer Society (ACS). (2003). *Cancer facts and figures—2003.* Atlanta: American Cancer Society.

Brenner, S., & Tamir, E. (2002). Early detection of melanoma: The best strategy for a favorable prognosis. *Clinics in Dermatology 20,* 203-211.

Fu, M.R., Anderson, C.M., McDaniel, R., & Armer, J. (2002). Patients' perceptions of fatigue in response to biochemotherapy for metastatic melanoma: A preliminary study. *Oncology Nursing Forum 29,* 961-966.

Greene, F.L., Page, D.L., Fleming, I.D., et al. (Eds.). (2002). *AJCC cancer staging handbook* (6th ed.) New York: Springer-Verlag, pp. 209-220.

Jerant, A.F., Johnson, J.T., Sheridan, C.M., & Caffrey, T.J. (2000). Early detection and treatment of skin cancer. *American Family Physician 62,* 357-374.

Longman, A.J. (1998). Nursing care of the client with skin cancer. In J.K. Itano & K.N. Taoka (Eds.). *Core curriculum for oncology nursing* (3rd ed.). Philadelphia: W.B. Saunders, pp. 552-560.

Rigel, D.S., & Carucci, J.A. (2000). Malignant melanoma: Prevention, early detection, and treatment in the 21st century. *CA: A Cancer Journal for Clinicians 50,* 215-236.

Saraiya, M., Hall, H.I., & Uhler, R.J. (2002). Sunburn prevalence among adults in the United States, 1999. *American Journal of Preventive Medicine 23,* 91-97.

Thompson, N., Bond, L.K., Vance, R.B., et al. (2001). Addressing treatment options in metastatic melanoma. *Cancer Practice 9,* 221-226.

29 Nursing Care of the Client with Head and Neck Cancer

ELLEN CARR

Theory

I. Introduction.
- **A.** Include cancers of the oral cavity, oropharynx, nasal cavity, paranasal sinuses, nasopharynx, larynx, hypopharynx, and salivary glands. Also cancers of the thyroid and parathyroid.
- **B.** Incidence is small in number (approximately 3% of all cancers) (National Cancer Institute [NCI], 2002a). Client coping with dysfunction and body image requires adaptation, support from nursing.
  - **1.** Incidence, staging, and treatment of cancer in this area depend on the specific location of the tumor.
  - **2.** Majority of head and neck tumors occur in the oral cavity (48%), larynx (25%), and oropharynx (10%) (Haggood, 2001).
- **C.** Epidemiology.
  - **1.** Usually occur in the 50- to 70-year age-group (Fang & Forastiere, 2001; Haggood, 2001).
  - **2.** More men than women are diagnosed with these cancers.
  - **3.** For specific head and neck cancers, risk factors listed in Box 29-1.
    - **a.** Tobacco use increases the risk of developing head and neck cancer 25-fold; excessive alcohol intake increases the risk of developing oral or pharyngeal cancer ninefold (Haggood, 2001).
    - **b.** Smokeless tobacco (snuff, chew), pipes, and cigars are also risk factors for head and neck cancer (Haggood, 2001; Harris, 2000).
- **D.** Histology of head and neck tumors—90% squamous cell; 10% adenocarcinoma (salivary glands), melanoma, sarcoma, or lymphoma (Fang & Forastiere, 2001).
  - **1.** Rapid cell turnover in head and neck tumors affects their initial development and growth. Relatively high mitotic rate of tumor cells also provides the basis for treatment strategies (i.e., high-dose cancer therapies) (Barasch & Peterson, 2003).
  - **2.** The oral mucosa has a high cell turnover rate and is home to diverse and complex microflora. Therefore the mucosa, when treated with chemotherapy or radiation, is highly susceptible to treatment-related toxic side effects (NCI, 2003a).
- **E.** Developments in care and treatment: reduced deformities, improved cosmetic effect because of prosthetic devices and surgical flaps (myocutaneous and free flaps).

BOX 29-1
RISKS FOR SPECIFIC HEAD AND NECK CANCERS

- Oral cavity—sun exposure (lip); human papillomavirus (HPV) infection.
- Salivary glands—radiation to the head and neck. This exposure can come from diagnostic x-rays or from radiation therapy (RT) for noncancerous conditions or cancer.
- Paranasal sinuses and nasal cavity—certain industrial exposures, such as wood or nickel dust inhalation. Tobacco and alcohol use may play less of a role in this type of cancer.
- Nasopharynx—Asian, particularly Chinese, ancestry; Epstein-Barr virus infection; occupational exposure to wood dust; consumption of certain preservatives or salted foods.
- Oropharynx—poor oral hygiene, mechanical irritation such as from poorly fitting dentures, and use of mouthwash that has a high alcohol content.
- Hypopharynx—Plummer-Vinson (also called Paterson-Kelly) syndrome, a rare disorder that results from nutritional deficiencies. This syndrome is characterized by severe anemia and leads to difficulty swallowing because of webs of tissue that grow across the upper part of the esophagus.
- Larynx—exposure to airborne particles of asbestos, especially in the workplace.
  Note: Those with previously diagnosed head and neck cancer are at risk to develop a new primary cancer, usually in the head and neck, esophagus, or lungs. Those who smoke are at higher risk for head and neck cancers.

Data from National Cancer Institute: *Head and neck cancer: questions and answers,* 2002. Retrieved February 9, 2003 http://cis.nci.nih.gov/fact/6_37.htm; National Institutes of Health (NIH) (U.S. Department of Health and Human Services, Public Health Service): *Information about detection, symptoms, diagnosis, and treatment of oral cancer.* NIH Publication No. 97-1574, 2002.

    1. Since the early 1970s, more conservative surgical technique and reconstruction have resulted in increasing quality of life—decreasing dysfunctions (airway, communication, swallowing).

F. Metastatic patterns.

    1. Head and neck cancer is a locally aggressive disease that can spread regionally to the lymphatics of the neck (Figure 29-1).

    2. Most clients present with stage III or IV disease (tumor is very large, has invaded adjacent tissue, or is a primary tumor that has spread to the lymphatics) (Harris, 2000; Figure 29-2).

    3. The incidence of local regional failure is as high as 60%; clinically detected distant metastasis occurs at a rate of 20% (Haggood, 2001).

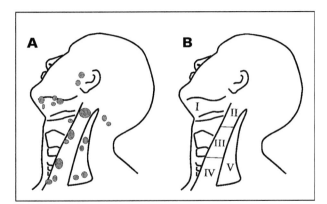

FIGURE 29-1 ■ **A,** Regional lymphatic pattern in the head and neck. **B,** Neck levels of the head and neck. (From Shah JP, Lydiatt W: Treatment of cancer of the head and neck, *CA: Cancer J Clin* 45[6]:357, 1995.)

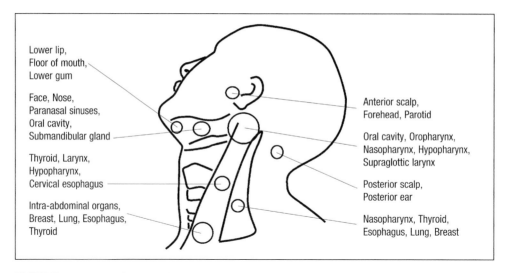

Lower lip,
Floor of mouth,
Lower gum

Face, Nose,
Paranasal sinuses,
Oral cavity,
Submandibular gland

Thyroid, Larynx,
Hypopharynx,
Cervical esophagus

Intra-abdominal organs,
Breast, Lung, Esophagus,
Thyroid

Anterior scalp,
Forehead, Parotid

Oral cavity, Oropharynx,
Nasopharynx, Hypopharynx,
Supraglottic larynx

Posterior scalp,
Posterior ear

Nasopharynx, Thyroid,
Esophagus, Lung, Breast

FIGURE 29-2 ▪ Likely sites of metastasis from various sites of the head and neck. (From Shah JP, Lydiatt W: Treatment of cancer of the head and neck, *CA: Cancer J Clin* 45[6]:357, 1995.)

4. Head and neck cancer tends to recur locally. One study reported that 16% of head and neck clients develop a second head and neck tumor within 9 years (second primary tumor site: 40% in head and neck area, 30% in lung, 9% in esophagus, 20% elsewhere) (Harris, 2000).
5. Most common sites of distant metastasis—lung, liver, bone.
   G. Trends in survival.
1. Since several specific cancer categories are grouped as head and neck cancers, each category has its own incidence/survival rates.
2. Survival rates.
   a. Oral and pharyngeal cancers somewhat better: 1-year survival = 84%; 5-year survival = 54% (American Cancer Society [ACS], 2002).
   b. Laryngeal cancer (all stages): 5-year survival = 65%. If local disease when detected, 83%; if regional disease when detected, 50%; if distant metastases when detected, 38% (ACS, 2002).
   c. Thyroid cancer overall 5-year survival rate is 95% (Haggood, 2001).
3. Smoking and drinking alcohol increase the risk of developing recurrent disease.
  II. Anatomy of the head and neck (Figure 29-3).
   A. Oral cavity—extends from the lips to the hard palate above and the circumvallate papillae below; structures include lips, buccal mucosa, floor of mouth, upper and lower alveoli, retromolar trigone, hard palate, and anterior two thirds of the tongue.
   B. Oropharynx—extends from the circumvallate papillae below and hard palate above to the level of the hyoid bone; structures include the base of tongue (posterior one third), soft palate, tonsils, and posterior pharyngeal wall.
   C. Nasal cavity and paranasal sinuses—include nasal vestibule; paired maxillary, ethmoid, and frontal sinuses; and a single sphenoid sinus.
   D. Nasopharynx—located below the base of skull and behind the nasal cavity; continuous with the posterior pharyngeal wall.

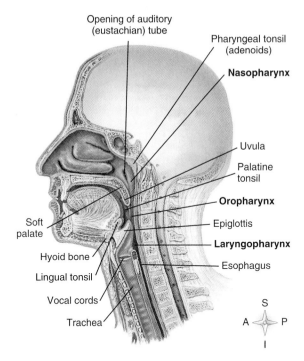

Opening of auditory
(eustachian) tube

Pharyngeal tonsil
(adenoids)

Nasopharynx

Uvula

Palatine
tonsil

Oropharynx

Soft
palate

Epiglottis

Laryngopharynx

Hyoid bone

Esophagus

Lingual tonsil

Vocal cords

Trachea

S

A ⟡ P

I

FIGURE 29-3 ■ Anatomy of the head and neck. (From Thibodeau G, Patton K: *Anatomy and physiology*, ed 6, St. Louis, 2003, Mosby.)

E. Larynx—extends from the epiglottis to the cricoid cartilage; protected by the thyroid cartilage, which encases it; subdivided into three areas.
  1. Supraglottis—below the base of tongue, extending to but not including the true vocal cord; includes epiglottis, aryepiglottic folds, arytenoid cartilages, and false vocal cords.
  2. Glottis—area of the true vocal cord.
  3. Subglottis—below the true vocal cord, extending to the cricoid cartilage.
F. Hypopharynx—extends from the hyoid bone to the lower border of the cricoid cartilage; structures include pyriform sinuses, postcricoid region, and the lower posterior pharyngeal wall.
G. Thyroid—at base of neck, below Adam's apple. Provides thyroid hormones to the system.
H. Parathyroid—located on the posterior thyroid. Most people have four glands (ranges from two to eight glands). Glands provide parathyroid hormone to the system.
I. Critical adjacent structures (Fang & Forastiere, 2001; Haggood, 2001; Harris, 2000; Sidransky, 2001).
  1. Regional lymph nodes of the neck drain the anatomic structures of the head and neck; area includes submental submaxillary, upper and lower jugular, posterior triangle (spinal accessory), and preauricular nodes (see Figure 29-1).
  2. Head and neck structures are contiguous with the lower aerodigestive tract—trachea, lungs, esophagus.
  3. The nasopharynx and paranasal sinuses are close to the brain.
III. Primary functions of the head and neck (Haggood, 2001; Harris, 2000; Sidransky, 2001).

A. Respiration—the upper respiratory tract is passageway for transporting air into the lungs. Respiratory process is as follows:
1. The diaphragm descends, increasing the intrathoracic pressure.
2. Negative pressure results in air entering the mouth and nose, where it is warmed, filtered, and humidified.
3. Air enters the upper air passageways of the pharynx, larynx, and trachea, then enters the lung.
4. The olfactory membrane lies along the superior part of each nostril as well as along the septum and superior turbinates. The olfactory cells within the membrane serve as receptors for the sense of smell.
B. Speech—is formed from sound waves created as air is expelled from the lungs, passing through the vocal cords. Speech is mechanically perfected through the following processes:
1. Phonation—achieved by the larynx.
2. Articulation—achieved by the lips, tongue, and soft palate.
3. Resonation—resonators (pharynx, mouth, nose, paranasal sinuses) create the tone and quality of speech.
C. Swallowing—26 muscles and six cranial nerves orchestrate the transport of food from the mouth to the stomach in four phases of swallowing (Harris, 2000; Sidransky, 2001).
1. Oral preparatory—in the oral cavity, bolus of food is chewed and combined with saliva.
   a. Taste receptors are on the tongue, soft palate, glossopalatine arch, and posterior wall of the pharynx.
2. Oral—tongue, using front/back movement, propels bolus into the pharynx.
3. Pharyngeal—bolus moves through the pharynx and is propelled toward the esophagus; the vocal cords close, and the larynx moves upward and forward, preventing aspiration.
4. Esophageal—bolus moves through the esophagus and enters the stomach.
D. Hormone regulation.
1. Thyroid: thyroid hormones serve as a growth factor in bone formation; regulate metabolism.
2. Parathyroid: parathyroid hormone regulates body's calcium.
IV. Functional changes associated with cancers of the head and neck (Haggood, 2001; Sidransky, 2001).
A. Respiration.
1. Head and neck cancer affects the structures of the upper airway, which transport warmed, filtered, and humidified air into the lungs.
2. When disease and treatment affect this area, the natural air-conditioning function of the upper air passageways is bypassed. The effect–cooling and dryness of the trachea and lungs–can lead to infection.
3. When upper airway is altered, sense of smell changes (e.g., inability to sniff).
B. Speech.
1. When larynx removed (all or part), results in loss of vibrating component for speech; thus sound waves cannot be produced (total laryngectomy) or are diminished (partial).
2. Surgery to the mouth, tongue, or palate causes changes in the person's ability to articulate clear, understandable speech.
3. Cancer or treatment of the nose or paranasal sinuses influences the tone and quality of the speech.

C. Swallowing.
  1. Supraglottic laryngectomy affects the pharyngeal phase of swallowing, decreasing protection of the glottis. Until swallowing techniques learned, aspiration is a risk.
  2. When structures in the oral cavity and oropharynx undergo extensive resections (requiring flap reconstruction), swallowing phases (oral preparatory and oral) change and may result in the following:
    a. Drooling of saliva.
    b. Decreased mastication.
    c. Aspiration.
    d. Pooling of food and fluids.
  3. Radiation therapy (RT) to this area causes decreased saliva production (xerostomia), with loss of lubrication of food bolus and taste changes.
D. Trismus (a restriction in opening the mouth) can be a side effect from radiation treatment (NCI, 2003b).
  1. The condition can affect the client's ability to eat a regular diet. It also can affect the following:
    a. Speech.
    b. Swallowing.
    c. Mastication.
    d. Adequate oral hygiene.
  2. Jaw exercises can help reduce the stiffness of trismus.
V. Principles of medical management.
  A. Screening and diagnosis.
    1. For early detection, no definitive screening examination established. However, thorough oral examination is recommended (ACS, 2002).
      a. Every 3 years for 20- to 40-year-olds.
      b. Every year for people older than 40 years.
    2. Those diagnosed with head and neck cancer are at an increased risk to develop other primary tumors because of prolonged exposure of the mucosal surface to carcinogens (NCI, 2002c).
      a. The initial workup includes evaluation to rule out multiple primary tumors.
  B. Evaluation of suspected head and neck tumors includes the following (Haggood, 2001; Harris, 2000; Sidransky, 2001):
    1. Thorough history and examination of all structures of the upper aerodigestive tract.
    2. History of specific risk factors (see Box 29-1).
    3. Signs and symptoms of disease (Box 29-2).
    4. Physical examination.
      a. Visualization.
      b. Mirror examination of the pharynx and larynx.
      c. Palpation via a bimanual examination to assess the oral cavity and upper neck.
    5. Radiologic studies (Table 29-1).
      a. Computed tomographic (CT) scan—to assist in determining the extent of the primary tumor and to identify metastasis to the cervical lymph nodes.
      b. Chest x-ray examination—to identify disease in the lung, a second primary tumor, or distant metastasis.
      c. Panorex—panoramic views to evaluate mandibular invasion from oral cavity and oropharyngeal lesions.

BOX 29-2
SIGNS AND SYMPTOMS OF HEAD AND NECK CANCERS*

Common Symptoms of Several Head and Neck Cancer Sites
- A lump or sore that does not heal
- A sore throat that does not go away
- Difficulty swallowing
- A change or hoarseness in the voice

Other Possible Symptoms
- Oral cavity
  - White or red patch on the gums, tongue, or lining of the mouth
  - Swelling of the jaw that causes dentures to fit poorly or become uncomfortable
  - Unusual bleeding or pain in the mouth
- Nasal cavity and sinuses
  - Sinuses that are blocked and do not clear
  - Chronic sinus infections that do not respond to treatment with antibiotics
  - Bleeding through the nose
  - Frequent headaches
  - Swelling or other trouble with the eyes
  - Pain in the upper teeth
  - Problems with dentures
- Salivary glands
  - Swelling under the chin or around the jawbone
  - Numbness or *paralysis* of the muscles in the face
  - Pain that does not go away in the face, chin, or neck
- Oropharynx and hypopharynx
  - Ear pain
- Nasopharynx
  - Trouble breathing or speaking
  - Frequent headaches
  - Pain or ringing in the ears, or trouble hearing
- Larynx
  - Pain when swallowing
  - Ear pain
- Metastatic squamous neck cancer
  - Pain in the neck or throat that does not go away

Modified from National Cancer Institute (NCI): *Head and neck cancer: questions and answers,* 2002. Retrieved February 19, 2003 from http://cis.nci.nih.gov/fact/6_37.htm; National Cancer Institute (NCI): *Head and neck cancer: treatment,* 2002. Retrieved February 19, 2003 http://www.nci.nih.gov/cancerinfo/treatment/head-and-neck; National Cancer Institute (NCI): *Nasopharyngeal cancer,* 2002. Retrieved February 19, 2003 http://www.nci.nih.gov/cancerinfo/pdq/treatment/nasopharyngeal/healthprofessional/; National Institutes of Health (NIH) (U.S. Department of Health and Human Services, Public Health Service): *Information about detection, symptoms, diagnosis, and treatment of oral cancer.* NIH Publication No. 97-1574, 2002; Neville BW, Day TA: Oral cancer and precancerous lesions, *CA: Cancer J Clin* 52:195-215, 2002.
*These symptoms may be caused by cancer or by other, less serious conditions. It is important to check with a physician or dentist about any of these symptoms.

    d. Magnetic resonance imaging (MRI) scan—superior to the CT scan in staging nasopharyngeal primaries.

    e. Cine-esophagography/barium swallow—to identify the extent of lesions in the oropharynx that may extend into the hypopharynx.

    f. Bone and liver scans—to evaluate distant metastasis among high-risk clients (bone pain or elevated liver enzyme levels).

TABLE 29-1
Diagnostic Procedures in Evaluation of Head and Neck Tumors

Description	Time Required	Sensations Experienced	Potential Side Effects/ Complications	Self-Care Measures	Symptoms to Report to Health Care Team
PANORAMIC X-RAY EXAMINATION (PANOREX) Examination of an entire dental arch viewed on one film To evaluate mandibular invasion	10 min	None	None	None	N/A
CINE-ESOPHAGOGRAPHY Video x-ray examination of oral and pharyngeal stages of swallowing To identify extension of lesions into hypopharynx	30 min	Vary, depending on degree of dysphagia	Aspiration	None	Temperature elevation Productive cough
BARIUM SWALLOW AND X-RAY EXAMINATION OF UPPER GASTROINTESTINAL TRACT To evaluate tumor invasion of hypopharynx and cervical esophagus	15 min	Chalky taste	Constipation secondary to use of barium	Assess bowel function Take laxative as needed Force fluids	No bowel movement within 3 days Abdominal distention
PANENDOSCOPY Surgical procedure in which a lighted scope is passed along the upper aerodigestive tract to inspect and obtain biopsy specimens from areas of the entire mucosa (includes bronchoscopy, esophagoscopy, laryngoscopy) To detect metastasis or second primary tumor	1 hr	Related to general anesthesia	Reactions to general anesthesia Airway obstruction Tracheoesophageal fistula Sore throat Aspiration Hemorrhage from biopsy site Pneumothorax	Deep breathe, turn, ambulate	Difficulty breathing Excessive bleeding Inability to swallow (nurse should check for return of gag reflex) Increased temperature, cough, or sputum production

Data from Haggood AS: Head and neck cancers. In Otto S, editor: *Oncology nursing*, ed 4, St Louis, 2001, Mosby, pp. 285-325; Harris L: Head and neck malignancies. In Yarbro CH, Frogge MH, Goodman M, Groenwald SL, editors: *Cancer nursing: principles and practice*, ed 5, Sudbury, Mass, 2000, Jones and Bartlett Publishers, pp. 1210-1243; Sidransky D: Cancers of the head and neck. In DeVita VT, Hellman S, Rosenberg SA, editors: *Cancer: principles and practice of oncology*, ed 6, Philadelphia. 2001, Lippincott Williams & Wilkins, pp. 789-914.
N/A, Not applicable.

6. Laboratory studies—complete blood count, chemistry studies, liver function tests.
7. Histologic diagnosis from the following:
    a. Fine-needle aspiration from suspicious neck nodes.
    b. Excisional biopsy of the lesion—to diagnose or to cure.
        (1) On small oral cavity, lip, or skin lesions.
        (2) As a rule, an open or excisional biopsy of suspicious neck nodes is contraindicated (to avoid seeding of the tumor).
            (a) Exception: when all other examinations fail to identify a primary site or when lymphoma is suspected.
    c. Incisional biopsy—taking a small sample of tumor along with adjoining normal tissue.
    d. Panendoscopy (passing an endoscope along the entire mucosa of the upper aerodigestive tract)—to examine and perform a biopsy on suspicious areas, determine the full extent of disease, and identify synchronous primary tumors.
C. Staging—TNM classification system developed by the American Joint Committee on Cancer (AJCC, 2002) (Table 29-2; Figure 29-4).
D. Treatment strategies—surgery and radiation are the primary treatment modalities for managing malignant head and neck tumors; chemotherapy is for recurrent and metastatic disease (Fang & Forastiere, 2001).
    1. Treatment is based on the T and N classification.
        a. For T1 and T2 lesions of the oral cavity, larynx, nose, and paranasal sinuses, treatment is surgery or radiation.
        b. For T3 and T4 tumors, treatment is combination therapy.

TABLE 29-2
Overview of Selected TNM Staging of Cancers of the Head and Neck

CLASSIFICATION

T = PRIMARY TUMOR

General: for All Sites

TX	Primary tumor cannot be assessed
T0	No evidence of primary tumor
Tis	Carcinoma in situ

Oral Cavity, Oropharynx

T1	Greatest diameter of primary tumor ≤2 cm
T2	>2 cm or ≤4 cm
T3	>4 cm
T4a or T4b	Massive tumor, with deep invasion into maxilla, mandible, pterygoid muscles, deep tongue muscle, skin, soft tissues of neck

Hypopharynx

T1	Tumor confined to one subsite of hypopharynx
T2	Tumor invades more than one subsite of hypopharynx or an adjacent site, without fixation of the hemilarynx
T3	Tumor invades more than one subsite of the hypopharynx or an adjacent site, with fixation of the hemilarynx
T4a or T4b	Tumor involves adjacent structures (e.g., cartilage or soft tissues of neck)

TABLE 29-2
Overview of Selected TNM Staging of Cancers of the Head and Neck—cont'd

Nasopharynx
T1	Tumor confined to one subsite
T2	Involvement of two subsites within nasopharynx
T3	Extension into nasal cavity or oropharynx
T4a or T4b	Invasion into skull and/or cranial nerve(s)

Larynx
Glottic
T1	Limited to true vocal cords; normal vocal cord mobility; may include anterior or posterior commissure
T2	Supraglottic or subglottic extension; normal or impaired mobility
T3	Confined to larynx proper; vocal cord fixation
T4a or T4b	Cartilage destruction and/or extension out of larynx to other tissues

Supraglottic
T1	Limited to subsite of supraglottis; normal vocal cord mobility
T2	Extension to glottis or adjacent supraglottic subsite; normal vocal cord mobility
T3	Confined to larynx proper; cord fixation and/or extension into hypopharynx or preepiglottic space
T4a or T4b	Massive tumor, cartilage destruction, and/or extension out of larynx

Subglottic
T1	Limited to subglottic region
T2	Extension to vocal cord(s)
T3	Limited to larynx; vocal cord fixation
T4a or T4b	Massive tumor; cartilage destruction and/or extension out of larynx

N = NODAL METASTASIS
NX	Nodes cannot be assessed
N0	No regional lymph node metastasis
N1	Single, ipsilateral node: ≤3 cm
N2A	Single, ipsilateral node: >3 cm or ≤6 cm
N2B	Multiple, ipsilateral nodes: all ≤6 cm
N3A	Ipsilateral nodes(s): one >6 cm
N3B	Bilateral nodes (each side subclassed)
N3C	Contralateral node(s), only

M = DISTANT METASTASIS
MX	Presence of distant metastasis cannot be assessed
M0	No distant metastasis
M1	Distant metastasis present

STAGE GROUPINGS
Stage I	T1, N0, M0
Stage II	T2, N0, M0
Stage III	T3, N0, M0; T1, T2, or T3 with N1, M0
Stage IV	T4a or T4b, N0 or N1, M0
	Any T, N2 or N3, M0
	Any T, any N, M1

Derived from AJCC Cancer Staging Manual, Sixth Edition. For a complete, official description of TNM, Stage Grouping and Histologic Grade for this site, please consult Greene F.L., Page D.L., Fleming, I.D., et al. *AJCC Cancer Staging Manual,* Sixth Edition. New York: Springer-Verlag, 2002.
Note: Changes to system include subcategories for T4 lesions (T4a: resectable; T4b: unresectable).

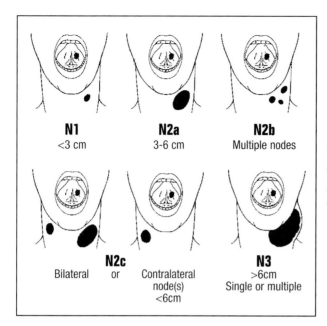

FIGURE 29-4 ■ Lymph node staging for the head and neck. (From Shah JP, Lydiatt W: Treatment of cancer of the head and neck, *CA: Cancer J Clin* 45[6]:358, 1995.)

   c. For N1, N2, and N3, see Table 29-2.
   d. For clinically negative neck nodes and a large primary lesion (T2, N0) of the oral cavity, oropharynx, hypopharynx, or larynx, treatment is either lymphadenectomy or radiation (because tumor cells can spread) (NCI, 2002c).
  2. Surgery.
   a. Common surgical procedures used in treating head and neck malignancies (Table 29-3).
  3. RT.
   a. Primary treatment to control the primary tumor and adjacent lymph nodes while maintaining structure and function; external beam dose range is 6000 to 7000 cGy (Haggood, 2001; Sidransky, 2001; Wang, 2000).
   b. Adjuvant treatment for stages III and IV disease and tumors that can spread toward the midline (e.g., oropharyngeal lesions); external beam dose is approximately 5000 cGy (Haggood, 2001; Sidransky, 2001; Wang, 2000).
   c. External beam RT occurs approximately 4 to 6 weeks after surgery.
   d. Preoperative radiation or permanently placed iodine-125 seeds may be used to debulk large or unresectable lesions.
     (1) Advantage: fewer wound complications.
     (2) Need to have preoperative dental evaluations, removal of diseased teeth, and prophylactic fluoride treatment.
     (3) After wounds heal (3 to 6 weeks), postoperative radiation started; treatment is for 6 to 7 weeks.
   e. For nasopharyngeal cancer, treatment is primarily radiation.
     (1) Surgery avoided since area is close to vital structures of the brain.
     (2) Carefully selected clients who experience treatment failure with RT may be treated with base of skull resection of tumor.

TABLE 29-3
Surgical Procedures for Head and Neck Cancer

Procedure	Physical Alteration	Nursing Implications
Laser	Little to none	Minimal bleeding
Composite resection	Resection of oral cavity/ oropharyngeal lesion in continuity with neck dissection Portion of mandible is resected Reconstruction with myocutaneous flaps is usually required, with resections of large amounts of tissue	May experience problems with speech (decreased articulation with tongue involvement), swallowing (impaired mastication, salivary drooling, aspiration), altered facial contour
Supraglottic laryngectomy	Resection of structures above the false vocal cords, including the epiglottis (preserves the true vocal cords)	Aspiration until swallowing techniques are learned Maintains a relatively normal voice
Hemilaryngectomy	Vertical excision of one true and one false cord and underlying cartilage	Hoarse voice Minimal or no swallowing problems
Total laryngectomy	Excision of the entire larynx from the hyoid bone to the second tracheal ring	Permanent tracheostomy Aphonia Decreased sense of smell Unable to perform Valsalva's maneuver
Maxillectomy	Partial or total en bloc resection of the cavity May include the ethmoid sinus, lateral nasal wall, palate, and floor of orbit	Preoperatively, maxillofacial prosthodontist makes dental obturator to fill the large surgical defect and to facilitate swallowing Requires daily care to cavity and placement of obturator
Orbital exenteration	Resection of orbit secondary to extension of maxillary sinus tumor or recurrent disease	Facial defect Unilateral vision loss Requires daily care and cleansing of cavity
Craniofacial/skull base resection	Surgical approach to inaccessible midfacial and extensive paranasal sinus and nasopharyngeal lesions	May have facial defect and cranial nerve (III, IV, V) deficits
Radical neck dissection	Resection of sternocleidomastoid muscle, jugular vein, spinal accessory nerve, and cervical lymph nodes	Shoulder droop Concave contour of neck
Modified neck dissection	Radical neck dissection with preservation of the sternocleidomastoid muscle, jugular vein, or spinal accessory nerve	Shoulder droop if spinal accessory nerve resected Concave contour of neck
Lymphadenectomy	Resection of lymph nodes in neck	Surgical scars

Modified from American Cancer Society (ACS): *All about laryngeal and hypopharyngeal cancer.* Retrieved February 19, 2003 http://www.cancer.org/docroot/CRI/CRI_2x.asp?sitearea=CRI&dt=23, 2003a; American Cancer Society (ACS): *Surgery for laryngectomy.* Retrieved February 19, 2003 http://www.cancer.org/docroot/CRI/content/ CRI_2_4_4X_Surgery_23.asp?sitearea, 2003; Haggood AS: Head and neck cancers. In Otto S, editor: *Oncology nursing,* ed 4, St Louis, 2001, Mosby, pp. 285-325; National Cancer Institute (NCI): *Head and neck cancer: treatment.* Retrieved February 19, 2003 http://www.nci.nih.gov/cancerinfo/treatment/head-and-neck, 2002; Sidransky D: Cancers of the head and neck. In DeVita VT, Heilman S, Rosenberg SA, editors: *Cancer: principles and practice of oncology,* ed 6, Philadelphia, 2001, Lippincott Williams & Wilkins, pp. 789-914.

    f. For lesions of the anterior and posterior tongue, floor of mouth, and nasal vestibule, treatment can be brachytherapy (implanted iridium-192 or cesium-137).

       (1) Maximizes dose to the tumor bed and minimizes exposure to surrounding tissue. (See Box 29-3 for side effects associated with RT to the head and neck region.)

    g. For metastatic thyroid cancer, use of iodine-191 ablation treatment (Staiduhar et al., 2000).

  4. Chemotherapy.

    a. Chemotherapy alone is not curative.

       (1) Reduces tumor volume or rids clinically detectable squamous cell carcinomas.

       (2) Treatment for recurrent or metastatic disease.

    b. As adjuvant and neoadjuvant therapy, single-agent or combination chemotherapy regimens: cisplatin (Platinol), bleomycin (Blenoxane), fluorouracil (5-Fluorouracil, 5-FU), paclitaxel (Taxol), and methotrexate (Mexate). Also for palliative therapy for recurrent or unresectable lesions (Fang & Forastiere, 2001; Haggood, 2001; Sidransky, 2001).

    c. Combination protocols of chemotherapy with RT because of sensitizing effect of chemotherapy.

       (1) Example: RADPLAT (protocol for mouth cancers; strategy is concurrent RT and cisplatin infusion to the tumor) (Sidransky, 2001).

  5. Palliative therapy.

    a. Surgery, radiation, and/or chemotherapy is used for unresectable lesions or recurrent tumors or when surgery is considered high risk.

    b. To relieve pain, bleeding, or obstruction; treatment may include short courses of radiation (3000 cGy over 2 to 3 weeks) (Haggood, 2001; Sidransky, 2001; Wang, 2000).

BOX 29-3
RADIATION THERAPY: SIDE EFFECTS

- Physical alterations
- Skin reactions
- Fatigue
- Anorexia
- Oral stomatitis
- Xerostomia
- Taste changes
- Pharyngitis

Modified from Huang HY, et al: Symptom profile of nasopharyngeal cancer clients during radiation therapy, *Cancer Pract* 8:274-281, 2000; Maher K: *Radiation therapy: toxicities and management.* In Yarbro CH, Frogge MH, Goodman M, Groenwald SL, editors: *Cancer nursing: principles and practice,* ed 5, Sudbury, MA, 2000, Jones and Bartlett Publishers, pp. 323-351; Sidransky D: Cancers of the head and neck. In DeVita VT, Hellman S, Rosenberg SA, editors: *Cancer: principles and practice of oncology,* ed 6, Philadelphia, 2001, Lippincott Williams & Wilkins, pp. 789-914.

Assessment

I. Initial and ongoing (see Section V.B. of Theory).

II. During treatment.

  A. Surgery (Clarke, 2002; Harris, 2000).

    1. Adequate airway: cleanliness of tracheostomy.

    2. Ability to communicate—use of paper and pen, Magic Slate, electronic communication device, picture board, or nonverbal cues.

    3. Ability to swallow.

    4. Range of motion of head, neck, and shoulders.

    5. Coping with anticipated and actual physical changes associated with surgical procedure.

    6. Skin and suture lines for areas of erythema, induration, and tenderness, which may be signs that fistula is forming.

    7. Understand surgical procedure, preoperative preparation, and postoperative care and rehabilitation.

  B. RT (Haggood, 2001; Sidransky, 2001).

    1. Skin integrity—color, tenderness, dryness, breakdown, pruritus.

    2. Fatigue—duration; activities that minimize or relieve fatigue.

    3. Appetite.

    4. Oral cavity inspection; assess for mucositis, infection, xerostomia, taste changes (Table 29-4).

      a. Oral mucositis (also called stomatitis) is an inflammation of the mouth and throat lining, a frequent side effect of radiation treatment in head and neck cancer clients (and of some chemotherapy treatments).

        (1) Inflammation appears as redness and swelling, with the client reporting pain caused by infection, bleeding.

        (2) Client can also have xerostomia (dry mouth because of decreased saliva).

        (3) Clinical assessment tools available, which provide grading criteria to rate changes in oral mucosa (Clarkson et al., 2004; NCI, 2003a).

          (a) Criterion is typically 1 to 4 (4 = severe symptoms).

          (b) Areas of assessment: lips, gingival and oral mucosa, tongue, teeth, saliva.

        (4) Mucositis after radiation: 6 to 8 weeks (mucositis after chemotherapy: 7 to 14 days).

    5. Pharyngitis, globus, dysphagia.

    6. Level of anxiety.

    7. Coping ability with body image changes.

    8. Understanding about RT.

    9. Self-care ability.

  C. Chemotherapy (Camp-Sorrell, 2000; Haggood, 2001; Sidransky, 2001).

    1. Nausea and vomiting; use and efficacy of antiemetics.

    2. Intake and output of fluids, daily weight, electrolyte levels including creatinine for renal function.

    3. Oral cavity inspection; assess for mucositis and infection.

    4. Monitor vital signs.

    5. Monitor blood counts; assess for infections, fever, and myalgias from neutropenia.

    6. Assess for bleeding from thrombocytopenia; fatigue from anemia.

    7. Understanding about chemotherapy.

    8. Self-care ability.

TABLE 29-4

Radiation Therapy for Cancer of the Head and Neck—Nursing Diagnoses and Implications

Nursing Diagnoses	Nursing Implications

Impaired skin integrity	1. Assess skin reactions.
	2. Instruct client and family to keep skin clean.
	  a. Avoid irritating treated skin.
	  b. When washing treated area, use only lukewarm water and mild soap; pat dry.
	  c. Do not rub, scrub, or scratch the skin in the treatment area.
	3. Instruct client to avoid shaving within area of treatment.
	4. Apply moisturizing lotion as directed for skin dryness.
	  a. Use skin care products that will not cause skin irritation.
	  b. If pruritus occurs, apply a thin layer of hydrocortisone cream.
	  c. Do not apply any skin lotions within 2 hr of a treatment.
	  d. Do not use any powders, creams, perfumes, deodorants, body oils, ointments, lotions, or home remedies in the treatment area for several weeks afterward unless approved by radiation oncologist/nurse.
	5. If moist desquamation occurs, use Burrow's compresses 3 or 4 times per day.
	6. Do not wear tight clothing over the area.
	7. Avoid putting anything that is hot or cold, such as heating pads or ice packs, on treated skin.
	8. Avoid exposing the radiated area to the sun during treatment.
	  a. Wear protective clothing (e.g., a hat with a broad brim, a shirt with long sleeves).
	  b. Use a sunscreen.

Activity intolerance	1. Assess level of fatigue. 2. Advise client to plan rest periods throughout the day. 3. Maintain nutritional intake. 4. Utilize resources to conserve energy. 5. Obtain assistance for chores and transportation as needed.
Imbalanced nutrition: less than body requirements related to anorexia	1. Assess appetite. 2. Monitor weight. 3. Recommend frequent, small meals. 4. Advise on use of nutrient-dense foods, such as nutritional supplements.

Impaired oral mucous membrane	1. Client needs thorough prophylactic dental assessment several weeks before radiation treatment begins (e.g., cleaning, filling of caries).
	2. Assess oral cavity: note presence of erythema, xerostomia, ulcerations, infections.
	3. Prevention: thorough and frequent mouth care.
	  a. As ordered by physician, perform systematic oral care at least every 4 hr (minimum: after meals and before bedtime) with soft toothbrush and rinse of normal saline or half normal saline/half baking soda. Use nonabrasive (waxed) dental floss.
	  b. Only for crusted areas, use half normal saline/half hydrogen peroxide. (Avoid daily use of hydrogen peroxide solution since frequent use can decrease wound healing.)
	  c. Use fluoridated toothpaste, or apply fluoride treatment recommended by dentist.
	  d. To gently cleanse the cavity, a gravity gavage or jet-spray dental cleansing system may be used.
	  e. Use a Toothette to remove mucous crusts that develop on immobile suture lines and flaps.

TABLE 29-4
Radiation Therapy for Cancer of the Head and Neck—Nursing Diagnoses and Implications—cont'd

Nursing Diagnoses	Nursing Implications

	f. To minimize drying of the mucosa, avoid lemon glycerin swabs and commercially prepared mouthwashes that contain alcohol.
	g. Avoid foods and fluids with high sugar content.
	h. Sip water frequently.
	i. Use saliva substitutes as needed.
	j. If wearing dentures, make sure they remain clean and well fitting.
	4. Once mucositis established:
	  a. Perform oral care with a half-and-half solution of peroxide and normal saline at least every 4 hr.
	  b. Remove excess secretions from the oral cavity; use, or instruct the client (if able to use), a tonsil-tip suction catheter.
	  c. Pain management: nonsteroidal antiinflammatories to begin; then opioids, if necessary.
	5. Recommend soft, nonspicy, nonacidic diet.
	  a. Choose foods that taste good and that are easy to eat.
	  b. To change food consistency, add fluids and use sauces/gravies to soften food.
	  c. Eat small, frequent meals.
	  d. Cut food into small, bite-sized pieces.
	  e. Use liquid food supplements (with adequate daily calories) that are easier to swallow than solids.
	  f. If swallowing after treatment will considerably decrease oral nutrition, consider the placement of a nasogastric tube, PEG (percutaneous esophageal gastrostomy) tube, or G-tube (gastric) to ensure adequate nutrition.
	6. Maintain hydration status.

Disturbed sensory perception: gustatory	1. Assess presence of taste changes. 2. Recommend experimenting with different food tastes. 3. Advise performing mouth care before meals. 4. Recommend chewing foods longer, to allow longer contact of food with taste receptors in mouth.

Impaired swallowing	1. Assess for pharyngitis.
	2. Monitor for infections.
	  a. Signs of infection: inflammation, swelling, redness.
	  b. Candidiasis is the most common clinical infection of the oropharynx in irradiated clients.
	    1) Topical treatments: antifungals, e.g., nystatin (Mycostatin), clotrimazole (Lotrimin).
	    2) Systemic treatments: ketoconazole (Nizoral), fluconazole (Diflucan).
	  c. Bacterial infections: treat with antibiotics, based on culture/sensitivity tests.
	3. Monitor weight.
	4. Use topical anesthetics or systemic analgesics as prescribed for pain.
	5. Recommend soft, nonspicy, nonacidic diet.
	6. Maintain hydration.

Continued.

TABLE 29-4

Radiation Therapy for Cancer of the Head and Neck—Nursing Diagnoses and Implications—cont'd

Nursing Diagnoses	Nursing Implications
PSYCHOSOCIAL ISSUES	
Anxiety	1. Assess level of anxiety. 2. Allow client and family to verbalize issues and concerns. 3. Provide education about illness and treatment.
Disturbed body image	1. Assess client's understanding about body image changes. 2. Provide education about changes and rehabilitative measures available. 3. Allow client and family to discuss issues and concerns about body image changes.
Deficient knowledge related to radiation therapy and self-care measures	1. Assess client's and family's understanding about radiation therapy and self-care measures. 2. Provide education about radiation therapy and self-care measures; utilize available multimedia client education tools: booklets, videos, audiotapes. 3. Evaluate comprehension of client education materials.

Data from American Cancer Society (ACS): *All about laryngeal and hypopharyngeal cancer.* Retrieved February 19, 2003 http://www.cancer.org/docroot/CRI/CRI_2x.asp?sitearea=CRI&dt=23, 2003; Barasch A, Peterson DE: Risk factors for ulcerative oral mucositis in cancer patients: Unanswered questions, *Oral Oncol* 39(2):91-100, 2003; Clarkson JE, Worthington HV, Eden OB: Interventions for preventing mucositis for patient with cancer receiving treatment. Cochrane Review. In *Cochrane Library Issue, Issue 1, 2004,* Chichester, UK, 2004, John Wiley & Sons, Ltd; Devine P, Doyle T: Brachytherapy for head and neck cancer: a case study, *Clin J Oncol Nurs* 5(20):55-57, 2001; Haggood AS: Head and neck cancers. In Otto S, editor: *Oncology nursing,* ed 4, St Louis, 2001, Mosby, pp. 285-325; Harris L: Head and neck malignancies. In Yarbro CH, Frogge MH, Goodman M, Groenwald SL, editors: *Cancer nursing: principles and practice,* ed 5, Sudbury, Mass, 2000, Jones and Bartlett Publishers, pp. 1210-1243; His RA, et al: Therapy for cancer of the base of the tongue: managing the side effects, *Cancer Pract* 8:264-267, 2000; Huang HY, Wilkie DJ, Schubert MM, Ting LL: Symptom profile of nasopharyngeal cancer clients during radiation therapy, *Cancer Pract* 8:274-281, 2000; Maher K: Radiation therapy: toxicities and management. In Yarbro CH, Frogge MH, Goodman M, Groenwald SL: *Cancer nursing: principles and practice,* ed 5, Sudbury, MA, 2000, Jones and Bartlett Publishers, pp. 323-351; National Cancer Institute (NCI): *Oral complications of chemotherapy and head/neck radiation.* Retrieved January 30, 2004. http://www.cancer.gov/cancerinfo/pdq/supportivecare/oralcomplications/HealthProfessional, 2003; National Cancer Institute (NCI): *Radiation therapy and you: a guide to self-health during cancer treatment.* Retrieved January 30, 2004 http://www.cancer.gov/cancerinfo/radiation-therapy-and-you/page5#, 2003; Rose P, Yates P: Quality of life experienced by clients receiving radiation treatment for cancers of the head and neck, *Cancer Nurs* 24:255-263, 2001; Rose-Ped A, et al: Complications of radiation therapy for head and neck cancers: the client's perspective, *Cancer Nurs* 25:461-467, 2003; Shih A, et al: A research review of the current treatments for radiation-induced oral mucositis in clients with head and neck cancer, *Oncol Nurs Forum* 29:1063-1080, 2002; Sidransky D: Cancers of the head and neck. In DeVita VT, Hellman S, Rosenberg SA, editors: *Cancer: principles and practice of oncology,* ed 6, Philadelphia, 2001, Lippincott Williams & Wilkins, pp. 789-914.

Nursing Diagnoses

I. Surgery.
    A. Ineffective airway clearance.
    B. Impaired verbal communication.
    C. Imbalanced nutrition: less than body requirements.
    D. Impaired physical mobility.
    E. Disturbed body image.
    F. Risk for impaired skin integrity.
    G. Deficient knowledge related to surgery and self-care measures.
II. RT (see Table 29-4).
III. Chemotherapy (Table 29-5).

TABLE 29-5
Chemotherapy for Cancers of the Head and Neck—Nursing Diagnoses and Implications

Nursing Diagnoses	Nursing Implications
Risk for deficient fluid volume related to nausea and vomiting	1. Assess for nausea and vomiting. 2. Instruct client to use antiemetics before chemotherapy and as needed 3. Monitor hydration status. 4. Encourage fluids. 5. Utilize nonpharmacologic measures to manage nausea and vomiting, e.g., relaxation exercises, distraction. 6. Encourage small, frequent meals. 7. Provide diet that is low in fat and nonsweet; encourage fluids. 8. Provide mouth care frequently during the day.
Risk for injury related to nephrotoxicity of cisplatin (Platinol)	1. Monitor laboratory values, electrolytes, especially creatinine and blood urea nitrogen levels. 2. Provide hydrating intravenous fluids and medications as ordered. 3. Monitor intake and output. 4. Encourage fluids. 5. Control nausea and vomiting.

Impaired oral mucous membrane	1. Assess oral cavity: tenderness, ulceration, bleeding, infections.
	2. Instruct client about mouth care:
	  a. Brush teeth after each meal.
	  b. Floss teeth at bedtime, if client normally practices flossing.
	  c. Perform frequent oral rinses with warm normal saline.
	3. Advise on diet consisting of nonspicy, nonacidic, room-temperature or cool foods.
	4. Maintain hydration.

Risk for infection related to neutropenia	1. Monitor blood counts: white blood count, neutrophils; assess for neutropenia.
	2. Institute neutropenia precautions when white blood cell count is decreased:
	  a. Monitor temperature: be alert for fever, chills, sweats, myalgias; report these occurrences.
	  b. Avoid crowds.
	  c. Avoid persons with colds or other respiratory infections.
	  d. Avoid sharing eating utensils, beverage containers.
	  e. Avoid handling animal excreta (i.e., litter box, bird cage).
	  f. Preserve and protect skin integrity.

Risk for injury related to thrombocytopenia	1. Monitor platelet count.
	2. Institute bleeding precautions when platelet count is decreased:
	  a. Assess skin, mucous membranes, bowel movements, urine, emesis, and secretions for signs of bleeding.
	  b. Assess signs of hemorrhage: hypotension, changes in consciousness, headache, vomiting, tachycardia.
	  c. Protect skin integrity: avoid venipuncture, intramuscular injections.
	  d. Perform mouth care; avoid traumatizing oral mucosa.
	  e. Institute bowel program to prevent constipation.
	  f. Avoid trauma to rectal tissues: avoid rectal medication, rectal thermometer, enemas.
	  g. Use electric razor.
	  h. Provide safe environment that eliminates hazards for injury.

Risk for activity intolerance related to anemia	1. Assess for fatigue. 2. Monitor blood counts: red blood cells, hematocrit.

Continued.

TABLE 29-5
Chemotherapy for Cancers of the Head and Neck—Nursing Diagnoses and Implications—cont'd

	3. Recommend measures to minimize fatigue: 　**a.** Pace activities. 　**b.** Plan rest periods during the day. **4.** Administer blood products as ordered. **5.** Ensure adequate nutritional intake.
Deficient knowledge related to chemotherapy and self-care measures	**1.** Assess level of understanding about chemotherapy. **2.** Provide information about chemotherapy: effects, side effects, and self-care measures as well as symptoms to report. **3.** Provide educational booklets, videotapes, and audiotapes as they are available. **4.** Evaluate comprehension of client education.

Data from American Cancer Society (ACS): *All about laryngeal and hypopharyngeal cancer.* Retrieved February 19, 2003 http://www.cancer.org/docroot/CRI/CRI_2x.asp?sitearea=CRI&dt=23, 2003a; Camp-Sorrell D: Chemotherapy: toxicity and management. In Yarbro CH, Frogge MH, Goodman M, Groenwald SL, editors: *Cancer nursing: principles and practice,* ed 5, Sudbury, Mass, 2000, Jones & Bartlett Publishers, pp. 444-486; Haggood AS: Head and neck cancers. In Otto S, editor: *Oncology nursing,* ed 4, St Louis, 2001, Mosby, pp. 285-325; Harris L: Head and neck malignancies. In Yarbro CH, Frogge MH, Goodman M, Groenwald SL, editors: *Cancer nursing: principles and practice,* ed 5, Sudbury, MA, 2000, Jones & Bartlett Publishers, pp. 1210-1243; National Cancer Institute (NCI): *Head and neck cancer: treatment.* Retrieved February 19, 2003 http://www.nci.nih.gov/cancerinfo/treatment/head-and-neck, 2002; Sidransky D: Cancers of the head and neck. In DeVita VT, Hellman S, Rosenberg SA, editors: *Cancer: principles and practice of oncology,* ed 6, Philadelphia, 2001, Lippincott Williams & Wilkins, pp. 789-914.

Outcome Identification (Haggood, 2001; Harris, 2000)

I. Client identifies type of cancer, rationale for treatment, alteration in anatomy and physiology that will result from treatment, and the specific side effects of treatment.

II. Client lists signs and symptoms and treatment of immediate and long-term side effects of disease and treatment.

III. Client discusses self-care measures to decrease incidence and severity of symptoms associated with disease and treatment.
  A. Refrains from or stops using tobacco and drinking alcoholic beverages.
  B. Maintains prophylactic oral care during and after radiation treatment (diseased teeth removed, daily fluoride treatments).
  C. Maintains high-residue diet and high fluid intake to prevent constipation. (After total laryngectomy, client may lose ability to do Valsalva's maneuver.)

IV. Client demonstrates self-care skills when disease and/or treatment affects structure or function.
  A. Wound care.
  B. Airway management.
    1. Perform tracheostomy care.
    2. Perform stoma care.
    3. Perform suctioning.
    4. Provide humidification via stoma.
  C. Nutritional care.
  D. Self-monitors for disease progression or recurrence.
    1. Demonstrates self-examination of the head and neck area.
    2. Lists symptoms to report—red areas (erythroplakia), white areas (leukoplakia), ulcers that do not heal in 2 weeks, larger lymph nodes or changes.

V. Client discusses coping strategies (ACS, 2003a; Haggood, 2001; Harris, 2000).
   A. Can be independent with activities of daily living and new skills (tracheostomy care, esophageal speech).
   B. Socialization with family and friends.
   C. Return to previous work or activities or occupational training for alternative work and leisure activities.
   D. Participation in support groups and informational systems to assist in problem solving, lifestyle changes, and adjustment (Lost Chord Club, I Quit Clinics, I Can Cope educational programs).
VI. Client describes plan for follow-up care.
   A. To monitor rehabilitation and detect recurrence or a second primary tumor.
      1. Cites schedule for clinical evaluation (e.g., year 1, every month; year 2; every 2 months; year 3, every 3 months; year 4, every 4 months; year 5, every 5 months; after 5 years, every year) (Staffel et al., 2001).
      2. List signs and symptoms of recurrence—pain, dysphagia, neck nodes enlargement, ulceration, bleeding, hemoptysis, airway obstruction, bone pain.
   B. To promote physical and psychosocial adjustment—use of physical therapist, occupational therapist, speech therapist, CanSurmount or Laryngectomy Club.
   C. To change lifestyles—enrolls in stop smoking and/or alcohol cessation programs.
VII. Client discusses community resources.
   A. Support groups and organizations.
      1. ACS-affiliated groups: Lost Chord Club, I Can Cope, CanSurmount.
      2. Other examples of support groups (with websites).
         a. International Association of Laryngectomees. www.larynxlink.com.
         b. SPOHNC—Support for People with Oral and Head and Neck Cancer. www.spohnc.org
         c. Head and Neck Cancer Community. www.headandneckcancer.org
   B. Medical supply providers: information about stoma bibs, shower shields, medications, other equipment.
   C. Medic-Alert Foundation International: 1-800-ID-ALERT (1-800-432-5378).

Planning and Implementation
General

I. Ongoing interventions that are collaborative, multidisciplinary, and systematic.
   A. Various disciplines involved in care: surgery, radiation oncology, medical oncology, nursing, social work, physical medicine, rehabilitation, speech and language pathology, nutrition, and others.
   B. Determine client goals and time frames to accomplish goals.
      1. Meet regularly; confer as a multidisciplinary team.
   C. Table 29-6 provides an example of a pathway to organize client-focused care involving many disciplines (Clarke, 2002).

Intervention: Surgery for Head and Neck Cancers

I. Preoperative preparation (Bauer, 2001; Clarke, 2002; Haggood, 2001; Harris, 2000).
   A. At time of diagnosis, initiate client and family preoperative teaching; discuss disease, treatment, side effects, and anticipated postoperative changes.
   B. Provide instruction about equipment (tracheostomy tube, drains, nasogastric tube, tonsil-tip suction catheter).

TABLE 29-6
Sample Head and Neck Client Pathway: Surgery Without a Tracheostomy*

	Presurgical	Day of Surgery	During Surgery	After Surgery	At Home
ASSESSMENT	■ A nurse will call to confirm your surgery. ■ A complete history and physical must be done by your physician or nurse practitioner before you have surgery. ■ If you become ill before your surgery, call your physician to decide if your surgery should be rescheduled.	■ Come to the operating room on the ____th floor of the main hospital building. ■ You will be given an identification bracelet. ■ Your vital signs will be taken and recorded. ■ An operating room nurse and an anesthesiologist will talk to you.	■ An anesthesiologist and/or nurse anesthetist will monitor your vital signs. POSTANESTHESIA CARE ■ After surgery, you will be transferred to the recovery room. ■ You may be transferred to the surgical intensive care unit for monitoring. ■ Your vital signs, comfort level, and incision will be monitored.	■ A nurse will monitor your vital signs and comfort level. ■ Your incision will be monitored and cleaned several times each day. ■ It is normal for your face and neck to be swollen; swelling may be present for a while. ■ Neck surgery may result in limited motion of your arm and shoulder. ■ Jaw surgery may result in difficulty opening your mouth.	■ A member of the head and neck team will call you 3-5 days following discharge to check on your progress. ■ Schedule follow-up appointments as instructed.
DIET	■ Please do not eat or drink anything, chew gum, or eat mints after midnight the night before your surgery. • Do not smoke or drink alcohol 5 days before surgery.	■ Please continue to not eat, drink, smoke, and chew gum.		■ Diet will be prescribed by your physician. ■ Your diet will change as your swallowing improves.	■ Follow the diet prescribed by the physician. ■ Notify the physician if you have any difficulty eating or drinking.
TESTS	■ During your preadmission testing. • Blood will be drawn.	■ You may have more blood tests done before surgery.	■ All tissue removed will be sent to pathology. (the laboratory) for	■ Blood work will be done as needed. ■ A swallowing x-ray may be	■ As ordered by physician

		examination by a physician (pathologist).	ordered. Other tests may be ordered as needed.	
TREATMENTS/ MEDICATIONS	• You will be asked for a urine specimen. • An electrocardiogram (ECG) and/or a chest x-ray may be performed. ▪ Avoid taking aspirin, Bufferin, ibuprofen, or Alka-Seltzer for 7–14 days before surgery. ▪ Bring list of all prescription and nonprescription medications and supplements (vitamins and herbal preparations) you are currently taking. ▪ Your physician will inform you of the need to take routine medications before surgery.	▪ Take medication with a sip of water *only if instructed by your physician.* ▪ An intravenous (IV) line will be started.	▪ IV fluids and antibiotics will be given during and after surgery. ▪ Ointment will be placed in your eyes. ▪ A catheter may be placed in your bladder.	▪ IV fluids and antibiotics will be continued as needed. ▪ You may have drains in your neck connected to suction. ▪ Antibiotics will be ordered. ▪ You may receive special mouth care. ▪ Pain medication will be given as needed.	▪ Prescriptions will be given for medications; have prescriptions for liquid pain medications filled at the pharmacy. ▪ Follow your instructions for wound, incision, and drain care.
ACTIVITY/ SAFETY	▪ Leave all valuables at home. ▪ Wear comfortable, loose-fitting clothes.	▪ You will be dressed in a hospital gown. ▪ You will be safely transported to the operating room. ▪ A registered nurse will be present and attend to your needs throughout and following the procedure.	▪ Safety straps will be in place. ▪ Special air stockings will be wrapped around your legs to prevent blood clots.	▪ The head of your bed will be raised to reduce swelling. ▪ You will be out of bed with assistance as tolerated. ▪ You will be encouraged to be as active as possible. ▪ Physical and occupational therapy may be ordered to assist with your activity.	▪ Follow your physician's instructions regarding restricted activity. ▪ Gradually increase your activity. ▪ It is important to balance activity with periods of rest.

(Continued)

TABLE 29-6
Sample Head and Neck Client Pathway: Surgery Without a Tracheostomy*—cont'd

	Presurgical	Day of Surgery	During Surgery	After Surgery	At Home
CONSULTANTS	■ Your physician will review your test results and may request further consultation to ensure that you are in the best possible condition for surgery. ■ You may be asked to obtain medical clearance from your internist or cardiologist. ■ You may be referred to a radiation oncologist. ■ You may be referred to a maxillofacial prosthodontist (dental specialist).		■ Medical specialists are available if your physician needs a consultation.	■ A dietitian will evaluate your nutritional needs. ■ A speech-language pathologist may evaluate your swallowing and communication needs. ■ Other consultants are available as needed.	■ Schedule appointments with consultants as directed by your physician.
TEACHING NEEDS	■ You will be scheduled for teaching with the nurse, social worker, and speech-language pathologist from the head and neck team. ■ The needs and questions	■ Any questions you have will be answered before surgery.	■ You will be in surgery for several hours; your family will be told when your surgery is over.	■ You will be instructed in the care of your wounds, drains, and any other equipment needed. ■ You may receive dietary/ swallowing instructions.	■ Notify the physician of the following: ● Increased redness or swelling around your wound/incision, or drainage from your wound/incision.

- you and your family have will be answered at this time.
- Hospital maps are available for your convenience.

POSTANESTHESIA CARE
- You will remain in the recovery room until you are ready to be transferred to the head and neck surgery unit.

- You will receive a discharge instruction sheet.

- Fever of 101° F (38.3° C)
- Unrelieved pain
- Difficulty swallowing
- Weight loss
- Difficulty breathing
- Avoid smoking and drinking alcohol.

DISCHARGE PLANNING
- Plans for your discharge will be an ongoing process during your hospitalization.
- Your expected length of stay is determined by your procedure and recovery.

- If needed, the social worker will arrange for a visiting nurse and equipment needs at home.
- The social worker will assist you with any financial concerns.

- Once you arrive at home, you may feel free to call 555-555-5555 where a nurse will be able to answer your questions.

SUPPORTIVE NEEDS
- A variety of staff is available to meet your emotional, social, and spiritual needs.

- You will be visited in the presurgical area by members of the head and neck team.

- Your family will be visited in the waiting area by members of the head and neck team.
- Your physician will keep your family informed about the progress of surgery.

- The social worker will assist you and your family with emotional, social, and spiritual needs.
- The hospital chaplain is available as needed.

- Your navigator guide is available to assist you as needed.

From Greater Baltimore Medical Center (GBMC): *Head and neck patient pathway: surgery without a tracheostomy* (brochure), Baltimore, 2000, GBMC. Copyright 2000 by GBMC.
*This document is intended as a guideline. Each client is an individual, and responses may vary. If you have any questions, please talk to your physician.

    C. As needed, provide counseling and support.

    D. Discuss economic and rehabilitation resources.

        1. If appropriate, arrange a preoperative and a postoperative visit with a Lost Chord or Laryngectomy Club member (contact ACS or local agencies).

    E. Preoperatively determine reading ability and plan for postoperative communication.

        1. Paper and pencil.

        2. Magic Slate.

        3. Picture board.

        4. Nonverbal cues.

        5. Electronic communication board or device.

 II. Postoperative interventions to maximize safety for client (Clarke, 2002; Haggood, 2001; Harris, 2000; Miller & Sessions, 2001; Smith, 2003).

    A. Place client in close proximity to nurses' station to monitor client with altered airway.

    B. For all tracheostomy clients, keep at the bedside an extra tracheostomy tube of the same size (inner and outer cannulas and obturator), scissors, and a tracheal dilator.

    C. At all times, keep the call bell within reach.

    D. Identify method of communication if client has a tracheostomy.

    E. Observe for signs and symptoms of delirium tremens in clients with recent history of alcohol abuse.

    F. Observe for aspiration in clients who have had a supraglottic laryngectomy (includes resection of structures in the oropharynx, or cranial nerve [IX, X, XII] deficits).

    G. For clients at risk for carotid rupture, implement carotid precautions (see Section IV.B.).

III. Postoperative interventions to decrease severity of symptoms.

    A. Manage airway (tracheostomy) (ACS, 2002; Clarke, 2002; Harris, 2000; Sidransky, 2001; Smith, 2003).

        1. Permanent tracheostomy (total laryngectomy) (Figure 29-6).

            a. Airway.

                (1) While client needs mechanical ventilation, use a cuffed tracheostomy tube; may remove by postoperative day 2 or 3.

                (2) If stoma begins to narrow, a laryngectomy tube may be used.

            b. Humidity.

                (1) Provide humidified air or oxygen via a tracheostomy collar to prevent mucosa drying and crusting of secretions.

                (2) To provide humidity, apply moistened 4×4 gauze pads over the stoma.

                (3) Advise that a stoma bib worn over the stoma helps lessen drying of mucosa.

                (4) Teach symptoms of inadequate humidity—thick, tenacious secretions that are difficult to expectorate.

            c. Stoma care.

                (1) Cleanse stoma with a half-and-half peroxide and normal saline solution.

                (2) Remove all mucous crusting twice each day and as needed.

                (3) Remove visible mucous plugs with a Kelly clamp.

                (4) Apply a thin layer of prescribed ointment around the stoma twice each day.

2. Temporary tracheostomy (ACS, 2003a; Harris, 2000; NCI, 2002c; Sidranksy, 2001).
   a. If mechanical ventilation is needed or if the client is at risk for aspiration, keep a cuffed tube inflated. (Tube is usually placed in the operating room and maintained for 5 days.)
   b. Physician usually changes initial tracheostomy tube to a noncuffed tube. (If the client is aspirating, maintain the cuffed tube.)
   c. As edema decreases, the client may be able to breathe without the tracheostomy tube.
      (1) Tube is downsized to a no. 4 or 5 or a fenestrated tube.
      (2) Tube is plugged for 24 hours.
      (3) If the client can breathe with the tube plugged for a prolonged time and can expectorate secretions through the mouth, the client's cannula can be removed.
      (4) Change the dressing over the stoma every day and as needed.
      (5) Until the wound has sealed, teach the client to place a finger over stoma dressing when coughing or speaking.
   d. For all tracheostomies, suctioning is based on the need for airway clearance.
      (1) To prevent hypoxemia and arrhythmia, hyperoxygenate and/or hyperinflate the lungs before and after suctioning.
      (2) To precipitate coughing and mobilize secretions if needed, instill 2 to 5 ml of normal saline solution into the tracheostomy to lavage and stimulate the trachea and bronchi.
      (3) To mobilize secretions and prevent atelectasis, use an incentive spirometer attached via a female adapter to a plastic tracheostomy tube and/or use chest physical therapy (as indicated).
      (4) Record the color, amount, and odor of sputum produced and how frequently suctioning is required.
B. Tracheostomy care (Cady, 2002; Clarke, 2002; Harris, 2000; Sidransky, 2001; Smith, 2003).
   1. Remove the inner cannula and cleanse off all mucus and crusts initially with a half-and-half solution of peroxide and normal saline every 4 to 8 hours, then twice daily and as needed.
   2. Replace soiled tracheostomy ties as needed. To determine tightness, allow one fingerbreadth ease underneath ties.
C. Wound care (Clarke, 2002; Harris, 2000).
   1. Every 3 to 4 hours, assess the surgical wounds, noting color (pink versus cyanotic), temperature, and capillary refill (immediately after blanching) of skin and muscle flaps.
   2. Avoid excessive pressure that interferes with flap perfusion and viability (e.g., tight tracheostomy ties, oxygen collars, hyperextension of the neck, and the client lying on the flap).
   3. Assess integrity of suture lines, both external and intraoral (if applicable); breakdown may be the first sign of wound infection or fistula formation.
   4. Clean external suture lines with a half-and-half solution of peroxide and normal saline; then apply prescribed ointment every 4 to 8 hours.
   5. If client has nasal surgery, a maxillectomy, and/or an orbital exenteration, as ordered by the physician, gently cleanse the cavities to remove accumulated crusts.
      a. Use a half-and-half solution of normal saline and sodium bicarbonate or normal saline solution alone.

      6. Assess wound drains for color, amount, and odor of drainage.

         a. If not prevented or treated early, clotting and air leaks can lead to wound infections.

   D. Oral care (ACS, 2003a; Harris, 2000; Sidransky, 2001).

      1. Prevention: thorough and frequent mouth care (see Table 29-4).

         a. As ordered by physician, perform systematic oral care at least every 4 hours with soft toothbrush and rinse of normal saline or half normal saline/half baking soda. Use nonabrasive (waxed) dental floss.

         b. Use fluoridated toothpaste, or apply fluoride treatment recommended by dentist.

         c. To gently cleanse the cavity, use a gravity gavage or jet-spray dental cleansing system.

   E. Nutrition (ACS, 2003a; McGuire, 2000).

      1. Assess nutritional status before surgery; 60% of head and neck clients initially present with malnutrition.

      2. Identify clients with nutritional deficiencies who require oral, enteral, or parenteral nutritional supplements.

         a. Greater than 10% body weight loss during any treatment phase.

         b. More than 20% below ideal body weight.

      3. Confer with physician regarding methods of nutritional support—enteral tube feedings, other methods.

      4. Assess client after surgery for swallowing dysfunction.

   F. Mobility (Miller & Sessions, 2001).

      1. If neck dissection, the spinal accessory nerve and the sternocleidomastoid muscles may be resected.

         a. Result: shoulder droop, atrophy of the trapezius muscle, forward curvature of the spine, and limited range of motion (approximately 90 degrees) of the shoulder.

         b. Treatment: after wound drains removed and client has progressed to resistive exercises, initiate passive and active range of motion shoulder exercises. Optimal goal: functional range of 150 degrees.

   G. Body image changes (Cady, 2002; Miller & Sessions, 2001; Sweed et al., 2002).

      1. Promote control of secretion and odors; teach wound, oral, and tracheostomy care.

      2. Encourage self-care activities (e.g., tracheostomy care, tube feeding, suctioning) and activities of daily living (e.g., grooming, hair combing, shaving, applying makeup).

      3. Encourage resocialization: progressive ambulation, social interactions, support group participation (e.g., Voice Masters, Lost Chord Club, I Can Cope, CanSurmount).

      4. Consult the social worker to assist with counseling and financial, vocational, and adjustment issues.

      5. Inform the client of resources to purchase tracheostomy covers, scarves, makeup, or other cosmetic assistance; consult ACS Look Good, Feel Better programs (e.g., hair care, scarves).

      6. Support clients and their families to grieve; allow them to voice concerns, fears, and anxieties.

   H. Other alterations in functioning related to disease and treatment (Cady, 2002; Harris, 2000; Maher, 2000; Miller & Sessions, 2001; National Institutes of Health [NIH], 2002).

      1. Loss of sense of smell and/or taste.

    2. Loss of ability to blow nose (may need suctioning with nasal congestion or a cold).

    3. Loss of ability to perform Valsalva's maneuver may predispose client to constipation; administer stool softeners.

    4. Loss of normal airway.

        a. Advise to wear Medic-Alert bracelet identifying client as a neck breather; for emergencies, carry cards and/or windshield stickers.

        b. Establish emergency plans with local emergency system (e.g., tape recorder at phone with prerecorded call for help).

        c. Teach the client, family, public, and professionals first aid for individuals with a laryngectomy.

    5. Loss of ability to blow air from the mouth (cannot extinguish candles on a birthday cake).

IV. Monitoring for unique side effects.

  A. Fistula formation (Harris, 2000; Sidransky, 2001).

    1. More common with preoperative radiation.

    2. Breakdown of suture lines (pharyngeal, tracheoesophageal) allows secretions to leak into the wounds or under skin flaps.

    3. Usually occurs 3 to 5 days after surgery.

    4. Observe for signs and symptoms—erythema, drainage, tenderness of the suture line; low-grade temperature of 100° to 101° F (38° to 38.3° C); fluctuance below the neck skin; local edema.

    5. To allow healing, maintain nothing by mouth (NPO) status.

    6. To promote granulation of wound, perform dressing changes and wound packing every 4 to 8 hours or as needed.

  B. Carotid artery rupture (Harris, 2000; Sidransky, 2001).

    1. Occurs in 3.5% of head and neck clients treated with radical surgery.

    2. Risk increases with RT or fistula formation.

    3. Clients with exposed carotid artery on "carotid precautions"; supplies placed at the bedside include the following:

        a. Three bath towels.

        b. Six packs of 4 × 4 sponges.

        c. Six 5 × 9 combine dressing pads.

        d. One cuffed tracheostomy tube.

        e. 10-ml syringe.

        f. Alcohol swabs.

        g. Four packs of 4-inch rolled gauze (e.g., Kling).

        h. Intravenous (IV) solutions (normal saline, lactated Ringer's).

        i. Type and crossmatch—stamped requisitions for 2 units of blood.

        j. Suction apparatus and setup.

        k. Arterial blood gases kit.

        l. Blood drawing equipment.

        m. Latex gloves, disposable gowns, goggles.

    4. Keep an intact heparin/saline lock in place.

    5. Place clients on stool softeners to avoid straining.

    6. Use wet-to-wet dressing changes to avoid debriding the artery.

    7. In the event of a rupture, do the following:

        a. Apply pressure if bleeding externally or pack gauze in mouth if bleeding internally, and call for assistance.

        b. Establish an airway.

        c. Inflate the cuff on the tracheostomy tube to prevent aspiration and to apply internal pressure on the artery.

    d. Suction oral and tracheal secretions.

    e. Infuse IV fluids, e.g., via the heparin/saline lock.

    f. Obtain blood from the blood bank, and determine arterial blood gas values.

    g. Call operating room personnel to alert them about the emergency.

    h. Prepare the client; transfer to the operating room.

    i. Initiate universal precautions (as quickly as possible).

    j. If the client is alert, provide supportive and explanatory information throughout the situation.

V. Interventions to enhance adaptation and rehabilitation.

  A. Communication (Dropkin, 2001; Haggood, 2001).

    1. Cancers in the oral cavity affect the function of articulation; therapy includes the following:

      a. Exercises to increase strength, range of motion, coordination, and accuracy of tongue movement.

      b. Use of oral prostheses to compensate for tissue loss and allow for greater contact of the tongue with the palate, creating more intelligible speech.

    2. Cancers in the larynx affect phonation; therapy includes the following:

      a. After a partial laryngectomy, exercises to improve voice quality, pitch, and loudness.

      b. After a total laryngectomy.

        (1) Use of artificial larynx that transmits sound into the vocal tract.

        (2) Use of esophageal speech—air is swallowed and trapped in the esophagus, then released, allowing air to vibrate against the walls of the esophagus.

        (3) Use of tracheoesophageal prosthesis—placement of a prosthesis in a surgically created tracheoesophageal fistula; sound is formed by air from the lungs, creating a better quality of esophageal speech (Schultz, 2002).

  B. Swallowing (Haggood, 2001; Harris, 2000).

    1. Surgeries in the head and neck can affect swallowing.

    2. Complete a thorough clinical evaluation of the oral preparatory and pharyngeal stages of swallowing.

    3. To assess the oral and pharyngeal stages of the swallow: a barium swallow and x-ray examination or cine-esophagography are performed.

    4. An individual swallowing plan is developed and includes the following (Harris, 2000):

      a. Compensatory strategies—postural changes that facilitate passage of food into the oral cavity and pharynx (head elevated); changes in food consistency (i.e., thin versus thick fluids, semisolid versus pureed foods).

      b. Indirect swallowing therapy—jaw and tongue range of motion exercises; adduction of tongue exercises to improve laryngeal closure.

      c. Direct swallowing therapy using supraglottic swallow.

        (1) Prepare the bolus of food in the oral preparatory phase.

        (2) Before initiating the swallow, hold breath to close vocal cords.

        (3) Swallow while still holding breath.

        (4) Cough while exhaling after the swallow to expectorate remaining food or fluids on top of vocal cords.

        (5) Repeat steps 3 and 4 (swallow/cough).

    5. To avoid aspiration, inflate the cuff on the tracheostomy tube partially or totally during meals and 30 minutes afterward.

    6. For some clients, removal of the tracheostomy tube improves swallowing by allowing the larynx to elevate.

    7. Until the client can take adequate amounts by mouth, enteral tube feedings are used to maintain nutritional requirements.

C. Client education and support (Cady, 2002; Dropkin, 2001; Haggood, 2001; Harris, 2000).

    1. Begin discharge teaching before surgery, and reinforce this teaching immediately after surgery; teaching includes care of the tracheostomy tube, stoma care, suctioning techniques, enteral/supplemental feeding, alternative methods of providing humidity (bedside humidifier at bedtime and as needed), swallowing techniques, and speech, occupational, and physical therapy.

    2. Teach self-examination of lips, mouth, and oral cavity and palpation of adjacent nodes to monitor disease progression or recurrence.

    3. Include discharge teaching about reducing risk factors to minimize risk of recurrence (e.g., use smoking cessation programs, Alcoholics Anonymous).

    4. Recommend a head and neck cancer support group to discuss fears and help clients and families cope with the disease and treatment.

    5. Provide literature and Internet websites to reinforce or augment teaching; sources: American Cancer Society, the International Association of Laryngectomies, the National Cancer Institute.

Intervention: Radiation Therapy for Head and Neck Cancer

I. See Table 29-4 for nursing diagnoses and implications.

Intervention: Chemotherapy for Head and Neck Cancer

I. See Table 29-5 for nursing diagnoses and implications.

Evaluation

The oncology nurse systematically and regularly evaluates the client's and/or family's responses to interventions to determine progress toward the achievement of expected outcomes. Relevant data are collected, and actual findings are compared with expected findings. Nursing diagnoses, outcomes, and plans of care are reviewed and revised as necessary.

REFERENCES

American Cancer Society (ACS). (2002). *Cancer facts and figures 2002.* Atlanta: American Cancer Society.

American Cancer Society (ACS). (2003a). *All about laryngeal and hypopharyngeal cancer.* Retrieved February 19, 2003 from the World Wide Web ACS website: http://www.cancer.org/docroot/CRI/CRI_2x.asp?sitearea=CRI&dt=23.

American Cancer Society (ACS). (2003b). *Surgery for laryngectomy.* Retrieved February 19, 2003 from the World Wide Web ACS website: http://www.cancer.org/docroot/CRI/content/CRI_2_4_4X_Surgery_23.asp?sitearea.

Barasch, A., & Peterson, D.E. (2003). Risk factors for ulcerative oral mucositis in cancer patients: Unanswered questions. *Oral Oncology 39*(2), 91-100.

Bauer, A.M. (2001). Current trends of surgical management of head and neck carcinomas. *Nursing Clinics of North America 36,* 501-506.

Cady, J. (2002). Laryngectomy: Beyond loss of voice—caring for the client as a whole. *Clinical Journal of Oncology Nursing 6*, 347-351.

Camp-Sorrell, D. (2000). Chemotherapy: Toxicity and management. In C.H. Yarbro, M.H. Frogge, M. Goodman, & S.L. Groenwald (Eds.). *Cancer nursing: Principles and practice* (5th ed.). Sudbury, MA: Jones and Bartlett Publishers, pp. 444-486.

Clarke, L.K. (2002). Pathways for head and neck surgery: A client-education tool. *Clinical Journal of Oncology Nursing 6*(2), 78-82.

Clarkson, J.E., Worthington, H.V., & Eden, O.B. (2004). Interventions for preventing mucositis for patient with cancer receiving treatment. Cochrane Review. In *Cochrane Library Issue, Issue 1, 2004*. Chichester, UK: John Wiley & Sons, Ltd.

Devine, P., & Doyle, T. (2001). Brachytherapy for head and neck cancer: A case study. *Clinical Journal of Oncology Nursing 5*(20), 55-57.

Dropkin, M.J. (2001). Anxiety, coping strategies, and coping behaviors in clients undergoing head and neck cancer surgery. *Cancer Nursing 24*, 143-148.

Fang, B., & Forastiere, A. (2001). Head and neck cancer. In J. Abraham & C. Allegra (Eds.). *Bethesda handbook of clinical oncology*. New York: Lippincott Williams & Wilkins, pp. 3-28.

Greene, F.L., Page, D.L., Fleming, I.D., et al. (Eds.). (2002). *AJCC cancer staging manual* (6th ed.). New York: Springer-Verlag.

Haggood, A.S. (2001). Head and neck cancers. In S. Otto (Ed). *Oncology nursing* (4th ed.). St. Louis: Mosby, pp. 285-325.

Harris, L. (2000). Head and neck malignancies. In C.H. Yarbro, M.H. Frogge, M. Goodman, & S.L. Groenwald (Eds.). *Cancer nursing: Principles and practice* (5th ed.). Sudbury, MA: Jones and Bartlett Publishers, pp. 1210-1243.

His, R.A., Witt, M.E., Jesse, M., et al. (2000). Therapy for cancer of the base of the tongue: Managing the side effects. *Cancer Practice 8*, 264-267.

Huang, H.Y., Wilkie, D.J., Schubert, M.M., & Ting., L.L. (2000). Symptom profile of nasopharyngeal cancer clients during radiation therapy. *Cancer Practice 8*, 274-281.

Maher, K. (2000). Radiation therapy: Toxicities and management. In C.H. Yarbro, M.H. Frogge, M. Goodman, & S.L. Groenwald. *Cancer nursing: Principles and practice* (5th ed.). Sudbury, MA: Jones and Bartlett Publishers, pp. 323-351.

McGuire, J. (2000). Nutritional care of surgical oncology clients. *Seminars in Oncology Nursing 16*, 128-134.

Miller, S.D., & Sessions, R.B. (2001). Rehabilitation after treatment for head and neck cancer. In V.T. DeVita,, S. Hellman, & S.A. Rosenberg (Eds.). *Cancer: Principles and practice of oncology* (5th ed.). Philadelphia: Lippincott Williams & Wilkins, pp. 907-916.

National Cancer Institute (NCI). (2002a). *Head and neck cancer: Questions and answers.* Retrieved February 19, 2003 from the World Wide Web Cancer Facts website: http://cis.nci.nih.gov/fact/6_37.htm.

National Cancer Institute (NCI). (2002b). *Head and neck cancer: Treatment.* Retrieved February 19, 2003 from the World Wide Web CancerNet (PDQ) websites for health professionals: http://www.nci.nih.gov/cancerinfo/treatment/head-and-neck.

National Cancer Institute (NCI). (2002c). *Hypopharyngeal cancer.* Retrieved February 19, 2003 from the World Wide Web CancerNet (PDQ) websites for health professionals: http://www.nci.nih.gov/cancerinfo/pdq/treatment/hypopharyngeal/healthprofessional/.

National Cancer Institute (NCI). (2002d). *Nasopharyngeal cancer.* Retrieved February 19, 2003 from the World Wide Web CancerNet (PDQ) websites for health professionals: http://www.nci.nih.gov/cancerinfo/pdq/treatment/nasopharyngeal/healthprofessional/.

National Cancer Institute (NCI). (2003a). *Oral complications of chemotherapy and head/neck radiation.* Retrieved January 30, 2004 from the World Wide Web CancerNet (PDQ) websites for health professionals: http://www.cancer.gov/cancerinfo/pdq/supportivecare/oralcomplications/healthprofessional.

National Cancer Institute (NCI). (2003b). *Radiation therapy and you: A guide to self-health during cancer treatment.* Retrieved January 30, 2004 from the World Wide Web: http://www.cancer.gov/cancerinfo/radiation-therapy-and-you/page5#.

National Institutes of Health (NIH) (U.S. Department of Health and Human Services, Public Health Service). (2002). *Information about detection, symptoms, diagnosis, and treatment of oral cancer.* NIH Publication No. 97-1574, 2002.

Neville, B.W., & Day, T.A. (2002). Oral cancer and precancerous lesions. *CA: A Cancer Journal for Clinicians 52*, 195-215.

Rose, P., & Yates, P. (2001). Quality of life experienced by clients receiving radiation treatment for cancers of the head and neck. *Cancer Nursing 24*, 255-263.

Rose-Ped, A., Bellm, L.A., Epstein, J.B., et al. (2003). Complications of radiation therapy for head and neck cancers: The client's perspective. *Cancer Nursing 25*, 461-467.

Schultz, P.N. (2002). Providing information to clients with a rare cancer: Using Internet discussion forums to address the needs of clients with medullary thyroid carcinoma. *Clinical Journal of Oncology Nursing 6*(4), 219-222.

Shih, A., Miaskowski, C., Dodd, M.J., et al. (2002). A research review of the current treatments for radiation-induced oral mucositis in clients with head and neck cancer. *Oncology Nursing Forum 29*, 1063-1080.

Sidransky, D. (2001). Cancers of the head and neck. In V.T. DeVita, S. Hellman, & S.A. Rosenberg (Eds.). *Cancer: Principles and practice of oncology* (6th ed.). Philadelphia: Lippincott Williams & Wilkins, pp. 789-914.

Smith, R.P. (2003). *Laryngeal cancer: The basics.* Retrieved February 19, 2003 from the World Wide Web OncoLink, The University of Pennsylvania Cancer Center website: http://www.oncolink.com/types/article.cfm?c=7&s=24&ss=185&id=9450.

Staffel, J.G., Denneny, J.C., Eibling, D.E., et al. (2001). *Primary otolaryngology care.* Alexandria, VA: American Academy of Otolaryngology—Head and Neck Surgery.

Staiduhar, K.I., Neithercut, J., Chu, E., et al. (2000). Thyroid cancer: Clients' experiences of receiving iodine-131 therapy. *Oncology Nursing Forum 27*, 1213-1218.

Sweed, M.R., Schiech, L., Barsevick, A., et al. (2002). Quality of life after esophagectomy for cancer. *Oncology Nursing Forum 29*, 1127-1131.

Wang, C.C. (2000). Cancer of the head and neck. In C.C. Wang (Ed.). *Clinical radiation oncology: Indications, techniques and results* (2nd ed.). New York: Wiley-Liss, p. 103.

30 Nursing Care of the Client with Cancers of the Neurologic System

SHIRLEY J. KERN

BRAIN TUMORS

Theory

I. Physiology and pathophysiology associated with brain tumors.
   A. Anatomy.
      1. Primary structures (Segal, 1998) (Figures 30-1 and 30-2).
         a. Cerebrum—two hemispheres consisting of pairs of lobes: frontal, temporal, parietal, occipital.
         b. Thalamus and hypothalamus located at the base of the cerebrum.
         c. Cerebellum—located in the posterior fossa at the back of the head below the occipital lobes.
         d. Brainstem—located at the base of the brain and the top of the spinal cord; consists of midbrain, pons, and medulla oblongata.
      2. Critical adjacent structures (Segal, 1998).
         a. Meninges—membranes that cover brain and spinal cord; outermost layer is the dura, a thick, whitish, inelastic covering.
         b. Ventricles—four connected cavities in the brain through which cerebrospinal fluid (CSF) flows (Figure 30-3).
            (1) CSF is a clear, colorless, odorless fluid that bathes the brain and spinal cord within the dural covering.
            (2) Blockage of CSF flow because of tumor growth can cause hydrocephalus.
         c. Cerebral blood vessels.
            (1) Two vertebral arteries and two internal carotid arteries supply blood to the brain.
            (2) Circle of Willis connects the anterior and posterior arteries to provide alternative routes if blood flow to a single vessel is blocked.
            (3) Venous drainage is accomplished via dural sinuses, vascular channels between the two layers of the dura.
         d. Blood-brain barrier.
            (1) Tighter junctions among the cells of the brain capillaries that selectively allow substances to cross neuronal membranes.
            (2) Movement across the barrier depends on particle size, lipid solubility, chemical dissociation, and protein-binding potential of the substance.

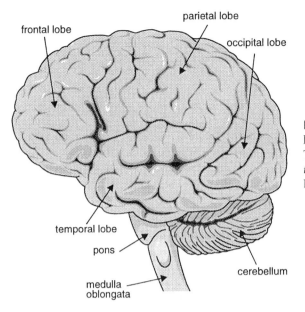

FIGURE 30-1 ■ Lobes of the cerebral hemispheres. (From American Brain Tumor Association: *A primer of brain tumors*, ed 7, Chicago, 1998, American Brain Tumor Association, p. 10.)

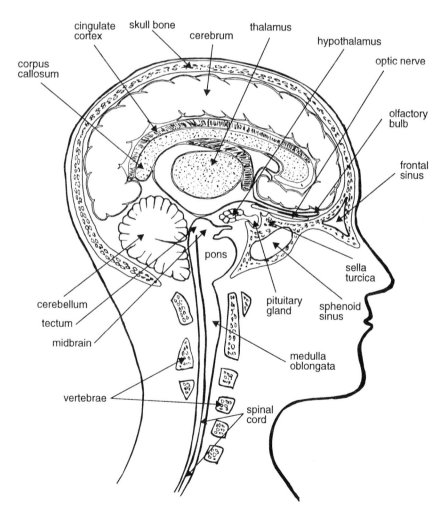

FIGURE 30-2 ■ Cross section of the brain. (From American Brain Tumor Association: *A primer of brain tumors*, ed 7, Chicago, 1998, American Brain Tumor Association, p. 14.)

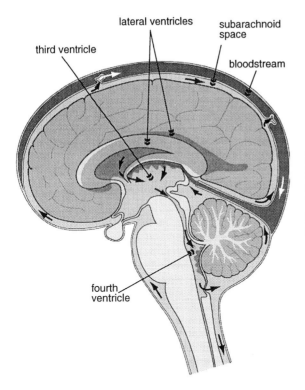

FIGURE 30-3 ■ Ventricles and cerebrospinal brain flow (*arrows* show direction). (From American Brain Tumor Association: *A primer of brain tumors*, ed 7, Chicago, 1998, American Brain Tumor Association, p. 25.)

    e. Skull.
       (1) Normally acts as a protective framework.
       (2) With malignant tumors, the skull's rigidity forces an increase in intracranial pressure (ICP) as the tumor grows and cerebral edema increases.
    f. Cranial nerves.
       (1) Twelve pairs—ten arise from the brainstem, and two arise from the cerebrum.
       (2) Peripheral nerves of the brain.
       (3) Tumors near the brainstem produce cranial nerve deficits.
  3. The most common primary malignant tumors tend to arise from support (glial) cells in the brain (Louis & Stemmer-Rachamimov, 2000).
    a. Astrocytes—connective tissue cells.
    b. Oligodendrocytes—cells that produce myelin.
    c. Ependyma—lining of the ventricles.
  4. Some tumors, more common in children, arise from primitive neuroectodermal cells. These are called primitive neuroectodermal cell tumors (PNETs) (Taylor & Rutka, 2000).
    a. Medulloblastomas.
    b. Ependymoblastomas.
    c. Pinealoblastomas.
  5. All these tumors occur within the structures of the brain.
B. Functions of the brain (Segal, 1998) (Figure 30-4).
  1. Frontal lobes.
    a. Personality.
    b. Intellect.
    c. Judgment.

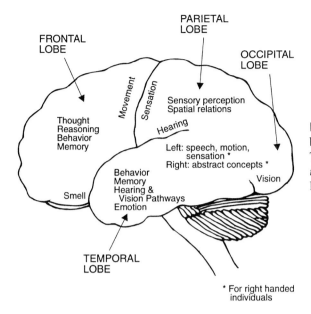

FIGURE 30-4 ■ Functions of the cerebral lobes. (From American Brain Tumor Association: *A primer of brain tumors*, ed 7, Chicago, 1998, American Brain Tumor Association, p. 26.)

    d. Abstract thinking.
    e. Mood and affect.
    f. Memory.
    g. Speech (in the left frontal lobe for most right-handed people).
2. Motor strip—at the conjunction of the frontal lobe with the parietal lobe.
    a. Right motor strip area controls motor function on the left side.
    b. Left motor strip area controls motor function on the right side.
3. Parietal lobes—sensory input.
    a. Pain.
    b. Temperature.
    c. Pinprick.
    d. Light touch.
    e. Proprioception.
    f. Two-point discrimination.
    g. Double simultaneous discrimination.
    h. Stereognosis.
    i. Graphesthesia.
4. Occipital lobes.
    a. Sight.
    b. Visual identification of objects.
5. Temporal lobes.
    a. Hearing.
    b. Memory.
    c. Receptive speech.
6. Cerebellum.
    a. Coordination.
    b. Balance.
7. Thalamus.
    a. Monitors sensory input.
    b. Acts as a relay station for sensory information.

8. Hypothalamus controls the following:
   a. Water balance.
   b. Sleep.
   c. Temperature.
   d. Appetite.
   e. Blood pressure.
   f. Coordination of overall patterns of activity.
9. Brainstem (pons, midbrain, medulla) controls the following:
   a. Blood pressure.
   b. Heartbeat.
   c. Respirations.

C. Changes associated with cancer (Wen & Black, 1999).
   1. Direct injury to brain tissue.
      a. Focal neurologic deficits specific to tumor location (see list of functions).
      b. Abnormal firing of neurons resulting in seizure activity.
   2. Cerebral edema.
      a. Compression of normal tissues from swelling around the tumor.
      b. Symptoms are more diffuse than focal.
         (1) Increased sleepiness.
         (2) Headaches, usually unilateral and worse in the morning.
         (3) Confusion.
         (4) Herniation.
            (a) Decreased level of consciousness.
            (b) Pupillary abnormalities or other cranial nerve dysfunctions.
            (c) Decorticate or decerebrate posturing.
            (d) Coma.
            (e) Irregular breathing.
            (f) Death.
   3. Hydrocephalus—resulting from blockage of CSF pathways caused by tumor growth and/or edema. Symptoms include the following:
      a. Headache.
      b. Loss of balance.
      c. Memory loss.
      d. Confusion.
      e. Urinary incontinence.
   4. Increased ICP related to tumor growth, edema, or hydrocephalus. See earlier descriptions for symptoms.

D. Histology.
   1. Astrocytomas—most common brain tumors (Enam et al., 2000).
      a. Grade I: pilocytic astrocytoma. Usually found in children. Also referred to as juvenile pilocytic astrocytoma (JPA).
      b. Grade II: astrocytoma—low-grade tumor with little evidence of malignant behavior.
      c. Grade III: anaplastic astrocytoma—tumor that exhibits nuclear pleomorphism, mitosis, or increased cellularity, which indicates a tendency for rapid growth.
      d. Grade IV: glioblastoma multiforme—a tumor with all the features of rapid growth plus necrosis. This is the most malignant of brain tumors and also the most common, accounting for about 45% to 50% of all gliomas.
   2. Oligodendrogliomas: comprise about 5% of all brain tumors (Louis & Stemmer-Rachamimov, 2000).

       a. Grades I and II are called oligodendrogliomas and are quite indolent.

       b. Grades III and IV are called anaplastic oligodendrogliomas and feature the more aggressive features of a malignant tumor.

  3. Medulloblastomas (Taylor & Rutka, 2000).

       a. Occur primarily in children.

       b. Start in the cerebellum.

       c. Metastasize to other areas of the central nervous system (CNS) through the CSF.

  4. Ependymomas (Taylor & Rutka, 2000).

       a. Arise from the lining of the ventricles.

       b. May be malignant or benign but are usually benign.

       c. Account for 2% to 8% of all CNS neoplasms and 6% to 12% of childhood intracranial tumors.

  5. Primary CNS lymphoma (Raizer & DeAngelis, 2000).

       a. Until 1974, only accounted for about 1% of all brain tumors. Since then, a threefold increase has been noted.

       b. More likely to occur in immunosuppressed individuals (transplant recipients and those who test human immunodeficiency virus [HIV] positive).

       c. Brain has no lymph tissue. Mechanism for development of CNS lymphomas is not understood.

  6. Mixed tumors (Louis & Stemmer-Rachamimov, 2000).

       a. More than one cell type.

       b. Usually astrocytes and oligodendrocytes.

       c. May be astrocytes and ependymal cells.

  7. Tumors of neuronal origin are quite rare and tend to be benign.

E. Presentation (Segal, 1998; Wen & Black, 1999).

  1. Seizure (35%) (Keles & Berger, 2000).

  2. Headache.

       a. Usually unilateral.

       b. Usually more severe when the person first awakens.

  3. Hemiparesis.

  4. Aphasias.

  5. Visual field cuts.

  6. Confusion.

F. Metastatic patterns (Gupta & Rutka, 2000).

  1. Recurrence is usually restricted to the CNS.

  2. Distant metastases rarely occur; when present, they occur in lung or bone.

G. Epidemiology (Jukich et al., 2001; Prados & Levin, 2000).

  1. Approximately 17,500 new primary brain tumors every year in the United States.

  2. More than 50% of primary brain tumors are malignant and infiltrate the brain substance.

  3. Brain tumor is the most common solid tumor in children.

  4. Incidence is increasing for unknown reasons. The following have been postulated:

       a. Better diagnostic procedures.

       b. Lengthening of the lifespan allows for a greater chance to develop brain tumors.

       c. Unknown environmental factors.

       d. Men are more likely than women to develop a malignant brain tumor (ratio of 1.5:1).

   e. Changes in coding/classification.

   f. Increase in CNS lymphoma because of HIV/AIDS (acquired immuno-deficiency syndrome).

 II. Principles of medical management.

  A. Screening and diagnostic procedures (Blake & Maravilla, 1999; Martin et al., 2000).

   1. Currently no screening tests to identify clients with brain tumors.

   2. CT (computed tomography) (Blake & Maravilla, 1999).

    a. Often used as initial study for clients suspected of having a brain tumor.

    b. Less expensive than magnetic resonance imaging (MRI).

    c. Malignant tumors are best visualized with contrast-enhanced scans.

   3. MRI (Martin et al., 2000).

    a. Provides the best imaging of brain tumors.

     (1) Contrast is used to enhance the area of tumor.

     (2) Shows the tumor on different planes: sagittal, axial, coronal.

     (3) Easier for the surgeon to identify critical structures.

     (4) Can see patterns of cerebral edema more clearly.

    b. Normally used in the following instances:

     (1) Preoperatively.

     (2) Postoperatively within 24 hours to assess residual tumor volume. Postoperative scan provides the baseline value to measure treatment effect.

     (3) For follow-up examination about every 3 months while undergoing treatment.

   4. Stereotactic biopsy (Spiegelmann & Friedman, 1999).

    a. Done when tumor cannot be surgically resected.

    b. Requires a special frame that can only be used on the head (Figure 30-5), unless the biopsy is being done in an intraoperative MRI unit.

    c. Provides a small sample of tissue with which to make a diagnosis.

    d. Sampling error is possible, so that the tumor may be read out as less malignant than it actually is.

   5. Surgical resection (LaCroix et al., 2001; Prados & Levin, 2000).

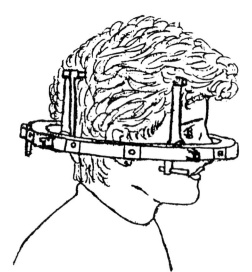

FIGURE 30-5 ■ Stereotactic frame used for stereotactic biopsy and radiosurgery.

    a. Subtotal—removal of a portion of the tumor for diagnostic purposes and to reduce mass effect.

    b. Gross total—removal of all visible tumor.

        (1) Diagnostic tissue sample.

        (2) Reduction of mass effect.

        (3) Theoretically improves response to treatment (smaller tumor burden).

        (4) Done only when surgery will not create a worsening of neurologic deficits.

B. Staging methods (Louis & Stemmer-Rachamimov, 2000; Segal, 1998).

    1. Size of tumor, location, and degree of malignancy are the best indicators of prognosis.

    2. TNM classification (primary tumor, regional lymph nodes, distant metastases).

        a. TNM classification is limited because two of the three indicators are usually not applicable to brain tumors.

        b. Tumor size: applicable.

        c. Node involvement: does not apply to brain tumors.

        d. Metastases outside the brain and spinal cord: extremely rare.

    3. WHO (World Health Organization) classification frequently used in clinical practice.

        a. Degree of malignancy is based on the grade of a tumor.

        b. The criteria to establish the grade are as follows:

            (1) Atypia (similarity to normal cells).

            (2) Mitotic index (rate of growth).

            (3) Necrosis (dead tumor cells in the center of the tumor indicating uncontrolled growth).

            (4) Infiltration (potential for invasion depending on whether it has a definitive margin).

            (5) Vascularity (blood supply).

        c. Four grades are assigned.

            (1) Grade I—biologically benign and most often associated with long-term survival. There is nearly a normal appearance when seen under the microscope, and the tumors grow slowly.

            (2) Grade II—can have a slightly abnormal appearance under the microscope. They are relatively slow growing and can invade adjacent normal tissue. They can recur and sometimes at a higher grade.

            (3) Grade III—considered malignant, but sometimes not a definite distinction between grades II and III. Abnormal cells are seen microscopically, and infiltration can take place into adjacent normal brain tissue.

            (4) Grade IV—considered the most malignant and most aggressive. There is rapid reproduction with many abnormal and heterogeneous cells seen under the microscope. Areas of necrosis are also seen. These are extremely infiltrative into normal brain tissue.

C. Standard therapies (Harsh IV, 1999).

    1. Surgery: see descriptions in diagnostic section.

        a. Clients may receive surgery two or three times for the following reasons:

            (1) Decrease tumor burden.

            (2) Differentiate tumor from treatment effects.

        (3) Restage tumor—lower-grade tumors may become more malignant over time.

    b. A biopsy may be indicated to restage tumor if a resection would do the following:

        (1) Increase or create neurologic deficit.

        (2) Be risky for the client because of other health concerns.

2. Radiotherapy—currently considered the most effective therapy for most malignant brain tumors.

    a. Standard (conventional) radiation (Bauman & Larson, 2000).

        (1) Given over 6 to 7 weeks.

        (2) Total dose ranges from 5500 to 6200 cGy—varies depending on tumor type.

        (3) Higher dose can result in severe long-term side effects (dementia, cognitive problems, radiation necrosis).

        (4) Radiate the tumor plus a 2- to 3-cm margin.

        (5) Whole-brain radiation is seldom used except for metastatic tumors.

    b. Stereotactic radiosurgery (Kondziolka et al., 2000).

        (1) Uses the same type of head frame used for stereotactic biopsy (see Figure 30-5).

        (2) The frame allows the radiation to be focused on the tumor.

        (3) Radiation is delivered in several arcs so that the tumor receives the full dose, but normal tissues are spared.

        (4) The dose is calculated depending on the tumor type, size of tumor, proximity to critical structures (e.g., the optic nerve) that can be easily damaged by high-dose radiation.

        (5) The dose is delivered in a single high-dose fraction.

        (6) Usually used in conjunction with or following standard radiation.

    c. Fractionated stereotactic radiotherapy (Kondziolka et al., 2000).

        (1) Uses a relocatable stereotactic frame so that several focused fractions can be delivered over several days (Figure 30-6).

        (2) Provides doses equivalent to the amount delivered by conventional radiation.

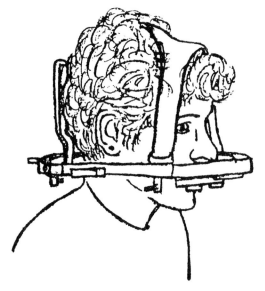

FIGURE 30-6 ■ Relocatable stereotactic frame used for fractionated stereotactic radiotherapy.

        (3) Spares normal tissue—reduction in side effects (hair loss, dementia, cognitive dysfunction).

        (4) May replace or augment conventional radiotherapy.

    d. Brachytherapy (Laperriere, 2000).

        (1) Implantation of radioactive seeds into the tumor bed.

        (2) Seeds are left in place for 3 or 4 days.

        (3) Many clients who receive brachytherapy develop severe radiation side effects.

        (4) Rarely used because of side effects.

        (5) With the development of stereotactic radiosurgery (SRS), many brachytherapy-eligible clients are likely being treated with radiosurgery.

3. Chemotherapy (Hall, 2002; Macdonald, 2001; Prados & Levin, 2000).

    a. Usually reserved as an adjunct to radiation.

    b. Chemotherapy agents are often used to control growth or reduce tumor burden, but the benefit is often short lived because of the resistance of tumor cells.

    c. Number of long-term survivors increases with the use of chemotherapy in high-grade tumors.

    d. Anaplastic oligodendrogliomas are more sensitive to chemotherapy than other tumors. Complete responses may occur.

    e. Commonly used drugs.

        (1) Carmustine (BCNU).

           (a) Used since the 1970s for brain tumors.

           (b) Lipid solubility allows it to pass the blood-brain barrier.

           (c) Can be given intravenously (IV) or in wafers that are implanted at the time of surgery.

        (2) PCV3—regimen using three drugs: procarbazine (Matulane), lomustine (CCNU), vincristine (Oncovin).

           (a) Used primarily for treating anaplastic oligodendrogliomas.

           (b) Also used as a standard regimen for treating other malignant gliomas by some cancer treatment centers.

        (3) Temozolomide (Temodar)—an oral, second-generation alkylating agent that can permeate the blood-brain barrier.

           (a) Approved by the U.S. Food and Drug Administration (FDA) in 1999 for the treatment of grade III anaplastic astrocytoma tumors but not approved for glioblastomas. Temozolomide frequently used, however, for glioblastomas and anaplastic oligodendrogliomas across the United States and in Europe.

           (b) In Europe, temozolomide was approved for all forms of glioma.

           (c) Myelosuppression is minimal and noncumulative, and clients describe good quality of life during this treatment.

4. Investigational modalities.

    a. Blood-brain barrier disruption (Doolittle et al., 2000).

        (1) Requires intraarterial infusion of mannitol or RMP-7 to open the barrier, then infusion of chemotherapy.

        (2) Initial results very promising for treatment of CNS lymphoma in clients who are not HIV positive. There is a survival time of approximately 44.5 months with this treatment protocol and it preserves cognitive functioning.

        (3) Appears to double median survival time for clients with malignant gliomas.

      b. Bone marrow transplant/stem cell rescue.
        (1) Pediatric protocols.
        (2) Clients with recurrent anaplastic oligodendrogliomas.
      c. Gene therapy—used primarily for malignant gliomas (Weyerbrock & Oldfield, 2000).
        (1) Herpes simplex virus.
        (2) Diphtheria toxin.
        (3) Large variety of vector systems and gene transfer concepts are being investigated.
      d. Immunotherapy—cells are taken from the client, grown in a laboratory, killed with radiation, and reinjected into the client, along with other drugs to stimulate the immune response. Clinical trials are currently still being conducted, but the efficacy of this approach already has been shown in a couple of pilot series.
  D. Trends in survival.
    1. Dependent on location, size, and accessibility of tumor.
    2. Use of multimodality therapy has increased the number of long-term survivors.
    3. Chemotherapy has been useful particularly with the following:
      a. Anaplastic oligodendroglioma—median survival has doubled from 2 years to about 4 years.
      b. Primary CNS lymphoma median survival (Raizer & DeAngelis, 2000).
        (1) No treatment—1 to 3 months.
        (2) Surgery—not indicated.
        (3) Radiation therapy (RT) in combination with chemotherapy—12 to 40 months, depending on the chemotherapy regimen.

Assessment

  I. Pertinent personal and family history (Wrensch et al., 2000).
    A. Risk factors are not known.
    B. Exposure to some environmental factors has been explored but not confirmed, for example:
      1. Vinyl chloride.
      2. Radiation.
      3. Petrochemical products.
      4. Inks and solvents.
      5. Hair dyes.
      6. Cellular telephones.
      7. High-power lines.
    C. Most common solid tumor of childhood.
    D. Incidence slightly higher in males.
    E. Although no hereditary pattern has been established for malignant tumors, they are more likely to occur in people with the following:
      1. Neurofibromatosis.
      2. Tuberous sclerosis.
      3. von Hippel–Lindau disease.
    F. Immunocompromised clients are at higher risk for primary CNS lymphoma.
  II. Pertinent medical history (Wrensch et al., 2000).
    A. Sudden onset of seizure activity.
    B. Headaches.

        1. Recent onset or more severe than usual.
        2. Usually unilateral.
        3. May be worse in the morning or awaken the client.
    C. Describes focal neurologic deficits.
    D. Family reports change in personality.
    E. Family reports episodes of memory loss or confusion.
  III. Physical examination (Wen & Black, 1999).
    A. Neurologic examination.
    B. Look for focal neurologic deficit.
  IV. Diagnostic evaluation (Blake & Maravilla, 1999; Martin et al., 2000).
    A. CT with and without contrast medium, or
    B. MRI with and without contrast medium.

Nursing Diagnoses

    I. Deficient knowledge related to tumor specifics, treatment options, and so on.
   II. Decreased intracranial adaptive capacity.
  III. Risk for activity intolerance.
  IV. Disturbed body image.
   V. Risk for caregiver role strain.
  VI. Interrupted family processes.
 VII. Risk for injury.
VIII. Sexual dysfunction.

Outcome Identification (Meyers, 2000; Shelton, 2000)

    I. Client identifies the tumor type.
   II. Client and caregivers describe treatment options.
  III. Client and caregivers identify resources for support and learning, such as the following:
    A. Members of the health care team.
    B. Brain tumor support groups.
    C. Other cancer support groups.
    D. American Brain Tumor Association.
    E. American Cancer Society.
    F. National Brain Tumor Foundation.
    G. The Brain Tumor Society.
  IV. Client's caregivers recognize signs and symptoms of increased ICP and seek assistance.
   V. Client and/or caregivers identify medications, know the correct doses, and describe possible side effects.
  VI. Client and caregivers identify reasons for decreased activity tolerance.
    A. Radiation.
    B. Chemotherapy.
    C. Cerebral edema.
    D. Hemiparesis.
    E. Steroid myopathy (from dexamethasone [Decadron] used to control cerebral edema).
    F. Poor balance.
 VII. Client and caregivers identify strategies to conserve energy and increase activity tolerance.
    A. Frequent rest periods.
    B. Gradual increase to normal activities.

    C. Physical therapy (PT) to improve muscular tone and develop balance compensation techniques.

  VIII. Client identifies methods for coping with body image disturbances.

    A. Hair loss from radiation, which will most likely be permanent.

      1. Wigs.

      2. Hats or scarves.

      3. Shaving the head.

    B. Neurologic deficits.

      1. Use of appliances and aids.

      2. Speech therapy, PT, occupational therapy (OT) sessions to enhance function.

  IX. Caregivers identify resources for respite and self-care.

  X. Family identifies changes in its structure and processes.

  XI. Family identifies resources to assist in coping with changes, such as the following:

    A. Social services.

    B. Psychologists and family counselors.

    C. Attorney to assist with estate planning and power of attorney issues if the client becomes unable to competently manage affairs.

    D. Child support group dealing with chronically ill parent, loss of parent.

  XII. If the client has seizures, the caregivers demonstrate first aid procedures for a person having seizures.

  XIII. Client and/or caregivers recognize the potential for injury when neurologic deficits interfere with balance, ambulation, driving, and ability to perform activities of daily living.

  XIV. Client and caregivers identify resources for assisting with safety issues.

    A. Physical therapy: balance compensation, strengthening.

    B. Occupational therapy: assistive devices, safety assessments.

    C. Speech therapy: speech and memory training.

  XV. Client and his/her sexual partner identify issues that may affect sexual function.

    A. Radiation in which the field includes the pituitary region.

    B. Need for birth control with chemotherapy regimens.

    C. Potential for sterility with certain chemotherapy agents.

    D. Fatigue.

    E. Neurologic deficits.

Planning and Implementation (Meyers, 2000; Shelton, 2000)

  I. Identify knowledge deficits related to brain tumor.

    A. Provide information in written and oral forms.

    B. Be available to answer questions.

    C. Provide information about other resources.

      1. American Brain Tumor Association
        2720 River Road, Suite 146
        Des Plaines, IL 60018-4110
        Patient Line: 1-800-886-2282
        www.abta.org

      2. National Brain Tumor Foundation
        414 Thirteenth Street, Suite 700
        Oakland, CA 94612
        1-800-934-CURE
        www.braintumor.org

   3. The Brain Tumor Society
      124 Watertown Street, Suite 3H
      Watertown, MA 02472
      1-800-770-8287
      www.tbts.org
II. Assess neurologic status for evidence of the following:
   A. Increasing ICP or cerebral edema.
   B. Progression of the tumor.
   C. Effectiveness of antiseizure medication.
   D. Effectiveness of steroid treatment.
   E. Side effects of medications.
III. Assess the client for evidence of activity intolerance.
   A. Counsel the client and family on available resources.
   B. Discuss methods for conserving energy.
IV. Identify resources for clients with body image disturbance.
V. Identify resources for a caregiver experiencing stress.
VI. Assess family processes.
   A. Identify altered processes.
   B. Provide information regarding resources and support.
VII. Assess the client for risk of injury.
   A. Poor balance.
   B. Seizures.
   C. Poor insight or judgment.
VIII. Counsel caregivers and client when safety concerns arise.
IX. Provide information regarding possibility of sexual dysfunction.
   A. Discuss effects of brain tumor and treatment.
   B. Provide information specific to the individual's situation.
      1. Use of birth control.
      2. Possibility of sterility.
      3. Banking of sperm or fertilized ova.
      4. Loss of menstrual cycling in women who lose pituitary function because of radiation.
      5. Alternative sexual positions.
      6. Loss of libido.

Evaluation

The oncology nurse systematically and regularly evaluates the client's and/or family's responses to interventions to determine progress toward the achievement of expected outcomes. Relevant data are collected, and actual findings are compared with expected findings. Nursing diagnoses, outcomes, and plans of care are reviewed and revised as necessary.

SPINAL CORD TUMORS

Theory

I. Physiology and pathophysiology associated with spinal cord tumors (Cooper et al., 2003; Fehlings & Rao, 2000; Segal, 1998).
   A. Anatomy.
      1. The spinal cord is an extension of the brain.

   a. Cord body begins at the brainstem and extends through the spinal foramina of vertebrae to the L1 to L2 vertebral level.
   b. Consists of 31 pairs of spinal nerves.
2. Critical adjacent structures.
   a. Vertebral column.
      (1) Thirty-three vertebrae joined by ligaments.
      (2) Bony structure encasing and protecting the cord.
      (3) Divisions—seven cervical, twelve thoracic, five lumbar, five sacral (fused), four coccygeal (fused).
   b. Intravertebral disks—cartilage pads separating vertebrae, allowing flexion of the cord.
   c. Meninges—layers of tissue that surround the spinal cord and brain.
   d. CSF—fluid that bathes and cushions the spinal cord; contained within the meninges.
   e. Vertebral blood vessels—supply from vertebral and spinal arteries.
3. Consist of same cell types as brain.
4. Malignant primary tumors tend to arise from intramedullary (within the spinal cord) support cells (Figure 30-7).
   a. Astrocytes.
   b. Ependymal cells.
5. Metastatic tumors are more likely to occur outside the dura (extradural) (Figure 30-7). The most frequent spinal metastases are from the following primary sites:
   a. Breast.
   b. Lung.
   c. Prostate.
6. Benign tumors are more likely to occur inside the dura but outside the spinal cord (extramedullary), such as the following (Figure 30-7).
   a. Meningiomas.
   b. Neurofibromas.
   c. Schwannomas.
B. Functions of the spinal cord.
   1. Motor function of the body from neck to toes.
   2. Sensory function of the body from the back of the head to the toes.
   3. Loss of function depends on the following:
      a. Site of tumor.
         (1) Cervical—neck, arms, hands.
         (2) Thoracic—chest to umbilicus.
         (3) Lumbar—hips to toes.
      b. Size of tumor.
C. Changes in function with spinal tumors.
   1. Growth of tumor creates cord compression as it enlarges.
   2. Can also compress spinal nerves and occlude blood vessels.
D. Histologic types (see Section I.A.4., 5, and 6 of Theory).
E. Presentation.
   1. Pain.
      a. Along spine.
      b. Radicular.
   2. Sensory impairment.
      a. Numbness or tingling.
      b. Usually unilateral and progressive.
   3. Motor impairment.

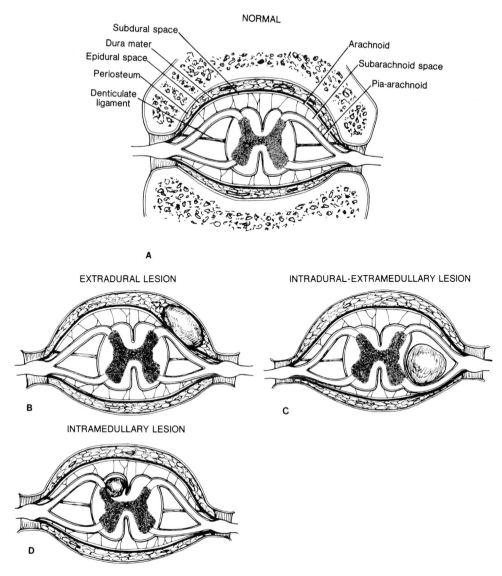

FIGURE 30-7 ■ Location of intraspinal tumors. **A,** Normal anatomy. **B,** Extradural lesion (metastases). **C,** Intradural-extramedullary lesion (neurofibroma). **D,** Intramedullary lesion (glioma). (From Borenstein DG, Wiesel SW, Boden SD: *Low back pain: Medical diagnosis and comprehensive management*, ed 2, Philadelphia, 1996, WB Saunders, p. 412.)

      a. Develops in conjunction with sensory impairment.
      b. Paresis, usually unilateral.
      c. Spasticity.
      d. Bladder and bowel dysfunction.
      e. Motor impairment is a late sign and may not be reversible with surgery.
   F. Metastatic patterns—primary spinal tumors tend not to metastasize distantly. They may invade dura and adjacent structures.
   G. Trends in epidemiology—no trends noted.
II. Principles of medical management (Cooper et al., 2003; Fehlings & Rao, 2000; Schwartz & McCormick, 2003; Segal, 1998).

A. Screening and diagnostic procedures.
   1. Spine films.
   2. CT—best for bony structures.
   3. MRI—best for defining soft tissues.
   4. Myelogram—aids in seeking source of spinal compression.
   5. Electromyography—detects muscular innervation dysfunctions peripherally.
B. Staging methods.
   1. Clinical neurologic status.
   2. Degree of malignancy of tumor.
   3. Invasion into adjacent structures.
   4. Status of systemic disease, if tumor is metastatic.
C. Treatment strategies.
   1. Extradural tumors.
      a. High-dose corticosteroids to reduce edema (e.g., dexamethasone [Decadron]).
      b. Radiation, if primary tumor is known and is radiosensitive.
      c. Surgery if tumor is not radiosensitive, neurologic status is deteriorating, or tumor type is not known, and if surgery will not put the client at risk for more severe neurologic deficit or other life-threatening complications.
   2. Intradural/extramedullary—surgical resection.
   3. Intradural/intramedullary.
      a. Surgical resection if possible.
      b. Malignant gliomas may require radiation and chemotherapy.
D. Trends in survival.
   1. Life expectancy is normal for clients with benign tumors that can be completely resected.
   2. Treatment for clients with malignant primary spinal cord tumors or metastatic tumors is palliative, and life expectancy is 1 to 2 years.

Assessment (Fehlings & Rao, 2000)

I. Pertinent personal and family history.
   A. History of neurofibromatosis.
   B. History of breast, lung, or prostate cancer.
   C. Describes localized or radicular neck or back pain.
   D. Describes sensory changes.
      1. Numbness and tingling.
      2. Unable to differentiate hot and cold.
      3. Loss of sensation of touch and/or pain.
   E. Describes decreased motor function.
   F. Describes loss of bowel or bladder control.
II. Physical examination.
   A. Neurologic assessment.
      1. Sensation.
      2. Movement and strength.
   B. Assess abdomen for the following:
      1. Signs of urinary retention.
      2. Bowel sounds.
      3. Hardness and distention.
   C. Attempt to elicit pain at site along spine.

Nursing Diagnoses

   I. Acute pain.
  II. Impaired urinary elimination.
 III. Bowel incontinence.
  IV. Impaired physical mobility.
   V. Disturbed tactile sensory perception.
  VI. Sexual dysfunction.

Outcome Identification

   I. Client identifies methods for pain control.
  II. Client describes signs and symptoms of bladder dysfunction.
 III. Client implements a bladder and/or bowel control program.
  IV. Client lists safety hazards related to decreased sensation and mobility.
   V. Client identifies resources for learning to compensate for loss of motor and sensory functions.
  VI. Client has access to information about sexual issues.

Planning and Implementation (Fehlings & Rao, 2000)

   I. Pain management.
   A. Develop pain control plan in conjunction with the client and family based on the following:
     1. Degree of pain.
     2. Degree of control with medications in use.
     3. Available alternatives.
     4. Expectation that surgery or radiation will help alleviate pain.
   B. Implement the plan, and assess.
  II. Urinary elimination.
   A. Assess the status of urinary elimination based on the following:
     1. Urinary retention.
     2. Potential for infection.
     3. Urinary incontinence with skin irritation.
   B. Develop a plan in conjunction with the client and family.
 III. Bowel elimination.
   A. Assess the status of bowel function.
   B. Develop a plan in conjunction with the client and family to do the following:
     1. Provide a routine for bowel elimination.
     2. Provide back-up strategies if incontinence occurs unexpectedly.
  IV. Provide the client and family with information about rehabilitation for sensory and motor loss.
   V. Counsel the client and family on safety hazards related to motor and sensory loss.
  VI. Provide information on sexuality issues as needed.

Evaluation

The oncology nurse systematically and regularly evaluates the client's and/or family's responses to interventions to determine progress toward the achievement of expected outcomes. Relevant data are collected, and actual findings are compared with expected findings. Nursing diagnoses, outcomes, and plans of care are reviewed and revised as necessary.

REFERENCES

Bauman, G.S., & Larson, D.A. (2000). Conventional radiation. In M. Bernstein & M.S. Berger (Eds.). *Neuro-oncology: The essentials.* New York: Thieme Medical Publishers, pp. 169-182.

Blake, L.C., & Maravilla, K.R. (1999). Computed tomography. In M.S. Berger & C.B. Wilson (Eds.). *The gliomas.* Philadelphia: W.B. Saunders, pp. 242-274.

Cooper, P.R., Wienecke, R.J., & White, B.T. (2003). Spinal meningiomas. In H.H. Batjer & C.M. Loftus (Eds.). *Textbook of neurological surgery: Principles and practice.* Philadelphia: Lippincott Williams & Wilkins, pp. 1857-1864.

Doolittle, N.D., Miner, M.E., Hall, W.A., et al. (2000). Safety and efficacy of a multicenter study using intraarterial chemotherapy in conjunction with osmotic opening of the blood-brain barrier for the treatment of patients with malignant brain tumors. *Cancer 88*(3), 637-647.

Enam, S.A., Rock, J.P., & Rosenblum, M.L. (2000). Malignant glioma. In M. Bernstein & M.S. Berger (Eds.). *Neuro-oncology: The essentials.* New York: Thieme Medical Publishers, pp. 309-318.

Fehlings, M.G., & Rao, S.C. (2000). Spinal cord and spinal cord tumors. In M. Bernstein & M.S. Berger (Eds.). *Neuro-oncology: The essentials.* New York: Thieme Medical Publishers, pp. 445-464.

Gupta, N., & Rutka, J.T. (2000). Molecular neuro-oncology. In M. Bernstein & M.S. Berger (Eds.). *Neuro-oncology: The essentials.* New York: Thieme Medical Publishers, pp. 30-41.

Hall, W.A. (2002). *Current issues in the management of malignant glioma. A CME monograph,* 1-16. San Antonio: Dannemiller Memorial Educational Foundation and Seiris Corp.

Harsh IV, G.R. (1999). Management of recurrent gliomas. In M.S. Berger & C.B. Wilson (Eds.). *The gliomas.* Philadelphia: W.B. Saunders, pp. 649-659.

Jukich, P.J., McCarthy, B.J., Surawicz, T.S., et al. (2001). Trends in incidence of primary brain tumors in the United States, 1985-1994. *Neuro-oncology 3,* 141-151.

Keles, G.E., & Berger, M.S. (2000). Functional mapping. In M. Bernstein & M.S. Berger (Eds.). *Neruo-oncology: The essentials.* New York: Thieme Medical Publishers, pp. 130-134.

Kondziolka, D., Flickinger, J.C., & Lunsford, L.D. (2000). Stereotactic radiosurgery and radiation therapy. In M. Bernstein & M.S. Berger (Eds.). *Neuro-oncology: The essentials.* New York: Thieme Medical Publishers, pp. 183-197.

LaCroix, M., Abi-Said, D., Fourney, D.R., et al. (2001). A multivariate analysis of 416 patients with glioblastoma multiforme: Prognosis, extent of resection, and survival. *Journal of Neurosurgery 95,* 190-198.

Laperriere, N.J. (2000). Brachytherapy. In M. Bernstein & M.S. Berger (Eds.). *Neuro-oncology: The essentials.* New York: Thieme Medical Publishers, pp. 198-204.

Louis, D.N., & Stemmer-Rachamimov, A.O. (2000). Pathology and classification. In M. Bernstein & M.S. Berger (Eds.). *Neuro-oncology: The essentials.* New York: Thieme Medical Publishers, pp. 18-29.

Macdonald, D.R. (2001). Temozolomide for recurrent high-grade glioma. *Seminars in Oncology 28*(4, Suppl. 13), 3-12.

Martin, A.J., Hall, W.A., Liu, H., et al. (2000). Brain tumor resection: Intraoperative monitoring with high-field strength MR imaging: Initial results. *Radiology 215*(1), 221-228.

Meyers, C.A. (2000). Quality of life of brain tumor patients. In M. Bernstein & M.S. Berger (Eds.). *Neuro-oncology: The essentials.* New York: Thieme Medical Publishers, pp. 466-472.

Prados, M.D., & Levin, V. (2000). Biology and treatment of malignant glioma. *Seminars in Oncology 27*(3, Suppl. 6), 1-10.

Raizer, J.J., & DeAngelis, L.M. (2000). Primary central nervous system lymphoma. In M. Bernstein & M.S. Berger (Eds.). *Neuro-oncology: The essentials.* New York: Thieme Medical Publishers, pp. 377-383.

Schwartz, T.H., & McCormick, P.C. (2003). Intramedullary tumors of the spinal cord. In H.H. Batjer & C.M. Loftus (Eds.). *Textbook of neurological surgery: Principles and practice.* Philadelphia: Lippincott Williams & Wilkins, pp. 1864-1872.

Segal, G. (1998). *A primer of brain tumors: A patient's reference manual.* Chicago: American Brain Tumor Association.

Shelton, B.K. (2000). Preventing crises in the patient with cancer. *Oncology Nursing Forum 27*(6), 905-913.

Spiegelmann, R., & Friedman, W. (1999). Closed biopsy techniques. In M.S. Berger & C.B. Wilson (Eds.). *The gliomas.* Philadelphia: W.B. Saunders, pp. 376-390.

Taylor, M.D., & Rutka, J.T. (2000). Pediatric posterior fossa tumors. In M. Bernstein & M.S. Berger (Eds.). *Neuro-oncology: The essentials.* New York: Thieme Medical Publishers, pp. 363-376.

Wen, P.Y., & Black, P.M. (1999). Clinical presentation, evaluation, and preoperative preparation of the patient. In M.S. Berger & C.B. Wilson (Eds.). *The gliomas.* Philadelphia: W.B. Saunders, pp. 328-336.

Weyerbrock, A., & Oldfield, E.H. (2000). Gene therapy. In M. Bernstein & M.S. Berger (Eds.). *Neuro-oncology: The essentials.* New York: Thieme Medical Publishers, pp. 273-288.

Wrensch, M.R., Minn, Y., & Bondy, M.L. (2000). Epidemiology. In M. Bernstein & M.S. Berger (Eds.). *Neuro-oncology: The essentials.* New York: Thieme Medical Publishers, pp. 2-17.

31 Nursing Care of the Client with Leukemia

MOLLY J. MORAN AND SUSAN EZZONE

Theory

I. Physiology of the hematologic system.
   A. Hematopoiesis is the process of blood cell formation (Figure 31-1) (Wujcik, 2000).
      1. Blood-forming organs include bone marrow, liver, spleen.
         a. Normal bone marrow is essential to develop immunity; maintain hemostasis; transport hemoglobin, oxygen, and carbon dioxide.
         b. Liver and spleen are primarily blood-forming organs in the fetus but are capable of blood cell production in response to demand or disease processes in an adult.
      2. Pluripotent progenitor cell (stem cell) originates in the bone marrow and is responsible for production of all hematopoietic cells.
         a. Pluripotent stem cell is capable of self-replication, proliferation, and differentiation into myeloid and lymphoid stem cells.
         b. Myeloid stem cell differentiates into hematopoietic cells including red blood cells (RBCs), white blood cells (WBCs; neutrophil, eosinophil, basophil, monocyte), platelets.
         c. Lymphoid stem cell differentiates into B and T lymphocytes, which are responsible for activities of the immune system.
II. Pathophysiology of leukemia (Wujcik, 2000).
   A. Leukemia—malignant disorder of blood cells and lymphatic tissue, most commonly involving the WBCs.
      1. Leukemic or malignant cells excessively proliferate, resulting in over-crowding of bone marrow and inability to produce normal-functioning hematopoietic cells.
      2. Leukemic cells are capable of infiltrating and accumulating in other organs (e.g., central nervous system [CNS], eyes, testes, skin). Organ involvement is most common in acute leukemia.
      3. Classification/description of leukemias (Tables 31-1, 31-2, and 31-3) based on predominant cell line affected and level of maturation reached.
      4. Symptoms of leukemia (Table 31-4) attributed to the following:
         a. Type of leukemia cell.
         b. Degree of leukemic cell burden.
         c. Degree of myelosuppression.
         d. Effects of organ involvement.
   B. Leukemia may occur in any phase of the life cycle and is treated over time, from months to years.

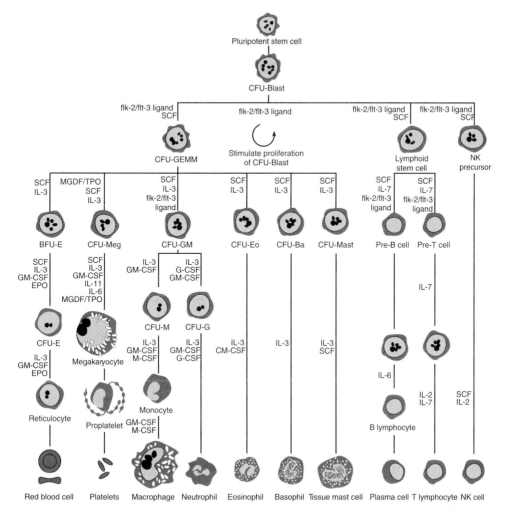

FIGURE 31-1 ■ Hematopoietic tree. All hematopoietic cells are derived from a common stem cell under the influence of various growth factors or combinations of growth factors. *BFU-E*, Erythrocyte burst-forming units; *CFU*, colony-forming units; *CFU-Ba*, basophil CFU; *CFU-Eo*, eosinophil CFU; *CFU-g*, granulocyte CFU; *CFU-GEMM*, granulocyte/erythroid/macrophage/megakaryocyte CFU; *CFU-GM*, granulocyte/macrophage CFU; *CFU-M*, macrophage CFU; *CFU-mast*, mast cell CFU; *CFU-Meg*, megakaryocyte CFU; *NK*, natural killer; *SCF*, stem cell factor; *IL-3*, interleukin-3; *GM-CSF*, granulocyte-macrophage colony-stimulating factor; *Epo*, erythropoietin; *IL-11*, interleukin-11; *IL-6*, interleukin-6; *MGDF*, megakaryocyte growth and development factor; *Tpo*, thrombopoietin; *M-CSF*, macrophage colony-stimulating factor; *G-CSF*, granulocyte colony-stimulating factor; *IL-7*, interleukin-7; *IL-2*, interleukin-2. (Reprinted from Hunt P, Foote MA: The new generation of recombinent human hematopoietic cytokines: *Curr Opin Biotech* 6:692, 1995.)

III. Epidemiology (Table 31-5).
   A. Approximately 33,440 cases of leukemia will be diagnosed in 2004 (acute cases slightly more than chronic) (American Cancer Society [ACS], 2004).
   B. Leukemia occurs in more adults than children (ACS, 2004).
   C. Acute lymphocytic leukemia (ALL) is the most common form of leukemia in children (Westlake & Bertolone, 2002).

TABLE 31-1
French American British (FAB) Classification System of Acute Leukemia

Myeloid	Lymphocytic
M0 Minimally differentiated	
M1 Undifferentiated myelocytic	L1, childhood (pre B- and T-cell)
M2 Myelocytic	L2, adult (pre B- and T-cell)
M3 Promyelocytic	L3, Burkitt's type (B-cell)
M4 Myelomonocytic	
M5 Monocytic	
M6 Erythroleukemia	
M7 Megakaryocytic	

From Wujcik D: Leukemia. In Yarbro CH, Frogge MH, Goodman M, Groenwald SL, editors: *Cancer nursing: principles and practice,* ed 5, Sudbury, Mass, 2000, Jones and Bartlett Publishers, p. 1247.

TABLE 31-2
Rai and Binet Staging Systems for Chronic Lymphocytic Leukemia

Stage	Extent of Disease	Risk	Median Survival (yr)
0	Lymphocytosis of bone marrow (≥40% of lymphocytes) and	Low	0
1	blood (>5000/μl)		
I	Stage 0 plus lymphadenopathy	Intermediate	7
II	Stage 0 or I plus splenomegaly and/or hepatomegaly	Intermediate	7
III	Stage 0, I, or II plus anemia (hemoglobin <11 g/dl)*	High	2
IV	Stage 0, I, or II plus thrombocytopenia (platelets <100,000/μl)*	High	2

From Foon KA: Chronic leukemia. In Mazza JJ, editor: *Manual of clinical hematology,* Philadelphia, 2002, Lippincott Williams & Wilkins, p. 231.
*Excluding anemia or thrombocytopenia caused by immunologic destruction of cells.

TABLE 31-3
Phases of Chronic Myelogenous Leukemia

Phase	Description
Chronic phase	Excessive proliferation and accumulation of mature granulocytes
	Absence of lymphadenopathy
	Splenomegaly
	Philadelphia chromosome (Ph[1]) present in 90% of persons
Accelerated phase	Progressive leukocytosis
	Increased myeloid precursors (including blasts); increased basophils
	Splenomegaly
	Weight loss
	Weakness
	Progressive chromosomal abnormalities
Blast crisis	Presence of 30%-40% blasts or promyelocytes in bone marrow
	Leukostasis
	Microvascular occlusion of the CNS or lungs
	Myeloblastic transformation more common than lymphoblastic
	Resembles AML

Data from Wujcik D: Leukemia. In Yarbro CH, Frogge MH, Goodman M, Groenwald SL, editors: *Cancer nursing: principles and practice,* ed 5, Sudbury, Mass, 2000, Jones and Bartlett Publishers, pp. 1256-1257.
CNS, Central nervous system; *AML,* acute myelogenous leukemia.

TABLE 31-4
Common Clinical Presentation of Leukemia

Diagnosis	Symptoms	Signs	WBC	Platelet	RBC	Other

AML	Fatigue
	Malaise
	Weight loss
	Fever
	Recurrent infections
	Unexplained bleeding
	Palpitations
	Dyspnea
	Anorexia
	Bone pain
	Neurologic complaints
	  Headache
	  Vomiting
	  Visual changes
	  Seizures
		Sudden onset
		Rapid downhill course
		Bone marrow failure
		Anemia
		Thrombocytopenia
		Neutropenia
		Hepatomegaly
		Organ infiltration
		Pale skin
			Myeloblasts
			Low
			Normal
			High
			
			Neutropenia
			ANC <1000 cells/mm^3
				Low	Low	Hyperuricemia
						Elevated lactate
						  dehydrogenase

ALL	Same as AML	Same as AML Lymphadenopathy Splenomegaly	Lymphoblasts Same as AML	Low	Low	
CML	Malaise Anorexia Weight loss Left upper quadrant pain Abdominal fullness Bone and joint pain Fever Night sweats	Insidious onset Pale skin Hepatomegaly Splenomegaly Bleeding disorders Anemia Peripheral blood leukocytosis	Mature myelocytes >100,000 cells/mm^3	Normal or high	Low	High serum B$_{12}$ level Low LAP level

(Continued)

TABLE 31-4
Common Clinical Presentation of Leukemia—cont'd

Diagnosis	Symptoms	Signs	WBC	Platelet	RBC	Other
CLL	Asymptomatic in early stages Recurrent infections Malaise Anorexia Fatigue Early satiety Abdominal discomfort	Insidious onset Splenomegaly Hepatomegaly Lymphadenopathy Anemia Thrombocytopenia Hypogammaglobulinemia Rashes	Small mature or immature lymphocytes B cells >20,000 cells/mm³ in early disease >100,000 cells/mm³ in advanced disease	Low	Low	

WBC, White blood cell; *RBC,* red blood cell; *AML,* acute myelogenous leukemia; *ALL,* acute lymphocytic leukemia; *ANC,* absolute neutrophil count; *CML,* chronic myelogenous leukemia; *LAP,* leukocyte alkaline phosphatase; *CLL,* chronic lymphocytic leukemia.

TABLE 31-5
Overall Remission and Survival Rates for Leukemia

Description	Median Age (yr)	Initial Remission Rate	Median Survival with Treatment
Acute myelogenous leukemia	50-60	60%-70%	10-15 mo
Acute lymphoblastic leukemia	4	Adults: 65%-85%; children: 90%	Adults: 2 yr; children: 5 yr
Chronic myelogenous leukemia	49	90%	3 yr
Chronic lymphocytic leukemia	60	90%	4-6 yr

From Wujcik D: Leukemia. In Yarbro CH, Frogge MH, Goodman, M, Groenwald SL, editors: *Cancer nursing: principles and practice*, ed 5, Sudbury, Mass, 2000, Jones and Bartlett Publishers, p. 1249.

    D. Acute myelogenous leukemia (AML) and chronic lymphocytic leukemia (CLL) are the most common forms in adults (ACS, 2004).
IV. Etiology and risk factors.
    A. Etiology unknown.
    B. Risk factors most often associated—exposure to chemicals and drugs (e.g., alkylating agents), genetic predisposition, exposure to radiation, viruses.
V. Principles of medical management.
    A. Acute leukemia.
      1. AML (also called acute nonlymphocytic leukemia [ANLL]).
        a. Induction—initial treatment with chemotherapy agents given at high doses to eradicate leukemia and achieve complete remission (CR) resulting in bone marrow repopulation with normal cells (<5% blasts) and normal blood counts.
          (1) Induction regimen usually includes cytarabine (cytosine arabinoside, AraC, Cytosar-U) plus an anthracycline. In children, other agents, such as etoposide (VP-16, Etopophos, VePesid) and thioguanine (6-thioguanine, 6-TG), may be added.
          (2) All-trans-retinoic acid (ATRA) is being used as initial treatment in acute promyelocytic leukemia (APL) (M3) along with an anthracycline-based cytotoxic chemotherapeutic agent. ATRA induces differentiation of cells, restoring growth of normal blood cells. In a small subset of clients with acute promyelocytic leukemia (APL), ATRA will not result in cell differentiation (Wujcik, 2000).
          (3) Arsenic trioxide (Trisenox)—U.S. Food and Drug Administration (FDA) approved for use in inducing remission and consolidation in clients with APL who have relapsed or who are refractory with ATRA and an anthracycline-based chemotherapeutic agent (Mayorga et al., 2002).
          (4) Intrathecal cytarabine or methotrexate (Mexate), with or without cranial radiation, is given if CNS leukemia is present. In children, cranial irradiation is incorporated into most protocols and is considered a standard part of treatment.
          (5) Long-term survival for children with M3 leukemia is improving with the use of ATRA and chemotherapy (Landier, 2002).
          (6) Cytokines—use of granulocyte colony-stimulating factors (G-CSFs) or granulocyte-macrophage colony-stimulating factors (GM-CSFs)

after completion of induction therapy is being studied to determine efficacy in modifying granulocytopenia in leukemia treatment. Has been shown to decrease infectious episodes in elderly clients with acute leukemia (Balducci & Carreca, 2002).

  b. Postremission therapy given to reduce leukemic cell population and achieve long-term, disease-free survival (DFS). Includes consolidation, intensification, maintenance, bone marrow transplantation (BMT).

    (1) Consolidation therapy—one or two cycles of the same chemotherapy agents used in the induction therapy. Usually given after remission occurs.

    (2) Intensification therapy—high-dose chemotherapy given immediately or within several months of induction therapy. Same chemotherapy agents may be used at higher doses, or different drugs thought to be cross resistant with induction therapy drugs may be used.

    (3) Maintenance therapy—lower doses of the same drugs used for induction therapy or different drugs given monthly for a prolonged time period to "maintain" a disease-free state. Maintenance therapy not currently recommended in treatment of AML.

      (a) ATRA is not used for maintenance therapy in acute promyelocytic leukemia (M3) because the drug becomes less effective with prolonged therapy (Wujcik, 2000).

    (4) BMT (O'Connell & Schmit-Pokorny, 1997).

      (a) Allogeneic or matched unrelated BMT has become standard therapy for treatment of AML in first remission with long-term DFS rates of 45% to 65%. Transplantation in second or subsequent remissions or relapse decreases DFS to approximately 20% or less. Interest is growing in the use of allogeneic peripheral blood stem cells for transplantation.

      (b) Interest is also growing in nonmyeloablative transplantation using less toxic preparative regimen. Nonmyeloablative transplant may be offered to clients who are elderly or clients with high-risk factors causing them to be ineligible for myeloablative transplantation. Graft-versus-host disease with graft-versus-tumor effect is intended to eradicate disease (Carell & Giralt, 2000).

      (c) Autologous bone marrow or peripheral blood stem cell transplantation is controversial, and further investigation is underway to evaluate risk of disease recurrence.

    (5) Gemtuzumab ozogamicin (Mylotarg)—approved by the FDA to treat clients (60 years of age and older) in first relapse with CD33+ AML and who are not candidates for cytotoxic chemotherapy (Sorokin, 2000).

2. Acute lymphocytic leukemia (ALL).

  a. Prognostic factors used to predict outcomes include cell morphology, age, WBC count at presentation, success of initial induction therapy, chromosomal abnormalities.

  b. Adults (Wujcik, 2000).

    (1) Initial treatment consists of protocol that includes vincristine (Oncovin), prednisone, anthracycline, cyclophosphamide (Cytoxan), with or without asparaginase (Elspar).

    (2) CNS prophylaxis includes intrathecal chemotherapy and/or high-dose systemic chemotherapy and possibly cranial irradiation.

(3) Postremission therapy options include short-term, relatively intensive chemotherapy followed by longer-term therapy at lower doses. Multiple drugs not previously administered may be given.

(4) BMT (O'Connell & Schmit-Pokorny, 1997).

(a) Allogeneic BMT from histocompatible leukocyte sibling human leukocyte antigen (HLA) donor should be considered for treatment of clients younger than age 50 years in first CR with high-risk ALL. Effect on DFS of transplantation in first CR remains to be determined.

(b) Interest is growing in nonmyeloablative transplantation using less toxic preparative regimen. Nonmyeloablative transplant may be offered to clients who are elderly or clients with high-risk factors causing them to be ineligible for myeloablative transplantation. Graft-versus-host disease with graft-versus-tumor effect is intended to eradicate disease (Carell & Giralt, 2000).

(c) Autologous BMT for treatment of ALL is optimally accomplished by collecting marrow during first CR. Various approaches have been used for marrow purging to remove residual leukemic cells. Wide variation in DFS exists because of differences in timing of transplantation and efforts to decrease residual leukemic cells.

c. Children (Westlake & Bertolone, 2002).

(1) Induction chemotherapy regimens consist of prednisone, vincristine, with asparaginase and/or daunorubicin (Cerubidine). Usually the four-drug regimen is limited to use in higher-risk clients because of toxicities.

(a) CNS treatment is given if CNS disease present or as prophylaxis. Treatment may consist of intrathecal methotrexate with or without radiation. Intrathecal therapy with methotrexate, cytarabine, and hydrocortisone may be given.

(2) Postremission (consolidation/intensification and maintenance) therapy continues for 2 to 3 years. Other agents that might be used in consolidation/intensification therapy include the following: cyclophosphamide, cytarabine, etoposide, ifosfamide (Ifex), methotrexate. Numerous drug combinations and schedules are used for maintenance. Low-risk ALL is treated with methotrexate and mercaptopurine (6-MP, Purinethol) with or without vincristine and prednisone. Additional drugs are used for intermediate and high-risk ALL.

(3) BMT.

(a) Allogeneic BMT for treatment of ALL in children should be considered if relapse occurs within 18 months of therapy or during therapy. Estimated DFS for clients transplanted in second CR is 40% to 62%.

(b) Autologous BMT for children with ALL generally is not a treatment option because most clients have high-risk disease, and transplantation in first CR is not possible.

B. Chronic leukemia (Wujcik, 2000).

1. Chronic myelogenous leukemia (CML).

a. Chronic phase.

(1) Two commonly used agents are hydroxyurea (Hydrea, Mylocel) and busulfan (Myleran). These oral agents are used to control

leukocytosis but do not eradicate disease or induce cytogenetic remission.

(2) Alpha-2a interferon is being used in chronic phase.

b. Accelerated phase of CML is treated with increasing doses of chemotherapy with generally poor results.

c. Blastic crisis (Wujcik, 2000).

(1) Transformation into lymphoid leukemia—treatment is similar to that for ALL using combinations of vincristine and prednisone.

(2) Transformation in myeloid leukemia—treatment is similar to that for AML and includes investigational protocols.

(3) Hydroxyurea may be given for palliation.

(4) Radiation therapy (RT) may be given for lytic bone lesions.

(5) CNS or meningeal disease may be treated with intrathecal methotrexate, cytarabine, or cranial irradiation.

d. Imatinib mesylate (Gleevec)—approved by the FDA for treating CML (chronic phase, accelerated phase, or blast crisis) after alpha-2a interferon failure (Broder, 2001).

e. BMT (O'Connell & Schmit-Pokorny, 1997).

(1) Allogeneic or syngeneic BMT may be used as effective treatment for CML and may result in long-term DFS. Controversy exists regarding optimal timing of undergoing BMT. According to the International Bone Marrow Transplant Registry (IBMTR) data, clients undergoing BMT in chronic phase have a 50% to 60% long-term DFS, whereas in accelerated and blastic phases, DFS is estimated to be 35% to 40% and 10% to 20%, respectively.

(2) Interest is growing in nonmyeloablative transplantation using less toxic preparative regimen. Nonmyeloablative transplant may be offered to clients who are elderly or clients with high-risk factors causing them to be ineligible for myeloablative transplantation. Graft-versus-host disease with graft-versus-tumor effect is intended to eradicate disease (Carell & Giralt, 2000).

(3) Autologous bone marrow or peripheral blood stem cell transplantation for treatment of chronic or transformed CML has been used with varying results. Stem cells are collected during the chronic phase of the disease with the intent to reinfuse the cells following myeloablative therapy.

2. Chronic lymphocytic leukemia (CLL) (Wujcik, 2000).

a. Treatment is delayed until the client is symptomatic, such as exhibiting signs of hemolytic anemia, cytopenia, lymphadenopathy that is painful and/or disfiguring, or symptomatic organomegaly.

b. Disease is followed by monitoring lymphocyte count.

c. Chlorambucil (Leukeran) is used to suppress production of well-differentiated, small lymphocytes.

d. Cyclophosphamide inhibits growth of less mature lymphocytes with limited effect on neutrophils and platelets.

e. Leukocytosis and immune-mediated cytopenias can be controlled by use of corticosteroids. Splenectomy may be used for symptom relief when steroids are no longer effective.

f. RT is effective treatment for lymphadenopathy and/or splenomegaly that is painful.

      g. Fludarabine (Fludara) has been approved for treatment of B-cell CLL.

      h. Newest treatment approach is the use of monoclonal antibody treatment—rituximab (Rituxan) for CD+ lymphocytes and alemtuzumab (Campath-1H) (Seeley & DeMeyer, 2002).

      i. BMT—clinical trials are currently underway to evaluate the use of myeloablative and nonmyeloablative stem cell transplantation for the treatment of CLL (Carell & Giralt, 2000).

    3. Hairy cell leukemia (Wujcik, 2000).

      a. Decision to treat is based on presence of symptomatic cytopenias, massive splenomegaly, or other complications.

      b. 10% of clients will never require treatment.

      c. Treatment options.

        (1) 2-Chlorodeoxyadenosine (2-CdA) (Cladribine).

        (2) Pentostatin (Nipent).

        (3) Alpha-interferon.

        (4) Splenectomy is rare but indicated when the client has low WBC count, splenomegaly, and minimal bone marrow involvement.

Assessment

I. Client history.

  A. Exposure to radiation.

    1. Previous treatment with RT.

    2. Accidental exposure through environmental sources of radiation.

    3. Exposure to radiation in the work setting.

  B. Exposure to chemicals.

    1. Previous treatment with antineoplastic agents (e.g., alkylating agents, etoposide).

    2. Previous treatment with medications such as chloramphenicol, phenylbutazone.

    3. Accidental or work-related exposure to chemicals (e.g., benzene).

  C. Exposure to viruses.

    1. Human immunodeficiency virus (HIV) associated with T-cell lymphocytic leukemia.

    2. Epstein-Barr virus (EBV).

  D. Genetic abnormalities.

    1. Down syndrome.

    2. Turner's syndrome.

    3. Bloom's syndrome.

    4. Klinefelter's syndrome.

    5. Fanconi's anemia.

    6. Neurofibromatosis.

    7. Ataxia telangiectasia.

  E. Family history of genetic abnormalities or cancer.

  F. Chief complaint (see Table 31-4, symptoms).

  G. Psychosocial profile.

II. Physical examination.

  A. Head and neck—pale mucous membranes, bleeding gums, lymphadenopathy.

  B. Abdomen—hepatomegaly, splenomegaly.

  C. Neurologic—headache, papilledema, meningismus, abnormal cranial nerve responses.

   D. Respiratory—abnormal lung sounds if pneumonia is present.
   E. Cardiovascular—tachycardia, murmurs.
   F. Musculoskeletal—joint pain and inflammation.
   G. Integumentary—bruising, ecchymoses, petechiae.
   H. Lymph nodes—cervical, supraclavicular, axillary, mediastinal, or inguinal lymphadenopathy.
   I. Genitourinary—urinary tract infections, hematuria, testicular mass, menorrhagia.
III. Diagnostic studies.
   A. Complete blood count with WBC differential (see Table 31-4 for values at diagnosis for each type of leukemia).
      1. Thrombocytopenia.
      2. Anemia.
      3. Abnormal differential.
         a. Neutropenia.
         b. Leukocytosis.
         c. Blasts.
   B. Other blood tests.
      1. Liver function tests (e.g., for elevated lactate dehydrogenase [LDH]).
      2. Uric acid (hyperuricemia).
   C. Bone marrow aspirate and biopsy.
      1. Cell morphology.
      2. Immunophenotype.
      3. Cellularity.
      4. Cytogenetic analysis (important for diagnosis and prognosis).
   D. Cerebrospinal studies.
      1. Increased protein.
      2. Decreased glucose.
      3. Leukemic cells.

Nursing Diagnoses

   I. Deficient knowledge related to type of leukemia and rationale for treatment.
  II. Risk for injury.
 III. Risk for infection.
  IV. Ineffective coping.
   V. Compromised family coping.

Outcome Identification

    I. Client and family describe the type of leukemia and rationale for treatment.
   II. Client and family list signs and symptoms of immediate and long-term effects of leukemia and treatment.
  III. Client lists self-care measures to decrease the incidence and severity of symptoms and complications associated with disease and treatment.
   IV. Client demonstrates skills in self-care necessary because of effects of disease and treatment.
    V. Client and family describe schedule and procedures for routine follow-up care, including blood work, bone marrow biopsy, and lumbar puncture.
   VI. Client and family list signs and symptoms of recurrent disease.
  VII. Client and family describe potential community resources available to assist with diagnosis, treatment, rehabilitation, survivorship.

Planning and Implementation

I. Interventions to decrease the incidence and severity of complications unique to leukemia.
   A. Myelosuppression (see Chapter 13).
   B. Septic shock (see Chapter 18).
   C. Disseminated intravascular coagulation (DIC) (see Chapter 18).
II. Interventions for management of unique side effects of disease or treatment.
   A. Myelosuppression (see Chapter 13).
   B. Septic shock (see Chapter 18).
   C. DIC (see Chapter 18).
   D. Tumor lysis syndrome (see Chapter 18).
   E. Mucositis (see Chapter 14).
   F. Leukostasis.
      1. Physiologic effect—increase in blood viscosity that may result in obstruction of the microcirculation or formation of thrombi of WBCs in small vessels, resulting in capillary plugging, vessel rupture, bleeding, and organ damage.
      2. Clients at risk—diagnosis of acute or chronic leukemia with a WBC count greater than 50,000 to 100,000/mm^3.
      3. Most common sites.
         a. Brain/CNS.
         b. Lung.
         c. Other organs may be involved.
      4. Most common signs.
         a. Increased intracranial pressure (see also Chapter 19).
         b. Respiratory distress.
         c. Other signs depend on organs involved.
      5. Most common complications.
         a. Pulmonary hemorrhage.
         b. Cerebral hemorrhage.
      6. Medical management.
         a. Initiation of chemotherapy to treat the disease process.
         b. Initiation of leukapheresis to temporarily decrease the WBC count.
         c. Administration of intravenous (IV) fluids.
         d. Initiation of cranial radiation if appropriate.
      7. Nursing interventions.
         a. Frequency of monitoring dependent on individual client and symptoms. General guidelines are as follows:
            (1) Perform neurologic examination every 2 to 4 hours when the WBC count is greater than 50,000 to 100,000/mm^3.
            (2) Monitor vital signs including blood pressure every 2 to 4 hours.
               (a) Assess respiratory rate, depth, effort, and effectiveness every 2 to 4 hours.
               (b) Auscultate lung sounds.
            (3) Monitor for signs of bleeding every 2 to 4 hours.
            (4) Interventions for management of myelosuppression (see Chapter 13).
            (5) Contact physician with any aberrant findings.
         b. Initiate safety measures as appropriate.
   G. Cerebellar toxicity.
   H. Chemotherapy-induced acral erythema (hand-foot syndrome).
   I. Retinoic acid syndrome.

   III. Interventions for management of vascular access devices (see Chapter 9).

   IV. Interventions for management of alterations in coping.

      A. Psychosocial issues (see Chapter 2).

      B. Altered body image and alopecia (see Chapter 3).

      C. Cultural issues (see Chapter 4).

      D. Survivorship issues (see Chapter 5).

   V. Interventions for management of sexuality concerns or abnormalities (see Chapter 6).

   VI. Interventions for supportive care related to death and dying issues (see Chapter 7).

   VII. Interventions for rehabilitation (see Chapter 8).

Evaluation

The oncology nurse systematically and regularly evaluates the client's and/or family's responses to interventions to determine progress toward the achievement of expected outcomes. Relevant data are collected, and actual findings are compared with expected findings. Nursing diagnoses, outcomes, and plans of care are reviewed and revised as necessary.

REFERENCES

American Cancer Society (ACS). (2004). *Cancer facts and figures—2004*. Atlanta: Author.

Balducci, L., & Carreca, I. (2002). The role of myelopoietic growth factors in managing cancer in the elderly. *Drugs 62*(Suppl. 1), 47-63.

Broder, B. (2001). *Understanding chronic myeloid leukemia: Current and new therapies*. East Hanover, NJ: Novartis Pharmaceuticals Corporation, pp. 1-12.

Carell, A.M., & Giralt, S. (2000). Novel preparative regimens II: Non-myeloablative regimens. In J.M. Rowe, H.M. Lazarus, & A.M. Carella (Eds.). *Handbook of bone marrow transplantation*. Malden, MA: Blackwell Science, pp. 95-110.

Foon, K. (2002). Chronic leukemia. In J.J. Mazza (Ed.). *Manual of clinical hematology* (3rd ed.). Philadelphia: Lippincott Williams & Wilkins, pp. 228-231.

Landier, W. (2002). Myeloid diseases. In C.R. Baggott, K.P. Kelly, D. Fochtman, & G.V. Foley (Eds). *Nursing care of children and aldolescents with cancer* (3rd ed.). Philadelphia: W.B. Saunders, pp. 491-502. .

Mayorga, J. Richardson-Hardin, C., & Dicke, K.A. (2002). Arsenic trioxide as effective therapy for relapsed acute promyelocytic leukemia. *Clinical Journal of Oncology Nursing 6*(6), 341-346.

O'Connell, S., & Schmit-Pokorny, K. (1997). Blood and marrow stem cell transplantation: Indications, procedure, process. In M.B. Whedon & D. Wujcik (Eds.). *Blood and marrow stem cell transplantation: Principles, practice and nursing insights*. Sudbury, MA: Jones and Bartlett Publishers, pp. 66-99.

Seeley, K., & DeMeyer, E. (2002). Nursing care of patients receiving Campath. *Clinical Journal of Oncology Nursing 6*(3), 138-143.

Sorokin, P. (2000). Mylotarg approved for patients with CD33+ acute myelogenous leukemia. *Clinical Journal of Oncology Nursing 4*(6), 279-280.

Westlake, S.K., & Bertolone, K.L. (2002). Acute lymphoblastic leukemia. In C.R. Baggott, K.P. Kelly, D. Fochtman, & G.V. Foley (Eds.). *Nursing care of children and adolescents with cancer* (3rd ed.). Philadelphia: W.B. Saunders, pp. 466-490.

Wujcik, D. (2000). Leukemia. In C.H. Yarbro, M.H. Frogge, M. Goodman, & S.L. Groenwald (Eds.). *Cancer nursing: Principles and practice* (5th ed.). Sudbury, MA: Jones and Bartlett Publishers, pp. 1244-1268.

32 Nursing Care of the Client with Lymphoma or Multiple Myeloma

RYAN R. IWAMOTO

Theory

I. Physiology of the lymphoid system.
   A. Primitive or pluripotent stem cell, located in the bone marrow, is progenitor for both myeloid and lymphoid cell lines (Armitage et al., 2001; Armitage & Weisenburger, 1998).
   B. Primary lymphoid tissues are the bone marrow and the thymus.
      1. Lymphocytes develop from committed lymphoid stem cells in the bone marrow.
      2. A portion migrates to the thymus.
         a. These cells proliferate and mature into T cells.
         b. In adults, T cells continue to proliferate peripherally.
      3. Lymphoid cells maturing in the bone marrow become B cells.
         a. Mature B cells, known as plasma cells, produce immune globulins (antibodies).
   C. Secondary lymphoid tissues.
      1. Lymph nodes, spleen, Waldeyer's ring (oropharyngeal lymphoid tissue).
      2. Groups of cells in the gut, called Peyer's patches.
      3. Lymphoid cells in the epithelium of the gut and respiratory tract called mucosa-associated lymphoid tissue (MALT).
      4. Distributed in interstitium and in most tissues, except in the central nervous system.
   D. Cells of the lymphoid system include the following:
      1. T cells and B cells.
      2. Monocytes (peripheral blood) and macrophages (tissues).
      3. Reticular supporting cells, which form the lymph node structure.
      4. Dendritic (Langerhans') cells, found in the skin as well as lymph nodes.
      5. See Chapter 21 for information on function of the immune system.
II. Malignancies of the lymphoid system.
   A. Hodgkin's disease.
      1. Incidence.
         a. Estimated 7880 new cases diagnosed and 1320 deaths from Hodgkin's disease in 2004 (Jemal et al., 2004).
         b. Slightly more men than women develop this disease.
         c. Age-related bimodal incidence: first peak occurs in third decade of life, and second peak occurs after age 50 years.
      2. Etiology: unclear, may be associated with viral etiology (Epstein-Barr virus) or immune disorder (Diehl et al., 2001).

3. Malignant cell is Reed-Sternberg cell (Dalla-Favera & Gaidano, 2001; Diehl et al., 2001; Yarbro, 2000).
   a. Cells express antigens characteristic of activated B and T cells.
   b. Cells also have characteristics of reticular cells.
   c. Hodgkin's disease may actually be a group of related diseases.
4. Clinical presentation (Diehl et al., 2001).
   a. Enlarged lymph nodes with or without systemic symptoms.
      (1) Cervical, supraclavicular, or mediastinal regions most common.
      (2) Tends to spread first to adjacent lymph nodes. Immune suppression before treatment is common.
   b. Systemic symptoms include fever, weight loss, and night sweats.
B. Non-Hodgkin's lymphoma (NHL).
   1. Incidence.
      a. Estimated 54,370 new cases diagnosed and 19,410 deaths from NHL in 2004 (Jemal et al., 2004).
      b. NHL accounts for 4% of new cancers and 4% of cancer-related deaths in men and women in the United States (Jemal et al., 2004).
   2. Etiology (Armitage et al., 2001).
      a. Cause of most cases of NHL is unknown.
      b. Immunodeficiency: inherited, acquired, solid organ transplantation.
      c. Infectious agents: Epstein-Barr virus associated with Burkitt's lymphoma.
      d. Environmental and occupational exposure to chemical, pesticides, and solvents.
   3. Malignancies of T and B lymphocytes (Armitage et al., 2001; Dalla-Favera & Gaidano, 2001; Yarbro, 2000).
      a. A collection of diseases rather than a single disease.
      b. Majority are B-cell neoplasms, some are T-cell neoplasms.
   4. Rarely diagnosed as a single involved lymph node or region.
      a. Most often presents as disseminated disease.
      b. Involvement of bone marrow, liver, or other extranodal site is common.
   5. Aggressiveness and prognosis vary among types.
C. Myeloma.
   1. Incidence.
      a. Estimated 15,270 new cases diagnosed and 11,070 deaths from multiple myeloma in 2004 (Jemal et al., 2004).
      b. Median age at onset is 68 years.
   2. Etiology (Munshi et al., 2001).
      a. Environmental exposure to ionizing radiation.
      b. Exposure to low-level radiation (e.g., radiologists, those employed in the nuclear industry or who handle radioactive materials).
      c. Exposure to metals (especially nickel), agricultural chemicals, benzene and petroleum products, aromatic hydrocarbons, and silicone.
      d. Hereditary and genetic factors.
   3. Malignancy of the plasma cell, a B cell that has differentiated to produce immunoglobulins (Munshi et al., 2001; Otto, 2001; Sheridan & Serrano, 2000; Yarbro, 2000).
      a. Although a solitary plasmacytoma can occur, multiple myeloma, by definition, is a systemic disease.
      b. Myeloma cells produce abnormally high blood levels of monoclonal immunoglobulins.
         (1) Referred to as M (monoclonal) protein.
         (2) Not effective in immune function.

      c. Myeloma cells also produce osteoclast-activating factor (possibly inter-leukin-1 beta).
         (1) Produces lytic bone lesions, resulting in a "punched out" appear-ance on radiographs and often in pathologic fractures.
         (2) Increases bone resorption, which can cause hypercalcemia.
    4. Clinical presentation.
      a. Occasionally diagnosed with routine laboratory tests as an elevated blood protein or anemia.
      b. Commonly presents with bone pain resulting from lytic lesions.
      c. Renal insufficiency is common owing to hypercalcemia, hyperviscos-ity, or deposits of amyloids or immunoglobulins.

III. Diagnostic measures.
  A. Hodgkin's disease (Diehl et al., 2001; Yarbro, 2000).
    1. Excisional lymph node biopsy is required.
    2. Diagnosis requires presence of Reed-Sternberg cells on pathologic exami-nation.
  B. Non-Hodgkin's lymphoma: excisional lymph node biopsy is required for diagnosis and differentiation of types of non-Hodgkin's lymphoma (Armitage et al., 2001; Yarbro, 2000).
  C. Multiple myeloma (Munshi et al., 2001; Sheridan & Serrano, 2000).
    1. Bone marrow biopsy demonstrates presence of more than 10% plasma cells.
    2. Serum protein immunoelectrophoresis demonstrates increased levels of heavy-chain M proteins.
    3. Urine protein immunoelectrophoresis demonstrates increased levels of light-chain M proteins (Bence Jones proteins).

IV. Classification.
  A. Hodgkin's disease.
    1. Pathologic classification and grade (Dalla-Favera & Gaidano, 2001; Diehl et al., 2001).
      a. Lymphocyte predominance, nodular.
      b. Lymphocyte predominance, diffuse.
      c. Mixed cellularity.
      d. Nodular sclerosis.
      e. Lymphocyte depletion.
    2. Staging.
      a. Hodgkin's disease is staged on the extent of disease and the presence or absence of systemic symptoms ("B" symptoms) (Diehl et al., 2001; Greene et al., 2002).
      b. Ann Arbor staging system.
         (1) Stage I—single lymph node region or structure.
         (2) Stage II—two or more lymph node regions, same side of diaphragm.
         (3) Stage III—lymph nodes on both sides of diaphragm.
         (4) Stage IV—extranodal sites.
         (5) If the client has fever, night sweats, or weight loss (>10% of body weight), "B" designation is added to stage. If the client does not have these symptoms, this is designated with the letter "A."
      c. Cotswald modifications to the Ann Arbor system.
         (1) Further subdivided stages based on bulk and location of disease and response to therapy.
      d. Staging workup is completed to determine extent of disease.

(1) History, physical, chest x-ray examination, and complete blood count (CBC).

(2) Computed tomography (CT) scans of the chest, abdomen, and pelvis.

(3) Lymphangiogram may be completed if the CT scan result is negative.

(4) Staging laparotomy should be completed only if results will alter the initial treatment plan.

3. Prognosis is related to pathologic classification, stage, age of the client, and response to treatment (Diehl et al., 2001).

   a. For early-stage disease, 10-year survival rates are near 90%.

   b. In treated, advanced disease, 10-year survival is more than 50%.

B. Non-Hodgkin's lymphoma.

1. Pathologic classification and grade.

   a. Revised European-American Classification of Lymphoid Neoplasms (REAL)/World Health Organization (WHO) (Armitage & Weisenburger, 1998; Harris et al., 1994; Jaffe et al., 2001) (Box 32-1).

      (1) Standard classification system for NHL and clinical trials in lymphoma.

      (2) Categorizes lymphoid malignancies using morphologic, immunophenotype, and genetic information.

      (3) Lists disease entities with varying aggressiveness and prognoses.

   b. International Working Formulation (IWF) divides lymphomas into grades (The International Non-Hodgkin's Lymphoma Prognostic Factors Project, 1993).

      (1) Low, intermediate, and high.

      (2) Low-grade lymphomas are indolent; intermediate and high-grade lymphomas are aggressive.

2. Ann Arbor staging with Cotswald modifications (Greene et al., 2002).

   a. Staging workup includes history, physical, chest x-ray examination, blood counts, other blood studies, abdominal-pelvic CT scans.

   b. Lymphangiogram may be performed.

   c. Bilateral bone marrow biopsy is required.

   d. Staging laparotomy is no longer recommended.

3. Prognosis depends on grade or aggressiveness of lymphoma and responsiveness to treatment.

   a. Low-grade lymphomas have an indolent course with prolonged survival (10 to 15 years) without aggressive therapy. Low-grade NHL is characterized by recurrences. Occasionally low-grade NHL can transform into high-grade NHL.

   b. Prognosis of aggressive histology lymphomas depends on tumor bulk, responsiveness to therapy, and the client's ability to tolerate treatment.

      (1) International Prognostic Index (IPI) (The International Non-Hodgkin's Lymphoma Prognostic Factors Project, 1993).

         (a) Predictive model of outcome for aggressive NHL.

         (b) Five risk factors were identified that predicted lower complete response, relapse-free survival, and overall survival (Table 32-1).

   c. Relapse may occur requiring biopsy and restaging.

C. Multiple myeloma.

1. Multiple myeloma (plasma cell myeloma/plasmacytoma) is included in the REAL/WHO classification system (Harris et al., 1994; Jaffe et al., 2001).

BOX 32-1
REAL/WHO CLASSIFICATION OF LYMPHOMAS

B-Cell Neoplasms
PRECURSOR B-CELL NEOPLASM
- Precursor B-lymphoblastic leukemia/lymphoma (precursor B-cell acute lymphoblastic leukemia)

MATURE (PERIPHERAL) B-CELL NEOPLASMS
- B-cell chronic lymphocytic leukemia/small lymphocytic lymphoma
- B-cell prolymphocytic leukemia
- Lymphoplasmacytic lymphoma
- Splenic marginal zone B-cell lymphoma (with or without villous lymphocytes)
- Hairy cell leukemia
- Plasma cell myeloma/plasmacytoma (multiple myeloma)
- Extranodal marginal zone B-cell lymphoma of MALT type
- Nodal marginal zone B-cell lymphoma (with or without monocytoid B cells)
- Follicular lymphoma
- Mantle cell lymphoma
- Diffuse large B-cell lymphoma
- Burkitt's lymphoma/Burkitt's cell leukemia

T-Cell and NK-Cell Neoplasms
PRECURSOR T-CELL NEOPLASM
- Precursor T-lymphoblastic lymphoma/leukemia (precursor T-cell acute lymphoblastic leukemia)

Mature (Peripheral) T-Cell and NK-Cell Neoplasms
- T-cell prolymphocytic leukemia
- T-cell granular lymphocytic leukemia
- Aggressive NK-cell leukemia
- Adult T-cell lymphoma/leukemia (HTLV1+)
- Extranodal NK-cell and T-cell lymphoma, nasal type
- Enteropathy-type T-cell lymphoma
- Hepatosplenic $\gamma\delta$ T-cell lymphoma
- Subcutaneous panniculitis-like T-cell lymphoma
- Mycosis fungoides/Sézary syndrome
- Anaplastic large cell lymphoma, T/null cell, primary cutaneous type
- Peripheral T-cell lymphoma, not otherwise characterized
- Angioimmunoblastic T-cell lymphoma
- Anaplastic large cell lymphoma, T/null cell, primary systemic type

Data from Armitage JO, Weisenburger D, for the Non-Hodgkin's Lymphoma Classification Project: new approach to classifying non-Hodgkin's lymphomas: clinical features of the major histologic subtypes, *J Clin Oncol* 16(8):2780-2795, 1998; Harris NL, Jaffe ES, Stein H, et al: A revised European-American classification of lymphoid neoplasms: A proposal from the International Lymphoma Study Group, *Blood* 84(5):1361-1392, 1994; Jaffe ES et al, editors: *World Health Organization classification of tumours. Pathology and genetics of tumours of haematopoietic and lymphoid tissues*, Lyon, 2001, IARC Press.
REAL, Revised European-American Classification of Lymphoid Neoplasms; *WHO*, World Health Organization. *MALT*, mucosa-associated lymphoid tissue; *NK*, natural killer.

2. Staging quantifies tumor volume on the basis of hemoglobin level, M proteins in urine and blood, serum calcium level, and presence of bone lesions.
3. Although median survival time from diagnosis is 10 years, most clients with multiple myeloma die of the disease.

TABLE 32-1
International Prognostic Index (IPI)

IPI Risk Factors	Favorable (0 points)	Unfavorable (1 point)*
Age (yr)	≤60	>60
Ann Arbor tumor stage	I or II	III or IV
Number of extranodal sites	≤1	>1
Performance status (ECOG)	0 or 1	≥2
Serum LDH level	Normal	Abnormal

IPI Risk	
Low	0-1
Intermediate	2
High intermediate	3
High	4-5

From The International Non-Hodgkin's Lymphoma Prognostic Factors Project: a predictive model for aggressive non-Hodgkin's lymphoma, *N Engl J Med* 329(14):987-994, 1993.
ECOG, Eastern Cooperative Oncology Group; *LDH,* lactate dehydrogenase.
*The unfavorable risk factors are summed to determine the IPI risk for lower complete response, relapse-free survival, and overall survival.

V. Treatment (Box 32-2).
  A. Hodgkin's disease (Diehl et al., 2001; Yarbro, 2000).
      1. Stage I or IIA.
          a. External beam radiation therapy (RT).
          b. Chemotherapy followed by RT.
              (1) ABVD (Adriamycin [doxorubicin], bleomycin, vinblastine, dacarbazine.
              (2) MOPP (mechlorethamine, Oncovin [vincristine], procarbazine, prednisone).
              (3) ABVD/MOPP in alternating cycles.
      2. Stage II.
          a. Chemotherapy followed by RT or chemotherapy alone.
          b. With bulky mediastinal disease—chemotherapy followed by RT.
      3. Advanced disease (stage III or IV): combination chemotherapy or chemotherapy followed by RT.
      4. Salvage therapy for clients who suffer a relapse after chemotherapy.
          a. No standard approach.
          b. Alternative chemotherapy (crossover to MOPP or ABVD if not previously used) or, if more than 1 year has passed since treatment, repeat previously used chemotherapy.
          c. Autologous marrow or peripheral blood stem cell (PBSC) transplantation following high-dose chemotherapy has produced complete remission rates of 40% to 70%.
  B. Non-Hodgkin's lymphoma (Armitage et al., 2001; National Comprehensive Cancer Network, 2002; Yarbro, 2000).
      1. Follicular (low-grade), stage I or II disease.
          a. RT (locoregional treatment).
          b. Monoclonal antibodies (rituximab [Rituxan]).

BOX 32-2
TREATMENT OF LYMPHOID MALIGNANCIES

Hodgkin's Disease
Radiation therapy
- External beam radiation therapy for stage I or IIA
- Radiation therapy following chemotherapy for stage II, III, IV, or bulky disease may be considered
Chemotherapy
- Combination chemotherapy for stages IIB, III, and IV
- ABVD Adriamycin [doxorubicin], bleomycin, vinblastine, dacarbazine) alone or in combination with MOPP (mechlorethamine, Oncovin (vincristine), procarbazine, prednisone)
Salvage therapy
- Alternative chemotherapy regimen, or
- Autologous bone marrow or peripheral blood stem cell (PBSC) transplant

Non-Hodgkin's Lymphoma
FOLLICULAR (LOW-GRADE) LYMPHOMA
Radiation therapy
- Stage I or II disease
Monoclonal antibodies
Rituximab
Chemotherapy
- Single-agent or combination chemotherapy regimens, including cyclophosphamide, doxorubicin, vincristine (Oncovin), prednisone (CHOP); other combination chemotherapy regimens for relapsed disease
Observation
- Asymptomatic disease
Salvage therapy
- Autologous PBSC, allogeneic PBSC, or bone marrow transplant

DIFFUSE LARGE B-CELL (INTERMEDIATE AND HIGH-GRADE/AGGRESSIVE) LYMPHOMA
Chemotherapy
- Combination chemotherapy regimens, including CHOP
Radiation therapy
- Stage I or II disease, used in combination with chemotherapy

SALVAGE THERAPY
- Other chemotherapy regimens, autologous PBSC, allogeneic PBSC, or bone marrow transplantation

Multiple Myeloma
Chemotherapy
- Melphalan and prednisone, or VAD (vincristine, doxorubicin [Adriamycin], dexamethasone)
- Interferon
- Autologous bone marrow transplant or PBSC transplant as consolidation for appropriate clients
Radiation therapy
- Palliative radiation therapy for symptomatic lesions
Salvage therapy
- Autologous PBSC, allogeneic PBSC, or bone marrow transplant

Data from Diehl V, Mauch PM, Harris NL: Hodgkin's disease. In DeVita V, Jr, Hellman S, Rosenberg S, editors: *Cancer: principles and practice of oncology*, ed 6, Philadelphia, 2001, Lippincott Williams & Wilkins, pp. 2339-2387; National Comprehensive Cancer Network: Non-Hodgkin's lymphoma. In *Practice guidelines in oncology-v.1.2002*, National Comprehensive Cancer Network, 2002, Rockledge, P; Otto S: Multiple myeloma. In Otto S, editor: *Oncology nursing*, ed 4, St Louis, 2001, Mosby, pp. 439-446; Sheridan C, Serrano M: Multiple myeloma. In Yarbro CH, Frogge MH, Goodman M, Groenwald, SL, editors: *Cancer nursing: principles and practice,* ed 5, Sudbury, Mass, 2000, Jones and Bartlett Publishers, pp. 1354-1370.

      c. Chemotherapy (single-agent or combination therapy).

      d. Observation until symptomatic.

  2. Diffuse large B-cell (intermediate and high-grade/aggressive) NHLs are considered systemic disease and treated with combination chemotherapy.

      a. Regimens generally include cyclophosphamide (Cytoxan), doxorubicin, vincristine, and prednisone given on a complex schedule.

      b. Other drugs including rituximab may also be used.

      c. In stage I or II disease, RT may be used with chemotherapy.

  3. Recurrent non-Hodgkin's lymphoma.

      a. Other chemotherapy regimens.

      b. Autologous PBSC, allogeneic PBSC, or bone marrow transplantation (Holmberg & Stewart, 2003).

C. Multiple myeloma (Munshi et al., 2001; Otto, 2001; Sheridan & Serrano, 2000).

  1. Chemotherapy for symptomatic disease.

      a. Melphalan (Alkeran) and prednisone, or vincristine, doxorubicin, dexamethasone (Decadron) (VAD) has shown excellent response rates.

      b. Interferon alpha inhibits plasma cell growth and may prove useful.

  2. RT for symptomatic lesions.

  3. Autologous PBSC transplantation has produced complete response in almost 50% of clients, up to 70 years of age, when used as consolidation.

  4. Allogeneic PBSC or bone marrow transplant has shown benefit, but the technique is limited because of age of clients and lack of appropriate donors.

  5. Bisphosphonates.

  6. Thalidomide (Thalomid).

Assessment

I. During diagnosis and staging.

  A. Personal and family history.

    1. Age.

      a. Hodgkin's disease is more common in young adults with a second peak in older adults.

      b. Non-Hodgkin's lymphoma incidence increases with age.

      c. Peak incidence of multiple myeloma is about 60 years of age.

    2. Family history of Hodgkin's disease in first-degree relatives increases risk.

    3. Personal history of immunosuppression increases risk of lymphoma (human immunodeficiency virus [HIV] disease, solid organ or other transplant).

    4. Symptoms prompting client to seek treatment.

      a. Enlarged lymph nodes.

      b. Presence of B symptoms.

        (1) Fever.

        (2) Night sweats.

        (3) Anorexia and/or weight loss.

        (4) Weakness, shortness of breath.

      c. Presence of pain, especially bone pain.

      d. Changes in urinary function from tumor-related ureteral obstruction.

B. Physical examination.
   1. Palpation of enlarged lymph nodes.
   2. Palpation of liver and spleen for enlargement.
   3. Neurologic examination for deficits.
C. Coping skills.
   1. Feelings about staging procedures and possible diagnosis.
   2. Coping strategies used in the past.
   3. Effectiveness of previous coping strategies.
D. Social situation.
   1. Ability to keep appointments for diagnosis and staging procedures.
      a. Transportation.
      b. Economic issues.
      c. Understanding of need for procedures.
   2. Additional stresses in home and family.
   3. Social support systems.
E. Knowledge of procedures and potential outcomes.
II. During treatment.
   A. Side effects of therapy (see Chapters 36 and 38).
      1. Laboratory values: neutropenia, thrombocytopenia, electrolyte abnormalities.
      2. Symptoms of infection or bleeding.
      3. Nutritional deficits, anorexia, nausea and vomiting.
      4. Fatigue.
   B. Symptoms of oncologic emergencies.
      1. Tumor lysis syndrome can occur during initial treatment of lymphoma (Lyden, 2000).
      2. Hypercalcemia associated with tumor lysis syndrome can occur (Myers, 2001).
      3. Clients with lymphoma or Hodgkin's disease who have mediastinal disease must be observed for superior vena cava syndrome (Sitton, 2000; Yarbro, 2000).
      4. Chapters 18 and 19 give specific assessment parameters for these emergencies.
   C. Presence of bone pain and effectiveness of measures to manage pain.
   D. Mobility and ability to perform activities of daily living.
   E. Body image and adaptation to illness.
III. Rehabilitation phase.
   A. Sexual or endocrine dysfunction.
   B. Symptoms of second malignancies.
      1. Treatment with alkylating agents or with high-dose combination chemotherapy increases risk of second malignancy.

Nursing Diagnoses (Daniel, 2001; Brant & Wickman, 2004)

I. During diagnosis and staging.
   A. Fear.
   B. Ineffective coping.
   C. Compromised family coping.
   D. Decisional conflict related to treatment options.
   E. Deficient knowledge related to diagnosis.
   F. Fatigue.

 II. During treatment.
  A. Deficient knowledge related to treatment.
  B. Impaired oral mucous membranes.
  C. Impaired skin integrity.
  D. Fatigue.
  E. Nausea.
  F. Risk for infection.
  G. Imbalanced nutrition: less than body requirements.
  H. Impaired physical mobility.
  I. Pain.
  J. Situational low self-esteem.
 III. During the rehabilitation phase.
  A. Sexual dysfunction.
  B. Fear.
  C. Deficient knowledge related to long-term side effects of treatment.
  D. Fatigue.
  E. Pain.

Outcome Identification

 I. During diagnosis and staging, the client and family will do the following:
  A. Communicate feelings about a potential diagnosis.
  B. Identify and use effective coping skills.
  C. Arrive on time and prepared for scheduled tests and procedures.
  D. Verbalize information about disease and treatment.
  E. Participate in treatment decisions.
 II. During the treatment phase, the client will do the following:
  A. Verbalize knowledge of treatment regimen.
  B. Identify measures to manage fatigue.
  C. List symptoms of infection.
  D. Describe situations requiring professional intervention.
  E. Discuss measures to enhance nutritional intake.
  F. Maintain active or passive motion within mobility limitations.
  G. Use effective strategies for pain management.
  H. Participate in measures to enhance self-esteem.
 III. During the rehabilitation phase, the client will do the following:
  A. Identify potential or actual alterations in sexual function related to disease and treatment.
  B. Demonstrate adaptive behaviors.
   1. Incorporate possibility of disease recurrence into lifestyle without being overwhelmed by threat.
   2. Participate in health maintenance behaviors.
  C. Identify measures to manage fatigue.

Planning and Implementation

 I. An individualized and holistic plan of care for the client with a lymphoid malignancy is developed to achieve outcomes related to identified nursing diagnoses (Brant & Wickman, 2004).
 II. The plan of care is developed and implemented in cooperation with the client, the client's family, and the multidisciplinary team.

III. Standards of care, care maps, or pathways, when available, provide a blueprint for client care.

IV. Appropriate nursing interventions for the client with lymphoid malignancy include, but are not limited to, the following:

  A. Encourage communication of feelings about disease and treatment.

  B. Refer to community resources (support groups, Leukemia & Lymphoma Society, American Cancer Society, I Can Cope, Multiple Myeloma Research Foundation).

  C. Explore coping options with the client and family and validate effective mechanisms.

  D. Develop a written schedule and specific instructions for preparation for tests and procedures.

  E. Provide culturally sensitive information. This information is provided in written format at an appropriate reading level or in an alternative format understandable to the client and family.

  F. Clarify and explain information verbally.

  G. Implement measures to assist the client in managing fatigue (see Chapter 1).

  H. Discuss effects of treatment and symptoms requiring professional intervention.

  I. Provide nutritional counseling to discuss measures to assist the client in maintaining nutritional intake (see Chapters 9 and 14).

  J. Encourage active participation in care.

  K. Assist the client in maintaining activity. (Inactivity increases the risk of bone resorption.)

  L. Provide pharmacologic and nonpharmacologic interventions to manage nausea and vomiting (see Chapters 10, 11, and 14).

  M. Provide pharmacologic and nonpharmacologic interventions to manage pain (see Chapters 1, 10, and 11).

  N. Encourage verbalization of feelings about changes in appearance.

  O. Provide information on measures to cope with appearance changes (e.g., wigs, scarves, hats for alopecia; Look Good, Feel Better program).

  P. Discuss options for sperm banking, when appropriate, before beginning treatment.

  Q. Refer to appropriate resources for sexual dysfunction, including gynecologist, fertility specialist, or sexuality counselor.

  R. Review symptoms of endocrine dysfunction that should be reported to the health care team.

Evaluation

The oncology nurse systematically and regularly evaluates the client's and/or family's responses to interventions to determine progress toward the achievement of expected outcomes. Relevant data are collected, and actual findings are compared with expected findings. Nursing diagnoses, outcomes, and plans of care are reviewed and revised as necessary.

REFERENCES

Brant, J.M., & Wickham, R.S. (Eds.) (2004). *Statement on the scope and standards of oncology nursing practice.* Pittsburgh: Oncology Nursing Society.

Armitage, J.O., Mauch, P.M., Harris, N.L., & Bierman, P. (2001). Non-Hodgkin's lymphoma. In V. DeVita, Jr., S. Hellman, & S. Rosenberg (Eds.). *Cancer: Principles and practice of oncology* (6th ed.). Philadelphia: Lippincott Williams & Wilkins pp. 2256-2316.

Armitage, J.O., Weisenburger, D., for the Non-Hodgkin's Lymphoma Classification Project. (1998). New approach to classifying non-Hodgkin's lymphomas: Clinical features of the major histologic subtypes. *Journal of Clinical Oncology 16*(8), 2780-2795.

Dalla-Favera, R., & Gaidano, G. (2001). Molecular biology of lymphomas. In V. DeVita, Jr., S. Hellman, & S. Rosenberg (Eds.). *Cancer: Principles and practice of oncology* (6th ed.). Philadelphia: Lippincott Williams & Wilkins. pp. 2215-2235.

Daniel, B.T. (2001). Malignant lymphoma. In S. Otto (Ed.). *Oncology nursing* (4th ed.). St. Louis: Mosby, pp. 416-438.

Diehl, V., Mauch, P.M., & Harris, N.L. (2001). Hodgkin's disease. In V. DeVita, Jr., S. Hellman, & S. Rosenberg (Eds.). *Cancer: Principles and practice of oncology* (6th ed.). Philadelphia: J.B. Lippincott, pp. 2339-2387.

Greene, F.L., Page, D.L., Fleming, I.D., et al. (Eds.). (2002). Lymphoid neoplasms. *American Joint Committee on Cancer (AJCC) Cancer Staging manual* (6th ed.). New York: Springer-Verlag.

Harris, N.L., Jaffe, E.S., Stein, H., et al. (1994). A revised European-American classification of lymphoid neoplasms: A proposal from the International Lymphoma Study Group. *Blood 84*(5), 1361-1392.

Holmberg, L.A., & Stewart, F.M. (2003). Hematopoietic stem cell transplantation for non-Hodgkin's lymphoma. *Oncology 17*(5), 627-640.

Jaffe, E.S., Harris, N.L., Stein, H., & Vardiman, J.W. (Eds.). (2001). *World Health Organization classification of tumours. Pathology and genetics of tumours of haematopoietic and lymphoid tissues.* Lyon: IARC Press.

Jemal, A., Tiwari, R.C., Murray, T., et al. (2004). Cancer statistics. *CA: A Cancer Journal for Clinicians 54*(1), 8-29.

Lyden, J. (2000). Tumor lysis syndrome. In C.H. Yarbro, M.H. Frogge, M. Goodman, & S.L. Groenwald (Eds.). *Cancer nursing: Principles and practice* (5th ed.). Sudbury, MA: Jones and Bartlett Publishers, pp. 920-930.

Munshi, N.C., Tricot, G., & Barlogie, B. (2001). Plasma cell neoplasm. In V. DeVita, Jr., S. Hellman, & S. Rosenberg (Eds.). *Cancer: Principles and practice of oncology* (6th ed.). Philadelphia: Lippincott Williams & Wilkins, pp. 2465-2499.

Myers, J.S. (2001). Oncologic complications. In S. Otto (Ed.). *Oncology nursing* (4th ed.). St. Louis: Mosby, pp. 498-581.

National Comprehensive Cancer Network. (2002). Non-Hodgkin's lymphoma. In *Practice guidelines in oncology-v.1.2002.* National Comprehensive Cancer Network, Rockledge, PA.

Otto, S. (2001). Multiple myeloma. In S. Otto (Ed.). *Oncology nursing* (4th ed.). St. Louis: Mosby, pp. 439-446.

Sheridan, C., & Serrano, M. (2000). Multiple myeloma. In C.H. Yarbro, M.H. Frogge, M. Goodman, & S.L. Groenwald (Eds.). *Cancer nursing: Principles and practice* (5th ed.). Sudbury, MA: Jones and Bartlett Publishers, pp. 1354-1370.

Sitton, E. (2000). Superior vena cava syndrome. In C.H. Yarbro, M.H. Frogge, M. Goodman, & S.L. Groenwald (Eds.). *Cancer nursing: Principles and practice* (5th ed.). Sudbury, MA: Jones and Bartlett Publishers, pp. 900-912.

The International Non-Hodgkin's Lymphoma Prognostic Factors Project. (1993). A predictive model for aggressive non-Hodgkin's lymphoma. *New England Journal of Medicine 329*(14), 987-994.

Yarbro, C.H. (2000). Malignant lymphomas. In C.H. Yarbro, M.H. Frogge, M. Goodman, & S.L. Groenwald (Eds.). *Cancer nursing: Principles and practice* (5th ed.). Sudbury, MA: Jones and Bartlett Publishers, pp. 1329-1353.

33 Nursing Care of the Client with Bone and Soft Tissue Cancers

ELLEN CARR

Theory

I. Classification.
  A. Classify sarcoma subtypes by cell histology rather than by location—more accurate (previously, classification systems have been based on site differences) (Demetri, 2002).
  B. No clear etiology for all sarcomas; now can subtype tissue of origin; sarcomas share mesodermal cellular origin (Brennan et al., 2001).
    1. Sarcomas originate from many tissue types—fat, nerve, muscle, joint, deep skin tissue.
    2. Sarcomas probably develop from aberrant malignant mesenchymal cells (National Cancer Institute [NCI], 2002d).
    3. Locations (Brennan et al., 2001) (Figure 33-1).
II. Common malignant bone and soft tissue cancers (with cell or tissue of origin) (Piasecki, 2000; Yasko et al., 2001) (Tables 33-1 to 33-3).
  A. Osteosarcoma (osseous tissue).
  B. Chondrosarcoma (cartilaginous tissue).
  C. Fibrosarcoma (fibrous tissue).
  D. Ewing's Family of Tumors (EFT) (reticuloendothelial tissue). Occur mainly during childhood (NCI, 2002c).
    1. Ewing's sarcoma of bone (60% to 80%) (NCI, 2002c).
    2. Extraosseous Ewing's (EOE) (8%) (NCI, 2002c).
    3. Primitive neuroectodermal tumor (PNET) (5%) (NCI, 2002c).
  E. Miscellaneous soft tissue sarcomas (Brennan et al., 2001).
    1. Liposarcoma (adipose tissue).
      a. Most develop in thigh or inside back of abdomen (American Cancer Society [ACS], 2003).
    2. Leiomyosarcoma (involuntary smooth muscle).
    3. Rhabdomyosarcoma (skeletal muscle).
    4. Angiosarcoma (vascular tissue).
    5. Malignant fibrous histiocytoma (histiocytic origin).
    6. Malignant peripheral nerve sheath tumors (nerve).
    7. Kaposi's sarcoma (immunosuppression, human herpesvirus type 8 [HHV-8]).
    8. Synovial sarcomas (synovial; joint).
    9. Extraskeletal chondrosarcoma (extraskeletal cartilage; osseous tumor).
III. Epidemiology.
  A. Incidence of primary malignant bone and soft tissue tumors is low (ACS, 2002).

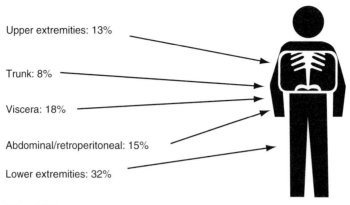

Upper extremities: 13%

Trunk: 8%

Viscera: 18%

Abdominal/retroperitoneal: 15%

Lower extremities: 32%

Other: 14%

FIGURE 33-1 ■ Sites of soft tissue sarcomas. (From Memorial Sloan-Kettering Cancer Center, 1982 to 2001. Based on admission records [n = 5000].) Memorial Sloan-Kettering Cancer Center (MSKCC). (2002). *Questions and answers about sarcoma.* Retrieved February 19, 2003 from the World Wide Web: http://www.mskcc.org/mskcc/html/444.cfm.

TABLE 33-1
Cancers of the Bone

Types of Cancer	Tissue of Origin	Common Locations	Common Ages (yr)
Osteosarcoma	Osteoid	Knees, upper legs, upper arms	10-25
Chondrosarcoma	Cartilage	*Pelvis,* upper legs, shoulders	50-60
Ewing's sarcoma	Immature nerve tissue, usually in bone marrow	Pelvis, upper legs, ribs, arms	10-20

From Cancer Information Service (CIS), NCI: *Cancer facts. Bone cancer: questions and answers,* 2002. Retrieved March 20, 2004 from the World Wide Web: http://cis.nci.nih.gov/fact/6_26.htm.

TABLE 33-2
Major Types of Soft Tissue Sarcomas in Adults

Tissue of Origin	Type of Cancer	Usual Location in the Body
Fibrous tissue	Fibrosarcoma	Arms, legs, trunk
	Malignant fibrous histiocytoma	Legs
	Dermatofibrosarcoma	Trunk
Fat	Liposarcoma	Arms, legs, trunk
Muscle		
Striated muscle	Rhabdomyosarcoma	Arms, legs
Smooth muscle	Leiomyosarcoma	Uterus, digestive tract
Blood vessels	Hemangiosarcoma	Arms, legs, trunk
	Kaposi's sarcoma	Legs, trunk
Lymph vessels	Lymphangiosarcoma	Arms
Synovial tissue (linings of joint cavities, tendon sheaths)	Synovial sarcoma	Legs
Peripheral nerves	Neurofibrosarcoma	Arms, legs, trunk
Cartilage and bone-forming tissue	Extraskeletal chondrosarcoma	Legs
	Extraskeletal osteosarcoma	Legs, trunk (not involving the bone)

From Cancer Information Service (CIS), NCI: *Cancer facts. Soft tissue sarcomas: questions and answers,* 2002. Retrieved March 20, 2004 from the World Wide Web: http://cis.nci.nih.gov/fact/6_12.htm.

TABLE 33-3
Major Types of Soft Tissue Sarcomas in Children

Tissue of Origin	Type of Cancer	Usual Location in the Body	Most Common Ages (yr)
MUSCLE			
Striated muscle	Rhabdomyosarcoma		
	Embryonal	Head and neck, genitourinary tract	Infant-4
	Alveolar	Arms, legs, head and neck	Infant-19
Smooth muscle	Leiomyosarcoma	Trunk	15-19
FIBROUS TISSUE	Fibrosarcoma	Arms, legs	15-19
	Malignant fibrous histiocytoma	Legs	15-19
	Dermatofibrosarcoma	Trunk	15-19
FAT	Liposarcoma	Arms, legs	15-19
BLOOD VESSELS	Infantile hemangiopericytoma	Arms, legs, trunk, head, neck	Infant-4
SYNOVIAL TISSUE (LININGS OF JOINT CAVITIES, TENDON SHEATHS)	Synovial sarcoma	Legs, arms, trunk	15-19
PERIPHERAL NERVES	Malignant peripheral nerve sheath tumors (also called neurofibrosarcomas, malignant schwannomas, neurogenic sarcomas)	Arms, legs, trunk	15-19
MUSCULAR NERVES	Alveolar soft part sarcoma	Arms, legs	Infant-19
CARTILAGE AND BONE-FORMING TISSUE	Extraskeletal myxoid chondrosarcoma	Legs	10-14
	Extraskeletal mesenchymal	Legs	10-14

From Cancer Information Service (CIS), NCI: *Cancer facts. Soft tissue sarcomas: questions and answers,* 2002. Retrieved March 20, 2004 from the World Wide Web: http://cis.nci.nih.gov/fact/6_12.htm.

1. Bone.
   a. 2004 estimates—2440 new cases; deaths—1300 (ACS, 2004).
   b. Account for fewer than 1% of all malignant tumors in the United States (U.S.) (NCI, 2002d).
2. Soft tissue.
   a. 2004 estimates—8680 new cases; incidence slightly higher for men. Deaths in 2004, 3660 (ACS, 2004).
   b. Account for fewer than 15% of all cancers in U.S. adults (Demetri, 2002).
   c. Five-year survival in adults is 90% if found early; 10% to 15% survival if found when metastasized (ACS, 2003).

IV. Risk factors.

 A. Bone—no definitive risk factors. The following factors suggested (Piasecki, 2000):

 1. Previous high-dose irradiation.

 2. Chemicals—vinyl chloride gas, arsenic, dioxin.

 3. Prior treatment with antineoplastic agents—melphalan (Alkeran), procarbazine (Matulane), nitrosoureas, chlorambucil (Leukeran).

 4. Immunosuppression.

 5. Familial, genetic connections.

 6. Preexisting bone conditions (e.g., Paget's disease).

 7. Skeletal maldevelopment.

 B. Soft tissue.

 1. Uncommon and diverse presentations do not suggest common risk factors. Most sarcomas develop in people with no known risk factors (Piasecki, 2000).

 2. Some suggested factors.

 a. History of treatment with radiation therapy (RT); e.g., treated for breast cancer.

 b. History of trauma.

 c. Genetic predisposition (ACS, 2002; Brennan et al., 2001).

 (1) Deoxyribonucleic acid (DNA) mutations are common in soft tissue sarcoma (acquired during life, rather than born with mutation) (NCI, 2002d).

 (2) Mutated tumor suppressor genes.

 (3) Those identified (ACS, 2003; NCI, 2002d).

 (a) Neurofibromatosis.

 (b) Gardner's syndrome.

 (c) Li-Fraumeni syndrome.

 (d) Inherited retinoblastoma.

 (4) Chemical exposure—asbestos, polyvinyl chloride gas, arsenic.

 (5) With Kaposi's sarcoma, exposure to HIV-positive saliva, blood, body fluids (Palella et al., 1998).

V. Pathophysiology and classification.

 A. Bone.

 1. From mesoderm and ectoderm; pseudocapsule contains tumor, then breaks through to surrounding tissue (called skip metastasis).

 2. Patterns of growth (Piasecki, 2000).

 a. Compress normal tissue.

 b. Resorption of bone by reactive osteoclasts.

 c. Destroy normal tissue (when malignant).

 3. Staging based on biologic behavior and tumor aggressiveness.

 a. When "A" stage lesions, present as intracompartmental.

 b. When "B" stage lesions, present as extracompartmental.

 4. Examples.

 a. Osteosarcoma (osteogenic sarcoma)—56% of all bone tumors (Otto, 2001).

 (1) Most often affects adolescents.

 (2) Males are affected more frequently than females (Piasecki, 2000).

 (3) Tumor cells are spindle shaped, from bone-forming mesenchyma in the medullary cavity. Reactive osteoclasts interact with normal bone to destroy it.

(4) Start in metaphysis of long bones (area of highest growth), especially in cases in knee region (Piasecki, 2000).

(5) Metastasize to the lung first; at diagnosis, 10% treated with surgery alone have 5-year survival; with adjuvant chemotherapy, 77% have 5-year survival (Piasecki, 2000).

b. Chondrosarcoma (Brennan et al., 2001).

(1) Occurs most often in adults ages 30 to 60 years (Piasecki, 2000).

(2) More often in men (Piasecki, 2000).

(3) Origin—malignant cartilaginous tumor cells from medullary canal or outside bone, destroying the bone.

(4) Commonly affect pelvis, femur, and shoulder.

(5) Often slow growing but can metastasize distantly.

c. Fibrosarcoma.

(1) Most often seen in adolescents and young adults.

(2) Commonly affects the femur and tibia.

(3) Arises from the medullary cavity, affects metaphyseal area.

(4) Constitutes fewer than 7% of all primary malignant bone cancers (Piasecki, 2000).

d. EFT (NCI, 2002c).

(1) Constitutes approximately 6% of all primary malignant bone cancers (Piasecki, 2000).

(2) Eighty percent diagnosed when 5 to 15 years old (Piasecki, 2000).

(3) Highly malignant (20% to 30% with metastases at time of diagnosis) (NCI, 2002c); origin in nonmesenchymal area of bone marrow; from shaft of long bones, pelvic bone, or chest wall.

(4) Most often affects pelvis and lower extremities; femoral diaphysis is the most common site.

(5) Spreads to adjacent tissue via many round cells; indistinct borders; necrotic and hemorrhagic areas are common.

(6) Metastasizes to lungs, lymph nodes, and other bones (NCI, 2002c).

(7) Associated with retinoblastoma and skeletal anomalies.

(8) Disease-free survivors—40% to 70% (because of multimodality therapies, precision in surgery [wide resections]) (Piasecki, 2000).

B. Soft tissue sarcomas.

1. Classified/staged by cell type, origin—connective tissue (fat, muscle, tendons, fibrous tissue) (Greene, 2002; Demetri, 2002; NCI, 2002a) (Box 33-1).

a. Identifying cell type, through careful pathology, is key (Couto, 2002).

2. Can appear anywhere because of the body's widespread connective tissue; most are found in the lower extremities or trunk.

3. Prognosis depends on tumor size, grade, resection margin (Stojadinovic et al., 2002).

4. When they metastasize, prognosis is poor.

VI. Treatments.

A. Overview (Brennan et al., 2001).

1. No standard set of guidelines, require multidisciplinary management (Demetri, 2002).

2. Goals.

a. Remove tumor.

b. Avoid amputation.

c. Preserve functioning.

d. For metastatic disease, palliative care.

BOX 33-1
STAGING SYSTEM FOR SARCOMA

- **T** stands for the size of the tumor.
  N stands for spread to lymph nodes (small bean-shaped collections of immune system cells found throughout the body that help fight infections and cancers).
  M is for metastasis (spread to distant organs).
- In soft tissue sarcomas, an additional factor, called histologic grade **(G)**, is used to stage the tumor. The histologic grade is based on how the sarcoma cells appear under the microscope.

To assign a stage, information about the tumor, its grade, lymph nodes, and metastasis is combined by a process called stage grouping. The stage is described by Roman numerals from I to IV with the letters A or B.

Histologic Grade
G1: Looks like normal tissue—tends to be slow growing
G2: Looks less like normal tissue—faster growing
G3: Only slightly looks like normal tissue—even faster growing
G4: Does not look at all like normal tissue—fastest growing

Tumor
T1: The sarcoma is less than 5 cm (2 inches)
T2: The sarcoma is 5 cm or greater
    a: The tumor is superficial—near the surface of the body
    b: The tumor is deep in the limb or abdomen

Lymph Nodes
N0: No lymph nodes have sarcoma cells in them
N1: Lymph nodes are present that have sarcoma cells in them

Metastasis
M0: No distant metastases (spread) of sarcoma are found
M1: Distant metastases of sarcoma are found

Stage Grouping for Soft Tissue Sarcomas
Stage IA: G1-2, T1a,b, N0, M0
The cancer is not too different from normal tissue. It is smaller than 5 cm (2 inches) and can be superficial or deep. It has not spread to lymph nodes or more distant sites.
Stage IB: G1-2, T2a, N0, M0
The cancer is not too different from normal tissue. It is larger than 5 cm (2 inches) and is superficial. It has not spread to lymph nodes or more distant sites.
Stage I sarcomas are low-grade cancers that can usually be cured. Five years after treatment, the chance of recurrence is only 20% and the survival rate is 99%.
Stage IIA: G1-2, T2b, N0, M0
The cancer is not too different from normal tissue. It is larger than 5 cm (2 inches) and is deep. It has not spread to lymph nodes or more distant sites.
Stage IIB: G3-4, T1a-b, N0, M0
The cancer looks very different from normal tissue and may contain many dividing cells. It is smaller than 5 cm (2 inches) and can be superficial or deep. It has not spread to lymph nodes or more distant sites.
Stage IIC: G3-4, T2a, N0, M0
The cancer looks very different from normal tissue and may contain many dividing cells. It is larger than 5 cm (2 inches) and is superficial. It has not spread to lymph nodes or more distant sites.
Stage II sarcomas are also often cured. Five years after treatment, the chance of recurrence is 35% and the survival rate is 82%.
Stage III: G3-4, T2b, N0, M0
The cancer looks very different from normal tissue and may contain many dividing cells. It is larger than 5 cm (2 inches) and is deep. It has not spread to lymph nodes or more distant sites.

BOX 33-1
STAGING SYSTEM FOR SARCOMA—cont'd

> Stage III sarcomas are large, deep, high-grade cancers and are less likely to be cured. Five years
> after treatment, the likelihood of recurrence is about 65% and the survival is only 50%.
> Stage IVA: any G, any T, N1, M0
> These cancers have spread to lymph nodes near the tumor.
> Stage IVB: any G, any T, any N, M1
> These cancers have spread to distant sites.
> Stage IV sarcomas are usually not curable.

Derived from AJCC Cancer Staging Manual, Sixth Edition. For a complete, official description of TNM, Stage Grouping
and Histologic Grade for this site, please consult Greene F.L., Page D.L., Fleming, I.D., et al. *AJCC Cancer Staging
Manual,* Sixth Edition. New York: Springer-Verlag, 2002.

    3. Treatments have improved because of development of better histologic
    assays via chromosomal translocations (Allander et al., 2001).
  B. Surgery.
    1. Surgical strategies for treatment based on histology, size, location, tumor
    grade, extent of disease, resectability (Demetri, 2002).
    2. Surgical strategies also depend on the following factors (Brennan et al.,
    2001):
      a. Treatment of choice with osteosarcoma, fibrosarcoma, chondrosar-
      coma.
      b. Amputation versus limb salvage issues: increased effort to salvage
      rather than amputate. The following issues affect the decision
      (Brennan et al., 2001):
        (1) Acceptable surgical margins.
        (2) Blood vessels and nerves involved with the tumor.
        (3) Age (in children younger than 10 years old, surgery affects limb
        growth).
        (4) If limb salvage, RT follows (typical strategy).
        (5) Amputation issues.
          (a) When tumor extends to incisional surface.
          (b) When location necessitates (e.g., tumor extends to vertebral
          body and pelvis).
          (c) Infection, skeletal immaturity.
          (d) Major neurovascular involvement (Brennan et al., 2001).
      c. For bone cancer, adjuvant chemotherapy has dramatically increased
      overall survival (55% to 80%) (Brennan et al., 2001).
      d. Reconstruction (Piasecki, 2000).
        (1) Bone autografts, allografts.
        (2) After soft tissue resection, three common methods.
          (a) Arthrodesis or fusion (with implants or grafts).
          (b) Arthroplasty for joints.
          (c) Allografts (since the 1960s)—bone, tendon, ligament, connec-
          tive tissue.
        (3) Tested for match, viral and bacterial contamination.
        (4) Method—bone frozen to accept graft.
        (5) Intercalary allograft placed between two segments of host bone;
        used for long bone grafts.
        (6) Issues—nonunion, infections, healing.

   C. Neoadjuvant radiotherapy.
     1. Soft tissue tumors can be radiosensitive and radioresponsive (Brennan et al., 2001).
     2. Usually external beam RT, before or after surgery.
       a. Used when tumor is localized.
       b. Used after surgical debulking or tumor removal.
     3. In some cases, brachytherapy is used alone or with external beam RT.
   D. Chemotherapy or immunotherapy.
     1. Used as an adjuvant or neoadjuvant with surgery (Sarcoma Meta-analysis Collaboration [SMAC], 2002).
     2. Since the addition of chemotherapy and immunotherapy as part of the multimodality approach to treatment, disease-free periods for clients have increased remarkably.
       a. Studies are small, and conclusions are difficult to generalize (Demetri, 2002).
       b. Outcomes show better local control, increased time to treatment failure, especially in EFT, rhabdomyosarcoma, and osteosarcomas (Demetri, 2002; Link et al., 1986; NCI, 2002b).
       c. In advanced tumors, sequential, single-agent protocols are more effective than complicated combination protocols (Demetri, 2002).
         (1) Exception: highly active antiretroviral therapy (HAART) for Kaposi's sarcoma (International Collaboration on HIV and Cancer [ICHC], 2000; NCI, 2002d).
       d. To date, localized administration to tumor site (cryoablation radiofrequency) has not been shown to be effective (Demetri, 2002).
       e. Targeted molecular therapies are promising (oncogene activation triggered by viruses or antibodies) (Demetri, 2002).
         (1) Example: identification of *CD117* expression associated with activation of *C-kit* receptors in gastrointestinal stromal tumors (Allandar et al., 2001).
     3. Common chemotherapeutic agents—doxorubicin (Adriamycin), cisplatin (Platinol), cyclophosphamide (Cytoxan), dacarbazine (DTIC-Dome), ifosfamide (Ifex), methotrexate (Mexate), vincristine (Oncovin) (Brennan et al., 2001; Demetri, 2002).
     4. Also, studies with topotecan (Hycamtin), vinblastine (Velban), paclitaxel (Taxol), docetaxel (Taxotere), gemcitabine (Gemzar), carboplatin (Paraplatin), dactinomycin (Cosmegen) (Demetri, 2002).
     5. Also used in palliation.
   E. Treatment of common malignant bone and soft tissue tumors.
     1. Osteosarcoma.
       a. Surgery.
       b. Multimodality.
         (1) Surgery.
         (2) Adjuvant radiotherapy (when tumor in axial location; for palliation).
         (3) Adjuvant chemotherapy and immunotherapy (National Institutes of Health [NIH], 2004a).
     2. Chondrosarcoma.
       a. Surgery.
     3. Fibrosarcoma.
       a. Surgery.
         (1) Radical surgery.
         (2) Amputation.
       b. Radiotherapy only for inoperable tumors.

4. EFT.
   a. Multimodality.
      (1) Surgery (for local control).
      (2) Radiotherapy (4500 to 5600 cGy for metastatic disease) (NCI, 2002c).
      (3) Chemotherapy (vincristine, doxorubicin, cyclophosphamide, ifosfamide/etoposide [Ifex/VP-16, Etopophos, VePesid]) (Brennan et al., 2001).
5. Miscellaneous soft tissue sarcomas (e.g., liposarcoma, leiomyosarcoma, rhabdomyosarcoma, angiosarcoma, malignant fibrous histiocytoma).
   a. Surgery.
      (1) Resection (thoracotomy) when spread to lung, provided that the primary tumor is controlled.
   b. Radiotherapy.
   c. Chemotherapy (NIH, 2004b).

Assessment

I. Osteosarcoma (Brennan et al., 2001).
   A. Clinical symptoms.
      1. Pain—onset, location, duration, quality; may be radicular; gradual onset, worse at night, increases with tumor burden.
      2. Swelling in affected area.
      3. Bone—rule out injury.
      4. If pathologic fracture, there can be acute, sudden pain.
   B. Physical examination.
      1. Mass visible, palpable; may be firm, nontender, warm.
      2. Size noted, bilateral comparison.
      3. Limited range of motion.
   C. Diagnostic data.
      1. Laboratory.
         a. Elevated serum alkaline phosphatase level because of increased osteoblastic activity (45% to 50% of clients) (Brennan et al., 2001; Piasecki, 2000).
      2. Radiographs (cannot see changes until tumor is advanced); three patterns of tumor (can occur isolated or together).
         a. Slow-growing tumor meets nontumor tissue.
         b. Moderately aggressive—extends into soft tissue.
         c. Aggressive, infiltrating—perpendicular striated (sunburst pattern).
      3. Other tests—magnetic resonance imaging (MRI), computed tomography (CT), fluoroscopy.
      4. Bone scan can show additional skeletal lesions.
   D. Staging.
      1. Biggest changes in staging identify subcategories, size/depth of tumors (AJCC, 2002) (Box 33-1).
II. Chondrosarcoma.
   A. Clinical symptoms.
      1. Dull, aching pain (like arthritis).
   B. Physical examination.
      1. Firm, swollen area; high-grade tumor can appear soft, viscous.
   C. Diagnostic data.
      1. Similar diagnostic studies as for osteosarcoma.

III. Fibrosarcoma (Brennan et al., 2001).
  A. Clinical symptoms.
   1. Pain in affected area.
  B. Physical examination.
   1. Swelling in affected area.
  C. Diagnostic data.
   1. On radiographs, usually seen within the bone; low-grade lesions have well-defined margins, high-grade lesions have poorly defined margins with a more moth-eaten pattern.
   2. Similar strategies as for osteosarcoma.
IV. EFT (Brennan et al., 2001; NCI, 2002c).
  A. Clinical symptoms.
   1. Symptom report can be vague; pain progressing, lump progressing; sometimes feel heat over lump.
   2. Flu-like symptoms, fever, fatigue.
   3. Anemia.
  B. Physical examination.
   1. Swelling, progressing in affected area.
  C. Diagnostic data.
   1. Appear onion-like on radiographs, from multiple layers of subperiosteal new bone reacting to tumor invading the bone cortex.
   2. Diagnosed after ruling out other malignant cell possibilities (e.g., rhabdomyosarcoma, lymphoma, neuroblastoma).
   3. Similar diagnostic studies as for osteosarcoma.
V. Soft tissue (Brennan et al., 2001; NCI, 2002d).
  A. Clinical symptoms.
   1. Starts as painless, swollen mass (>5 cm) unless affecting blood vessels or nerves.
   2. Only 50% of soft tissue sarcomas found in early stages (Memorial Sloan-Kettering Cancer Center [MSKCC], 2002).
   3. Tumor infiltrates can be distant from the site of origin.
   4. Pain (worsening) in one third of cases (MSKCC, 2002). In time, variety of presenting symptoms—peripheral neuralgias, vascular ischemia, paralysis, bowel obstruction; but often no symptoms reported.
  B. Physical examination.
   1. Depending on origin—lung, nerve, mobility affected.
  C. Diagnostic data.
   1. Tissue/cells from incisional, frozen, needle biopsies.
   2. MRI, CT.
   3. New technologies that offer more precision—electron microscope examination, immunohistochemical staining, DNA analysis, ultrasound (for size and density).
   4. Smaller lesions are usually benign (ACS, 2003).
   5. Lesions may recur after resection, reappearing deeper and larger, more aggressive with metastasis.
   6. Staging is not standard; grading system is based on mitotic activity (ACS, 2003).
VI. Metastatic disease.
  A. Spread from primary lesions to lung, breast, colon, pancreas, kidney, thyroid, prostate, stomach, testis (ACS, 2003; MSKCC, 2002).
  B. To evaluate spread—CT of chest and regional lymph nodes.

    C. Sarcomas frequently metastasize to lung.

    D. Other early metastatic sites—spine, ribs, pelvis (90% in axial skeleton) (ACS, 2003).

    E. Presents as dull aching pain, increasing at night.

    F. Palliative therapies include surgery, radiotherapy, chemotherapy.

VII. Miscellaneous assessment issues.

    A. Phantom limb pain or sensation (Piasecki, 2000).

      1. One to four weeks postoperatively; usually resolves in a few months.

      2. Client is aware of itching, pressure, tingling, severe cramping, throbbing, burning pain.

      3. Usually tripped by fatigue, stress, excitement, other stimuli.

      4. Greater when the amputation site is more proximal.

    B. Preoperative care when client will lose limb.

      1. For anticipated amputation, many psychologic needs (especially with adolescents). Among issues to address: anxiety; depression; grief about lost limb—physical as well as emotional and social losses; altered body image; fear of disability; coping with deformity; short-term loss of independence and self-sufficiency.

      2. Rehabilitation plan after surgery. Awareness of possible symptoms after surgery: phantom limb sensation, pain (throbbing, burning), itching pressure, tingling, severe cramping.

      3. Visit from amputee can be helpful—shares how to master his/her prosthesis and deal with emotional issues and change.

    C. Postoperative care when client has lost limb.

      1. Immediate postoperative management.

        a. Observe drainage from site; also for redness, hemorrhage, increased pain, tenderness and swelling, blisters, abrasions.

        b. If need for stump care, do the following:

          (1) Elevate stump (usually at least 24 hours) to prevent edema and promote venous return.

          (2) Frequent wrapping of stump with elastic bandages or stump shrinkers.

          (3) Dangling and transfer to chair after day of surgery.

        c. Assist client into prone position 3 or 4 times per day for 15 minutes minimum to prevent hip contractures.

        d. Teach client and family self-care of stump, prosthesis, and so on.

        e. Coordination of collaborative services (physical therapy, social services, occupational therapy, etc.).

    D. If limb salvage, postoperative management.

      1. Neurovascular checks distal to surgical site.

      2. Monitor for blood loss and anemia from extensive tumor resection and reconstruction.

      3. Monitor wound site for signs of infection.

      4. Manage pain.

      5. Coordinate rehabilitation plan.

Nursing Diagnoses (North American Nursing Diagnosis Association [NANDA], 2001) (Box 33-2)

  I. Impaired physical mobility.

 II. Anxiety.

BOX 33-2
COMMON NURSING DIAGNOSES AND INTERVENTIONS

Impaired Physical Mobility
1. Per schedule, position and turn carefully; maintain proper body alignment
2. As directed from physician and physical therapist, follow and encourage daily exercise, active and passive range of motion; intentionally increase strength and endurance; steadily increase frequency and ambulate in steadily larger physical area
3. Boost energy level with periods for adequate rest, well-balanced nutrition

Anxiety
1. Emphasize anxiety is normal; validate emotional stress; provide sounding board to keep focused, provide constructive problem solving, explore previous strategies that have decreased anxiety
2. Provide simple and clear information, concrete answers to concerns that cause anxiety: How will I cope? How will I function? Who will help me? When can I anticipate caring for myself?
3. Encourage adaptive behaviors; reinforce mastery of specific concrete tasks toward self-care and independence

Disturbed Body Image
1. Before surgery, explore values, expectations, methods of coping; after surgery, revisit those topics
2. Provide environment to continue to identify and to express feelings
3. Know support system—current and expanded (those who have had similar diagnoses and surgeries); mobilize support system to boost self-esteem, coping skills, ability to adjust; set realistic goals; adapt to changed self

Ineffective Coping
1. Provide a supportive, encouraging environment for client to verbalize concerns; be an active listener
2. Encourage independence in activities of daily living
3. Assess previous skills—expand repertoire to new coping skills: acquire knowledge, learn relaxation techniques, develop new relationships, identify new roles, recognize ways to maintain emotional equilibrium

Risk for Infection
1. Assess wound site for signs and symptoms of infection (redness, swelling, warmth, pain); assess client for systemic signs and symptoms of infection (fever, chills, aches, malaise)
2. Encourage adequate fluid intake, nutrition, rest
3. For dressing changes (per policy, practice aseptic or clean technique)
4. Protect vulnerable wound sites to prevent further trauma and injury

Impaired Skin Integrity
1. Provide regular and comprehensive skin assessment
2. Protect skin: keep skin clean and dry, apply skin preparations, avoid bumping/breaking of skin
3. Encourage and provide adequate fluid intake, well-balanced meals with adequate calories and protein
4. Proactively avoid decubitus ulcers: skin care; repositioning, vigilant hygiene; if decubiti develop, apply medication, change dressings, debride wounds, as ordered

Acute or Chronic Pain
1. Thorough assessment
2. Be proactive with pain medication before exercise and ambulation sessions
3. For effective pain management, also address depression, sleep, anxiety
4. Accompany effective pain medication protocols with adequate sleep and rest, nutrition, exercise
5. Apply nonpharmacologic strategies for pain control that can be effective: massage, heat/ice packs, ointment, relaxation techniques

III. Disturbed body image.
IV. Ineffective coping.
 V. Risk for infection.
VI. Acute or chronic pain.

Outcome Identification (Otto, 2001; Piasecki, 2000)

   I. Client describes symptoms that prompt a physician visit.
  II. Client describes the disease state, plan of care, and actions to maintain health.
 III. Client identifies strategies and resources to cope.
  IV. Client remains free of infection, anemia, and delayed wound healing.
   V. Client communicates pain (e.g., quality, source, intensity) to the health care providers.
  VI. Client identifies means to maintain fluid and nutritional balance.
 VII. Client maintains muscle tone, range of motion, levels of activity, mobilization, weight bearing; incorporates prosthesis if applicable.
VIII. Client identifies ways to maintain adequate elimination.
  IX. Client describes alterations in sexual function and feelings.
   X. Client identifies and practices ways to conserve energy, optimize ventilatory functioning.
  XI. Client describes signs and symptoms of altered circulation.

Planning and Implementation

   I. The nurse provides information and teaching (Piasecki, 2000). Teaching is amplified with information from the web (see selected list of websites, Box 33-3).
  II. Preoperative teaching is provided, which may include information on immobilization; wound care; risk for infection; implants; drains; postsurgical or delayed prosthetic fitting (if applicable); issues of endurance, muscle tone; psychosocial issues of depression, anxiety, fear, body image, self-esteem; and physical therapy (e.g., gait training, muscle development, motor function, lifestyle changes).
 III. The nurse provides counseling and teaches strategies to the client/family to assist them to cope with, for example, anxieties, fears, and body image and sexuality issues. Assistance in identifying resources and sources of social support is also provided (Otto, 2001; Piasecki, 2000).

Evaluation

The oncology nurse systematically and regularly evaluates the client's and/or family's responses to interventions to determine progress toward the achievement of expected outcomes. Relevant data are collected, and actual findings are compared with expected findings. Nursing diagnoses, outcomes, and plans of care are reviewed and revised as necessary.

BOX 33-3
SELECTED WEBSITES AND RESOURCES

American Cancer Society (ACS). *Bone cancer.*
http://www.cancer.org/docroot/CRI/content/CRI_2_4_1X_What_Is_bone_cancer_2.asp?site
area=CRI
American Cancer Society (ACS). *Cancer reference information: Sarcoma.* http://www.cancer.org/
downloads/CRI/2002_Sarcoma_Adult_Soft_Tissue.pdf
Bone Cancer International, Inc.
http://www.bonecancer.to/toc.html
CancerBacUp
http://www.cancerbacup.org.uk/Cancertype/ Bone
CancerIndex.org
http://www.cancerindex.org/clinks2c.htm
The Cure Our Children Foundation
http://www.cureourchildren.org/
Memorial Sloan-Kettering Cancer Center. *Bone cancer.*
http://www.mskcc.org/mskcc/html/1365.cfm
National Cancer Institute (NCI). *Adult soft tissue sarcoma.*
http://www.nci.nih.gov/cancerinfo/pdq/treatment/adult-soft-tissue sarcoma/healthprofessional
National Cancer Institute (NCI). *Childhood rhabdomyosarcoma.*
http://www.nci.nih.gov/cancerinfo/pdq/treatment/childrhabdomyosarcoma/healthprofessional/
#Section1
National Cancer Institute (NCI). *Ewing's family of tumors.*
http://www.nci.nih.gov/cancerinfo/pdq/treatment/ewings/healthprofessional/#Section1
Oncolink
http://www.oncolink.com/types/ types.cfm?c=1
Osteosarcoma Online
http://iucc.iu.edu/osteosarcoma/
Pediatric Oncology Resource Center/ACOR (Association of Cancer Online Resources)
http://www.acor.org/ped-onc/hp/ bonepages.html
The Sarcoma Alliance
http://www.sarcomaalliance.org/
The Sarcoma Foundation of America
http://www.curesarcoma.org/
What you need to know about cancer
http://cancer.about.com/cs/bonecancer/

REFERENCES

Allander, S.V., Nupponen, N.N., Ringner M., et al. (2001). Gastrointestinal stromal tumors with KIT mutations exhibit a remarkably homogeneous gene expression profile. *Cancer Research 61,* 8624-8628.

American Cancer Society (ACS). (2004). *Cancer facts and figures—2004.* Atlanta: Author.

American Cancer Society (ACS). (2003). *Cancer reference information: Sarcoma.* Retrieved February 19, 2003 from the World Wide Web: http://www.cancer.org/downloads/CRI/2002_Sarcoma_Adult_Soft_Tissue.pdf.

Brennan, M., Alektia, K., & Maki, R. (2001). Sarcomas of soft tissue and bone. In V.T. DeVita, S. Hellman, & S.A. Rosenberg (Eds.). *Cancer: Principles and practice of oncology* (6th ed.). Philadelphia: Lippincott Williams & Wilkins, pp. 1841-1891.

Cancer Information Service (CIS), NCI. (2002a). *Cancer facts. Bone cancer: Questions and answers.* Retrieved March 20, 2004 from the World Wide Web: http://cis.nci.nih.gov/fact/6_26.htm.

Cancer Information Service (CIS), NCI. (2002b). *Cancer facts. Soft tissue sarcomas: Questions and answers.* Retrieved March 20, 2004 from the World Wide Web: http://cis.nci.nih.gov/fact/6_12.htm.

Couto, S. (2002). *Soft tissue sarcoma: Diagnosing and treating soft tissue sarcomas.* Retrieved February 19, 2003 from the CancerSource.com. website on the World Wide Web: http://www.cancersourcern.com/search/getcontent.cfm?DiseaseID=26&Contentid=22684.

Demetri, G. (2002). *Management of soft tissue sarcomas. Program and abstracts of the Scripps Cancer Center's Annual Conference: Clinical hematology and oncology 2002;* February 16-19, 2002; La Jolla, CA.

Greene, F.L., Page, D.L., Fleming, I.D., et al. (Eds.). (2002). Musculoskeletal sites. *AJCC Cancer staging manual* (6thed.). New York: Springer-Verlag, pp. 211-228.

International Collaboration on HIV and Cancer (ICHC). (2000). Highly active antiretroviral therapy and incidence of cancer in human immunodeficiency virus infected adults. *Journal of the National Cancer Institute 92,* 1823-1830.

Link, M.P., Goorin, A.M., Miser, A.W., et al. (1986). The effect of adjuvant chemotherapy on relapse-free survival in patients with osteosarcoma of the extremity. *New England Journal of Medicine 314,* 1600-1606.

Memorial Sloan-Kettering Cancer Center (MSKCC). (2002). *Questions and answers about sarcoma.* Retrieved February 19, 2003 from the World Wide Web: http://www.mskcc.org/mskcc/html/439.cfm and http://www.mskcc.org/mskcc/html/444.cfm.

National Cancer Institute (NCI). (2002a). *Adult soft tissue sarcoma.* Retrieved March 20, 2004 from the World Wide Web CancerNet (PDQ) websites for health professionals: http://www.nci.nih.gov/cancerinfo/pdq/treatment/adult-soft-tissue-sarcoma/healthprofessional.

National Cancer Institute (NCI). (2002b). *Childhood rhabdomyosarcoma.* Retrieved February 19, 2003 from the World Wide Web CancerNet (PDQ) websites for health professionals: http://www.nci.nih.gov/cancerinfo/pdq/treatment/childrhabdomyosarcoma/healthprofessional/#Section1.

National Cancer Institute (NCI). (2002c). *Ewing's family of tumors.* Retrieved February 19, 2003 from the World Wide Web CancerNet (PDQ) websites for health professionals: http://www.nci.nih.gov/cancerinfo/pdq/treatment/ewings/healthprofessional/#Section1.

National Cancer Institute (NCI). (2002d). *Soft tissue sarcoma.* Retrieved February 19, 2003 from the World Wide Web CancerNet (PDQ) websites for health professionals: http://www.cancer.gov/cancer_information/cancer_type/soft_tissue_sarcoma.

National Institutes of Health (NIH) Clinical Trials.gov. (2004a). *Osteosarcoma.* Retrieved March 20, 2004 from the World Wide Web: http://clinicaltrials.gov/ct/gui/search?term=sarcoma&submit=Search.

National Institutes of Health (NIH) Clinical Trials.gov. (2004b). *Soft tissue sarcoma.* Retrieved March 20, 2004 from the World Wide Web: http://clinicaltrials.gov/ct/gui/search?term=sarcoma&submit=Search.

North American Nursing Diagnosis Association (NANDA). (2001). *Nursing diagnoses: Definitions and classification, 2001-2003.* Philadelphia: North American Nursing Diagnosis Association.

Otto, S. (2001). Pediatric cancers. In S. Otto (Ed.). *Oncology nursing* (4th ed.). St. Louis: Mosby, pp. 477-497.

Palella, F.J., Jr., Delaney, K.M., Moorman, A.C., et al. (1998). Declining morbidity and mortality among patients with advanced human immunodeficiency virus infection. *New England Journal of Medicine 338,* 853-860.

Piasecki, P. (2000). Bone and soft tissue sarcoma. In C.H. Yarbro, M.H. Frogge, M. Goodman, & S.L. Groenwald (Eds.). *Cancer nursing: Principles and practice* (5th ed.). Sudbury, MA: Jones and Bartlett Publishers, pp. 323-351.

Sarcoma Meta-analysis Collaboration (SMAC). (2002). *Adjuvant chemotherapy for localized resectable soft tissue sarcoma in adults (Cochrane Review). The Cochrane Library, 2.* Chichester, UK: John Wiley & Sons.

Stojadinovic, A., Leung, D.H.Y., Allen, P., et al. (2002). Primary adult soft tissue sarcoma: Time-dependent influence of prognostic variables. *Journal of Clinical Oncology 21,* 4344-4352.

Yasko, A., Patel, R., Pollack, A., & Pollock, R. (2001). Sarcomas of soft tissue and bone. In R.E. Lenhard, R.T. Osteen, & T. Gansler (Eds.). *Clinical oncology.* Atlanta: American Cancer Society, pp. 611-632.

34 Nursing Care of the Client with HIV-Related Cancers

THERESA A. MORAN

Theory

I. Human immunodeficiency virus (HIV) as a predisposing factor to certain cancers.
  A. Definition of HIV.
  1. Cytopathic retrovirus member of lentivirus family (Casey et al., 1996).
    a. Transmitted through body fluids.
    b. Long incubation and gradual progression are typical.
    c. Causes chronic disease in host.
  2. Structure (Casey et al., 1996).
    a. *p24* protein core surrounds the ribonucleic acid (RNA) genome.
    b. Bilayered lipid envelope.
    c. Surface antigens—gp120, gp41.
      (1) gp120—attracted to CD4 surface marker on host cells.
      (2) Human cell with most abundant CD4—T lymphocyte; CD4 cell surface marker also found on macrophages, monocytes, microglial cells, Langerhans' cells, and dendritic cells.
    d. In order to replicate, the virus uses reverse transcriptase, an enzyme that mediates transcription of viral RNA to deoxyribonucleic acid (DNA) in infected cell.
  B. Immunologic structures.
  1. T lymphocytes.
    a. Stem cells from bone marrow mature in thymus, acquire surface markers, seed peripheral lymphoid tissue, and are found in the general circulation; approximately 80% of circulating lymphocytes are T cells (Casey et al., 1996).
    b. Composed of CD4+ cells, also known as T4+ cells or helper cells, and CD8+ cells, also known as T8+ cells or suppressor cells. CD4+ cells responsible for "turning on" immune response, and CD8+ cells responsible for "turning off" immune response through the use of lymphokines/cytokines. Generally, CD4+ and CD8+ cells exist in a 2:1 ratio, with twice as many CD4+ cells as CD8+ cells (Casey et al., 1996).
    c. Pivotal in cell-mediated immunity; regulates overall immune response (Casey et al., 1996).
    d. Protects against intracellular parasites and tumors; provides immunosurveillance; responsible for graft rejection; displays memory effect.
    e. CD4+/T4 helper cells are primary HIV targets (Casey et al., 1996).

   2. B lymphocytes.
     a. Believed to mature in bone marrow; found in general circulation and also seed peripheral lymphoid germinal centers; 12% to 15% of circulating lymphocytes are B cells (Casey et al., 1996).
     b. Pivotal in humoral immunity.
     c. When stimulated, B cells produce plasma cells, which in turn produce antigen-specific antibody (Casey et al., 1996).
     d. Protect against bacterial and viral infections.
     e. B memory cells provide anamnestic effect (store template of specific antibodies).
   3. Lymphoid organs and circulation.
     a. Primary organs—bone marrow and thymus (Casey et al., 1996).
     b. Also included—lymphatic vessels, lymph nodes, spleen, liver (Casey et al., 1996).
     c. Nonencapsulated clusters of lymphoid tissue are found around lining of aerodigestive tract.
     d. Lymph nodes are located at junction of lymphatic channels (Casey et al., 1996).
       (1) Small and bean shaped; store T and B cells and macrophages.
       (2) Lymphadenopathy (increase in size of lymph nodes) occurs when immune response invoked by presence of antigen.
   4. Natural killer (NK) cells.
     a. Relatively small population of lymphocytes distinct from T and B cells. Are large granular lymphocytes that originate in the bone marrow (Casey et al., 1996; Kaplan & Northfelt, 1999).
     b. Primary function is cytotoxicity; target tumor and virally infected cells. Can also produce an array of cytokines that affect immune responses, including interferon-alpha (IFN-α).
     c. Nonspecific action; no specific memory function.
C. Physiologic basis of HIV infection and HIV-related cancers.
   1. HIV effect on CD4+ lymphocytes (Kaplan & Northfelt, 1999).
     a. HIV binds to CD4 surface marker on T cells.
     b. Fusion and release of viral RNA into host cells.
     c. Viral RNA is transcribed to DNA through action of reverse transcriptase and is integrated into host nuclear DNA; viral particles also are found in host cell cytoplasm.
     d. May remain dormant for variable period, or immediate viral production by infected cell may occur.
     e. Protease enzyme required for assembly of new virus.
     f. Newly produced virion buds from surface of infected cell and infects other cells.
     g. Host cells eventually are depleted.
   2. HIV effect on immune system.
     a. Progressive infection leads to qualitative and quantitative T4-lymphocyte dysfunction, with resultant defect in both cellular and humoral immunity as immunoregulatory function of T4 cells is gradually impaired (Kaplan & Northfelt, 1999).
       (1) Progressive destruction of CD4+ (helper) T cells results from viral replication in host.
       (2) HIV may cause polyclonal B-cell activity (also may be due to coinfection with Epstein-Barr virus [EBV]) (Cingolani et al., 2000; Scadden, 2000).

(3) Both cellular and humoral immunity impaired. Chronically stimulated B cells can lead to mutations that may result in malignant clone, or in polyclonal malignancy (Cingolani et al., 2000; Scadden, 2000).

(4) Impaired cellular immunity means impaired immune surveillance and allows for proliferation of malignantly transformed cells.

(5) No conclusive data exist about quantitative changes in the T4 cell count and stage of disease. However, a CD4+ count of less than 200 cells/mm^3 is associated with increased incidence of opportunistic infections, and some malignancies (Kaplan & Northfelt, 1999).

   b. Cofactors in disease progression.

(1) Definitive role of specific cofactors in disease progression is controversial; may be difficult to distinguish between comorbid infection and true causal relationship (Casey et al., 1996; Cingolani et al., 2000).

(2) Infectious cofactors may include presence of cytomegalovirus (CMV), EBV, and other viruses (Cingolani et al., 2000).

(3) Lifestyle factors may also influence course of infection; risk for disease progression increases in presence of inadequate nutrition, general poor health, smoking, activities that may result in infection with other strains of HIV (Casey et al., 1996; Cingolani et al., 2000).

3. Clinical staging and classification of HIV infection.

   a. Infection with HIV produces a continuum of changes in health status.

   b. Clinical status may change rapidly in either direction.

   c. Knowledge of disease stage guides selection of therapeutic intervention and psychosocial support.

   d. Two major systems for classifying HIV disease—Centers for Disease Control (CDC) system and Walter Reed system.

(1) CDC classification system (Table 34-1) (Casey et al., 1996).

(a) Considers both laboratory and clinical parameters.

(b) Provides surveillance definition to guide epidemiologic data collection and serves as framework for stratifying levels of illness.

TABLE 34-1
Centers for Disease Control Classification System for HIV Infection*

	Category A	Category B	Category C
	Asymptomatic; persistent generalized lymphadeno-pathy; or acute retroviral syndrome	Conditions not usually seen in immunocompetent people (e.g., oral thrush)	AIDS-defining illnesses (e.g., KS, invasive cervical cancer, lymphoma)
CD4 COUNT			
>500	A1	B1	**C1**
200-499	A2	B2	**C2**
0-199	**A3**	**B3**	**C3**

KS, Kaposi's sarcoma; *CDC*, Centers for Disease Control and Prevention; *HIV*, human immunodeficiency virus; *AIDS*, acquired immunodeficiency syndrome.
*CDC 1993 Classification System for HIV Infection uses two indices—CD4 count and clinical condition- to classify/stage disease in HIV+ persons. By definition, individuals with CD4 count less than 200 qualify for AIDS diagnosis, as well as those diagnosed with category C ("AIDS-defining") conditions (i.e., the categories in bold type).

TABLE 34-2
Walter Reed Staging System for HIV Infection

Stage	HIV Antibody Status	Chronic Lymphadenopathy	CD4 Count	Skin Test	Oral Thrush	Opportunistic Infections
0	Negative	—	>400	WNL	—	—
1	Positive	—	>400	WNL	—	—
2	Positive	Present	>400	WNL	—	—
3	Positive	+/–	<400	WNL	—	—
4	Positive	+/–	<400	Partial anergy	—	—
5	Positive	+/–	<400	Complete anergy	Yes	—
6	Positive	+/–	<400	Partial/complete anergy	+/–	Yes

HIV, Human immunodeficiency virus; *WNL*, within normal limits; +/–, may or may not be present.

      (2) Walter Reed staging system (Table 34-2) (Casey et al., 1996).
         (a) Based on clinical presentation of individual client.
         (b) Designed to correlate with progressive immune dysfunction.
         (c) Excludes neurologic symptoms.
   4. Malignant disease as a result of HIV infection.
     a. Impaired immune surveillance function and chronically stimulated B cells may result in growth of malignantly transformed cells (Casey et al., 1996; Kaplan & Northfelt, 1999).
     b. B-cell lymphoma—most frequently diagnosed malignant disease in HIV-infected clients. Since the advent of highly active antiretroviral therapy (HAART), incidence of Kaposi's sarcoma has declined dramatically (Casey et al., 1996; Kaplan & Northfelt, 1999).
     c. Confounding factors in clients with HIV disease are abnormal sites of presentation, poor duration of response to therapy, and presence of comorbid opportunistic infection.
     d. HIV-infected women are at increased risk for cervical dysplasia and for rapid progression to cervical cancer; diagnosis and staging are same as in non–HIV-positive disease in women, with the difference being the aggressiveness of the histology (Casey et al., 1996; Kaplan & Northfelt, 1999).
II. HAART and the incidence of HIV-related malignancies.
  A. Kaposi's sarcoma (KS).
    1. Spectrum of tumors in the context of HIV infection varies by risk group and has been dramatically influenced by HAART (Cattelan et al., 2001; Grulich et al., 2001).
    2. Incidence of KS already on the decline in the United States even before introduction of HAART; since then KS has become a relative rarity (Biggar, 2001; Kirk et al., 2001; Rabkin, 2000).
    3. Estimates of reduction of KS in HIV-infected persons are as much as eightyfold; however, in areas where HAART is not available, such as sub-Saharan Africa, KS remains a major problem and in some areas the major cancer diagnosis.
  B. Primary central nervous system lymphoma (PCNSL).
    1. Generally a complication of advanced HIV disease. Typically clients have a CD4 count of less than 100 cells/mm^3 and often less than 50 cells/mm^3.

Much less common, this subset of non-Hodgkin's lymphoma (NHL) has also undergone a dramatic change in incidence since the advent of HAART (Grulich et al., 2001).

2. Unlike systemic NHL, PCNSLs are uniformly associated with EBV. Felt that EBV latent gene expression is readily targeted by cytotoxic T lymphocytes and that this may account for decline in incidence of PCNSL with successful control of HIV-induced immune destruction with HAART (Grulich et al., 2001).

C. Systemic NHL.

1. Less dramatically reduced by HAART. Overall estimated twofold to sevenfold decline (Grulich et al., 2001; Kirk et al., 2001; Ratner et al., 2001).

2. In one European study, incidence of all subtypes of lymphoma significantly declined from 30.7 cases/100 patient-years in 1994 to 2.5 cases/100 patient-years in 1998. This decline was statistically significant. Was felt to be result of HAART becoming readily available. Greatest decline observed in immunoblastic lymphoma and PCNSL. However, during this same period the proportion of new acquired immunodeficiency syndrome (AIDS) cases secondary to lymphoma increased significantly from less than 4% in 1994 to 16% in 1998, also statistically significant (Rabkin, 2000).

3. The fact that a decline was only seen in specific subsets of NHL, specifically immunoblastic lymphoma and PCNSL, while the incidence of Burkitt's lymphoma and Hodgkin's disease remained unchanged, suggested to the authors the possible variable involvement of immune function in tumor development (Grulich et al., 2001; Kirk et al., 2001; Ratner et al., 2001).

III. HIV-related malignancies.

A. HIV-related lymphoma.

1. Definition/pathogenesis—traditionally considered a late manifestation of HIV infection, occurring in the setting of significant immune suppression with CD4 cells below $200/mm^3$.

a. Found equally in all subpopulations of HIV-infected persons. Reflects same epidemiologic characteristics as non–HIV-related lymphoma.

b. Characteristics specific to HIV include lower CD4 counts, older age, and lack of HAART-related lymphoma.

c. Majority of clients present with B-cell tumors of intermediate or high-grade histologic type. May be either systemic (i.e., involving the body) or primary central nervous system (CNS; i.e., involving only the CNS); no other organs/tissues involved. If there is involvement of sites outside the CNS, the client is considered to have systemic disease with CNS involvement (Levine et al., 2000).

d. In systemic disease, extranodal involvement is common; the most commonly affected sites are gastrointestinal (GI) tract, CNS, and bone marrow (Levine et al., 2000; van Baarle et al., 2001).

e. Appears to be a unique and identifiable pattern of involvement related to histologic subsets of NHL. Large cell lymphomas tend to be found in the GI tract, whereas small cell lymphomas are more likely to involve the bone marrow and meninges (Levine et al., 2000; van Baarle et al., 2001).

f. Primary effusion lymphoma (body cavity lymphoma), a distinct presentation associated with human herpesvirus type 8 (HHV-8) (Karcher & Alkan, 1997).

    g. Hodgkin's disease, multiple myeloma, and B-cell acute lymphocytic leukemia are examples of other lymphoid malignancies that have been diagnosed in HIV-infected persons. Although strongly suspected, no causal relationship has yet been identified (Lyter et al., 1995; Selik et al., 1995).

2. Cause.

    a. Exact cause unknown. In HIV-related PCNSL, EBV is consistently present. Thought that EBV latent genes are expressed, which are known to dysregulate cell growth control, and can result in transformation of B lymphocytes (Levine et al., 2000; Scadden, 2000; van Baarle et al., 2001).

    b. Systemic lymphomas seem to have more complex pathophysiology.

        (1) EBV present in 33% to 67% (depending on the report) and latent gene expression not consistently observed.

        (2) Those without EBV have range of other genetic abnormalities, including *Bcl-6* rearrangement, *C-myc* rearrangement, and *p53* mutations. Mutations appear to be histologically determined (i.e., small cell lymphoma commonly associated with *C-myc* rearrangements, but not *Bcl-6* and rarely *p53* mutations) (Levine et al., 2000; Scadden, 2000; van Baarle et al., 2001).

    c. In addition, B-cell growth kinetics appear to be altered in the presence of HIV infection, which results clinically in lymphadenopathy and hypergammaglobulinemia. May directly contribute to the process through antigenic drive (Levine et al., 2000).

    d. Finally, genetic analyses of client cohorts have begun to reveal host-related factors relevant to the risk of lymphoma. Some appear to be promotional and some protective. There may be a time when genomic analysis of host-pathogen interaction is used as a screening tool or to plan preventive strategies (Levine et al., 2000; van Baarle et al., 2001).

    e. Role of HHV-8 in development of primary effusion lymphomas still being investigated. The exact mechanism of pathology remains unknown, but it is known that in body cavity lymphomas, also known as primary effusion lymphomas, genomic material has been incorporated from both HHV-8 and EBV into their DNA (Groves et al., 2001).

3. Detection and diagnosis.

    a. Need to confirm HIV positivity—diagnosis of HIV infection usually made on basis of positive antibody test.

        (1) Enzyme-linked immunosorbent assay (ELISA) test for antibody to HIV is used for screening—high sensitivity and specificity in populations at risk.

        (2) If ELISA test positive, test repeated; if second test positive, confirmatory Western blot conducted on same specimen.

        (3) Other tests to demonstrate infection with HIV—polymerase chain reaction (PCR; a gene amplification technique) or viral culture.

    b. Diagnosis of HIV-related lymphoma—similar to testing done for same conditions when not related to HIV infection; because of wide variance in presenting symptoms, workup in HIV-infected person may be more aggressive or comprehensive than in uninfected person.

        (1) Brain biopsy may be performed to establish a diagnosis of malignancy versus opportunistic infections; constitutional symptoms such as night sweats may be related to infection with *Mycobacterium avium-intracellulare*. CNS symptoms may be related to cerebral toxoplasmosis (Grulich et al., 2001; Kaplan & Northfelt, 1999).

(2) In the absence of brain biopsy, diagnosis of PCNSL is a diagnosis of exclusion. Client may be treated for toxoplasmosis. If client demonstrates a response, then he/she is presumed to have toxoplasmosis. If no response demonstrated then client is presumed to have PCNSL, antibiotics are discontinued, and a trial of radiotherapy may be undertaken without tissue biopsy. The likelihood of a client having toxoplasmosis in the presence of a negative toxoplasmosis titer is very low. If possible, a biopsy is always preferable (Grulich et al., 2001; Kaplan & Northfelt, 1999).

4. Appearance and metastasis—wide array of possible clinical presentations. CNS, GI tract, and bone marrow involvement are more frequent in HIV-infected persons; virtually every organ system may be involved.
   a. CNS lesions may cause changes in cognitive function, memory loss, decreased attention span, headaches, personality change, focal neurologic deficits, or generalized seizure activity.
   b. GI tract lesions may cause malabsorption, diarrhea, constipation, or focal or diffuse abdominal discomfort or may present as an asymptomatic abdominal mass (Levine et al., 2000).
   c. Clients with primary effusion lymphomas present with effusions (pericardial, pleural, or ascites) and no discrete mass.
   d. Blood counts are usually normal despite bone marrow involvement.
5. Staging methods and procedures.
   a. Staging for HIV-related lymphoma typically follows the same schema as for non–HIV-related lymphoma (i.e., the Ann Arbor staging system; see Chapter 32) (Kaplan & Northfelt, 1999).
   b. Because HIV-related malignancies may present at abnormal sites, diagnostic imaging and/or endoscopic examinations may be more extensive than in HIV-negative persons.
6. Standard therapies.
   a. Treatment of HIV-related cancers based on approaches used for uninfected persons. However, underlying immune deficiency, presence of other opportunistic infections, polypharmacy, and generalized poor health status may require dose reduction, scheduling modifications, and/or selection of alternative approaches.
   b. Surgery.
      (1) Rarely used; exceptions include excisional or incisional biopsy in clients with HIV-related NHL.
   c. Chemotherapy.
      (1) Dose adjustment may be indicated based on CD4 count, treatment-related side effects, response, concomitant infections.
      (2) HIV-related lymphoma is treated with combination chemotherapy, using agents such as cyclophosphamide (Cytoxan), vincristine (Oncovin), methotrexate (Mexate), etoposide (VP-16, Vepesid), cytosine arabinoside (Ara-C, Cytosar), bleomycin (Blenoxane), and steroids. Use of methotrexate, bleomycin, Adriamycin (doxorubicin), cyclophosphamide, Oncovin (vincristine), and dexamethasone (M-BACOD) is common (Kaplan et al., 1997; Ratner et al., 2001).
         (a) PCNSL is usually resistant to systemic chemotherapy because few agents cross the blood-brain barrier. Exceptions are high-dose methotrexate (>3 g/m^2) and high-dose cytarabine (Ara-C) (>2 g/m^2) (Kaplan & Northfelt, 1999).

(b) Intrathecal administration of chemotherapy may be considered to treat lymphomatous meningitis; not useful in bulky disease.

(c) Use of concomitant HAART plus chemotherapy has been demonstrated to be tolerable; however, caution should be used when using chemotherapy together with zidovudine (AZT), which may cause significant bone marrow compromise.

(d) Ongoing studies are evaluating usefulness of stem cell transplant in HIV-positive clients with NHL or Hodgkin's disease (Little et al., 2000).

(e) Use of colony-stimulating factors and prophylactic antibiotics has resulted in decreased number of febrile episodes and hospitalizations. Use of HAART has improved median survival (Kaplan et al., 1991; Tam et al., 2002).

  d. Radiotherapy.

    (1) Role of radiotherapy in HIV-related lymphoma is one of palliation or consolidation (e.g., involved-field radiotherapy after chemotherapy). May be used to attempt to control otherwise unresponsive disease. In high-grade tumors, the response may be short lived. In low-grade tumors, which are slow growing to start with, there may be good control of symptoms that may be of longer duration (Kaplan & Northfelt, 1999).

  e. Biologic response modifiers—being evaluated as treatment for the underlying HIV infection, but they generally are not used to treat HIV-related lymphomas.

  f. Combined-modality treatment is not well documented as therapy for HIV-related malignancies; synergistic therapeutic effects and side effects must be weighed carefully.

7. Nursing management.

  a. Clients with HIV-related malignancies respond similarly to aggressive symptom management, including antiemetic therapy, as their non–HIV-related counterparts; because of polypharmacy, monitor carefully for drug-drug interactions.

  b. Need to thoroughly assess clients with fevers, respiratory symptoms, or GI symptoms for possible opportunistic infections.

  c. Client should be educated regarding the signs and symptoms of infection, dehydration, when to seek medical attention, neutropenic/thrombocytopenic precautions, and the importance of taking medication on time.

  d. Clients with HIV-related NHL typically present with bulky disease and are at risk for tumor lysis syndrome with their first chemotherapy treatment; frequent electrolyte monitoring is indicated in this population.

  e. A thorough psychosocial assessment of all clients should be performed.

8. Prognosis.

  a. Survival in persons with HIV-related malignancies depends on multiple factors, including HAART, the degree of immunosuppression, presence of opportunistic infection(s), nutritional status, location of presenting lesion, lifestyle, and availability and accessibility of adequate care (Grulich et al., 2001; Levine et al., 2000; Rabkin et al., 1999).

  b. Factors associated with shorter survival of clients with AIDS-related lymphomas include CD4 cell count below 100 cells/mm^3, stage III or

IV disease, age older than 35 years, history of injection drug use, and elevated lactate dehydrogenase (LDH). The International Prognostic Index (IPI) for aggressive lymphoma has also been validated in clients with AIDS-related lymphoma.

    c. Median survival time ranges from 4 to 10 months. Shortest survival time is with CNS primary tumor (median, 1 to 2 months); longest survival time is with low-grade lymphomas (1 to 4 years). Survival influenced by HAART, supportive care, and prophylactic interventions (Levine et al., 2000).

B. HIV-related KS.

  1. Definition/pathogenesis—soft tissue malignancy characterized by malignant growth of reticuloendothelial cell origin in HIV-infected persons (Grulich et al., 2001; Jacobson & Armenian, 1995; Kaplan & Northfelt, 1999).

  2. Cause.

    a. Before HIV, endemic KS occurred in geographic regions, such as Mediterranean basin and sub-Saharan Africa. Persons receiving immunosuppressive agents after organ transplant also at risk (transplant-associated KS) (Grulich et al., 2001; Jacobson & Armenian, 1995).

    b. In clients with HIV-related KS (epidemic KS), malignantly transformed cells reproduce unchecked as a result of underlying immune defect (Grulich et al., 2001; Jacobson & Armenian, 1995; Kaplan & Northfelt, 1999).

      (1) Disproportionate risk for KS among select immunodeficient populations raised suspicion of secondary infectious factor.

        (a) Confirmed by identification of HHV-8, also known as KS herpesvirus (KSHV).

        (b) Compelling evidence now exists for causative association of KSHV with KS (Boshoff & Chang, 2001; Chang et al., 1994; Gannem, 1997).

        (c) KSHV infection is necessary but not sufficient for KS. Its malignant potential appears to be quite low outside the setting of immune compromise (Boshoff & Chang, 2001; Chang et al., 1994; Chatlynne & Ablashi, 1999).

      (2) KSHV genome encodes a number of gene products. Host response to the virus appears to be critical in determining clinical outcome of infection, including tumor development (Boshoff & Chang, 2001; Chatlynne & Ablashi, 1999; Harrington et al., 1997).

      (3) HIV-associated *tat* gene product can enhance KSHV replication and increase expression of various chemokines. May thereby directly potentiate KSHV effects and indirectly contribute to oncogenesis (Harrington et al., 1997).

  3. Detection and diagnosis.

    a. Need to confirm HIV positivity—diagnosis of HIV infection usually made on basis of positive antibody test.

      (1) ELISA test for antibody to HIV is used for screening—high sensitivity and specificity in populations at risk.

      (2) If ELISA test positive, test repeated; if second test positive, confirmatory Western blot conducted on same specimen.

      (3) Other tests to demonstrate infection with HIV—PCR (a gene amplification technique) or viral culture.

    b. Diagnosis of HIV-related KS—similar to testing done for same condition when not related to HIV infection; because of wide variance in presenting symptoms, workup in HIV-infected person may be more aggressive or comprehensive than in uninfected person.

    c. Once tissue diagnosis of KS lesions confirmed, physician may elect not to perform a biopsy of new skin lesions; biopsy of visceral lesions may be done if the risk/benefit ratio permits.

4. Appearance and metastasis of HIV-related KS.

    a. Classic presentation includes skin lesions, ranging from pink to purple to brownish, flat or raised, usually painless (unless in a sensitive area), and do not blanch with pressure (Grulich et al., 2001; Kaplan & Northfelt, 1999).

    b. HIV-related KS may present as skin lesions or may first appear in any other organ system, including the oral cavity (Grulich et al., 2001; Jacobson & Armenian, 1995; Kaplan & Northfelt, 1999).

    c. Classic KS is typically indolent, whereas HIV-related KS may be very aggressive and progress rapidly (Grulich et al., 2001; Jacobson & Armenian, 1995; Kaplan & Northfelt, 1999).

5. Staging methods and procedures.

    a. No universally accepted staging system for HIV-related KS identified; schemas used include parameters of cutaneous, lymph node, and visceral involvement and the occurrence of "B symptoms" (fever, night sweats, unintentional weight loss).

    b. Because HIV-related malignancies may present at abnormal sites, diagnostic imaging and/or endoscopic examinations may be more extensive than in HIV-negative persons. However, in KS, diagnosing asymptomatic disease is of little benefit.

6. Standard therapies.

    a. Treatment of HIV-related cancers based on approaches used for uninfected persons. However, underlying immune deficiency, presence of other opportunistic infections, polypharmacy, and generalized poor health status may require dose reduction, scheduling modifications, and/or selection of alternative approaches.

    b. Surgery.

        (1) Rarely used in the treatment of KS. Exceptions include removal of lesions that interfere with function or cause significant pain.

    c. Chemotherapy.

        (1) Dose adjustment may be indicated based on CD4 count, treatment-related side effects, response, concomitant infections.

        (2) HIV-related KS most effectively treated with HAART (up to 86% response rate, with durable responses that generally increase over time). If recurrent or persistent, may be treated with single-agent chemotherapy or less frequently with combination chemotherapy. Treatment of HIV-related KS is palliative, not curative, and watchful waiting is an acceptable option (Biggar, 2001; Cattelan et al., 2001; Grulich et al., 2001).

            (a) Tumor treatment may be locally applied for those with limited, accessible lesions. Liquid nitrogen and intralesional vinblastine (Velban) are two agents that may be used.

            (b) Liposomal doxorubicin (Doxil) or daunorubicin (DaunoXome) is the preferred therapy. Studies have shown equivalent therapeutic response with decreased toxicities (Gill et al., 1996;

Harrison et al., 1995; Northfelt et al., 1998; Presant et al., 1993).

(c) Paclitaxel (Taxol) is a highly active and generally well-tolerated agent for KS (Gill et al., 1999; Welles et al., 1998).

(d) Combination approaches including vinca alkaloids (especially vincristine; doxorubicin (Adriamycin) and bleomycin (Blenoxane) are less commonly used (Gill et al., 1990; Northfelt et al., 1998).

(e) Because of the vascular nature of KS lesions, antiangiogenic compounds are a natural strategy for treatment, and trials are ongoing. These trials, which include thalidomide (Thalomid), fumagillin, metastat (a matrix metalloproteinase inhibitor), have all shown regression in early studies, and further research is needed and ongoing.

d. Radiotherapy.

(1) KS lesions are typically radiosensitive.

(a) Effective short- to moderate-term local control may be achieved, especially for cosmetic effects or relief of lymphedema caused by lymphatic lesions. Permanent alteration in the radiated skin and lymphatics may result with subsequent persistent edema and tissue breakdown (Kaplan & Northfelt, 1999).

(b) Aggressive nature of epidemic KS precludes radiotherapy with curative intent.

e. Biologic response modifiers.

(1) IFN-α, with or without concomitant zidovudine, has been approved as treatment for HIV-related KS; the efficacy of other biologic response modifiers is being evaluated (Kaplan & Northfelt, 1999).

(2) Other biologic response modifiers are being evaluated as treatment for the underlying HIV infection.

f. Combined-modality treatment is not well documented as therapy for HIV-related malignancies; synergistic effects and toxicities must be weighed carefully.

7. Nursing management.

a. Clients with HIV-related malignancies respond similarly to aggressive symptom management, including antiemetic therapy, as their non–HIV-related counterparts; because of polypharmacy, monitor carefully for drug-drug interactions.

b. Need to thoroughly assess clients with fevers, respiratory symptoms, or GI symptoms for possible opportunistic infections.

c. Client should be educated regarding the signs and symptoms of infection, dehydration, when to seek medical attention, neutropenic/thrombocytopenic precautions, and the importance of taking medication on time.

d. Clients receiving vinca alkaloids for treatment of their KS may experience severe jaw pain; this neuropathy has been reported in non-HIV clients but seems to occur more frequently in the HIV population. Continued use of the vinca alkaloid may result in permanent nerve damage.

e. Self-image may be an issue for clients with KS; since the lesions may be obvious, camouflaging these lesions with make-up may be useful.

  f. A thorough psychosocial assessment of all clients should be performed.
  8. Prognosis.
   a. Survival in persons with HIV-related malignancies depends on multiple factors, including HAART, the degree of immunosuppression, presence of opportunistic infection(s), nutritional status, location of presenting lesion, lifestyle, and availability and accessibility of adequate care (Grulich et al., 2001; Levine et al., 2000; Rabkin et al., 1999).
   b. Survival for clients with KS has increased dramatically in the era of HAART.
    (1) With prophylactic and supportive intervention, clients with HIV-related KS have survived for several years (Biggar, 2001; Grulich et al., 2001; Rabkin, 2000).
   c. In clients with GI tract lesions or B symptoms, survival time is shorter.
   d. Clients with prior or comorbid major opportunistic infection have the worst prognosis, with median survival time of less than 1 year.
 C. Other malignancies.
  1. NHL and KS have been causally linked to HIV infection, and in 1993 squamous cell carcinoma (SCC) of the cervix was added to the list of HIV-related malignancies, not because an increased incidence of this cancer had been documented, but because of the incidence of human papillomavirus (HPV) and cervical dysplasia found in women infected with HIV.
  2. Although there appears to be an increased incidence of SCC of the anus and Hodgkin's disease in the HIV population, no causal relationship has been established.
  3. HIV-infected clients are also at risk for other age- and behavior-associated malignancies.
  4. All clients should be screened appropriately.

Assessment

  I. Clients at risk for HIV-related cancers (Flaskerud & Ungvarski, 1995; Halloran & Hughes, 1991; McMahon & Coyne, 1989).
 A. Individuals identified as HIV positive.
 B. Risks for infection with HIV are highest among people who meet the following criteria:
  1. Been sexually active with more than one partner since 1978.
  2. Shared needles to inject illegal substances or had sex with someone who does.
  3. Received blood or blood products or organ transplant between 1978 and 1985.
  4. Been born to HIV-infected mothers.
  5. Been exposed to HIV in other ways, such as through an accidental needle stick.
 II. Pertinent history—requires tact and sensitivity on the part of the nurse when inquiring about sensitive topics, such as sexuality and illicit drug use (Casey et al., 1996; Halloran & Hughes, 1991).
 A. Inquire about sexual and drug use history (Casey et al., 1996; Flaskerud & Ungvarski, 1995).
  1. Unprotected (i.e., without a condom) vaginal or rectal intercourse (highest risk).

2. Sharing of needles for drug injection, especially in areas of high incidence of HIV infection (major risk); persons with substance abuse disorders may also be at high risk for sexual transmission from engaging in high-risk sex while intoxicated or in "survival sex" (engaging in sex to obtain money, drugs, food, or other needs).

3. Homosexual or bisexual males may be reluctant to acknowledge sexual activity with other males; use tact and a nonjudgmental approach.

4. Women may be unaware of bisexual behavior of partner or deny such behavior.

5. History of one or more sexually transmitted diseases (syphilis, gonorrhea, herpes, chlamydia, hepatitis, genital warts) indicates higher risk.

B. Inquire about history of blood, blood product, or organ transplantation (Casey et al., 1996; Flaskerud & Ungvarski, 1995; Halloran & Hughes, 1991).

1. Since 1985, all blood and blood products in United States tested for presence of HIV antibodies; transfusions received in other countries may not have been tested.

2. Since the early 1980s, clotting factors used by persons with hemophilia have been treated to kill HIV.

C. Among children, determine HIV status of mother; children born to mothers infected with HIV have a 30% to 50% chance of being infected if the mother does not receive prenatal antiretroviral therapy.

D. Inquire about changes in mental status, memory, attention span, or personality; family members or significant others may recognize these changes before the client does; include these findings in data collection.

E. Ask if the person has been tested for the presence of HIV antibody and what the result was.

1. Because of social stigma attached to HIV infection and discrimination against HIV-infected people, the person may be reluctant to acknowledge having been tested or the result.

2. Explain that information about HIV status may be important in determining a diagnosis and treatment plan.

3. Legal restrictions and requirements relative to HIV infection vary among states; the ethical obligation of the nurse to maintain client confidentiality is universal.

III. Physical examination.

A. Signs and symptoms may vary in intensity, may wax and wane over time, but are usually progressive.

B. Inspect the skin.

1. Include gingiva and oral cavity, skinfolds, plantar surfaces, scalp, sclera and nares; KS lesions can appear anywhere on the body.

2. Integumentary changes in a client known to be infected with HIV may indicate opportunistic infection and should be noted. If the person performing the physical examination is not the primary caregiver, the primary caregiver should then be notified, and/or the client should be referred for further workup.

3. KS lesions may be purple to pink to brown, flat or raised; they do not blanch with pressure and are usually painless unless in a sensitive anatomic area.

4. Despite appearance, KS lesions do not bleed easily.

5. Lymphedema may result from obstruction of lymph flow by neoplastic growth.

C. Assess the thorax and abdomen.
1. Lesions in the lungs can cause rales, wheezes, or cacophonous breath sounds. There may be decreased breath sounds in the client with an effusion.
2. Cardiac involvement occurs and can cause muffled heart tones or other abnormal heart sounds, palpitations, or chest pain.
3. Evaluate abdomen for tenderness, masses, hyperactive bowel sounds, hepatic or splenic enlargement, and ascites.
D. Neurologic and mental status examination can reveal changes caused by CNS lesions, opportunistic infections, HIV-related dementia, or medication.
1. Obtain baseline examination for comparison.
2. Assess cranial nerves, including pupillary response, extraocular movements, gag reflex. Observe client while walking to assess gait and note any signs of ataxia. Note appearance, behavior, speech, affect, sensorimotor activity; elicit complaints such as chronic headache, light-headedness, dizziness, photophobia, syncope, paresthesias.
3. Findings may vary day to day. Include findings obtained from family, caregiver, and significant others.
E. Other signs and symptoms to assess—unintentional weight loss, diarrhea or constipation, fever, chills, night sweats, lymphadenopathy.
IV. Evaluation of laboratory data.
A. Laboratory studies related to neoplastic processes are the same as those for clients with same pathology who are not infected with HIV.
1. Hematologic values may be skewed in presence of HIV bone marrow invasion; white cell count or platelet count may be elevated or reduced.
2. Schedule of routine testing may differ from that used among non–HIV-infected individuals.
B. Studies to monitor HIV infection.
1. In the absence of HAART, estimated that CD4/T4-lymphocyte count decreases over time at a median rate of 10 cells per month as a result of progressive destruction of T4 cells by HIV; may be used to quantify the relative immunocompetence of the host, with lower values reflecting decreased immune response. Chemotherapy will also cause a decrease in the CD4 count.
2. Virally infected cells produce β_2-microglobulin; increasing serum levels indicate progressive infection.
3. HIV core antigen *p24* serum levels increase with progressive infection.
   a. Levels of β_2-microglobulin and *p24* may decrease in end-stage disease.
   b. Decreases may be due to depletion of target cell population rather than to improvement of immune function.
4. Viral load refers to the amount of HIV RNA detectable in peripheral blood; there are two laboratory methods (PCR and branched DNA), which are not interchangeable.
   a. Viral load assays have been demonstrated to be reliable predictors of therapeutic response to antiretroviral therapy.
   b. Viral load assays do not measure virus that may be harbored in anatomic sites other than the peripheral blood (e.g., CNS, lymphatic system).

Nursing Diagnoses

I. Risk for infection.
II. Disturbed body image.

III. Decisional conflict.
IV. Fatigue.
 V. Imbalanced nutrition: less than body requirements.
VI. Disturbed thought processes.

Outcome Identification

 I. Risk for infection because of treatment of malignancy.
   A. Client identifies signs and symptoms of infection and course of action to take—for example, monitoring body temperature and notifying primary care provider of any temperature higher than institutional protocol.
   B. Client identifies self-care measures to decrease risk of infection—for example, neutropenia precautions, maintenance of adequate rest and nutrition.
 II. Disturbed body image.
   A. Client identifies cause of body image disturbance—public KS lesions, bulky lymphadenopathy, surgical scar, side effects of therapy; together with care provider, develops strategies to deal with disturbed body image—for example, methods of camouflaging specific area, referral to therapist for counseling.
   B. Client identifies self-care measures to decrease incidence and severity of symptoms associated with disease and treatment—for example, maintenance of adequate rest and nutrition, monitoring body temperature, scheduling of activities to minimize fatigue, use of appropriate skin care techniques, use of prescribed antiemetic agents, or other techniques for symptom management.
   C. Client and significant other identify immediate and long-term side effects of disease and treatment that may contribute to disturbed body image—for example, exacerbation of immune suppression by myelotoxic therapies, side effects specific to agents used, skin changes caused by radiotherapy.
 III. Decisional conflict.
   A. Client identifies the presence of HIV infection, specific malignancy, and rationale for treatment.
   B. Client and significant other are provided with the opportunity to learn about the new diagnosis and to have all questions answered in order to be able to make an informed decision regarding treatment.
   C. Client and significant other list signs and symptoms of recurrent disease—growth of old or appearance of new KS lesions, increasing lymphadenopathy or lymphedema, return or exacerbation of sensorimotor changes, increase in rate of weight loss, change in elimination pattern, exacerbation of prior symptoms; and have the ability and knowledge to seek medical attention.
   D. Client and significant other identify community resources to meet demands of disease, treatment, and survivorship—local AIDS service organizations, church or civic organizations, American Cancer Society, hospice organizations, self-help groups such as Alcoholics Anonymous or Narcotics Anonymous when appropriate, local credit bureau.
 IV. Fatigue.
   A. Client identifies self-care measures to decrease incidence and severity of fatigue—for example, maintenance of adequate rest and nutrition, planning one's activities, relying on friends/family to complete tasks.
   B. Client is aware that there can be metabolic reasons for fatigue and has blood work done regularly, and client is aware that blood transfusions and exogenous erythropoietin may help improve fatigue.

V. Imbalanced nutrition: less than body requirements.
  A. Client identifies self-care measures to maintain adequate nutrition—for example, planning small frequent meals, premedicating with antiemetics, use of appetite stimulants, nutrition consult, prepacking meals.
VI. Disturbed thought processes.
  A. Client identifies that some premedications and/or treatment may result in disturbed thought process and plans appropriately—for example, avoids decision making that day, has friend/family accompany him/her to appointment, avoids driving.
  B. Client identifies that depression is a normal response to being diagnosed with a malignancy and identifies self-care measures in response to depression—for example, seeking medical or psychiatric attention.

Planning and Implementation

I. Interventions to maximize safety for client and significant other.
  A. Ensure environmental safety for clients experiencing sensorimotor changes (e.g., provide adequate lighting, especially at night).
  B. Instruct client about avoidance of potential environmental sources of opportunistic infection, such as animal waste from pets or uncooked, undercooked, or improperly stored food.
  C. Teach techniques to reduce possibility of HIV transmission.
    1. HIV is transmitted through blood and semen; use a latex condom with a recommended water-based lubricant to reduce risk (petroleum-based lubricants or cosmetic creams weaken the condom, increasing the chance of breakage during use) during every episode of vaginal, rectal, or oral intercourse.
    2. Do not share toothbrushes, razors, other personal care items.
    3. For cleanup of emesis or other body fluid spills, wear gloves and use a solution of one part household bleach to 10 parts water.
    4. Insist that health care workers and volunteer caregivers follow universal precautions as recommended by the CDC to reduce the risk of occupational exposure to HIV (Table 34-3).

TABLE 34-3
Body Fluids in Universal Precautions (CDC)

Body Fluids for Which Universal Precautions Apply	Body Fluids for Which Universal Precautions DO NOT Apply (unless contaminated by blood)
Blood; any secretion or excretion contaminated with blood	Urine
Cerebrospinal fluid	Feces
Semen; vaginal secretions	Vomitus
Synovial fluid	Perspiration
Amniotic fluid	Nasal secretions
Pericardial fluid	Tears
Pleural fluid	Sputum or saliva (except in dental practice)
Peritoneal fluid	

CDC, Centers for Disease Control and Prevention.

II. Interventions to decrease incidence and severity of symptoms associated with disease or treatment.
   A. Teach (or refer for teaching) ways to enhance appearance, such as use of covering cosmetics to hide KS lesions in cosmetically sensitive areas; use of scarves or other clothing to cover swollen lymph nodes; use of clothing appropriate to changing body mass with weight loss.
   B. Instruct the client to avoid the use of aspirin, which may interfere with platelet function, and instead to use acetaminophen to control fevers, minor aches and pains. Nonsteroidal antiinflammatory agents also affect platelet function, and the client should check with the primary care provider before taking them.
   C. Encourage establishment of regular rest periods and scheduled activities in accordance with energy level.
   D. Monitor nutritional status.
      1. Teach techniques to enhance nutritional intake (e.g., use of supplements, keeping ready-to-eat foods available, eating smaller and more frequent meals).
      2. Provide or encourage frequent oral hygiene.
   E. Teach appropriate techniques for skin care in areas being treated with radiotherapy (see Chapter 36).
   F. Assess knowledge or use of experimental and/or alternative treatment regimens.
      1. Determine and assess client knowledge of any contraindications that may exist between prescribed therapies and those obtained outside usual health care channels.
      2. Some experimental agents become available before receiving full Food and Drug Administration approval through "parallel track" programs, which allow use of drugs outside the clinical trial setting.
      3. Alternative therapies available through various sources (e.g., "buyers' clubs") may be used by clients.
         a. Ascertain all treatment regimens client is using, regardless of the source.
         b. Monitor interactions among multiple forms of therapy.
         c. Assist client with the process of evaluating alternative therapies in terms of effectiveness, side effects, costs, and safety.

III. Interventions to monitor for sequelae of disease and treatment.
   A. Provide teaching about myelotoxic side effects of chemotherapy and signs and symptoms of infection, such as acute temperature elevation, appearance of suppurative lesions, bleeding.
   B. Assess anorectal skin integrity in clients with diarrhea; teach appropriate skin care.
   C. Instruct client to report any signs or symptoms of neuropathy, including changes in sense of touch, peripheral numbness or tingling, difficulty with fine motor movement or walking (may be a medication side effect or caused by HIV infection).

IV. Interventions to monitor response to medical management.
   A. Assess and document location, appearance, size of KS lesions, lymphadenopathy, organomegaly, or other tumor effects (e.g., abdominal masses, oral lesions, ascites).
   B. Monitor for changes in size or appearance of the previously noted abnormalities.
   C. Obtain baseline and ongoing evaluation of mental status, performance status, and self-care ability.

D. Assess nutritional status, and document changes.
   1. Maintain serial record of body weight, with client wearing approximately same clothing with each recording.
   2. Document presence of dysphagia, odynophagia, changes in appetite or taste, or diarrhea that may be the result of oral lesions or a side effect of treatment.

V. Interventions to enhance adaptation and rehabilitation.
   A. Use notes, phone calls, or other reminders for appointments and medication administration times (may also use a pillbox with built-in alarm).
      1. Provide written instructions with frequent repetition and reinforcement included.
      2. Provide instruction to caregivers and significant others if client experiences mental status changes.
   B. Refer client and significant others to community agencies, civic organizations, or churches for assistance with social entitlement programs, peer support, and other available services such as home meal delivery.
   C. Refer for physical and/or occupational therapy for assistance in learning adaptive techniques to cope with sensorimotor deficits.
   D. Encourage discussion about client's wishes for use of resuscitative measures.
      1. Facilitate decision-making process by establishing atmosphere of trust and acceptance, providing accurate information, respecting client's choices.
      2. Ensure that client's wishes are properly documented and communicated to health care providers.

VI. Interventions to incorporate client and significant other in care.
   A. Recognize that the client's family of choice may differ from biologic family of origin.
      1. Determine and follow the client's expressed wishes regarding who is to receive what kind of information, who will be allowed visitation in hospital, and which terms to use to describe relationship (e.g., lover, partner, friend).
      2. Assist or refer for assistance with execution of durable power of attorney, will, and other necessary legal documentation.
   B. Assess resources and coping strategies of client and significant other.
      1. Determine past experience with HIV disease; in areas of high incidence, multiple losses may occur without adequate time for effective grieving.
      2. Consider that the significant other with HIV disease may experience symptoms that limit ability to provide care.
      3. Recognize that a significant other who is not infected with HIV may experience feelings of guilt, uncertainty about own health, concern for the future.
      4. Monitor for indications of maladaptive coping strategies, especially if history of substance use disorder is present; assist with learning alternative behaviors to manage stress and cope.
      5. Assess knowledge and/or use of alternative therapies.
   C. Include persons identified by the client as significant others in teaching and care decisions when appropriate.

Evaluation

The oncology nurse systematically and regularly evaluates the client's and/or family's responses to interventions to determine progress toward the achievement of expected outcomes. Relevant data are collected, and actual findings are compared with expected findings. Nursing diagnoses, outcomes, and plans of care are reviewed and revised as necessary.

REFERENCES

Biggar, R.J. (2001). AIDS-related cancers in the era of highly active antiretroviral therapy. *Oncology 15,* 439-448.

Boshoff, C., & Chang, Y. (2001). Kaposi's sarcoma-associated herpes virus: A new DNA tumor virus. *Annual Review of Medicine 52,* 453-470.

Casey, K., Cohen, E., & Hughes, A. (Eds.). (1996). *Core curriculum in HIV/AIDS nursing.* Philadelphia: Nursecom.

Cattelan, A., Calabro, M., Gasperini, P., et al. (2001). Acquired immunodeficiency syndrome-related Kaposi's sarcoma regression after highly active antiretroviral therapy: Biologic correlates of clinical outcome. *Journal of National Cancer Institute Monograph 28,* 44-49.

Chang, Y., Cesarman, E., Pessin, M.S., et al. (1994). Identification of a herpes virus-like DNA sequence in AIDS-associated Kaposi's sarcoma. *Science 266,* 1865-1869.

Chatlynne, L.G., & Ablashi, E.V. (1999). Seroepidemiology of Kaposi's sarcoma-associated herpes virus (KSHV). *Seminars in Cancer Biology 3,* 175-185.

Cingolani, A., Gastaldi, R., Fassone, L., et al. (2000). Epstein-Barr virus infection is predictive of CNS involvement in systemic AIDS-related non-Hodgkin's lymphomas. *Journal of Clinical Oncology 18,* 3325-3330.

Flaskerud, J.H., & Ungvarski, P.J. (Eds.). (1995). *HIV/AIDS: A guide to nursing care* (3rd ed.). Philadelphia: W.B. Saunders.

Gannem, D. (1997). KSHV and Kaposi's sarcoma: The end of the beginning? *Cell 91,* 157-160.

Gill, P.S., Rarick, M.U., Espina, B., et al. (1990). Advanced acquired immune deficiency syndrome-related Kaposi's sarcoma: Results of pilot studies using combination chemotherapy. *Cancer 65,* 1074-1078.

Gill, P.S., Tulpule, A., Espina, B.M., et al. (1999). Paclitaxel is safe and effective in the treatment of advanced AIDS-related Kaposi's sarcoma. *Journal of Clinical Oncology 17,* 1876-1883.

Gill, P.S., Wernz, J., Scadden, D.T., et al. (1996). Randomized phase III trial of liposomal daunorubicin versus doxorubicin, bleomycin, and vincristine in AIDS-related Kaposi's sarcoma. *Journal of Clinical Oncology 14,* 2353-2364.

Groves, A., Cotter, M., Subramania, C., et al. (2001). The latency associated nuclear antigen encoded by Kaposi's sarcoma-associated herpesvirus activate two major essential Epstein-Barr virus latent promoters. *Journal Virology 75:* 9446-9457.

Grulich, A.E., Li, Y., & McDonald, A.M. (2001). Decreasing rates of Kaposi's sarcoma and non-Hodgkin's lymphoma in the era of potent combination anti-retoviral therapy. *AIDS 15,* 629-633.

Halloran, J.P., & Hughes, A.M. (1991). Knowledge deficit related to prevention and early detection of HIV disease. In J.C. McNally, E.T. Somerville, C. Miaskowski, & M. Rostad (Eds.). *Guidelines for oncology nursing practice* (2nd ed.). Philadelphia: W.B. Saunders, pp. 47-54.

Harrington, W., Jr., Sieczkowski, L., Sosa, C., et al. (1997). Activation of HHV-8 by HIV-1 tat. *Lancet 349,* 774-775.

Harrison, M., Tomlinson, D., & Stewart, S. (1995). Liposomal-entrapped doxorubicin: An active agent in AIDS-related Kaposi's sarcoma. *Journal of Clinical Oncology 13,* 914-920.

Jacobson, L.P., & Armenian, H.K. (1995). An integrated approach to the epidemiology of Kaposi's sarcoma. *Current Opinion in Oncology 7,* 450-455.

Kaplan, L.D., Kahn, J.O., Crowe, S., et al. (1991). Clinical and virologic effects of recombinant human granulocyte-macrophage colony stimulating factor in patients receiving chemotherapy for HIV associated non-Hodgkin's lymphoma: Results of a randomized trial. *Journal of Clinical Oncology 9,* 929-940.

Kaplan, L.D., & Northfelt, D.W. (1999). Malignancies associated with AIDS. In M.A. Sande & P.A. Volberding (Eds.). *The medical management of AIDS (6th ed.).* Philadelphia: W.B. Saunders, pp. 467-497.

Kaplan, L.D., Straus, D.J., Testa, M.A., et al. (1997). Low-dose compared with standard-dose m-BACOD chemotherapy for non-Hodgkin's lymphoma associated with human immunodeficiency virus infection. *New England Journal of Medicine 336,* 1641-1648.

Karcher, D.S., & Alkan, S. (1997). Human herpesvirus-8-associated body cavity-based lymphoma in human immunodeficiency virus-infected patients: A unique B-cell neoplasm. *Human Pathology 28,* 801-808.

Kirk, O., Pedersen, C., & Cozzi-Lepri, A. (2001). Non-Hodgkin's lymphoma in HIV-infected patients in the era of highly active antiretroviral therapy. *Blood 98*, 3406-3412.

Levine, A.M., Senevirante, L., Espina, B.M., et al. (2000). Evolving characteristics of AIDS-related lymphoma. *Blood 96*, 4084-4090.

Little, R.F., Yarchoan, R., & Wilson, W.H. (2000). Systemic chemotherapy for HIV-associated lymphoma in the era of highly active antiretroviral therapy. *Current Opinion in Oncology 12*, 438-444.

Lyter, D.W., Bryant, J., Thackeray, R., et al. (1995). Incidence of HIV-related and non-related malignancies in a large cohort of homosexual men. *Journal of Clinical Oncology 13*(10), 2540-2546.

McMahon, K.M., & Coyne, N. (1989). Symptom management in patients with AIDS. *Seminars in Oncology Nursing 5*(4), 289-301.

Northfelt, D.W., Dezube, B.J., Thommes, J.A., et al. (1998). Pegylated-liposomal doxorubicin versus doxorubicin, bleomycin, and vincristine in the treatment of AIDS-related Kaposi's sarcoma: Results of a randomized phase III clinical trial. *Journal of Clinical Oncology 16*, 2445-2451.

Presant, C.A., Scolaro, M., Kennedy, P., et al. (1993). Liposomal daunorubicin treatment of HIV-associated Kaposi's sarcoma. *Lancet 341*, 1242-1243.

Rabkin, C.S. (2000). AIDS and cancer in the era of highly active antiretroviral therapy (HAART). *European Journal of Cancer 37*, 1316-1319.

Rabkin, C.S., Testa, M.A., Huang, J., & VonRoenn, J.H. (1999). Kaposi's sarcoma and non-Hodgkin's lymphoma incidence trends in AIDS Clinical Trial Group study participants. *Journal of Acquired Immune Deficiency Syndromes and Human Retrovirology 21*(Suppl.1), S31-S33.

Ratner, L., Lee, J., Tang, S., et al. (2001). Chemotherapy for human immunodeficiency virus-associated non-Hodgkin's lymphoma in combination with highly active antiretroviral therapy. *Journal of Clinical Oncology 19*, 2171-2178.

Scadden, D.T. (2000). Epstein-Barr virus, the CNS, and AIDS-related lymphomas: As close as flame to smoke. *Journal of Clinical Oncology 18*, 3323-3324.

Selik, R.M., Chu, S.Y., & Ward, J.W. (1995). Trends in infections and cancers among persons dying of HIV infection in the U.S. from 1987-1992. *Annals of Internal Medicine 123*, 933-936.

Tam, H., Zhang, Z., Jacobson, L.P., et al. (2002). Effect of highly active antiretroviral therapy on survival among HIV-infected men with Kaposi's sarcoma or non-Hodgkin lymphoma, *International Journal of Cancer 98*, 916-922.

van Baarle, D., Hovenkamp, E., & Callan, M.F. (2001). Dysfunctional Epstein-Barr virus (EBV)-specific CD8+ T lymphocytes and increased EBV load in HIV-1 infected individuals progressing to AIDS-related non-Hodgkin's lymphoma. *Blood 98*, 146-155.

Welles, L., Saville, M.W., Lietzau, J., et al. (1998). Phase II trial with dose titration of paclitaxel for the therapy of human immunodeficiency virus-associated Kaposi's sarcoma. *Journal of Clinical Oncology 16*, 1112-1121.

THOMAS J. SZOPA

Theory

I. Principles of surgery (Rosenberg, 2001).
   A. Surgery is the treatment of choice for malignant tumors that meet the following criteria:
      1. Have low growth fractions and long cell-cycle times.
      2. Are confined locally and/or regionally.
   B. Surgery is planned to do the following:
      1. Remove the malignant tumor and a margin of adjacent normal tissue.
      2. Remove the malignant tumor with attention to postprocedure quality of life issues, including structural, functional, and cosmetic changes.
   C. The type and extent of a surgical procedure are based on the following:
      1. Tumor size, physical location, and ease of surgical access.
      2. Impact on local neighboring organs and structure.
      3. Impact of the client's physical and emotional status on surgical outcomes and risk of complications.
      4. Client's preference of available surgical options.
   D. Surgical procedures include strategies to decrease the local and systemic spread of cancer (Cady, 2001).
      1. Ligation of local blood vessels and local and regional draining lymphatics.
      2. Irrigation of wounds with cytotoxic agents.
      3. Changing surgical gloves frequently.
      4. Cleaning surgical instruments with cytotoxic solutions.
      5. Using a "no-touch" technique with tumor tissue.
II. Role of surgery in cancer care (Frogge & Cunning, 2000; Rosenberg, 2001).
   A. Establish a tissue diagnosis.
      1. Incisional biopsy (Table 35-1).
      2. Excisional biopsy (see Table 35-1).
      3. Needle biopsy (see Table 35-1).
         a. Fine-needle aspiration.
         b. Core—helpful in determining invasiveness of disease and hormone receptor status.
         c. Sentinel node biopsy—performed along with lymphatic mapping to identify the first (sentinel) node that drains the primary tumor site and localization of the tumor's nodal drainage system. Prognosis is directly related to the sentinel node status and requires less invasive procedures for study of a tumor's lymph node drainage status and extent of disease (Zervos & Burak, 2002).

    B. Determine the stage of disease.

       1. Obtain multiple biopsies to identify and determine the extent of disease.

       2. Remove tumor along with affected organs or tissues.

       3. Mark residual tumor on affected organs to assist in subsequent cancer treatment planning and delivery.

    C. Treat disease (Jennings, 2001; Mintzer, 1999).

       1. Primary treatment—removal of the malignant tumor and a margin of adjacent normal tissue.

       2. Adjuvant treatment—removal of tissues to decrease the risk of cancer incidence, progression, or recurrence.

          a. Cytoreductive surgery—reduction of the tumor volume to improve the effect of other cancer treatment modalities.

TABLE 35-1
Surgical Procedures

Type of Procedure	Uses in Cancer Care	Advantages	Disadvantages
Incisional biopsy	Obtain tissue for pathologic examination	Simple method to obtain diagnosis	Additional, more extensive surgical procedure generally performed to remove tumor
Excisional biopsy	Establish tissue diagnosis and tumor removal	Quick, simple removal of tumor at biopsy time; may not require hospitalization; decreased cost; minimal cosmetic effects	Tumor cells may be implanted along surgical path and incision, resulting in local recurrence
Needle biopsy ■ Fine-needle aspiration ■ Core biopsy ■ Sentinel node biopsy	Obtain tissue for pathologic examination; determine stage	Simple to perform, reliable, inexpensive; performed with client under local anesthesia on outpatient basis; result obtained very quickly	Risk of injury to adjacent structures; risk of tumor cell implantation along needle track and recurrence
Diagnostic laparotomy	Determine stage and extent of disease	Provides more accurate diagnostic information for treatment planning	Major surgical procedure with risk for postoperative complications; requires hospital stay; costly; multiple lifestyle disruptions
Local excision	■ Primary treatment ■ Cytoreductive surgery ■ Removal of solitary metastasis ■ Palliative treatment	Minimal tissue removal with little effect on functional status and appearance; may not require hospital stay or short hospital stay	Risk of microscopic residual disease left in tissue, resulting in local recurrence
Wide excision	■ Primary treatment ■ Cytoreductive surgery ■ Palliative treatment	Eliminates visible and microscopic disease locally and in adjacent tissue that has increased risk for disease spread	Longer, more involved rehabilitation required; may cause major changes in functional ability and appearance; may require reconstructive procedures

(Continued)

TABLE 35-1
Surgical Procedures—cont'd

Type of Procedure	Uses in Cancer Care	Advantages	Disadvantages
Laser	■ Primary treatment ■ Cytoreductive surgery ■ Palliative treatment	Can be used in all body systems; decreased blood loss and need for blood products; decreased local recurrence rates; minimal side effects, including minimal pain during and after surgery; decreased wound drainage; earlier return of functional ability, reduced incidence of functional disabilities; minimal preparation time and easy to deliver treatment; decreased procedure time; decreased or eliminated hospital stay; may be repeated on recurrent tumor; may perform immediate graft; may be performed when traditional surgery is contraindicated (e.g., because of location of tumor; client is a poor surgical risk as a result of health status)	None noted
Photodynamic therapy	Primary treatment	More precise in locating cancer cells, particularly when all sites of disease are unknown; decreased risks and variety of side effects compared with traditional surgery	Photosensitivity for 4-6 wk, causing possible lifestyle disruptions
Stereotaxis	■ Obtain biopsy ■ Primary treatment ■ Cytoreductive surgery ■ Implantation of radioactive sources, hyperthermia, or chemotherapeutic agents ■ Perform thalamotomy for intractable cancer pain or tremor	Minimize tissue exposed and affected; less trauma to brain tissue than traditional approaches with decreased neurologic deficits; shorter hospital stay and reduced hospitalization costs; lower mortality and morbidity	Use dependent on size and location of tumor, and current expertise and technology in imaging modalities and computer technology; neurologic side effects dependent on size and location of tumor

TABLE 35-1
Surgical Procedures—cont'd

Type of Procedure	Uses in Cancer Care	Advantages	Disadvantages
Laparoscopic and endoscopic surgery	■ Establish tissue diagnosis ■ Determine stage ■ Primary treatment	Decreased postoperative pain and procedure-related complications; earlier recovery and return to activities of daily living; shorter hospital stay with decreased treatment costs	Use dependent on size and location of primary tumor and existence of regional disease; anatomic defects may limit access and use; data inconclusive on long-term effect on prognosis
Radiofrequency ablation	■ Primary treatment ■ Cytoreductive surgery ■ Palliative treatment	Performed on outpatient basis; decreased pain and postoperative complications, earlier recovery, used in clients unable to tolerate more invasive or traditional procedures	Use dependent on size and location of tumor

    b. Prophylactic surgery—removal of nonvital organs that have an extremely high risk of subsequent cancer (Table 35-2).
3. Salvage treatment—use of an extensive surgical approach to treat local disease recurrence after the use of a less extensive primary approach (Table 35-3).
4. Palliative treatment—use of procedures to promote client comfort and quality of life without the goal of cure of disease (Dunn, 2002; Easson et al., 2001; McCahill & Ferrell, 2002).
    a. Examples—bone stabilization, relief of obstruction, removal of solitary metastasis, therapy for oncologic emergencies, ablative surgery, management of cancer pain.
    b. Benefit of palliative treatment depends on the biologic pace of the cancer, projected life expectancy, and expected primary treatment outcome.

TABLE 35-2
Surgical Procedures to Prevent Cancer

Primary Health Issue	Related Cancer	Prophylactic Procedure
Cryptorchidism	Testicular	Orchiopexy
Polyposis coli	Colon	Colectomy
Familial colon cancer	Colon	Colectomy
Ulcerative colitis	Colon	Colectomy
Multiple endocrine neoplasia, types II and III	Medullary cancer of the thyroid	Thyroidectomy
Familial breast cancer	Breast	Mastectomy
Familial ovarian cancer	Ovary	Oophorectomy

TABLE 35-3
Examples of Salvage Therapy

Cancer Site	Primary Conservative Approach	Salvage Approach
Breast	Lumpectomy and RT	Mastectomy
Bladder	Primary RT	Radical cystectomy
Early glottic carcinoma	Primary RT	Hemilaryngectomy
Prostate	Primary RT	Radical prostatectomy

RT, Radiation therapy.

5. Combination treatment—use of surgery with other treatment modalities to improve tumor resectability; decrease the extent of tissue removed; limit the change in physical appearance and functional ability; and improve treatment outcomes (Beddar et al., 2002).
   a. Examples—preoperative chemotherapy, radiation therapy (RT), or immunotherapy; intraoperative chemotherapy or RT; and postoperative chemotherapy, RT, or immunotherapy.
   b. Risk of type and severity of side effects experienced increases with each additional treatment modality used (Drake & Oishi, 1995).
      (1) Chemotherapy may affect wound healing (methotrexate [Mexate]); renal function (cisplatin [Platinol]); cardiac function (doxorubicin [Adriamycin]); or pulmonary function (bleomycin [Blenoxane]).
      (2) RT may affect wound healing in the treatment field or function of organs within the treatment field (pulmonary fibrosis).
   c. Current research issues.
      (1) Timing of combination therapies.
      (2) Sequencing of combination therapies.
      (3) Identifying combination therapies most effective in controlling cancer with minimal untoward effects.
   D. Place therapeutic and supportive hardware, such as a gastrostomy tube; hyperalimentation lines; ventricular reservoir; external or implantable vascular access catheters, ports, and pumps; and radioactive implants.
   E. Assess response to treatment by "second-look" procedures.
      1. Procedure performed within a predetermined time frame after initial therapy.
      2. Sites and volume of residual tumor are identified and resected if possible.
   F. Reconstruct affected body parts.
      1. Repair or reduce anatomic defects from cancer surgery to improve function and/or cosmetic appearance.
      2. Examples—fecal or urinary diversion, breast reconstruction, fistula excision, skin flap development, prosthesis placement.
III. Types and classifications of surgery (see Table 35-1).
   A. Surgical extent.
      1. Local excision—removal of cancer with a small margin of normal tissue.
      2. Wide excision—removal of cancer, tissue containing primary lymph nodes, contiguous structures involved, contiguous structures at high risk for tumor spread.
   B. Electrosurgery—use of electric current for cell destruction.
   C. Cryosurgery—use of liquid nitrogen to freeze tissue to result in cell destruction.

D. Chemosurgery—use of combined topical chemotherapy and layer-by-layer surgical removal of abnormal tissue.

E. Laser (light amplification by stimulated emission of radiation) surgery (see Table 35-1).

    1. Contact tip or "laser scalpel" provides a focused form of energy within a precise location and depth of tissue (Werner et al., 2002).

    2. Photodynamic therapy—intravenous (IV) injection of a light-sensitizing agent (hematoporphyrin derivative [HPD]) with uptake by cancer cells, followed by exposure to laser light within 24 to 48 hours of injection (see Table 35-1).

        a. Results in fluorescence of cancer cells and cell death.

        b. Used for determining extent of disease and response to treatment.

F. Stereotactic surgery (Chang & Adler, 2001)—method of precisely locating specific sites within, based on three-dimensional coordinates (see Table 35-1).

    1. Treatment planning and intervention incorporate the following:

        a. A head frame that provides for rigid skull fixation.

        b. An arc quadrant that attaches to the head frame, providing direction to treatment instrumentation to the localized intracranial target.

        c. Stereotactic data acquisition and processing system that includes the use of various imaging modalities and computer technology to process information regarding the geometric configuration, volume, and extent of the tumor.

        d. A surgical tool to be used to treat the tumor.

G. Laparoscopic resection (Bickert & Frickel, 2002)—the use of a laparoscope to visualize, reach, and remove tumor through several small incisions (see Table 35-1).

H. Endoscopy (Carrion & Seigne, 2002)—use of endoscope to visualize, take tissue samples, or remove tumor.

I. Radiofrequency ablation—the localized application of thermal energy that destroys tumor by heating to temperatures exceeding 122° F (50° C) causing protein denaturation and thermal coagulation (Iannitti et al., 2002; Zagoria et al., 2002).

IV. Safety measures in the delivery of surgery.

A. Aseptic techniques are used to reduce the risks of infection.

    1. Skin preparation to specific surgical site.

    2. Sterile techniques during procedures.

    3. Wound dressings.

B. Type of anesthesia is selected based on client preference, previous response to anesthesia, physical and mental history, type and duration of procedure, surgical site, and positioning during the surgical procedure.

C. Electrical hazards are prevented by proper grounding plate placement within the operating room and by checking electrical cords, plugs, and outlets.

D. Informed consent is obtained.

    1. The nature of and reason for surgery are explained.

    2. All available options and risks associated with each option are discussed.

    3. Risks of the surgical procedure and administration of anesthesia are described.

    4. Potential benefits and outcomes of the treatment are explained.

E. Client is prepared for the surgery.

    1. Delivery of specific operative site or system preparations, such as bowel preparations, medications, or nutritional interventions.

2. Positioning during the surgical procedure to prevent joint damage, muscle stretch or strain, and pressure ulcers.

Assessment (Frogge & Cunning, 2000; Marek & Boehnlein, 2003; Pfifer, 2001)

I. Pertinent personal history.
   A. Factors that may increase the incidence of complications of surgery.
      1. Presence of preexisting cardiovascular, pulmonary, renal, neurologic, musculoskeletal, gastrointestinal (GI), or liver disease.
      2. Previous surgical history—type of surgery; experience with anesthetic agents, blood transfusions, and surgical complications.
      3. Lifestyle activities, such as tobacco use, alcohol ingestion, illegal medications use, or abuse of over-the-counter medications.
      4. Previous cancer therapy and the length of time since therapy was completed.
      5. Present medications.
      6. Allergies.
      7. Physiologic changes of aging (Table 35-4).
   B. Factors that may influence discharge planning.
      1. Home environment.
      2. Financial status.
      3. Self-care capabilities.
      4. Anticipated changes in self-care capabilities resulting from surgery.
      5. Support personnel or services available and patterns of use.
      6. Employment status and type of work.
II. Physical examination.
   A. Cardiovascular—heart rate and rhythm, blood pressure, presence and quality of regional pulses, color and temperature of regional extremities.
   B. Pulmonary—respiratory rate, depth, and rhythm; lung expansion; posture.

TABLE 35-4
Physiologic Changes Related to the Aging Process That Can Affect Surgery

Physiologic Changes	Effects	Potential Postoperative Complications
CARDIOVASCULAR		
↓Elasticity of blood vessels	↓Circulation to vital organs	Shock (hypotension), thrombosis with pulmonary emboli, delayed wound healing, postoperative confusion, hypervolemia, decreased response to stress
↓Cardiac output	Slower blood flow	
↓Peripheral circulation	↑Blood pressure	
RESPIRATORY		
↓Elasticity of lungs and chest wall	↓Vital capacity	Aspiration, atelectasis, pneumonia, postoperative confusion
↑Residual lung volume	↓Alveolar volume	
↓Forced expiratory volume	↓Gas exchange	Difficulty maintaining airway
↓Ciliary action	↓Cough reflex	Difficult intubation
Fewer alveolar capillaries	↓Hyperextension of neck	
Arthritic changes of cervical spine		
Tenacious sputum		

TABLE 35-4
Physiologic Changes Related to the Aging Process That Can Affect Surgery—cont'd

Physiologic Changes	Effects	Potential Postoperative Complications
URINARY		
↓Glomerular filtration rate	↓Kidney function	Prolonged response to anesthesia and drugs, overhydration with intravenous fluids, hyperkalemia, urinary tract infection, urinary incontinence
↓Bladder muscle tone	Stasis of urine in bladder	
↓Bladder capacity	Loss of urinary control	
Weakened perineal muscles		Incomplete bladder emptying, urinary retention, urinary frequency
Benign prostatic hypertrophy		
MUSCULOSKELETAL		
↓Muscle mass	↓Activity	Atelectasis, pneumonia, thrombophlebitis, pulmonary embolism, constipation, fecal impaction, positioning difficulty
Loss of bone mass	Skeletal instability	
Osteoporosis	Hip and vertebral fractures	
Arthritis	↓Range of motion	
GASTROINTESTINAL		
↓Intestinal motility	Retention of feces	Aspiration, ileus, constipation or fecal impaction
IMMUNE SYSTEM		
Fewer killer T cells	↓Ability to protect against invasion by pathogenic microorganisms	Delayed wound healing, wound infection, wound dehiscence, pneumonia, urinary tract infection
↓Response to foreign antigens		
NEUROLOGIC		
Cerebral atherosclerosis	↓Cerebral blood flow	Cerebrovascular accident
	↓Thermoregulatory ability	Intraoperative and postoperative hypothermia
Benign hyperthermia	↓Vasoconstriction, lower core temperature	Delayed shivering, delayed recovery from anesthetics
↓Basal metabolic rate		
Impaired thermoregulatory ability	↑Cardiac workload, hypoxia	
INTEGUMENTARY		
↓Elasticity	↓Protective function	Pressure ulcers, bruising
Small vessel fragility	Dehydration	Hypothermia
↓Lean body mass	Impaired vascular circulation	Delayed wound healing
↑Overall body fat		Delayed recovery from anesthetics because of storage in adipose tissue
↓Subcutaneous tissue	↓Tissue nutrition	
	↑Sensitivity to cold environments	
METABOLIC		
Electrolyte imbalances	Hyperkalemia, hypokalemia	Confusion, dysrhythmias, delayed wound healing, wound dehiscence or evisceration
↓Gamma globulin level		
↓Plasma proteins	↓Inflammatory response	

From Marek J, Boehnlein M: Preoperative nursing. In Phipps W, Monahan F, Sands J, et al, editors: *Medical-surgical nursing: health and illness perspectives*, ed 7, St Louis, 2003, Mosby, pp. 376-377.

C. Renal—color and odor of urine, urinary elimination patterns, previous urinary output.
D. GI—color, consistency, and caliber of stool; bowel elimination patterns.
E. Mobility—muscle strength and endurance, range of motion; gait; activity level.
F. Nutrition—weight; skin turgor; amount, content, and patterns of nutritional intake.
G. Comfort level.
III. Psychosocial examination.
   A. Explore client's and family's concerns.
     1. Meaning attached to the loss of body part and/or functioning.
     2. Expectations related to the procedure, such as pain, disability, or survival.
     3. Perceived impact of surgery on lifestyle and relationships.
   B. Assess the client's and family's current level of coping.
     1. Coping strategies used in previous illnesses or times of stress.
     2. Support systems available and patterns of use.
     3. Community resources available and patterns of use.
IV. Critical laboratory and diagnostic data unique to surgery.
   A. Cardiovascular—electrocardiogram (ECG).
   B. Hematologic—complete blood count, prothrombin time, partial thromboplastin time.
   C. Hepatic—liver function studies.
   D. Renal—urinalysis, blood urea nitrogen, creatinine, electrolytes.
   E. Pulmonary—chest x-ray examination.
   F. Nutritional—serum albumin.

Nursing Diagnoses

I. Acute pain.
II. Impaired skin integrity.
III. Ineffective airway clearance.
IV. Imbalanced nutrition: less than body requirements.
V. Deficient knowledge related to type of and rationale for surgical procedure, potential immediate and long-term complications of surgery, and so on.
VI. Anxiety.

Outcome Identification

I. Client and family describe the type of and rationale for surgery.
II. Client and family list potential immediate and long-term complications of the surgery.
III. Client describes self-care measures to decrease the incidence and severity of complications of surgery.
IV. Client demonstrates new self-care skills demanded by structural or functional effects of surgery.
V. Client and family describe schedule and procedures for routine follow-up care.
VI. Client and family list changes in condition that should be reported to the health care team.
   A. Signs and symptoms of infection.
   B. Persistent nausea, vomiting, or decrease in appetite.
   C. Poor wound healing.
   D. Changes in bowel or bladder patterns.

    E. Changes in location or increased severity of pain or intolerance to discomfort.

    F. Inability to resume functional ability within anticipated time frame.

VII. Client and family identify potential community resources to meet unique demands of therapy and rehabilitation.

Planning and Implementation (Boehnlein & Marek, 2003; Frogge & Cunning, 2000; Lefor, 1999)

   I. Interventions to maximize safety for the client and family.

     A. Implement the preoperative medical preparation regimen as ordered.

       1. Dietary restrictions.

       2. Bowel preparation.

       3. Skin preparation.

     B. Use aseptic or clean technique, as indicated, for invasive procedures such as insertion of tubes, drains, or IV lines.

  II. Interventions to decrease incidence and severity of complications unique to surgery.

     A. Ineffective airway clearance.

       1. Teach turning, coughing, and deep breathing (TCDB) techniques to the client and family, and schedule activities postoperatively.

       2. Demonstrate use of incentive spirometry.

       3. Use suction devices to assist the client to remove mucus or sputum.

     B. Impaired skin integrity.

       1. Assist the client to turn and shift positions in bed every 2 hours.

       2. Massage uninjured areas gently.

       3. Use mattress overlays, such as therapeutic foam mattress, alternating air mattress, or water mattress or specialty beds, such as low-airflow, air-fluidized, or kinetic therapy, for high-risk clients.

       4. Establish a schedule for changing the surgical dressing.

       5. Use protective film, hydrocolloid barriers, and/or collection devices around drains or tubes with copious drainage.

       6. Encourage early ambulation.

     C. Acute pain.

       1. Teach splinting of incision during TCDB or with movement.

       2. Use nonpharmacologic methods for pain control.

         a. Progressive muscle relaxation.

         b. Guided imagery.

         c. Music.

         d. Massage.

         e. Diversional activities.

       3. Administer analgesic and antiemetic medications as ordered by the physician.

     D. Anxiety.

       1. Allow the client and family to discuss feelings, fears, and concerns.

       2. Provide client and family teaching.

         a. Plan of care and rationale for procedures.

         b. Anticipated care settings, equipment, and experiences related to surgery.

         c. Self-care strategies to prevent or minimize complications of surgery.

       3. Encourage use of coping strategies that have been effective in the past during times of stress.

4. Initiate referrals for physical and psychosocial support based on client and family risk factors (nutritional services, social service, respiratory therapy, rehabilitative service, etc.).

5. Allow for adequate rest periods between care activities.

III. Interventions to monitor for unique complications of surgery.

A. Ineffective airway clearance.

1. Assess the client on a routine basis for changes in respiratory effort, rate, and rhythm and for subjective responses to breathing.

2. Inspect chest wall for symmetric movement, use of accessory muscles, diaphragmatic breathing, and sternal retraction.

3. Auscultate lungs for adventitious or absent breath sounds.

B. Impaired skin integrity.

1. Assess incision site for redness, swelling, increased drainage, discomfort, and approximation of surgical margins.

2. Assess bony prominences for an area remaining red 30 minutes or longer after pressure is relieved.

C. Imbalanced nutrition: less than body requirements.

1. Assess for return of bowel sounds.

2. Assess for physical signs of dehydration—color and moisture of mucous membranes; skin turgor.

3. Assess fluid loss via incisional or fistula wounds, urinary output, and tube drainage or drain output.

4. Assess intake/output ratio.

5. Weigh the client daily.

6. Evaluate tolerance to progressive diet—appetite, amount and type of foods eaten, responses to eating.

7. Monitor laboratory parameters of nutritional status.

IV. Interventions to enhance adaptation and rehabilitation (Pfifer, 2001).

A. Implement postoperative teaching plan that includes changes in self-care activities and activities resulting from surgery, progressive return to maximal level of activity, anticipated discharge medications, wound management, proper use of assistive or prosthetic devices, community resources available for home care, plans for follow-up care, contact person if questions arise, and changes in condition to report to the health care team.

B. Include the multidisciplinary team in providing for client's and family's needs in postoperative care and discharge planning: nutritional support, rehabilitative services (physical, occupational, and/or speech therapy), respiratory therapy, social work/case management, spiritual care, and so on.

C. Involve the client and family in assessment, planning, and evaluation of care through transition periods.

D. Instruct the client and family about rehabilitation programs available, such as physical and occupational therapy, speech therapy, ostomy outpatient clinics, and prosthetic fitting services.

E. Refer the client and family to support programs available, such as Reach to Recovery, ReCon Group, Voicemasters, Make Today Count, International Association of Laryngectomees, and United Ostomy Association chapters.

F. Refer the client and family to professional counselors as indicated.

Evaluation

The oncology nurse systematically and regularly evaluates the client's and/or family's responses to interventions to determine progress toward the achievement of

expected outcomes. Relevant data are collected, and actual findings are compared with expected findings. Nursing diagnoses, outcomes, and plans of care are reviewed and revised as necessary.

REFERENCES

Beddar, A.S., Domanovic, M.A., Kubu, M.L., & Ellis, R. (2002). Mobile linear accelerators for intraoperative radiation therapy. *Association of Operating Room Nurses 74*(5), 700-705.

Bickert, D., & Frickel, D. (2002). Laparoscopic radical prostatectomy. *Association of Operating Room Nurses 75*(4), 762-782.

Boehnlein, M.J., & Marek, J.F. (2003). Postoperative nursing. In W. Phipps, F. Monahan, J. Sands, et al. (Eds.). *Medical surgical nursing—Health & illness perspectives* (7th ed.). St. Louis: Mosby, pp. 427-454.

Cady, B. (2001). Fundamentals of contemporary surgical oncology: Biologic principles and the threshold concept govern treatment and outcomes. *Journal of the American College of Surgeons 192*(6), 777-792.

Carrion, R., & Seigne, J. (2002). Surgical management of bladder carcinoma. *Cancer Control 9*(4), 284-292.

Chang, S., & Adler, J. (2001). Current status and optimal use of radiosurgery. *Oncology 15,* 209-221.

Drake, D.B., & Oishi, S.N. (1995). Wound healing considerations in chemotherapy and radiation therapy. *Clinics in Plastic Surgery 22*(1), 31-37.

Dunn, G.P. (2002). Surgical palliation in advanced disease: Recent developments. *Current Oncology Representative 4*(3), 233-241.

Easson, A.M., Asch, M., & Swallow, C.J. (2001). Palliative general surgical procedures. *Surgical Oncology Clinics of North America 10*(1), 161-184.

Frogge, M., & Cunning, S. (2000). Surgical therapy. In C.H. Yarbro, M.H. Frogge, M. Goodman, & S.L. Groenwald (Eds.). *Cancer nursing: Principles and practice* (5th ed.). Sudbury, MA: Jones and Bartlett Publishers, pp. 272-285.

Iannitti, D., Dupuy, D., Mayo-Smith, W., & Murphy, B. (2002). Hepatic radiofrequency ablation. *Archives of Surgery 137*(4), 422-430.

Jennings, M. (Ed.). (2001). Treatment advances in surgical oncology. *Nursing Clinics of North America 36*(3), 499-623.

Lefor, A.T. (1999). Perioperative management of the patient with cancer. *Chest 115*(5, Suppl.), 165S-171S.

Marek, J., & Boehnlein, M. (2003). Preoperative nursing. In W. Phipps, F. Monahan, J. Sands, et al. (Eds.). *Medical surgical nursing—Health & illness perspectives* (7th ed.). St. Louis: Mosby, pp. 361-390.

McCahill, L., & Ferrell, B. (2002). Palliative surgery for cancer pain. *Western Journal of Medicine 176*(2), 107-110.

Mintzer, D. (1999). The changing role of surgery in the diagnosis and treatment of cancer. *American Journal of Medicine 106*(1), 81-89.

Pfifer, K. (2001). Surgery. In S. Otto (Ed.). *Oncology nursing* (4th ed.). St. Louis: Mosby, pp. 585-594.

Rosenberg, S. (2001). Principles of cancer management: Surgical oncology. In V. DeVita, Jr., S. Hellman, & S. Rosenberg (Eds.). *Cancer: Principles and practice of oncology* (6th ed.). Philadelphia: Lippincott Williams & Wilkins, pp. 253-264.

Werner, J., Dunne, A., Folz, B., & Lippert, B. (2002). Transoral laser microsurgery in carcinomas of the oral cavity, pharynx and larynx. *Cancer Control 9*(50), 379-386.

Zagoria, R., Chen, M., Shen, P., & Levine, E. (2002). Complication from radiofrequency ablation of liver metastases. *American Surgeon 68*(2), 204-209.

Zervos, E., & Burak, W. (2002). Lymphatic mapping in solid neoplasms: State of the art. *Cancer Control 9*(3), 189-202.

36 Nursing Implications of Radiation Therapy

MARY ELLYN WITT*

Theory

I. Principles of radiation—energy emitted and transferred through matter or space.
   A. Radiation physics is the study of radiation energy and its effect on cellular biology.
      1. Ionizing radiation is used in the treatment of cancer based on the ability of the radiation to interact with the atoms and molecules of the tumor cells to produce specific harmful biologic effects to either the molecules of the cell or the cell environment (Hilderley, 2000).
      2. X-rays, gamma rays, and cosmic radiation are ionizing radiation.
      3. Forms of ionizing radiation.
         a. Electromagnetic: radiation in the form of energy waves. Includes photons (x-rays, gamma rays).
         b. Particulate: radiation in the form of subatomic particles. Includes electrons, protons, neutrons, alpha particles, and beta particles.
   B. Radiobiology is the study of events that occur after ionizing radiation is absorbed by a living organism or cell.
      1. Biologic effects of ionizing radiation.
         a. Cellular targets—the target, or most critical site for radiation damage, is deoxyribonucleic acid (DNA). Radiation-induced DNA damage includes single and double strand breaks as well as the formation of cross links. The mechanism of DNA damage differs among the various radiation types (Mundt & Roeske, 2003).
         b. Biologic response to radiation is affected by the level of DNA damage, oxygen effect (well-oxygenated tumors show greater response), and sensitivity of the cell to the radiation (Dunne-Daly, 1999).
      2. Normal tissue and tumor are affected by ionizing radiation. Time in which biologic changes appear and the nature and severity of effects depend on the amount of radiation absorbed, fractionation, and rate at which it is administered. Acute- and late-responding tissues are affected differently by the biologic effect and radiosensitivity.
         a. Biologic effect of fractionation on tumors and normal tissue depends on four factors known as the four "R's" of radiobiology.
            (1) Repair—normal tissue is spared by divided doses because it has greater repair of sublethal damage and repopulation abilities than dosed tumor tissue.

---

*ACKNOWLEDGMENT: The author would like to acknowledge Ellen Sitton, who was the author of this chapter in the previous editions. This fourth edition is an update of her previous work.

(2) Reassortment or redistribution of cells within the cell cycle occurs after a dose of fractionated radiation. Redistribution brings more of the cells into mitosis, the most sensitive phase of the cell cycle (after G$_2$), with each successive radiation dose.

(3) Reoxygenation occurs because the decreased tumor burden leads to better blood flow patterns in the tumor.

(4) Repopulation involves the replacement of dead or dying cells through cell multiplication (Dunne-Daly, 1999; Hellman, 2001; Maher, 2000).

   b. Radiosensitivity—all normal and cancer cells are vulnerable to effects of radiation and may be injured or destroyed by radiation therapy (RT). Cells vary in sensitivity to radiation. Generally, rapidly dividing cells, both normal and cancer cells, are most sensitive (e.g., mucosa) and are referred to as radiosensitive. Nondividing or slowly dividing cells are generally less radiosensitive, or radioresistant (e.g., muscle cells, neurons) (Table 36-1).

C. Principles behind treatment of cancer with radiation and control of side effects.

   1. A course of RT is planned to deliver a dose high enough to destroy the tumor in the primary site and surrounding lymph nodes at risk for cancer while not exceeding the tolerance of the normal tissues in the radiation field (or portal).

   2. Side effects and sequelae of RT are generally the result of the effect of radiation on normal tissues. All normal tissues have a limit with regard to the amount of radiation they can receive and still remain functional.

      a. Early side effects occur during RT or weeks or months after RT and generally heal after the RT course. They are usually exhibited first by tissues with rapidly proliferating cells (e.g., gastrointestinal [GI] mucosa, bone marrow). These tissues are considered acute-responding tissues and generally demonstrate early side effects. The severity of this early response to irradiation is not a predictor of severity of late response.

TABLE 36-1
Relative Radiosensitivity of Various Tumors and Tissues

Tumors	Relative Radiosensitivity	Tissues of Origin
Lymphoma, leukemia, seminoma, dysgerminoma	High	Lymphoid, hematopoietic (marrow), spermatogenic epithelium, ovarian follicular epithelium
Squamous cell cancer of the oropharyngeal, glottis, bladder, skin, and cervical epithelia; adeno-carcinomas of alimentary tract	Fairly high	Oropharyngeal stratified epithelium, sebaceous gland epithelium, urinary bladder epithelium, optic lens epithelium, gastric gland epithelium, colon epithelium, breast epithelium
Breast, salivary gland tumors, hepatomas, renal cancer, pancreatic cancer, chondrosarcoma, osteogenic sarcoma	Fairly low	Mature cartilage of bone tissue, salivary gland epithelium, renal epithelium, hepatic epithelium, chondrocytes, osteocytes
Rhabdomyosarcoma, leiomyosarcoma, ganglioneurofibrosarcoma	Low	Muscle tissue, neuronal tissue

Modified from Rubin P, Siemann D: Principles of radiation oncology and cancer radiotherapy. In Rubin P, editor: *Clinical oncology: a multidisciplinary approach for physicians and students,* ed 7, Philadelphia, 1993, WB Saunders, p. 75.

     b. Subacute-responding tissues show few, if any, early effects but demonstrate damage in weeks to months after RT.

     c. Late effects occur months to years after RT and are permanent. Tissues composed of slowly proliferating cells develop injury slowly (e.g., central and peripheral nervous system, kidney, dermis, cartilage, bone).

     d. Late-responding tissues (e.g., spinal cord, peripheral nerves, kidney, dermis, cartilage, bone) generally demonstrate little evidence of early effects and show late effects months to years after RT (Table 36-2). The risk of a second malignancy following radiation is low. Sarcoma is the most common radiation-induced second primary malignancy (Mundt & Roeske, 2003).

   D. Tissue response to fractionation.

     1. External beam irradiation—a total dose tolerated by the tissues in the irradiated field is prescribed and is fractionated, or divided, into daily doses (usually 180 to 200 cGy/day). High dose per fraction and large total doses have been shown to be related to increased severity of late effects.

     2. Radioactive source therapy—a total dose tolerated by the tissues in the irradiated area is prescribed. This dose may be given over several days as a continuous application (low dose rate [LDR]) or in a single or several doses over several minutes (high dose rate [HDR]).

     3. Excessive prolongation of treatment allows surviving tumor cells to proliferate during treatment.

II. RT fundamentals.

   A. More than 60% of clients treated for cancer are treated with RT during the course of the disease (Dunne-Daly, 1999; Maher, 2000).

   B. The goal of RT is to destroy or inactivate cancer cells while preserving the integrity of normal tissue within the treatment field (Dunne-Daly, 1999).

   C. Aims of radiation treatments.

     1. Cure. Purpose—kill all cells in a malignant tumor capable of cell division while limiting the dose to the normal tissues, for example, early prostate cancer. The client is expected to have a normal life span and systematic follow-up evaluation for late effects of RT.

     2. Control. Purpose—limit the growth and spread of disease, for example, advanced non–small cell lung cancer. The client is expected to have a period of symptom-free time.

     3. Adjuvant. Purpose—radiation often precedes or follows definitive surgery to ensure local control, for example, breast radiation after lumpectomy.

TABLE 36-2
Response to Radiation: Acute/Late Responding

Acute-Responding Tissues	Subacute-Responding Tissues	Late-Responding Tissues
Bone marrow, ovary, testis, lymph node, salivary gland, small bowel, stomach, colon, oral mucosa, larynx, esophagus, arterioles, skin, bladder, capillaries, vagina	Lung, liver, kidney, heart, spinal cord, brain	Lymph vessels, thyroid, pituitary, breast, bone cartilage, pancreas, uterus, bile ducts

Data from Hall EJ, Cox JD: Physical and biologic basis of radiation therapy. In Cox JD, editor: *Moss' radiation oncology: rationale, technique, results,* ed 7, St Louis, 1994, Mosby, pp. 3-65.

4. Palliation. Purpose—improve quality of life by reducing or relieving symptoms or impending complications (e.g., relief of pain from bony metastasis, treatment of impending cord compression, relief of superior vena cava syndrome, decreasing obstruction, reduction/relief of symptoms from brain metastasis). Life span is not expected to be extended (Dow et al., 1997; Maher, 2000).

D. Methods of delivery of RT.
  1. Local treatment.
    a. External beam treatment machines in radiation oncology (teletherapy).
      (1) Linear accelerator (may treat with x-rays and/or electrons).
        (a) X-rays: intermediate to deep treatment (depth of penetration varies with energy).
        (b) Electron beam: shallow treatment (spares deeper tissues; depth of penetration varies with energy; high skin doses).
      (2) Cobalt-60.
        (a) Radioactive source: emission of gamma rays.
    b. Radioactive source therapy: brachytherapy.
      (1) Beta particles and gamma rays from sealed radioactive sources (Table 36-3).
  2. Systemic treatment.
    a. Radioactive source therapy: radiopharmaceutical therapy.
      (1) Beta particles and gamma rays from unsealed radioactive sources (Nicolaou, 1999) (See Table 36-3).

E. Progress and innovations in radiation oncology.
  1. Combined-modality treatment.
    a. RT and chemotherapy (pre-RT, concurrent, post-RT).
    b. Intraoperative RT.
    c. Radioimmunotherapy (RIT).
    d. Hyperthermia and RT.
  2. Three-dimensional–conformal RT (e.g., six-field conformal prostate RT).
  3. Intensity-modulated RT (IMRT).
  4. Radiopharmaceuticals for metastatic bone pain, for example, strontium-89.
  5. HDR and LDR brachytherapy.
  6. Arc RT (e.g., stereotactic radiosurgery).

TABLE 36-3
Radioisotopes and Their Properties

Radioisotope	Symbol	Half-Life	Type
Cesium-137	^{137}Cs	30 yr	Beta, gamma
Gold-198	^{198}Au	2.7 days	Beta, gamma
Iodine-125	^{125}I	60 days	Beta, gamma
Iodine-131	^{131}I	8 days	Beta, gamma
Iridium-192	^{192}Ir	74.4 days	Beta, gamma
Phosphorus-32	^{32}P	14.3 days	Beta
Radium-226	^{226}Ra	1620 yr	Alpha, gamma
Strontium-90	^{90}Sr	28.1 yr	Beta

From National Council on Radiation Protection and Measurements: *Protection against radiation from brachytherapy sources. Report no. 40*, Bethesda, Md, 1972, National Council on Radiation Protection and Measurements.

7. Gamma knife.
8. Altered fractionation (e.g., twice daily fractionation, HDR).
9. Total body irradiation.
10. Total skin electron irradiation.
11. Particle beam therapy (e.g., neutron therapy, proton therapy). Few machines available in the United States.
12. Chemical modification (radiosensitizers, radioprotectors). 5-Fluorouracil is a chemotherapy agent that is a radiosensitizer. Amifostine (Ethyol) is an example of a radioprotector.
13. Intravascular brachytherapy for restenosis of cardiac stent.
14. Partial breast irradiation (Boelsen & Jamar, 2000; Dow et al., 1997; Mundt & Roeske, 2003; Vicini et al., 2003; Witt et al., 2003).

III. Teletherapy (external beam RT).
   A. Precise dose delivered to the client from outside the body.
   B. Treatment process.
   1. Client consultation.
   2. Simulation—x-ray examination made to simulate treatment volume, facilitating decisions for treatment position and treatment field(s). Immobilization devices as needed. Treatment marks placed on skin or immobilization device (e.g., mask). Computed tomography (CT), magnetic resonance imaging (MRI), and other modalities are used for tumor localization to plan fields.
   3. Treatment planning by radiation oncologist and physicist. Treatment plan based on pathology of tumor, location, radiosensitivity of tumor and normal tissue in treatment volume. CT or MRI from simulation used to plan and prescribe treatment. Prescription will include daily and total dose of radiation, specific instructions on beam delivery, and number of radiation fields to be treated.
   4. Client education.
   5. Client treatment, evaluation of client status and side effects during treatment course, and long-term follow-up (Behrend, 2000).

IV. Radioactive source therapy.
   A. Radioactivity.
   1. Definition—radioactivity, or radioactive decay, is the spontaneous emission of highly energetic particles (alpha and/or beta) or rays (gamma) from the nuclei of an element (radioisotope).
      a. Alpha particles—large particles; not used in brachytherapy.
      b. Beta (β) particles—characteristics similar to electrons; less penetrating than gamma rays.
      c. Gamma (γ) rays—same as x-rays; penetrating (Hilderley, 2000).
   2. Energy—each radioactive element radiates energy as particles and/or rays that are characteristic for that element. Some elements emit particles and/or rays with energies that are more penetrating than others and therefore require more shielding to absorb the radiation. Shielding is measured in centimeters of lead (Pb). Half-value layer (HVL) blocks one half of the radiation.
   3. Half-life—proportion of atoms that disintegrate in a given time is predictable. The time required for one half of the atoms of a given quantity of radioactive material to decay is the physical half-life. Important in unsealed source RT (Table 36-3).
   4. Units of measurement (Box 36-1).
      a. RT—radiation-absorbed dose; gray (Gy), rad.

BOX 36-1
UNITS OF MEASUREMENT

Absorbed Dose (gray, rad)
1 Gy = 100 rad
100 cGy = 100 rad
Therapeutic doses are prescribed in Gy or cGy

Dose Equivalent (Sievert, rem)
1 Sv = 100 rem
Badge readings are in mrem (millirem)

Activity (Becquerel, Curie)
$1 Bq = 2.7 \times 10^{-11} Ci = 1 dps$
$1 Ci = 3.7 \times 10^{10} dps$

dps, Disintegration per second.

(1) Gray—more common unit used for absorbed dose in Europe, becoming more universal. Centigray (cGy)—unit of absorbed radiation dose equal to one hundredth of a Gray.
(2) Rad—more common unit used in United States.
(3) 1 Gy = 100 cGy = 100 rad.
   b. Radiation protection—dose equivalent; Sievert measure, roentgen-equivalent–man (REM).
   c. Radioactive material—activity; Becquerel, Curie (Dow et al., 1997).
B. Treatment with radioactive sources (Figure 36-1).
   1. Selection of type and method depends on client and disease factors.
      a. Sealed sources (brachytherapy).
         (1) Dose rate—LDR, HDR.
         (2) Type—intracavitary, interstitial, intraluminal.

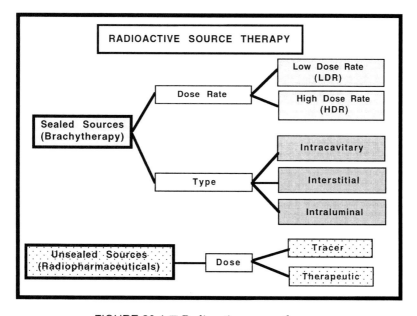

FIGURE 36-1 ■ Radioactive source therapy.

  b. Unsealed sources (radiopharmaceutical therapy).
    (1) Dose—therapeutic dose (tracer dose for diagnostic tests).
  2. Sealed sources (brachytherapy)—treatment of tumors with radioactive sources placed either temporarily or permanently adjacent to the tumor (intracavitary or surface application), into the tumor (interstitial application), or into a lumen (intraluminal).
    a. Primary advantage: ability to deliver high dose of radiation to small volume of tumor while delivering limited dose to adjacent normal tissues. Can be delivered over a period of several days (e.g., LDR) or in a few minutes (e.g., HDR).
    b. Radioactive material is sealed in a container and never comes in direct contact with the client.
      (1) Energy of radiation penetrates through container to treat client.
      (2) When sealed source removed from client, client no longer requires radiation precautions.
      (3) Sealed sources used for LDR and HDR brachytherapy.
    c. LDR remote afterloading device uses computer-controlled loading and unloading of sources from the client from outside the client's room.
      (1) Reduces exposure to staff to negligible amount near zero.
      (2) Physician prescribes treatment in number of hours that the sources are loaded in the client.
      (3) Each treatment generally lasts several days.
    d. HDR machines—remote afterloading devices; generally use one highly radioactive computer-controlled source to treat clients.
      (1) May only be used where adequate shielding is available.
      (2) Each treatment lasts only a few minutes.
      (3) Client is not radioactive after source is removed.
    e. Principles of time, distance, and shielding utilized to minimize exposure to the staff and visitors.
  3. Unsealed sources (radiopharmaceutical therapy)—radioactive materials administered intravenously (IV), orally, or into a body cavity. Result in uptake of radioactive element into various parts of the body, depending on element and form in which administered. Radioactivity may be distributed fairly uniformly over the body or may concentrate in specific organs (Dow et al., 1997; Dunne-Daly, 1999).
    a. Therapeutic dose—a dose of radiation high enough to treat the tumor. Aim is to deliver a predetermined dose to an organ or area of the body to treat the area with radiation.
    b. Tracer dose—used for diagnostic tests (e.g., bone, liver, thyroid scans). Dose is very low, and client is generally released from the hospital after the test.
V. Radiation safety and protection.
  A. Dose limitation—radiation protection (Table 36-4).
    1. Dose limits are applied to all individuals. Different limits are applied to occupationally exposed radiation workers.
      a. ALARA (as low as reasonably achievable)—the best radiation protection guide is to keep radiation exposure as low as reasonably achievable. Radiation should be continually monitored and controlled.
      b. EDE (effective dose equivalent)—exposure to ionizing radiation from artificial sources is controlled by law.
  B. Radiation monitoring.
    1. Personnel monitoring—individuals working in a restricted area should wear a personal monitor to measure radiation dose (e.g., film badge or dosimeter).

TABLE 36-4
Recommendations Regarding Limits for Exposure to Ionizing Radiation

Class of Individual	Effective Dose Limits
Occupational workers*	
Annual	50 mSv
Cumulative	10 mSv × age
Public (annual)	
Continuous or frequent exposure*	1 mSv
Infrequent exposure*	5 mSv
Embryo-fetus exposures (monthly)	
Equivalent dose limit	0.5 mSv
Negligible individual dose (annual)*	0.01 mSv

From National Council on Radiation Protection and Measurements: *Limitation of exposure to ionizing radiation. Report no. 116*, Bethesda, Md, 1993, National Council on Radiation Protection and Measurements.
mSv, Millisievert.
*Sum of external and internal exposures, but excluding doses from natural sources.

      a. Film badge contains small photographic film; worn on the trunk of the body.
        (1) Badges are read and exchanged monthly.
        (2) Workers should never wear a badge belonging to someone else because doing so does not allow determination of how much exposure each person received.
      b. Dosimeter, such as the Luxel Dosimeter, worn in same manner, but measures radiation exposure from x-ray, beta, and gamma radiation through a thin layer of aluminum oxide.
        (1) Dosimeters are available to measure radiation exposure; they can be read at the time of exposure.
    2. Survey meters (e.g., Geiger counter)—used for surveying the client, room, trash, linen, and so on after brachytherapy or radiopharmaceutical therapy.
  C. Radiation safety.
    1. Essential considerations in minimizing exposure to radiation—time, distance, shielding.
      a. Time—minimize the amount of time spent near radioactive sources. Work quickly and efficiently. Rotate staff responsibilities.
      b. Distance—intensity of radiation decreases rapidly as the distance increases.
        (1) Doubling the distance decreases exposure to one fourth the exposure received at the original distance (e.g., exposure of 40 mrem/hr at 1 meter is 10 mrem/hr at 2 meters).
        (2) Staff should work as far away from the source as possible and never touch a source (use long-handled forceps for dislodged sources).
      c. Shielding—the type of shielding and its thickness depend on the type and energy of radioactive source.

Assessment

  I. Factors that influence effective communication.
    A. Barriers to learning (e.g., language, hearing deficit, visual problems).
    B. Cultural issues.

    C. Developmental stage.

    D. Acute physical problems, for example, pain or dyspnea.

  II. History and physical assessment.

    A. Cancer history (personal and family).

    B. Previous and current cancer treatment.

    C. Intercurrent disease; especially any condition involving tissues included in the radiation treatment volume.

    D. Relevant laboratory data (e.g., white blood count [WBC], hemoglobin, hematocrit levels) and diagnostic data (e.g., results of CT scans, pathology examination, staging).

    E. Current symptoms and other medical conditions (e.g., pregnancy, restricted range of motion).

    F. Weight.

    G. Current medications.

  III. Psychosocial assessment.

    A. Coping patterns.

    B. Support systems and client's ability to meet transportation and care needs during treatment and follow-up care.

    C. Knowledge and perceptions regarding treatment.

  IV. Factors influencing side effects of RT.

    A. Site of radiation field (tissues to be irradiated).

    B. Time-dose-volume relationship (length of treatment, fractionation, volume of tissue irradiated).

    C. Radiosensitivity of tissues in treatment volume and potential early and late side effects.

    D. Radiation type and energy, including depth of treatment prescribed.

    E. Nutritional status.

    F. Client adherence to recommended care during RT.

    G. Individual differences among clients.

Nursing Diagnoses

  I. Table 36-5 lists common, potential nursing diagnoses for specific sites of irradiation.

  II. Commonly used nursing diagnoses.

    A. Fear.

    B. Deficient knowledge related to potential side effects of RT.

    C. Imbalanced nutrition: less than body requirements.

    D. Fatigue.

    E. Acute pain.

    F. Ineffective role performance.

    G. Delayed growth and development.

Outcome Identification

  I. Client and family describe state of the disease, therapy, and potential side effects of RT.

  II. Client and family participate in decision-making process regarding the plan of care and life activities as appropriate.

  III. Client participates in self-care measures to minimize occurrence, severity, and complications of side effects of RT.

  IV. Client and family participate in measures to minimize fear and anxiety associated with treatment.

TABLE 36-5
Potential Nursing Diagnoses for Specific Sites

Site of Irradiation	Potential Nursing Diagnoses
Skin	Impaired skin integrity related to radiation-induced changes
	Disturbed body image related to treatment lines, radiation-induced changes, tattoos
Head and neck	Impaired oral mucous membranes related to radiation-induced changes
	Imbalanced nutrition: less than body requirements, related to mucositis, xerostomia, altered taste sensation, radiation caries
	Impaired physical mobility (temporomandibular joint) related to trismus
	Impaired verbal communication related to vocal cord irradiation, mucositis, xerostomia
Central nervous system	Risk for injury related to radiation-induced increased intracranial edema
	Disturbed body image related to alopecia
Chest	Imbalanced nutrition: less than body requirements, related to esophagitis
	Risk for infection related to leukopenia
	Risk for injury related to thrombocytopenia
	Ineffective breathing pattern related to radiation pneumonitis and/or fibrosis
	Decreased cardiac output related to cardiotoxicity
	Impaired physical mobility (shoulder joint) related to radiation fibrosis
Abdomen	Imbalanced nutrition: less than body requirements, related to gastritis, nausea, vomiting
	Diarrhea
	Risk for infection related to leukopenia
	Risk for injury related to thrombocytopenia
	Acute pain related to radiation hepatitis
	Risk for deficient fluid volume related to radiation nephritis
Pelvis	Diarrhea
	Risk for infection related to leukopenia
	Risk for injury related to thrombocytopenia
	Impaired urinary elimination related to radiation cystitis
	Sexual dysfunction
	Ineffective sexuality patterns

  V. Client and family report signs and symptoms of early and late side effects of RT to a member of the health care team.
 VI. Client and family identify appropriate community and personal resources for information and services.
VII. Client and family describe follow-up plan.

Planning and Implementation

  I. Client education and interventions to incorporate client and family in care.
 II. Interventions to minimize side effects of RT (Table 36-6).
   A. Note incidence and severity of side effects.
   B. Perform nursing assessments and interventions related to area treated.
III. Interventions to maximize radiation protection and safety with sealed- and unsealed-source RT.
   A. Exposure—utilize principles of time, distance, and shielding to minimize exposure.

TABLE 36-6
Side Effects of Radiation Therapy

Site	Potential Early Effects	Potential Intermediate/Late Effects	Nursing Considerations
Skin	Erythema, pigmentation, dry desquamation, moist desquamation, alopecia	Fibrosis, atrophy, telangiectasis, altered pigmentation, slow healing of trauma, carcinogenesis	*Early effects:* nonmoist reaction: wash with mild soap and water and use aloe vera–based product for comfort; avoid perfume, deodorant, and shaving with razor over radiation site (Olsen et al., 2001) Moist desquamation: wash with saline or wound cleanser and use hydrogel dressing. Observe for increased reaction in skinfolds and with electrons Observe for increased expected reaction if client has had chemotherapy that enhances skin reaction (e.g., doxorubicin [Adriamycin], dactinomycin [Actinomycin D, Cosmegen]) *Early and late effects:* protect skin from chemical, mechanical, thermal irritants/injury and from sun (see Chapter 12)
Bone marrow	Myelosuppression (especially leukopenia, thrombocytopenia)		Large treatment areas covering significant amounts of bone marrow →increased myelosuppression (see Chapter 13)
Spine		Lhermitte's sign; significantly damages growth in axial spine in children	*Late:* radiation to growing bone decreases growth; monitor growth and development patterns after RT in children; assess neurologic and sensory functions
Brain	Alopecia, somnolence	Hypothyroidism (if pituitary gland is in field)	*Early:* use mild shampoo Moisturizing skin creams (aloe vera based preferred) as needed Plan for alopecia (generally temporary) (see Chapter 3) *Late:* assess neurologic and sensory function
HEAD AND NECK			
Mucosa	Mucositis	Pale mucosa, telangiectasia	Pretreatment dental evaluation Avoid chemical, thermal, and mechanical irritants to mucosa (Shih et al., 2002)
Salivary glands	Xerostomia	Xerostomia, dental caries	Dental prophylaxis and fluoride program; assess for signs/symptoms of hypothyroidism
Teeth		Radiation dental caries	See Chapter 14 for mucositis, xerostomia, and taste alterations and interventions
Tongue, taste buds	Changes in taste		
Larynx	Laryngitis		

Site	Acute effects	Late effects	Nursing interventions
Thyroid		Hypothyroidism	
Bone (mandible)		Osteoradionecrosis	
CHEST			
Lung	Radiation pneumonitis	Radiation pneumonitis, pulmonary fibrosis	Assess breathing. Assess nutritional status (see Chapter 14). See Chapter 16 for pulmonary toxicity.
Heart		Pericarditis, pancarditis, myocardial infarction	See Chapter 17 for cardiovascular toxicity
Esophagus	Esophagitis, dysphagia	Stricture, fistula	See Chapter 14 for dysphagia
ABDOMEN			
Small bowel	Diarrhea, fat malabsorption, nausea and vomiting	Small bowel obstruction, stricture	Antidiarrheal and antiemetic use. Assess nutritional status. Low-residue diet. Adequate fluids (see Chapter 15 for diarrhea, bowel obstruction). See Chapter 14 for nausea, vomiting
Stomach	Gastritis, nausea and vomiting 1-2 hr after treatment		
PELVIS			
Bladder	Radiation cystitis	Fibrosis	Assess bladder function, bladder analgesic use (see Chapter 15)
Large bowel, rectum	Diarrhea, nausea and vomiting, inflammation of hemorrhoids, tenesmus	Bowel ulceration, inflammation	Antidiarrheal use (see Chapter 15)
Ovaries	Premature menopause	Ovarian failure, especially if older than 25 yr; altered sexuality	Family planning issues; before treatment, suggest consultation with fertility specialist regarding current methods of egg preservation
Testes		Azoospermia	Discuss sperm banking before treatment if azoospermia anticipated; evaluate impact on client (see Chapter 6)
Vagina	Inflammation, dryness, dyspareunia	Dryness, stenosis, vaginal shortening, dyspareunia	Water-based lubricants (women). Vaginal dilator after treatment
Penis	Inflammation	Erectile dysfunction, urethral stenosis	Assess potency before RT (men)
ALL SITES			
	Fatigue	Carcinogenesis	Fatigue reduction strategies; follow-up assessment (see Chapter 1 for fatigue interventions)

RT, Radiation therapy.

      1. Remote afterloading—sources automatically withdrawn from the client and kept in a safe in the machine while staff and visitors are present. Negligible radiation exposure to staff and visitors.

B. Unsealed sources—blood and body fluids become radioactive.
      1. Inpatient rooms are specially prepared by radiation safety staff; plastic covers and absorbent floor coverings.
      2. Client may use the toilet and flush it three times after each use to dilute radioactive urine, stool, or vomitus.
      3. Everything exposed to the client's body fluids is potentially contaminated with radiation. Client uses disposable dishes. Linens and wastes kept in containers in the room and monitored for radiation before being removed.
      4. Staff wears gowns and gloves. Before leaving room, staff washes hands with the gloves on and then again after they are removed.

C. Sealed sources—accountability for all sources must be maintained.
      1. Shielded container is placed in room in the event of a dislodged source. Long forceps are used to place sources in the lead container.
      2. Dressings at implant site are changed by the physician only.
      3. Linens and wastes are kept in containers in the room and surveyed by a survey meter (e.g., Geiger counter) for radiation before being removed.
      4. Client and room are surveyed on removal of the sources.

D. Shielding—room designation for brachytherapy and radiopharmaceutical therapy depends on facility and radioactive material being used. Many institutions have specially shielded rooms. Clients generally are in a private room.

E. Shielding (portable)—portable shields may be placed by radiation safety officer (RSO) or designee at the bedside. Staff should stand behind the shield if possible when radioactive sources are in the client.

F. Exposure rate.
      1. Measurements of exposure rate are generally done at 1 meter from the client, on the nonclient side of a portable shield, and at the door of the room by the RSO or designee.
      2. Measurement of exposure rates in uncontrolled areas (e.g., room next door) may also be done.

G. Exposure—client movement within the room may be restricted during the procedure.
      1. Unless specifically ordered by the physician, client is to remain in room.
      2. Some clients may be out of bed but may be instructed to stay behind the shields unless using the bathroom. Clients remain in bed when visitors are present.

H. Radiation signs and instructions—radiation warning signs are posted on the door, chart, and client's armband. Information regarding source, exposure rate, specific instructions to nurses and visitors is generally placed in the chart.

I. Contamination or lost sealed source—in the event of possible contamination or loss of a source, the RSO and radiation oncology or nuclear medicine physician are notified immediately.

J. Time—minimize amount of time personnel are in room.
      1. Personnel are also rotated when radioactive sources cannot be remotely afterloaded.
      2. Visitors are restricted in amount of time spent in room.

K. Distance—visitors and personnel (when possible) remain 6 feet from client and behind the shield.

   L. Children (under the age of 18 years) and pregnant visitors and staff are not to enter the room when radioactivity is present.
   M. Discharge.
       1. Release of clients containing radioactive elements is very carefully controlled.
       2. Limitations on the quantity of radioactivity and exposure at 1 meter.
       3. Instructions must be given to the client and significant others (Behrend, 2000; Dow et al., 1997).
IV. Interventions to monitor for late effects of RT (Fieler, 1997).
 V. Communication of the client's responses with the health care team.
VI. Documentation of interventions and the client's responses.

Evaluation

The oncology nurse systematically and regularly evaluates the client's and/or family's responses to interventions to determine progress toward the achievement of expected outcomes. Relevant data are collected, and actual findings are compared with expected findings. Nursing diagnoses, outcomes, and plans of care are reviewed and revised as necessary.

ADDITIONAL RESOURCES

American Cancer Society
1-800-ACS-2345
website: www.cancer.org

American Society for Therapeutic Radiology and Oncology (ASTRO)
1-800-962-7876
website: www.astro.org

National Cancer Institute
1-800-4-CANCER
website: http://cancernet.nci.nih.gov

REFERENCES

Behrend, S.W. (2000). Radiation therapy treatment planning. In C.H. Yarbro, M.H. Frogge, M. Goodman, & S. Groenwald (Eds.). *Cancer nursing: Principles and practice* (5th ed.). Sudbury, MA: Jones and Bartlett Publishers, pp. 300-322.

Boelsen, R., & Jamar, S. (2000). Advances in radiation oncology. *Oncology Nursing Updates 7,* 1-11.

Dow, K.H., Bucholtz, J.D., Iwamoto, R., et al. (Eds.). (1997). *Nursing care in radiation oncology* (2nd ed.). Philadelphia: W.B. Saunders.

Dunne-Daly, C.F. (1999). Principles of radiotherapy and radiobiology. *Seminars in Oncology Nursing 15*(4), 250-259.

Fieler, V. (1997). Side effects and quality of life in patients receiving high–dose rate brachytherapy. *Oncology Nursing Forum 24*(3), 545-553.

Hall, E.J., & Cox, J.D. (1994). Physical and biologic basis of radiation therapy. In J.D. Cox (Ed.). *Moss' radiation oncology: Rationale, technique, results* (7th ed.). St Louis: Mosby–Year Book, pp. 3-65.

Hellman, S. (2001). Principles of cancer management: Radiation therapy. In V. DeVita, Jr., S. Hellman, & S. Rosenberg (Eds.). *Cancer: Principles and practice of oncology* (6th ed.). Philadelphia: Lippincott Williams & Wilkins, pp. 265-288.

Hilderley, L. (2000). Principles of radiation therapy. In C.H. Yarbro, M. Goodman, M.H. Frogge, & S. Groenwald (Eds.). *Cancer nursing: Principles and practice* (5th ed.). Sudbary, MA: Jones and Bartlett Publishers, pp. 286-299.

Maher, K. (2000). Radiation therapy: Toxicities and management. In C.H. Yarbro, M.H. Frogge, M. Goodman, & S. Groenwald (Eds.). *Cancer nursing: Principles and practice* (5th ed.). Sudbury, MA: Jones and Bartlett Publishers, pp. 323-351.

Mundt, A.J., & Roeske, J. (2003). Principles of radiation oncology. In E. Vokes & H. Golomb (Eds.). *Oncologic therapies* (2nd ed.). New York: Springer, pp. 9-17.

National Council on Radiation Protection and Measurements. (1993). *Limitation of exposure to ionizing radiation. Report no. 116.* Bethesda, MD: National Council on Radiation Protection and Measurements.

National Council on Radiation Protection and Measurements. (1972). *Protection against radiation from brachytherapy sources. Report no. 40.* Bethesda, MD: National Council on Radiation Protection and Measurements.

Nicolaou, N. (1999). Radiation therapy treatment planning and delivery. *Seminars in Oncology Nursing 15*(4), 260-269.

Olsen, D., Raub, W., Bradley, C., et al. (2001). The effect of aloe vera gel/mild soap versus mild soap alone in preventing skin reactions in patients undergoing radiation therapy. *Oncology Nursing Forum 28*(3), 543-547.

Rubin, P., & Siemann, D. (1993). Principles of radiation oncology and cancer radiotherapy. In P. Rubin (Ed.). *Clinical oncology: A multidisciplinary approach for physicians and students* (7th ed.). Philadelphia: W.B. Saunders, pp. 71-90.

Shih, A., Miaskowski, C., Dodd, M., et al. (2002). A research review of the current treatments for radiation-induced oral mucositis in patients with head and neck cancer. *Oncology Nursing Forum 29*(7), 1063-1078.

Vicini, F., Remouchanps, V., Wallace, M., et al. (2003). Ongoing clinical experience utilizing 3D conformal external beam radiotherapy to deliver partial-breast irradiation in patients with early-stage breast cancer treated with breast conserving therapy. *International Journal of Radiation Oncology, Biology, Physics 57*(5), 1247-1253.

Witt, M.E., Haas, M., Marrinan, M., & Brown, C. (2003). Understanding stereotactic radiosurgery for intracranial tumors, seed implants for prostate cancer, and intravascular radiotherapy for cardiac restenosis. *Cancer Nursing 26*(6), 494-502.

37 Nursing Implications of Biotherapy and Molecular Targeted Therapy

DANIELLE M. GALE

Theory

I. Definition.
  A. Biotherapy—treatment with agents derived from biologic sources and/or those agents able to affect biologic responses.
  B. Biologic response modifiers—agents or approaches that change the relationship between the tumor and host by modifying the biologic response of the host to tumor cells with a resultant therapeutic effect.
  C. Biologic response modifiers differ from chemotherapy agents in that most biologic agents are cytokines, proteins with low molecular weights having a short range of action on cells that are located near the cells that produce them (the cytokines) to stimulate immune responses (Rieger, 1999).
  D. Molecular targeted therapy (MTT)—agents or approaches that target cell membrane receptors, signaling pathways and proteins, enzymatic activity, and regulatory cell growth controls that are aberrant or more abundant in malignant cells than normal cells (Figure 37-1). This leads to a higher therapeutic index and a lower toxicity profile than conventional therapy (Gemmill & Idell, 2003). Approaches include monoclonal antibodies (MAbs) and vaccines, which are also considered biologic therapy. Other molecular targeted approaches, such as tyrosine kinase (TK) and proteasome inhibitors, are not generally considered biologic therapy.
  E. The focus of this chapter will be biologic and molecular targeted agents approved by the U.S. Food and Drug Administration (FDA) for the treatment of cancers.
II. Goals and approaches.
  A. Diagnosis of cancer.
    1. MAbs are used in the differential diagnosis of cancer.
      a. Classification of leukemias/lymphomas (recognition of cell surface markers).
      b. Identification of tumors with light microscopy.
    2. Radiolabeled MAbs (low-dose radioisotopes tagged to MAbs) are used to detect tumors using special scans.
  B. Treatment of cancer.
    1. Curative intent.
      a. Primary treatment.
        (1) Single agent (e.g., interferon-alpha) for the treatment of chronic myelogenous leukemia (Cuaron & Thompson, 2001).

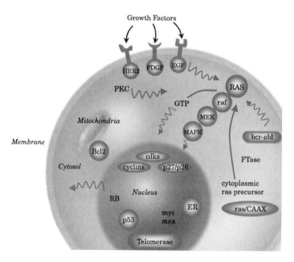

FIGURE 37-1 ■ Potential targets for molecular therapy. (From Gibbs JB: Mechanism-based target identification and drug discovery in cancer research, *Science* 287:1969-1973, 2000.)

    (2) Combination therapy, for example, CHOP (cyclophosphamide, doxorubicin, Oncovin [vincristine], prednisone) plus rituximab (Rituxan) for high-grade lymphoma (Coiffier et al., 2002).
  b. Adjuvant therapy.
    (1) After surgery to maintain the disease-free interval (e.g., interferon-alpha after surgery in clients with melanoma).
    (2) Many agents not FDA approved but under study in the adjuvant setting include the following:
      (a) Imatinib mesylate (Gleevec).
      (b) Trastuzumab (Herceptin).
      (c) Iodine-131 (I-131) tositumomab (Bexxar).
2. Control or stabilization of disease.
3. Maintenance therapy.
  a. After chemotherapy to maintain remissions and/or decrease the recurrence of disease (e.g., interferon-alpha after chemotherapy in a client with multiple myeloma and/or in lymphoma, or rituximab after chemotherapy).
4. Combination therapy.
  a. With other biologic agents (e.g., hematopoietic growth factors used in stimulation of dendritic cells [DCs]).
  b. Chemotherapy (synergistic effects of MAbs, such as rituximab and trastuzumab with many chemotherapeutic agents).
  c. After surgery.
  d. Radiotherapy.
C. Supportive therapy.
  1. Hematopoietic growth factors after antineoplastic therapy to decrease the incidence and severity of neutropenia, anemia, and thrombocytopenia.
D. Investigational.
  1. The use of biotherapy in many cancers and clinical situations remains under investigation. Many applications currently supported in the literature have not received regulatory (FDA) approval.

III. Types of agents and indications. Table 37-1 lists complete information on mechanism of action, indications, side effects, and key nursing considerations for FDA-approved agents only (Brown et al., 2001).

    A. Cytokines—generic term for proteins released by cells that affect the function of other cells. Many agents pleotrophic, that is, possess multiple effects.

        1. Interferons (IFNs).

            a. Family of glycoprotein hormones with immunomodulatory, antiproliferative, and antiviral effects.

            b. Numerous types of IFN available for commercial use (Cuaron & Thompson, 2001). Types of IFN are not the same, cannot be substituted for each other, and include the following:

                (1) IFN-alpha (IFN-α) (Alferon, Roferon-A, Intron A, Infergen).

                (2) IFN-gamma (IFN-γ) (Actimmune).

                (3) IFN-beta (IFN-β) (Betaseron, Avonex).

        2. Interleukins (ILs).

            a. "Between leukocytes," protein molecules responsible for the signaling and communication among cells of the immune system.

            b. Named numerically in order of their discovery with 18 isolated but only two FDA approved.

            c. Regulatory approval (see Table 37-1).

                (1) IL-2 (Aldesleukin, Proleukin) (Gale & Sorokin, 2001).

                (2) IL-11 (oprelvekin [Neumega]) (see 3. Hematopoietic growth factors, below).

            d. ILs under study as antitumor agents include the following:

                (1) IL-4—stimulates growth of resting B cells and mast cells.

                (2) IL-6—effect on hematopoiesis, differentiation effects on T and B cells, increases production of acute-phase proteins. Also under study for mucositis.

                (3) IL-12—facilitates T-helper 1 responses, enhances lytic activity of natural killer (NK) cells, increase-secretion of IFN-γ, augments specific cytotoxic T-lymphocyte response.

        3. Hematopoietic growth factors.

            a. Family of glycoprotein molecules that regulate the reproduction, maturation, and functional activity of blood cells (also see Chapter 10).

            b. Initial agents approved had short half-life, requiring frequent administration; newly approved agents are pegylated, requiring less frequent dosing (Ozer et al., 2000).

            c. Regulatory approval.

                (1) Granulocyte-colony stimulating factor (G-CSF) (filgrastim [Neupogen], pegfilgrastim [Neulasta]) indicated for chemotherapy-induced neutropenia (Bedell, 2003).

                (2) Granulocyte-macrophage CSF (GM-CSF) (sargramostim [Leukine]) indicated for chemotherapy-induced neutropenia.

                (3) Erythropoietin (EPO) (epoetin alfa [Epogen, Procrit], darbepoetin alfa [Aranesp]) indicated for chemotherapy-induced anemia.

                (4) IL-11 (oprelvekin [Neumega]) indicated for chemotherapy-induced thrombocytopenia (Wujcik, 2001).

                (5) Hematopoietic growth factors being studied in manufacture of vaccines and stimulation of DCs.

        4. Tumor necrosis factor (TNF) under study.

            a. Monokine (protein produced by activated monocytes) that causes the hemorrhagic necrosis of cancer cells; mediator of septic shock.

            b. Regulatory approval: remains investigational.

TABLE 37-1
FDA-Approved Biologic and Molecular Targeted Agents

Agent	Actions	Uses	Common Side Effects	Nursing Considerations

Interleukin-2 (IL-2)	Supports growth and maturation of subpopulations of T cells
	Stimulates activity of NK (natural killer) cells and cytotoxic T cells
	Induces proliferation of other lymphokines
		IL-2 (Aldesleukin, Proleukin) is FDA approved for treatment of metastatic renal cell carcinoma, melanoma, HIV	Capillary leak syndrome
			Tachycardia
			Hypotension
			Hypovolemia
			Pulmonary edema
			Peripheral edema
			Fatigue
			GI
			  Nausea and vomiting
			  Anorexia
			  Diarrhea
			CNS changes
			Skin changes
			  Erythema
			  Dry desquamation
			  Rash
			Altered laboratory tests values
			  Hepatic
			  Hematologic
			  Hypocalcemia
			  Hypomagnesemia
				Medicate with acetaminophen and/or NSAIDs (if kidney function is adequate) as needed
				Monitor:
				  Orthostatic BP/pulse
				  Daily weights
				  Input and output
				  Perform skin care
				Maintain:
				  Fluid balance
				  Nutritional status (Mavroukakis et al., 2001)

Interferon-alpha (IFN-α)	Antiviral activity, antiproliferative activities, immunomodulatory activities	Interferon-α 2a (Roferon-A) is FDA approved for hairy cell leukemia, acquired immunodeficiency syndrome (AIDS)–related Kaposi's sarcoma, treatment of chronic myelogenous leukemia (CML), hepatitis C
		Interferon-α 2b (Intron A) is FDA approved for hairy cell leukemia, AIDS-related Kaposi's sarcoma, condyloma acuminatum, chronic hepatitis B (in adults and children) and C, and adjuvant therapy for clients with melanoma with high risk of recurrence
		Use of interferon-α also shown efficacious in other diseases, such as renal cell cancer, metastatic melanoma, and other hematologic malignancies, but these uses remain investigational (Cuaron & Thompson, 2001)
			Acute
			Flulike syndrome (headaches, fever, chills, arthralgia, myalgia)
			Nausea and vomiting
			Chronic
			Fatigue
			Neurologic
			  Decreased short-term memory
			  Decreased concentration/attention span
			  Decreased ability to perform mathematic calculations
			GI
			  Taste changes
			  Anorexia
			  Weight loss
			Integumentary
			  Dry skin
			  Pruritus
			  Partial alopecia
			Hematologic
			  Neutropenia
			  Thrombocytopenia
				Chills usually occur 3-6 hr after administration
				Premedicate with acetaminophen and repeat every 4 hr as needed (not to exceed 3 g/24 hr)
				Fever occurs 30-90 min after onset of chills, and peaks of 104° F (40° C) are not uncommon
				Fevers and chills may decrease in severity over time
				Fatigue, anorexia, and malaise may continue to worsen over time and may be dose limiting
				Monitor neurologic and mental status at every visit
				Antidepressant therapy may be beneficial
				If neurotoxicity occurs, drug may need to be discontinued
				Maintaining adequate hydration with fluids (IV if necessary) may lessen side effects such as fatigue and malaise
				Institute measures to maintain weight early

Tyrosine kinase inhibitors

Agent	Action	Indication	Side effects	Dosage / Nursing considerations
Imatinib mesylate	Small molecule antagonist with activity against tyrosine kinases by blocking binding site for ATP, preventing transduction of signals to the nucleus that induces cellular proliferation and apoptosis	Imatinib mesylate (Gleevec) indicated for CML with Philadelphia chromosome–positive disease (first line and relapsed) and in GI stromal tumors (GIST)	Most common side effects: mild to moderate edema, nausea, vomiting, muscle cramps, bone pain, diarrhea, rash. Less common side effects: anemia, neutropenia, thrombocytopenia, liver toxicity, drug interactions (Kantarjian & Talpaz, 2001)	Dosage: oral tablets available, 100 mg or 400 mg. In CML: Chronic—400 mg/day; Accelerated or blast crisis—600 mg/day. In GIST: 400 mg or 600 mg per day; Administration can continue until disease progression. *Special considerations*: Take with food to decrease GI upset. Monitor weight and for signs of fluid retention—if present, diuretics and/or dose adjustments may be needed. CBC should be performed weekly for first month, then biweekly for 1 mo, and periodically thereafter. Monitor liver function periodically. Metabolized via cytochrome P-450 pathway; drug interactions possible with acetaminophen, digoxin, anticoagulants, anticonvulsants, and oral contraceptives (see full prescribing information for complete list [Novartis, 2003])
Gefitinib	An anilinoquinazoline that inhibits intracellular phosphorylation of tyrosine kinases associated with transmembrane receptors, including HER1-EGFR (epidermal growth factor receptor), thereby inhibiting tumor cells' growth and proliferation	Gefitinib (Iressa) is FDA approved for treatment of clients with advanced NSCLC who have failed previous chemotherapy treatments containing a platinum and docetaxel	Most common side effects: mild to moderate diarrhea, acneiform rash and skin reactions, nausea and vomiting. Less common but serious and sometimes fatal side effect is interstitial lung disease (2% Japan, 0.3% United States)	Dosage: oral tablets (250-mg tablet with or without food daily). Monitor for signs and symptoms of pulmonary distress: SOB, wheezing, difficulty breathing; and teach to report to health care provider (HCP). Monitor bowel movements, and treat with loperamide as needed. Teach clients to wear sunscreen and hats and limit sun exposure while receiving EGFR inhibitors since sunlight can exacerbate skin reactions. Teach that rash may be a sign of response and treat with over-the-counter products, e.g., Gold Bond powder, diphenhydramine lotion, Aveeno baths, Sween cream (Krozely, 2004)
Bortezomib	Proteasome inhibitor that blocks activity of proteasomes, enzymes that play a critical role in regulating cell function and growth	Bortezomib (Velcade) is FDA approved for clients with multiple myeloma who have received two prior therapies and have demonstrated disease progression from the last therapy	Most common adverse events: nausea, fatigue, diarrhea, constipation, thrombocytopenia, fever, peripheral neuropathy, vomiting (Tariman, 2003)	Dosage: IV injection, 1.3 mg/m² by IV push twice weekly for 2 wk on days 1, 4, 8, and 11 followed by a 10-day rest period before next cycle. Monitor closely for neuropathy. Monitor CBC periodically

Monoclonal antibodies (MAbs)

Agent	Action	Indication	Side effects	Dosage / Nursing considerations
Unconjugated MAbs	Action specific for targeted antigen. Main actions the result of immune system activation through complement-dependent cytotoxicity (CDC), antibody-dependent cellular cytotoxicity (ADCC), and/or stimulating apoptosis (programmed cell death)	Variety of tumor types	Side effects related to immune stimulation with subsequent cytokine cascade and loss of any healthy cells expressing targeted antigen. Anaphylaxis may occur with any MAb but is more likely to occur with murine products, such as tositumomab or ibritumomab; symptoms include cyanosis, hypoxia, severe rigors, wheezing, back pain, hypertension (HTN) or hypotension	Vary by agent but most common is infusion-related reactions, which is seen with most unconjugated MAbs. Management: Need for premedication varies by agent; see individual agents. Always administer as an infusion, never as an IV push or bolus. Baseline vital signs should be obtained and repeated at periodic intervals throughout the infusions. Should infusion-related reactions occur, stop or slow the infusion depending on severity of reaction; stop if severe or anaphylaxis is suspected

(Continued)

TABLE 37-1

FDA-Approved Biologic and Molecular Targeted Agents—cont'd

Agent	Actions	Uses	Common Side Effects	Nursing Considerations
Rituximab	Chimeric MAbs that target CD20, a protein expressed on surface of normal and malignant B cells	Rituximab (Rituxan) is FDA approved for treatment of relapsed or refractory, low-grade or follicular, CD20-positive, B-cell non-Hodgkin's lymphoma (NHL); as an initial treatment for bulky NHL; retreatment of low-grade or follicular lymphoma Contraindicated in clients with known anaphylaxis or IgE-mediated hypersensitivity to murine proteins or any component of this product (Genentech, 2002)	Adverse events: usually mild to moderate, predominantly an infusion-related symptom complex seen most frequently with first infusion (fevers, chills, rigors, hypotension, bronchospasm) Other common side effects: nausea, pruritus, headache, asthenia, myalgia Less common side effects: hypersensitivity reactions (non–IgE mediated), angioedema, bronchospasm, throat irritation, rhinitis, urticaria, rash, vomiting, dizziness, HTN With rituximab treatment, severe infusion reactions and tumor lysis have been observed in clients with high circulating white blood counts (>25,000)	For fevers and chills, administer acetaminophen For rigors, meperidine or other narcotic agent may be helpful along with blankets and warm liquids For hypotension, administer IV fluids May restart infusion after side effects have resolved, at a slower rate under close nursing supervision (DiJulio, 2001) Premedication with acetaminophen and diphenhydramine recommended Since transient hypotension may occur, consideration should be given to withholding antihypertensive medications 12 hr before rituximab infusion Dosage: 375 mg/m² × 4-8 doses Retreatment dose: 375 mg/m² × 4 doses Always administer as an infusion, never as a push or bolus Start first infusions at 50 mg/hr increasing by 50 mg/hr every 30 min to a maximum rate of 400 mg/hr If first dose is well tolerated, subsequent infusions may be started at 100 mg/hr, increasing by 100 mg/hr to a maximum rate of 400 mg/hr See above for more on infusion-related reaction management Treat bronchospasm with bronchodilators and/or oxygen May restart infusion after symptoms have resolved at one half the previous rate under close supervision Monitor after treatment for tumor lysis syndrome (electrolytes, kidney function) in those clients at high risk
Trastuzumab	Humanized MAbs that target the HER2 protein, found on many cells in low numbers but over-expressed on 25%-30% of those with breast cancer	Trastuzumab (Herceptin) is FDA approved for first-line use in combination with paclitaxel for treatment of HER-2 protein overexpressing metastatic breast cancer and as a single agent second line for those who have received one or more chemotherapy regimens for their metastatic breast cancer (Genentech, 2002)	Most common side effect: infusion-related symptom complex, mild to moderate in severity (fevers, chills, rigors); more common with first and decreasing in incidence and severity with subsequent infusions Other less common side effects: nausea, vomiting, pain (at tumor sites), headaches, dizziness, dyspnea, hypotension, rash, asthenia; cardiotoxicity may occur, especially in those with advanced age who receive trastuzumab concurrently with doxorubicin and cyclophosphamide	Premedication not recommended Always administer as an infusion, never as a push or bolus Dosage: 4 mg/kg loading dose followed by 2 mg/kg weekly dose Administer first infusion over 90 min and subsequent infusions over 30 min See above for more on infusion-related reaction management Baseline cardiac assessment to evaluate left ventricular function is recommended before start of therapy and repeated at periodic intervals during trastuzumab therapy; any signs or symptoms of cardiac dysfunction, such as dyspnea, SOB, edema, weight gain or increased pulse, BP, or respirations, should be reported to the HCP
Alemtuzumab	Humanized MAb that targets CD52, a glycoprotein expressed on the surface of normal and malignant B and T lymphocytes, NK cells, monocytes,	Alemtuzumab (Campath) is FDA approved for treatment of B-cell chronic lymphocytic leukemia (B-CLL) in clients who have been treated with alkylating agents and who have failed fludarabine therapy	Most common side effect: infusion-related events, resulting in discontinuation of therapy in 6% of clients (fevers, chills, nausea, vomiting, hypotension) Other common side effects: neutropenia, anemia, thrombocytopenia, infections,	Never administer more than 30-mg single dose or 90-mg cumulative dose per week Administer as a 2-hr infusion, never as a push or bolus Premedicate with first dose and at dose escalations with diphenhydramine and acetaminophen Monitor vital signs during infusion

	macrophages, and tissues of male reproductive system	fatigue, skeletal pain, anorexia, asthenia, HTN, tachycardia, SVT, headaches, dysesthesia, dizziness, marrow hypoplasia Serious, and in rare cases fatal, pancytopenia/marrow hypoplasia, autoimmune thrombocytopenia purpura (AITP), and autoimmune hemolytic anemia (AHA) have occurred with alemtuzumab as well as serious infusion-related reactions and serious, sometimes fatal, infections	Given 3 times per week by IV infusion or subcutaneous injection (under study) During therapy and until 2 mo after therapy or CD4+ count is >200 cells/µl, whichever occurs later, antiinfective prophylaxis should be administered (e.g., trimethoprim-sulfamethoxazole DS, twice daily 3 times per week, and famciclovir, 250 mg twice daily); antifungal agent may also be prescribed Initiate therapy at a dose of 3 mg daily; once tolerated may escalate dose to 10 mg/day, then 30 mg/day as tolerated to a maintenance dose of 30 mg/day 3 times per week on alternate days for up to 12 wk. If therapy is interrupted >7 days, initiate therapy at 3 mg and resume escalation as above CBC should be monitored, and dose modifications based on hematologic toxicity are recommended (Lynn et al., 2003; Seeley & DeMeyer, 2002)
Cetuximab	Chimeric MAb that targets HER1-EGFR (epidermal growth factor receptor) By binding with HER1, it blocks ability to initiate receptor activation and downstream signaling in tumor cell	Severe infusion reactions were seen in 3% of clients, rarely with fatal outcomes, with 90% seen with first infusion; if a severe reaction occurs, immediately interrupt and permanently discontinue treatment **Other serious reactions** Dermatologic toxicity (1%) Interstitial lung disease (0.5%) Fever (5%) Sepsis (3%) Kidney failure (2%) Pulmonary embolus (1%) Dehydration (5%) Diarrhea (6%) Most common adverse events when given with irinotecan Rash (88%) Asthenia/malaise (73%) Diarrhea (72%) Nausea (29%) Abdominal pain (45%) Vomiting (41%)	See above for more on infusion-related reaction management Dosage: as monotherapy or in combination with irinotecan Cetuximab, 400 mg/m² loading/initial dose as a 120-min IV infusion (maximum infusion rate 5 ml/min) Weekly maintenance dose: 250 mg/m² infused over 60 min (maximum infusion rate, 5 ml/min) Premedication with an H₁ antagonist (e.g., 50 mg of diphenhydramine IV) recommended Use a low protein-binding 0.22 micron in-line filter Never administer as an IV push or bolus Can be administered via an infusion pump or syringe pump Should be piggybacked in following the cetuximab infusion; 1-hr observation period recommended **Dose modification** Severe acneiform rash; first occurrence—delay infusion 1-2 wk; if improves, continue at 250 mg/m²; if no improvement seen, discontinue therapy Second occurrence—delay infusion 1-2 wk; if improvement seen, reduce dose to 20 mg/m²; if no improvement seen, discontinue Third occurrence—delay infusion 1-2 wk; if improvement seen, reduce dose to 150 mg/m²; if no improvement, discontinue Fourth occurrence—discontinue **Special considerations** Teach clients to wear sunscreen and hats and limit sun exposure while receiving cetuximab since sunlight can exacerbate skin reactions; EGR receptor testing should be performed Monitor bowel movements and treat with loperamide as needed Teach that rash may be a sign of response and treat with over-the-counter products, e.g., Gold Bond powder, diphenhydramine lotion, Aveeno baths, Sween cream (Krozely, 2004)

Cetuximab (Erbitux) is indicated to be used in combination with irinotecan for the treatment of EGF-expressing, metastatic colorectal carcinoma in clients who are refractory to rinotecan-based chemotherapy

No contraindication (AstraZeneca, 2004)

Contraindicated in clients who have active systemic infections, underlying immunodeficiency, or known type I hypersensitivity or anaphylactic reactions to alemtuzumab or one of its components (Berlex, 2002)

(Continued)

TABLE 37-1

FDA-Approved Biologic and Molecular Targeted Agents—cont'd

Agent	Actions	Uses	Common Side Effects	Nursing Considerations
Bevacizumab	Humanized MAb that binds to the ligand VEGF (vascular endothelial growth factor), a key mediator in angiogenesis (Muehlbauer, 2003); first antiangiogenic agent FDA approved	Bevacizumab (Avastin) used in combination with IV 5-fluorouracil-based chemotherapy is indicated for first-line treatment of clients with metastatic carcinoma of colon or rectum No contraindications Safety in children has not been established Since angiogenesis is critical to fetal development its inhibition during bevacizumab therapy is likely to result in adverse effects on pregnancy even though there are no adequate or well-controlled studies in pregnant women Women should not breastfeed during bevacizumab therapy (Idec Pharmaceuticals Corp., 2004)	Most serious but rare adverse events GI perforations (2%) Wound healing complications (1%) Hemorrhage: two patterns: Minor hemorrhage grade 1 epistaxis, nosebleeds) Serious hemorrhagic events seen in NSCLC (bevacizumab not indicated in lung cancer) Hypertension (60%-67% any grade, 7% severe HTN) well controlled with standard HTN medications in most clients Proteinuria (nephritic syndrome, 0.5%) Congestive heart failure (CHF) in 2% of all clients; most common in those receiving concurrent anthracyclines and/or those with history of receiving left chest wall radiation	Dosage: bevacizumab, 5 mg/kg as an IV infusion every 14 days until disease progression; first infusion over 90 min; if well tolerated, second infusion may be given over 60 min, and if well tolerated, all subsequent infusions may be given over 30 min Should never be given as an IV push or bolus Should be given as an IV push or bolus Never administer or mix with dextrose solutions No premedications recommended *Special considerations* Bevacizumab therapy should not be initiated for at least 28 days following major surgery Bevacizumab therapy should be suspended at least several weeks before elective surgery and not resumed until the incision is fully healed BP monitoring should be done every 2-3 wk during therapy and for at least 4 mo after therapy completion Clients should be monitored for development and worsening of proteinuria with serial urinalysis Clients with a 2+ or higher dipstick should undergo further testing with a 24-hr collection Dose modifications: none recommended with bevacizumab Bevacizumab therapy should be permanently discontinued in clients who develop GI perforations, wound dehiscence requiring medical intervention, serious bleeding, nephrotic syndrome, or hypertensive crisis Temporary suspension of bevacizumab is recommended in clients with moderate to severe proteinuria and severe HTN not controlled with medical management Vary by agent, target, and toxin; see below
Conjugated MAbs	Allow delivery of a potent toxin to the targeted tumor cell; less reliance on host effectors mechanisms since toxin usually causes cell death	Variety of tumor types	Side effects related to targeted cells affected, normal and cancerous, and toxin-related side effects	
Gemtuzumab ozogamicin	Humanized MAb conjugated with calicheamicin, a potent antitumor antibiotic that targets CD33, a protein expressed on surface of leukemia blast cells and immature myeloid cells; antibody is internalized once binding occurs, releasing toxin,	Gemtuzumab ozogamicin (Mylotarg) is approved for treatment of clients with CD33-positive acute myeloid leukemia in first relapse who are 60 yr of age or older and who are not considered candidates for chemotherapy Contraindicated in clients with known hypersensitivity to gemtuzumab ozogamicin or any of its parts, and	Severe myelosuppression occurs with all clients at the recommended dose, including neutropenia, thrombocytopenia, and anemia Fevers and chills also common, and a post-infusion symptom complex includes fevers, chills, and less commonly hypotension and dyspnea Infection and hepatotoxicity, including severe venoocclusive disease, has been reported	Use low protein-binding 1.2-micron filter Protect drug from light Administer as a 2-hr infusion, never as an IV push or bolus Premedicate with diphenhydramine and acetaminophen repeating the acetaminophen × 2 at 4-hr intervals after treatment Hydrate, and consider premedication with allopurinol Two 9 mg/m² doses 14 days apart (first 9 mg/m² on day 1 and next 9 mg/m² on day 14) with no dose modification for hematologic toxicity Vital signs should be monitored during infusion and for 4 hr following the infusion

Drug	Description	Indications/Contraindications	Adverse Effects	Nursing Implications
	resulting in DNA strand breaks and cell death (Wyeth-Ayerst Labs, 2000)	may cause fetal harm when administered to pregnant women Note: not recommended for clients with WBC >30,000 because of increased risk of pulmonary events	Less commonly bleeding, mucositis, and transient, usually reversible, abnormalities of liver function were observed	Monitor after infusion for tumor lysis syndrome (electrolytes and kidney function) CBC and liver functions should be monitored periodically
Ibritumomab tiuxetan	Murine-conjugated MAb with either radionucleotide indium-111 (for imaging) or yttrium-90 (for treatment with beta radiation) attached to a murine monoclonal that targets CD20 on normal and malignant B cell; tiuxetan is the linker-chelator agent (Hendrix et al., 2002)	Ibritumomab tiuxetan (Zevalin) is FDA approved for follicular NHL clients refractory to rituximab and for treatment of clients with relapsed or refractory low-grade, follicular or transformed B-cell NHL Contraindicated in clients with known anaphylaxis or IgE-mediated hypersensitivity to murine proteins or any component of this product (Idec Pharmaceuticals Corp., 2002)	Most serious adverse effects: infections, allergic reactions (bronchospasms, angioedema), hemorrhage while thrombocytopenic (resulting in deaths) Grade 3 or 4 adverse events seen in 89% of clients included thrombocytopenia and neutropenia Other common toxicities included anemia, nausea, vomiting, abdominal pain, diarrhea, increased cough, dyspnea, dizziness, arthralgia, anorexia, anxiety, and ecchymosis Secondary malignancies have been seen in 2% of clients treated	Do not give to clients with >25% bone marrow involvement and/or impaired bone marrow reserve, platelet count <100,000 cells/mm^3, neutrophil count <1500/mm^3, hypocellular bone marrow, or clients with a history of failed stem cell collection Day 1—rituximab (250 mg/m^2 over 4 hr) followed by In-111 ibritumomab tiuxetan (over 10 min) Assess biodistribution with 1-3 images 24-120 hr later Day 7-9 (any day × 1) rituximab (250 mg/m^2 over 4 hr) followed by Y-90 ibritumomab tiuxetan over 10 min, with dosage figured by platelet count:Normal: >150,000 cells/mm^3—0.4 mCi/kg; 100-140,000 cells/mm^3—0.3 mCi/kg CBC (including platelet counts) should be monitored weekly until levels recover (usually by 8-10 wk after therapy) Beta radiation does not require special shielding once injected into client Clients should be instructed to do the following: Clean spilled urine and dispose of material contaminated with body fluids so others will not handle (flush down toilet or place in plastic bag) Wash hands after using the toilet Use condoms during sexual relations for 1 wk Avoid pregnancy for 1 yr Discontinue breastfeeding during therapy (Hendrix, 2004)
Iodine-131 tositumomab	Murine-conjugated MAb with iodine-131 (beta radiation) that targets CD20 on normal and malignant B cells	Iodine-131 tositumomab (Bexxar) is indicated for treatment of clients with CD20-positive, follicular NHL, with and without transformation, whose disease is refractory to rituximab and has relapsed following chemotherapy The iodine-131 tositumomab therapeutic regimen is not indicated for initial treatment of clients with CD20-positive NHL Contraindicated in clients with known anaphylaxis or IgE-mediated hypersensitivity to murine proteins or any component of this product (Glaxo-SmithKline, 2003)	Most common adverse events Myelosuppression Myelodysplasia/acute leukemia Other less common adverse events Thyroid dysfunction/hypothyroidism (9.1%-17.4%) HAMA (10 %) (human antimouse antigens) Fevers/infections Asthenia/fatigue	Do not give to clients with >25% bone marrow involvement and/or impaired bone marrow reserve, platelet count <100,000 cells/mm^3, neutrophil count <1500/mm^3, hypocellular bone marrow, or clients with a history of failed stem cell collection In addition clients should have the following: Negative pregnancy test if childbearing age Normal renal function—serum creatinine <1.5 times the upper limit of normal Iodine-131 tositumomab therapeutic regimen—dosimetric step Day 0: two infusions 450 mg of tositumomab I-131 tositumomab (5 mCi, 35 mg) Scan no. 1—day 2, 3, or 4 Scan no. 2—day 6 or 7 Scan no. 3—therapeutic step day 7-14 (1 day only) Two infusions 450 mg of tositumomab I-131 tositumomab (dose 65 or 75 cGy total body dose of radiation, 35 mg) Thyroid protection Potassium iodide solution, Lugol's solution, or potassium tablets daily start at least 24 hr before dosimetric doses and continue 2 wk after therapeutic dose (Glaxo SmithKline, 2003)

(Continued)

TABLE 37-1

FDA-Approved Biologic and Molecular Targeted Agents—cont'd

Agent	Actions	Uses	Common Side Effects	Nursing Considerations
				Special considerations Radioactive components need to be ordered and administered by a licensed individual and in a licensed facility Clients emit radioactivity for a few days to a couple of weeks after iodine-131 tositumomab and should be instructed to limit radiation exposure to close contacts by doing the following: Not sleeping in the same bed Not driving together in the car for long periods of time No sexual intercourse
Retinoids	Tretinoin—all-trans retinoic acid Vitamin A derivatives with biologic effects in vision, growth, reproduction, epithelial cell differentiation, immune functions	Tretinoin is FDA approved for treatment of acute promyelocytic leukemia	Common side effects: teratogenesis, headaches, irritability, alopecia, arthralgias (joint and muscle pain), fatigue, dryness of the eyes and mucosa, skin changes including dryness, desquamation, sun sensitivity	Dosage: 45 mg/m²/day Given as two evenly divided doses until a complete remission is obtained Discontinue 30 days after complete remission or after 90 days of treatment Take with food to enhance absorption Should not be used during pregnancy, and women of childbearing age should practice effective contraception Protective measures should be used when out in the sun; liberal use of skin and lip lubricants Acetaminophen and NSAIDs for arthralgias (Spratto & Woods, 2001)
Fusion proteins	Direct cytocidal action or toxin to cells that express the targeted receptor Denileukin diftitox: recombinant DNA-derived cytotoxic protein composed of amino acid sequences for the diphtheria toxin fragments A and B-His followed by the sequences for interleukin-2 (Ligand Pharmaceuticals, 1999)	Denileukin diftitox (Dab389IL-2, ONTAK) is FDA approved for treatment of clients with persistent or recurrent cutaneous T-cell lymphoma whose malignant cells express the CD25 component of the IL-2 receptor Contraindicated in clients with known hypersensitivity to denileukin diftitox or any components of this product: diphtheria toxin, IL-2, or excipients	Acute hypersensitivity reactions were seen in 69% of clients during or within 24 hr of the infusion, one half on the first day of dosing regardless of treatment cycle, including hypotension, back pain, dyspnea, vasodilation, rash, chest pain or tightness, tachycardia, dysphagia or laryngismus, syncope, allergic reaction (1%), or anaphylaxis (1%) Vascular leak syndrome was reported with hypotension, edema, and hypoalbuminemia in one third of clients Other common side effects: infections, diarrhea, decreased lymphocyte counts, hypoalbuminemia, elevated transaminases, rashes	Never administer as an IV bolus Administer 9 or 18 mcg/kg/day IV over at least 15 min for 5 consecutive days every 21 days Do not use an in-line filter to administer Weight, BP, liver enzymes, serum albumin levels, and development of edema should be monitored during and after therapy For reactions, slow or stop infusion depending on severity of reaction Administration of IV antihistamines, corticosteroids, and epinephrine may also be required to treat hypersensitivity reactions and should be kept on hand along with resuscitative equipment (Walker & Dang, 2004)

FDA, Food and Drug Administration; *HIV,* human immunodeficiency virus; *GI,* gastrointestinal; *CNS,* central nervous system; *NSAIDs,* nonsteroidal antinflammatory drugs; *IV,* intravenous; *ATP,* adenosine triphosphate; *CBC,* complete blood count; *NSCLC,* non–small cell lung cancer; *IgE,* immunoglobulin E; *SOB,* shortness of breath; *BP,* blood pressure; *SVT,* supraventricular tachycardia; *EGFR,* epidermal growth factor receptor, *NS,* normal saline; *DNA,* deoxyribonucleic acid.

B. MAbs.
1. Highly specific antibodies produced from a single clone of cells.
2. May be murine (100% murine, momab), chimeric (30% murine with 70% human, ximab), humanized (about 95% human with 5% murine, zumab) (Figure 37-2).
3. Unconjugated MAbs are specific for an antigen found on the surface of cells and activate the immune system to kill cancer cells through complement-dependent cytotoxicity (CDC), antibody-dependent cellular cytotoxicity (ADCC), and/or stimulating apoptosis (programmed cell death). Side effects are usually due to immune stimulation and resulting cytokine cascade, resulting in flulike symptoms and infusion-related reactions.
4. Conjugated MAbs target specific antigens on the surface of cells but also have anticancer agents attached to them, such as toxins, chemotherapeutic agents, or a radioactive isotope. Side effects are related more to the toxin attached and, with radioactive isotopes, may include toxicity to nearby cells as well (Cheson, 2001; DiJulio, 2001; Rieger et al., 2001).
5. Regulatory approval for use in radiolabeled scans for the detection of disease includes the following:
   a. Satumomab pendetide (OncoScint CR/OV).
   b. Capromab pendetide (ProstaScint).
6. Unconjugated MAbs regulatory approved for therapeutic use in oncology.
   a. Rituximab (Rituxan).
   b. Trastuzumab (Herceptin).
   c. Alemtuzumab (Campath).
   d. Cetuximab (Erbitux).
   e. Bevacizumab (Avastin).
7. Conjugated MAbs regulatory approved for therapeutic use in oncology.
   a. Gemtuzumab ozogamicin (Mylotarg).
   b. Ibritumomab tiuxetan (Zevalin).
   c. Iodine-131 (I-131) tositumomab (Bexxar).
8. MAbs under study for use in oncology (Schmidt & Wood, 2003).
   a. HU1D10—targets HLA-DR on B cells (non-Hodgkin's lymphoma [NHL], chronic lymphocytic leukemia [CLL]).

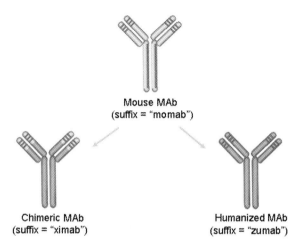

FIGURE 37-2 ■ Monoclonal antibodies. (Courtesy of Genentech BioOncology, Inc.)

    b. ABX-EGF (Abgenix)—targets HER1-EGFR (human epidermal growth factor receptor-1 protein–epidermal growth factor receptors).

    c. Epratuzumab—targets CD22 on B cells (NHL).

    d. BL22—conjugated with immunotoxin to target CD22 (hairy cell leukemia, CLL).

    e. LMB-2—conjugated, targets Tac antigen CD25 (CLL, T-cell leukemias, Hodgkin's disease).

    f. Edrecolomab—targets protein 17-1A (colorectal cancer).

    g. Oregovomab—targets oncofetal protein CA 125 (ovarian cancer).

C. Fusion proteins.

    1. Fusion proteins direct cytocidal action or toxin to cells, which express the targeted receptor.

    2. Regulatory approved agent denileukin diftitox (Dab389IL-2, ONTAK) (Rosenberg, 2000).

D. Effector cells.

    1. Immune cells (e.g., lymphocytes) removed from the client by pheresis or from the tumor during surgery, grown outside the body, and readministered as an intravenous (IV) infusion.

        a. Lymphokine-activated killer (LAK) cells.

        b. Tumor-derived activated cells (TDACs).

        c. Autolymphocyte therapy (ALT).

        d. T-cell receptor–activated T cells (TRACs).

        e. Anti-CD3/anti-CD28 coactivated T cells (COACTs).

        f. Antigen-specific cytotoxic T lymphocytes (CTLs).

        g. Dendritic cells (DCs) can be used subcutaneously, intradermal.

        h. BiAbs (combine specificity of two MAbs into one protein).

        i. T cells with chimeric receptors (T bodies).

    2. Regulatory approval—remain investigational (Rosenberg, 2000).

E. Immunomodulators.

    1. Agents that nonspecifically stimulate the immune system (e.g., bacillus Calmette-Guerin [BCG] [Immucyst, Pacis, TheraCys, TICE BCG], levamisole [Ergamisol]).

    2. Regulatory agencies have given approval for levamisole used as adjuvant therapy in combination with fluorouracil (5-FU, 5-fluorouracil) for the treatment of colon cancer (Dukes' C classification) and BCG administered as an intravesical instillation for the treatment of bladder cancer (Rosenberg, 2000).

F. Retinoids.

    1. Vitamin A derivatives that have a significant role in vision, growth, reproduction, epithelial cell differentiation, and immune function.

    2. Regulatory approval has been granted for tretinoin (Vesanoid) for the treatment of clients with acute promyelocytic leukemia (APL).

G. Vaccines.

    1. Active-specific immunotherapy (ASI)—goal to mobilize the immune system into attacking existing cancer cells by targeting tumor-associated antigens (TAAs), which are predominantly located on cancer cells.

    2. Many types of vaccines under clinical investigation in many tumor types for past 20 years; none regulatory approved.

        a. Peptide/protein TAAs stimulate strong immune responses.

        b. Recombinant viral (poxvirus, adenovirus)/bacterial—through recombinant techniques tumor antigen genes introduced into viruses that attract antigen-presenting cells (APCs) when injected into client.

    c. Cellular vaccines (whole-cell and tumor lysate).
       (1) Autologous—from the client's own tumor, first require many steps.
       (2) Allogeneic—use multiple tumor cell lines.
    d. Deoxyribonucleic acid (DNA) vaccines—use DNA-infected cells injected into muscles.
    e. DC-based vaccines.
       (1) DCs are excellent APCs.
       (2) Many methods used to load with TAAs.
       (3) Cytokines used to optimize the immune response (IL-2, IL-12, IL-7, IL-15, IFN-α, Flt-3 ligand) (Muehlbauer & Schwartzentruber, 2003).
H. Molecular targeted therapies (Figure 37-3).
    1. Tyrosine kinase inhibitors (TKIs)—oral agents, small molecule inhibitors (Gale, 2003).
      a. Imatinib mesylate—targets TK of Bcr-Abl in CML (chronic myeloid leukemia), KIT in GIST (gastrointestinal stromal tumors), and PDGFR (platelet-derived growth factor receptor) (Kantarjian & Talpaz, 2001).
      b. Gefitinib (Iressa)—an anilinoquinazoline that inhibits phosphorylation of TKs associated with the transmembrane receptor HER1-EGFR, overexpressed in many cancers, including non–small cell lung cancer (NSCLC), for which it is approved.
      c. Other TKIs under study include erlotinib HCl (Tarceva, HER1) for NSCLC, canertinib (pan-HER), EKG-569 (HER1, HER2), and GW572016 (HER1, HER2) (Gale, 2003).
      d. Common side effects of HER1 inhibitors—rash, diarrhea, nausea.
      e. Other small molecule inhibitors under investigation include farnesyl transferase inhibitors (FTIs). Farnesylation is a critical step in the Ras/Raf pathway, which is overmutated in cancers.
       (1) Tipifarnib (Zarnestra, R115777),
       (2) Lornafarnib (SCH66336), and
       (3) BMS 214662.
    2. Proteasome inhibitors.

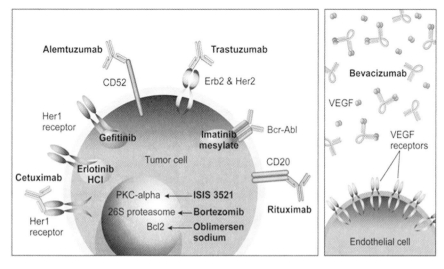

FIGURE 37-3 ■ Selected target therapies. *VEGF,* Vascular endothelial growth factor. (Courtesy of Genentech BioOncology, Inc.)

      a. Bortezomib (Velcade) blocks activity of proteasomes, which can lead to cell death. FDA approved in multiple myeloma.

      b. Under study—PS-341 in hematologic malignancies.

    3. Cell-cycle inhibitors under study.

      a. Flavorpiridol (HMR 1275) inhibits cyclin-dependent kinases.

    4. Antisense oligonucleotides under study.

      a. Oblimersen, G3139 (Genasense) targets Bcl-2 in many tumor types.

      b. ISIS-5132 inhibits Raf-1, a protein kinase involved in activating TK-mediated signaling.

  I. Gene therapy considered investigational. Three general approaches.

    1. Tumor directed—gene introduced into tumor cells to destroy them.

    2. Immunotherapy—active or adoptive.

    3. Delivery of genes done by viral and nonviral vectors (Liu, 2003).

IV. Production of biologic agents.

  A. Recombinant DNA technology.

    1. Technique for the production of large amounts of pure protein through insertion of the genetic sequence coding for that protein into an expression system (e.g., bacteria, yeast, mammalian cells).

  B. Hybridoma technology.

    1. Technique for the production of large amounts of pure immunoglobulin (e.g., MAbs). Classic technique fused murine myeloma cells with murine lymphocytes to produce hybridomas (Rieger, 2001).

  C. Gene therapy.

    1. Technique in which a functioning gene is inserted into a client's cells to reverse an acquired genetic defect or to add a new function to the cell.

  D. Growth of effector cells ex vivo.

    1. LAK cells.

    2. TDACs.

V. Rationale for biotherapy.

  A. Theory of immune surveillance.

    1. An intact immune system is able to recognize cancer cells as different from normal cells and can destroy the cancer cells.

    2. Cancer cells are constantly produced by the body and destroyed by the functioning immune system.

    3. Cancer develops when the immune system does not function properly or is unable to recognize cancer cells as foreign (Brown et al., 2001).

VI. Mechanisms of action.

  A. Biologic effects are mediated through attachment to cell surface receptors.

  B. Biologic agents are pleiotropic (possessing more than one biologic effect).

  C. Administration of one biologic agent often stimulates or suppresses the production of other biologic agents in vivo.

  D. Mechanisms of action for a biologic agent in a given disease are not generally well understood and most likely differ for use of the same agent (e.g., IFN) in different diseases.

  E. Classification.

    1. Agents that augment, modulate, or restore the immune response of the host.

    2. Agents that have direct antitumor activity (cytotoxic or antiproliferative mechanisms of action).

    3. Agents that have other biologic effects, such as affecting the differentiation or maturation of cells or the ability of the tumor cell to metastasize or survive (Rieger, 2001).

    4. MTTs—agents that target cell membrane receptors, signaling pathways and proteins, enzymatic activity, and regulatory cell growth controls that are aberrant or more abundant in malignant cells than normal cells; may or may not be biologic agents.

VII. Safety measures in the delivery of biotherapy.

    A. Aseptic techniques should be used when preparing and administering biologic agents.

    B. Most biologic agents are natural body proteins; however, there are few published studies on the mutagenicity and carcinogenicity of these agents.

        1. Universal precautions are recommended.

        2. Generation of aerosols and direct skin contact with agents fused to chemotherapeutic agents should be avoided (see Chapter 39).

        3. Use isotope-specific guidelines for radioisotopes attached to MAbs (see Chapter 36).

        4. The U.S. Occupational Safety and Health Administration (OSHA) has identified IFNs as hazardous agents that must be handled according to the OSHA guidelines for cytotoxic agents (Brown et al., 2001).

    C. Consult pharmacy resource personnel and product literature for specific information regarding preparation, storage, administration guidelines and special precautions, and disposal.

    D. Institutional guidelines pertaining to investigational protocols should be consulted when biologic agents are given as part of a clinical research protocol.

Assessment

    I. Pertinent personal history.

    A. Assess current medications, especially those that may be contraindicated with biologic agents.

        1. Aspirin.

        2. Steroids. Contraindicated with IL-2.

        3. Nonsteroidal antiinflammatory drugs (NSAIDs).

        4. Medications that may alter mentation or coagulation.

        5. Immunosuppressants.

        6. Antihypertensive therapy.

        7. Herbs such as the following:

            a. *Astragalus* (antiviral) also is considered an immunostimulant.

            b. Cat's claw *(Uncaria tomentosa)* has risk of renal failure.

            c. Chaparral *(Larrea divaricata)* has risk of liver failure.

            d. Echinacea *(Echinacea* species) may alter immunosuppressant effects of cancer chemotherapy, corticosteroids.

            e. Red clover *(Trifolium pratense)* should not be used by those with a history of breast cancer.

            f. St. John's wort *(Hypericum perforatum)* may interfere with immunosuppressants.

            g. Turmeric *(Curcuma domestica)* may interfere with immunosuppressants (Decker & Myers, 2001).

    B. Disease status—type and stage of cancer.

    C. Assess for chronic illnesses that may be exacerbated by side effects associated with biologic therapy—heart disease, diabetes, neurologic or psychiatric disorders, pulmonary disease, hypertension, psoriasis.

    D. Assess history of, and response to, prior cancer therapies.

    E. Allergies.

    II. Physical examination.

        A. Before initiation of therapy (to serve as a baseline for comparison) and at regular intervals during the course of therapy to evaluate tolerance to therapy, the client should have a thorough physical assessment by body system.

           1. Cardiovascular—heart rate and rhythm, abnormal heart sounds, blood pressure, and orthostatic blood pressure with agents known to cause hypotension.

           2. Pulmonary—respiratory rate, breath sounds, shortness of breath, cyanosis, clubbing.

           3. Gastrointestinal (GI)/nutritional—weight, eating patterns, abdominal girth, mucositis, xerostomia.

           4. Musculoskeletal—range of motion, functional status, presence and patterns of arthralgias.

           5. Neurologic—affect, orientation, memory, attention span, social engagement, sensory perception.

           6. Integumentary—erythema, rash, lesions, injection site reactions, dryness, decreased turgor, alopecia.

           7. General—presence of fever and flulike symptoms, fatigue.

   III. Psychosocial examination.

        A. Assess baseline mental status.

        B. Assess current social structure, including support systems, primary caretaker, housing and living arrangements, and work status.

        C. Assess type, number, and effectiveness of previous coping strategies used by client and family.

        D. Determine response to illness and emotional state.

        E. Assess ability to perform self-care activities (especially important if therapy is to be administered in the ambulatory setting).

        F. Consider financial status—need for referral to social worker or access to pharmaceutical company reimbursement assistance programs.

        G. Assess cultural factors and health-related beliefs.

   IV. Evaluation of laboratory data.

        A. Hematologic—white blood count, differential, hemoglobin and hematocrit levels, platelet count.

        B. Renal function—blood urea nitrogen (BUN) and creatinine levels.

        C. Liver function—lactate dehydrogenase (LDH), alkaline phosphatase, serum glutamic-oxaloacetic transaminase (SGOT), serum glutamate pyruvic transaminase (SGPT), bilirubin levels.

        D. Nutritional parameters—electrolytes, protein, albumin levels.

        E. Diagnostic and staging results.

    V. Client's and family's perceptions of treatment goals and demands.

        A. Treatment goals (e.g., diagnostic, therapeutic, supportive, or investigational).

        B. Requirements of treatment, such as length of hospitalization, follow-up clinic visits, laboratory and diagnostic test requirements, and financial obligations.

        C. Expected side effects of biotherapy.

        D. Self-care skills required (Rieger, 2001).

Nursing Diagnoses

    I. Risk for imbalanced body temperature.

   II. Fatigue.

  III. Deficient knowledge related to type of biologic agent and potential side effects.

    IV. Impaired memory.
     V. Risk for impaired skin integrity.
    VI. Imbalanced nutrition: less than body requirements.
   VII. Acute pain.

Outcome Identification

     I. Client and family describe the type of, and rationale for, treatment with biologic
         therapy.
    II. Client and family receive culturally competent care.
   III. Client and family list potential immediate and long-term complications of bio-
         therapy—constitutional symptoms, bone pain, fatigue, anorexia, weight loss or
         gain, somnolence, confusion, psychosis, chest pain, hypotension, irregular
         heartbeats, shortness of breath, decreased urinary output, allergic reaction.
    IV. Client and family describe self-care measures to decrease incidence and sever-
         ity of side effects associated with biologic therapy.
     V. Client and family demonstrate self-care skills required to administer biotherapy
         (e.g., medication self-administration, use of ambulatory infusion pumps, care of
         venous access devices).
    VI. Client and family verbalize changes in condition that should be reported to the
         health care team.
         A. Fever uncontrolled with acetaminophen or unrelated to normal response to
             therapy (i.e., fevers with IL-2 >8 hours after dose).
         B. Weight gain greater than 10 pounds in 1 week or 3 pounds in 1 day.
         C. Weight loss of more than 10% of body weight over several months.
         D. Shortness of breath at rest or extreme shortness of breath with exertion.
         E. Dizziness, chest pain, or irregular heartbeats.
         F. Marked changes in volume of urinary output.
         G. Overwhelming fatigue that impairs activities of daily living (ADLs).
         H. Significant changes in mental status (e.g., depression, confusion, psychosis);
             allergic reactions or intense inflammatory reactions at the injection site.
         I. Rash.
   VII. Client and family identify potential community resources to meet unique
         demands of therapy and rehabilitation.

Planning and Implementation

     I. Dosing and administration of biologic agents.
         A. Use aseptic procedures for mixing and administering biologic agents.
         B. Identify the location of emergency equipment and supplies (with adminis-
             tration of MAbs; these should be located at the bedside).
         C. Obtain baseline pulse, respirations, blood pressure, and temperature values
             before administration of biotherapy.
         D. Administer premedications (e.g., acetaminophen, diphenhydramine
             [Benadryl]) as ordered by the physician.
         E. Perform dosage calculation.
             1. Standardized total dose.
             2. Per body surface area or per kilogram of body weight.
             3. Adjustments in dose based on the following:
                 a. Organ function (e.g., renal, hematologic).
                 b. Toxicity grading (e.g., for fatigue, mental status changes, hematologic
                     values).

    F. Identify issues related to stability, compatibility with other drugs, and filterability that are unique to biologic agents.
       1. Most biologic agents are stored refrigerated, not frozen.
       2. Some are administered with albumin to ensure stability.
       3. Agents should not be shaken during reconstitution to avoid denaturing the biologic protein.
    G. Consider common routes of administration.
       1. Subcutaneous.
       2. Intramuscular.
       3. IV (e.g., bolus infusion, continuous infusion).
       4. Additional routes of administration may include intralesional, intravesicular, intraarterial, intraperitoneal, intracavitary, intrathecal, topical, intralymphatic, and oral (Rieger, 2001).

II. Interventions to monitor for unique complications of biologic therapy.
    A. Monitor orthostatic blood pressure and pulse rate with agents known to cause hypotension.
    B. Monitor fever patterns to differentiate normal responses to treatment from septic spikes.
    C. Evaluate symptoms for frequency, severity, duration, and effects on ADLs. Most biotherapy-related side effects are more severe with higher doses, and they tend to affect the quality of life.
       1. Overwhelming fatigue.
       2. Weight loss or gain of 10 pounds or more in 1 week.
       3. Marked mental status changes, such as excessive somnolence, psychosis, or confusion.
       4. Cardiac symptoms, such as chest pain, arrhythmias, and symptomatic hypotension.
       5. Other symptoms—increased dyspnea, oliguria, edema, severe allergic or local inflammatory reaction.
    D. Observe client for adherence to outpatient regimen.
    E. Monitor critical changes in laboratory test values as ordered by the physician (Jassack, 2002).

III. Interventions to decrease the incidence and severity of complications unique to biologic therapy.
    A. Impaired skin integrity.
       1. Bathe in shower or bath with tepid water, and avoid scrubbing skin.
       2. Apply lubricants (water-based lotions or creams) to skin after bathing and at regular intervals during the day.
       3. Encourage measures to maintain skin integrity, such as position changes, weight shifts, getting out of bed, ambulation, and pressure-relieving devices.
    B. Mental status changes.
       1. Assess, at regular intervals, mental status and potential for injury (e.g., risk of falling).
       2. Teach family to monitor for subtle behavioral changes and report to a member of the health care team.
       3. Maintain a safe physical environment.
       4. Evaluate the impact of mental status changes on functional status, judgment, and independence in ADLs.
    C. Capillary leak syndrome (movement of fluid from the vascular bed into tissues)—end results are edema, weight gain, hypotension, and decreased urinary output; seen with IL-2 (Aldesleukin, Proleukin) and sargramostim (GM-CSF, Leukine) at high doses.

    1. Administer supportive medical therapy, such as albumin, diuretics, fluids, and vasopressors, as ordered by the physician (Mavroukakis et al., 2001).

    2. Instruct the client to change positions from lying to sitting to standing slowly to avoid dizziness.

    3. Report significant changes to physician.

       a. Urinary output less than 30 ml/hr.

       b. Symptomatic hypotension.

       c. Dyspnea.

       d. Weight gain greater than 10 pounds in 1 week.

D. Fatigue (see Chapter 1).

E. Flulike symptoms.

    1. Monitor temperature and fever patterns.

    2. Use comfort measures to control fever and chills (e.g., warm blankets or clothing, warm beverages).

    3. Medicate round-the-clock with agents such as acetaminophen to control symptoms.

    4. Monitor vital signs at regular intervals and adjust as needed based on client status (e.g., elderly, those with underlying cardiac or pulmonary problems) (Shelton, 2001).

F. Hypersensitivity versus allergic reactions.

    1. Hypersensitivity reactions more common with MAbs. Usually seen with first infusion.

    2. Stop administration of MAbs.

    3. Administer fluids and emergency medications (e.g., diphenhydramine, epinephrine [Adrenalin], methylprednisolone [Solu-Medrol], albuterol [Proventil, Ventolin] nebulizer treatments) as ordered.

    4. Monitor vital signs every 5 minutes until stable.

    5. If hypersensitivity reactions suspected may consider premedication with steroids and reintroduction of agent at a slower infusion rate.

    6. If true allergic reaction is seen, reintroduction of agent not usually recommended (Rieger, 2001).

G. Infusion-related reactions.

    1. Very common with MAbs, especially with first infusion.

    2. Usually caused by cytokine cascade, not immunogenic reaction against MAb.

    3. Slow or stop the infusion depending on the severity of the reaction.

    4. Administer fluids and emergency medications (e.g., diphenhydramine, epinephrine, methylprednisolone) as ordered.

    5. Monitor vital signs.

    6. Consider reintroduction of agent once client fully recovered to baseline, at a rate 50% of rate at which the reaction occurred, and dose escalate very slowly.

    7. Premedication with acetaminophen and diphenhydramine is recommended with some agents to decrease the severity of infusion-related reactions.

H. Subcutaneous injection precautions.

    1. Allow drug to come to room temperature.

    2. Prepare site (rotate injection sites frequently) with antiseptic.

    3. Use small-gauge needle, and inject slowly at a 90-degree angle.

    4. Do not aspirate, rub, or apply undue pressure.

    5. Assess site for signs and symptoms of infection and inflammation. If present notify health care provider and treat per orders (antibiotics may be

ordered); application of warm compresses for 20 minutes four times daily may provide comfort (Rieger, 2001).

IV. Client and family education.
   A. Teach strategies to manage acute effects of therapy—infusion-related reactions, nausea, flulike symptoms (see Chapters 12 and 14).
   B. Teach strategies to manage chronic side effects of therapy—fatigue, mental status changes, anorexia (see Chapters 1, 12, and 14).
   C. Teach the client and family needed self-care skills for receiving biologic therapy in the ambulatory setting.
   D. Provide literature available for commercially available biologic agents.
   E. Discuss changes in lifestyle resulting from side effects of therapy and continued need for follow-up care.
   F. Teach client and family signs and symptoms of untoward reactions related to biotherapy administration that should be reported to a member of the health care team.
   G. Use client logs to document the incidence and severity of side effects and the type and effectiveness of self-care strategies used (Rumsey, 2001).

Evaluation

The oncology nurse systematically and regularly evaluates the client's and/or family's responses to interventions to determine progress toward the achievement of expected outcomes. Relevant data are collected, and actual findings are compared with expected findings. Nursing diagnoses, outcomes, and plans of care are reviewed and revised as necessary.

REFERENCES

AstraZeneca Pharmaceuticals LP. (2004). Erbitux (cetuximab). *Full prescribing information.* Wilmington, DE.

Bedell, C. (2003). Pegfilgrastim for chemotherapy-induced neutropenia. *Clinical Journal of Oncology Nursing* 7(1), 55, 56, 63, 64.

Berlex, Oncology (2002). Campath (alemtuzumab). *Full prescribing information.* Richmond, CA.

Brown, K.A., Esper, P., Kelleher, L.O., et al. (Eds.). (2001). *Chemotherapy and biotherapy: Guidelines and recommendations for practice.* Pittsburgh:Oncology Nursing Society

Cheson, B.D. (Ed.). (2001). *New frontiers in cancer therapy: Monoclonal antibody therapy of hematologic malignancies.* Abingdon, Oxford, United Kingdom: Darwin Scientific Publishing Limited.

Cheson, B.D. (Ed.). (2001). New frontiers in cancer therapy: monoclonal antibody therapy of hematologic malignancies, Abingdon, Oxford, United Kingdom. Darwin Scientific Publishing Limited.

Coiffier, B., LePage, E., Briere, J., et al. (2002). CHOP chemotherapy plus rituximab compared to CHOP alone in elderly patients with diffuse large B-cell lymphoma. *New England Journal of Medicine 346,* 235-242.

Cuaron, L., & Thompson, J. (2001). The interferons. In P.T. Rieger (Ed.). *Biotherapy: A comprehensive overview* (2nd ed.). Sudbury, MA: Jones and Bartlett Publishers, pp. 123-195.

Decker, G.M., & Myers, J. (2001). Commonly used herbs: Implications for clinical practice. *Clinical Journal of Oncology Nursing 5*(2), 2-13.

DiJulio, J.E. (2001). Monoclonal antibodies: Overview and use in hematologic malignancies. In P.T. Rieger (Ed.). *Biotherapy: A comprehensive overview* (2nd ed.). Sudbury, MA: Jones and Bartlett Publishers, pp. 283-316.

Gale, D.M. (2003). Molecular targets in cancer therapy. *Seminars in Oncology Nursing 19*(3), 193-205.

Gale, D.M., & Sorokin, P. (2001). The interleukins. In P.T Rieger (Ed.). *Biotherapy: A comprehensive overview* (2nd ed.). Sudbury, MA: Jones and Bartlett Publishers, pp. 195-244.

Glaxo SmithKline. (2003). Bexxar (Iodine-131 tositumomab). *Full prescribing information.* Philadelphia.

Gemmill, R., & Idell, C.S. (2003). Biological advances for new treatment approaches. *Seminars in Oncology Nursing 19*(3), 162-168.

Genentech. (2002). Herceptin (trastuzumab). *Full prescribing information.* South San Francisco.

Genentech. (2002). Rituxan (rituximab). *Full prescribing information.* South San Francisco.

Gibbs, J.B. (2000). Mechanism-based target identification and drug discovery in cancer research. *Science 287,* 1969-1973.

Hendrix, C. (2004). Radiation safety guidelines for radioimmunotherapy with yttrium 90 ibritumomab tiuxetan. *Clinical Journal of Oncology Nursing 8*(1), 31-34.

Hendrix, C.S., De Leon, C., & Dillman, R.O. (2002). Radioimmunotherapy for non-Hodgkin's lymphoma with yttrium 90 ibritumomab tiuxetan. *Clinical Journal of Oncology Nursing 6*(3), 144-148.

IDEC Pharmaceuticals Corp. (2004). Avastin (bevacizumab). *Full prescribing information.* South San Francisco, CA: Genentech.

IDEC Pharmaceuticals Corp. (2002). Zevalin (ibritumomab tiuxetan). *Full prescribing information.* San Diego: Author.

Jassack, P.F. (Ed.). (2002). *Oncology supportive care quarterly: Focused on nursing issues in the care of oncology patients 1*(1).

Kantarjian, H.M., & Talpaz, M. (2001). Imatinib mesylate: Clinical results in Philadelphia chromsome positive leukemia. *Seminars in Oncology 28*(Suppl. 17), 9-18.

Krozely, P. (2004). Epidermal growth factor receptor tyrosine kinase inhibitors: Evolving role in the treatment of solid tumors. *Clinical Journal of Oncology Nursing 8*(2), 163-168.

Ligand Pharmaceuticals. (1999). ONTAK (denileukin diftitox). *Full prescribing information.* San Diego: Author.

Liu, K. (2003). Breakthroughs in cancer gene therapy. *Seminars in Oncology Nursing 19*(3), 217-226.

Lynn, A., Williams, M.L., Sickler, J., & Burgess, S. (2003). Treatment of chronic lymphocytic leukemia with alemtuzumab: A review for nurses. *Oncology Nursing Forum 30*(4), 689-696.

Mavroukakis, S.A., Muehlbauer, P.M., White, R.L, & Schwartzentruber, D.J. (2001). Clinical pathways for managing patients receiving interleukin 2. *Clinical Journal of Oncology Nursing 5*(5), 207-217.

Muehlbauer, P.M. (2003). Anti-angiogenesis in cancer therapy. *Seminars in Oncology Nursing 19*(3), 180-192.

Muehlbauer, P.M., & Schwartzentruber, D.J. (2003). Cancer vaccines. *Seminars in Oncology Nursing 19*(3), 206-216.

Novartis. (2003). Gleevec (imatinib mesylate). *Full prescribing information.* East Hanover, NJ: Author.

Ozer, H., Armitage, J.O., Bennett, C.L., et al. (2000). 2000 update of recommendations for the use of hematopoietic colony-stimulating factors: Evidence-based clinical practice guidelines. *Journal of Clinical Oncology 18,* 3558-3585.

Rieger, P.T. (Ed.). (2001). *Biotherapy: A comprehensive overview* (2nd ed). Sudbury, MA: Jones and Bartlett Publishers.

Rieger, P.T. (1999). *Clinical handbook for biotherapy.* Sudbury, MA: Jones and Bartlett Publishers.

Rieger, P.T., Green, M., & Murray, J.L. (2001). Monoclonal antibodies: Applications in solid tumors and other disease. In P.T. Rieger (Ed.). *Biotherapy: A comprehensive overview* (2nd ed.). Sudbury, MA: Jones and Bartlett Publishers, pp. 317-356.

Rosenberg, S.A. (Ed.). (2000). *Principles and practice of biologic therapy of cancer* (3rd ed.). Philadelphia: J.B. Lippincott.

Rumsey, K.A. (2001). Patient education. In P.T. Rieger (Ed.). *Biotherapy: A comprehensive overview* (2nd ed.). Sudbury, MA: Jones and Bartlett Publishers, pp. 623-646.

Schmidt, K.V., & Wood, B.A. (2003). Trends in cancer therapy: Role of monoclonal antibodies. *Seminars in Oncology Nursing 19*(3), 169-179.

Seeley, K., & DeMeyer, E. (2002). Nursing care of patients receiving Campath. *Clinical Journal of Oncology Nursing 6*(3), 138-143.

Shelton B.K. (2001). Flu-like syndrome. In P.T. Rieger (Ed.). *Biotherapy: A comprehensive overview* (2nd ed.). Sudbury, MA: Jones and Bartlett Publishers, pp. 519-546.

Spratto, G.R., & Woods, A.L. (2001). *PDR: Nurse's drug handbook.* Montvale, NJ: Delmar Publications and Medical Economics Co., pp. 1321-1324.

Tariman, J.D. (2003). Understanding novel therapeutic agents for multiple myeloma. *Clinical Journal of Oncology Nursing 7*(5), 521-528.

Walker, P., & Dang, N.H. (2004). Denileukin diftitox as novel targeted therapy in non-Hodgkin's lymphoma. *Clinical Journal of Oncology Nursing 8*(2), 169-174.

Wujcik, D. (2001). Hematopoietic growth factors. In P.T. Rieger (Ed.). *Biotherapy: A comprehensive overview* (2nd ed.). Sudbury, MA: Jones and Bartlett Publishers, pp. 245-282.

Wyeth-Ayerst Labs. (2000). Mylotarg (gemtuzumab ozogamicin). *Full prescribing information.* Philadelphia.

38 Nursing Implications of Antineoplastic Therapy

SUSAN VOGT TEMPLE AND BARBARA C. PONIATOWSKI

Theory

I. Principles of cancer chemotherapy.
   A. Cancer chemotherapy is the treatment of choice for malignancies of the hematopoietic system and as systemic therapy for solid tumors, including solid tumors that have metastasized regionally or distally (Chu & DeVita, 2001).
   B. The application of antineoplastic agents to the treatment of cancer is based on concepts of cellular kinetics, which include the cell cycle, cell-cycle time, growth fraction, and tumor burden (Chu & DeVita, 2001; Tortorice, 2000).
      1. Cell cycle—a five-stage process of reproduction that occurs in both normal and malignant cells (Vermeulen et al., 2003) (Figure 38-1).
         a. Gap 0 (G_0), or resting phase.
            (1) Cells are not dividing and are temporarily out of the cell cycle.
            (2) Cellular activity continues to occur except reproduction.
            (3) Duration of time in G_0 phase is highly variable.
         b. Gap 1 (G_1): postmitotic phase, or interphase.
            (1) As cells are activated they enter the cell cycle at the G_1 phase.
            (2) Enzymes necessary for deoxyribonucleic acid (DNA) synthesis are produced.
            (3) Protein and ribonucleic acid (RNA) synthesis also occurs.
            (4) Duration of time in G_1 is variable, lasting from hours to days.
         c. Synthesis (S).
            (1) Cellular DNA is duplicated in preparation for DNA division.
            (2) Duration of time in the S phase is approximately 10 to 20 hours.
         d. Gap 2 (G_2), or premitotic phase.
            (1) Further protein and RNA synthesis occurs.
            (2) Precursors of the mitotic spindle apparatus are produced.
            (3) Duration of time in G_2 is short, ranging from 2 to 10 hours.
         e. Mitosis (M).
            (1) Cellular division occurs in four phases—prophase, metaphase, anaphase, telophase.
                (a) Prophase—nuclear membrane breaks down, and chromosomes clump.
                (b) Metaphase—chromosomes align in the middle of the cell.
                (c) Anaphase—chromosomes segregate to the centriole.

---

*Susan Vogt Temple and Barbara C. Poniatowski are full-time employees of GlaxoSmithKline (GSK). The views and opinions expressed therein are those of the authors/editors and do not necessarily reflect those of GSK.

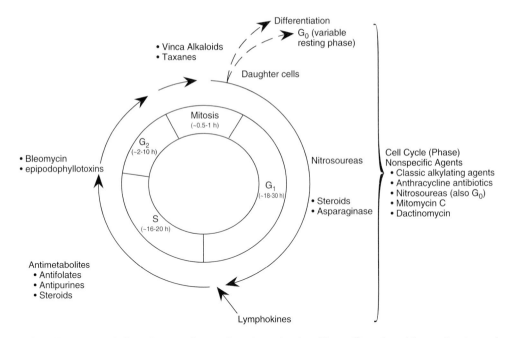

FIGURE 38-1 ■ Cell-cycle specificity of antineoplastics. The cell cycle with mechanism of action of select chemotherapeutic agents. (Reprinted with permission from GlaxoSmithKline Oncology, 2003. Property of GlaxoSmithKline Oncology; modified from DiPero J, Talbert R, Yee G: *Pharmacotherapy. A pathophysiologic approach,* ed 4, Stamford, Conn, 1999, Appleton & Lange.)

        (d) Telophase—cellular division occurs with the production of two daughter cells.

     (2) Duration of time in M phase is approximately 30 to 60 minutes (Gribbon & Loescher, 2000; Kastan & Skapek, 2001).

  2. Cell-cycle time—the amount of time required for a cell to move from one mitosis to another mitosis.

    a. The length of the total cell cycle varies with the specific type of cell; the length of the G_0 phase is the major determinant of the cell-cycle time.

    b. A shorter cell-cycle time results in higher cell kill with exposure to cell cycle–specific agents.

    c. Continuous infusion of cell cycle–specific agents results in exposure of a greater number of cells and in a higher cell kill in tumors with short cell-cycle times.

  3. Growth fraction of tumor—the percentage of cells actively dividing at a given point of time.

    a. A higher growth fraction results in a higher cell kill with exposure to cell cycle–specific agents.

    b. Tumors with a greater fraction of cells in G_0 are more sensitive to cell cycle–nonspecific agents.

  4. Tumor burden—the number of cells present in the tumor.

    a. Cancers with a small tumor burden are usually more sensitive to antineoplastic therapy.

    b. As the tumor burden increases, the growth rate slows, and the number of cells actively dividing decreases.

    c. The higher the tumor cell burden, the greater probability of heterogeneity of tumor cells and emergence of drug-resistant clones (Chu & DeVita, 2001; Tortorice, 2000).

C. Approaches to chemotherapy.
  1. Single-agent chemotherapy.
    a. Ongoing use of single-agent chemotherapy increases the probability of resistant clones.
    b. Most common application is in the relapse setting.
  2. Combination chemotherapy—the use of two or more antineoplastic agents to produce additive or synergistic results against tumor cells.
    a. Combining agents with actions in different phases of the cell cycle increases the number of cells exposed to cytotoxic effects during a given treatment cycle.
    b. Combining agents, in which one agent modulates the toxicity of another agent.
    c. Combining agents may decrease the incidence and severity of side effects of therapy.
    d. Effective in clients with large tumors containing a small number of proliferating cells. Agent kills a high proportion of tumor cells and stimulates (recruits) remaining tumor cells to enter the proliferative phase. Additional agents kill newly proliferating cells.
    e. Combining agents decreases the possibility of drug resistance.
    f. Criteria for selection of antineoplastic agents for combination therapy.
      (1) Demonstrate cytotoxic activity when used alone to treat a specific cancer.
      (2) Possess different, nonoverlapping toxicities.
      (3) Exhibit toxicities that occur at different points of time from the treatment.
      (4) Exhibit biologic effects that result in enhanced cytotoxicity.
  3. Regional chemotherapy—method of delivering higher doses of chemotherapy to the specific site of the tumor, such as the liver, bladder, peritoneal cavity, pleural space, while reducing the intensity of systemic toxicity.
  4. High-dose chemotherapy administered with supportive therapy (e.g., granulocyte/granulocyte-macrophage colony stimulating factors for neutropenia) or with an antidote to diminish toxicity (e.g., high-dose methotrexate [Mexate] with leucovorin rescue, ifosfamide [Ifex] with mesna [Mesnex]) (Chu & DeVita, 2001; Tortorice, 2000).
D. Factors influencing the response to antineoplastic agents.
  1. Characteristics of the tumor.
    a. Location.
    b. Size/tumor burden.
    c. Growth rate/fraction.
    d. Presence of resistant cells.
    e. Ratio of sensitivity of malignant cells and normal target cells.
    f. Hormone receptor status.
    g. Adequate blood supply with adequate drug uptake.
  2. Characteristics of the client.
    a. Physical status, including performance status, age, comorbidities, prior therapies.
    b. Psychosocial status.
  3. Administration schedule.
    a. Bolus.
    b. Continuous infusion.
    c. Combined modality therapy (Tortorice, 2000).

II. Roles of chemotherapy in cancer care.
  A. Cure.
    1. Single-treatment modality—for example, acute lymphocytic leukemia in children, Hodgkin's disease, lymphosarcoma, Burkitt's lymphoma, testicular carcinoma, gestational trophoblastic tumors, non-Hodgkin's lymphoma (in children), diffuse large cell lymphoma, Ewing's sarcoma.
    2. Combined-treatment modality (e.g., Wilms' tumor, osteogenic sarcoma, rhabdomyosarcoma).
  B. Control.
    1. Goal is to extend the length and quality of life when hope of cure is not realistic.
    2. Examples—breast cancer, chronic lymphocytic leukemia, chronic and acute myelogenous leukemia, small cell carcinoma of the lung, prostatic cancer, multiple myeloma, gastric carcinoma, endometrial carcinoma, non-Hodgkin's lymphoma (indolent), hairy cell leukemia, ovarian carcinoma, neuroblastoma, colorectal cancer, liver cancer, soft tissue sarcomas.
  C. Palliation.
    1. Goal is to improve comfort when neither cure nor control is possible.
    2. Relief of tumor-related symptoms (Chu & DeVita, 2001).
III. Types and classifications of chemotherapy. Antineoplastic agents are classified according to the phase of action during the cell cycle, mechanism of action, biochemical structure, or physiologic action.
  A. Phase of action during the cell cycle.
    1. Cell cycle–specific agents.
      a. Major cytotoxic effects are exerted on cells actively dividing at specific phases throughout the cell cycle.
      b. Agents are not active against cells in the resting phase (G_0).
      c. Agents are schedule dependent and most effective if administered in divided doses or by continuous infusion.
      d. Cytotoxic effects occur during the cell cycle and are expressed when cell repair or division is attempted.
    2. Cell cycle–nonspecific agents.
      a. Major cytotoxic effects are exerted on cells at any phase, including G_0, in the cell cycle.
      b. Agents are dose dependent and most effective if administered by bolus doses because the number of cells affected is proportional to the amount of drug given.
      c. Cytotoxic effects occur during the cell cycle and are expressed when cell division is attempted (Brown et al., 2001).
  B. Biochemical structure, mechanism of action, or derivation (Box 38-1).
    1. Alkylating agents.
      a. Mechanisms of action—interfere with DNA replication through cross linking of DNA strands, DNA strand breaking, and abnormal base pairing of proteins.
      b. Most agents are cell cycle nonspecific.
      c. Major toxicities occur in the hematopoietic, gastrointestinal (GI), and reproductive systems (Grochow, 2001) (Table 38-1).
    2. Nitrosoureas (considered a subgroup of alkylating agents).
      a. Mechanisms of action—interfere with DNA replication and repair.
      b. Nitrosoureas are non–cross resistant to other alkylating agents.
      c. Most agents are cell cycle nonspecific.
      d. Most agents cross the blood-brain barrier.

BOX 38-1
CLASSIFICATIONS OF ANTINEOPLASTIC AGENTS

Antimetabolites
5-Azacytidine
5-Fluorouracil (5-FU)
6-Thioguanine (6-TG, Thioguanine)
6-Mercaptopurine (6-MP, Purinethol)
Cladribine (2CdA, Leustatin)
Cytosine arabinoside (Ara-C, Cytosar,
    cytarabine)
Floxuridine (FUDR)
Fludarabine (Fludara)
Gemcitabine (Gemzar)
Capecitabine (Xeloda)
Methotrexate (Mexate, MTX)
Deoxycoformycin (pentostatin, Nipent)

Alkylating Agents—Platins
Carboplatin (Paraplatin)
Cisplatin (Platinol)
Oxaliplatin (Eloxatin)

Alkylating Agents—Nonplatins
Altretamine (hexamethylmelamine,
    Hexalen)
Busulfan (Myleran)
Chlorambucil (Leukeran)
Cyclophosphamide (Cytoxan)
Dacarbazine (DTIC-Dome)
Ifosfamide (Ifex)
Mechlorethamine (nitrogen mustard,
    Mustargen)
Melphalan (Alkeran)
Triethylenethiophosphoramide
    (thiotepa)

Antitumor Antibiotics—Anthracyclines
Daunorubicin (Cerubidine)
Doxorubicin (Adriamycin)
Epirubicin (Ellence)
Idarubicin (Idamycin)

Antitumor Antibiotics
Bleomycin (Blenoxane)
Dactinomycin (actinomycin D,
    Cosmegen)
Mitomycin-C (Mitomycin)
Mitoxantrone (Novantrone)
Plicamycin (Mithracin)

**Antitumor Antibiotics—Liposomal
Formulations**
Doxorubicin hydrochloride liposome (Doxil)
Daunorubicin citrate liposomal
    (DaunoXome)

**Nitrosoureas (also considered
alkylating agents)**
Carmustine (BCNU)
Chlorozotocin
Streptozocin (Zanosar)
Lomustine (CCNU)

Plant Alkaloids—Vincas
Vinblastine (Velban)
Vincristine (Oncovin)
Vinorelbine (Navelbine)

**Plant Alkaloids—
Epipodophyllotoxins**
Etoposide (VP-16, VePesid, Etopophos)
Teniposide (VM 26, Vumon)

Plant Alkaloids—Taxanes
Paclitaxel (Taxol)
Docetaxel (Taxotere)

**Topoisomerase I Inhibitors—
Camptothecins**
Irinotecan (Camptosar, CPT-11)
Topotecan hydrochloride (Hycamtin)

Glucocorticoids
Prednisone
Hydrocortisone
Methylprednisolone (Solu-Medrol)
Dexamethasone (Decadron)

Hormones
Estrogens
    Chlorotrianisene (TACE)
    Diethylstilbestrol (DES)
    Estramustine (Emcyt)
    Estratab
    Estradiol
Nonsteroidal aromatase inhibitor
    Anastrozole (Arimidex)
Steroidal aromatase inactivator
    Exemestane (Aromasin)
Nonsteroidal selective aromatase
    inhibitor
    Letrozole (Femara)
Antiestrogen
    Tamoxifen (Nolvadex)
Estrogen antagonist
    Fulvestrant (Faslodex)
Progestins
    Medroxyprogesterone acetate
        (Depo-Provera)
    Megestrol acetate (Megace)

Continued

BOX 38-1
CLASSIFICATIONS OF ANTINEOPLASTIC AGENTS—cont'd

LHRH analogues
  Leuprolide (Lupron)
  Goserelin acetate (Zoladex)
Nonsteroidal antiandrogens
  Bicalutamide (Casodex)
  Flutamide (Eulexin)

Miscellaneous Agents
Amsacrine (m-AMSA)
L-asparaginase (Elspar)

Hydroxyurea (Hydrea, Mylocel)
Procarbazine (Matulane)
Pegaspargase (Oncaspar)
Imatinib mesylate (Gleevec, STI-571)

Data from Berg D: Oxaliplatin: A novel platinum analog with activity in colorectal cancer, *Oncol Nurs Forum* 30(6):957-966, 2003; Brown K et al, editors: *Chemotherapy and biotherapy guidelines and recommendations for practice,* Pittsburgh, 2001, Oncology Nursing Society; Lonning P, Pfister C, Martoni A, Zamagni C: Pharmacokinetics of third-generation aromatase inhibitors, *Semin Oncol* 30(4, Suppl 14):23-32, 2003; Miller W: Aromatase inhibitors: Mechanism of action and role in the treatment of breast cancer, *Semin Oncol* 30(4, Suppl 14):3-11, 2003; Tortorice P: Chemotherapy: Principles of therapy. In Yarbro CH, Frogge MH, Goodman M, & Groenwald SL, editors: *Cancer nursing: principles and practice,* ed 5, Sudbury, Mass, 2000, Jones and Bartlett Publishers, pp 353-384; Versea L, Rosenzweig M: Hormonal therapy for breast cancer: Focus on fulvestrant, *Clin J Oncol Nurs* 7(3):307-311, 2003.
LHRH, Luteinizing hormone releasing hormone.

TABLE 38-1
Potential Side Effects of Chemotherapy

System	Side Effects
Hematopoietic	Neutropenia
	Thrombocytopenia
	Anemia
Gastrointestinal	Anorexia
	Nausea
	Vomiting
	Mucositis
	Stomatitis
	Diarrhea
	Constipation
	Pancreatitis
	Hepatic toxicity
Integumentary	Dermatitis
	Hyperpigmentation
	Alopecia
	Nail changes
	Radiation recall
	Rash, urticaria
Genitourinary	Cystitis
	Hemorrhagic cystitis
	Acute renal failure
	Chronic renal insufficiency
Cardiovascular	Cardiac toxicity
	Venous fibrosis
	Phlebitis
	Extravasation

TABLE 38-1
Potential Side Effects of Chemotherapy—cont'd

System	Side Effects
Neurologic	Central neurotoxicity
	Ototoxicity
	Metabolic encephalopathy
	Peripheral neuropathy
Pulmonary	Fibrosis
	Pneumonitis
	Edema
Reproductive	Infertility
	Changes in libido
	Erectile dysfunction
	Amenorrhea
Mood alterations	Anxiety
	Depression
	Euphoria
Metabolic alterations	Hypocalcemia
	Hypercalcemia
	Hypoglycemia
	Hyperglycemia
	Hyperphosphatemia
	Hyperuricemia
	Hypokalemia
	Hyperkalemia
	Hypomagnesemia
Latent effects	Cognitive dysfunction
	Learning disabilities
	Changes in memory
	Secondary malignancies
Other	Hypersensitivity
	Fatigue
	Ocular toxicity

Data from Brown K et al, editors: *Chemotherapy and biotherapy guidelines and recommendations for practice,* Pittsburgh, 2001, Oncology Nursing Society; Camp-Sorrell D: Chemotherapy: toxicity management. In Yarbro CH, Frogge MH, Goodman M, & Groenwald SL, editors: *Cancer nursing: principles and practice,* ed 5, Sudbury, Mass, 2000, Jones and Bartlett Publishers.

    e. Major toxicities occur in the hematopoietic and GI systems (Brown et al., 2001).
  3. Antimetabolites.
    a. Mechanisms of action—inhibit protein synthesis, substitute erroneous metabolites or structural analogues during DNA synthesis, and inhibit DNA synthesis.
    b. Most agents are cell cycle specific, S phase.
    c. Major toxicities occur in the hematopoietic and GI systems (Gutheil & Finucane, 2001).
  4. Antitumor antibiotics.
    a. Mechanisms of action—interfere with RNA and DNA synthesis.
    b. Most agents are cell cycle nonspecific.
    c. Major toxicities occur in the hematopoietic, GI, reproductive, and cardiac systems (cumulative doses) (Riggs, 2001; Verweij et al., 2001) (see Table 38-4).

5. Plant alkaloids.
   a. Mechanisms of action—mitotic spindle poison.
   b. Most agents are cell cycle specific, M phase, but may have activity in G_1 and S phases.
   c. Major toxicities occur in the hematopoietic, integumentary, neurologic, and reproductive systems; also hypersensitivity reactions (Rowinsky & Donehower, 2001; Rowinsky & Tolcher, 2001a) (see Table 38-4).
6. Topoisomerase I inhibitors.
   a. Mechanism of action—prevent realigning of DNA strands, maintaining single-strand DNA breaks.
   b. Major toxicities occur in hematopoietic and GI systems (Rowinsky & Tolcher, 2001b; Takimoto & Arbuck, 2001).
7. Hormonal agents.
   a. Mechanism of action—alter the internal/extracellular environment.
   b. Most agents are cell cycle nonspecific.
   c. Major toxicities—sexual/reproductive, GI, mood and sleep pattern changes (see Table 38-4).
8. Miscellaneous agents.
   a. Mechanisms of action—poorly understood.
   b. Variety of toxic effects (Brown et al., 2001; Tortorice, 2000).
IV. Chemoprotective agents.
   A. New agents designed to protect against specific toxic effects of chemotherapy.
      1. Dexrazoxane (Zinecard).
         a. Cardioprotective agent against doxorubicin.
         b. For cumulative dose greater than 300 mg/m².
         c. Administer 30 minutes before doxorubicin.
         d. Dose-limiting toxicity: myelosuppression in conjunction with chemotherapy.
      2. Amifostine (Ethyol).
         a. Cytoprotective agent for toxic effects of cisplatin-related renal toxicities.
         b. Administer 30 minutes before cisplatin.
         c. Side effects.
            (1) Frequent occurrence of transient hypotension.
               (a) Hold antihypertensive agents 24 hours before amifostine administration.
               (b) Frequent assessment of blood pressure: at baseline, during infusion, and post infusion.
               (c) Stop infusion if systolic blood pressure falls below established threshold levels.
            (2) Nausea, vomiting.
               (a) Administer antiemetics (e.g., serotonin inhibitor and steroid) before amifostine (Brown et al., 2001; Tortorice, 2000).
V. Routes of administration—advantages of each route, potential complications, and nursing implications are presented in Table 38-2.

Assessment

I. Pertinent personal and family history.
   A. Type of cancer and phase of cancer trajectory.
   B. Previous cancer therapy and time interval since last therapy.

TABLE 38-2
Routes of Administration of Antineoplastic Agents

Route	Advantages	Disadvantages	Complications	Nursing Implications
Oral	Ease of administration	Inconsistency of absorption	Drug-specific complications	Teach compliance with medication schedule Teach client techniques for handling drugs
Subcutaneous/ intramuscular	Ease of administration Decreased side effects	Requires adequate muscle mass and tissue for absorption Inconsistent absorption	Infection Bleeding	Evaluate platelet count before administration Use smallest gauge needle possible Prepare injection site with an antiseptic solution Assess injection site for signs and symptoms of infection
Intravenous	Consistent absorption Required for vesicants	Sclerosing of veins over time	Infection Phlebitis	Check for blood return before, during, and after drug administration
Intraarterial	Increased doses to tumor with decreased systemic side effects	Requires surgical procedure or special radiography for catheter and/or port placement	Bleeding Embolism Pain	Monitor for signs/symptoms of bleeding Monitor prothrombin time (PT), activated partial thromboplastin time (aPTT) Monitor catheter site
Intrathecal/ intraventricular	More consistent drug levels in cerebrospinal fluid	Requires lumbar puncture or surgical placement of reservoir or implanted pump Pump occlusion/ malfunction Requires additional education for nurse, client, family Nurse practice act may not allow nurse to administer agents via intrathecal/ intraventricular route	Increased intracranial pressure Headaches Confusion Lethargy Nausea/vomiting Seizures Infection	Observe site for signs of infection Monitor reservoir or pump functioning Assess client for headache or signs of increased intracranial pressure
Intraperitoneal	Direct exposure of intraabdominal surfaces to drug	Requires placement of Tenckhoff catheter or intraperitoneal port	Abdominal pain Abdominal distention Bleeding Ileus Intestinal perforation Infection Nausea	Warm chemotherapy solution to body temperature Check patency of catheter or port Instill drug/solution according to protocol—infuse, dwell, and drain or continuous infusion Reposition client according to protocol to allow for intraperitoneal distribution
Intravesicular	Direct exposure of bladder surfaces to drug	Requires insertion of indwelling catheter	Urinary tract infection Cystitis Bladder contracture Urinary urgency Allergic drug reactions	Maintain sterile technique when inserting indwelling catheter Instill solution, clamp catheter for 1 hr, and unclamp to drain according to protocol

Continued

TABLE 38-2
Routes of Administration of Antineoplastic Agents—cont'd

Route	Advantages	Disadvantages	Complications	Nursing Implications
Intrapleural	Sclerosing of pleural lining	Requires insertion of a thoracotomy tube Nurse practice act may not allow nurse to administer drug via intrapleural route	Pain Infection	Monitor for complete drainage from pleural space before instillation of drug Following instillation, clamp tubing and reposition client every 10-15 min × 2 hr for adequate distribution of the drug Attach tubing to suction according to protocol Assess client for pain; provide analgesia Assess client for anxiety; provide emotional support

Data from Brown K et al, editors: *Chemotherapy and biotherapy guidelines and recommendations for practice,* Pittsburgh, 2001, Oncology Nursing Society; Goodman M: Chemotherapy: principles of administration. In Yarbro CH, Frogge MH, Goodman M, & Groenwald SL, editors: *Cancer nursing: Principles and practice,* ed 5, Sudbury, Mass, 2000, Jones and Bartlett Publishers, pp. 385-4443.

     1. Attitudes of the client and family toward previous therapy.
     2. Side effects experienced and their severity.
     3. Self-care measures used to minimize side effects.
     4. Effectiveness of measures in reducing the incidence and severity of side effects.
   C. Dietary intake.
   D. Alternative/complementary therapy use.
   E. Knowledge of rationale for, and goals of, treatment; agents to be given; potential side effects; and relative risks and benefits of treatment.
II. Physical examination.
   A. Renal—intake and output, color of urinary output, patterns of urinary elimination.
   B. GI system.
     1. Oral cavity—cleanliness; moisture; integrity of lips, gums, teeth, oral mucosa, and tongue.
     2. Bowel—presence of bowel sounds; consistency, color, and caliber of stool; patterns of bowel elimination.
     3. Rectum—integrity of perirectal and perineal tissue; presence of hemorrhoids, redness, or pain.
   C. Hematologic system.
     1. Color of skin and mucous membranes; presence of bruising or petechiae.
     2. Activity intolerance.
     3. Presence of signs and symptoms of infection.
   D. Neurologic system.
     1. Preexisting deficits.
     2. Behavioral and cognitive functioning.
     3. Objective and subjective toxicities.
     4. Subsequent functional impairment.
   E. Pulmonary system.
     1. Skin and mucous membrane color.

      2. Respiratory rate, depth, rhythm, cough.

      3. Use of accessory muscles.

   F. Performance status.

III. Psychosocial examination.

   A. Previous responses to stressors and effective coping mechanisms used.

   B. Level of independence and responsibility, desire, and ability for self-care.

   C. Support systems and personnel available to the client and family.

IV. Laboratory/diagnostic data.

   A. Complete blood count with differential.

   B. Creatinine, blood urea nitrogen (BUN), liver function tests (LFTs).

   C. Electrolyte levels (Brown et al., 2001; Goodman, 2000; Gullatte, 2001).

   D. Other pertinent data specific to chemotherapy agents (e.g., ejection fraction, pulmonary function testing).

Nursing Diagnoses

   I. Deficient knowledge related to chemotherapy protocol, names of agents, potential side effects.

  II. Imbalanced nutrition: less than body requirements.

  III. Risk for infection.

  IV. Impaired oral mucous membrane.

  V. Sexual dysfunction.

  VI. Fatigue.

 VII. Disturbed body image.

VIII. Constipation.

  IX. Diarrhea.

  X. Nausea.

Outcome Identification

   I. Client describes the chemotherapy protocol—names of agents, routes, methods, schedules of administration, and schedules for routine laboratory and physical examination follow-up visits.

  II. Client and family list potential immediate and long-term side effects of the antineoplastic agents.

  III. Client and family describe self-care measures to decrease the incidence and severity of complications of therapy.

  IV. Client and family list changes that should be reported immediately to the health care team.

   A. Signs and symptoms of infection—for example, temperature of 100.5° F (38.1° C) or higher, pain, swelling, redness, pus, chills, rigors, cough, change in cough, sore throat, diarrhea.

   B. Nausea or vomiting that persists and is unrelieved by usual methods; inability to maintain oral intake.

   C. Unusual bleeding or bruising.

   D. Stomatitis.

   E. Reduced urine output.

   F. Acute changes in mental or emotional status.

   G. Diarrhea or constipation unrelieved by usual control methods.

  V. Client and family identify community resources to meet potential demands of treatment and rehabilitation.

VI. Client and family demonstrate competence in self-care skills demanded by the treatment plan (e.g., care of venous access devices, implanted ports, or intracavitary catheters).

Planning and Implementation

I. Interventions to maximize safe administration of chemotherapy to client.
   A. Review orders—compare with formal drug protocol or reference source; check for completeness (e.g., schedule, route, admixture solution).
   B. Determine drug dosage.
      1. Verify actual height and weight on day of administration.
      2. Calculate body surface area (BSA) or appropriate dose calculation (i.e., area under the curve [AUC]).
      3. Recalculate drug dosage, and check against order.
   C. Review drugs to be administered and potential side effects and toxicities.
   D. Review and/or obtain orders for other medications, intravenous (IV) fluids (e.g., antiemetics; prehydration and posthydration).
   E. Check current laboratory test values.
   F. Verify that informed consent has been obtained if required.
   G. Assess the client.
      1. Previous experience with chemotherapy.
      2. Understanding and acceptance of the treatment plan.
      3. Resolution of prior cycle toxicities/side effects.
   H. Conduct client and family teaching (e.g., chemotherapy administration procedures, antiemetic schedule, self-care measures for potential side effects).
   I. Prepare drugs as needed, following safe handling procedures (see Chapter 39).
   J. Double-check chemotherapy order with second registered nurse (RN), pharmacist, or other licensed health care provider; BSA/dose calculation; and appropriate laboratory values.
   K. Obtain appropriate material.
      1. Emergency equipment.
      2. Agents for management of extravasation and/or anaphylaxis as indicated.
      3. Spill kit.
   L. Select site for venipuncture if peripheral administration is to be performed.
      1. Select distal sites before proximal sites.
      2. Evaluate general condition of veins.
      3. Note type of medications to be infused.
      4. Avoid sites where damage to underlying tendons or nerves is more likely to occur—for example, antecubital region, wrist, dorsal surface of the hand; areas with recent venipuncture sites, sclerosed veins; or areas of previous surgery, such as skin grafts, side of mastectomy, lumpectomy, node dissection, or partial amputation.
   M. Monitor central or peripheral IV administration.
      1. Verify presence of blood return before, during, and after administration of therapy.
      2. Observe for signs and symptoms of infiltration.
   N. Administer prechemotherapy hydration, antiemetics, and other medications if ordered.
   O. Administer chemotherapy drugs according to agency policy, following safe handling procedures (see Chapter 39), and according to the five rights.

  1. Right medication.
  2. Right time.
  3. Right route.
  4. Right dose.
  5. Right client.
  P. Assess the client for signs of infiltration (burning, pain, swelling, redness).
  Q. Flush the IV with appropriate solution after administering each agent and at completion of the infusion.
  R. Remove the needle or IV catheter, or inject heparin into the central line or device as needed.
  1. Apply an adhesive bandage to the peripheral IV site.
  2. Have the client elevate the extremity for 3 to 5 minutes after the needle is withdrawn.
  3. Apply gentle pressure to the site to reduce local bleeding.
  S. Document medication administration, infusion site, client education, and client response according to agency policy (Brown et al., 2001; Goodman, 2000; Gullatte, 2001).
II. Interventions to minimize risk of extravasation.
  A. Obtain appropriate materials and agents for management of extravasation as indicated (Table 38-3).
  1. Extravasation—infiltration or leakage of an IV antineoplastic agent into the local tissues.
    a. Irritants—agents that cause a local inflammatory reaction but do not cause tissue necrosis (see Table 38-3).
    b. Vesicants—agents that have the potential to cause cellular damage or tissue destruction if leakage into subcutaneous tissue occurs (see Table 38-3).
      (1) Instruct the client to report pain, burning, or other sensations with the infusion.
      (2) Administer vesicants in larger veins of the arm, midway between the wrist and elbow.
      (3) Assess patency every 2 to 3 ml when administering IV push and every 5 minutes for piggyback infusion.
    c. If extravasation occurs or is suspected, do the following:
      (1) Discontinue infusion, leaving needle or IV catheter in place.
      (2) Aspirate residual medication and blood from the IV tubing.
      (3) If recommended, instill the IV antidote and then remove the needle (see Table 38-3).
      (4) If no IV antidote is recommended, remove the needle.
        (a) Avoid applying pressure to the area to decrease spread of drug infiltrate.
        (b) Apply a sterile dressing; use heat or cold compresses as indicated.
        (c) Elevate the affected extremity to decrease swelling.
      (5) Notify the physician of extravasation; arrange follow-up.
      (6) Document extravasation in medical record to include date, time, needle size and type, site, method of administration, medications administered, sequence of antineoplastic agents, approximate amount of agent extravasated, subjective symptoms reported by client, nursing assessment of site, nursing interventions, notification of physician and interventions, instructions given to client, follow-up measures, and signature (Brown et al., 2001; Goodman, 2000).

TABLE 38-3
Agents Associated with Extravasation/Tissue Injury

Agent	Antidote	Type
Amsacrine (m-AMSA)	None	Vesicant
Bleomycin (Blenoxane)	None	Vesicant/irritant
Carboplatin (Paraplatin)	Unknown	Irritant
Carmustine (BCNU, BiCNU)	Unknown	Vesicant
Cisplatin (Platinol)	Sodium thiosulfate	Vesicant if >20 ml of 0.5mg/ml concentration extravasates
Dacarbazine (DTIC-Dome)	None	Irritant
Dactinomycin (actinomycin D)	None	Vesicant
Daunorubicin (Cerubidine)	None	Vesicant
Doxorubicin (Adriamycin)	None	Vesicant
Liposomal doxorubicin (Doxil)	None	Irritant
Epirubicin (Ellence)	None	Vesicant
Etoposide (VePesid, VP-16)	None	Vesicant/irritant
Idarubicin (Idamycin)	None	Vesicant
Ifosfamide (Ifex)	Unknown	Irritant
Mechlorethamine (Mustargen)	Isotonic sodium thiosulfate	Vesicant
Melphalan (Alkeran)	None	Vesicant
Mitomycin (Mutamycin)	None	Vesicant
Mitoxantrone (Novantrone)	Unknown	Vesicant (ulceration rare unless infiltrated in concentrated dose)
Paclitaxel (Taxol)	None	Vesicant/irritant
Plicamycin (Mithracin)	None	Vesicant
Streptozocin (Zanosar)	None	Vesicant
Teniposide (VM 26)	None	Irritant
Vinblastine (Velban)	None	Vesicant
Vincristine (Oncovin)	None	Vesicant
Vindesine (Eldisine)	None	Vesicant
Vinorelbine (Navelbine)	None	Vesicant

Data from Clamon G: Extravasation. In Perry M, editor: *The chemotherapy source book,* ed 3, Philadelphia, 2001, Lippincott Williams & Wilkins, pp. 432-435; Hood A, Reeck M: Dermatologic toxicity. In Perry M, editor: *The chemotherapy source book,* ed 3, Philadelphia, 2001, Lippincott Williams & Wilkins, pp. 424-432.

III. Interventions to decrease the incidence and severity of complications of chemotherapy.
   A. See the following chapters for interventions for common complications of chemotherapy: fatigue (see Chapter 1); anxiety (see Chapter 2); alopecia, disturbed body image (see Chapter 3); reproductive issues, sexual dysfunction (see Chapter 6); neuropathies, alterations in mental status (see Chapter 12); myelosuppression (see Chapter 13); anorexia, mucositis, nausea and vomiting, taste alterations, electrolyte imbalances (see Chapter 14); pulmonary toxicity, anemia (see Chapter 16); cardiovascular toxicity (see Chapter 17).
   B. Interventions for specific complications of selected antineoplastic agents are presented in Table 38-4.

TABLE 38-4
Specific Toxicities and Nursing Interventions for Selected Chemotherapeutic Agents

Toxicity	Chemotherapeutic Agents	Nursing Interventions

Hypersensitivity	Asparaginase
	Paclitaxel
	Bleomycin
	Carboplatin
	Cisplatin
	Docetaxel
	Liposomal
	  doxorubicin
	  hydrochloride
		Identify clients at risk—clients with previous allergic
		  reactions to this or other medications; cycle of therapy
		Assess for early signs of hypersensitivity—urticaria,
		  pruritus, generalized uneasiness, hypertension, pro-
		  gressing to more severe reactions, including shortness
		  of breath, chest pain, back pain, hypotension, bron-
		  chospasm, cyanosis, rigors, chills
		Taxane reactions generally occur at onset of first and/or
		  second infusion; platin reactions generally occur after
		  six infusions and during infusion
		Assess for signs of anaphylactic-type reactions
		Supportive care as indicated
		Premedicate as ordered
		Bleomycin test dose in lymphoma clients (may not be
		  predictive of reaction before first dose)

Pulmonary injury
  (pulmonary
  toxicity pre-
  senting as pneu-
  monitis that may
  progress to pul-
  monary fibrosis)
	Bleomycin
	Mitomycin
	Cyclophosphamide
	Methotrexate
	Cytosine arabinoside
	Carmustine
	Procarbazine
		Monitor cumulative dose of bleomycin, which should not
		  exceed 400 units; doses above this limit significantly
		  increase risk of pulmonary toxicity
		Assess for signs of pulmonary toxicity—dry persistent
		  cough, dyspnea, tachypnea, cyanosis, basilar rales
		Pulmonary toilet/ adequate exercise
		Higher levels of Fio_2 increase bleomycin toxicity potential

Renal toxicity	Cisplatin
	High-dose
	  methotrexate
		Monitor creatinine, BUN, urinary output
		Avoid other nephrotoxic agents
		Provide adequate hydration/diuresis
		Premedicate with chemoprotective agent if ordered for
		  cisplatin

Ototoxicity	Cisplatin	Teach client to report tinnitus Monitor dose levels; risk increases with dosage >60-75 mg/m^2 Refer client for audiograms if indicated

Hemorrhagic
  cystitis
	Cyclophosphamide
	Ifosfamide
		Ensure adequate fluid intake >3000 ml/day unless
		  contraindicated
		Void every 2-4 hr during day and every 4 hr at night
		Assess for signs of cystitis
		Administer mesna/continuous bladder irrigation (CBI) as
		  ordered
		Oral doses of cyclophosphamide should be given early in
		  the day.

Cardiotoxicity mani-
  fested by ECG
  changes, CHF,
  cardiomyopathy
	Doxorubicin
	Daunorubicin
	Epirubicin
	Idarubicin
	Cyclophosphamide
	  (high dose)
	5-Fluorouracil
	Capecitabine
	Mitoxantrone
		Monitor cumulative doses of agents; maximal cumulative
		  dose is 550 mg/m^2 for doxorubicin—doses above this
		  significantly increase risk for cardiotoxicity; maximal
		  cumulative dose for doxorubicin is 450 mg/m^2 if client
		  received or is concurrently receiving radiation to
		  mediastinum or cyclophosphamide
		Assess for signs of cardiotoxicity, including ECG
		  changes; signs of CHF, including weight gain, pedal
		  edema, shortness of breath, JVD
		Mitoxantrone—risk not as great as with daunorubicin
		  and doxorubicin; increased risk with cumulative doses
		  >125 mg/m^2

Continued

TABLE 38-4

Specific Toxicities and Nursing Interventions for Selected Chemotherapeutic Agents—cont'd

Toxicity	Chemotherapeutic Agents	Nursing Interventions
Diarrhea	Irinotecan	Early and late diarrhea that can be dose limiting Early diarrhea occurs within 24 hr of administration and is generally cholinergic; treatment may include atropine Late diarrhea occurs >24 hr after dose and is managed with loperamide on schedule recommended by manufacturer
Peripheral neuropathy	Paclitaxel Cisplatin Oxaliplatin Carboplatin	Sensory and motor nerve changes; stocking-glove distribution of dysesthesia Appears in distal extremities of hands/feet and progresses proximally Loss of sense includes proprioception, vibration, pain, temperature, and touch
Hypotension	Etoposide	Rapid infusion may precipitate hypotension; administer over 30-60 min Monitor blood pressure
Neurotoxicity (central)	Ifosfamide Methotrexate Vincristine Cytarabine Intrathecal Administration	Monitor creatinine, BUN, and albumin; risk of neurotoxicity increases with decreased renal function and low albumin Neurologic checks every 4 hr for clients at risk Teach clients and families to report early signs of neurotoxicity
Neurotoxicity (peripheral)	Paclitaxel Docetaxel Vincristine Vinorelbine Vinblastine Cisplatin	Assess for numbness of hands and feet; footdrop, slapping gait, tingling of fingertips and toes, decreased fine and gross motor abilities Monitor for constipation as a potential early sign of neurotoxicity Teach client to report symptoms of neurotoxicity

Data from Brown K et al, editors: *Chemotherapy and biotherapy guidelines and recommendations for practice,* Pittsburgh, 2001, Oncology Nursing Society; Camp-Sorrell D: Chemotherapy: toxicity management. In Yarbro CH, Frogge MH, Goodman M, & Groenwald SL, editors: *Cancer nursing: principles and practice,* ed 5, Sudbury, Mass, 2000, Jones and Bartlett Publishers, pp. 444-486; Singer M: Cardiotoxicity and capecitabine: a case report, *Clin J Oncol Nurs* 7(1):72-75, 2003; Weiss R: Hypersensitivity reactions. In Perry M, editor: *The chemotherapy source book,* ed 3, Philadelphia, 2001, Lippincott Williams & Wilkins, pp. 436-452.
BUN, Blood urea nitrogen; *ECG,* electrocardiogram; *CHF,* congestive heart failure; *JVD,* jugular vein distention.

Evaluation

The oncology nurse systematically and regularly evaluates the client's and/or family's responses to interventions to determine progress toward the achievement of expected outcomes. Relevant data are collected, and actual findings are compared with expected findings. Nursing diagnoses, outcomes, and plans of care are reviewed and revised as necessary.

REFERENCES

Berg, D. (2003). Oxaliplatin: A novel platinum analog with activity in colorectal cancer. *Oncology Nursing Forum 30*(6), 957-966.
Brown, K., Esper, P., Kelleher, L., et al. (Eds.). (2001). *Chemotherapy and biotherapy guidelines and recommendations for practice.* Pittsburgh: Oncology Nursing Society.

Camp-Sorrell, D. (2000). Chemotherapy: Toxicity management. In C.H. Yarbro, M. H. Frogge, M. Goodman, & S.L. Groenwald (Eds.). *Cancer nursing: Principles and practice* (5th ed.). Sudbury, MA: Jones and Bartlett Publishers, pp. 444-486.

Chu, E., & DeVita, V.T. (2001). Principles of cancer management: Chemotherapy. In V. T. DeVita, S. Hellman, & S.A. Rosenberg (Eds.). *Cancer: Principles and practice of oncology* (6th ed.). Philadelphia: Lippincott Williams & Wilkins, pp. 289-306.

Clamon, G. (2001). Extravasation. In M. Perry (Ed.). *The chemotherapy source book* (3rd ed.). Philadelphia: Lippincott Williams & Wilkins, pp. 432-435.

Goodman, M. (2000). Chemotherapy: Principles of administration. In C.H. Yarbro, M.H. Frogge, M. Goodman, & S.L. Groenwald (Eds.). *Cancer nursing: Principles and practice* (5th ed.). Sudbury, MA: Jones and Bartlett Publishers, pp. 385-443.

Gribbon, J., & Loescher, L. (2000). Biology of cancer. In C. Yarbro, M.H. Frogge, M. Goodman, & S. Groenwald (Eds.). *Cancer nursing: Principles and practice* (5th ed.). Sudbury, MA: Jones and Bartlett Publishers, pp. 17-34.

Grochow, L. (2001). Covalent DNA-binding drugs. In M. Perry (Ed.). *The chemotherapy source book* (3rd ed.). Philadelphia: Lippincott Williams & Wilkins, pp. 192-207.

Gullatte, M. (2001). Principles and standards of chemotherapy administration. In M. Gullatte (Ed.). *Clinical guide to antineoplastic therapy: A chemotherapy handbook.* Pittsburgh: Oncology Nursing Society, pp. 31-45.

Gutheil, J., & Finucane, D. (2001). Antimetabolites. In M. Perry (Ed.). *The chemotherapy source book* (3rd ed.). Philadelphia: Lippincott Williams & Wilkins, pp. 208-226.

Hood, A., & Reeck, M. (2001). Dermatologic injury. In M. Perry (Ed.). *The chemotherapy source book* (3rd ed.). Philadelphia: Lippincott Williams & Wilkins, pp. 424-432.

Kastan, M., & Skapek, S. (2001). Molecular biology of cancer: The cell cycle. In V.T DeVita, S. Hellman, & S.A. Rosenberg (Eds.). *Cancer: Principles and practice of oncology* (6th ed.). Philadelphia: Lippincott Williams & Wilkins, pp. 91-109.

Lonning, P., Pfister, C., Martoni, A., & Zamagni, C. (2003). Pharmacokinetics of third-generation aromatase inhibitors. *Seminars in Oncology 30*(4, Suppl. 14), 23-32.

Miller, W. (2003). Aromatase inhibitors: Mechanism of action and role in the treatment of breast cancer. *Seminars in Oncology 30*(4, Suppl. 14), 3-11.

Riggs, C. (2001). Antitumor antibiotics and related compounds. In M. Perry (Ed.). *The chemotherapy source book* (3rd ed.). Philadelphia: Lippincott Williams & Wilkins, pp. 227-252.

Rowinsky, E., & Donehower, R. (2001). Antimicrotubule agents. In B. Chabner & D. Longo (Eds.). *Cancer chemotherapy and biotherapy: Principles and practice* (3rd ed.). Philadelphia: Lippincott Williams & Wilkins, pp. 329-372.

Rowinsky, E., & Tolcher, A. (2001a). Microtubule-targeting drugs. In M. Perry (Ed.). *The chemotherapy source book* (3rd ed.). Philadelphia: Lippincott Williams & Wilkins, pp. 252-277.

Rowinsky, E., & Tolcher, A. (2001b). Topoisomerase-I-targeting drugs. In M. Perry (Ed.). *The chemotherapy source book* (3rd ed.). Philadelphia: Lippincott Williams & Wilkins, pp. 289-304.

Singer, M. (2003). Cardiotoxicity and capecitabine: A case report. *Clinical Journal of Oncology Nursing 7*(1), 73-75.

Takimoto, C., & Arbuck, S. (2001). Topoisomerase I targeting agents: The camptothecins. In B. Chabner & D. Longo (Eds.). *Cancer chemotherapy and biotherapy: Principles and practice* (3rd ed.). Philadelphia: Lippincott Williams & Wilkins, pp. 579-646.

Tortorice, P. (2000). Chemotherapy: Principles of therapy. In C.H. Yarbro., M.H. Frogge, M. Goodman & S.L. Groenwald (Eds.). *Cancer nursing: Principles and practice* (5th ed.). Sudbury, MA: Jones and Bartlett Publishers, pp. 353-384.

Vermeulen, K., Van Brockstaele, D., & Berneman, Z. (2003). The cell cycle: A review of regulation, deregulation and therapeutic targets in cancer. *Cell Proliferation 36*(3), 131-149.

Versea, L., & Rosenzweig, M. (2003). Hormonal therapy for breast cancer: Focus on fulvestrant. *Clinical Journal of Oncology Nursing 7*(3), 307-311.

Verweij, J. Sparreboom, A., & Nooter, K. (2001). Antitumor antibiotics. In B. Chabner & D. Longo (Eds.). *Cancer chemotherapy and biotherapy: Principles and practice* (3rd ed.). Philadelphia: Lippincott Williams & Wilkins, pp. 482-537.

Weiss, R. (2001). Hypersensitivity reactions. In M. Perry (Ed.). *The chemotherapy source book* (3rd ed.). Philadelphia: Lippincott Williams & Wilkins, pp. 436-452.

39 Principles of Preparation, Administration, and Disposal of Hazardous Drugs

JEAN M. ELLSWORTH-WOLK AND JAN HAWTHORNE MAXSON

Theory

I. Exposure to hazardous drugs poses a potential health risk to personnel who prepare, handle, administer, and dispose of these drugs.
   A. Definition: hazardous drugs possess any one of the following characteristics: genotoxicity, carcinogenicity, teratogenicity, or fertility impairment (American Society of Health-System Pharmacists [ASHP], 1990; Occupational Safety and Health Administration [OSHA], 1999).
   B. Categories may include antineoplastic or cytotoxic agents, biologic agents, antiviral agents, or immunosuppressive agents.
   C. Potential routes of exposure.
      1. Direct contact—skin and mucous membrane contact and absorption, inhalation, or ingestion (e.g., contaminated food), accidental needle stick (Polovich, 2003).
      2. Indirect contact—body fluids and excreta of clients who have received antineoplastic agents within the past 48 hours (Welch & Silveira, 1997).
   D. Potential effects of exposure to hazardous drugs.
      1. Short term—occur within hours or days after exposure (Polovich, 2003).
         a. Contact dermatitis, alopecia, local skin or mucous membrane irritation, blurred vision, allergic responses, dizziness, gastrointestinal (GI) tract problems, headache.
      2. Long term—occur within months or years after exposure (Polovich, 2003).
         a. Liver damage.
         b. Chromosomal abnormalities.
         c. Increased risk of cancer.
         d. Reproductive risks.
II. Institutional responsibilities with respect to hazardous drugs.
   A. Define agency policies and procedures about use of hazardous drugs consistent with professional and federal recommendations to minimize risks to personnel (OSHA, 1999).
   B. Orient and update annually all agency personnel who may come in contact with hazardous drugs about the potential risks of hazardous drugs and agency policies and procedures (Polovich, 2003).

C. Review agency policies and procedures about hazardous drugs at periodic intervals.

D. Include compliance to policies and procedures as a component of the agency's quality assurance and performance improvement program.

E. Develop a monitoring system for reviewing incident reports involving hazardous drugs.

F. Develop an employment medical surveillance program for monitoring the effects of acute and chronic exposure, including medical history, physical examination, laboratory studies, and biologic monitoring (Polovich, 2003).

G. Material safety data sheets (MSDSs) to be readily available in the workplace to all employees working with hazardous chemicals (OSHA, 1999).

H. Allow all employees who are pregnant, who are trying to conceive (male and female) or breastfeeding, or who have other medical reasons for not being exposed to hazardous drugs to elect to refrain from preparing or administering those agents or caring for clients during their treatment with them (Brown et al., 2001; Polovich, 2003).

Assessment

I. Previous health history of personnel.
   A. Personal history of cancer.
   B. Family history of cancer.
   C. Personal risk factors for cancer.
   D. Presence of signs and symptoms of site-specific cancers.
   E. Reproductive history (Polovich, 2003).
II. Physical and psychosocial examination—examination as defined by agency policy.

Nursing Diagnosis

I. Risk for injury related to handling hazardous drugs.

Outcome Identification

I. Nurse discusses potential risks related to handling hazardous drugs.
II. Nurse describes procedures designed to minimize exposure to hazardous drugs.
III. Nurse documents accidental exposure to hazardous drugs according to agency policy.
IV. Nurse recognizes professional and federal resources for monitoring changes in potential risks from, and recommendations regarding exposure to, hazardous drugs.

Planning and Implementation

I. Interventions to minimize risk of exposure during preparation. (Drug preparers should be specially trained.)
   A. Follow the manufacturer's recommendations for preparation.
   B. Determine a dedicated environment for drug preparation.
      1. Prepare antineoplastic agents in a centralized area.
      2. Prohibit eating, drinking, smoking, and applying cosmetics in the work area (OSHA, 1999).

C. Obtain and maintain special equipment for drug preparation.
   1. Prepare hazardous drugs, including oral drugs that must be compounded or crushed, in a class II (type B) or class III biologic safety cabinet (BSC) for maximal protection (ASHP, 1990 OSHA, 1999).
      a. Hood should be vented outside if feasible.
      b. Blower should be operated 24 hours per day, 7 days per week (AHSP, 1990).
      c. Hood should be serviced at regular intervals according to manufacturer's recommendations and must be recertified every 6 months (ASHP, 1990
      d. "When asepsis is not required, a class I BSC or an isolator intended for containment applications (containment isolator) may be sufficient." A type I BSC may be appropriate for crushing or compounding of oral preparations. "The exhaust from these [BSC] cabinets should be HEPA-filtered and whenever feasible exhausted to the outdoors" (National Institute for Occupational Safety and Health [NIOSH], 2004).
   2. Use a disposable, plastic-backed, absorbent pad underneath work area to minimize contamination by droplets or spills (AHSP, 1990).
      a. Pads are changed (at a minimum) at the completion of drug preparation or at the end of the shift.
      b. Pads are changed immediately after a contamination.
   3. Wear protective clothing during preparation of hazardous drugs.
      a. Disposable, long-sleeved gown made of lint-free, low-permeability fabric with knitted or elastic cuffs and a closed front (AHSP, 1990; OSHA, 1999).
      b. Disposable, surgical latex, nitrile, polyurethane or neoprene (0.007 to 0.009 inch), nonpowdered gloves with cuffs long enough to tuck over the cuffs of the gown (ASHP, 1990; Connor et al., 1999; Gross & Groce, 1998; OSHA, 1999).
         (1) Gloves should be inspected before use for visible tears (Polovich, 2003).
         (2) Double gloving recommended (NIOSH, 2004).
         (3) Gloves should be discarded immediately after a puncture, a tear, contamination, or 60 minutes of use (Polovich, 2003).
      c. Plastic face shield or splash goggles when splashes, sprays, or aerosols may be generated.
D. Follow special procedures when preparing drugs (ASHP, 1990; Brown et al., 2001; OSHA, 1999; Polovich, 2003).
   1. Wash hands thoroughly before and after preparation of hazardous drugs.
   2. Use needles, syringes, tubing, and connectors with Luer-Lok attachments
   3. Use special care when preparing agents packaged in ampules.
      a. Clear all fluid from the neck of the ampule. (Tap the stem of the ampule to clear all fluid from the neck of the ampule.)
      b. Wrap a sterile gauze pad around the neck of the ampule.
      c. Use a snapping motion to break off the top of the ampule, breaking it away from your body.
      d. Remove cap from syringe with filter needle. Insert tip of needle into the ampule, which is upright on a flat surface, and withdraw fluid into the syringe.
      e. Change needle before administration.
      f. Discard excess solution from ampule into a sealed waste vial or according to agency policy.

4. Use special care when reconstituting agents packaged in vials.
   a. Employ a multiuse dispensing pin or an 18-or 19-gauge needle with a hydrophobic filter or dispensing pin.
   b. Create negative pressure in the vial when adding diluent by aspirating a volume of air slightly larger than that of the volume of diluent added.
   c. Add diluent slowly.
   d. Allow diluent to run slowly down the side of the vial.
   e. Withdraw dose of agent into syringe.
   f. Allow air pressure to equalize between the vial and syringe before removing the needle.
5. Expel air from a syringe or tubing containing hazardous drugs slowly onto a sterile gauze pad contained in a sealable plastic bag.
6. Prime all tubing with intravenous (IV) solution before adding hazardous drug.
7. Consider use of a closed-system device for drug preparation and administration (Connor et al., 2002).
8. Place on each container a label that states "Hazardous Drug: Handle with Gloves, Dispose of Properly" (ASHP, 1990; OSHA, 1999; Polovich, 2003).
9. Wipe outside of the container with a moist gauze and ports with alcohol swabs before placing the container in a sealable bag for transport (Polovich, 2003).
10. Hazardous drugs should be transported to the administration area in sealed plastic bags that have been appropriately labeled.
11. Gowns, gloves, and preparation equipment should be discarded in appropriately labeled puncture-proof container.

II. Interventions to minimize exposure to hazardous drugs during administration.
   A. Wear personal protective equipment (PPE) during administration (ASHP, 1990; OSHA, 1999; Polovich, 2003).
      1. Disposable, long-sleeved gown made of lint-free, low-permeability fabric with knitted or elastic cuffs and a closed front.
         a. Gowns should be changed when leaving the client area or immediately if contaminated (Polovich, 2003).
      2. Good-quality disposable, surgical latex, nitrile, polyurethane or neoprene, nonpowdered gloves with cuffs long enough to tuck over the cuffs of gown (ASHP, 1990; Gross & Groce, 1998; OSHA, 1999; Polovich, 2003).
         a. Gloves should be inspected for visible defects before each use (Polovich, 2003).
         b. Double gloving recommended (NIOSH, 2004).
         c. Change gloves after each use, tear, puncture, or contamination or after 30 minutes of use (Brown et al., 2001).
   B. Consider using safe handling guidelines for biologic agents (other than interferon, which is classified hazardous [OSHA, 1999]) to maintain consistency of nursing practice and because of limited occupational exposure data (Estes, 2002). (See also Chapter 37, Nursing Implications of Biotherapy and Molecular Targeted Therapy.)
   C. Use gloves when handling oral agents (Polovich, 2003).
   D. Face shield should be used if there is a risk for splashing, such as with intracavitary instillation (Polovich, 2003).
   E. Prepare agents for infusion over an absorbent, plastic-backed pad.
      1. Spiking of bag should be done in a BSC or using a dry spike extension and backflow technique (Polovich, 2003).

2. Place a plastic-backed absorbent pad under the connection site and client's arm during infusion or injection (ASHP, 1990; Brown et al., 2001; OSHA, 1999).

3. Do not expel air or prime needle of intramuscular (IM) or subcutaneous injection syringe (Polovich, 2003).

4. Wrap sterile gauze around injection ports during IV push procedures (ASHP, 1990; Gullo, 1995; OSHA, 1999; Welch & Silveira, 1997).

F. Wash hands thoroughly after administering antineoplastic agents.

III. Interventions to minimize exposure to hazardous drugs during disposal (ASHP, 1990; OSHA, 1999; Polovich, 2003).

A. Place contaminated materials along with PPE in a sealable plastic bag and dispose of in a puncture-proof, leak-proof container labeled as "Hazardous Waste." The lid should be kept closed at all times.

B. Dispose of syringes and needles, without recapping, directly into puncture-proof container designed for hazardous waste.

C. Handle residual contaminated fluid from intracavitary administration as hazardous, and place in a sealed, leak-proof container labeled "Hazardous."

D. Wash hands after disposal of hazardous drugs and equipment used to prepare or administer.

E. Don gloves, and decontaminate equipment used during administration (infusion pump, bedside table) using appropriate solution (Polovich, 2003).

IV. Interventions to minimize the incidence and severity of exposure to hazardous drugs.

A. Direct contact.

1. Wash exposed areas with copious amounts of water or special solution (OSHA, 1999).

a. Wash exposed skin thoroughly with soap (nongermicidal) and water.

b. Flood involved eye while holding the eyelid open with water or an isotonic eye wash for at least 15 minutes.

2. Seek medical evaluation as soon as possible after an accidental exposure.

3. Complete an incident report according to institutional policies and procedures.

B. Accidental spill.

1. Obtain a spill kit, which is clearly labeled and readily available in all areas where storage, transportation, preparation, and/or administration of chemotherapy occurs. Contents of spill kit include the following (ASHP, 1990; Brown et al., 2001; OSHA, 1999; Polovich, 2003):

a. Protective clothing—NIOSH–approved respirator, splash goggles or safety goggles, two pairs of disposable gloves (inner latex gloves, outer utility gloves), disposable low-permeability coveralls or gown, shoe covers.

b. Special equipment—two sealable, thick, plastic hazardous waste disposal bags; absorbent, plastic-backed sheets or spill pads; 250-ml and 1-L spill control pillows; small scoop to collect broken glass fragments; disposable toweling; puncture-resistant container; plastic scraper; two disposal bags; a hazardous waste label.

2. Wear PPE.

3. Absorb liquids with a spill pad or sheet.

4. Remove powdered agents with a damp, disposable gauze pad or soft toweling.

5. Collect glass fragments in scoop.

6. Dispose of all contaminated materials in a sealed, thick, plastic bag labeled with a chemotherapy-warning label.
7. Wash the contaminated area.
   a. Wash with detergent three times, and rinse with water (OSHA, 1999).
   b. Consider use of two-step inactivator system of 2% sodium hypochlorite and 1% sodium thiosulfate. Commercially available as Surface Safe manufactured by SuperGen (Dorr, 2001).
8. To clean a spill on carpet, use absorbent powder to absorb spill, use vacuum cleaner reserved for hazardous spill (Polovich, 2003).
9. Complete an incident report according to institutional practices and procedures.

C. Environmental contamination following preparation and administration.
   1. Regular surface decontamination of BSC and administration equipment and environment should be done with appropriate solution (Connor et al., 1999; Polovich, 2003).
   2. A two-step deactivation system of sodium hypochlorite (bleach solution) and sodium thiosulfate results in the chemical degradation and mutagenic inactivation of many commonly used chemotherapy drugs (Connor et al., 1999; Dorr, 2001; Polovich, 2003).

V. Interventions to minimize risk of indirect exposure from body fluids of clients who have received antineoplastic agents within the past 48 hours.
   A. Forty-eight hours is standard time frame recommended for precautions to be implemented (ASHP, 1990; OSHA, 1999), but because of differences in hazardous drug excretion time, a drug-specific time frame may be preferred (Polovich, 2003).
   B. Wear protective clothing (gloves, gowns) when handling urine, stool, blood, or emesis. Wear gown and goggles if splashing of body fluids is expected, and avoid splattering body fluids during disposal (ASHP, 1990; OSHA, 1999).
   C. Place linen contaminated with body fluids in a specially marked laundry bag placed inside a labeled impervious bag. The laundry bag and its contents should be prewashed, and then the linens should be added to other laundry for a second wash (Polovich, 2003).
   D. Consider other measures to reduce exposure from body fluids.
      1. Limiting transfers of contaminated fluids from one container to another, using closed systems of drainage collection, and so on (Polovich, 2003).
   E. Consideration of double flushing of toilets for 48 hours following hazardous drug administration (Polovich, 2003).

Evaluation

The oncology nurse systematically and regularly evaluates his/her clinical practice to determine progress toward the achievement of expected outcomes. Relevant data are collected, and actual findings are compared with expected findings. Nursing diagnoses, outcomes, and quality monitoring programs are reviewed and revised as necessary.

INTERNET RESOURCES

Hazardous Drugs/Antineoplastic Drugs
website: www.osha-slc.gov/SLTC/hazardousdrugs/index.html.

National Institute of Health Recommendations for the Safe Handling of Cytotoxic Drugs
website: www.nih.gov/od/ors/ds/pubs/cyto/index.htm.

Occupational Hazards Related to Antineoplastic Agents—Review Agents
website: www.uth.tmc.edu/schools/sph/an_agents/decon.htm.

OSHA: Hazardous Drugs
website: www.osha-slc.gov/SLTC/hazardousmedications/index.html.

OSHA Technical Manual, Section VI, Chapter 2: Controlling Occupational Exposure to
   Hazardous Drugs
website: www.osha-slc.gov/dts/osta/otm/otm_vi/otm_vi_2.html.

REFERENCES

American Society of Health-System Pharmacists (ASHP). (1990). ASHP technical assistance
   bulletin on handling cytotoxic and hazardous drugs. *American Journal of Hospital Pharmacy*
   47, 1003-1049.

Brown, K.A., Esper, P., Kelleher, L.O., et al. (Eds.). (2001). *Chemotherapy and biotherapy guidelines*
   and recommendations for practice. Pittsburgh: Oncology Nursing Society.

Connor, T.H., Anderson, R.W., Sessink, P.J., & Spivey, S.M. (2002). Effectiveness of a closed system device in containing surface contamination with cyclophosphamide and ifosfamide in
   an IV admixture area. *American Journal of Health-System Pharmacists 59*, 68-72.

Connor, T.H., Anderson, R.W., Sessink, P.J., et al. (1999). Surface contamination with antineoplastic agents in six cancer treatment centers in Canada and the United States. *American*
   Journal of Health-System Pharmacists 56, 1427-1432.

Dorr, R.T. (2001). Achieving safe handling of cytotoxic agents: What is being done? Paper presented at the 2001 Annual Congress of the Oncology Nursing Society, San Diego. Retrieved
   February 10, 2003 from the World Wide Web: http/www.macmcm.com/ons/ons200102.htm.

Estes, J.M. (2002). Handling and disposal of monoclonal antibodies. *Clinical Journal of Oncology*
   Nursing, 6 290-291.

Gross, E.R., & Groce, D.F. (1998). An evaluation of nitrile gloves as an alternative to natural
   rubber latex for handling chemotherapeutic agents. *Journal of Oncology Pharmacy Practice 4*,
   165-168.

Gullo, S.M. (1995). Safe handling of antineoplastic drugs: Translating the recommendations
   into practice. *Oncology Nursing Forum 22*, 517-525.

National Institute for Occupational Safety and Health (NIOSH). (2004). *Preventing occupational*
   exposures to antineoplastic and other hazardous drugs in healthcare settings. Retrieved March 25,
   2004, from http://www.cdc.gov/niosh/docs/2004-HazDrugAlert/

Occupational Safety and Health Administration (OSHA). (1999). Controlling occupational
   exposure to hazardous drugs (*OSHA technical manual* [TED 1-0.15A], Section VI, Chapter 2).
   Washington, D.C.: Occupational Safety and Health Administration.

Polovich, M. (Ed.). (2003). *Safe handling of hazardous drugs.* Pittsburgh: Oncology Nursing
   Society

Welch, J., & Silveira, J.M. (Eds.). (1997). *Safe handling of cytotoxic drugs.* Pittsburgh: Oncology
   Nursing Society.

40 Nursing Implications of Hematopoietic Stem Cell Transplantation

TERRY WIKLE SHAPIRO

Theory

I. Principles of hematopoietic stem cell transplantation (HSCT) (Mangan, 2000; O'Connell & Schmit-Pokorny, 1997; Secola, 2001).

  A. Many malignancies exhibit a dose-related response to chemotherapy or radiation therapy (RT); increasing the dose raises the number of cells that are destroyed.

    1. The dose of chemotherapy or RT that can be delivered is limited by the degree of marrow toxicity.

    2. Bone marrow or stem cells from either the client (autograft) or a donor (allograft) are infused, and they engraft to "rescue" the client's hematopoietic function from the toxic effects of antineoplastic therapy or RT. Box 40-1 outlines sources of autografts and allografts.

    3. Therefore high doses of antineoplastic therapy or RT may be administered to treat more aggressive, higher-risk diseases.

  B. Nonmyeloablative HSCT, or "mini" HSCT (Alcindor et al., 2000).

    1. Immunotherapy whereby the client receives lower doses of chemotherapy and often total body irradiation followed by marrow or peripheral blood stem cells from an allogeneic donor.

    2. Objective of this transplant is to induce an immunologic response known as "graft versus tumor" (GVT).

    3. Currently reserved for older clients (>60 years) or those with comorbidities since the risk of acute toxicities from the lowered doses of chemoradiotherapy is less.

  C. Process of bone marrow transplantation (Alcindor et al., 2000; Blume & Thomas, 2000; Kapustay & Buchsel, 2000; Kline & Bertolone, 1998; Secola, 2001; Thomas et al., 1999; Whedon & Wujcik, 1997) (Figure 40-1).

    1. Marrow source is identified (see Box 40-1).

      a. Allografting.

        (1) Allografting involves transplanting marrow, peripheral blood stem cells (PBSCs), or umbilical cord blood (UCB) to a recipient who is genetically different.

        (2) Allografting, using a monozygotic twin as a donor, is termed a *syngeneic transplant*.

        (3) The most common and preferred situation is for hematopoietic stem cells (HSCs) to be donated by a six-out-of-six (6/6) antigen, human leukocyte antigen (HLA)–matched sibling.

BOX 40-1
SOURCES OF MARROW/STEM CELLS

Allografts
MATCHED SIBLING DONOR
Bone marrow
Peripheral blood stem cells
Umbilical cord blood

IDENTICAL TWIN DONOR
Bone marrow
Peripheral blood stem cells
Umbilical cord blood

PARTIALLY MATCHED FAMILY MEMBER
Bone marrow
Peripheral blood stem cells
Umbilical cord blood

MATCHED UNRELATED DONOR
Bone marrow
Peripheral blood stem cells
Umbilical cord blood

Autografts
Autologous bone marrow
Autologous peripheral blood stem cells
Autologous umbilical cord blood (rare)

Data from Applebaum F: The use of bone marrow and peripheral blood stem cell transplantation in the treatment of cancer, *CA: Cancer J Clin* 46(3):143-164, 1996; Bahtia V, Portor DL: Novel approaches to allogeneic stem cell therapy, *Expert Opin Biol Ther* 1(1):3-15, 2001; Blume K, Thomas ED: A review of autologous hematopoietic cell transplantation, *Biol Blood Marrow Transplant* 6:1-12, 2000; Buchsel PC, Kapustay P: Peripheral stem cell transplantation. In Miaskowski C, Buchsel P, editors: *Oncology nursing: assessment and clinical care*, St Louis, 1999, Mosby, pp. 187-208; Shapiro TJW, Rust D, Davis D, editors: *A clinical guide to bone marrow and stem cell transplantation*, Sudbury, Mass, 1997, Jones and Bartlett Publishers.

(4) Partially matched family members or matched unrelated donors from a volunteer panel may also be used as donors.

(5) UCB may be used as a source of allogeneic stem cells in the related, matched sibling as well as in the unrelated donor situation.

(6) Allografts are indicated for some congenital abnormalities of bone marrow function or in cases when there is disease involving the marrow not amenable to cure with standard treatment (e.g., leukemias). Box 40-2 shows diseases treated with allogeneic transplantation.

(7) "Mini," or nonmyeloablative, HSCTs are used in the allogeneic transplant setting when the client is older, has preexisting comorbidities, and has a disease that will benefit from the GVT immunologic effect.

b. Autografting (Blume & Thomas, 2000; Mangan, 2000).

(1) Autografting involves transplanting marrow or PBSCs back into the person from whom the blood cells originated.

(2) Because marrow or stem cell sources for allografting cannot always be found or because it may be too risky, autologous bone marrow or PBSC transplantation is used as a method for treating a number of malignant disorders.

(3) Using autologous marrow or PBSCs is not feasible for clients who have a deficiency of their functional bone marrow, as is the case with aplastic anemia, inborn errors of metabolism, and immunodeficiency states.

(4) May be used in circumstances in which autologous marrow or PBSCs are preferable to using an allogeneic source of stem cells (e.g., to avoid graft-versus-host disease [GVHD], in situations in

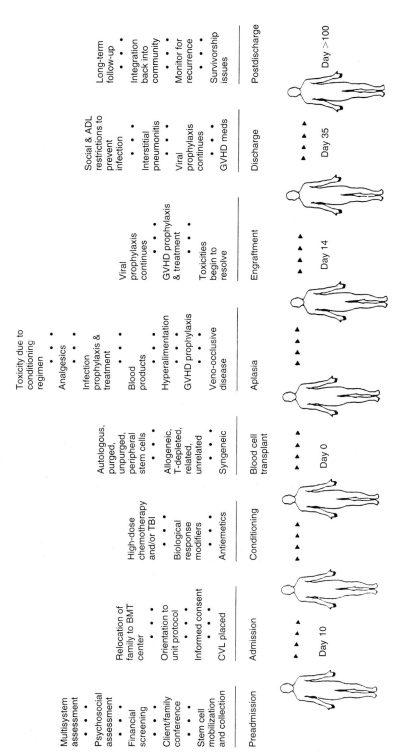

FIGURE 40-1 ■ Usual stages of the inpatient transplant process. *BMT*, Bone marrow transplant; *CVL*, central venous line, *TBI*, total body irradiation; *GVHD*, graft-versus-host disease; *ADL*, activities of daily living. (Modified from Ford R, Eisenberg S: Bone marrow transplant: Recent advances and nursing implications, *Nurs Clin North Am* 25[2]:406, 1990.)

BOX 40-2
DISEASES TREATED WITH ALLOGRAFTING OF HEMATOPOIETIC STEM CELLS

Leukemias—Syndromes
Acute myelogenous leukemia
Acute lymphoblastic leukemia
Chronic myelogenous leukemia
Myelodysplastic syndromes
Acute myelofibroids

Bone Marrow Failure
Severe aplastic anemia
Fanconi's anemia
Reticular dysgenesis

Lymphoproliferative Disorders
Hodgkin's disease
Non-Hodgkin's lymphoma
Multiple myeloma
Chronic lymphocytic leukemia

Immunodeficiencies
Severe combined immunodeficiency
Wiskott-Aldrich syndrome
Miscellaneous immunodeficiencies

Hematologic Disorders
β-Thalassemia
Sickle cell anemia
Congenital neutropenia
Osteoporosis

Nonhematologic Genetic Disorders
I-cell disease
Mucopolysaccharidosis
Leukodystrophy
Miscellaneous metabolic disorders

Data from Applebaum F: The use of bone marrow and peripheral blood stem cell transplantation in the treatment of cancer, *CA: Cancer J Clin* 46(3):143-164, 1996; Buchsel PC, Kapustay P: Peripheral stem cell transplantation. In Miaskowski C, Buchsel P, editors: *Oncology nursing: assessment and clinical care,* St Louis, 1999, Mosby, pp. 187-208; Kapustay PM, Buchsel PC: Process, complications, and management of peripheral blood stem cell transplantation. In Buchsel PC, Kapustay PM, editors: *Stem cell transplantation: a clinical textbook,* Pittsburgh, 2000, Oncology Nursing Society; Shapiro TJW, Rust D, Davis D, editors: *A clinical guide to bone marrow and stem cell transplantation,* Sudbury, Mass, 1997, Jones and Bartlett Publishers; Whedon MB, Wujcik D, editors: *Blood and marrow stem cell transplantation: principles, practice, and nursing insights,* ed 2, Sudbury, Mass, 1997, Jones and Bartlett Publishers.

which marrow contamination with malignant cells is unlikely, and when there is no evidence of an immunologic, antitumor effect [GVT] with allogeneic transplant).

(5) In older clients (>50 years of age), autografting may also be considered more desirable because of the high morbidity and mortality associated with allografting and GVHD.

(6) Most frequently used in the setting of high-risk solid tumors (e.g., sarcoma, neuroblastoma, brain tumors) in which the chance for cure is relatively low with standard or conventional doses of chemotherapy. In this case, autografting is considered a marrow or stem cell "rescue." Box 40-3 shows diseases treated with autologous transplantation.

(7) In some autografting situations, it is questioned whether a low (undetectable) level of tumor cells persisting in the infused cells may promote relapse. However, routine purging, even in diseases that involve the marrow, is unproven. Research in this area continues.

(8) PBSCs are most commonly used as an autografting source, but are especially used in cases of prior pelvic irradiation, marrow fibrosis, unacceptable anesthesia risk, or when early engraftment is desired.

(9) Autologous HSCT has recently been found to be effective in some autoimmune diseases since it allows for high doses of immunosuppressive therapy to be administered. Few autologous HSCTs have been done for these diseases; studies are not definitive. More research is needed.

BOX 40-3
DISEASES TREATED WITH AUTOGRAFTING OF HEMATOPOIETIC STEM CELLS

Leukemias—Syndromes
Acute myelogenous leukemia
Acute lymphoblastic leukemia
Chronic myelogenous leukemia

Lymphoproliferative Disorders
Hodgkin's disease
Non-Hodgkin's lymphoma
Multiple myeloma
Chronic lymphocytic leukemia

Solid Tumors
Neuroblastoma
Ewing's sarcoma

Hepatoblastoma
Testicular cancer
Osteosarcoma
Cerebral tumors
Others

Autoimmune Diseases
Systemic lupus
Rheumatoid arthritis

Data from Applebaum F: The use of bone marrow and peripheral blood stem cell transplantation in the treatment of cancer, *CA: Cancer J Clin* 46(3):143-164, 1996; Buchsel PC, Kapustay P: Peripheral stem cell transplantation. In Miaskowski C, Buchsel P, editors: *Oncology nursing: assessment and clinical care,* St Louis, 1999, Mosby, pp. 187-208; Kapustay PM, Buchsel PC: Process, complications, and management of peripheral blood stem cell transplantation. In Buchsel PC, Kapustay PM, editors: *Stem cell transplantation: A clinical textbook,* Pittsburgh, 2000, Oncology Nursing Society; Shapiro TJW, Rust D, Davis D, editors: *A clinical guide to bone marrow and stem cell transplantation,* Sudbury, Mass, 1997, Jones and Bartlett Publishers; Whedon MB, Wujcik D, editors: *Blood and marrow stem cell transplantation: principles, practice, and nursing insight,* ed 2, Sudbury, Mass, 1997, Jones and Bartlett Publishers.

    c. A bone marrow aspirate and biopsy are performed on the client before HSCT to determine if the client is in remission or has malignant cells present.

      (1) Optimally, clients are transplanted in the interval as near to complete remission as possible, when their disease is considered "chemoresponsive."

      (2) For clients using autologous donation, marrow with malignant cells cannot be harvested; PBSCs may be used instead, but the risk of posttransplant relapse is high.

      (3) Autologous PBSCs may also be harvested as a backup for clients whose risk of allogeneic rejection is high.

    d. In the allogeneic client, histocompatibility testing is done to determine if the client and donor are genetically compatible (Morishima et al., 2002; National Marrow Donor Program [NMDP] website).

      (1) HLA testing—major histocompatibility complex encoded by genes (one pair from each parent) present on chromosome 6.

        (a) Major loci of importance are HLA-A, HLA-B, and HLA-DR.

        (b) Results of allogeneic transplant are related to the degree of histocompatibility between the donor and recipient.

        (c) Clients without an HLA-matched, related donor have approximately a 50% chance of finding an HLA-matched, unrelated volunteer donor or donated UCB donor from the National Marrow Donor Registry. Minority clients are less likely to find an HLA-compatible donor. Use of matched unrelated donors is less successful because of higher incidence of GVHD.

      (2) Further deoxyribonucleic acid (DNA) testing of the HLA-DR is also performed to determine the degree of histocompatibility between donor and recipient.

  2. Marrow recipient is prepared with dose-intense (marrow ablative) therapy (Figures 40-2 and 40-3).

    a. Conditioning protocol is established based on the primary disease and type of transplant.

    b. Goals of pretransplant conditioning regimen are as follows:

      (1) To eradicate remaining malignancy in the recipient.

      (2) To suppress the immune system of the recipient to allow for marrow engraftment (allografts only).

      (3) To open spaces within the marrow compartment for newly infused marrow to engraft.

    c. Conditioning regimen may include high-dose chemotherapy alone or in combination with total lymph node or total body irradiation.

    d. Conditioning regimen is usually completed several days before marrow transplant or infusion.

  3. Marrow or PBSCs from donor (allogeneic) or client (autologous) are harvested and processed (Blume & Thomas, 2000; Callahan et al., 2000; Kline & Bertolone, 1998).

    a. Bone marrow harvesting is performed with the client under general or regional anesthesia.

      (1) Two to four punctures are made in the posterior iliac crests bilaterally.

      (2) Approximately 10 ml/kg of the recipient's weight is aspirated.

      (3) Marrow is then filtered to remove bone and fat particles.

      (4) Processed marrow is placed in a blood administration bag for cryopreservation (autologous) or immediate infusion (allogeneic).

      (5) Matched, unrelated donor marrow is generally processed at the donor's local hospital and then is transferred to the recipient's transplant center, unless the marrow is T-cell depleted.

    b. PBSCs are generally collected following stem cell mobilization with hematopoietic growth factors or chemotherapy or both.

      (1) Cells are collected, usually via a centrally placed pheresis catheter, using a special cell separator and are then cryopreserved.

      (2) After the client has completed the conditioning regimen, the cells are thawed and reinfused.

    c. Stem cells from an umbilical cord may be used if a match is found through the Cord Blood Registry or if the baby is believed to be a match with a family member who requires an allogeneic transplant.

      (1) Related and unrelated cord blood cells are harvested at birth from volunteer donors and are cryopreserved at a designated cord blood bank.

      (2) The cells are transported to the recipient's transplant center, thawed, and infused on the day of transplant.

      (3) At present, cord blood transplants are generally reserved for clients weighing less than 60 kg, although studies are currently underway using multiple, matched cord blood units for larger clients (Callahan et al., 2000; Kline & Bertolone, 1998).

    d. Some centers are using a variety of experimental techniques to purge autologous marrow of possible tumor contaminants.

      (1) Purging may be performed using monoclonal antibodies, chemotherapy, or physical means (centrifugation).

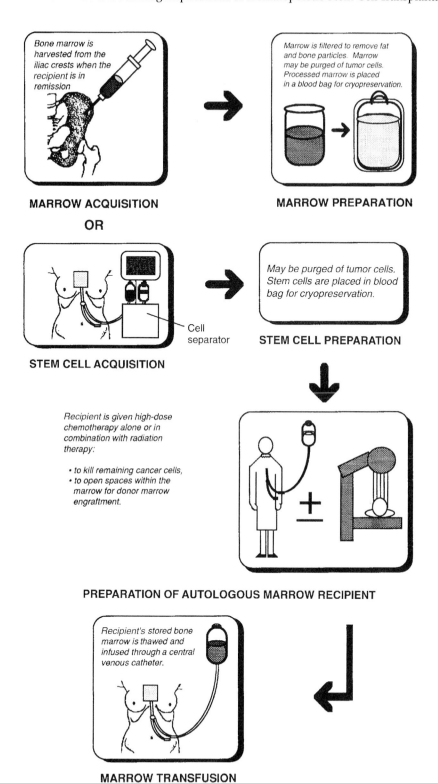

FIGURE 40-2 ■ Preparation of the recipient for an autologous hematopoietic stem cell transplant (HSCT).

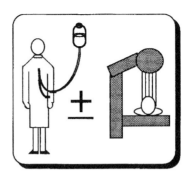

Recipient is given high-dose chemotherapy alone or in combination with radiation therapy:

• to kill remaining cancer cells,
• to suppress the immune system, and
• to open spaces within the marrow for donor marrow engraftment.

PREPARATION OF ALLOGENEIC MARROW RECIPIENT

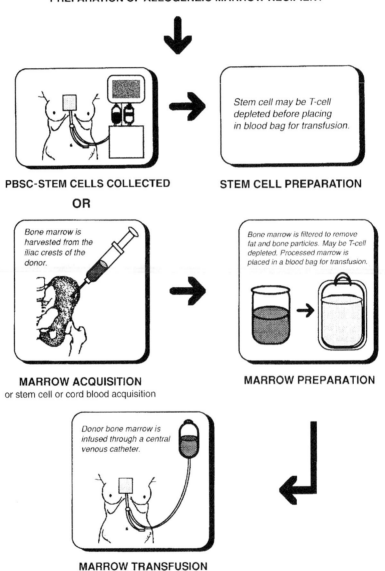

Stem cell may be T-cell depleted before placing in blood bag for transfusion.

PBSC-STEM CELLS COLLECTED   **STEM CELL PREPARATION**

OR

Bone marrow is harvested from the iliac crests of the donor.

Bone marrow is filtered to remove fat and bone particles. May be T-cell depleted. Processed marrow is placed in a blood bag for transfusion.

MARROW ACQUISITION   **MARROW PREPARATION**
or stem cell or cord blood acquisition

Donor bone marrow is infused through a central venous catheter.

MARROW TRANSFUSION

FIGURE 40-3 ■ Preparation of the recipient for an allogeneic hematopoietic stem cell transplant (HSCT). *PBSC,* Peripheral blood stem cell.

(2) Purging may damage the marrow, thus increasing the risk of delayed engraftment.

4. Marrow HSCs are infused through a central venous catheter.

a. With autologous marrow or autologous stem cell transplant, the cells are thawed at the client's bedside and reinfused.

b. With allogeneic marrow transplant, freshly harvested marrow is brought to the client's room and infused.

c. If allogeneic cord blood is used, the cells are thawed at the client's bedside and reinfused.

5. Client is supported through the period of marrow aplasia (10 to 30 days), and preventive measures to decrease potential complications (e.g., infection, GVHD) of bone marrow transplantation are instituted. See Table 40-1 for preventive measures for bone marrow transplantation–associated complication control practices.

II. Role of bone marrow transplantation.

A. Cure—because of the aggressive nature of the therapy, each client is evaluated with curative intent.

B. Palliation—few clients are treated to prolong life for a short period of time.

III. Marrow source.

A. Type of transplant is based on marrow source (see Box 40-1).

1. Autologous—client receives own bone marrow or PBSCs that were harvested before the pretransplant conditioning.

2. Allogeneic—client receives bone marrow, PBSCs, or UCB from a healthy, related or unrelated donor.

TABLE 40-1
Preventive Measures for Bone Marrow Transplantation–Associated Complications

Complication	Information	Preventive Measures	Nursing Implications

Graft-versus-host disease (GVHD)	Results from engraftment of immunocompetent donor T lymphocytes reacting against immunoincompetent recipient tissues (skin, gastrointestinal [GI] tract, liver)
	 Occurs in 30%-60% of allogeneic bone marrow transplant recipients
	 Risk is increased when donor is not a 6/6 HLA antigen match or when a matched unrelated donor is used
	 Can be either acute or chronic
		Depletion of T cells from marrow
		 Preventive immunosuppressive agents
		 Cyclosporine A
		   IV: Sandimmune
		   oral: Neoral
		 High-dose steroids
		 Antithymocyte globulin
		 Muromonab-CD3 (OKT-3)
		 Azathioprine (Imuran)
		 Thalidomide (Thalomid)
		 Monoclonal antibodies
		   FK506 (Tacrolimus)
		 Mycophenolate mofetil (MMF) (Cellcept)
		 Methotrexate (Mexate)
		 Rapamycin (Sirolimus)
			Monitor for delayed marrow engraftment
			 Monitor for prolonged lymphopenia and neutropenia
			 Evaluate cyclosporine or tacrolimus levels, and notify practitioner of significant abnormalities
			 Monitor for side effects of immunosuppressive agents
			 Monitor for signs of infection
			 Maintain skin integrity
			 Maintain client's functional capacity
			 Monitor for signs of hemolytic-uremic syndrome

Continued

TABLE 40-1
Preventive Measures for Bone Marrow Transplantation–Associated Complications—cont'd

Complication	Information	Preventive Measures	Nursing Implications
Pulmonary interstitial pneumonitis	Occurs most frequently in clients >30 yr of age, with history of chest irradiation or previous bleomycin therapy; and CMV positive Causative agents Cytomegalovirus *Aspergillus* *Pneumocystis carinii* 5% Other 15%	Use of cytomegalovirus (CMV)–seronegative blood products when donor and recipient are CMV seronegative Use of filtered air system Antimicrobial therapy Ganciclovir (Cytovene) Foscarnet (Foscavir) Intravenous immunoglobulin Trimethoprim and sulfamethoxazole (Septra) Aerosolized or intra-venous (IV) pentamidine (NebuPent, Pentacari-nat, Pentam 300) Ribavirin (Rebetol)	Monitor for side effects of antimicrobial therapy Implement turn, cough, and deep-breathe routine Encourage activity
Venoocclusive disease	Damage to the small venules of the liver from pretransplant conditioning regimen Occurs in 5%-54% of clients; most common in clients undergoing matched, unrelated donor transplants and those with pretransplant liver enzyme elevations or previous radiation to abdomen	Ursodiol (Actigall) Heparin Strict fluid management	Monitor liver function studies Monitor for weight gain Evaluate abdominal pain Monitor renal function

Data from Brockstein BE et al: Cardiac and pulmonary toxicity in patients undergoing high-dose chemotherapy for lymphomas and breast cancer: Prognostic factors, *Bone Marrow Transplant* 25(8):885-894, 2000; Chao N, editor: *Graft versus host disease*, Austin, Tex, 1999, RG Landis Co; Dykewicz CA et al.: Guideline for preventing opportunistic infection among hematopoietic stem cell transplant recipients. Recommendations of the CDC, Infectious Diseases Society of America, and the American Society of Blood and Marrow Transplantation, *Biol Blood Marrow Transplant* 6:659-727, 2000; Kapustay PM, Buchsel PC: Process, complications, and management of peripheral blood stem cell transplantation. In Buchsel PC, Kapustay PM, editors: *Stem cell transplantation: A clinical textbook*, Pittsburgh, 2000, Oncology Nursing Press; Shapiro TJW et al., editors: *A clinical guide to bone marrow and stem cell transplantation*, Sudbury, Mass, 1997, Jones and Bartlett Publishers.

      3. Syngeneic—client receives bone marrow or PBSCs from a genetically identical twin.

  B. Factors affecting source of donor marrow.

      1. Primary disease to be treated.

      2. Availability of a histocompatible donor.

      3. Age of the client.

Assessment

I. Pertinent personal history.
  A. Diagnosis (see Boxes 40-2 and 40-3 for conditions commonly treated with HSCT) (Applebaum, 1996; Bahtia & Portor, 2001; Blume & Thomas, 2000; Secola, 2001; Shapiro et al., 1997).
  B. Clients with malignancies that are at high risk for recurrence after standard therapy are selected for bone marrow transplantation. However, these malignancies must demonstrate a response to either antineoplastic therapy or RT.
  C. Factors that may increase the incidence of complications of marrow transplantation (Blume & Thomas, 2000; Loerzel & Hassey Dow, 2003; Shapiro et al., 1997).
    1. Amount of previous cancer therapy, length of time since last therapy, response to past therapy, and length of disease-free interval.
    2. Underlying kidney, lung, liver, or cardiac dysfunction.
    3. Previous infections and response to therapy.
    4. Age—older clients (>17 years) are more likely to develop transplant-related complications.
    5. Psychosocial dysfunction.
II. Physical examination.
  A. Pulmonary—respiratory rate, depth, and rhythm; lung expansion; adventitious breath sounds.
  B. Renal—color and odor of urine and urinary output, edema, weight gain.
  C. Mobility—muscle strength and endurance, range of motion, gait, activity level.
  D. Nutrition—weight; skin turgor; amount, content, and patterns of nutritional intake.
  E. Comfort level—pain rating, anxiety, ability to rest.
  F. Cardiovascular—heart rate and rhythm, heart sounds, blood pressure.
  G. Gastrointestinal (GI)—color, consistency, and caliber of stool; abdominal pain; distention; bowel sounds.
  H. Genitourinary—color of urine, suppleness of bladder, condition of perineum.
  I. Integumentary—color and intactness of skin, condition of oral mucous membranes, dental evaluation, condition of perineum and rectum.
  J. Neurologic—mental status, orientation, sensation, reflexes.
III. Psychosocial examination.
  A. Psychologic evaluation.
    1. Feelings on decision to have bone marrow transplant.
    2. Understanding of aggressiveness of treatment, goals of therapy, and chances of survival.
    3. Number, type, effectiveness of coping mechanisms used in past stressful situations by client and family members.
    4. Perceptions of client and family about isolation, prolonged hospitalization, living will, use of life-support technology, and potential death or survival.
    5. Caregiver's ability to comprehend role.
  B. Social evaluation.
    1. Previous roles and responsibilities within the family and community.
    2. Type, number, and history of use of support systems within the family and community.
    3. Financial status—employment, insurance coverage, resources for daily living needs.
    4. Eligibility for community resources.

IV. Critical laboratory and diagnostic data unique to marrow transplantation (Shapiro et al., 1997).
   A. Hematologic—complete blood count, differential, platelet count, coagulation studies, type and crossmatch with marrow donor.
   B. Hepatic—lactic acid dehydrogenase (LDH) and bilirubin levels.
   C. Renal—electrolyte, blood urea nitrogen (BUN), creatinine, cyclosporine A levels, tacrolimus (FK-506) levels, viral urine cultures, electron microscopy.
   D. Cardiovascular—electrocardiogram, cardiac ejection fraction.
   E. Pulmonary—chest x-ray examination, pulmonary function tests; arterial blood gases, oxygen saturation (pulse oximetry).
   F. Immune—antibody titers for cytomegalovirus (CMV), CMV antigenemia studies, human herpesvirus type 6 antibody and ribonucleic acid (RNA) studies, herpesvirus titers, Epstein-Barr virus panel, toxoplasmosis, hepatitis B surface antigen, immunoglobulin levels, human immunodeficiency virus (HIV) antibody, hepatitis C antigen.
   G. Infectious disease—blood cultures for bacteria and fungi; urine and stool cultures for bacteria, fungi, and viruses; blood for buffy coat; CMV antigenemia studies; human herpesvirus type 6 RNA studies; respiratory and sputum cultures for bacteria, fungi, viruses, *Legionella*, acid-fast bacilli (AFB); stool and urine for electron microscopy cultures and stains for *Pneumocystis carinii* pneumonia (PCP), respiratory syncytial virus (RSV) nasal culture.

Nursing Diagnoses

I. Anxiety.
II. Risk for infection.
III. Risk for imbalanced body temperature.
IV. Acute pain.
V. Risk for imbalanced fluid volume.
VI. Impaired oral mucous membrane.
VII. Impaired tissue integrity.
VIII. Impaired social interaction.
IX. Diarrhea.

Outcome Identification (Kapustay & Buchsel, 2000; Schmit-Pokorny et al., 2003)

I. Client and family describe the rationale for HSCT.
II. Client participates in self-care strategies to decrease the risk and severity of predictable side effects of HSCT.
III. Client and family describe recommended changes in self-care, lifestyle, and social interactions to minimize the effects of bone marrow transplantation on health.
IV. Client and family discuss strategies to maintain valued roles and relationships during the transplant and posttransplant periods.
V. Client and family list community resources available for assistance and support.
VI. Client and family discuss the rationale, schedule, and procedures required for continued follow-up care after bone marrow transplantation.

Planning and Implementation

I. Interventions to maximize safety for the client and family.
   A. Maintain aseptic techniques and the level of protective isolation identified by the HSCT program (see Table 40-1 for general guidelines).

    B. Implement the conditioning regimen ordered by the physician or other provider.

    C. Teach the client and family strategies to decrease risk of infection, bleeding, and injury during period of aplasia following bone marrow or stem cell or cord blood infusion.

II. Interventions to decrease the incidence and severity of complications unique to bone marrow transplantation.

    A. Anxiety.

        1. Assess changes in and perceived contributing factors to anxiety levels in client and family.

        2. Provide a thorough orientation to the inpatient and outpatient bone marrow transplant units and procedures common to bone marrow transplantation.

        3. Implement strategies to encourage the client and family to express concerns about bone marrow transplantation demands.

        4. Consult with the occupational therapist to develop a plan for diversional activities during isolation.

        5. Teach new anxiety-relieving strategies as desired or needed by client and family.

        6. Asses the caregiver's ability to implement care demands.

    B. Risk for infection (see Chapter 13). Table 40-2 outlines common opportunistic infections and their time of occurrence after transplant (Kapustay & Buchsel, 2000; Shapiro et al., 1997).

TABLE 40-2
Infectious Complications and Occurrence in HSCT Recipients

Organism	Common Site
FIRST MO AFTER TRANSPLANT	
VIRAL	
Herpes simplex virus (HSV)	Oral, esophageal, skin, GI tract, and genital
Respiratory syncytial virus (RSV)	Sinopulmonary
Epstein-Barr virus (EBV)	Oral, esophageal, skin, GI tract
Human herpesvirus type 6 (HHV6)	Pulmonary, CNS, GI tract
BACTERIAL	
Gram-positive organisms *(Staphylococcus epidermidis, S. aureus,* streptococci)	Skin, blood, sinopulmonary
Gram-negative organisms (*Escherichia coli, Pseudomonas aeruginosa, Klebsiella)*	GI, blood, oral, perirectal
FUNGAL	
Candida (C. albicans, C. glabrata, C. krusei)	Oral, esophageal, skin
Aspergillus fumigatus, A. flavus	Sinopulmonary, skin
1-4 MO AFTER TRANSPLANT	
VIRAL	
Cytomegalovirus (CMV)	Pulmonary, hepatic, GI
Enteric viruses (rotavirus, coxsackievirus, adenovirus)	Pulmonary, urinary, GI, hepatic
RSV	Sinopulmonary
Parainfluenza virus	Pulmonary
HHV6, human polyoma virus	Genitourinary

Continued

TABLE 40-2
Infectious Complications and Occurrence in HSCT Recipients—cont'd

Organism	Common Site
BACTERIAL	
Gram-positive organisms	Sinopulmonary, skin, venous access devices
FUNGAL	
Candida species	Oral, hepatosplenic, integument
Aspergillus species	Sinopulmonary, CNS, skin
Mucormycosis	Sinopulmonary
Coccidioidomycosis	Sinopulmonary
Cryptococcus neoformans	Pulmonary, CNS
PROTOZOA	
Pneumocystis carinii	Pulmonary
Toxoplasma gondii	Pulmonary, CNS
4-12 MO AFTER TRANSPLANT	
VIRAL	
CMV, echoviruses, RSV, varicella-zoster virus (VZV), human polyoma virus	Integument, pulmonary, hepatic, genitourinary
BACTERIAL	
Gram-positive organisms (*Streptococcus pneumoniae, Haemophilus influenzae,* pneumococci)	Sinopulmonary, blood Sinopulmonary
FUNGAL	
Aspergillosis	Sinopulmonary
Coccidioidomycosis	Sinopulmonary
PROTOZOA	
Pneumocystis carinii	Pulmonary
Toxoplasma gondii	Pulmonary, CNS
>12 MO AFTER TRANSPLANT	
VIRAL	
VZV	Integument
CMV	Pulmonary, hepatic
BACTERIAL	
Gram-positive organisms (streptococci, *H. influenzae,* encapsulated bacteria)	Sinopulmonary, blood

Data from Dykewicz CA et al.: Guideline for preventing opportunistic infection among hematopoietic stem cell transplant recipients. Recommendations of the CDC, Infectious Diseases Society of America, and the American Society of Blood and Marrow Transplantation, *Biol Blood Marrow Transplant* 6:659-727, 2000; Kapustay PM, Buchsel PC: Process, complications, and management of peripheral blood stem cell transplantation. In Buchsel PC, Kapustay PM, editors: *Stem cell transplantation: a clinical textbook,* Pittsburgh, 2000, Oncology Nursing Society; Shapiro TJW et al, editors: *A clinical guide to bone marrow and stem cell transplantation,* Sudbury, Mass, 1997, Jones and Bartlett Publishers; Whedon MB, Wujcik D, editors: *Blood and marrow stem cell transplantation: principles, practice, and nursing insights,* ed 2, Sudbury, Mass, 1997, Jones and Bartlett Publishers.

HSCT, Hematopoietic stem cell transplant; *GI,* gastrointestinal; *CNS,* central nervous system.

1. Notify the physician of initial temperature greater than 101° F (38.3° C) or other symptoms indicative of infection.
2. Teach the client and family strategies to decrease the risk of endogenous infections.
   a. Meticulous hand washing.
   b. Routine oral and perineal care.
   c. Skin care.
3. Teach the client and family strategies to decrease risk of exogenous infections (Dykewicz et al., 2000).
   a. Restrict visitors with suspected or known infections.
   b. Limit visitation of children (especially school-aged children).
   c. Place the client on a sterile or low-microbial diet.
   d. Avoid invasive procedures (e.g., peripheral intravenous [IV] catheter, intramuscular injections, urinary catheterization, rectal examinations, rectal temperatures).
   e. Recommend influenza vaccine for all close contact individuals.
4. Administer prophylactic antimicrobial therapy as ordered.
   a. Fluconazole (Diflucan), itraconazole (Sporanox), clotrimazole (Lotrimin, Mycelex), or nystatin (Mycostatin) to prevent fungal infection.
   b. Trimethoprim-sulfamethoxazole (Septra, Bactrim) or pentamidine (NebuPent, Pentacarinat, Pentam 300) for prevention of PCP.
   c. Acyclovir (Aciclovir, Zovirax) for prevention of herpesvirus infection and CMV.
   d. Ganciclovir (Cytovene) or foscarnet (Foscavir) for prevention of CMV and other viral infections.
   e. IV immunoglobulin for prevention of CMV infection.
   f. Oral nonabsorbable antibiotics or ciprofloxacin (Cipro) for decontamination of the GI tract of endogenous bacteria.
5. Administer hematopoietic growth factors as ordered.
6. Perform routine surveillance cultures for bacteria, fungi, and viruses and antigenemia studies.
7. Transfuse CMV-seronegative blood products or leukopoor-filtered blood products to clients who are seronegative for CMV.

C. Risk for injury.
1. For clients receiving high-dose cyclophosphamide (Cytoxan), hemorrhagic cystitis is a potential complication.
   a. Administer continuous bladder irrigation (CBI) as ordered.
   b. If CBI is not used, administer hydration, push oral fluids, and have the client void every hour for 6 hours following cyclophosphamide administration.
   c. Administer mesna (Mesnex), a uroprotectorant, as ordered.
   d. Administer antispasmodics and analgesics as ordered.

D. Alteration in comfort related to keratitis (corneal irritation).
1. Provide sunglasses and darken the room to relieve discomfort.
2. Discourage the client from rubbing eyes—use mittens.
3. Administer artificial tears, steroid eye drops, and analgesics as ordered.

E. Altered oral mucous membrane (see Chapter 14).

III. Interventions to monitor for unique complications of bone marrow transplantation.
A. GVHD (Table 40-3) (Chao, 1999; Chen et al., 2002; Cimiotti, 2002; Ferrara & Antin, 1999).

TABLE 40-3
Clinical Staging and Grading of Acute GVHD

Staging by Organ		
Organ	**Stage**	**Parameters**
RASH		
Skin	I	<25% BSA
	II	25%-50% BSA
	III	Generalized erythroderma
	IV	Bullae and desquamation
TOTAL BILIRUBIN (MG/DL)		
Liver	I	2-3.5
	II	3.5-8
	III	8-15
	IV	>15
VOLUME OF DIARRHEA (ML/24 HR)		
Gut	I	Adult: 500-1000 ml/day
		Pediatric: 10-15 ml/kg/day
	II	Adult: 1000-1500 ml/day
		Pediatric: 15-20 ml/kg/day
	III	Adult: 1500-2000 ml/day
		Pediatric: 20-30 ml/kg/day
	IV	Adult: >2000 ml/day
		Pediatric: >30 ml/kg/day

Overall Clinical Grade

Grade	Description
0	Stage I clinical skin GVHD
I	Stage II clinical skin GVHD
II	Stage II-III clinical skin GVHD and stage II-IV clinical liver and/or gut GVHD; only one system stage III or greater
III	Stage II-IV clinical skin GVHD (with grade 2 or higher histology) and stage II-IV clinical liver and/or gut GVHD; only one system stage III or greater
IV	Stage II-IV clinical skin GVHD (with grade 2 or higher histology) and stage II-IV clinical liver and/or gut GVHD; two or more systems stage III or higher

Data from Chao N, editor: *Graft versus host disease*, Austin, Tex, 1999, RG Landis Co; Ferrara JLM, Antin JH: The pathophysiology of graft versus host disease. In Thomas ED et al., editors: *Hematopoietic cell transplantation*, ed 2, Malden, Mass, 1999, Blackwell Science, pp. 305-315; Kapustay PM, Buchsel PC: Process, complications, and management of peripheral blood stem cell transplantation. In Buchsel PC, Kapustay PM, editors: *Stem cell transplantation: A clinical textbook*, Pittsburgh, 2000, Oncology Nursing Press; Shapiro TJW et al, editors: *A clinical guide to bone marrow and stem cell transplantation*, Sudbury, Mass, 1997, Jones and Bartlett Publishers.
GVHD, Graft-versus-host disease; *BSA*, body surface area.

1. Monitor condition of skin (erythema, rash), especially on the palms of hands and soles of feet.
2. Evaluate changes in liver function study results.
3. Monitor the amount, consistency, frequency, and color of stool.

B. Hepatic venoocclusive disease (Box 40-4) (Kapustay & Buchsel, 2000; Williams & Vickers, 2000).

1. Weigh the client every day; notify the medical practitioner of weight gain greater than 5 pounds.

BOX 40-4
RISK FACTORS FOR THE DEVELOPMENT OF VENOOCCLUSIVE DISEASE

- Pretransplant chemotherapy
- Abdominal radiation
- Pretransplant hepatotoxic drug therapy (e.g., amphotericin)
- Elevated transaminases before conditioning regimen
- Human leukocyte antigen (HLA)–mismatched or unrelated allogeneic transplant
- Vancomycin (Vancocin, Vancoled) or acyclovir (Aciclovir, Zovirax) therapy (as markers of infection)
- Viral hepatitis
- Metastatic liver disease
- Karnofsky score <90% before transplant
- Second transplant

Data from Kapustay PM, Buchsel PC: Process, complications, and management of peripheral blood stem cell transplantation. In Buchsel PC, Kapustay PM, editors: *Stem cell transplantation: a clinical textbook*, Pittsburgh, 2000, Oncology Nursing Society; Shapiro TJW et al, editors: *A clinical guide to bone marrow and stem cell transplantation*, Sudbury, Mass, 1997, Jones and Bartlett Publishers; Williams DB, Vickers CR: Hepatic complications. In K. Atkinson (Ed.). *Clinical bone marrow and blood cell transplantation*, ed 2, New York, 2000, Cambridge University Press, pp. 912-924.

    2. Monitor location of pain (right upper quadrant).
    3. Evaluate for elevation in serum bilirubin.
    4. Evaluate changes in mental status.
    5. Measure abdominal girth every day if other parameters indicate possible venoocclusive disease.
    6. Skin care for clients with hyperbilirubinemia.
    7. Evaluate level of abdominal pain.
  C. Pulmonary interstitial pneumonitis (Brockstein et al., 2000; Shapiro, 1997).
    1. Monitor temperature.
    2. Assess for presence of cough, chest pain, or adventitious breath sounds.
    3. Evaluate activity tolerance.
IV. Interventions to enhance adaptation and rehabilitation.
  A. Implement a program of range of motion and isometric exercises during the isolation period, especially if the client is taking high-dose steroids.
  B. Initiate client and family teaching about care of the central venous catheter early in the course of hospitalization.
  C. Encourage the client, donor, and significant other to express concerns related to the transplant experience.
  D. Discuss potential changes in lifestyle and social interaction required immediately after discharge from the hospital.
  E. Long-term follow-up (Buchsel & Kapustay, 1997; Saleh & Brockopp, 2001; Schmit-Pokorny et al., 2003).
    1. Educate client and family members on common outpatient problems after HSCT.
    2. Common problems include fatigue, weight loss, sexual dysfunction, cataracts, chronic GVHD, herpes zoster virus, depression, isolation.
    3. Ensure that survivorship issues are addressed through long-term follow-up program.
      a. Life-long evaluation of allogeneic recipient for chronic GVHD.
      b. Address fertility issues.
      c. Reentry back into community and work.
      d. Delayed organ dysfunction (pulmonary, cardiac, renal dysfunction).

Evaluation

The oncology nurse systematically and regularly evaluates the client's and/or family's responses to interventions in order to determine progress toward the achievement of expected outcomes. Relevant data are collected, and actual findings are compared with expected findings. Nursing diagnoses, outcomes, and plans of care are reviewed and revised as necessary.

REFERENCES

Alcindor, T., Gorgun, G., Miller, K., et al. (2000). Engraftment and immunologic effects of a less novel myeloablative allogeneic transplant conditioning regimen of continuous infusion Pentostatin, photopheresis, and low dose TBI. *Blood 96*(11), 327a.

Applebaum, F. (1996). The use of bone marrow and peripheral blood stem cell transplantation in the treatment of cancer. *CA: A Cancer Journal for Clinicians 46*(3), 143-164.

Bahtia, V., & Portor, D.L. (2001). Novel approaches to allogeneic stem cell therapy. *Expert Opinions in Biologic Therapy 1*(1), 3-15.

Blume, K., & Thomas, E.D. (2000). A review of autologous hematopoietic cell transplantation. *Biology of Blood and Marrow Transplantation 6*, 1-12.

Brockstein, B.E., Smiley, C., Al-Sadir, J., & Williams, S.F. (2000). Cardiac and pulmonary toxicity in patients undergoing high-dose chemotherapy for lymphomas and breast cancer: Prognostic factors. *Bone Marrow Transplantation 25*(8), 885-894.

Buchsel, P.C., & Kapustay, P. (1997). Models of ambulatory care for blood cell and bone marrow transplantation. In M.B. Whedon & D.Wujcik (Eds). *Blood and marrow stem cell transplantation: Principles, practice, and nursing insights* (2nd ed.). Sudbury, MA: Jones and Bartlett Publishers, pp. 525-561.

Buchsel, P.C., & Kapustay, P. (1999). Peripheral stem cell transplantation. In C. Miaskowski & P. Buchsel (Eds.). *Oncology nursing: Assessment and clinical care.* St. Louis: Mosby, pp. 187-208.

Callahan, T., Johnson, A., Frey, M., & Kurtzberg, J. (2000). State of the art umbilical cord blood transplantation. *Journal of Pediatric Oncology Nursing 17*(2), 126-127.

Chao, N. (Ed.) (1999). *Graft versus host disease.* Austin, TX: R.G. Landis Co.

Chen, B., Cui, X., Liu, C., & Chao, N. (2002). Prevention of graft versus host disease while preserving graft versus leukemia effect after selective depletion of host reactive T-cells by photodynamic cell purging process. *Blood 99*(9), 3083-3088.

Cimiotti, J. (2002). Peripheral blood stem cell transplantation and graft versus host disease: A case study. *Journal of Pediatric Oncology Nursing 19*(5), 182-187.

Dykewicz, C.A., Jaffe, H.W., & Kaplan, J.E. (2000). Guideline for preventing opportunistic infections among hematopoietic stem cell transplant recipients. Recommendations of the CDC, Infectious Diseases Society of America, and the American Society of Blood and Marrow Transplantation. *Biology of Blood and Marrow Transplantation 6*, 659-727.

Ferrara, J.L.M., & Antin, J.H. (1999). The pathophysiology of graft versus host disease. In E.D. Thomas, K.G. Blume, & S.J. Forman (Eds.). *Hematopoietic cell transplantation* (2nd ed.). Malden, MA: Blackwell Science, pp. 305-315.

Kapustay, P.M., & Buchsel, P.C. (2000). Process, complications, and management of peripheral blood stem cell transplantation. In P.C. Buchsel & P.M. Kapustay (Eds.). *Stem cell transplantation: A clinical textbook.* Pittsburgh: Oncology Nursing Society, pp. 5.1, 5.28.

Kline, R.M., & Bertolone, S.J. (1998). Umbilical cord blood transplantation: Providing a donor for everyone needing a bone marrow transplant? *Southern Medical Journal 91*, 821-828.

Loerzel, V.W., & Hassey Dow, K. (2003). Cardiac toxicity related to cancer treatment. *Clinical Journal of Oncology Nursing 7*(5), 557-572.

Mangan, K.F. (2000). Choice of conditioning regimens. In E.D. Ball, J. Lister, & P.Law (Eds.). *Hematopoietic stem cell therapy.* New York: Churchill Livingstone, pp. 403-413.

Morishima, Y., Sasazuki, T., Inoko, H., et al. (2002). The clinical significance of human leukocyte antigen (HLA) allele compatibility in patients receiving a marrow transplant from serologically HLA-A, HLA-B, and HLA-DR matched unrelated donors. *Blood 99*, 4200-4206.

National Marrow Donor Program (NMDP) website. www.nmdpresearch.org.

O'Connell, S.A., & Schmit-Pokorny, K. (1997). Pulmonary and cardiac complications. In M.B. Whedon & D. Wujcik (Eds.). *Blood and marrow stem cell transplantation: Principles, practice, and nursing insights* (2nd ed.). Sudbury, MA: Jones and Bartlett Publishers, pp. 66-99.

Saleh, U., & Brockopp, D. (2001). Quality of life one year following bone marrow transplantation: Psychometric evaluation of quality of life in BMT survivors tool. *Journal of Pediatric Oncology Nursing 19*(2), 1457-1458.

Schmit-Pokorny, K., Franco, T., Frappier, B., & Vyhlidal, R.C. (2003). The cooperative care model: An innovative approach to deliver blood and stem cell transplant care. *Clinical Journal of Oncology Nursing 7*(5), 509-514.

Secola, R. (2001). Hematopoietic stem cell transplantation: A glimpse of the past and view of the future. *Journal of Pediatric Oncology Nursing 18*(4), 171-177.

Shapiro, T.J. (1997). Pulmonary and cardiac complications. In M.B.Whedon & D. Wujcik (Eds.). *Blood and marrow stem cell transplantation: Principles, practice, and nursing insights* (2nd ed.). Sudbury, MA: Jones and Bartlett Publishers, pp. 266-297.

Shapiro, T.J.W., Rust, D., & Davis, D. (Eds.). (1997). *A clinical guide to bone marrow and stem cell transplantation.* Sudbury, MA: Jones and Bartlett Publishers.

Thomas, E.D., Blume, K.G., & Forman, S.J. (Eds.). (1999). *Hematopoietic stem cell transplantation* (2nd ed.). Malden, MA: Blackwell Science.

Whedon, M.B., & Wujcik, D. (Eds.). (1997). *Blood and marrow stem cell transplantation: Principles, practice, and nursing insights* (2nd ed.). Sudbury, MA: Jones and Bartlett Publishers.

Williams, D.B., & Vickers, C.R. (2000). Hepatic complications. In K. Atkinson (Ed.) *Clinical bone marrow and blood stem cell transplantation* (2nd ed.). New York: Cambridge University Press, pp. 912-924.

41 Complementary and Alternative Medicines

PAUL JAY ROSS

Theory

I. Definition—therapies that are considered outside the realm of conventional (allopathic, bio-, scientific, orthodox, Western) medicine, yet claim physiologic and/or psychologic benefits ranging from cancer cure to symptom relief. These treatment modalities are characterized as *alternative, complementary,* or *integrative,* depending on whether clients view them as supplements to or replacements for conventional medicine. Their context of use, whether practiced singly, sequentially, or in conjunction with others, also shapes how they are understood by researchers, health care practitioners, and their clients.

  A. *Alternative therapies* are used instead of conventional treatments.

    1. Understood by their proponents to have qualities (cost, availability, familiarity, effectiveness, tradition, cultural or ethnic association, side-effect profile) that are superior or preferred to those of conventional therapy.

  B. *Complementary therapies* are more often associated with treatments that supplement, or even enhance, conventional interventions.

    1. Often focus on client-defined outcomes that have only vague biomedical equivalents (blood cleansing or detoxifying attributes) or are not adequately addressed by conventional medicine (e.g., quality of life, psychospiritual needs).

    2. Commonly viewed as effective, safe, "natural," and/or nontoxic supportive therapies that combat the rigors and ill effects of biomedicine.

  C. *Integrative therapies* are a subset of complementary therapies with strong suggestive scientific evidence of safety and effectiveness.

    1. More readily combined with conventional regimens by health care providers (Shapiro & Safer, 2002).

  D. *Complementary and alternative medicine* (CAM) describes the entire domain.

    1. CAM is widely used by those with cancer—numerous studies suggest more than 50% use these modalities (Richardson et al., 2000; Sparber et al., 2000).

    2. A major concern is that there are relatively few well-designed studies to evaluate whether these therapies are safe and effective for the medical conditions for which they are promoted.

II. Features.

  A. Mechanism of action is described in common-sense terms.

    1. Highlights cancer as a symptom of body imbalance (Ross, 2000).

    2. Enables clients to "see for themselves" what works for *them.*

  B. Contrasted with conventional medicine, which is often viewed as impersonal, paternalistic, dangerous, and overly regulated.

1. Suspicion and cynicism are directed to government regulatory bodies (Food and Drug Administration [FDA]), "big business" (pharmaceutical companies), and "self-serving" professional organizations (American Medical Association).
2. CAM—virtually unregulated, drawn from a diffuse knowledge base, easily accessed, and personally evaluated—is commonly appreciated as a counterbalance to the slow and drawn-out deliberations of an overly conservative and bureaucratic medical "establishment" (Ross, 2000).

C. Emphasis is on client-directed strategies, psychosocial as well as physical needs, global and diverse approaches to health care, equal relationship between healer and client, proactive and enhanced opportunities for desirable (client-defined) outcomes (Cauffield, 2000).

D. Administered in the following situations:
   1. Home settings (e.g., folk medicines, herbal and dietary supplements).
   2. Specialty facilities.
      a. Within the United States (e.g., the Livingston-Wheeler Clinic in California, which offers a regimen of vaccines, antibiotics, a restrictive diet, and cleansing enemas; the Burzynski Research Institute in Texas, which treats with antineoplastons—synthetic protein–based infusions originally derived from urine).
      b. Internationally (e.g., the Centro Hospitaliario Internacional Pacifico SA [CHIPSA], Center for Integrative Medicine in Mexico, which provides an array of regimens, including Laetrile, a compound derived from apricot kernels, and Coley toxins, an immunotherapy centered on injections of inactive bacterial cultures; the Immuno-Augmentative Clinic in Grand Bahamas, which features daily injections of "proteins and tumor antibodies").
   3. With formal hospital approval. A significant and increasing number of major teaching and research hospitals—for example, Memorial Sloan-Kettering, Stanford, Duke—have CAM or integrative medicine departments and clinics that offer a range of modalities including music therapy, healing touch, medical Qigong, guided imagery, and energy healing.
      a. Growing number of CAM therapies are reimbursed by third-party payers (Wolsko et al., 2002).

E. Easily accessed through informal social networks, the Internet, and specialty (e.g., health food store, herbalists) and broad-based (e.g., discount variety) local and national retailers (*Consumer Reports*, 2000).

F. Advocated by popular electronic and print media, informal social networks, and a variety of practitioners, including folk healers, academics, and conventional health care providers.
   1. Is increasingly consumer driven. Mass marketing is both a cause and effect of the popularity of CAM (Etkin & McMillen, 2003; Etkin & Ross, 2002).

G. Promises positive, definitive outcomes.
   1. Claims of efficacy commonly based on anecdotes, testimonials, and personal experience (Ross, 2000).
      a. Efficacy is "evidenced" through reference to long historical use and/or "native traditions" that describe individuals as "in tune with nature" and free of the corrupting (and polluting) influences of urban lifestyles.
   2. Practices are not subjected to scientific scrutiny (i.e., clinically and otherwise empirically tested and reviewed in reputable peer-reviewed journals); but there is increasing interest (e.g., National Center for Complementary

and Alternative Medicine [NCCAM], National Cancer Institute [NCI], National Institutes of Health [NIH], FDA) in funding, investigating, and publishing research on CAM. CAM proponents often make selective use of ambiguous scientific evidence and/or draw from basic (acontextual) research to equate association with effectiveness (Ross, 2000).

  3. Inconsistent and inconsequential surveillance of CAM use compromises an understanding of side-effect profiles (Ernst, 2001).

    a. There is little formal mechanism for reporting CAM side effects or impartially tracking specific CAM use over time.

    b. This reinforces the association of CAM with natural and safe practice.

  4. Lack of acceptance by conventional medicine is frequently dismissed as evidence of conspiracy and bureaucratic inefficiency (Montbriand, 1999).

  H. Used by an ever-increasing number of clients with cancer (Etkin & Ross, 2002; Richardson et al., 2000).

    1. CAM users represent all sociocultural, economic, and other demographic segments.

    2. CAM therapies used at any time along the cancer continuum—at diagnosis, at recurrence, with localized or metastasized disease, when asymptomatic, and/or for palliation in advanced disease.

    3. Primarily used as an adjunct to conventional treatment regimens.

      a. Little evidence to suggest that CAM use displaces, or results in the delay of, conventional options.

      b. Current practice trend is to integrate CAM with conventional medicine (Sparber et al., 2000).

    4. Results in more attention to CAM from conventional health care professionals.

      a. There is a proliferation of nursing and medical school curricula, journals, research, education efforts, and resources (e.g., specialty Internet sites, clinical trials, NCCAM).

    5. More attention is devoted to public policy and client safeguards by health care program accrediting agencies, state and federal regulations, scopes of practice, and medical and personal liabilities (Boyer, 2002; Cohen & Eisenberg, 2002).

      a. Both the Joint Commission on Accreditation of Healthcare Organizations (JCAHO) and the American College of Surgeons Commission on Cancer (COC) stipulate that health care facilities address and regulate CAM use.

III. Major categories of CAM.

  A. Nutritional and dietary regimens.

    1. Rationale.

      a. If diet can prevent cancer, it may also cure cancer.

        (1) Includes both familiar (e.g., broccoli) and exotic foods (e.g., green tea), single supplements (e.g., "pharmafoods," such as garlic, soy), and complete diets (e.g., macrobiotics).

        (2) Cautions—potential interactions (e.g., soy isoflavones and tamoxifen (Nolvadex) and restrictive diets (e.g., wheatgrass diet, juicing and fasting) (Brown et al., 2001; Kumar, 2002).

      b. Dietary elements function as antioxidants, destroy malignant cells, and enhance cell differentiation.

        (1) Includes lycopene, Gerson diet, and megavitamin therapy (vitamins A, C, E).

      (2) Ongoing clinical trials include examinations of low-fat diets, macrobiotics, melatonin, selenium, vitamin E, and soy (genistein) (NIH, 2003).

      (3) Cautions—antioxidants may interfere with radiation and chemotherapy (e.g., anthracyclines, alkylating agents), be hepatotoxic (vitamin A), have anticoagulant effects (vitamins C, E), and compromise diagnostic tests (vitamin C) (Conklin, 2000; Decker, 2003; Weiger et al., 2002).

B. Traditional and folk medicines.

  1. Rationale—valid understandings of pathology and physiology exist that differ from conventional medical paradigms. Practices are time honored (Ross, 2000).

    a. Include well-integrated classical systems (e.g., traditional Chinese medicine [TCM], Ayurveda) and others fostered by cultural and ethnic identity (e.g., Hawaiian lomi lomi).

    b. Emphasis is on cultural context and includes transcultural practices, such as ingestion or topical applications (e.g., mixtures of animal parts and/or botanicals), mind-body techniques (e.g., meditation), and spiritual/supernatural associations (e.g., icons, amulets).

    c. Ongoing clinical trials include examinations of TCM (e.g., huang lian) (NIH, 2003).

    d. Cautions—rationales cannot be transposed to other cultural contexts; these approaches are difficult to monitor and are the least amenable to critique.

C. Pharmacologic and biologic treatments.

  1. Rationale—often borrowed piecemeal from conventional medicine. Draw selectively on basic research to support claims for immune boosting and detoxifying agents.

    a. These often are highly controversial approaches that feature special diets, vitamins, minerals, and enzymes that target the immune system (e.g., immunoaugmentative therapy, antineoplaston therapy, enzyme and amino acid infusions, Coley toxins, Di Bella therapy, Greek cancer cure, 714-X).

    b. Another common objective is to purge body "toxins" (e.g., colonic irrigations, coffee enemas, chelation therapy, shark or bovine cartilage infusions).

    c. Some aim to control symptoms (e.g., hydrazine sulfate for cachexia).

    d. Others are offered as cures (e.g., Laetrile [amygdalin, vitamin B_{17}]).

    e. Ongoing clinical trials include examinations of the Gonzalez regimen, antineoplaston therapy, shark cartilage, and hyperbaric oxygen (NIH, 2003).

    f. Cautions—most often adopted as alternative therapies either before or after conventional approaches. Little evidence of efficacy. Many have serious safety concerns (e.g., hepatotoxicity, interactions with other drugs) (Ernst, 2001).

D. Botanical ("herbal") medicines.

  1. Rationale—botanicals are natural medicines that have been time tested. Many current drugs are based in botanical analogues (e.g., vinca alkaloids, taxoids).

    a. Includes herbs that are part of an ethnic "traditional" pharmacopoeia (e.g., Native American, Chinese), as well as products that are "discovered" to have medicinal properties not related to a traditional use—for example, injections of mistletoe or Iscador (Boik, 2001).

    (1) Available as single products (e.g., aloe vera) or as plant mixtures (e.g., Essiac, PC-SPEC, many TCMs).

    (2) Used as *preventives* (e.g., cat's claw and echinacea to ward off infections, grape seed and green tea to reduce overall cancer risk), *treatments* (e.g., aloe vera for liver and prostate cancer, blue-green algae as an immune system stimulant, noni as a general cancer remedy, milk thistle as a liver protectant and for prostate cancer, chaparral as a blood purifier and general cancer cure, Essiac for breast cancer), and *supportive therapies* (e.g., chamomile and ginger for nausea, ginseng for energy, kava-kava and valerian for insomnia) (American Cancer Society, 2002; Decker & Myers, 2001; Rosenthal, 2000; Ross, 2000).

  b. Many claims of efficacy focus on immunostimulatory aspects (e.g., Essiac, Iscador) as well as the promotion of general well-being (e.g., noni [Etkin & McMillen, 2003]).

  c. There is little evidence to support the use of botanicals. Studies often focus on purified extracts and individual constituents rather than on the whole-plant and complex mixtures that are actually consumed.

    (1) There is no within-industry standardization to ensure consistency of source, preparation, and activity.

    (2) Because herbal and dietary supplements (HDSs) are not under the purview of the FDA, there is virtually no regulation for safety, product quality, and health claims (Ross, 2000).

  d. Ongoing clinical trials include examinations of green tea, curcumin, flaxseed, ginger, ginkgo, grape seed extract, milk thistle extract (silymarin), noni, mistletoe, red clover, and St. John's wort (NIH, 2003).

  e. Cautions—botanicals may interact with one another and with conventional medicines, including chemotherapy (Weiger et al., 2002). Clients may also develop allergies to botanical products. Some apparently present little risk when taken alone (e.g., cascara, green tea, prickly ash bark), but others can be highly toxic (e.g., pau d'arco, chaparral, comfrey) (Ernst, 2001; Kumar, 2002; Montbriand, 1999).

    (1) Antiplatelet or anticoagulant activity (e.g., ginkgo, ginseng, green tea, chamomile, feverfew) (Kumar, 2002).

    (2) Hepatotoxicity (e.g., chaparral, kava-kava) (Kumar, 2002).

    (3) Interaction with chemotherapy (e.g., St. John's wort with etoposide (VP-16)) (Decker & Myers, 2001).

    (4) Alter immunosuppressants (e.g., echinacea with cyclosporine [Neoral, Sandimmune], corticosteroids) (Decker & Myers, 2001).

E. Mind-body-spirit techniques (see Chapter 11).

  1. Rationale—a person's emotions influence the course of disease.

  a. Includes practices that range from reducing stress and disease risk (e.g., yoga, biofeedback, support groups, music therapy) to specific visualization of healing (e.g., forming mental images of white blood cells engulfing cancer cells).

  b. Ongoing clinical trials include examinations of music therapy, massage, prayer, and mindfulness-based art therapy (NIH, 2003).

  c. Cautions—least invasive and sufficiently benign for use in conventional biomedical settings. Some concern that therapeutic failure can result in self-blame (Cassileth, 1998; Ross, 2000).

F. Manual healing and physical touch methods (see Chapter 11).

  1. Rationale—the course of disease is influenced by energies or forces that can be physically manipulated.

    a. Range from acupuncture and chiropractic to the therapeutic and/or healing touch practices taught by nurses. Evidence exists that these practices are efficacious in limited settings.

    b. Ongoing clinical trials include examinations of acupressure as a chemotherapy antiemetic, and acupuncture to help control symptoms associated with colorectal cancers (NIH, 2003).

    c. Cautions—limited risks. Several practices are offered to clients in the conventional health care settings (e.g., acupuncture, acupressure, healing touch).

Assessment

I. Relevant client history.

    A. Demographics—age, gender, education, residence, economic status, ethnic and other cultural identity.

      1. CAM users are characterized as well-educated, affluent people who wish to participate in their own health care, rather than as clients who are "marginalized, desperate, and medically naïve" (Jonas, 1997; Ross, 2000).

      2. For some cultural groups, CAM practices are an integral part of their health values and beliefs.

      3. Appeal is sufficiently broad to anticipate that all clients find some CAM practices relevant.

    B. Perspective on disease etiology and treatment.

      1. Ethnic and cultural identity helps shape care decisions (Etkin et al., 1999).

        a. Client-driven care defines what clients expect, how they assess efficacy, and what they want from health care.

      2. Contrasting experience of conventional medicine.

        a. CAM users value holistic, personal care—with a focus on quality of life and on the client rather than the "tumor"—as an alternative to the reductionistic perspective of biomedicine.

        b. Intimidated by, or fearful of, conventional therapy; attracted to "natural," "low-tech," and easily explained modalities.

        c. Distrust of "established medicine," bureaucracies, and complex regulations.

        d. Dissatisfaction with ambiguity and uncertain outcomes.

          (1) Use of CAM is not directly related to stage of disease progression or prognosis.

          (2) Conventional medicine does not target all symptoms.

          (3) Discussions of statistical probabilities confuse clients.

        e. Desire to participate in care decisions and avoid an orchestrated "one-size-fits-all" health care delivery.

Nursing Diagnoses

  I. Deficient knowledge related to cancer treatment and its effects and CAM practices.

  II. Decisional conflict.

  III. Effective management of therapeutic regimen.

Outcome Identification

I. Client describes prescribed conventional treatment and its effects.

    A. Client identifies CAM practices used to health care providers.

II. Client verbalizes positive and negative aspects of choices and alternative actions.
   A. Client expresses satisfaction with choices made.
III. Client manages his/her treatment regimen.

Planning and Implementation

I. Interventions to provide for a well-informed client.
   A. Encourage open communication about conventional therapy options and CAM.
      1. Support an informal dialogue initiated by nurses, clients, and/or their families.
         a. Success depends on building rapport, ensuring a culturally sensitive and nonjudgmental social and professional environment.
         b. Recognize that quick dismissals of CAM may shut down further communication.
         c. Document all CAM therapies used by client.
         d. Acknowledge that disclosure of CAM use is an ongoing process that is shaped by client's health concerns and rapport with the health care team.
            (1) Client disclosure of CAM use at time of admission is likely to be understated (Ross, 2000).
      2. Explain conventional therapies in a way that client understands.
         a. Attraction of CAM practices is that they are conveyed easily, are comprehensible, and are persuasive.
      3. Seek to comprehend why conventional medicine may not satisfy client (e.g., lack of psychosocial support, poor symptom control, inconvenience, lack of understanding).
         a. Discussion must include what the client values and expects.
      4. Explore client's rationales for using CAM or contemplating CAM use (e.g., accessibility, dissatisfaction with conventional therapies, social pressure, agency and empowerment).
      5. Emphasize and support the client's right to choose among therapeutic options.
         a. Therapeutic objectives for client may not be the same as the health care team.
   B. Support the need for a well-informed health care team.
      1. Familiarity with professional and popular educational resources (including Internet sites; see Table 41-1)
      2. Knowledge about CAM sources (including health food vendors).
      3. Recognition that clients are important sources of information about alternatives.
      4. Awareness that CAM may reflect cultural preferences and is an integral component of a client's family and social identity.
         a. Family, friends, and coworkers are significant sources of CAM.
      5. Recognition that clients may deny use of CAM out of fear of losing conventional medical services.
         a. Clients may consider the subject matter of CAM irrelevant to the health care team.
      6. Able to effectively discuss CAM from a scientific, evidence-based perspective.
         a. The failure to offer objective information about safety and efficacy compromises client-initiated dialogue about CAM.

TABLE 41-1
Internet Resource Sites

Site	Web Address
American Cancer Society: Complementary and Alternative Therapies	www.cancer.org
CancerSource: Complementary & Integrative Therapies	http://cit.cancersource.com/
Dunn, Steven: CancerGuide	www.cancerguide.org
Longwood Herbal Task Force	www.mcp.edu/herbal
M.D. Anderson Cancer Center: Complementary/Integrative Medicine	www.mdanderson.org/departments/CIMER
Memorial Sloan-Kettering Cancer Center: About Herbs, Botanicals & Other Products	www.mskcc.org/aboutherbs
National Center for Complementary and Alternative Medicine	http://nccam.nih.gov
Natural Medicines Comprehensive Database	www.naturaldatabase.com
NCCAM Cam on PubMed	www.nlm.nih.gov/nccam/camonpubmed.html
NCI cancer.gov: Complementary and Alternative Medicine	www.cancer.gov/cancerinfo/treatment/cam
NIH ClinicalTrials.gov: Linking Patients to Medical Research	www.clinicaltrials.gov
Quackwatch	www.quackwatch.org
Rosenthal Center for Complementary and Alternative Medicine: Carol Ann Schwartz, Cancer Initiative	www.rosenthal.hs.columbia.edu/cancer/info/infosheets.html

C. Ability to differentiate CAM practices that interfere with conventional medicine from those that complement it.
   1. Practices that should be given primary attention include those that risk harm (e.g., provide antagonistic or other undesirable biophysical results, cause delay or termination of biomedical treatment).
      a. All ingested CAM agents potentially risk interactions with conventional medications.
   2. Incorporate the popular and compatible features of CAM into conventional regimens, for example, more personalized attention and better access to providers (Shapiro & Safer, 2002).
      a. Identifying why alternatives are sought since it may suggest more effective conventional interventions.

Evaluation

The oncology nurse systematically and regularly evaluates the client's and/or family's responses to interventions to determine progress toward achieving expected outcomes. Relevant data are collected, and actual findings are compared with expected findings. Nursing diagnoses, outcomes, and plans of care are reviewed and revised as necessary.

REFERENCES

American Cancer Society. (2002). *Complementary and alternative cancer methods handbook.* Atlanta: American Cancer Society.

Boik, J. (2001). *Natural compounds in cancer therapy.* Princeton, MN: Oregon Medical Press.

Boyer, E. (2002). Issues in the management of dietary supplement use among hospitalized patients [Electronic version]. *International Journal of Medical Toxicology 5*(1), 1-7.

Brown, J., Byers, T., Thompson, K., et al. (2001). Nutrition during and after cancer treatment: A guide for informed choices by cancer survivors. *CA: A Cancer Journal for Clinicians 51*(3), 153-181.

Cassileth, B.R. (1998). *The alternative medicine handbook.* New York: W.W. Norton & Co.

Cauffield, J.S. (2000). The psychosocial aspects of complementary and alternative medicine. *Pharmacotherapy 20*(11), 1289-1294.

Cohen, M., & Eisenberg, D. (2002). Potential physician malpractice liability associated with complementary and integrative medical therapies. *Annals of Internal Medicine 136*(8), 596-603.

Conklin, K.A. (2000). Dietary antioxidants during cancer chemotherapy: Impact on chemotherapeutic effectiveness and development of side effects. *Nutrition and Cancer 37*(1), 1-18.

Consumer Reports. (2000). The mainstreaming of alternative medicine. May, 17-25.

Decker, G.M. (2003). Commonly used vitamin supplements: Implications for clinical practice. A special insert. *Clinical Journal of Oncology Nursing 7*(2), pp. 1-28.

Decker, G.M., & Myers, J. (2001). Commonly used herbs: Implications for clinical practice. A special insert. *Clinical Journal of Oncology Nursing 5*(2), pp. 64 a-64 p.

Ernst, E. (2001). *The desktop guide to complementary and alternative medicine.* London: Harcourt Publishers Ltd.

Etkin, N.L., Dixon, A., Nishimoto, P., & Ross, P.J. (1999). Medicinal foods in multiethnic Hawaii. In A. Guerci (Ed.). *Anthropology, nutrition, and health.* Genoa: Erga Edzioni.

Etkin, N.L., & McMillen, H. (2003). The ethnobotany of Noni: Dwelling in the land between La au Lapa au and testimonials. In S.C. Nelson (Ed.). *CTAHR proceedings.* Honolulu: College of Tropical Agriculture and Human Resources. University of Hawaii, pp. 11-16.

Etkin, N.L., & Ross, P.J. (2002). Polypharmacy and the elderly cancer patient: Rethinking "noncompliance." In A. Guerci & S. Consigliere (Eds.). *Living old age: The Western world and modernization.* Genoa: Erga Edzioni.

Jonas, W. (1997). Researching alternative medicine. *Nature Medicine 3*, 824-827.

Kumar, N.B. (2002). *Integrative nutritional therapies for cancer.* St. Louis: Facts & Comparisons.

Montbriand, M.J. (1999). Past and present herbs used to treat cancer: Medicine, magic or poison? *Oncology Nursing Forum 26*(1), 49-62.

National Institutes of Health (NIH). (2003). Linking patients to medical research. Retrieved February 2003 from the World Wide Web: http://www.clinicaltrials.gov.

Richardson, M.A., Sanders, T., Palmer, J., et al. (2000). Complementary/alternative medicine use in a comprehensive cancer center and the implications for oncology. *Journal of Clinical Oncology 18*(13), 2505-2514.

Rosenthal, D.S. (2000). *American Cancer Society's guide to complementary and alternative cancer methods.* Atlanta: Health Content Products.

Ross, P.J. (2000). Complementary and alternative medicine. In V. Fieler & P. Hanson (Eds.). *Oncology nursing in the home.* Pittsburgh: Oncology Nursing Society, pp. 201-228.

Shapiro, D., & Safer, M. (2002). Integrating complementary therapies into a traditional oncology practice. *Oncology Issues 17*(1), 35-40.

Sparber, A., Bauer, L., Curt, G., et al. (2000). Use of complementary medicine by adult patients participating in cancer clinical trials. *Oncology Nursing Forum 27*(4), 623-630.

Weiger, W.A., Smith, M., Boon, H., et al. (2002). Advising patients who seek complementary and alternative medical therapies for cancer. *Annals of Internal Medicine 137*(11), 889-903.

Wolsko, P., Eisenberg, D., Davis, R., et al. (2002). Insurance coverage, medical conditions, and visits to alternative medical providers: Results of a national survey. *Annals of Internal Medicine 162*(3), 281-289.

PART SEVEN

HEALTH PROMOTION

42 Epidemiology and Prevention of Cancer

SHARON J. OLSEN

Theory

I. Cancer epidemiology.
  A. Definition.
  1. Study of the distribution and determinants of cancer in population groups.
  2. Assists in development of population-based risk profiles.
  B. Global cancer statistics (National Cancer Institute [NCI], 2003a; World Health Organization [WHO], 2003).
  1. Among developed and developing countries, an estimated 5.3 million men and 4.7 million women were diagnosed with cancer and 6.2 million died in 2000.
  2. According to WHO the following will occur:
    a. Cancer rates will increase by 50% to 15 million new cases in 2020 primarily because of steadily aging populations, increases in smoking prevalence, and the worldwide adoption of unhealthy lifestyles.
    b. Annual death toll from tobacco use alone will climb to 10 million people in 2020, double what it is now.
  3. The three leading cancer killers worldwide are lung (responsible for 17.8% of all cancer deaths), stomach (10.4%), and liver (8.8%) cancers.
  4. Industrial nations with the highest overall cancer rates include the United States, Italy, Australia, Germany, the Netherlands, Canada, and France.
  5. Developing countries with the lowest cancer rates are in northern Africa and southern and eastern Asia (a complete list of cancer rates by countries can be found at http://www-dep.iarc.fr/).
  C. Cancer statistics in the United States (Jemal et al., 2004).
  1. Cancer incidence—the number of new cancers of a specific site/type occurring in a specified population during 1 year.
    a. Usually expressed as the number of cancers per 100,000.
    b. Published annually by the American Cancer Society (ACS) at http://www.cancer.org/docroot/home/index.asp.
    c. In 2004, the ACS estimated 1,368,030 new cancer cases (Jemal et al., 2004).
      (1) Does not include carcinoma in situ for any site except urinary bladder.
      (2) Does not include basal and squamous cell skin cancers since more than 1 million basal and squamous cell skin cancers are expected in 2004.
  2. Cancer prevalence—the number or percent of people alive on a certain date in a population who previously had a diagnosis of cancer.
    a. Includes new (incidence) and preexisting cases and is a function of both past incidence and survival.

    b. Information on prevalence used for health planning, resource allocation, and an estimate of cancer survivorship.

       (1) As of January 1, 2000, the NCI estimated that approximately 9.6 million Americans with a history of cancer were alive in various stages of disease or nondisease.

          (a) Sixty-one percent of survivors are over age 65 years.

          (b) About 14% were diagnosed more than 20 years ago.

          (c) Current average ages of male and female cancer survivors are 69 and 64 years, respectively.

3. Cancer mortality—number of deaths attributed to cancer during a specified time period in a defined population.

    a. In 2004, 563,700 Americans were expected to die of cancer (more than 1540 per day).

    b. Cancer is the second leading cause of death in the United States..

    c. One of every four U.S. deaths is due to cancer.

4. Case-fatality—number of persons among all those who have a form of cancer who die of it during a specified period of time.

    a. Provides a measure of the aggressiveness of cancer or of the success of medical intervention.

    b. For example, lung cancer accounts for 32% of the cancer deaths in men, or the overall 5-year survival rate for lung cancer is about 15%.

5. Cancer survival—generally reported as 5-year relative survival rates, which represent persons who are living 5 years after diagnosis, whether disease free, in remission, or undergoing treatment.

    a. Five-year survival rate for all cancers combined is 63%.

6. Trends from 2000 to 2001.

    a. Overall cancer incidence and mortality decreased slightly between 1992 and 2000.

       (1) Incidence stabilized in men but increased by 0.4% in women.

       (2) Mortality declined by 1.5% for men but stabilized for women.

    b. Prostate cancers (PCs) experienced the most dramatic decreases in incidence, 3% per year.

    c. Liver and intrahepatic cancers showed the most dramatic increase: 3.9% per year.

    d. Other cancers demonstrating increased incidence rates over that time frame include female breast, kidney/renal, melanoma of the skin, and thyroid.

    e. Reductions in cancer incidence rates were noted in Hodgkin's disease, stomach, leukemia, male lung cancer, uterine cancer, and PC.

7. Minority statistics.

    a. Socioeconomic disparities and unequal access to medical care may underlie many of the differences associated with race/ethnicity.

       (1) Data on race and ethnicity are currently more available than are data on socioeconomic status (SES) and therefore serve to highlight existing disparities.

    b. Mortality rates.

       (1) Statistics for mortality also vary by race. Rates from 1996 to 2000 are as follows (per 100,000 population) (Ries et al., 2003).

          (a) African American: male, 356.2; female, 198.6.

          (b) Caucasian: male, 249.5; female, 166.9.

          (c) Hispanic: male, 176.7; female, 112.4.

(d) Asian and Pacific Islander: male, 154.8; female, 102.

(e) American Indians/Alaskan Natives: male, 172.3; female, 115.8.

(2) African American men have a cancer mortality rate about 43% higher than Caucasians.

(3) African American women have a cancer mortality rate about 20% higher than Caucasian women.

(4) Death rate for lung cancer is about 27% higher for African Americans than for Caucasians.

(5) The prostate cancer (PC) mortality rate for African American men is more than twice that of Caucasian men.

c. Incidence rates.

(1) Statistics for incidence of all cancers vary by race. Rates from 1996 to 2000 are as follows (per 100,000 population) (Ries, et al., 2003):

(a) African American: males 696.8; females 406.3.

(b) Caucasian: males 555.9; females 431.8.

(c) Asian and Pacific Islander: males 392.0; females 306.9.

(d) Hispanic: males 419.3; females 312.2.

(e) Native Americans/Alaskan Natives: males 259.0; females 229.2).

(2) For lung cancer in African American men, rates are about 50% higher than in Caucasian men.

(3) Native Hawaiian men have elevated rates of lung cancer compared with Caucasian men.

(4) Alaskan Native men and women experience higher rates of cancers of the colon and rectum than Caucasians.

(5) Vietnamese women in the United States have a cervical cancer incidence rate more than 5 times greater than Caucasian women.

(6) Hispanic women experience elevated rates of cervical cancer.

(7) Asian and Pacific Islanders have twice the stomach and liver cancer incidence and mortality of Caucasians.

8. Cancer rates relative to select demographic variables.

a. Age—incidence of most cancers increases with age.

b. Gender—cancer is more common in males than females.

c. Geography—major incidence and mortality differences exist in different locations.

(1) Migratory data demonstrate adoption of the cancer pattern of the area to which migration occurs, suggesting lifestyle and behavioral factors as well as environmental ones as causative or exacerbating.

d. SES—cancer rates correlate with SES but not in a consistent fashion.

(1) Low SES correlates with increased risk of lung cancer, cervical cancer, stomach cancer, and cancer of the head and neck.

(a) Increased tobacco use among poorer populations.

(b) More advanced disease presentations are evident in rural and lower SES groups (CDC, 2002).

(2) High SES increases the risk of breast, prostate, and colon cancers.

(3) Economic, social, and cultural factors can create barriers to accessing information and preventive services.

9. Recent statistics for five most common cancers (Jemal et al., 2004; NCI, 2001).

a. Lung.

(1) Women.

(a) Second most common cancer among women, accounts for 12% of all female cancer cases and rates are declining slowly.

(b) Most common cause of cancer-related death in women; accounts for 25% of all female cancer deaths.

(c) An estimated 80,660 new cases and 68,510 deaths are expected in the United States in 2004.

(d) Lung cancer rate per 100,000 varies by ethnicity.

    (i) Japanese (15).

    (ii) Korean, Filipino, Hispanic, and Chinese women (16 to 25).

    (iii) Vietnamese, Caucasian, Hawaiian, and African American women (31 to 44).

    (iv) Alaskan Natives (51).

(2) Men.

(a) Second leading cause of new cancer cases, accounts for 14% of all male cancers and rates are declining.

(b) Most common cause of cancer-related death and accounts for about 30% of all male cancers.

(c) Estimated 93,110 new cases and 91,930 deaths are expected in the United States in 2004.

(d) Age-adjusted lung cancer incidence rates (per 100,000) range from a low of about 14 among American Indians to a high of 117 among African Americans, an eightfold difference.

    (i) Between these two extremes, rates fall into two groups in the following ranges: 42 to 53 for Hispanics, Japanese, Chinese, Filipinos, and Koreans; 71 to 89 for Vietnamese, Caucasians, Alaskan Natives, and Native Hawaiians.

(3) Both genders.

(a) Five-year survival rates for Caucasians (15%, all stages) minimally exceed those of African Americans (12%).

(b) Risk factors: cigarette smoking, radon exposure.

b. Breast cancer.

(1) Women.

(a) Most common cancer among women, accounts for 32% of all female cancer cases and 15% of all female cancer deaths.

(b) Research suggests that one in eight to one in nine women will develop breast cancer in her lifetime.

(c) Estimated 215,990 new cases and 40,110 deaths are expected in the United States in 2004.

(d) Highest age-adjusted mortality occurs among African American women, followed by Caucasian and Hawaiian women.

    (i) Higher breast cancer mortality among African American women is related to the fact that relative to Caucasian women, a larger percentage of their breast cancers are diagnosed at a later, less treatable stage.

(e) Five-year survival rate for Caucasians (88%, all stages) exceeds that for African American women (73%).

(2) Men.

(a) Rare disease that accounts for less than 1% of all male cancers and less than 1% of all diagnosed breast cancers.

(b) Estimated 1450 new cases and 470 deaths are expected in the United States in 2004.

(c) Unlike breast cancer in women, where rates have stabilized and seem to be decreasing, incidence in men younger than age 40 years seems to be substantially increasing.

(d) Median age at diagnosis in men in most series is 68 years compared with 63 years in women.

(3) Risk factors.

(a) Female gender; increasing age; early menarche; late menopause; nulliparity; older age at first live birth; family history of breast cancer; personal history of proliferative benign breast disease; history of radiation exposure; *BRCA1, BRCA2, p53,* or *PTEN* (phosphatase and tensin homologue deleted on chromosome 10) mutations.

c. Prostate cancer.

(1) One fifth of all U.S. men will be diagnosed in their lifetime; fortunately, only 3% will die of this disease.

(2) Estimated 230,110 new cases in the United States in 2004.

(a) Number of new cases is expected to reach 380,000 by 2025 because of the aging male population.

(3) Second leading cause of death from cancer among U.S. men.

(a) Seventh leading cause of death in the United States.

(b) Estimated 29,900 deaths are expected in the United States in 2004.

(4) For the 5-year period ending in 2000, NCI statistics show an average annual incidence rate of 277/100,000 African American men, compared with 168/100,000 Caucasian men.

(a) Discrepancy in death rates over the same period is even greater: 73 PC deaths per 100,000 African American men versus 30 per 100,000 Caucasian men (Reynolds, 2003).

(5) The Selenium and Vitamin E Cancer Prevention Trial (SELECT): a clinical trial to determine if 7 to 12 years of daily selenium and/or vitamin E supplements reduce risk of developing PC.

(a) Funded by NCI. Began August 2001 with accrual for 5 years. See http://www.cancer.gov/select.

(6) Risk factors—increasing age; family history of PC; African American heritage; high-fat diet.

(a) African American Hereditary Prostate Cancer Study has been established to find genes involved in hereditary PC. See http://www.genome.gov/10000831.

d. Colorectal cancer (CRC).

(1) Third most common malignant neoplasm worldwide and second leading cause of cancer deaths (irrespective of gender) in the United States.

(2) Estimates for 2004: 146,940 new cases and 56,730 deaths in the United States (colon and rectal cancer cases).

(3) About 6% of Americans are expected to develop the disease within their lifetime.

(4) Between 1985 and 1995, incidence rates in the United States declined by 1.8% per year, but stabilized during 1995 to 1999.

(5) Over the past 15 years, the mortality rate declined by 1.7% per year.

(6) Overall 5-year survival rate is 62.1%. Despite advances in surgical technique and adjuvant therapy, there has been only a modest improvement in survival for clients who present with advanced CRC.

      (7) CRC risk begins to increase after age 40 years and rises sharply at the ages of 50 to 55 years; the risk doubles with each succeeding decade and continues to rise exponentially.

      (8) Nearly 9 out of 10 colon cancer cases and deaths could be prevented if everyone 50 years or older would lead a healthy lifestyle and have regualar screening (ACS, 2002).

      (9) Risk factors: age; diets that are high in fat and calories and low in fiber; polyps; familial polyposis; women with a history of cancer of the ovary, uterus, or breast; personal history of CRC; family history; ulcerative colitis.

    e. Pancreatic cancer.

      (1) U.S. 2004 estimates: 31,860 new cases; 31,270 deaths.

      (2) Fourth most common cause of cancer death among men and women.

      (3) African Americans have appreciably higher rates than Caucasians.

      (4) Survival rates are dismal.

        (a) One-year relative survival is 20% to 30%.

        (b) Five-year survival is approximately 5%.

        (c) Majority of clients are diagnosed with advanced disease, and, in general, no standard treatment appreciably alters its rapidly progressive, fatal course.

      (5) Risk factors: germline mutations in *p16* and *BRCA2* have been implicated in a small fraction of cases; chronic pancreatitis; cigarette smoking (current smokers have 2 to 3 times the risk of non-smokers); studies of dietary factors suggest associations with consumption of smoked or processed meats or with animal foods in general and lower risk with consumption of fruits and vegetables; colonization by *Helicobacter pylori;* history of diabetes mellitus.

  10. For the most up-to-date national cancer statistics, see http://www.cancer.org; http://www.cancer.gov.

II. Cancer prevention.

  A. According to the Institute of Medicine's recent report, "Fulfilling the Potential of Cancer Prevention and Early Detection" (Curry et al., 2003), "the US is failing to take advantage of proven methods of preventing cancer."

    1. The institute reports that if sustained efforts were made to help people change their behavior, such as ceasing smoking, and systems were in place to enable them to take advantage of cancer detection procedures, 60,000 cancer deaths and about 100,000 new cancer cases annually could be prevented by 2015.

    2. Behavior modifications that will save the most lives from cancer include helping people stop smoking, maintain a healthy diet, keep their weight under control, stimulate physical activity, and moderate their alcohol consumption.

  B. Definitions.

    1. Primary prevention.

      a. Involves the identification of genetic, biologic, and environmental factors that are etiologic or pathogenic in the development of cancer, and subsequent complete or significant interference with their effects on carcinogenesis (see http://www.cancer.gov/cancerinfo/pdq/prevention).

      b. Interventions that focus on reducing the risk of cancer in individuals and groups.

(1) Educating clients about risk reduction behaviors related to the following:
   (a) Eliminating or limiting exposure to causative factors, such as sun and tobacco.
   (b) Promoting protective factors (including health-promoting activities), such as eating a diet high in fruits, vegetables, and whole grains and wearing protective clothing and sunscreens when in the sun.
(2) Chemoprevention.
   (a) Use of natural or synthetic substances to reduce the risk of developing cancer or to reduce the chance that cancer will recur.
   (b) For example, nonsteroidal antiinflammatory drugs, including celecoxib (Celebrex), piroxicam (Feldene), sulindac (Clinoril), and aspirin, may prevent adenoma formation or cause adenomatous polyps to regress in individuals with prior CRC or adenomatous polyps and in the setting of familial adenomatous polyposis.
(3) Prophylactic surgery.
   (a) Surgical removal of organs to prevent disease.
   (b) For example, bilateral prophylactic oophorectomy has been judged effective in reducing ovarian cancer occurrence in women at increased risk for inherited ovarian cancer and removal of adenomatous polyps may reduce the risk of CRC.
2. Risk—the likelihood that exposure to a certain factor will influence the chance of developing a particular cancer based on the national average.
  a. Types of risk.
   (1) Absolute risk—a measure of cancer occurrence in terms of cancer incidence and mortality.
     (a) For example, absolute risk can be expressed either as the number of cases per a specified number of women—most commonly 100,000.
        (i) Because this number is based on averages, it is important to recognize that the number cannot be applied to any individual.
        (ii) It is an overestimate for women with few risk factors and an underestimate for women with several.
        (iii) It also varies according to ethnic background and is modified by age.
   (2) Relative risk—an estimate of one group's increased probability of developing a certain cancer based on exposure to one or more risk factors compared with a reference or unexposed group.
     (a) Higher the relative risk, the greater the risk of developing that specific cancer.
     (b) Relative risk numbers derived through studies or analyses that involve comparing two groups that, as a whole, are closely matched in terms of distributions of age, weight, health histories, and so on.
        (i) One group will have a certain risk factor, and those in the other will not.
        (ii) Researchers determine how many in each group develop cancer over a certain number of years.

(c) Relative risk is also known as risk ratio, hazard ratio, or odds ratio.

(d) For example, if 2% of the women in the first group and 3.5% of those in the second group develop breast cancer, those in the second group are said to have 1.75 times the risk of the first group.

    (i) Thus that risk factor is said to increase the risk of breast cancer by 75%.

    (ii) Sometimes relative risk is reported as a range—for example, hormone replacement therapy (HRT) increases the risk of breast cancer by 30% to 70%. This means that some studies have found that HRT increases breast cancer by 30%, others by 70%.

(3) Attributable risk—the amount of disease in a population that could be avoided by reducing risk factors in individuals and in terms of cost to society.

(a) Relates more to public policy than to individual health.

(b) For example, it was hypothesized that if every woman in the world were to have a baby before age 25 years, 17% of the world's breast cancer would be eliminated.

    (i) Public health authorities who were considering encouraging this practice would have to weigh the possible advantages of early pregnancy against the problems of young parenthood and increased population growth.

(4) Cumulative risk—the total amount of risk over time. For example, a woman has a one in eight to one in nine risk for developing breast cancer in her lifetime.

b. Risk factor—an identifiable trait or habit (e.g., personal behavior, genetic makeup or exposure) that is statistically associated with an increased susceptibility for disease, disability, or death (e.g., early menarche, late onset of menopause, and *BRCA1* gene inheritance are risk factors for breast cancer).

c. Risk assessment—the procedure by which the probability of developing a disease, disability, or death is predicted through analysis of individual characteristics known as risk factors. Purposes include the following:

(1) Assist in diagnosis.

(2) Help establish patterns of inheritance.

(3) Assist in identification of persons at risk.

(4) Contribute to the biologic understanding of cancer.

(5) Educate clients to alter or change risk factors to decrease risk for cancer.

(6) Risk assessment for breast cancer may be assessed using a tool adapted from the Gail model, which is available through the NCI. See http://bcra.nci.nih.gov/brc/q1.htm.

(a) After completing a brief questionnaire, a woman will receive an estimate of her chances of being diagnosed with breast cancer within the next 5 years.

C. Important theoretic principles.

1. Cancer is caused by complex interactions between genes and a variety of external factors.

a. At conception, inherited cancers and rare familial cancer syndromes present with an overexpressed oncogene or disabled tumor suppressor gene.

(1) Subsequent exposures or genetic events appear to be necessary to trigger cancer.

(2) About 10% of cancers are believed to be heritable.

b. In the more common nonfamilial cancers, environmentally induced mutations send a somatic cell down a pathway to cancer.

c. Sporadic cancers generally result from the accumulation of discrete genome changes that occur over time, perhaps 10 to 30 years.

2. Mechanisms of carcinogenesis predict that individual susceptibility to cancer may result from several factors, including the following:

a. Differences in the metabolism of carcinogenic chemicals (uptake, activation, detoxification).

b. Incompetent deoxyribonucleic acid (DNA) repair mechanisms.

c. The presence of inherited or acquired alterations in proto-oncogenes or tumor suppressor genes.

d. Impaired nutritional status.

e. Circulating hormonal factors.

f. Immunologic factors.

g. Occupational and environmental exposures.

3. Recognizing risk factors identifies individuals at greater risk for cancer and provides the opportunity to intervene early to prevent disease.

a. Three-generation family history (pedigree) review and analysis combined with a thorough social, health, and occupational exposure assessment is central to early risk identification.

4. Changes in lifestyle have the potential to reduce cancer risks.

a. Evidence suggests that as much as 50% or more of cancer incidence can be prevented through smoking cessation and changed dietary habits.

5. Reducing exposure to carcinogens may reduce cancer risk.

D. Recent cancer prevention research findings.

1. Lung cancer.

a. Overall findings of the Alpha-Tocopherol, Beta-Carotene Trial, and the Beta-Carotene and Retinol Efficacy Trial (CARET) indicate that pharmacologic doses of β-carotene (β-carotene at 20 mg/day in the former trial and β-carotene at 30 mg/day plus retinol at 25,000 international units/day in the latter trial) increase lung cancer risk in groups who are characterized by smoking and asbestos exposure (NCI, 1997).

2. Breast cancer.

a. Tamoxifen (Nolvadex).

(1) The Breast Cancer Prevention Trial randomly assigned more than 13,000 women with a 5-year risk of breast cancer of 1.7% or more to tamoxifen or placebo.

(a) After a mean follow-up period of 4 years, tamoxifen (Novaldex) had reduced the incidence of breast cancer by 49% as compared with the incidence with placebo (Fisher et al., 1998).

(2) Currently the only drug approved by the U.S. Food and Drug Administration (FDA) for reducing the risk of breast cancer.

(3) Clinical trials are now comparing the efficacy of raloxifene (Evista) with that of tamoxifen in reducing the risk of breast cancer.

b. Higher plasma levels of folate and possibly vitamin B_6 may reduce the risk of developing breast cancer.

(1) Deficient folate status can result in abnormal DNA synthesis because of misincorporation of uracil into DNA, leading to chromosome breaks and disruption of DNA repair.

(2) Alcohol is a known folate antagonist.

(3) Achieving adequate circulating levels of folate may be particularly important for women at higher risk of developing breast cancer because of higher alcohol consumption (Zhang et al., 2003).

3. Prostate cancer (PC).

a. No consistently agreed on methods for prevention.

b. Prostate Cancer Prevention Trial (PCPT) found that finasteride (Propecia) delayed or reduced the cumulative incidence of PC but also appeared to increase the risk of high-grade PC.

(1) Researchers concluded that finasteride was not an attractive agent for the chemoprevention of PC (Thompson et al., 2003).

c. Selenium was used as a dietary supplement in the Nutritional Prevention of Cancer Trial and was associated with a reduction in PC incidence.

(1) Potential action includes a beneficial scavenger of DNA-damaging oxygen free radicals, a potent inducer of apoptosis that eliminates damaged, potentially cancerous cells or prompts cells to initiate DNA repair.

d. Lycopene—several studies have found an inverse association between PC and the intake of tomatoes and tomato-based products, the major dietary source of lycopene.

4. Colorectal cancer (CRC).

a. Nonsteroidal antiinflammatory drugs, including celecoxib, piroxicam, sulindac, and aspirin, may prevent adenoma formation or cause adenomatous polyps to regress in individuals with prior CRC or adenomatous polyps and in the setting of familial adenomatous polyposis (Janne & Mayer, 2000).

b. Calcium—research involving the Nurses' Health Study (NHS) and the Health Professionals Follow-up Study (HPFS) concluded higher calcium intake was associated with a reduced risk of distal colon cancer (Wu et al., 2003).

(1) Calcium may inhibit colon carcinogenesis by binding bile acids and fatty acids in the bowel lumen or by directly inhibiting the proliferation of colonic epithelial cells (Janne & Mayer, 2000).

c. Selenium—low levels are associated with risk of CRC.

d. Diets low in folate appear to increase risk for colorectal adenomas and carcinomas (Janne & Mayer, 2000).

(1) Nurses Health Study (NHS): supplementation with folate (as a multivitamin) was protective against CRC. Greatest risk reduction among women taking high daily doses of folate (more than 400 micrograms daily). Risk reduction (RR, 0.25) was statistically significant only after 15 years of use (Giovannucci et al., 1998).

e. Fiber.

(1) A case control study of more than 38,000 individuals found that people who had the highest amounts of fiber in their diets (36 grams/day or more) had the lowest incidence of colon adenomas (Ulrike, 2003).

(2) A prospective cohort study of more than 500,000 individuals in 10 countries found that people who ate the most fiber (averaging 33 g/day) had a 25% lower incidence of CRC than those who ate about 12 g/day (Bingham et al., 2003).

(3) Most important sources of fiber were fruits and grains/cereals, not fiber from vegetables and legumes (Ulrike, 2003).

5. Pancreatic cancer.
   a. Contaminants—the bacterial contaminant *Helicobacter pylori* is linked to gastric and pancreatic cancer.
   b. In the NHS cohort, women who reported more than 20 years of regular aspirin use had a 58% increased risk of pancreatic cancer compared with women who were never regular users, and the higher the aspirin dose, the higher the observed incidence of cancer (Schernhammer et al., 2004).
6. Cervical cancer.
   a. Five types of human papillomavirus (HPV-16, -18, -31, -33, -45) are responsible for most cervical cancers.
   b. Preliminary evidence suggests a vaccine against HPV-16 using empty-viral capsids, called "viruslike particles," reduces the risk of acquiring transient and persistent HPV-16 infections and cervical neoplasia.
      (1) HPV-16–vaccinated women are protected not only from preinvasive diseases associated with HPV-16 infection but also from persistent HPV-16 infection and transient HPV-16 infection with efficacy rates of 100%, 100%, and 91%, respectively (Koutsky et al., 2002).
      (2) Vaccine not only prevents cervical cancer from developing but also prevents its causative agent from residing in the genital tract where it can infect new sexual partners.
      (3) If women were vaccinated against these types of HPV before they became sexually active, there should be a reduction of at least 85% in the risk of cancer and a decline of 44% to 70% in the frequency of abnormal Papanicolaou smears attributable to HPV (Crum, 2002).
7. Skin cancer.
   a. The Actinic Keratosis Trial found retinol (25,000 international units/day) can prevent development of a first new squamous cell carcinoma or a first new basal cell carcinoma of the skin.
   b. Use of tanning beds and lamps increases the risk of basal cell carcinoma and squamous cell carcinoma, which together account for more than 1 million new U.S. cancer cases each year (Karagas et al., 2002).

Assessment

I. Identify lifestyle risk factors.
   A. Tobacco use.
      1. Single most important cause of cancer mortality in the United States.
         a. Accounts for at least 30% of all cancer deaths.
         b. Accounts for at least 90% of lung cancer cases.
      2. In 2000, 26% of adult men and 22% of adult women were current smokers.
      3. Associated cancers of the lung, trachea, bronchus, larynx, pharynx, oral cavity, esophagus (squamous cell), bladder, pancreas, kidney, and cervix. Also linked with colorectal adenomas.
      4. Risk of cancer from tobacco is concentrated in the 30% to 40% of the adult population who are current or former smokers.
         a. Tobacco exposure accounts for about 60% of their overall cancer risk.
      5. Cigarettes are the most important cause of tobacco-related cancer.
      6. Other forms of tobacco, notably chewing tobacco and snuff, are also established carcinogens.

7. Environmental tobacco smoke (secondhand/sidestream smoke).
   a. Approximately 30% of all lung cancers caused by factors other than smoking are attributable to environmental tobacco smoke exposure.
   b. Known impact on children includes increased risk of bronchitis, pneumonia, fluid in middle ear, asthma attacks, respiratory tract irritation, and reduced lung function.
8. Synergistic effect with alcohol: increases risk of cancers of the mouth, throat, larynx, and esophagus.
9. Evidence is strong that tobacco addiction is almost always acquired in adolescence.
10. Smokers who quit before age 50 years halve the risk of dying within 15 years compared with those who continue to smoke.
    a. Risk of dying is reduced substantially among quitters after age 70 years.
    b. Risk of lung cancer is 30% to 50% lower than continuing smokers after 10 years of cessation.
    c. Former smokers lower risks of cervical and bladder cancers.

B. Alcohol consumption.
   1. Contributes to about 3% of cancer mortality.
   2. Contributes to cancer of the esophagus, liver, pharynx, stomach, colon, breast.
   3. Synergistic effect with tobacco.
   4. As few as one or two drinks per day may contribute to breast and perhaps colon and rectal cancer.

C. Diet.
   1. Accounts for 20% to 42% of cancer deaths.
   2. Epidemiologic, experimental (animal), and clinical investigations suggest that diets high in total fat, protein, calories, alcohol, and meat (both red and white) and low in calcium and folate are associated with an increased incidence of CRC.
   3. Dietary fat and breast cancer association is controversial.
   4. High-fiber diet (in particular, one high in fruits and vegetables) appears protective for cancers of the lung, colon, rectum, bladder, oral cavity, stomach, cervix, and esophagus.
   5. In a study of 42,254 women who ate the largest amounts of healthy foods (fruits, vegetables, whole grains, low-fat dairy products, lean meats and poultry), death rates from cancer, heart disease, and stroke were about 30% lower compared with those consuming very little of these foods (Kant et al., 2000).
   6. Overweight and obesity might account for 20% of all cancer deaths in U.S. women and 14% in U.S. men.
      a. That means 90,000 cancer deaths could be prevented annually if Americans maintained a healthy body weight.
      b. Overweight, defined as a body mass index above 25 kg/m^2, is estimated to be responsible for almost 10% of cancers.
      c. The United States has a bona fide obesity epidemic (Calle et al., 2003).
   7. Nutrients modulate cancer in a number of ways (Go et al., 2003).
      a. Inhibiting phase 1 drug metabolizing enzymes through the cytochrome P450 superfamily.
      b. Modifying carcinogen detoxification through phase 2 drug metabolizing enzymes.
      c. Scavenging reactive DNA agents and enhancing DNA repair mechanisms.

    d. Interacting with signal transduction.

    e. Inhibiting angiogenesis.

    f. Suppressing abnormal proliferative characteristics, either by influencing apoptosis or cell-cycle checkpoint activities.

II. Identify occupational and physical environment risks.

  A. Occupational cancer risks.

    1. Account for about 4% of cancers.

    2. Introduction of effective regulation of workplace exposures, in the middle years of the twentieth century, is believed to have reduced these risks substantially.

    3. Asbestos: single most important known occupational carcinogen.

      a. Asbestos-related lung cancer and mesothelioma peaked during the middle to late 1980s because of extensive occupational exposure in shipyards during World War II.

      b. Occupational exposures to asbestos fibers, environmental smoke, and/or radon have a synergistic role in elevating risk of smoking-related lung cancer.

    4. Special population concerns.

      a. Blue collar workers—tend to have higher smoking rates that increase risks associated with occupational exposures.

      b. African Americans—discriminatory work assignments have historically resulted in placement in more hazardous jobs: steel, rubber, and chemical industries.

      c. Steel workers—increased lung cancer rates.

      d. Rubber workers—increased PC rates.

      e. Chemical workers—increased bladder cancer rates.

      f. Miners—increased exposure to uranium and radon with a subsequent increase in gastric cancer and birth defects.

    5. Resources.

      a. National Toxicology Program provides information about potentially toxic chemicals to health regulatory and research agencies.

        (1) Evaluates exposures that may be carcinogenic.

        (2) Publishes reports on carcinogens every 2 years; offers numerous fact sheets. See http://ntp-server.niehs.nih.gov/default.html.

      b. International Agency for Research on Cancer is part of the WHO.

        (1) Its mission is to coordinate and conduct research on the causes of human cancer and the mechanisms of carcinogenesis and to develop scientific strategies for cancer control. See http://www.iarc.fr/.

      c. Environmental Protection Agency programs address air pollution, chemicals, pesticides, toxic waste. See http://www.epa.gov/.

      d. National Institute for Occupational Safety and Health, a part of the Centers for Disease Control, focuses on workplace safety and a variety of health-related topics. See http://www.cdc.gov/niosh/homepage.html.

  B. Environmental risk factors.

    1. Account for about 2% of cancer deaths.

    2. Sun exposure: several kinds of skin cancer seem linked to sun exposure, fair skin, and family history.

      a. Basal cell carcinoma: most common skin cancer; is rarely deadly; influenced by both long-term and intermittent sun exposure.

      b. Squamous cell carcinoma: often begins with small scaly lesions called solar keratoses, or actinic keratoses. Linked to cumulative time in the sun. Both squamous and basal cell cancers typically found on the head, neck, and arms, areas of the body most frequently exposed to sunlight.

   c. New cases of melanoma increased 126% between 1973 and 1995; about 6% each year.

     (1) Melanoma seems to be linked to intermittent sun exposure and sunburn—in other words, recreational sun exposure, especially sunbathing.

     (2) Risk factors include a large number of moles, irregularly shaped or pigmented moles, and a history of sunburn, especially during childhood.

  3. Electromagnetic field (EMF) exposures (Heath, 1996).

   a. Relationship to carcinogenesis is inconclusive.

   b. Some evidence for contribution to childhood leukemia.

  4. Contribution of cellular telephones, microwaves, and other wireless systems to cancer remains unclear.

  5. Radon gas (inhalable radioactive particles).

   a. Most is naturally occurring but can be associated with radioactive waste.

   b. Domestic exposure (in the home, etc.) can increase risk for lung cancer.

III. Identify biologic risk factors.

  A. Viral exposures (Wong et al., 2002).

   1. Associated with 15% of all cancers worldwide.

   2. Hepatocellular carcinoma accounts for about 80% of virus-linked cancers to date.

   3. Human immunodeficiency virus (HIV) infection results in immunosuppression that increases risk of Kaposi's sarcoma and B-cell lymphomas.

   4. Epstein-Barr virus (EBV).

    a. A herpesvirus.

    b. Endemic in human population since more than 90% of adults worldwide are seropositive.

    c. Causes infectious mononucleosis.

    d. Closely associated with Burkitt's lymphoma, nasopharyngeal cancers, undifferentiated parotid carcinoma, a subset of clients with Hodgkin's disease, and a variety of B-cell lymphoma.

    e. Associated with undifferentiated gastric carcinomas and most recently with aggressive human breast cancers.

   5. Human papillomavirus (HPV).

    a. Cervical cancer.

     (1) More than 20 types of papillomaviruses have now been identified, and five are associated with cervical cancer.

     (2) HPV type 16 (HPV-16) is leading candidate in the pathogenesis of preinvasive and invasive cervical neoplasia.

    b. Oral cancer.

     (1) HPV-16 detected in a substantial proportion of squamous cell carcinomas of the soft palate, tonsils, and base of the tongue.

     (2) HPV-16 detected in 90% of all HPV-associated head and neck squamous cell carcinomas and 50% of all oropharyngeal head and neck squamous cell carcinomas.

   6. Evidence supports causal relationship between human T-cell lymphotropic virus–1 (HTLV-1) and certain T-cell leukemias.

  B. Familial and genetic contributions.

   1. Most cancer appears to be autosomal dominant.

   2. Inherited genetic mutations account for 5% to 20% of cancers.

   3. Gene-gene and/or gene-environment interactions determine expression.
   4. Associated phenotypes (observable characteristics) include early age of onset; tumor bilaterality; multiple primaries; and multiple family members with similar or syndrome-associated cancers.
   5. Inherited cancer cannot be prevented, but preventing or eliminating contact with risk-enhancing lifestyle and environmental exposures is important.
IV. Identify iatrogenic risks.
   A. Hormonal agents.
      1. Hormone replacement therapy (HRT) (Rossouw et al., 2002).
         a. Combined estrogen/progesterone HRT given to postmenopausal women increases risk of breast cancer but may reduce risk of CRC.
         b. Observational studies suggest that HRT halves the risk of coronary heart disease and osteoporosis but increases the risk of breast cancer by 30% to 40%.
         c. Estrogens may prevent CRC by decreasing the production of secondary bile acids, by decreasing the production of insulin-like growth factor I, by exerting direct effects on the colorectal epithelium, or by a combination of these mechanisms.
         d. The Cancer Prevention Study II found a significant decrease in mortality from colon cancer with the use of HRT (RR, 0.71); the effect was stronger in women currently using HRT (RR, 0.55) and for those who had received continuous HRT therapy for more than 11 years (RR, 0.54).
         e. Estrogen alone increases risk of uterine cancer.
      2. Tamoxifen.
         a. Currently approved by FDA for use to reduce risk of breast cancer.
         b. After 4 years of follow-up, high-risk women participating in the Breast Cancer Prevention Trial experienced a 49% reduction in the incidence of breast cancer compared with placebo.
         c. Tamoxifen found to also reduce benign breast disease by 28%.
            (1) Disorders affected included adenosis, cysts, duct ectasia, fibrocystic disease, hyperplasia, metaplasia, fibroadenoma, and fibrosis (Tan-Chiu et al., 2003).
         d. The Study of Tamoxifen And Raloxifene (STAR) trial is currently underway to compare effectiveness of tamoxifen with raloxifene for reducing risk of breast cancer. See http://www.nsabp.pitt.edu/STAR/Index.html.
      3. Oral contraceptive use appears to cause a very small increase in risk of breast cancer but to reduce the risk of cancer of ovary and uterus.
      4. Estrogen exposure in the fetus (from diethylstilbestrol) is associated with vaginal cancer in adulthood.
   B. Anabolic steroids may be associated with liver cancer.
   C. Certain fertility drugs (i.e., menotropins [Pergonal]) may increase the risk for ovarian cancer.
   D. Growth hormones given to children may increase risk for leukemia.
   E. Immunosuppressive agents (for organ recipients) increase the risk of non-Hodgkin's lymphoma.
   F. Antineoplastic agents (especially alkylating agents) increase the risk of secondary cancers.
V. Assess combination risk factors to identify subpopulations at greatest risk.
   A. Synergistic effects of carcinogens (e.g., alcohol and tobacco).
   B. Hereditary predisposition and lifestyle choices (e.g., pigmented nevi syndrome and sun exposure).

VI. Assess other contributing factors.
  A. Socioeconomic status (SES).
   1. Correlations between SES and cancer exist but are not consistent.
   2. Low SES correlates with increased risk of cancers of the lung, cervix, stomach, and head and neck.
   3. High SES increases risk of breast, prostate, and colon cancers.
  B. Illiteracy (Davis et al., 2002).
   1. One in five Americans has low literacy skills; another 27% are marginally literate.
   2. Limits capacity to obtain, process, and understand both written and verbal cancer-related health education messages that recommend prevention, screening, and early detection.
  C. Unemployment, poor or substandard housing, inadequate or substandard nutritional status.
   1. May place day-to-day survival priorities over prevention, screening, and early detection.
   2. May modify immune status and increase exposures to risk factors.
  D. Inadequate access to health care and/or health insurance.
   1. Compromises access to high-quality and consistent screening, early detection, and follow-up care, which often results in detection of cancers too advanced for optimal outcomes.
  E. Motivation for preventive behavior (health belief model).
   1. Perceived susceptibility to cancer—evidence indicates that individuals at risk often are unaware of their risks (ask "How likely do you feel you are to develop cancer?").
   2. Perceived severity of cancer (ask "How serious do you feel cancer is?").
   3. Perceived benefits of preventive behavior (ask "Do you think you can decrease your risk for cancer by not smoking [or the habit in question]?").
   4. Perceived barriers to preventive action (ask "What problems do you think you may have lowering the fat content in your diet [or the behavior in question]?").

Nursing Diagnosis

I. Ineffective health maintenance related to insufficient knowledge of cancer prevention activities.

Outcome Identification

I. Client will assume responsibility for own wellness as measured by the following:
  A. Describing personal risk factors for cancer based on family history, age, exposures, and lifestyle.
  B. Stating intent to adopt behavioral strategies for reducing cancer risk or risks (e.g., smoking cessation, dietary modification, weight reduction, exercise, safe sex practices).

Planning and Implentation

I. Identify and personalize cancer risks.
  A. Risk assessment via three-generation family pedigree development and analysis.

  B. Comprehensive occupational and health history and analysis.

  C. Physical examination.

II. Facilitate lifestyle change.

  A. Smoking cessation (Agency for Health Care Policy and Research, 1996; NCI, 2003; Sargent & DiFranza, 2003).

   1. Act as a role model by not smoking.

   2. Ask about and record the tobacco-use status of every client.

   3. Assess willingness and readiness to quit.

   4. Advise every smoker to quit.

    a. Be clear. (Say, "I think it is important for you to quit smoking now, and I will help you.")

    b. Speak strongly. (Say, "As your clinician, I need you to know that quitting smoking is the most important thing you can do to protect your current and future health.")

    c. Personalize your advice. (Say, "You've already had one heart attack.")

    d. Mention the impact of smoking on children or others in the household. (Say, "You know your children need you.")

   5. Assist the client with a quit plan. Advise the smoker to do the following:

    a. Set a quit date, ideally within 2 weeks.

    b. Inform friends, family, and coworkers of plans to quit, and ask for support.

    c. Remove cigarettes from home, car, and workplace, and avoid smoking in these places.

    d. Review previous quit attempts—what helped, what led to relapse.

    e. Anticipate challenges, particularly during the critical first few weeks, including nicotine withdrawal.

   6. Give advice on successful quitting.

    a. Total abstinence is essential—not even a single puff.

    b. Drinking alcohol is strongly associated with relapse.

    c. Having other smokers in the household hinders successful quitting.

   7. Encourage use of nicotine replacement therapy.

    a. Both the nicotine patch and nicotine gum are effective pharmacotherapies for smoking cessation.

    b. Nicotine patch may be easier to use than the gum in most clinical settings.

   8. Keep culturally and educationally appropriate materials on cessation techniques readily available.

   9. Follow up.

   10. Counsel for relapse.

   11. Reinforce abstinence.

  B. Avoid sun exposure (Table 42-1).

  C. Eat healthy; exercise regularly and control weight (see Table 42-1).

  D. Limit viral exposures (HIV, HPV).

   1. Advocate for abstinence or monogamy.

   2. Encourage safe sex and condom use.

   3. Counsel against intravenous (IV) drug use, or educate about and facilitate access to sterile needle and syringe programs.

   4. Advocate that preventing pregnancy in infected women avoids fetal exposure.

  E. Avoid occupational carcinogen exposures, use protective clothing and/or devices, and follow safety procedures when exposure is mandatory.

  F. Encourage participation in chemoprevention trials.

TABLE 42-1
Evidence-Based Cancer Prevention Recommendations

DIETARY RECOMMENDATIONS	**THE 5 A DAY FOR BETTER HEALTH PROGRAM**
	▪ Officially launched in 1991, it is jointly sponsored by NCI and the Produce for Better Health Foundation, a nonprofit consumer education foundation representing the fresh, frozen, dried, canned, and juice fruit and vegetable industry.
	▪ The program recommends children ages 2-6 yr consume five servings of fruits and vegetables daily. Children over the age of 6 yr should eat six servings; active women and teens should eat seven, and active teen boys and men should eat nine, according to program guidelines.
	
	ACS (ACS, 2002, p. 10)
	▪ Eat a variety of healthful foods, with an emphasis on plant sources.
	  ● Eat five or more servings of a variety of vegetables and fruit each day.
	  ● Choose whole grains in preference to processed (refined) grains and sugars.
	  ● Limit consumption of red meats, especially high-fat and processed meats.
	  ● Choose foods that help maintain a healthful weight.
	▪ Maintain a healthful weight throughout life.
	  ● Balance caloric intake with physical activity.
	  ● Lose weight if currently overweight or obese.
	▪ If you drink alcoholic beverages, limit consumption.

VITAMIN SUPPLEMENTATION	**THE U.S. PREVENTIVE SERVICES TASK FORCE** (USPSTF, June 2003) ▪ The evidence is insufficient to recommend for or against the use of supplements of vitamins A, C, or E; multivitamins with folic acid; or antioxidant combinations for the prevention of cancer or cardiovascular disease. ▪ Recommends against the use of β-carotene supplements, either alone or in combination, for the prevention of cancer or cardiovascular disease.
PHYSICAL ACTIVITY	**ACS** (ACS, 2002, p. 10) ▪ Adopt a physically active lifestyle. ▪ *Adults:* engage in at least moderate activity for 30 min or more on 5 or more days of the week; 45 min or more of moderate to vigorous activity on 5 or more days per week may further enhance reductions in the risk of breast and colon cancer. ▪ *Children and adolescents:* engage in at least 60 min per day of moderate to vigorous physical activity at least 5 days per week.
LUNG CANCER PREVENTION	**AMERICAN COLLEGE OF CHEST PHYSICIANS** (Dragnev et al., 2003) ▪ For all individuals, smoking prevention should be strongly encouraged to decrease the risk of lung cancer. ▪ For all individuals, school-based and community-based interventions that are aimed at reducing tobacco exposure should be recommended, including a "life skills training" approach that is aimed at reducing tobacco, alcohol, and illicit drug use; campaigns with brief recurring antismoking messages; high tobacco excise taxes; and restrictions on smoking in the workplace. ▪ Smokers should be identified since smoking cessation reduces the risk of lung cancer.

TABLE 42-1
Evidence-Based Cancer Prevention Recommendations—cont'd

LUNG CANCER
PREVENTION—cont'd   **AMERICAN COLLEGE OF CHEST PHYSICIANS** (Dragnev et al., 2003)
- Current smokers should be advised to quit smoking, and, when appropriate, clinicians should prescribe and monitor pharmacotherapy. Individuals who smoke and want to quit also should have access to psychosocial treatment and behavioral modification therapies as indicated. There is sufficient-to-strong evidence that indicates these practices will help to increase long-term smoking abstinence rates.
- Individuals who are at risk for lung cancer and were treated with β-carotene, retinol, isotretinoin, or N-acetyl-cysteine for lung cancer prevention did not experience clinical benefit. There is also evidence that the use of β-carotene and isotretinoin for lung cancer chemoprevention in high-risk individuals may increase the risk for lung cancer, especially in individuals who continue to smoke. These agents should not be used outside of a clinical trial for primary, secondary, or tertiary lung cancer prevention.
- For individuals at risk for lung cancer and for clients with a history of lung cancer there are not yet sufficient data to recommend the use of any agent either alone or in combination for primary, secondary, or tertiary lung cancer chemoprevention outside of a clinical trial.

U.S. DEPARTMENT OF HEALTH AND HUMAN SERVICES (U.S. Department of Health and Human Services, Public Health Services, 2000)
- Evidence-based smoking cessation strategies were developed titled *Treating tobacco use and dependence.* Rockville, MD: U.S. Department of Health and Human Services, Public Health Service; http://guideline.gov/.

WHO (World Health Organization, 2003)
- 192 member nations unanimously adopted the Framework Convention on Tobacco Control, which required that countries impose severe restrictions on tobacco advertising, sponsorship, and promotion. The agreement also established new labeling—such as a large warning that will cover 30% of cigarette packages—and imposed both new clean indoor air controls and legislation to clamp down on tobacco smuggling. The United States has adopted this treaty, but ratification by Congress and the president is pending.

BREAST CANCER
PREVENTION   **USPSTF** (USPSTF, July 2002a)
- Recommends against routine use of tamoxifen or raloxifene for the primary prevention of breast cancer in women at low or average risk for breast cancer.
- Recommends that clinicians discuss chemoprevention with women at high risk for breast cancer and at low risk for adverse effects of chemoprevention. Clinicians should inform clients of the potential benefits and harms of chemoprevention.

GYNECOLOGIC
CANCERS   **USPSTF** (USPSTF, July 2002b)
- There is insufficient evidence to recommend for or against routine counseling of women about measures for the primary prevention of gynecologic cancers.
- Clinicians counseling women about contraceptive practices should include information on the potential benefits of the following with respect to gynecologic cancers: oral contraceptives, barrier contraceptives, tubal sterilization.

(Continued)

TABLE 42-1
Evidence-Based Cancer Prevention Recommendations—cont'd

GYNECOLOGIC CANCERS—cont'd	**USPSTF** (USPSTF, July 2002b) ■ Clinicians should promote maintaining desirable body weight, smoking cessation, and safe sex practices. These measures may reduce the incidence of certain gynecologic cancers and have other positive health benefits.
SKIN CANCER PREVENTION	**USPSTF** (USPSTF, October 2003) ■ Evidence is insufficient to recommend for or against routine counseling by primary care clinicians to prevent skin cancer. ACS (ACS, 2002, p. 23) ■ Avoid direct exposure to the sun between the hours of 10 AM and 4 PM, when ultraviolet rays are the most intense. ■ Wear hats with a brim wide enough to shade face, ears, and neck, as well as clothing that covers as much as possible of the arms, legs, and torso. ■ Cover exposed skin with a sunscreen lotion with a sun protection factor (SPF) of 15 or higher. ■ Avoid tanning beds and sun lamps, which provide an additional source of UV radiation.

NCI, National Cancer Institute; *ACS*, American Cancer Society; *UV*, ultraviolet.

III. Rationale.
   A. The Institute of Medicine reports that if sustained efforts were made to help people change their behavior, such as quitting smoking, and systems were in place to enable them to take advantage of cancer detection procedures, 60,000 cancer deaths and about 100,000 new cancer cases annually could be prevented by 2015.
   B. Behavior modifications that will save the most lives from cancer include helping people stop smoking, maintain a healthy diet, keep their weight under control, stimulate physical activity, and moderate their alcohol consumption.

Evaluation

The oncology nurse systematically and regularly evaluates the client's and/or family's responses to interventions to determine progress toward the achievement of expected outcomes. Relevant data are collected, and actual findings are compared with expected findings. Nursing diagnoses, outcomes, and plans of care are reviewed and revised as necessary.

REFERENCES

Agency for Health Care Policy and Research. (1996). Smoking cessation: Information for specialists. Publication 96-0694, No. 18. Rockville, MD: USDHHS, PHS, AHCPR, CDCP.

American Cancer Society (ACS). (2002). *Cancer prevention & early detection: Facts & figures 2003.* Atlanta: American Cancer Society.

Bingham, S.A., Day, N.E., Luben, R., et al. (2003). Dietary fibre in food and protection against colorectal cancer in the European Prospective Investigation into Cancer and Nutrition (EPIC): An observational study. *Lancet 361*(9368), 1496-1501.

Calle, E.E., Rodriquez, C., Walker-Thurmond, K., & Thun, M.J. (2003). Overweight, obesity, and mortality from cancer in a prospectively studied cohort of US adults. *New England Journal of Medicine 348*(17), 1625-1638.

Centers for Disease Control and Prevention (CDC). (2002). *US mortality public use data tape.* Atlanta: CDC.

Crum, C.P. (2002). The beginning of the end for cervical cancer? *New England Journal of Medicine 347*(21), 1703-1705.

Curry, S.J., Byers, T., & Hewitt, M. (2003). *Fulfilling the potential of cancer prevention and early detection. National Cancer Policy Board, Institute of Medicine National Research council of the National Academies.* Washington, D.C.: National Academies Press.

Davis, T.C., Williams, M.V., Marin, E., et al. (2002). Health literacy and cancer communication. *CA: A Cancer Journal for Clinicians 52*(3), 134-149.

Dragnev, K.H., Stover, D., & Dmitrovsky, E. (2003). Lung cancer prevention: The guidelines. *Chest 123*(1 Suppl.): 60S-71S.

Fisher, B., Costantino, J.P., Wickerham, D.L., et al. (1998). Tamoxifen for prevention of breast cancer: Report of the National Surgical Adjuvant Breast and Bowel Project P-1 Study. *Journal of the National Cancer Institute 90*(18), 1371-1388.

Giovannucci, E., Stampfer, M.J., Colditz, G.A., et al. (1998). Multivitamin use, folate, and colon cancer in women in the Nurses' Health Study. *Annuals of Internal Medicine* 129(7):517-524.

Go, W.L.W., Butrum, R.R., & Wong, D.A. (2003). Diet, nutrition and cancer prevention: The postgenomic era. *Journal of Nutrition 133,* 3830S-3836S.

Heath, C.W. (1996). Electromagnetic field exposure and cancer: A review of epidemiologic evidence. *CA: A Cancer Journal for Clinicians 46*(1), 29-44.

Janne, P.A., & Mayer, R.J. (2000). Chemoprevention of colorectal cancer. *New England Journal of Medicine 342*(26), 1960-1968.

Jemal, A., Tiwari, R.C., Murray, T., et al. (2004). Cancer statistics, 2004. *CA: A Cancer Journal for Clinicians 54*(1), 9-29.

Kant, A.K., Schatzkin, A., Graubard, B.I., & Schairer, B. (2000). A prospective study of diet quality and mortality in women. *Journal of the American Medical Association 283*(16), 2109-2115.

Karagas, M.R., Stannard, V.A., Mott, L.A., et al. (2002). Use of tanning devices and risk of basal cell and squamous cell skin cancers. *Journal of the National Cancer Institute 94*(3), 224-226.

Koutsky, L.A., Anlt, K.A., & Wheeler, C.M. (2002). A controlled trial of a human papillomavirus type 16 vaccine. *New England Journal of Medicine 347*(21), 1645-1651.

National Cancer Institute (NCI). (April 2001). *NCI, DCCPS, Surveillance Research Program, Cancer Statistics Branch, Surveillance, Epidemiology, and End Results Program Public-Use Data Tapes 1973-1998.* NIH, Bethesda, MD.

National Cancer Institute (NCI). (2003). Prevention and cessation of cigarette smoking: Control of tobacco use. Retrieved October 30, 2003 from the World Wide Web: http://www.cancer.gov/cancerinfo/pdq/prevention/control-of-tobacco-use.

National Cancer Institute (NCI). (1997). Questions and answers about beta carotene chemoprevention trials. Retrieved October 30, 2003 from the World Wide Web: http://cis.nci.nih.gov/fact/4_13.htm.

Reis, L.A., Eisner, M., Kosary C., et al. (2003). SEER cancer statistics review, 1975-2000. Bethesda, MD: National Cancer Institute.

Reynolds, T. (2003). Study seeks to clarify genetic basis of prostate cancer in African Americans. *Journal of the National Cancer Institute 95*(18), 1356-1357.

Rossouw, J.E., Anderson, G.L., Prentice, R.L., et al. (2002). Risks and benefits of estrogen plus progestin in healthy postmenopausal women: Principal results from the Women's Health Initiative randomized clinical trial. *Journal of the American Medical Association 288*(3), 321-333.

Sargent, J.D., & DiFranza, J.R. (2003). Tobacco control for clinicians who treat adolescents. *CA: A Cancer Journal for Clinicians 53*(2), 102-123.

Schernhammer, E.S., Kang, J.H., Chan, A.T., et al. (2004). A prospective study of aspirin use and the risk of pancreatic cancer in women. *Journal of the National Cancer Institute 96*(1), 22-28.

Tan-Chiu, E., Wang, J., Constantino, J.P., et al. (2003). Effects of tamoxifen on benign breast disease in women at high risk for breast cancer. *Journal of the National Cancer Institute 95*(4), 302-307.

Thompson, I.M., Goodman, P.J., Tangen, C.M., et al. (2003). The influence of finasteride on the development of prostate cancer. *New England Journal of Medicine 349*(3), 215-224.

Ulrike, P. (2003). Dietary fibre and colorectal adenoma in a colorectal cancer early detection programme. *Lancet 361*(9368), 1491-1495.

U.S. Department of Health and Human Services, Public Health Services. (2000). *Treating tobacco use and dependence.* Rockville, MD: US Department of Health and Human Services, Public Health Service; http://guideline.gov/.

U.S. Preventive Services Task Force (USPSTF). (July 2002a). Breast cancer—chemoprevention. Retrieved October 30, 2003 from the World Wide Web: http://www.ahcpr.gov/clinic/uspstf/uspsbrpv.htm.

U.S. Preventive Services Task Force (USPSTF). (July 2002b). Counseling—gynecological cancers. Retrieved October 30, 2003 from the World Wide Web: http://www.ahcpr.gov/clinic/uspstf/uspsgyca.htm.

U.S. Preventive Services Task Force (USPSTF). (June 2003). Routine vitamin supplementation to prevent cancer and cardiovascular disease, June 2003. Retrieved October 30, 2003 from the World Wide Web: http://www.ahcpr.gov/clinic/uspstf/uspsvita.htm.

U.S. Preventive Services Task Force (USPSTF). (October 2003). Skin cancer counseling. Retrieved October 30, 2003 from the World Wide Web: http://www.ahcpr.gov/clinic/uspstf/uspsskco.htm.

Wong, M., Pagano, J.S., Schuller, J.T., et al. (2002). New associations of human papillomavirus, simian virus 40, and Epstein-Barr virus with human cancer. *Journal of the National Cancer Institute 94*(24), 1832-1836.

World Health Organization (WHO). (April 2003). Global cancer rates could increase by 50% to 15 million by 2020. Retrieved May 14, 2003 from the World Wide Web: http://www.who.int/mediacentre/releases/2003/pr27/en/print.html.

Wu, K., Willett, W.C., Fuchs, C.S., et al. (2003). Calcium intake and risk of colon cancer in women and men. *Journal of the National Cancer Institute 94*(6), 437-446.

Zhang, S.M., Willett, W.C., Selhub, J., et al. (2003). Plasma folate, vit B_6, vit B_{12}, homocysteine and risk of breast cancer. *Journal of the National Cancer Institute 95*(5), 373-380.

43 Early Detection of Cancer

CANDIS MORRISON

Theory

I. Rationale.
   A. The best and most effective treatment for cancer is prevention.
   B. Early detection of cancer and effective therapy can result in decreased morbidity and mortality.
   C. Development of risk profiles and use of screening guidelines enhance screening efficacy and decrease costs.

II. Definitions.
   A. Secondary prevention.
      1. Allows for interventions that can prevent, postpone, or attenuate the symptomatic clinical state by identification of the potential for development of a disease or existence of a disease while the individual is asymptomatic.
      2. Emphasizes early diagnosis through application of screening and diagnostic examinations and tests and prompt treatment to halt the pathologic process, thereby shortening its duration and severity and enabling the person to return to a former state of health at the earliest time possible.
      3. Employs selective screening strategies to detect preclinical disease in the asymptomatic person at a time when the disease is presumed to be localized, for the purpose of decreasing morbidity and mortality.
   B. Surveillance.
      1. Regular ongoing monitoring of people who have already been identified as being at high risk.
      2. Based on established guidelines.
   C. Risk.
      1. Likelihood that exposure to a certain factor will influence the chance of developing a particular cancer, based on the national average (see Chapter 42).
   D. Diagnosis.
      1. Clinical problem-solving process applied to symptomatic clients or those asymptomatic clients with abnormal screening tests.

III. Screening.
   A. Although there are more than 100 different cancers, most lack proven screening interventions.
      1. Cancers of the breast, cervix, colorectal area, prostate, skin, and testes have widely accepted screening interventions.
      2. Only breast, cervix, and colorectal cancers have met the criteria for acceptance by the U.S Preventive Services Task Force (USPSTF, 2002).

B. Principles of screening tests.

    1. Utility screening tests are used to do the following:

        a. Identify asymptomatic persons with risk factors for disease.

        b. Detect occult disease and permit early treatment.

        c. Reassure clients found free of disease, with or without risk factors.

        d. Direct clients to genetic counseling in familial conditions when appropriate.

    2. Attributes of screening tests.

        a. Sensitivity—measure of the probability that a test result will be positive if the disease being investigated is present.

        b. Specificity—measure of the probability that a test result will be negative if the disease being investigated is not present.

        c. Predictive value.

            (1) Positive predictive value—the percentage of persons with a positive screening test result who actually have the disease.

            (2) Negative predictive value—the percentage of persons with a negative screening test result who clearly do not have the disease.

        d. Ease of administration.

        e. Acceptability to clients.

            (1) The following test characteristics serve to enhance compliance and utilization and minimize short- or long-term side effects.

                (a) Safe (has few potential complications).

                (b) Convenient (preferably readily available during health care visits).

                (c) Relatively low cost (Rimer et al., 2001).

    3. Characteristics of disease that may justify risks and costs associated with any screening program.

        a. It is sufficiently common to justify the effort to detect it.

        b. It is highly prevalent in a preclinical state.

        c. Mortality and morbidity are substantial.

        d. An effective screening test with high sensitivity and specificity is available.

        e. Effective treatment is available (and acceptable) to alter the natural history of the disease.

        f. There is a presymptomatic period during which detection and treatment may occur.

        g. Presymptomatic treatment improves outcomes (Rimer et al., 2001).

    4. Characteristics of the population.

        a. Sufficiently high prevalence of disease.

        b. Accessible to screening.

        c. Likely to comply with subsequently recommended diagnostic tests and treatment (Rimer et al., 2001).

    5. Screening biases.

        a. Biases invalidate comparisons of stage distribution or survival between series of asymptomatic screen-detected and symptomatic screen-detected disease.

            (1) Well-designed, randomized trials generally control for these biases (Rimer et al., 2001).

        b. Types of biases.

            (1) Lead-time bias.

                (a) Occurs when disease is detected earlier but the detection does not affect mortality. Survival time appears to be longer but actually is not.

(b) Appearance of improved survival in cases where diagnosis is made by a screening procedure. Results in an earlier diagnosis because of the screening procedure. Lengthens the interval from diagnosis to death rather than lengthening life.

(c) This bias is most notable when short follow-up periods, such as 5-year survival rates, are used.

(d) Determined by the sensitivity of the test, testing interval, and duration of the preclinical stage (Rimer et al., 2001).

(2) Length bias.

(a) At any point in time, a population consists of persons with aggressive, symptomatic disease and symptomatic, less aggressive disease.

(b) Screening identifies both, but, because a greater proportion has less aggressive disease, it appears that survival is lengthened because the average lifespan observed increases.

(c) Improved survival in the screened population derives, at least in part, from the growth properties of the tumor rather than from the benefits of the screening (Rimer et al., 2001).

(3) Selection bias.

(a) Occurs if clients undergoing screening have better health habits than the general population or have lower mortality or longer survival because they are more resistant to the disease or more compliant with therapy (Rimer et al., 2001).

6. Outcome measures in cancer screening.

   a. Short-term measures.

   (1) Number of individuals in the target population offered screening.

   (2) Number and proportion of individuals in the target population who received screening.

   (3) Number and proportion of the target population examined by multiple screens.

   (4) Number or prevalence of preclinical cancers detected in persons with abnormal screens brought to definitive diagnosis or follow-up.

   (5) Cost per cancer detected.

   (6) Sensitivity and specificity of the screening test.

   (7) Positive and negative predictive values of the screening test.

   b. Long-term measures.

   (1) Stage distribution of detected cancers.

   (2) Case-fatality rate of screened individuals.

   (3) Site-specific cancer mortality rate of screened target population.

   (4) Total costs.

   (5) Impact of early detection on quality of life (positive and negative); for example, prostate-specific antigen (PSA) screening controversy based on the fact that a causal relationship between screening and decreased mortality has not been proven, nor has the value of aggressive therapy versus watchful waiting been proven (Carroll et al., 2001).

C. Types of screening.

1. Mass screening—screen an entire population (e.g., for phenylketonuria [PKU]).

2. Selective or prescriptive screening—high-risk populations, looking for a specific problem or condition (e.g., for *BRCA1* gene, Tay-Sachs disease, sickle cell anemia, myelomeningocele).

3. Single screening—for a single defect or condition (e.g., for hypertension).

    4. Multiple screening—two or more defects or conditions (e.g., school vision and hearing screening).

    5. Multiphasic screening—profile over time (e.g., Denver Developmental Screening Test).

    6. Combinations.

        a. Multiple or mass screening (e.g., health fairs for height, weight, blood pressure, hematocrit level).

        b. Selective and mass screening (e.g., vision or hearing).

        c. Selective and single screening (e.g., sickle cell anemia).

        d. Multiphasic and mass screening (e.g., Denver Developmental Screening Test).

        e. Multiphasic and selective screening (e.g., vision).

  D. Screening modalities for early detection of cancer.

    1. Radiographs.

    2. Cytologic specimens.

    3. Tumor markers (Table 43-1).

        a. Substances that may be detected in higher than normal quantities in fluids or tissues of some clients with cancer.

        b. Produced by tumor itself or body's reaction to the cancer.

        c. Generally used in conjunction with other modality (i.e., radiographs).

        d. Problems with tumor marker use.

           (1) Not elevated in every person with the cancer (especially in early stages of the disease).

           (2) May be elevated in persons with benign conditions.

           (3) Many markers not specific to a particular type of cancer since the marker can be elevated by more than one type of cancer (National Cancer Institute [NCI], 1998).

TABLE 43-1
Characteristics of the Most Commonly Used Tumor Markers

Marker	Utility	Comments
Prostate-specific antigen (PSA)	Useful in monitoring effectiveness of prostate cancer treatment and in evaluating for recurrence after treatment has ended	May be elevated in men with benign prostate conditions and thus cannot distinguish between these and malignant conditions.
Prostatic acid phosphatase (PAP)	Not used as frequently as PSA to diagnosis prostate cancer	Elevations also associated with testicular cancer, leukemia, non-Hodgkin's lymphoma, and nonmalignant conditions, such as Paget's disease, osteoporosis, cirrhosis, pulmonary embolism, and hyperparathyroidism.
CA 125	Elevated in ovarian cancer and some nonmalignant conditions	Used to monitor treatment for ovarian cancer or to detect recurrence. Not all ovarian cancers produce CA 125. May also be elevated in nonmalignant conditions: endometriosis, pelvic inflammatory disease, peritonitis, pancreatitis, liver disease, and any condition that inflames the pleura. Also, menstruation and pregnancy can elevate this marker.

TABLE 43-1
Characteristics of the Most Commonly Used Tumor Markers—cont'd

Marker	Utility	Comments
Carcinoembryonic antigen (CEA)	Colorectal cancer; other cancers can also produce elevated levels—melanoma, lymphoma, lung, breast, pancreas, stomach, bladder, kidney, cervix, thyroid, liver, ovary	Monitoring colorectal cancer (especially when disease has metastasized). Used after treatment to check for recurrence. Mild elevations common in smokers. Elevations seen in nonmalignant conditions such as inflammatory bowel disease, pancreatitis, liver disease.
α-Fetoprotein (α-FP)	Normally produced by the developing fetus; elevation in adult suggests either primary liver or germ cell cancer	Rare elevations seen with stomach cancer. Noncancerous conditions can cause elevations—hepatitis, ataxia-telangiectasia, Wiskott-Aldrich syndrome.
Human chorionic gonadotropin (HCG)	Normally produced by the placenta during pregnancy; used to screen for choriocarcinoma; elevations may also indicate cancer of the testis, ovary, liver, stomach, pancreas, and lung	Marijuana use may elevate levels of this marker.
CA 19-9	Colorectal cancer and other GI malignancies, such as pancreatic, stomach, and bile duct cancer	In pancreatic cancer, higher levels are associated with more advanced disease. Noncancerous conditions that may produce elevations of CA 19-9 include pancreatitis, gallstones, cholecystitis, and cirrhosis.
CA 15-3	Advanced breast cancer	Rarely elevated in early-stage breast cancers. May be elevated with benign breast or ovarian disease, pelvic inflammatory disease and hepatitis, pregnancy and lactation.
CA 27-29	Breast cancer; may also be elevated in cancers of the colon, stomach, kidney, lung, pancreas, ovary, uterus, and liver	Check for recurrence of stage II and III breast cancer. Nonmalignant conditions (pregnancy, endometriosis, ovarian cysts, kidney and liver disease, benign breast disease).
Lactate dehydrogenase (LDH)	Most cancers	Almost all cancers cause elevations of LDH; thus cannot be used in diagnosis but may be a helpful monitoring test. Elevations from nonmalignant conditions (heart failure, lung or liver disease, hypothyroidism, anemia).
Neuron-specific enolase (NSE)	Small cell lung cancer (SCLC); neuroblastoma; Wilms' tumor; melanoma; cancers of thyroid, kidney, testicle, and pancreas	Greatest utility in clients with neuroblastoma and SCLC in whom this marker can provide data about extent of disease, prognosis, and response to therapy.

From National Cancer Institute (NCI). (1998). Tumor markers. Retrieved November 30, 2003 from the World Wide Web: http://cis.nci.nih.gov/fact.
GI, Gastrointestinal.

E. Recommendations for cancer screening may differ among organizations because of different organizational values, timing of guideline updates, and the manner in which they evaluate data (Rathorre et al., 2000).

F. Recommendations for specific cancers.

   1. Breast cancer.

      a. Mortality.

         (1) Estimated at 40,110 in 2004; second only to lung cancer (68,510).

         (2) Age-adjusted mortality stable between 1973 and 1991. Thereafter, a reduction of about 2% per year possibly attributed to improved treatments and screening (Jemal et al., 2004).

      b. Risk.

         (1) Lifetime risk estimated at one in eight to one in nine women based on life expectancy of 85 years (Jemal et al., 2002).

      c. Modalities used for early diagnosis. No one modality alone is sufficient (NCI, 2002).

         (1) Screening mammography.

         (2) Clinical breast examination.

         (3) Breast self-examination.

         (4) Biopsy of abnormalities found on screening.

         (5) Gail model.

            (a) Tool to assess 5-year and lifetime risk of developing invasive breast cancer based on characteristics of age, menarche age, age at first live birth, number of first-degree relatives with breast cancer, number of previous benign breast biopsies, atypical hyperplasia in a previous breast biopsy, and race.

            (b) Based on average age of 60 years for women in the United States (Gail et al., 1989).

         (6) Genetic testing for *BRCA1* and *BRCA2* mutations that are responsible for the majority of hereditary breast cancers (only about 5% to 7% of all breast cancers) is available, although it is not currently recommended for the general population by any cancer organization. This testing may be offered to family members of clients with features indicating an increased likelihood of a *BRCA* mutation.

            (a) Multiple cases of early breast cancer in family.

            (b) Ovarian cancer (with a family history of breast cancer).

            (c) Breast and ovarian cancer in the same woman.

            (d) Bilateral breast cancer.

            (e) Ashkenazi Jewish heritage.

            (f) Male breast cancer (Jardines et al., 2003).

         (7) Screening recommendations (Table 43-2).

   2. Colorectal cancer.

      a. Mortality.

         (1) Estimated 56,730 deaths from colorectal cancer in the United States in 2004 (Jemal et al., 2004).

      b. Risk.

         (1) Third most frequently diagnosed cancer in the United States.

         (2) Estimated 106,370 cases of colon cancer and 40,570 new cases of rectal cancer in the United States in 2004 (Jemal et al., 2004).

      c. Modalities for early diagnosis.

         (1) Screening begins at age 50 years in asymptomatic persons without family history.

TABLE 43-2
Screening Recommendations

Agency/Organization	Population	Test and Schedule
BREAST CANCER		
ACS	Women starting at age 20 yr	Breast self-examination (BSE) monthly
		Clinical breast examination (CBE):
		ages 20-39 yr, every 3 yr; annually thereafter
		Mammography annually ages 40 yr and thereafter
NCCN	Normal-risk women	Ages 20-39 yr:
		CBE every 1-3 yr
		Periodic BSE encouraged
		Ages 40 yr and older:
		Annual CBE
		Annual mammography
		Periodic BSE encouraged
	High-risk women	
	Women who have received prior thoracic irradiation initiate screening 8-10 yr after radiation exposure or at age 40 yr (if comes first)	Ages 25 yr and older
		CBE every 6-12 mo
		Annual mammography
		Periodic BSE encouraged
	Women over 35 yr with a 5-yr risk of invasive breast cancer ≥1.7% (based on Gail model)	CBE every 6-12 mo
		Annual mammography
		Periodic BSE encouraged
	Women with strong family history or genetic predisposition defined as:	Option of chemoprevention (i.e., tamoxifen) (Nolvadex)
	Family has >2 breast cancer cases and one or more cases of ovarian cancer *or*	Annual mammography and CBE 5-10 yr before age of cancer onset in index case
	Family has >3 breast cancer cases diagnosed before 50 yr *or*	Annual mammography and CBE starting at age 25 yr for those with genetic predisposition
	Family has sister pairs diagnosed before 50 yrs with two breast cancers, two ovarian cancers, or one cancer of each type in pair	
COLORECTAL CANCER		
ACS	Both genders, starting at age 50 yr	Fecal occult blood test (FOBT) annually, *or*
		Flexible sigmoidoscopy (flex sig) every 5 yr, *or*
		FOBT yearly and flex sig every 5 yr, *or*
		Double-contrast barium enema (DCBE) every 5 yr (yearly FOBT recommended), *or*
		Colonoscopy every 10 yr (yearly FOBT recommended)
NCCN	Normal risk, age ≥50yr asymptomatic, negative family history	FOBT annually with flexible sigmoidoscopy every 5 yr, *or*
		Colonoscopy every 10 yr *or*
		DCBE every 5 yr
	Patients with inflammatory bowel disease	
	Left-sided colitis	Screening begins 15 yr after onset of symptoms

(Continued)

TABLE 43-2
Screening Recommendations—cont'd

Agency/Organization	Population	Test and Schedule
NCCN—*cont'd*	Pancolitis	Screening begins 8 yrs after onset of symptoms. Screening for both consists of colonoscopy every 1-2 yr, including 4-quadrant biopsy every 10 cm. Additional sampling of strictures, masses, and polyps
PROSTATE CANCER		
ACS	Men age 50 yr and above	Digital rectal examination (DRE) and prostate-specific antigen (PSA) annually in men with a life expectancy of at least 10 yr
NCCN	Normal risk: age greater than 50 yr and life expectancy >10 yr	DRE and PSA annually starting at age 50 yr
	High risk: African American and/or positive family history and life expectancy greater than 10 yr	DRE and PSA annually starting at age 45 yr
	For men with elevations of PSA (4-10 ng/ml)	Percent-free PSA or transrectal ultrasound-guided biopsy (TRUS)
CERVICAL CANCER		
ACS	Screening should begin within 3 yr of initiation of vaginal intercourse (no later than 21 yr of age)	Pap smear yearly with conventional test or every 2 yr using liquid-based Pap tests; starting at age 30 yr, women who have had two normal consecutive tests may be screened every 2-3 yr; women 70 yr and over with three or more normal tests and no abnormal Pap tests in the past 10 yr may elect to discontinue screening
American College of Obstetricians and Gynecologists	Women with one or more high-risk factors associated with the development of cervical intraepithelial neoplasia (CIN)	Pap smears as frequently as 2-6 mo
NCCN	Women with normal histology or CIN I on biopsy	Pap test at 6 mo (possibly with human papillomavirus DNA testing)
	Women with CIN II or III on cervical biopsy	Cold-knife conization, LEEP, cryotherapy, or laser ablation
	Women with high-grade squamous intraepithelial lesions on Pap test	Colposcopy and cold-knife conization or LEEP to obtain tissue for evaluation
NCI, U.S. Preventive Services Task Force, and the Society of Thoracic Radiology	Asymptomatic persons	Screening not recommended

From Aberle, D.R. et al.: A consensus statement of the Society of Thoracic Radiology: Screening for lung cancer with helical computed tomography. *J Thorac Imag*, 2001, 16: 65-68; American Cancer Society (ACS): Breast cancer facts and figures 2003-2004. Retrieved January 5, 2004 from the World Wide Web: http://www.cancer.org/docroot/STT/content/STT_lx_Breast_Cancer_Facts_Figures_2003_2004.asp; American College of Obstetrician-Gynecologists (ACOG). ACOG Practice Bulletin: *Clinical Management Guidelines for obstetrician-gynecologists*, 102(2): 7-27, 2003; Ginsberg, R., et al.: Lung cancer surgical practice guidelines: Society of Surgical Oncology practice guidelines, 1997, *Oncology* 11, 892-895; Jemal A, et al. Cancer statistics, *CA: A Cancer Journal for Clinicians, 2003*, 53, 5-26; National Comprehensive Cancer Network (NCCN). *Practice guidelines in oncology, 2*. Washington, D.C., 2003, National Comprehensive Cancer Network; U.S. Preventive Services Task Force (USPSTF): *Guide to clinical preventive services*. Washington, D.C., 2002, U.S. Department of Health and Human Services, Public Health Service, Agency for Health Care Policy and Research.
ACS, American Cancer Society; *NCI*, National Cancer Institute; *NCCN*, National Comprehensive Cancer Network; *DNA*, deoxyribonucleic acid, *LEEP*, Loop electrosurgical excision procedure.

(2) Fecal occult blood test (FOBT).
  (a) Must evaluate any positive test.
  (b) Prescribed diet.
  (c) Three consecutive stool specimens.
  (d) Not by rectal examination (use stool cards).
(3) Flexible sigmoidoscopy using 60-cm or longer scope.
(4) Colonoscopy.
(5) Genetic screening—adenomatous polyposis coli (APC) testing.
  (a) Colorectal cancer with an early age of onset, *or*
  (b) Clustering of same or related cancers in close relative (colorectal, ovarian, endometrial, duodenal, stomach, small bowel, ureteral, renal pelvis, sebaceous adenomas, or sebaceous carcinomas), *or*
  (c) Multiple colorectal carcinomas or more than 10 adenomas in same person, *or*
  (d) Family with known hereditary syndrome associated with cancer regardless of known genetic mutation (National Comprehensive Cancer Network [NCCN], 2003).
(6) Biopsy of polyps.
(7) Insufficient data on virtual colonoscopy to permit recommendation regarding its use (NCCN, 2003).
  d. Screening recommendations (see Table 43-2).
3. Prostate cancer.
  a. Mortality.
    (1) Estimated 29,900 deaths in 2004 (Jemal et al., 2004).
  b. Risk.
    (1) Most commonly diagnosed cancer in American men and second leading cause of cancer deaths.
    (2) American men have about a one in six chance of developing this cancer (USPSTF, 2002).
    (3) The estimated number of new cases was 230,110 in 2004 (Jemal et al., 2004).
    (4) African American men and men with a father or brother with prostate cancer are at higher risk (USPSTF, 2002).
  c. Modalities for early diagnosis. More than 70% of prostate cancers are diagnosed in organ-confined state at diagnosis.
    (1) Digital rectal examination (DRE).
    (2) Serum PSA.
      (a) A glycoprotein secreted by prostatic epithelial cells.
      (b) PSA more than 4 ng/ml increases chance of positive prostate biopsy to almost 25% (NCCN, 2003).
      (c) PSA alone can provide nearly 90% specificity.
      (d) Must follow velocity of change, as well as absolute PSA quantity.
    (3) Biopsy indicated for PSA more than 4 ng/ml that is rising (USPSTF, 2002).
  d. Screening recommendations (see Table 43-2).
4. Cervical cancer.
  a. Mortality.
    (1) Estimated 3900 expected deaths in 2004 (Jemal et al., 2004).
    (2) Since 1950 dramatic decreases in death rates attributed to screening and early detection (Jemal et al., 2003).

    b. Risk.
        (1) Estimated 10,520 new cases expected in the United States in 2004 (Jemal et al., 2004).
    c. Modalities for early diagnosis.
        (1) Papanicolaou (Pap) smear.
        (2) Pelvic examination.
        (3) Biopsy of any grossly visible abnormalities.
        (4) Colposcopy is primary method for evaluation of abnormal Pap tests.
            (a) Involves viewing the cervix though a long–focal length, dissecting-type microscope at a magnification of 10 to 16 times.
            (b) Acetic acid (4%) is applied before viewing, which allows a directed biopsy.
    d. Screening recommendations (see Table 43-2).
  5. Lung cancer.
    a. Mortality.
        (1) Number one cancer killer in the United States for both genders (Jemal et al., 2004).
        (2) Estimated death rate approximately 160,440 in 2004 (Jemal et al., 2004).
    b. Risk.
        (1) Estimated 173,770 new cases expected in the United States in 2004 (Jemal et al., 2004).
    c. Modalities for early diagnosis.
        (1) Chest x-ray.
        (2) Sputum cytology.
            (a) More effective in cases of squamous cell carcinoma than in adenocarcinoma (Melamed, 2000).
            (b) Clinical trials show no difference in lung cancer cases detected or mortality when sputum cytology added to chest x-ray (Melamed, 2000).
        (3) Only therapy associated with high cure rate of lung cancer is surgical resection of early disease.

Assessment

  I. Cancer-related evaluation.
    A. Client assessment.
      1. Components necessary for client's individual risk profile.
        a. History.
           (1) Demographic—age, gender, race, date and place of birth, occupation, insurance coverage.
           (2) Chief complaint—reason for seeking examination. If related to a symptom, a complete symptom analysis is mandatory.
           (3) History of present illness.
               (a) Onset of symptom.
               (b) Location of pain.
               (c) Duration.
               (d) Characteristics.
               (e) Aggravating factors.
               (f) Relieving factors.
               (g) Timing.

(4) Allergies, current medications.

(5) Past medical history—previous state of health, previous cancer and/or cancer treatment, chronic illnesses, surgeries, hospitalizations.

(6) Family history—medical and cancer history in relatives.

(7) Occupational history (see Chapter 42).

(8) Social history (e.g., smoking, drinking, drug use, sexual habits, exercise).

(9) Review of systems.

    (a) Weight—present, usual, recent gain or loss.

    (b) Performance status—previous and present level of activity; note any weakness, fatigue, malaise.

    (c) Skin—changes in warts or moles; bleeding; change in sensation, any new lesions.

    (d) Head and neck—pain; tenderness; difficulty swallowing or chewing; hoarseness; discharge from eyes, ears, nose.

    (e) Lymphatic—lymphadenopathy, lymph node tenderness.

    (f) Respiratory—cough, pain, dyspnea, hemoptysis, shortness of breath.

    (g) Cardiac—hypertension, dyspnea, orthopnea, chest pain.

    (h) Gastrointestinal—change in appetite, pain, nausea, vomiting, change in bowel pattern.

    (i) Genitourinary—change in urinary pattern, hematuria, change in force or caliber of stream, pain.

    (j) Gynecologic—discharge, nonmenstrual or intermenstrual bleeding, bloating, enlarged abdominal girth.

    (k) Endocrine—flushing, sweating, tachycardia, palpitations, polyuria, polydipsia, appetite disturbance.

    (l) Hematologic—bruising, anemia, petechiae, purpura, bleeding disorder, anemia, fatigue, fever, infections, night sweats.

    (m) Musculoskeletal—pain, stiffness, limitation of movement.

    (n) Neurologic—headache; vertigo; seizures; visual disturbances; sensory, motor, or cognitive deficits.

    (o) Immune system—fever, chills, frequent infections (particularly respiratory).

  b. Risk factors (see Chapter 42).

B. Cancer-directed physical examination.

  1. Even in the absence of symptoms, the complete procedure should include examination of the skin, mouth, lymph nodes, breasts, cervix, pelvis, testicles, rectum, and prostate.

  2. Frequency.

    a. Cancer checkup every 3 years in asymptomatic individuals under 40 years of age.

    b. Annual checkups for those over 40 years of age.

  3. Remaining examination is directed by presence of abnormal findings.

  4. Specific foci.

    a. Skin.

      (1) Inspection of all cutaneous and mucous membrane surfaces.

      (2) Sun-exposed areas, such as face, chest, back, arms, legs, scalp, interdigital webs, and axillae; palms of hands and soles of feet deserve particular attention.

      (3) Regularity of color and surface, scaling, or bleeding.

b. Oral cavity.
  (1) Inspection for color and integrity of mucous membranes, tongue, lesions or plaques. Include area under tongue.
  (2) Palpation for masses and tenderness.

c. Breasts.
  (1) Clinical breast examination consists of systematic steps.
    (a) Inspection for asymmetry, dimpling, skin changes, irregular venous pattern, nipple direction, and nipple discharge.
    (b) Palpation for supraclavicular and infraclavicular nodes and for axillary tenderness, masses, and nodules.

d. Female genitalia.
  (1) Inspection for masses, asymmetry, lesions, discharge, and bleeding.
  (2) External palpation for masses, tenderness, shape and consistency of abdominal organs, including uterus, ovaries, and colon.
  (3) Pelvic examination—note mucosal integrity and color; presence of lesions, bleeding, or friability; discharge; constriction; nodules; masses.
  (4) Rectal examination—note external lesions, sphincter tone, masses, tenderness, constriction, bleeding.
  (5) Stool for occult blood.

e. Male genitalia.
  (1) Inspection for masses, shape of scrotum, cutaneous lesions, or nodules.
  (2) Palpation for tenderness, masses, consistency, contour, scrotal contents (testes, epididymis), and inguinal adenopathy.
  (3) Palpation of prostate gland for nodules, masses, tenderness, size, texture, and firmness.
  (4) Rectal examination (DRE)—note external lesions, masses, sphincter tone, constriction, masses, tenderness, and bleeding.
  (5) Stool for occult blood.

C. Screening and diagnostic tests (see Table 43-2).

Nursing Diagnoses

I. Deficient knowledge regarding recommendations for cancer screening and early detection.

II. Health-seeking behaviors: participation in appropriate cancer screening and early detection tests and evaluations.

Outcome Identification

I. Client identifies personal risk factors for cancer.
  A. Client discusses recommendations for cancer screening and early detection.

II. Client participates in cancer screening and early detection activities as recommended.

Planning and Implementation

I. Improve participation in screening programs.
  A. Target high-risk groups (e.g., elderly, socioeconomically disadvantaged) within respective community.

  B. Personalize potential participant's risk by use of health history and risk profiles.

  C. Use media resources to publicize benefits of screening and early detection.

 II. Enhance quality of screening programs.

  A. Collect data to evaluate control of screening.

   1. Number screened.

   2. Proportion of population screened once, twice, or more.

   3. Detected prevalence of preclinical disease.

   4. Percentage of false-positive and false-negative results.

   5. Cost per case.

   6. Proportion of positive findings brought to diagnosis and treatment.

   7. Costs of follow-up of false-positive results.

III. Implement client education.

  A. Teach screening recommendations, and monitor compliance.

  B. Initiate public education on early detection in schools and workplaces.

  C. Teach and monitor self-examination procedures (see Table 43-2).

  D. Teach "seven warning signals of cancer" (mnemonic CAUTION).

   1. **C**hange in bowel or bladder habits.

   2. **A** sore that does not heal.

   3. **U**nusual bleeding or discharge.

   4. **T**hickening or lump in breast or elsewhere.

   5. **I**ndigestion or difficulty swallowing.

   6. **O**bvious change in wart or mole.

   7. **N**agging cough or hoarseness.

IV. Provide education and follow-up care for clients with positive screening test results.

  A. Identify resources for cancer education and information.

  B. Facilitate referral for further evaluation.

  C. Reinforce importance of timely evaluation.

  D. Discuss implications of positive screening test results, and describe confirmatory evaluation.

Evaluation

The oncology nurse systematically and regularly evaluates the client's and/or family's responses to interventions to determine progress toward the achievement of expected outcomes. Relevant data are collected, and actual findings are compared with expected findings. Nursing diagnoses, outcomes, and plans of care are reviewed and revised as necessary.

REFERENCES

Aberle, D.R., Gamsu, G., Henschke, C.I., et al. (2001). A consensus statement of the Society of Thoracic Radiology: Screening for lung cancer with helical computed tomography. *Journal of Thoracic Imaging 16*, 65-68.

American Cancer Society (ACS). (2003). Breast cancer facts and figures 2003-2004. Retrieved January 5, 2004 from the World Wide Web: http://www.cancer.org/docroot/STT/content/STT_1x_Breast_Cancer_Facts_Figures_2003-2004.asp.

American College of Obstetrician-Gynecologists (ACOG). (2003). *ACOG Practice Bulletin: Clinical Management Guidelines for Obstetrician-Gynecologists 102*(2), 7-27.

Carroll, R.R., Lee, K.K., Fuks, Z.Y., & Kantoff, P.W. (2001). Cancer of the prostate. In V.T. DeVita, S. Hellman, & S.A. Rosenberg (Eds.). *Cancer: Principles and practice of oncology* (6th ed). Philadelphia: Lippincott Williams & Wilkins, pp. 1411-1479.

Gail, M.H., Brinton, L.A., Byar, D.P., et al. (1989). Projecting individualized probabilities of developing breast cancer for white females who are being examined annually. *Journal of the National Cancer Institute 20*(81), 1870-1886.

Ginsberg, R., Roth, J., & Fergusson, M. (1997). Lung cancer surgical practice guidelines: Society of Surgical Oncology practice guidelines. *Oncology 11*, 892-895.

Jardines, L., Haffty, B.G., Doroshow, J.H., et al. (2003). Breast cancer overview. Risk factors, screening, genetic testing, and prevention. In R. Pazdur, L.R. Coia, W.J. Hoskins, & L.D. Wagman (Eds.). *Cancer management: A multidisciplinary approach* (7th ed.). Philadelphia: F.A. Davis Co., pp. 163-214.

Jemal, A., Tiwari, R.C., Murray, T. et al. (2004). Cancer statistics, 2004. *CA: A Cancer Journal for Clinicians 54*, 8-29.

Jemal, A., Murray, T., Samuels, A. et al. (2003). Cancer statistics, 2003. *CA: A Cancer Journal for Clinicians 53*, 5-26.

Melamed, M.R. (2000). Lung cancer screening results in the National Cancer Institute New York study. *Cancer 89*(11, Suppl.), 2356-2362.

National Cancer Institute (NCI). (2002). *SEER Program public use data tapes 1973-1999*. Bethesda, MD: National Cancer Institute.

National Cancer Institute (NCI). (1998). Tumor markers. Retrieved November 30, 2003 from the World Wide Web: http://cis.nci.nih.gov/fact.

National Comprehensive Cancer Network (NCCN). (2003). *Practice guidelines in oncology, 2*. Jenkintown, PA: National Comprehensive Cancer Network.

Rathorre, S.S., McGreevey, J.D., & Schulman, K.A. (2000). Mandated coverage for cancer-screening services: Whose guidelines do states follow? *American Journal of Preventive Medicine 19*, 71-78.

Rimer, B.K., Schildkraut, J., & Hiatt, R.A. (2001). Cancer screening. In V.T. DeVita, S. Hellman, & S.A. Rosenberg (Eds.). *Cancer: Principles and practice of oncology* (6th ed.). Philadelphia: Lippincott Williams & Wilkins, pp. 627-640.

U.S. Preventive Services Task Force (USPSTF). (2002). *Guide to clinical preventive services*. Washington, D.C.: U.S. Department of Health and Human Services, Public Health Service, Agency for Health Care Policy and Research.

PART EIGHT

PROFESSIONAL PERFORMANCE

44 Application of the *Statement on the Scope and Standards of Oncology Nursing Practice* and Evidence-Based Practice

LINDA U. KREBS

STANDARDS OF ONCOLOGY NURSING PRACTICE

I. Overview.
   A. Originally developed in 1979 by the Oncology Nursing Society in collaboration with the American Nurses Association, the Standards were revised in 1987, 1996, and 2004.
   B. Applicable to all roles and settings in which oncology nurses care for clients.
   C. Emphasize the importance of the following:
      1. Interdisciplinary and intradisciplinary collaboration and collegiality.
      2. Ethical practice.
      3. Recognition of diversity and the need for cultural competence.
      4. Ensuring quality cancer care.
      5. Appropriate resource utilization (Brant & Wickham, 2004).
   D. Serve as a powerful guide for ensuring quality cancer care (Dorsett, 2000).
   E. Indicate to society at large that oncology nursing is able to define and control the quality of oncology nursing practice (Nelson, 2003).
II. Definitions.
   A. Standard—authoritative statement that is enunciated and promulgated by the profession by which the quality of practice, service, or education can be judged (Brant & Wickham, 2004).
   B. Client/patient—the individual, family, group, or community for whom the nurse provides specifically planned services (Brant & Wickham, 2004).
III. Components of each standard.
   A. Standard statement.
   B. Rationale—explanation of the underlying reason for the standard.
   C. Measurement criteria—relevant, measurable indicators that demonstrate compliance with the standard.
IV. Standards of Care (Box 44-1).
   A. Encompass the professional nursing actions and activities as carried out by the oncology nurse and include the following:
      1. Assessment.
      2. Diagnosis.

BOX 44-1
STANDARDS OF CARE

Standard I. Assessment
The oncology nurse systematically and continually collects data regarding the health status of the patient.

Standard II. Diagnosis
The oncology nurse analyzes assessment data to determine nursing diagnoses.

Standard III. Outcome Identification
The oncology nurse identifies expected outcomes individualized to the patient.

Standard IV. Planning
The oncology nurse develops an individualized and holistic plan of care that prescribes interventions to attain expected outcomes.

Standard V. Implementation
The oncology nurse implements the plan of care to achieve the identified expected outcomes for the patient.

Standard VI. Evaluation
The oncology nurse systematically and regularly evaluates the patient's response to interventions in order to determine progress toward achievement of expected outcomes.

Reprinted from Brant, JM & Wickham, RS, editors: *Statement on the scope and standards of oncology nursing practice,* Pittsburgh, 2004, Oncology Nursing Society, pp. 15-31.

      3. Outcome identification.
      4. Planning.
      5. Implementation.
      6. Evaluation (Brant & Wickham, 2004).
  B. Address each of the 14 high-incidence problem areas common to clients cared for by oncology nurses and include the following:
      1. Health promotion.
      2. Patient/family education.
      3. Coping.
      4. Comfort.
      5. Nutrition.
      6. Complementary and alternative medicine
      7. Protective mechanisms.
      8. Mobility.
      9. Gastrointestinal and urinary function.
      10. Sexuality.
      11. Cardiopulmonary function.
      12. Oncologic emergencies
      13. Palliative and end-of-life care
      14. Survivorship (Brant & Wickham, 2004).
  C. Purpose.
      1. For the nurse generalist.
         a. Serve as a guide for providing quality cancer care within the framework of the nursing process by ensuring the following:
            (1) Data collection is systematic, culturally competent, continuous, collected from multiple sources, documented, and communicated with members of the multidisciplinary cancer care team.

(2) Nursing diagnoses are derived from interpretation of presenting data and reflect the client's actual or potential health problems.

(3) Identified outcomes are derived from the nursing diagnoses and are individualized to the client's needs.

(4) The plan of care is derived from current knowledge of the nursing, biologic, social, behavioral, cultural, and physical sciences.

(5) The plan of care reflects the client's priorities and prescribed nursing strategies to achieve health promotion, maintenance, and restoration.

(6) The plan of care is implemented in concordance with the client.

(7) The client actively participates in all aspects of plan development, implementation, and evaluation.

(8) Client progress is assessed jointly by the nurse and client.

(9) Evaluation of client outcomes directs reassessment and revision of the plan of care.

    b. Facilitates professional development by doing the following:

(1) Identifying gaps in the knowledge base.

(2) Determining range of practice for which one is prepared.

  2. In oncology nursing practice, Standards of Care do the following:

    a. Provide a basis for the development of job descriptions, performance appraisals, evaluation instruments, and peer review.

    b. Present a basis for quality assessment and quality improvement.

    c. Generate research questions.

    d. Stimulate research to validate practice.

    e. Provide a basis for program evaluation.

    f. Promote intradisciplinary and interdisciplinary collaboration.

    g. Provide a basis for organizational policies, procedures, and protocols.

  3. For the client, standards ensure the following:

    a. Participation in health restoration, promotion, and maintenance.

    b. Quality of care consistent with existing standards.

V. Standards of Professional Performance (Box 44-2).

  A. Encompass the actions and activities that describe competent behaviors of the oncology nurse's role as a professional nurse and include the following:

    1. Quality of care.

    2. Practice evaluation

    3. Education.

    4. Collegiality.

    5. Ethics.

    6. Collaboration.

    7. Research.

    8. Resource utilization

    9. Leadership (Brant & Wickham, 2004).

VI. Examples of application of the Standards of Care and Standards of Professional Performance in oncology nursing practice.

  A. Application of Standard of Care III (Outcome Identification) to guide development of institution-specific plans of care for various aspects of the 14 high-incidence problem areas. For example:

    1. The potential for chemotherapy-induced mucositis provides an example of a care plan developed in relation to the high-incidence problem area, protective mechanisms (Box 44-3).

      a. An appropriate nursing diagnosis is "impaired oral mucous membranes related to effects of chemotherapy" (North American Nursing Diagnosis Association [NANDA], 2001).

BOX 44-2
STANDARDS OF PROFESSIONAL PERFORMANCE

Standard I. Quality of Care
The oncology nurse systematically evaluates the quality of care and effectiveness of oncology nursing practice within all practice settings.

Standard II. Practice Evaluation
The oncology nurse consistently evaluates his or her own nursing practice in relation to job-specific performance expectations, statewide regulatory requirements, and national oncology nursing professional standards.

Standard III. Education
The oncology nurse acquires and improves his or her knowledge base related to cancer care and oncology nursing that fosters enhanced competence and critical thinking skills.

Standard IV. Collegiality
The oncology nurse contributes to the professional development of unlicensed and licensed peers and interdisciplinary colleagues.

Standard V. Ethics
The oncology nurse uses ethical principles as a basis for decision making and patient advocacy.

Standard VI. Collaboration
The oncology nurse partners with patients, families, the interdisciplinary team, and community resources to provide optimal care.

Standard VII. Research
The oncology nurse contributes to the scientific base of nursing practice, education, and management via multiple venues: identifying clinical dilemmas and problems appropriate for rigorous study, collecting data, critiquing existing research, and making use of research.

Standard VIII. Resource Utilization
The oncology nurse considers factors related to safety, effectiveness, and cost in planning and delivering care to patients.

Standard IX. Leadership
The oncology nurse anticipates the dynamic nature of cancer care and readies herself or himself and colleagues for an evolving future.

Reprinted from Brant, JM & Wickham, RS, editors: *Statement on the scope and standards of oncology nursing practice*, Pittsburgh, 2004, Oncology Nursing Society, pp 33-42.

B. Application of Standard of Professional Performance I (Quality of Care) as a framework for an institutional quality improvement program (Box 44-4).
   1. Use the measurement criteria of each standard of care as a statement of acceptable practice.
   2. Use the 14 high-incidence problem areas for identification of potential indicators (well-defined, measurable dimensions of the quality and appropriateness of an important aspect of the client's care, which can include measurable care processes, clinical events, complications, or outcomes) that can be used to monitor oncology nursing care.
   3. Determine a threshold (a preestablished aggregate level of performance that should be achieved) for action.
   4. Collect data that monitor the quality and effectiveness of oncology nursing care.
   5. Analyze data to identify areas for improvement of care.

BOX 44-3
INSTITUTION-SPECIFIC CARE PLAN FOR THE CLIENT WITH POTENTIAL OR ACTUAL CHEMOTHERAPY-INDUCED MUCOSITIS

Nursing Diagnosis
Impaired oral mucous membrane related to effects of chemotherapy.

Expected Outcomes
1. The client/caregiver lists measures to prevent or minimize mucositis.
2. The client/caregiver identifies the signs and symptoms of mucositis and its related complications (e.g., infection, bleeding, pain).
3. The client/caregiver identifies an appropriate member of the health care team to contact if initial signs and symptoms of mucositis or its complications occur.
4. The client/caregiver describes self-care measures to prevent and/or manage mucositis and its potential complications.

Nursing Interventions
1. Assess oral cavity using mucositis grading system.
   a. Assess and document condition of oral mucosa every day (every shift if mucositis present).
   b. Recognize early signs and symptoms of oral mucositis (mild redness and swelling along gum line, sensation of mild burning and dryness).
   c. Assess for white patches *(Candida,* herpetic vesicles, raised yellow lesions).
   d. Assess entire mouth: mucous membranes, lips, tongue, gingiva, teeth.
   e. Assess for use of dentures, dental appliances.
2. Plan care based on stage/grade of mucositis.
   a. Preventive/potential.
   b. Mild/moderate.
   c. Severe.
3. Initiate/follow mouth care guidelines according to identified stage/grade of mucositis.
   a. Preventive/potential.
      i. Use a soft toothbrush.
      ii. Floss daily if platelet count >50,000.
      iii. Use sodium bicarbonate/salt mix (2:1), 1 tsp. in 8 oz. H_2O after meals and at bedtime.
      iv. Instruct client to avoid cigarettes; alcohol; citrus; hot, spicy, or coarse food.
      v. Avoid alcohol-based mouthwashes and lemon-glycerin swabs (because of drying effects).
   b. Mild/moderate.
      i. Include all components identified for those at potential risk.
      ii. Increase sodium bicarbonate/salt water mouth rinses to every 2 hours.
      iii. Culture any suspicious lesions.
      iv. Apply water-soluble lubricant to lips.
      v. Use dentures only during meals.
      vi. Obtain an order for a topical analgesic for relief of pain.
      vii. Obtain an order for topical antifungal if white patches and/or sore throat related to *Candida.*
      viii. Monitor fluid and nutrition intake.
      ix. Encourage high-calorie supplements.
   c. Severe.
      i. Include all components outlined for those at mild/moderate risk.
      ii. Add mouth rinse of Peredex, 15 ml three times daily swish and spit in addition to every 2 hours sodium bicarbonate/salt water mouth rinses.
      iii. Use sponge-tip applicator in place of soft toothbrush.
      iv. Remove and do not use dentures.
      v. Consider total parenteral nutrition (TPN) if unable to eat or drink.
      vi. Continue topical analgesics, and add parenteral analgesia as needed.
      vii. Continue topical antifungal, if indicated, or add systemic antifungal.

(Continued)

BOX 44-3

INSTITUTION-SPECIFIC CARE PLAN FOR THE CLIENT WITH POTENTIAL OR ACTUAL CHEMOTHERAPY-INDUCED MUCOSITIS—cont'd

4. Teach client/caregiver the following:
   a. Rationale for oral mucous membrane changes caused by chemotherapy.
   b. Oral evaluation at least once daily using a flashlight and mirror.
   c. Importance of keeping mouth clean and moist.
   d. Signs/symptoms of oral mucous membrane changes including those reportable to the health care team (e.g., bleeding, mouth pain, infection, ulcerations, redness, white patches, difficulty swallowing).
   e. Avoid use of alcohol (including alcohol-containing mouthwashes), tobacco products, and hot, spicy, and/or acidic drinks or foods.
   f. Rationale and measures to maintain adequate nutritional and fluid status.
   g. Mouth care procedures based on stage/grade (potential, mild/moderate, severe) of oral mucous membrane changes.
   h. Rationale and use of topical analgesics for mouth pain.
   i. Rationale and use of antibiotics for infections (if indicated).
   j. Rationale and use of antifungal agents for fungal infections (if indicated).
5. Reinforce client teaching every shift.
6. Assist client with oral care and rinses as needed.
7. Document the following:
   a. All pertinent information on flow sheet and Kardex.
   b. Client/family education on Multidisciplinary Teaching Sheet.

Modified with permission from Brackett, H: *Stomatitis competency,* Denver, 2000, University of Colorado Hospital.

BOX 44-4

QUALITY IMPROVEMENT PROJECT: SELF-CARE OF CENTRAL VENOUS CATHETER (CVC)

Standard III (Outcome Identification, Patient and Family Education)
"The client describes self-care measures and appropriate actions for highly predictable problems, oncologic emergencies, and problems associated with the disease, treatment, and side effects of therapy" (Brant & Wickham, 2004, p. 22).

Indicator
Before discharge with a CVC, 100% of patients/designated caregivers are able to demonstrate independent self-care management of the CVC, including the following:
1. Performing catheter flush with appropriate solution (i.e., heparin or normal saline)
2. Replacing catheter locking cap
3. Changing CVC dressing
4. Identifying potential or actual problems that must be reported to the health care team
5. Articulating phone number to be called to report any problem or concern

Monitoring for Occurrences
For a 2-month period, all patients discharged with a CVC will be assessed on items 1 through 5, as identified above, within 24 hours of discharge and then will be reassessed at the next outpatient clinic visit or hospital readmission. Results of the assessment will be documented on the CVC Client Monitoring Tool by the oncology clinical nurse specialist/educator.

Analysis of Findings
Data will be compiled, analyzed, and submitted to the multidisciplinary Oncology Oversight Committee for review and recommendations. In the event the threshold for action is reached, a report, including analysis of the problem, planned corrective actions, and a timetable for remonitoring, will be submitted to the multidisciplinary Quality Improvement Committee.

Modified from Volker, D: Application of the standards of practice and education. In Itano JK, Taoka KN, editors: *Core curriculum for oncology nursing,* ed 2, Philadelphia, 1998, WB Saunders, p. 719.

   6. Formulate recommendations to improve client outcomes and satisfaction with care.
   7. Implement recommendations and evaluate effectiveness.
 C. Application of Standards of Care and Standards of Professional Performance to education.
   1. Use the Standards of Care and Standards of Professional Performance to develop curricular content outlines for generalist oncology nursing education, staff development, and continuing education programs.
   2. Use the measurement criteria as learner objectives for nurse and client education (Box 44-5).
 D. Application of Standards of Care and Standards of Professional Performance to management.
   1. Use the Standards of Care and Standards of Professional Performance as a framework for development of staff performance evaluation instruments (Table 44-1).
   2. Use Standard of Professional Performance VIII (Resource Utilization) to justify resources required for the practice of oncology nursing.
 E. Application of Standard of Professional Performance VII (Research) to facilitate conduct of oncology nursing research.
   1. Use the measurement criteria identified to outline staff nurse roles and responsibilities in oncology nursing research.
   2. Conduct research related to use of the standards to identify the following:
     a. Which nursing interventions promote optimal client outcomes.
     b. The need for any additional high-incidence problem areas beyond the 14 identified.

BOX 44-5
USE OF STANDARD OF CARE MEASUREMENT CRITERIA FOR PATIENT EDUCATION

Use Standard of Care III (Outcome Identification) Measurement Criteria for Nutrition to develop learner objectives for teaching the patient with imbalanced nutrition, less than body requirements related to nausea and vomiting from chemotherapy.

Goal
The patient will manage his/her nutritional status in a manner that meets his/her goal of maximizing health maintenance and restoration during chemotherapy.

Learning Objectives
The patient will do the following:
1. Identify and differentiate between foods and nutritional fluids that are well tolerated and those that are distasteful, are unappetizing, or cause discomfort.
2. Describe measures that support adequate nutritional intake.
3. Choose alternative nutritional foods and fluids to replace those no longer appetizing or tolerated (may include altering texture, consistency, or flavor).
4. Delineate changes in eating habits (e.g., type of food, timing of meals, portion sizes) and environment (i.e., where meals/foods are eaten) to maintain adequate oral intake.
5. Designate specific dietary modifications that are congruent with sociocultural practices and lifestyle.
6. Describe measures to mange nausea and vomiting to minimize nutritional loss.
7. Identify a member of the health care team to notify if nutritional intake becomes inadequate or questions about dietary intake arise.

Modified from Brant, JM & Wickham, RS, editors: *Statement on the scope and standards of oncology nursing practice*, Pittsburgh, 2004, Oncology Nursing Society, pp 20, 21, 23, 24.

TABLE 44-1
Education Component of an Oncology Staff: Nurse Performance Evaluation Tool

STANDARD OF PROFESSIONAL PERFORMANCE III (EDUCATION)
The oncology nurse acquires and improves his or her knowledge base related to cancer care and oncology nursing that fosters enhanced competence and critical thinking skills.

RATING SCALE
1: Performance below standard
2: Performance meets standard
3: Performance exceeds standard

Measurement Criteria	Rating			Comments
	1	2	3	
Identifies deficits in knowledge and pursues venues (e.g., formal education, clinical experiences, continuing education) to enhance learning.				
Uses credible, evidence-based oncology educational resources and cites references accordingly.				
Sees information outside of oncology sources and evaluates application to cancer care.				
Integrates new knowledge and behaviors into practice setting				
Develops mentoring, publishing, and presentation skills as appropriate.				

Reprinted from Brant JM & Wickham RS, editors: *Statement on the scope and standards of oncology nursing practice*, Pittsburgh, 2004, Oncology Nursing Society, pp 35-36.

        c. Whether valid and reliable measurement instruments exist for research related to the standards.
   3. Use standards to identify possible oncology nursing–related research questions such as the following:
        a. What are the best methods to facilitate communication between clients and health care providers about living with cancer?
        b. How does the oncology nurse encourage active client participation in planning and evaluating care?

EVIDENCE-BASED PRACTICE (EBP)

  I. Overview.
    A. Has its basis in evidence-based medicine, which was first developed as a method for clinical learning in the 1980s at McMaster University in Hamilton, Ontario, Canada.
    B. The primary goal of EBP in oncology nursing is to guide nursing interventions in order to enhance the quality and outcomes of cancer care as well as provide care that is cost effective (Mast, 2000).
  II. Definition—multiple definitions exist; among them are the following:
    A. "The use of current best evidence in making decisions" (Goode, 2003, p. 7).
    B. "The conscientious, explicit, and judicious use of current best evidence in making decisions about the care of individual patients....integrating individ-

ual clinical expertise with the best available external evidence from systematic research" (Sackett et al., 1996, p. 71).

C. "...a systematic appraisal of the best evidence available in the context of the prevailing values and resources available" (Muir Gray, 2001, p. 12).

D. "Evidence-based oncology nursing is predicated on the notion that clinical practices and protocols should be defined by using authoritative evidence derived from well-designed clinical trials" (Jassak, 2001, p. 3).

III. The oncology nursing profession has mandated the inclusion of EBP in its standards. For the oncology nurse generalist, these mandates are a component of each of the six Standards of Care and also include the following:

A. Standard of Professional Performance VII (Research)—"the oncology nurse contributes to the scientific base of nursing practice, education, and management via multiple venues: identifying clinical dilemmas and problems appropriate for rigorous study, collecting data, critiquing existing research, and making use of research" (Brant & Wickham, p. 39).

B. ONS Standards of Oncology Nursing Education: Oncology Generalist Level Education.

1. Standard II (Resources). The standard states, "Educational materials specific to oncology nursing are peer-reviewed, evidence-based, current, available, and accessible to the faculty and students" (Jacobs, 2002, p. 2).

2. Standard V (Student: The Oncology Nurse Generalist). The standard states that the graduate of a generic nursing program should be able to assume nursing care responsibilities that include the following:

a. Using research evidence to collect and analyze client-related data.

b. Development and evaluation of an evidence-based plan of care.

c. Participation in oncology nursing research through identification of research questions, implementing research findings, and/or evaluating outcomes of interventions (Jacobs, 2002, p. 4).

IV. Need for EBP is based on changing health care practices, populations, and information, including the following:

A. An aging population that will require different methods and increased levels of care in their later years.

B. Evolving technology and knowledge, providing new methods and insights into oncology practice and nursing interventions.

C. Client expectations of knowledgeable health care providers and state of the art cancer care.

D. Professional expectations of understanding and utilizing new knowledge/technologic advances.

E. Costs and limits of health care and health care resources (Muir Gray, 2001).

V. Using evidence to inform clinical practice is a multistep process and includes the following:

A. Precise description of the client or clinical problem.

B. Identification of information needed to solve the problem.

C. Efficient search of the literature for relevant studies.

1. Data sources for EBP include but are not limited to the following:

a. Research-based evidence.

(1) Prospective, randomized controlled trials.

(2) Observational studies.

(3) Descriptive studies.

(4) Correlational studies.

       b. Theoretic evidence.
         (1) Propositions based on empiric knowledge.
         (2) Propositions based on nonempiric knowledge.
       c. Nonresearch evidence.
         (1) Retrospective or concurrent chart review.
         (2) Quality improvement and risk data.
         (3) Cost-effective analysis.
         (4) Benchmarking data.
         (5) International, national, and local standards of care.
         (6) Case reports/clinical expertise.
         (7) Principles of pathophysiology.
         (8) Infection control data.
         (9) Regulatory and legal data (Cooke & Grant, 2002; Goode, 2003; Rutledge & Grant, 2002).
   D. Evaluation of these studies for validity.
     1. Studies may range from meta-analysis and integrative reviews to case reports (Cooke & Grant, 2002).
     2. Studies may include both qualitative and quantitative research (Mast, 2000).
   E. Identification of the clinical relevance or "message."
   F. Development of a clinical protocol to guide client care.
   G. Implementation of the protocol.
   H. Evaluation or audit of processes and outcomes (Cope, 2003; Flemming & Fenton, 2002; Muir Gray, 2001).
VI. Mooney (2001) identified steps for developing EBP, including the following:
   A. Making a commitment to using EBP within the individual health care setting.
     1. Including overcoming the "research-practice gap," or disparity between new knowledge that is available for nursing interventions and the use of that knowledge in practice (Thompson, 2003).
     2. Identifying and overcoming the barriers that may create this gap.
       a. Personal (e.g., lack of knowledge, mentors, role models, resources, time, interest, ability to effect change).
       b. Professional (e.g., job responsibilities, decreased time).
       c. Organizational (e.g., inadequate support, resources, time allocated for EBP).
   B. Identifying and incorporating the necessary skills for developing EBP, including such skills as knowing how to do the following:
     1. Visualize "the big picture."
     2. Remain flexible.
     3. Think critically.
     4. Be a lifelong learner.
   C. Improving professional skills that promote building relationships, taking a leadership role, and taking an active role in the multidisciplinary health care team.
   D. Gaining knowledge about how to integrate current best evidence into oncology nursing practice through learning how to do the following:
     1. Critically evaluate evidence.
     2. Conduct a literature search.
     3. Determine the relevance of findings to the nurse's client and practice.
   E. Influencing others to adopt new ideas and interventions, based on valid evidence, into oncology practice.

VII. Potential research roles of the oncology nurse generalist that can facilitate EBP include the following:

A. Identification of practice problems through observation of client populations and quality improvement activities; focus of the practice problem may include the following:

1. Developing and testing interventions designed to improve client outcomes, such as the ability to perform central venous catheter care after one-to-one teaching compared with the effect of group teaching, or the impact of oral care protocol after the administration of mucosa-toxic chemotherapy.

2. Identifying variables associated with specific client problems or needs, such as pattern of diarrhea and perineal skin breakdown after the administration of high-dose cytosine arabinoside (Ara-C).

3. Describing the characteristics of a given situation, such as nonnursing tasks assigned to nurses in the outpatient clinic or content of change-of-shift reports.

B. Participation in evaluation of existing research/clinical evidence.

C. Collaboration with other health care providers/nurse researchers to identify and implement a potential solution to a specific clinical problem.

D. Participation in research activities under the guidance of a qualified researcher that can lead to changes in practice.

1. Conceptualization and design of a research study.
   a. Establishing the clinical significance of the problem.
   b. Identifying important clinical variables and client eligibility criteria.
   c. Assessing the feasibility of the methods and procedures proposed for the study.

2. Implementation of the research protocol.
   a. Enrolling clients.
   b. Implementing protocol-specific orders.
   c. Observing client responses and toxicities.
   d. Collecting data.
   e. Educating clients, caregivers, and other health care team members.

E. Participation in clinical trials to provide evidence for EBP.

1. Roles may include those noted above in section D.2.

2. Multiple types of clinical trials focusing on the following:
   a. Prevention/early detection.
   b. Diagnosis.
   c. Treatment.
   d. Supportive care.
   e. Quality of life.

3. Clinical trials process consists of four phases of investigation, three before U.S. Food and Drug Administration (FDA) approval and the fourth following approval.
   a. Phase I trials determine the maximal tolerated dose (MTD) and drug toxicities.
   b. Phase II trials focus on the specific tumor type or types for which the treatment appears promising.
   c. Phase III trials determine the following:
      (1) The effects of treatment relative to the natural history of the disease.
      (2) Whether a new treatment is as effective as the standard therapy but is associated with less morbidity.

d. Phase IV trials are implemented after FDA approval and evaluate new indications for a drug or device and also collect further data related to client use (Green et al., 2003; Klimaszewski et al., 2000; Krebs, 2004).

VIII. Critiquing research reports for potential use in EBP is essential.

    A. Research reports should be critiqued in order to do the following:

        1. Evaluate the believability of the results.

        2. Decide if the study is applicable to one's practice setting.

        3. Identify whether the study can be replicated for one's practice, if needed or desired.

        4. Decide if the findings are consistent with other findings on the topic.

        5. Identify whether the findings are ready for practice implementation.

        6. Decide what, if any, new knowledge can be gained from the research (Oman, 2003).

    B. Burns and Grove (2003) suggest the following steps for evaluating a research report.

        1. Review and critique the entire report, not just individual components.

        2. Closely review how the report is laid out (e.g., contains all the necessary components in a logical order) and the information presented.

        3. Identify whether the information is of value to nursing practice.

        4. Objectively identify the study's strengths and weaknesses.

    C. Guidelines and exact questions for completing the critique will vary depending on the type of methodology employed but include evaluation of the following areas:

        1. Problem or purpose.

            a. Is the purpose explicitly stated, including identifying research variables and nature of the population to be studied?

            b. Does the problem have significance to nursing, and is the projected significance clearly delineated?

            c. Are formally stated hypotheses included, and do they relate directly to the research problem (Burns & Grove, 2003; Bush, 2001; Oman, 2003)?

        2. Theoretic framework.

            a. Is a theoretic framework identified?

            b. Does the framework support the hypothesis, research statement, or question (Burns & Grove, 2003; Bush, 2001; Oman, 2003)?

        3. Design or method.

            a. Is the design used to conduct the study compatible with the research problem?

                (1) Qualitative research.

                    (a) Purpose—to describe and explore phenomena or to gain understanding.

                    (b) Characteristics—process focused, subjective, and not generalizable.

                    (c) Types—descriptive, surveys, phenomenology, content analysis.

                (2) Quantitative research.

                    (a) Purpose—to describe relationships and cause and effect and to identify facts.

                    (b) Characteristics—outcome focused, objective, generalizable.

                    (c) Types—quasiexperimental, experimental, correlational.

b. Is the method adequate to answer the question or phenomenon under study? Should a more rigorous design be used (Burns & Grove, 2003; Bush, 2001; Oman, 2003)?

4. Sampling.
   a. Is the selection of participants clearly identified? For a qualitative study, was purposive sampling undertaken?
   b. Was the selection of participants appropriate for the research purpose and method?
   c. Is the sample representative of the larger population (Burns & Grove, 2003; Bush, 2001; Oman, 2003)?

5. Data collection.
   a. Are data collection criteria clearly identified?
   b. Are data collection procedures explicitly defined?
   c. Are data collection instruments appropriate for research problem and proposed methodology?
   d. Are the instruments used for data collection valid and reliable? Is this information clearly presented?
   e. Is protection of human subjects, including protected health information, addressed?
   f. For qualitative research, is saturation of data described (Burns & Grove, 2003; Bush, 2001; Oman, 2003)?

6. Data analysis—will differ depending on whether a qualitative or quantitative method is used.
   a. Qualitative.
      (1) Does the researcher address the issues of credibility, auditability, and fittingness of the data?
      (2) Is the data analysis strategy compatible with the study purpose?
      (3) Are the findings presented in a manner that allows the reader to verify the researcher's theoretic conclusions?
      (4) Do the conclusions, implications, and recommendations reflect the findings of the study?
      (5) Would a quantitative approach be more appropriate (Burns & Grove, 2003; Bush, 2001; Oman, 2003)?
   b. Quantitative.
      (1) Does the report include the appropriate statistics?
      (2) Was there an appropriate amount of statistical data reported?
      (3) Were the results of any statistical tests significant, and was this information adequately reported?
      (4) Could the study have been strengthened by including qualitative data (Burns & Grove, 2003; Bush, 2001; Oman, 2003)?

7. Findings, implications, and recommendations.
   a. Are important results presented, and is their interpretation consistent with the results?
   b. Are implications related to nursing practice presented?
   c. Are specific limitations of the research study presented?
   d. Are the identified implications appropriate in relation to the specified limitations?
   e. Are specific recommendations for future research presented, and are they consistent with the findings and similar research (Burns & Grove, 2003; Bush, 2001; Oman, 2003)?

IX. Before implementation of research findings into nursing practice, the following types of questions should be asked:
  A. Are the resources and institutional support adequate to implement the findings?
  B. Are the results clinically significant?
  C. Can the results be generalized?
  D. Are the implementation strategies discussed by the researcher desirable and feasible in practice?
  E. Can the outcome of implementing the findings be measured?

X. Barnsteiner and Prevost (2002) have identified five strategies that will facilitate implementation of EBP.
  A. Change colleagues' viewpoints about research/research findings to make them seem valuable and usable.
  B. Increase knowledge about EBP process.
  C. Harness new knowledge through utilization of resources that synthesize knowledge for clinical application, including the following:
    1. The Cochrane Collaboration: http://www.cochrane.org.
    2. Agency for Healthcare Research and Quality (AHRQ): http://www.ahcpr.gov/.
    3. National Guidelines Clearing House: http://www.guideline.gov/.
    4. Online Journal of Knowledge Synthesis for Nursing: *www.stti.iupui.edu.*
    5. Evidence-Based Healthcare Information: *www.mlanet.org.*
    6. Oncology Nursing Society evidence-based online resource center: http://www.ons.org.
  D. Consider both the positive and negative possibilities of changing practices based on the evidence (i.e., cost, available resources, staff utilization).
  E. Institute system changes to incorporate EBP into the organizational culture.

TABLE 44-2
Research Priorities

National Institute of Nursing Research 2004 Priorities (NINR, 2004)	ONS Year 2000 Research Priorities (Ropka et al., 2002)

1. Chronic illnesses or conditions
  a. Chronic illness self-management and quality of life
2. Behavioral changes and interventions
  a. Decreasing low birth weight infants among minority populations
  b. Enhancing health promotion among minority men
3. Responding to compelling public health concerns
  a. End of life: bridging life and death
  b. Nursing research training and centers
	1. Pain
	2. Quality of life
	3. Early detection
	4. Prevention/risk detection
	5. Neutropenia/immunosuppression
	6. Hospice/end of life
	7. Oncologic emergencies
	8. Suffering
	9. Fatigue
	10. Ethical issues

Data from National Institute of Nursing Research (NINR). (n.d.). 2004 areas of research opportunity. Retrieved October 30, 2004 from the World Wide Web: http://nih.gov/ninr/research/dea/2004AoRO.html; Ropka ME, et al: Year 2000 Oncology Nursing Society Research Priorities Survey, *Oncol Nurs Forum* 29:481-491, 2002. *ONS,* Oncology Nursing Society.

XI. To further implementation of EBP, knowledge of national research priorities can focus research applications and provide potential sources of evidence (Table 44-2).

    A. National Institute of Nursing Research (NINR) for 2004 (NINR, 2004).

    B. Oncology Nursing Society 2000 Research Priorities Survey (Ropka et al., 2002).

REFERENCES

Barnsteiner, J., & Prevost, S. (2002). How to implement evidence-based practice: Some tried and true pointers. *Reflections on Nursing Leadership,* Second Quarter, 18-21, 43.

Brant, J.M., & Wickham, R.S. (Eds.) (2004). *Statement on the scope and standards of oncology nursing practice.* Pittsburgh: Oncology Nursing Society.

Burns, N., & Grove, S.K. (2003). *Understanding nursing research* (3rd ed.). Philadelphia: W.B. Saunders.

Bush, C.T. (2001). Understanding the scientific method and nursing research. In K.K. Chitty (Ed.). *Professional nursing: Concepts & challenges* (3rd ed.). Philadelphia: W.B. Saunders, pp. 275-303.

Cooke, L., & Grant, M. (2002). Support for evidence-based practice. *Seminars in Oncology Nursing 18,* 71-78.

Cope, D. (2003). Evidence-based practice: Making it happen in your clinical setting. *Clinical Journal of Oncology Nursing 7,* 97-98.

Dorsett, D.S. (2000). Quality of care. In C. Yarbro, M.H. Frogge, M. Goodman, & S. Groenwald (Eds.). *Cancer nursing: Principles and practice* (5th ed.). Sudbury, MA: Jones and Bartlett Publishers, pp. 1581-1608.

Flemming, K., & Fenton, M. (2002). Making sense of research evidence to inform decision making. In C. Thompson & D. Dowding (Eds.). *Clinical decision making and judgment in nursing.* Edinburgh: Churchill Livingstone, pp.109-129.

Goode, C.J. (2003). Evidence-based practice. In K.S. Oman, M.E. Krugman, & R.M. Fink (Eds.). *Nursing research secrets.* Philadelphia: Hanley & Belfus, pp. 7-14.

Green, S., Benedetti, J., & Crowley, J.E. (2003). *Interdisciplinary statistics: Clinical trials in oncology* (2nd ed.). Boca Raton, FL: Chapman & Hall/C.R.C.

Jacobs, L.A. (Ed.) (2002). *Standards of oncology nursing education: Generalist and advanced practice levels* (3rd ed.). Pittsburgh: Oncology Nursing Society.

Jassak, P.F. (2001). Introduction: Evidence-based oncology nursing practice: Improving patient outcomes in the next millennium. *Oncology Nursing Forum 28*(2, Suppl.), 3-4.

Klimaszewski, A.D., Aiken, J.L., Bacon, M.A., et al. (Eds.). (2000). *Manual for clinical trials nursing.* Pittsburgh: Oncology Nursing Society.

Krebs, L.U. (2004). Research and clinical trials. In P. Buchsel & C.H. Yarbro (Eds.). *Administrative issues and concepts in ambulatory care* (2nd ed.). Sudbury, MA: Jones and Bartlett Publishers, pp. 327-349.

Mast, M. (2000). Evidence-based practice: What it is, what it isn't. *ONS News 15*(6), 1, 4, 5.

Mooney, K. (2001). Advocating for quality cancer care: Making evidence-based practice a reality. *Oncology Nursing Forum 28*(2, Suppl.), 17-21.

Muir Gray, J.A. (2001). *Evidence-based healthcare* (2nd ed.). London: Churchill Livingstone.

National Institute of Nursing Research (NINR). (n.d.). 2004 areas of research opportunity. Retrieved October 30, 2004 from the World Wide Web: http://nih.gov/ninr/research/dea/2004AoRO.html.

Nelson, N. (2003). Image of nursing: Influences of the present. In J. Zerwekh & J.C. Claborn (Eds.). *Nursing today: Transitions and trends.* St. Louis: W.B. Saunders, pp. 49-78.

North American Nursing Diagnosis Association (NANDA). (2001). *Nursing diagnoses: Definitions and clarifications, 2001-2003.* Philadelphia: NANDA.

Oman, K.S. (2003). Reading, understanding, and critiquing research reports. In K.S. Oman, M.E. Krugman, & R.M. Fink (Eds.). *Nursing research secrets.* Philadelphia: Hanley & Belfus, pp. 37-45.

Ropka, M.E., Guterbock, T., Krebs, L.U., et al. (2002). Year 2000 Oncology Nursing Society research priorities survey. *Oncology Nursing Forum 29,* 481-491.

Rutledge, D.N., & Grant, M. (2002). Introduction. *Seminars in Oncology Nursing 18,* 1-2.

Sackett, D.L., Rosenberg, W.M., Gray, J.A., et al. (1996). Evidence-based medicine: What it is and what it isn't. *British Medical Journal 312,* 71-72.

Thompson, C.J. (2003). Overcoming the research-practice gap. In K.S. Oman, M.E. Krugman, & R.M. Fink (Eds.). *Nursing research secrets.* Philadelphia: Hanley & Belfus, pp. 15-24.

45 The Education Process

PATRICIA AGRE

I. Educational theory should be the basis for any formal (and many informal) educational interventions, whether they are aimed at an individual client (patient, staff nurse) or a community. A few of the many theories that can be useful for formulating teaching strategies are listed below. For others, see Bahn (2001), Gage and Berliner (1998), Glanz et al. (2002), and Zemke (2002).

A. Behavioral learning theory (operant conditioning, classical conditioning) posits that learning is based on observable behaviors that are reinforced to increase the strength of the behavior (Merriam & Caffarella, 1999). Examples of behavioral interventions are relaxation techniques, biofeedback, and visual imagery. Behavioral interventions are often used to help pediatric cancer clients cope with painful procedures; adult cancer clients can use them to reduce stress, pain, and anxiety and to increase coping ability.

B. Cognitive learning theory describes the internal process that leads to learning (Blackmore, 1996; Merriam & Caffarella, 1999). It requires attention and encoding for information to be retrieved and applied. An example of cognitive learning is the creation of a mnemonic for symptoms that should trigger a phone call to the physician/health care provider. A client's ability to differentiate systemic from local treatment demonstrates cognitive learning.

C. Social learning theory describes learning that takes place based on watching and imitating others (Bandura, 1977). Examples are the use of client-to-client volunteers. "I went through what you're going through and look how well I look now."

D. Motivational learning theory results from personal (internal) cues (e.g., "I want to be here for my children, so I've got to stop smoking") or environmental (external) cues (e.g., "I have to stop smoking because my workplace is nonsmoking and I hate sneaking out for a cigarette") (Wlodkowski, 1998).

E. Adult learning theory (andragogy) describes the adult learner as someone who is self-directed, independent, and problem centered (Knowles, 1970). Learning is based on past experience. An example of an adult learning experience would be an independent Internet search for information related to a new cancer diagnosis.

II. Client education.

A. Needs assessment (Lorig, 1996b; Soriano, 1995; Witkin & Altschuld, 1995).

1. Questions to be answered.

a. What does the client know? Ask what the client understands about his/her diagnosis, tests, treatment, needed self-care, and follow-up.

b. What does the client want to know? This may be different from what the nurse thinks the client wants to know (Griffiths & Leek, 1995).

c. Are there any cultural or religious beliefs or practices that might impact the teaching/learning process (Joint Commission on the Accreditation of Healthcare Organizations [JCAHO], 2004; Leininger, 2002)? For example, alternative botanicals may be a traditional and important part of the client's belief system, but these botanicals may interfere with chemotherapy drugs.

  d. What language does the client speak? If the nurse does not speak the same language, what is the alternative teaching plan?

  e. Does the client have a physical (e.g., hearing, vision, mobility, dexterity) or cognitive (e.g., stroke, confusion, somnolence) impairment that might impede learning?

  f. Does the client have a preferred learning style (e.g., visual, aural, or kinesthetic—seeing, hearing, doing; global or analytical—big picture, component parts) (Flannery, 1993; Wislock, 1993)?

  2. Methods (Lorig, 1996b; Soriano, 1995).

  a. Individual assessment—ask specific questions (e.g., what is the most important thing you want to learn now? Will your arthritis cause difficulties in giving yourself an injection?).

  b. Community assessment before development of targeted client education program/materials.

  (1) Survey or checklist (Lorig, 1996b).

  (2) Interested-party analysis (Lorig, 1996b).

  (3) Interview and key informant (Soriano, 1995).

  (4) Focus group (Soriano, 1995).

  3. Nursing diagnosis—based on the needs assessment and leads to the goals and objectives of teaching plan (North American Nursing Diagnosis Association [NANDA], 2001).

B. Goals and objectives (also called outcome criteria, outcome objectives) (Bellevue Community College, 2002; Landau, 2001; Ritchie, 1996).

  1. Goals.

  a. Do not specify how, when, or by whom they will be achieved.

  b. Provide a global view of intended outcomes; for example, the client will be able to care for himself/herself after discharge.

  2. Objectives (Lorig, 1996a).

  a. State "who" will do "what" by "when." (Effective objectives are "SMART"—specific, measurable, attainable, realistic, timed.)

  b. Provide specific assessment criteria; for example, the client will demonstrate correct technique for wound care before discharge.

C. Teaching plan.

  1. Decide who will do the teaching (e.g., staff nurse, client educator, client-to-client volunteer).

  2. Decide how it will be taught, based on client's preference and availability of alternative methods (e.g., one-on-one, group, video, computer, print, combination).

  3. Prepare for teaching by reviewing the literature (professional journal articles or recent textbooks), standards of care, and hospital procedure manuals and consulting experts (e.g., advanced practice nurses, physicians).

  4. Organize and practice all teaching sessions before doing the teaching.

  5. Plan the teaching to coincide with a teachable moment when the learner might be most likely to be receptive to the message (e.g., smoking cessation for family members when a client is diagnosed with lung cancer; self-care skills before discharge; cancer screening to coincide with a public awareness campaign).

D. Evaluation.

  1. Determine how to measure learning (e.g., learner explains in own words, return demonstration, quiz, behavior change).

2. Document learning outcomes (e.g., client can state the side effects of the medication; client can demonstrate correct catheter care technique) on care plan, documentation form, or nursing notes.
3. Reassess and reinforce teaching/learning at next available opportunity.

III. Family education—family members or significant others may have the same or different learning needs. Addressing these learning needs is especially important if the family member or significant other has a role in caring for the client at home.
   A. Do a needs assessment with, or independent of, the client.
   B. Identify overlapping and separate needs.
   C. Obtain client's permission to include family in teaching (Health Insurance Portability and Accountability Act [HIPAA]).
   D. Schedule teaching sessions when family can be available.
   E. Assess learning; reinforce as necessary.
   F. Document as indicated by needs and relationship with client (e.g., care provider, helper).

IV. Staff education (Abruzzese, 1996; Swansburg, 1995).
   A. Categories of staff learning needs assessment.
      1. Orientation for new staff nurses.
      2. Global needs assessment for all staff nurses.
      3. Individual needs assessment for all staff nurses.
      4. Targeted needs assessment for learning objectives related to critical events, new or revised policies/procedures, new treatments, and so on.
   B. Methods for assessing staff learning needs.
      1. Intuition (e.g., new staff nurses must understand hospital policies; staff nurses must be informed when nursing policies or procedures change).
      2. Self-assessment (e.g., nurses evaluate their own learning needs based on the type of client for whom they will provide care; nurses identify learning needs based on interest).
      3. Diagnostic methods (e.g., nurses are tested for competence in specific areas; nurses are observed in practice).
      4. Performance analysis (e.g., information is obtained from quality improvement and incident reports; infection control data are analyzed).
   C. Teaching plan.
      1. Use principles of adult learning (Avillion & Abruzzese, 1996; Knowles, 1970).
         a. Adults should understand why they must learn something.
         b. Adults should be self-directed.
         c. Teaching plan should take prior learning and experience into account.
         d. Educators should create a learning environment and culture.
      2. Determine objectives of teaching (e.g., nurse will demonstrate venipuncture technique; nurse will identify components of a client's admission assessment).
      3. Determine teaching method (e.g., class, one-on-one, print or computer, self-directed or teacher directed, games and simulations, grand rounds, panels and seminars, case studies, CD-ROM and World Wide Web).
      4. Establish evaluation criteria (e.g., test, observation, dialogue, learner satisfaction, performance improvement, client satisfaction).

V. Community education (Anderson & McFarlane, 2000; Clement-Stone et al., 2002; Glanz et al., 2002).
   A. Community health nursing.
      1. Community can be defined geographically (e.g., New York City, state of Missouri), by ethnic or religious group (e.g., African Americans, born-again

Christians), and by interest or characteristics (e.g., sexual orientation, occupation), among many others.

2. The role of the nurse in community health is defined by many organizations, including the American Nurses Association (http://www.ana.org), the American Public Health Association (http://www.apha.org), and state and local departments of health. Many definitions include the word "populations" as the target of nursing interventions.

B. *Healthy People Initiative* (U.S. Department of Health, Education, and Welfare, 1979) and *Healthy People 2010* (U.S. Department of Health and Human Services, 2000) have established national priorities to improve health and reduce health disparity (http://odphp.osophs.dhhs.gov/pubs/HP2000/2010.htm).

C. Models for health education and promotion.

1. Models of individual health behavior.

   a. Health belief model (Janz et al., 2002; Pierce & Nalle, 2002; Rosenstock, 1974) states that people change behavior based on perceived susceptibility to a condition, its perceived severity, the perceived benefits to reducing risk behaviors, and the perceived barriers to reducing the risk.

   b. Theory of reasoned action (Montano & Kasprzyk, 2002; Pierce & Nalle, 2002) proposes that variables such as demographics, attitudes, and personality traits affect health beliefs and motivations.

   c. Social cognitive theory (Bandura, 1977) (see I.C. above).

2. Models of community health behavior change.

   a. PRECEDE-PROCEED (Green & Kreuter, 2000) has nine phases—social diagnosis, epidemiologic diagnosis, behavioral and environmental diagnosis, educational and organizational diagnosis, and administrative and policy diagnosis are identified (PRECEDE) followed by plan implementation, process evaluation, impact evaluation, and outcome evaluation (PROCEED).

   b. Diffusion of innovations (Oldenburg & Parcel, 2002) identifies stages of change (awareness, interest, trial, decision, adoption) and places people on a continuum (innovators, early adopters, early majority, late majority, laggers).

D. Community assessment.

1. Identifies pertinent information.

   a. Descriptive data (e.g., demographics, history, ethnicity, values and beliefs, physical environment, health and social services).

   b. Illness prevalence data.

   c. Health learning needs (e.g., human immunodeficiency virus [HIV] and acquired immunodeficiency syndrome [AIDS] prevention, smoking prevention in teens).

2. Analyzes the data.

   a. Identifies common health problems (e.g., high incidence of heart disease, tuberculosis).

   b. Develops a community health diagnosis; for example, senior citizens are at risk for social isolation because of lack of public transportation.

E. Intervention.

1. Generally aimed at primary, secondary, or tertiary prevention.

2. Nurse works with community (e.g., key informants, leaders, health care community, schools) to prioritize and develop interventions to meet health needs identified in assessment.

3. Plan is implemented using community resources, advocates, agencies.

    F. Evaluation.
       1. Intervention is evaluated for impact on identified health need.
       2. Intervention may be modified for ongoing health needs (e.g., is it cost-effective, were objectives met, what are the long-term implications of continuing/not continuing the intervention?).

REFERENCES

Abruzzese, R.S. (Ed.). (1996). *Nursing staff development: Strategies for success* (2nd ed.). St. Louis: Mosby.

Anderson, E.T., & McFarlane, J. (Eds.). (2000). *Community as partner: Theory and practice in nursing* (3rd ed.). Philadelphia: Lippincott.

Avillion, A., & Abruzzese, R.S. (1996). Conceptual foundations of nursing staff development. In R.S. Abruzzese (Ed.). *Nursing staff development: Strategies for success* (2nd ed.). St. Louis: Mosby, pp. 30-43.

Bahn, D. (2001). Social learning theory: Its application in the context of nurse education. *Nurse Education Today 21*, 110-117.

Bandura, A. (1977). Self-efficacy: Toward a unifying theory of behavioral change. *Psychological Review 84*(2), 191-215.

Bellevue Community College. (2002). Moving to outcomes. Retrieved November 21, 2003 from the World Wide Web: http://www.bcc.ctc.edu/frc/bcclearning/outcomes/versus.htm.

Blackmore, J. (1996). Pedagogy: Learning styles. Retrieved November 20, 2003 from the World Wide Web: http://www.cyg.net/~jblackmo/dig.ib/styl-a.html.

Clement-Stone, S., McGuire, S.L., & Eigsti, D.G. (Eds.). (2002). *Comprehensive community health nursing: Family, aggregate, & community practice* (6th ed.). St. Louis: Mosby.

Flannery, D.D. (1993). Global and analytical ways of processing information. In D.D. Flannery (Ed.). *Applying cognitive learning theory to adult learning.* San Francisco: Jossey-Bass Publisher, pp. 15-24.

Gage, N.L., & Berliner, D.C. (1998). *Educational psychology* (6th ed.). Boston: Houghton Mifflin Co.

Glanz, K., Rimer, B.K. , & Lewis, F.M. (Eds.) (2002). *Health behavior and health education: Theory, research, and practice* (3rd ed.). San Francisco: Jossey-Bass Publisher.

Green, L.W., & Kreuter, M.W. (2000). *Health promotion planning: An educational and environmental approach* (2nd ed.). Mountain View, CA: Mayfield Publishing Co.

Griffiths, M., & Leek, C. (1995). Patient education needs: Opinions of oncology nurses and their patients. *Oncology Nursing Forum 22*, 139-144.

Janz, N.K., Champion, V.L., & Strecher, V.J. (2002). The health belief model. In K. Glanz, B.K. Rimer, & F.M. Lewis (Eds.). *Health behavior and health education: Theory, research, and practice* (3rd ed.). San Francisco: Jossey-Bass Publisher, pp. 45-66.

Joint Commission on the Accreditation of Healthcare Organizations (JCAHO). (2004). *CAMH: Comprehensive accreditation manual for hospitals: The official handbook.* http://www.jcaho.org.

Knowles, M.S. (1970). *The modern practice of adult education: From pedagogy to andragogy* (2nd ed.). New York: Adult Education Company.

Landau, V. (2001) *Developing an effective online class.* Retrieved October 11, 2004 from the World Wide Web: http:// www.roundworldmedia.com/cvc/module4/notes4.html.

Leininger, M.M. (2002). Theory of culture care diversity and universality. In J.B. George (Ed.). *Nursing theories* (5th ed.). Upper Saddle River, NJ: Prentice Hall, pp. 489-518.

Lorig, K. (1996a). How do I get from a needs assessment to a program? Program planning and implementation. In K. Lorig (Ed.). *Patient education: A practical approach* (2nd ed.). Thousand Oaks, CA: Sage Publications, pp. 67-96.

Lorig, K. (1996b). How do I know what patients want and need? Needs assessment. In K. Lorig (Ed.). *Patient education: A practical approach* (2nd ed.). Thousand Oaks, CA: Sage Publications, pp. 1-18.

Merriam, S.B., & Caffarella, R.S. (1999). Key theories of learning. In *Learning in adulthood* (2nd ed.). San Francisco: Jossey-Bass Publisher, pp. 251-256.

Montano, D., & Kasprzyk, D. (2002). The theory of reasoned action and the theory of planned behavior. In K. Glanz, B. K. Rimer, & F. M. Lewis (Eds.). *Health behavior and health education: Theory, research, and practice* (3rd ed.). San Francisco: Jossey-Bass Publisher, pp. 67-98.

North American Nursing Diagnosis Association (NANDA). (2001). *Nursing diagnoses: Definitions and classification 2001-2003*. Philadelphia: NANDA.

Oldenburg, B.F., & Parcel, G.S. (2002). Diffusion of innovations. In K.Glanz, B.K. Rimer, & F.M. Lewis (Eds.). *Health behavior and health education: Theory, research, and practice* (3rd ed.). San Francisco: Jossey-Bass Publisher, pp. 312-344.

Pierce, J.U., & Nalle, M. (2002). Theoretical models for health education and health promotion. In S. Clement-Stone, S.L. McGuire, & D.G. Eigsti (Eds.). *Comprehensive community health nursing: Family, aggregate, & community practice* (6th ed.). St. Louis: Mosby, pp. 379-399.

Ritchie, D. (1996). Understanding objectives. Retrieved November 21, 2003 from the World Wide Web: http://edweb.sdsu.edu/courses/EDTEC540/objectives/Difference.html

Rosenstock, I.M. (1974). Historical origins of the health belief model. *Health Education Monographs 2*, 328-335.

Soriano, F.I. (1995). Assessment methods. In *Conducting needs assessments: A multidisciplinary approach*. Thousand Oaks, CA: Sage Publications, pp. 15-34.

Swansburg, R.C . (1995). *Nursing staff development: A component of human resource development*. Sudbury, MA: Jones and Bartlett Publishers.

U.S. Department of Health and Human Services. (2000). *Healthy people 2010*. Retrieved November 24, 2003 from the World Wide Web: http://odphp.osophs.dhhs.gov/pubs/HP2000/2010.htm.

U.S. Department of Health, Education, and Welfare. (1979) *Healthy People: The Surgeon General's Report on Health Promotion and Disease Prevention*. Bethesda, MD.

Wislock, R.F. (1993). What are perceptual modalities and how do they contribute to learning? In D.D. Flannery (Ed.). *Applying cognitive learning theory to adult learning*. San Francisco: Jossey-Bass Publisher, pp. 5-13.

Witkin, B.R., & Altschuld, J.W. (1995). *Planning and conducting needs assessments: A practical guide*. Thousand Oaks, CA: Sage Publications.

Wlodkowski, R.J. (1998). *Enhancing adult motivation to learn: A comprehensive guide for teaching all adults*. San Francisco: Jossey-Bass Publisher.

Zemke, R. (2002). Who needs learning theory anyway? *Training 39*(9), 86-90.

46 Legal Issues Influencing Cancer Care

MARY MAGEE GULLATTE

I. Definition: pertaining to a law, conformity with a given law or statute.
II. Primary sources of law affecting health-related issues include the following (Pozgar & Santucci, 2002; www.law.com):
   A. Statutes—written laws enacted by legislatures that encompass the rules of society and are signed by a president or governor.
   B. Common law—court-made law that serves as the basis for most malpractice litigation.
   C. Administrative law—law made by administrative agencies appointed by the executive branch of government.
III. Purposes—concern over legal issues in the area of health care results from a need to do the following:
   A. Protect the rights of citizens, both the public and professionals.
   B. Delineate the responsibilities of recipients and providers of health care.
   C. Delineate the scope of practice for health care professionals and institutions.
   D. Ensure the provision of reasonable and customary health care.
IV. Sources used in legal decision making relevant to oncology nursing practice.
   A. Professional documents used to establish minimal acceptable standards of practice and health care.
      1. Nurse practice acts.
         a. Provide definition and role of nursing by state.
         b. Regulate the practice of nursing.
         c. Delineate requirements and specifications of licensure.
         d. Establish a board of nursing.
         e. Provide a mechanism for due process and penalties.
      2. Professional standards of practice (www.ons.org and www.ana.org).
         a. *American Nurses Association (ANA) Standards of Nursing Practice.*
         b. State nurse scope and practice standards.
         c. *Oncology Nursing Society (ONS) Statement on the Scope and Standards of Oncology Nursing Practice.*
         d. *ONS Standards of Oncology Education: Patient/Significant other and public.*
         e. *ONS Standards of Oncology Nursing Education: Generalist and Advanced Practice Levels.*
   B. Agency or institutional policies and procedures.
      1. Regulations override institutional policies.
      2. Statutes override regulations.
   C. Requirements of accrediting, governing, and regulatory agencies.
      1. Joint Commission on Accreditation of Healthcare Organizations (JCAHO).
      2. American College of Surgeons (ACS)—Commission on Cancer.

3. Occupational Safety and Health Administration (OSHA)—safety standards.
4. Centers for Disease Control and Prevention (CDC)—cancer-related standards.
5. Department of Health and Human Services (DHHS).
6. National Institutes of Health (NIH).
7. Centers for Medicare and Medicaid (CMS).
8. State department of human resources (DHR).
9. Emergency Medical Treatment and Active Labor Act (EMTALA)—requires that a physician (or other individual identified by hospital bylaws, rules, and regulations or another board-approved document) certify, before transfer, that a client is stable and that the benefits of transfer outweigh the risks of keeping said client in the originating facility (Buppert, 2003).
10. Agency for Healthcare Research and Quality (AHRQ)—established a national client safety database to improve quality and safety of client care (Cavanaugh, 2001).

D. Client rights (Table 46-1) (Annas, 1992).
1. American Hospital Association (AHA)—Patient's Bill of Rights.
2. JCAHO—standards of care related to client rights.
3. Right of self-determination.
4. Informed consent documents.
5. Security of individual health information: Health Insurance Portability and Accountability Act (HIPAA) (http://aspe.hhs.gov/admnsimp).

E. Client safety.
1. Institute of Medicine (IOM) (Kohn et al., 2000).
   a. Quality of Health Care in America Project launched in 1998—10-year initiative to improve health care quality over the ensuing decade; hence the following directives were established:
      (1) Review and synthesize findings in the literature pertaining to quality of care provided in the health care system.

TABLE 46-1
Client Rights Organizations

Organization	Goals/Objectives	National Office
American Civil Liberties Union (ACLU)	Actively protects the constitutional rights of citizens, rights to privacy, equal protection, confidentiality, access to records, and equal access to care	ACLU 125 Broad Street, 18th Floor New York, NY 10004 www.aclu.org
American Society of Law and Medicine	Professional continuing education related to current trends in health law Journals: *Law, Medicine and Health Care; American Journal of Law and Medicine*	American Society of Law and Medicine 765 Commonwealth Avenue Suite 1634 Boston, MA 02215 http://www.aslme.org/
Children in Hospitals, Inc.	Helps parents stay with and support their children during hospitalization Publishes a newsletter	Children in Hospitals, Inc. 31 Wilshire Park Needham, MA 02192

TABLE 46-1
Client Rights Organizations—cont'd

Organization	Goals/Objectives	National Office
Citizen Advocacy Center (CAC)	A support program for public members who serve on health care regulatory boards and governing bodies as representatives of the consumer interest. Provides research, training, technical support, and networking opportunities for public members	Citizen Advocacy Center 1400 Sixteenth Street, NW Suite 330 Washington, DC 20036 http://www.cacenter.org
Concern for Dying and Society for the Right to Die (formerly the Euthanasia Educational Council)	Provides information and support for those interested in exercising their rights as clients, especially the right to refuse medical treatment Developed the living will *Right to Die:* an annual updated collection of all state living will laws	Concern for Dying/ Society for the Right to Die 250 W. 57th Street New York, NY 10107
The Hemlock Society (End-of-Life Choices)	Promotes legislation to legalize physician-assisted suicide and distributes literature on the subject	The Hemlock Society (End-of-Life Choices) End-of-Life Choices PO Box 101810 Denver, CO 80246 http://www.hemlock.org/index.jsp
Law, Medicine and Ethics Program	Education, research, and advocacy in health law, with emphasis on client rights, health care regulation, and medical ethics	Law, Medicine and Ethics Program Boston University Schools of Medicine and Public Health 80 E. Concord Street Boston, MA 02118 www.bumc.bu.edu
The National Hospice and Palliative Care Organization	Information center about hospices Publishes a national directory and provides information	National Hospice & Palliative Care Organization (NHPCO) 1700 Diagonal Road Suite 625 Alexandria, VA 22314 www.nho.org
National Health Law Program	Legal services and backup center, specializing in health law, Medicaid, and access issues for the poor Publishes a newsletter	National Health Law Program 2639 South La Cienega Boulevard Los Angeles, CA 90034-2675 http://www.healthlaw.org
People's Medical Society	Provides information on issues regarding client rights Membership organization for consumers of medical services	People's Medical Society P.O. Box 868 Allentown, PA 18105-0868 www.peoplesmed.org
Public Citizen Health Research Group	Ralph Nader–affiliated consumer advocacy group Concerned with issues of medical care, drug safety, medical device safety, physician competence, and consumer health care issues	Public Citizen Health Research Group 1600 20th Street, NW Washington, DC 20009 http://www.citizen.org/hrg

Data from Annas GJ: *The rights of patients: the basic ACLU guide to patients rights,* ed 2 (rev), Totowa, NJ, 1992, Humana Press; Annas GJ: *The rights of patients*, ed 3, Carbondale, 2004, Southern Illinois University Press.

(2) Develop a communications strategy for raising the awareness of the general public and key stakeholders of quality of care concerns and opportunities for improvement.

(3) Articulate a policy framework that will provide positive incentives to improve quality and foster accountability.

(4) Identify characteristics and factors that enable or encourage providers, health care organizations, health plans, and communities to continuously improve the quality of care.

(5) Develop a research agenda in areas of continued uncertainty.

2. IOM report of suggested client deaths caused by medical errors may be as high as 98,000 (AHA, 1999). This report prompted an IOM Quality of Health Care in America Project committee to lay out a four-tiered approach to improve client safety (Kohn et al., 2000).

a. Establish a national focus to create leadership, research, tools, and protocols to enhance the knowledge base about safety.

b. Identify and learn from errors through immediate and strong mandatory reporting efforts with encouraging of voluntary efforts, with the aim of making sure that system continues to be made safer for clients.

c. Raise standards and expectations for improvements in safety through the actions of oversight organizations, group purchases, and professional groups.

d. Create safety systems inside health care organizations through the implementation of safe practices at the point of care delivery.

3. JCAHO 2004 National Patient Safety Goals (NPSGs) (JCAHO, 2004). The first NPSGs were approved in July 2002. As of January 1, 2004, all JCAHO-accredited health care organizations are surveyed for implementation of the following seven requirements or acceptable alternatives as appropriate to the services provided:

a. Improve the accuracy of client identification (use at least two client identifiers).

b. Improve the effectiveness of communication among caregivers (eliminate unapproved abbreviations).

c. Improve the safety of using high-alert medications (e.g., chemotherapy).

d. Eliminate wrong-site, wrong-client, wrong-procedure surgery.

e. Improve the safety of using volumetric infusion pumps (eliminate free flow).

f. Improve the effectiveness of clinical alarms.

g. Reduce the risk of health care–acquired infections.

(1) Comply with CDC hand hygiene guidelines.

(2) Manage as sentinel events all identified cases of unanticipated death or major permanent loss of function associated with a health care–acquired infection.

F. Client and proxy agreements.

1. Living wills.

2. Directives for organ and tissue donation.

3. Directives for withholding or withdrawing life-support measures.

4. Durable power of attorney.

5. Advance directives for medical care.

V. Individual and professional nurse accountability.

A. Individual nurse is responsible for professional nursing practice.

B. "Respondeat superior" renders employer liable and responsible for the actions of the employee.

VI. Liability (Garner, 2001; Stromborg & Christensen, 2001; www.law.com).
   A. Negligence—deviation from the acceptable standard of care that a reasonable person would use in a specific situation.
   B. Malpractice—deviation from a professional standard of care.
   C. Duty—care relationship between client and provider.
   D. Breach of duty—failure to meet an acceptable standard of care.
   E. Defamation—the act of harming the reputation of another by making false statements to a third person.
   F. False imprisonment—a restraint of a person in a bounded area without justification or consent.
   G. Slander—a defamatory statement expressed in a transitory form, especially speech.
   H. Proximate cause—the cause that directly produces an event and without which the event would not have occurred.
   I. Civil—of or pertaining to private rights and remedies that are sought by action or suit, but distinct from criminal proceedings.
   J. Assault—the threat of, or use of, force on another that causes that person to have a reasonable apprehension of imminent harmful or offensive contact.
VII. Litigations involving oncology nurses include the following:
   A. Medication errors by omission or commission.
   B. Failure to follow acceptable standard of care, resulting in client harm.
   C. Incomplete or absent documentation in medical record.
   D. Inadequate referral or follow-up.
   E. Lack of teaching.
   F. Insufficient discharge planning.
   G. Failure to follow through on assessed client need.
   H. Failure to monitor clients in restraints—including use of side rails to restrain.
   I. Failure to educate.
VIII. Potential actions resulting from legal allegations.
   A. Out-of-court settlement, which may include monetary or other restitution.
   B. Trial by jury resulting in monetary restitution, imprisonment, public service payback, or loss of licensure if found guilty; admissible evidence includes medical records, sworn testimony, and expert witness.
   C. Agency or institutional sanctions.
   D. Professional sanctions by state board of nursing.
IX. Prudent action by nurses to ensure "reasonable or customary care" is rendered to the client and is documented in the medical record.
   A. Demonstrate knowledge of and adherence to professional standards and procedures as determined by self-evaluation and peer review.
   B. Participate in policy review and revisions within the agency, private practice, and professional organizations.
   C. Maintain current knowledge of personal and institutional liability.
   D. Maintain adequate individual and agency liability insurance coverage.
   E. Keep diligent records with respect to the following:
      1. Accuracy of entries.
      2. Timeliness of charting.
      3. Accurate and timely filing of incident reports according to agency policy.
      4. Referrals and follow-up care.
      5. Avoidance of dangerous abbreviations in medical orders and documentation.
      6. Minimal use of verbal orders.

  X. Cancer legislation—current legislative issues related to cancer care focus on the following:
- **A.** Prevention and early detection of disease.
- **B.** Research and clinical trials.
- **C.** Evaluation of complementary and alternative treatments.
- **D.** Investigation using human subjects (NIH).
- **E.** Health disparities and unequal treatment (Smedley et al., 2003).
- **F.** Health issues of women.
- **G.** Environmental hazards.
- **H.** Occupational hazards.
- **I.** Access to health care.
- **J.** Economics of cancer.
- **K.** Research ethics (Griffin-Sobel, 2002).
- **L.** Cancer research funding.
- **M.** Cancer genomics (Offit, 1998).
- **N.** Cloning.

 XI. Issues pertinent to oncology nursing practice.
- **A.** Ownership of human cells and tissues.
- **B.** Right to self-determination and autonomy.
- **C.** Withholding care to terminally ill clients (Scanlon, 2003).
- **D.** Withdrawing medical treatment (Jennett, 2002).
- **E.** Occupational and environmental hazards.
- **F.** Human subject research.
- **G.** Complementary and alternative treatments.
- **H.** Addictions among nurses (www.nnsa.com).
- **I.** Informed consent—explicit versus implied.
- **J.** Advance directives.
- **K.** Quality of life and survivorship.
- **L.** Political reform related to access to health care for all.
- **M.** Palliative care (Kuebler & Esper, 2002).
- **N.** End-of-life care, as defined by the World Health Organization (WHO, 1998), is the "active, total care of patients whose disease is not responsive to curative treatment."
- **O.** Health Insurance Portability and Accountability Act of 1996 (HIPAA) (Follansbee, 2002).
- **P.** Telenurse practice (Larson-Dahn, 2001).
- **Q.** Cross-cultural and racial issues in end-of-life care (Kagawa-Singer & Blackhall, 2001; Phipps et al., 2003).
- **R.** Complying with HIPAA (www.hhs.gov/ocr/hipaa), the DHHS issued rules requiring health care providers to provide plain language notices to clients on how to protect client medical information, for example, how it may be used and disclosed. The rules apply to all covered entities that transmit client data electronically for health care claims or equivalent encounters. Included in this information are the following (Reiling, 2002):
  - **1.** Health care payment and remittance advice.
  - **2.** Coordination of benefits.
  - **3.** Health care claims status reports.
  - **4.** Health plan eligibility and disenrollments.
  - **5.** Health plan eligibility information transmissions.
  - **6.** Health care premiums.
  - **7.** Referral certifications and authorizations.

8. The first reports of injuries.

9. Health claim attachments.

S. Unequal treatment—confronting racial and ethnic disparities in health care (Smedley et al., 2003).

XII. Issues pertinent to advanced oncology nursing practice.

A. Verbal orders and presigned controlled-substance slips (know individual state laws).

B. E-health network services (electronic transactions: teleconsultations, videotaping procedures and consultations, interstate teleconsultations) (Rich & Edelstein, 2001).

C. Medicare reimbursement for telehealth (www.cms.gov)—under Medicare, telehealth payments are available to clinicians for client services if the service is one of the following: a professional consultation, office or other outpatient visit, individual psychotherapy or pharmacologic management; via telecommunication systems (excluding fax, telephone, or e-mail) for a beneficiary; a case originating from a rural site designated as a health care shortage area (Buppert, 2002).

D. "Noncompete" agreement with sponsoring/collaborating physician.

E. Delegation to unlicensed assistive personnel.

XIII. Nurse managers—a wide range of legal issues confront the nurse manager, including the following:

A. The reduction of professional nursing staff and the issue of liability; recommendations to reduce liability include the following responsibilities:

1. Communicate inadequate number of professional nursing staff.

2. Define the system to objectively measure acuity.

3. Define the number and skill mix of staff needed to provide safe client care.

4. Identify equipment and supply needs.

5. Initiate client care standards.

6. Document the impact of an inadequate number of professional nursing staff on client care.

7. Ensure that "reasonable" efforts have been taken to address the staffing problem.

8. Define job description and competency for use of unlicensed assistive personnel (UAP).

9. Ongoing documentation of staff competency.

B. Temporary staff and agency nurse liability—ostensible agency or apparent authority (client believes a health care worker is an employee of the health care agency); recommendations to reduce liability of the health care agency with respect to acts of independent contractors include the following responsibilities:

1. Verify credentials, such as nursing licensure, malpractice insurance, and cardiopulmonary resuscitation.

2. Orient to hospital and care unit.

3. Review health care agency policies and procedures.

4. Validate competency.

5. Identify professional as a contract nurse.

6. Evaluate care given.

7. Contract with a limited number of reputable per diem agencies.

C. Labor relations—collective bargaining: (ANA, 2003).

1. Taft-Hartley Act exempted nonprofit hospitals from jurisdiction of the National Labor Relations Board (NLRB), www.nlrb.gov.

   2. Hospitals became subject to the NLRB after 1974.
   3. Solicitation for union member—a "no solicitation" rule is often in effect to inhibit union solicitation within the health care agency.
   4. Recommendations for maintaining a union-free workplace include the following:
      a. Fair labor practices.
      b. Wide range of benefits.
      c. Avoidance of discrimination on basis of gender, race, color, creed, national origin, physical challenge, or lifestyle.
      d. Equitable hiring and promotion practices.
      e. Fair and competitive wages.
      f. Open line of communications between management and labor.
D. Impaired health care professionals (addictions) (American Nurses Association [ANA], 1985; National Council of State Boards of Nursing [NCSBN], 2000; Sloan & Vernarec, 2001; Trinkoff & Zhou, 2000).
   1. State boards of nursing report the degree of impairment is unclear; however, Loeb (1992) reported an estimated 7% of all nurses are impaired by alcohol or drugs. Factors contributing to increased substance abuse among nurses include job stress, rotating shifts, staff shortages, anxiety, and depression (Badzek et al., 1998).
   2. Factors contributing to chemical dependency among nurses (Jack, 1990)—job-related stress, easy access to controlled substances, inadequate narcotic control on nursing unit, financial concerns, home situations, failure of colleagues to report suspicious behaviors.
   3. Educate nurses about addiction: International Nurses Society on Addictions (IntNSA)—to advance excellence in "addictions nursing practice" through advocacy, collaboration, education, research, and policy development; www.intnsa.org.
   4. Management responsibilities.
      a. Establish policy on impaired professionals.
      b. Investigate suspected abuse promptly.
      c. Protect client and health care agency from harm and liability.
      d. Notify board of nursing and document actions.
      e. Offer support through peer or employee assistance programs.
      f. Provide reentry support.
      g. Investigate state nursing association peer assistance options (NCSBN, 2000).
      h. Quality health care in America (Kohn et al., 2000).
         (1) Medical device safety.
         (2) Medication safety.
         (3) Medical error reporting.
E. Create a culture of caring and staff and client satisfaction.
F. Understand national and state laws and statutes pertaining to employment.
   1. Sexual harassment.
   2. Workers compensation.
   3. Equal employment opportunity.
G. Counsel, support, and refer to legal counsel nurses who have been named in a lawsuit.
H. Create a culture of risk prevention and nonpunitive reporting of errors.
I. Conduct a failure mode, effect, and criticality analysis (FMECA) (JCAHO, 2004) to look at problem-prone systems and processes to prevent errors.

INTERNET RESOURCES

Agency for Health Care Policy Research (AHCPR)
website: http://www.guideline.gov
American Medical Association
website: http://www.ama-assn.org
American Nurses Association
websites: www.ana.org and http://www.nursingworld.org
Association of Community Cancer Centers
website: www.accc-cancer.org
Centers for Disease Control and Prevention
website: www.cdc.gov
Centers for Medicare and Medicaid
website: www.cms.hhs.gov
International Nurses Society on Addictions
website: www.intnsa.org
The Leapfrog Group
website: www.leapfrog.org
National Council of State Board of Nurses
website: www.ncsbn.org
National Institutes of Health
website: www.nih.gov
National Labor Relations Board
website: www.nlrb.gov
National Nurses Society on Addiction
website: www.nnsa.org
Oncology Nursing Society
website: www.ons.org
U.S. Department of Health and Human Services
Web site: www.hhs.gov

REFERENCES

American Hospital Association (AHA). (1999). *Hospital statistics*. Chicago: Author.
American Nurses Association (ANA). (2001). *Code of ethics for nurses with interpretive statements*. Washington, DC: Author.
American Nurses Association (ANA). (2003). Workplace issues: Organizing & collective bargaining. Website: http://nursingworld.org.
Annas, G.J. (1992). *The rights of patients: The basic ACLU guide to patient rights* (2nd rev. ed.). Totowa, NJ: Humana Press.
Annas, G.J. (2004). *The rights of patients* (3rd ed.). Carbondale: Southern Illinois University Press.
Badzek, L., Mitchell, K., Marra, S., & Bower, M. (1998). Administrative ethics and confidentiality privacy issues. *Online Journal of Issues in Nursing*, Retrieved February 27, 2003, from the World Wide Web, www.nursingworld.org, p. 6.
Buppert, C. (2002). How can I expand my practice to include: Telehealth? Ask the experts about legal/professional issues for advanced practice nurses from Medscape. Retrieved March 30, 2004 from the World Wide Web: www.medscape.com.
Buppert, C. (2003). Will the new EMTALA regulations restrict NPs from seeing patients in the emergency room? Ask the experts about legal/professional issues for advanced practice nurses from Medscape Nurses. Retrieved March 30, 2004 from the World Wide Web: www.medscape.com.
Cavanaugh, M. (2001). New regulations focus on medical errors. *RN 64*, 74.
Follansbee, N. (2002). Implications of the Health Information Portability and Accountability Act. *Journal of Nursing Administration 32*, 42-47.

Garner, B. (Ed.). (2001). *Black's law dictionary* (2nd pocket ed.). St. Paul, MN: West Group.

Griffin-Sobel, J. (2002). Ethics in research. *Gastroenterology Nursing 25,* 172-173.

Jack, L. (1990). *The core curriculum of addictions—nursing. National Nursing Society on Addictions.* Akokie, IL: Midwest Education Association. Name change: International Nurses Society on Addictions, Raleigh, NC.

Jennett, B. (2002). *The vegetative state: Medical facts, ethical and legal dilemmas.* Cambridge, United Kingdom: Cambridge University Press.

Joint Commission on Accreditation of Healthcare Organizations (JCAHO). (2004). National patient safety goals. Retrieved April 12, 2004 from the World Wide Web: http://www.jcaho.org.

Kagawa-Singer, M., & Blackhall, L. (2001). Negotiating cross-cultural issues at the end-of-life: "You got to go where he lives." *Journal of the American Medical Association 286,* 2993-3001.

Kohn, L., Corrigan, J., & Donaldson, M. (2000). *To err is human: Building a safer health system. Institute of Medicine.* Washington, DC: National Academy Press, pp. 1-30.

Kuebler, K., & Esper, P. (Eds.). (2002). *Palliative practices from A-Z for the bedside clinician.* Pittsburgh: Oncology Nursing Society.

Larson-Dahn, M. (2001). Tele-Nurse practice: Quality of care and patient outcomes. *Journal of Nursing Administration 31,* 145-152.

Law.com. (n.d.). Retrieved April 12, 2004 from the World Wide Web: http://www.dictionary.law.com.

Loeb, S. (Ed.). (1992). *Nurses handbook of law and ethics.* Springhouse, PA: Springhouse.

National Council of State Boards of Nursing (NCSBN). (2000). HIPDB and NPDB questions and answers. Retrieved November 9, 2000 from the World Wide Web: www.ncsbn.org/files/hipdb/hipdbqa.asp.

Offit, K. (1998). *Clinical cancer genetics: Risk counseling and management.* New York: John Wiley & Sons.

Phipps, E., True, G., Harris, D., et al. (2003). Approaching the end-of-life: Attitudes, preferences, and behaviors of African-American and white patients and their family caregivers. *Journal of Clinical Oncology 21,* 549-554.

Pozgar, G.D., & Santucci, N.M. (2002). *Legal aspects of health care administration.* Gaithersburg, MD: Aspen Publishers.

Reiling, R.B. (2002). Legal issues in complying with HIPAA: How oncology programs can untangle the "Privacy Notice." *Oncology Issues 17,* 31-32.

Rich, J.P., & Edelstein, S.A. (2001). E-health and oncology: A legal perspective. *Oncology Issues 16,* 15-17.

Scanlon, C. (2003). Ethical concerns in end-of-life care. *American Journal of Nursing 103,* 48-55.

Sloan, A., & Vernarec, E. (2001). Impaired nurses: Reclaiming careers. *RN 64,* 58-64.

Smedley, B., Stith, A., & Nelson, A. (2003). *Unequal treatment: Confronting racial and ethnic disparities in health care.* Washington, DC: National Academies Press.

Stromborg, M., & Christensen, A. (2001). Legal issues in chemotherapy administration. In M. Gullatte (Ed.). *Clinical guide to antineoplastic therapy: A chemotherapy handbook.* Pittsburgh: Oncology Nursing Society, pp. 281-295.

Trinkoff, A.M., Zhou, Q., Storr, C.L., & Soeken, K.L. (2000). Workplace access, negative proscriptions, job strain, and substance use in registered nurses. *Nursing Research 49,* 83-90.

World Health Organization (WHO). (1998). Symptom relief in terminal illness. Geneva: WHO; www.who.org.

47 Selected Ethical Issues in Cancer Care

PAULA NELSON-MARTEN AND JACQUELINE J. GLOVER

I. Introduction to clinical ethics (Nelson-Marten & Braaten, 2001).
  A. Ethical dilemmas occur daily in oncology nursing practice.
  B. An understanding of clinical ethics is important for the oncology nurse so he/she can apply this knowledge in daily nursing practice and advocate for clients and families to enhance care and quality of life.
  C. As scientific and technologic advances increase in health care and are used more widely, ethical issues will be noted more often.
  D. The terms *morals* and *ethics* are used interchangeably, but each term has a distinct meaning and derivation.
    1. Morals—taken from the Latin word *mores*, which means customs.
      a. Values or rules that are based on an individual's conscience and cultural and religious beliefs.
      b. Serve as guide to right/wrong behavior.
    2. Ethics—derived from the Greek term *ethos*, which means conduct, customs, and character.
      a. The study of how one determines right and wrong.
      b. A process for deciding the best course of action when faced with choices that are in conflict. Involves principles to guide thinking and facilitate reasoning.
  E. Ethical codes provide guidance for oncology nursing practice. American Nurses Association (ANA) Code for Ethics provides a framework for ethical nursing practice. The newest version (2001) is available online (www.nursingworld.org).
    1. ANA Code of Ethics makes values of nursing explicit and lists moral obligations and duties.
    2. Nine provisions in the code with interpretative statements for each. Provisions are as follows:
      a. Practices with compassion/respect.
      b. Primary commitment is the client.
      c. Promotes health and safety.
      d. Responsible for individual nursing practice.
      e. Owes same duties to self as others.
      f. Establishes/maintains health care environments.
      g. Advances the profession through practice, education, administration, and knowledge development.
      h. Collaborates to meet health needs.
      i. Responsible for maintaining the profession.
II. Ethical knowledge base.
  A. Ethical theories.

1. Organizing frameworks that help assess right and wrong in particular circumstances.
2. Ethical theories are not mutually exclusive claims to moral truth; rather they are important but partial contributions to a comprehensive, although necessarily fragmented, moral vision (Arras & Steinbock, 1995).

B. Two major types of ethical theories.
1. Utilitarianism: Jeremy Bentham (1748-1832) and John Stuart Mill (1806-1873) credited with this theory.
   a. Holds that actions are right in proportion as they tend to promote happiness; wrong as they tend to produce the reverse of happiness.
   b. Is a consequentialist theory in that it judges the rightness or wrongness of an action by the consequences of what will happen if the action is or is not performed.
2. Deontologic theories (formalism).
   a. Based on a calculation of duties (the Greek word for duty is "deon") rather than on consequences.
   b. Begin with assumption that what makes an action right or wrong is some intrinsic property of the action itself.
   c. Famous deontologic moral theorist Immanuel Kant (1724-1804): the end never justifies the means. If you want to know if a proposed action is morally permissible, the right question to ask is not "What are the likely consequences?" but "Can I, as a rational agent, consistently will that everyone in a similar situation should act this way?" (similar to a universal golden rule) or alternatively, "Is this action in accord with the requirement to treat other people as ends in themselves and not merely as means?"

C. Many approaches to health care ethics.
1. Principle based. Best exemplified in the work of Beauchamp and Childress (2001), *Principles of Biomedical Ethics.*
   a. This approach involves analyzing how the various principles apply in a given situation and determining how they should be balanced.
   b. Five core ethical principles identified.
      (1) Respect for persons or respect for autonomy (self-rule)—honor client confidences, practice shared decision making, communicate honestly.
      (2) Nonmaleficence (not harming)—ensure that anticipated treatment benefits outweigh any anticipated harms, offer only potentially therapeutic interventions.
      (3) Beneficence (promoting good)—act in the best interests of others.
      (4) Justice (fairness)—allocate scarce resources fairly, abide by institutional and/or insurance allocation policies.
      (5) Veracity—the obligation to tell the truth.
2. Casuistry. Case-based approach to ethical decision making.
   a. Focuses on practical decision making in particular cases and uses paradigm cases for comparison.
3. Ethics of care.
   a. Emphasizes importance of focusing on the client in the context of his/her relationships. Focuses on emotional commitment and a willingness to act unselfishly for the benefit of others. Emphasizes sympathy, compassion, fidelity, discernment, and love. Has its roots in a theologic ethics of love and, more recently, in some feminist writings.

      4. Virtue-based ethics.
         a. Emphasizes the agents who perform actions and make choices. Presumes that morally appropriate decisions occur as a result of being decided by morally sensitive and skilled people. Virtue theorists focus on the education and development of the agent making the decision.
      5. Narrative-based ethics.
         a. Puts emphasis on learning the client's story. The client's illness is the telling of a story that requires empathy and compassion. Narrative ethics can increase sensitivity to details of a case.
   D. Framework of ethical decision making (Scanlon & Glover, 1995).
      1. Step 1. Identify an ethical issue.
      2. Step 2. Gather relevant information/facts.
      3. Step 3. Describe the values at stake.
      4. Step 4. Identify a range of options.
      5. Step 5. Make a choice.
      6. Step 6. Give reasons to support choices.
      7. Step 7. Evaluate how the dilemma could have been prevented.
III. Issues in clinical practice for oncology nurses.
   A. Communication.
      1. Shared decision making between health care professionals and clients requires open and ongoing communication about all aspects of client care from the most mundane aspects of hospital or clinic policies and procedures to diagnosis and prognosis, treatment alternatives, and the effects of illness on the lives of clients and their families.
      2. Communication is two-way. Nurses have to be effective listeners as well as effective communicators of information.
   B. Informed consent is an important ethical and legal consideration.
      1. Definition—ethical and legal concept that requires health care professionals to provide sufficient information about the client's condition and the recommended treatments—its benefits, risks, and alternatives—to enable the client to make a responsible decision to accept or reject the recommendations.
      2. Purpose.
         a. Enable autonomous choice.
         b. Promote good client care as defined by the client.
         c. Protect client from harm.
         d. Ensure responsible medical and nursing professional actions.
         e. Avoid exploitation.
         f. Encourage self-scrutiny by health care professionals.
      3. Elements.
         a. Decision-making capacity.
            (1) Possession of a set of values and goals. Ability to do the following:
               (a) Understand information and communicate.
               (b) Reason and deliberate about one's choices.
            (2) Mental status testing may be inadequate to determine decision-making capacity. Client may have deficits in one or more of the following and still have decision-making capacity (orientation, attention span, immediate recall, long-term memory, calculating ability).
            (3) Clients who have depression, other mental illnesses, dementia, retardation, or other types of disabilities may still possess decision-making capacity; assessment is required.

> > (4) Decision-making capacity is not absolute or permanent. Clients may possess sufficient understanding and reasoning ability to make some decisions but not others; decision-making capacity is task specific.
> > > (a) Clients may have decision-making capacity at one time but not another (i.e., elderly clients with sundowner effect).
> > > (b) Competency versus decision-making capacity. Incompetency is determined by a court, and decision-making capacity is a clinical judgment.
> > > (c) Helpful questions to determine decision-making capacity (Moss, 2003).
> > > > (i) Can the client understand what is wrong with him/her and what are the proposed procedures and treatments?
> > > > (ii) Can the client understand the benefits and risks of the proposed procedures or treatment and the benefits and risks of the alternative procedures and treatments, including nontreatment?
> > > > (iii) Is the client able to reason and make a decision using the clinical information that has been disclosed to him/her and to incorporate his/her personal values and wishes?
> > > > (iv) Is the client able to explain why he/she made the health care decision that he/she did, and is the explanation consistent with his/her stated values and wishes?
> > (5) If a client lacks capacity, turn to a medical power of attorney representative that the client has appointed, or if none is available, appoint an appropriate proxy according to state law.
> > (6) Nurses should be familiar with their particular state laws. Next of kin are not always the legally appropriate proxies for incapacitated clients.
> **b.** Disclosure.
> > (1) Reasonable person standard—disclose what an ordinary person in the client's position would consider significant in deciding whether or not to consent to the procedure or treatment.
> > (2) Subjective standard—what this particular client needs or wants to know in order to make a decision.
> **c.** Comprehension.
> > (1) Information should be explained in a way that the client can understand. Pictures and diagrams are often helpful.
> **d.** Voluntarism. Coercion or undue pressure influence is unacceptable.
> **e.** Authorization. The client must make a clear and unambiguous choice as evidenced by the client's oral or written agreement.

4. Barriers to obtaining informed consent.
> **a.** Inadequate time allowed for discussion.
> **b.** Failure to check the client's understanding and to improve knowledge as needed.
> **c.** Failure to acknowledge uncertainty.
> **d.** Framing of information in such a way that biases are present or the client is pressured into a decision.
> **e.** Language barriers.
> **f.** Altered level of consciousness—confusion, disorientation, medication side effects, disease processes.
> **g.** Failure to address vulnerability, for example, feelings of loss of control, loss of power, and/or helplessness.

5. Exceptions to the requirement to obtain informed consent.
   a. Emergencies. Consent is implied in an emergency when there is an immediate threat to the client's life or permanent functioning.
   b. Waiver of consent. The client waives his/her right to disclosure and authorizes someone else to receive information.
   c. Legal requirements, for example, police orders for alcohol levels or statutory requirements for screening.
   d. Therapeutic privilege (rarely, if ever, justified)—the withholding of information based on possible harm of the information to the client.
6. The role of the nurse in informed consent.
   a. Disclosure. Physicians are responsible for explaining medical treatments and procedures.
      (1) Reinforce and clarify information presented.
      (2) Notify physician if unable to validate understanding.
      (3) Inform physician of possible medication administration that may interfere with comprehension.
      (4) Ascertain documentation of informed consent in the medical record.
   b. Advocacy.
      (1) Solicit and understand the client's value system.
      (2) Respect the right of the client to choose.
      (3) Encourage the client to ask questions and actively participate in decision making.
      (4) Assess and report anxiety and/or ambivalence related to the procedure or treatment.
      (5) Ensure client confidentiality.
      (6) The nurse should identify his/her own biases and prevent biases from compromising nursing care.
      (7) When a registered nurse (RN) has convictions that would impede quality care, he/she should be removed from the direct care of the client in question.
      (8) The RN must be first and foremost the advocate for the client and must be willing to address any intervention, act, or policy that has the potential to violate the client's rights.
C. Communicating bad news (Buckman, 1992).
   1. Definition of bad news. Any news that drastically and negatively alters the client's view of his/her future.
   2. Six-step protocol.
      a. Step 1: Getting started; getting the physical context right, where the meeting is held, and the right people there.
      b. Step 2: Finding out how much the client knows.
      c. Step 3: Finding out how much the client wants to know.
      d. Step 4: Sharing the information—aligning and educating.
      e. Step 5: Responding to the client's feelings.
      f. Step 6: Planning and follow-through.
D. Obligation to minimize pain and suffering.
E. Privacy and confidentiality.
   1. Important for respect of clients.
   2. Privacy includes protection of the client from having to reveal personal information that is not needed in the health care context and protection of the client from viewing by others.
   3. Confidentiality includes protecting information about a client that is critical in the health care context but should not be revealed to others outside this context.

      4. Justifiable breaches in confidentiality.

        a. Client's consent to disclose.

        b. Disclosure required by law (i.e., communicable diseases).

        c. Imminent, severe, and likely harm to self or a third party—duty to warn.

      5. Privacy and confidentiality requirements emphasized under the new federal law—Health Insurance Portability and Accountability Act (HIPAA) of 1996 (HIPAA, 1996).

  F. Genetic testing (Ahronheim et al., 2000).

      1. Raises particular concerns about confidentiality because of feared discrimination by insurance companies and employers.

      2. Raises issues of uncertainty. Tests may be marketed before reliable information about what the results mean for the client; consider referral to genetic counselors with particular expertise.

      3. Testing implicates other family members. Discuss sharing results with others before testing is done.

IV. Issues in clinical research for oncology nurses.

  A. Several important issues in clinical research that may involve ethical issues for the oncology nurse.

  B. Clinical trials. Research studies conducted with people who volunteer to take part. Are planned investigations to determine effective prevention methods and/or treatments for given conditions (http://cis.nci.nih.gov).

      1. Several types: prevention, screening, diagnostic, treatment, supportive care or quality of life, and genetic studies.

      2. Sponsored by governmental agencies and private organizations.

        a. The National Cancer Institute (NCI) sponsors clinical trials through the following groups:

          (1) Cancer centers at research institutions.

          (2) Clinical Trials Cooperative Group.

          (3) Clinical Trials Support Unit (CTSU) that makes phase III trials available to physicians and clients in the United States and Canada.

          (4) Community Clinical Oncology Program (CCOP).

        b. A minority-based community clinical oncology program encourages minority populations to participate in clinical trials.

        c. Private organizations include pharmaceutical as well as biotechnology companies that sponsor trials of their own drugs or products.

      3. Clinical trials may include one or several modalities, such as chemotherapy, radiation therapy, surgery, hormonal therapy, immunotherapy, gene therapy, or alternative therapies for symptom management (Rosse & Garcia, 2001).

  C. Clinical trials are conducted in a series of steps. For treatment trials these steps are called phases. Other types of clinical trials (screening, prevention, diagnostic, supportive, genetic) do not generally have phases.

      1. Phase I trials—first step in testing a new approach in humans. Assist in determining safe drug levels and/or schedules of a new drug using human subjects.

      2. Phase II trials—study the safety and effectiveness of an agent or intervention and evaluate its effect on the human body. Generally focus on a particular type of cancer.

      3. Phase III trials—compare the current standard therapy with a new agent or intervention to determine if one of the therapies is superior to the other for treating a particular type of cancer. Usually involve a large number of participants.

    4. Phase IV trials—less common than phases I, II, and III. Conducted to determine long-term safety and effectiveness of a treatment or intervention. Large numbers of participants are needed for a phase IV trial.

D. Risks and benefits of a clinical trial.

    1. Possible risks.

       a. Side effects that are not expected or that are worse than the standard care.

       b. New drugs or therapies may not be superior to standard care.

       c. If the trial is randomized the participant cannot choose the arm of the study he/she is in.

       d. Insurance may not cover all the involved costs.

       e. Involvement in the trial may include more health care visits than standard care.

    2. Benefits.

       a. Access to a new drug or therapy that is only available in the clinical trial.

       b. The new drug or therapy may be more effective than standard care.

       c. The participant may benefit from the drug or therapy under study.

       d. Clinical trial participants may receive more health care attention than that received with standard care.

       e. Results of the clinical trial may be helpful to other clients in the future.

E. Protecting participants.

    1. Determining which study a client receives.

    2. Role of the institutional review board (IRB).

       a. Protects the rights and welfare of participants in research by determining that risks to participants are minimized and if risks are reasonable in relation to anticipated benefits, if any, and the importance of the knowledge that may reasonably be expected to result.

       b. If the selection of participants is equitable.

       c. Informed consent will be sought from each prospective participant.

       d. Informed consent will be documented.

       e. The research plan makes adequate provision for monitoring the data collected to ensure the safety of participants.

       f. Provisions exist to protect the privacy of participants.

       g. Provisions exist to protect the confidentiality of data.

    3. Data and Safety Monitoring Board (DSMB).

       a. Role of the DSMB: to monitor client safety in large clinical trials (phase III). Usually composed of individuals who are not connected to the trial and who review the trial data periodically with these two questions in mind—are there any expected or severely toxic effects? What is the treatment outcome of the trial so far?

       b. DSMB will provide a summary report back to the IRB of the institution or institutions involved in the study. The report will include toxicities to trial participants.

    4. Eligibility criteria.

    5. Informed consent. This is of particular significance and is explained above in Section III. Issues in clinical practice for oncology nurses.

F. Potential ethical issues in oncology clinical trials (Works, 2000).

    1. Exclusion criteria. All clinical trials have specific exclusion criteria. These criteria may bar individuals from participation.

2. Inclusion of minorities. Many times clinical trials are not representative of minority populations. How much time and effort should be spent trying to attract minority populations to a trial?

3. Client perspective. Client may believe that a clinical trial is best hope for a cure. Client and family need to participate in open, frank discussion with all issues presented regarding prognosis, outcomes, and so on.

4. Clinical perspective. Ongoing debate regarding exclusion criteria—should it be relaxed or rigid? When criteria are restrictive, it takes more time to enroll enough clients to complete a trial.

5. Ethics of randomization. Randomized trials may create a conflict of interest for the physician and his/her dual roles of physician and clinical investigator. A physician may believe that one arm of the trial may be better for the client. In a randomized trial, the client will be put in one arm of the study and the treatment may not be the most effective for the particular client.

6. Cost issues. Insurance companies may deny payment or be reluctant to approve payment for participation in a clinical trial. Drugs for the clinical trial may be free, but tests and visits required by the protocol may be out-of-pocket expenses.
   a. Oncology nurse should advocate for the client and family in regard to financial issues.
   b. Can be very time consuming for the nurse to be involved.

G. Role of the nurse in clinical trials.
   1. Client advocate for all issues related to the trial and participation.
   2. Ensure that informed consent is obtained and documented.
   3. Assess and document the response to the treatment or intervention.
   4. Manage symptoms related to the treatment or intervention.
   5. Ensure confidentiality and anonymity.
   6. Ensure that client selection is appropriate with phase criteria.
   7. Ensure client confidentiality.

H. Obligations of the clinical researcher.
   1. Obtain IRB approval for most educational and health care agencies and all institutions receiving U.S. Department of Health & Human Services funds.
   2. Maintain separation between practice and research.
   3. Obtain informed consent.
   4. Ensure confidentiality.
   5. Ensure anonymity when appropriate to the research design.
   6. Ensure that participant selection is congruent with phase criteria.

I. Role of the nurse in clinical research.
   1. Manage symptoms related to the treatment or intervention.
   2. Provide physical and psychosocial care.
   3. Collaborate with the research team.
   4. Maintain current knowledge of the treatment or interventions.
   5. Encourage client autonomy throughout the research period.
   6. Maintain integrity of the study.
   7. Provide accurate documentation.
   8. Advocate for the client at all times.

J. Websites relevant to oncology clinical trials.
   1. www.cancer.gov/clinical trials.
   2. www.cancerwatch.org and type in "clinical trials" under "search for."

V. Ethical issues in palliative care and end-of-life care.

   A. Distinction among curative care, palliative care, and end-of-life care (Beltran & Coluzzi, 1997).

   1. Curative care.

   a. Type of care typically given by the health care system in the United States.

   b. Primary goal is to reverse the disease process and to prolong life.

   c. Secondary goal is symptom control.

   d. Approximately 30% of medical interventions result in curative care.

   2. Palliative care.

   a. Type of care that focuses on the management of chronic illness.

   b. Good supportive symptom management is the cornerstone of palliative care.

   c. Approximately 70% of current medical treatments are palliative in nature.

   d. Beltran and Coluzzi (1997) note that active palliative care can include curative therapies with the goal of restoration rather than curing.

   3. End-of-life care.

   a. Type of care given at the end of life is comfort care.

   b. Comfort care is best delivered through hospice.

   c. Primary goal includes symptom control/comfort and psychosocial, medical, and spiritual support.

   d. Secondary goal includes a good death for the client, support for the family, and possible prolongation of life.

   B. Advance directives. Since the passage of the federal Patient Self-Determination Act (PSDA), effective December 1, 1991, all health care institutions receiving federal funds are required to give clients written information about their right to participate in their own health care decisions and to complete advance directives (PSDA, 1994).

   1. Living will.

   a. Written document that directs a person's physician to withhold or withdraw life-prolonging interventions (e.g., cardiopulmonary resuscitation [CPR], kidney dialysis, feeding tubes, breathing machines) if he/she is terminally ill or (in some states) permanently unconscious.

   b. Instructs person's physician to provide only those treatments that will relieve pain and provide comfort.

   c. State laws differ regarding when a living will is valid and what provisions are acceptable. Some states require special documentation of desires related to the medical provision of hydration and nutrition.

   d. Role of the nurse.

   (1) Educate the client and family regarding the use of a living will.

   (2) Refer the client to an appropriate resource for initiating a living will.

   (3) Ensure that the health care team is aware of the existence and content of a living will.

   2. Medical power of attorney.

   a. Written document that allows a person to name another individual to make health care decisions for him/her if he/she is unable to make them.

   b. Some states include special provisions about what kinds of decisions a medical power of attorney representative can make and under what circumstances.

      c. Role of the nurse.

         (1) Educate the client and family regarding the opportunity to establish a medical power of attorney for health care.

         (2) Refer the client to appropriate resource to initiate the necessary legal documents.

         (3) Promote communication between the health care team and the person who is the medical power of attorney representative.

C. Do not resuscitate (DNR) orders.

  1. A physician's order not to perform CPR in the event that a client's pulse and/or respirations cease.

  2. Some people consider DNRs to be a kind of advance directive because clients must indicate their wishes before CPR is necessary. However, DNRs are different in that they are physicians' orders and must be written by a physician, based on the values and preferences of the client as expressed by a client with capacity or his/her legal representative.

  3. Many states have laws that allow for out-of-hospital DNRs that are respected by emergency medical professionals.

  4. It is critical to discuss goals of treatment with clients with potentially life-limiting illnesses, and a discussion of the provision of CPR is an important part of this discussion, but not the only part. The provision of all therapies should be guided by the client's values, goals, and preferences.

  5. Role of the nurse.

    a. Ensure that a clear understanding exists among the physician, client, and family members regarding resuscitation orders.

    b. Promote independent decision making throughout treatment by encouraging clients and family members to communicate openly with the health care team.

    c. Ensure proper documentation and appropriate renewal procedures of resuscitation orders according to institutional policies.

    d. Respect cultural values regarding death and dying.

    e. Validate emotional responses of clients and family members to resuscitation orders.

    f. Refer the client and family to other appropriate resources (pastoral care, support services, social services).

    g. Be an advocate for the client and family.

D. Common distinctions in end-of-life care. Nurse needs to look at both ethical and moral issues; to weigh the benefits and burdens of particular treatments and take into consideration the client's values and preferences.

  1. Extraordinary versus ordinary. Historically a distinction between treatments that are morally required and treatments that are not, based on the degree of burden. Efforts to identify such treatments independent of particular circumstances are misguided, for example, regarding all medical provision of hydration and nutrition as "ordinary" and thus required and all ventilators as "extraordinary" and thus morally optional.

  2. Withholding versus withdrawing. Foregoing life-sustaining therapies includes both withholding and withdrawing. Both are justified according to the proportion of benefits and burdens and client's values and preferences. A belief that it is justified to withhold treatments but not to withdraw them is misguided. If there is sufficient justification not to start a treatment, there is also sufficient justification to stop a treatment and perhaps more justification based on a trial of therapy that has proven ineffective. This distinction can have the perverse consequence of people not starting treatments in the face of uncertainty, because they are afraid that they cannot be stopped. There is no ethical and legal difference between the two.

3. Foreseen versus intended. Also known as the principle of double effect. Treatments that have multiple possible consequences (some good and some bad) may still be justified if the bad consequences are not intended but only foreseen to occur (i.e., adequate pain treatment is justified even if one possible consequence of high doses of pain medication is the possible shortening of the client's life; in this instance, relief of pain is both the intended and foreseen consequence—possibly hastening death is only foreseen).

4. Active versus passive. Historically used to help distinguish between actions that are not justified in leading to a client's death (boluses of potassium) and omissions (sometimes referred to as "allowing to die") that are justified. Not very helpful when it comes to common decisions about withdrawing life-sustaining technologies such as ventilators in the intensive care unit (ICU) since withdrawing a ventilator is an action that is universally regarded as justifiable based on proportion of benefits and burdens and client's values and preferences.

E. Potential palliative options of last resort.

1. Clients experiencing end-of-life care illnesses may also endure a great deal of pain and suffering. Although suffering can be multidimensional (physical, psychologic, social, or spiritual) in nature, it often is physical and relates to the amount of pain the individual is experiencing. Often clients request assistance in dealing with pain and suffering. Sometimes these requests are ethical but not legal, and they may or may not be current standards of medical or nursing practice.

2. The American Nurses Association developed six position statements in 1997 to serve as guidelines for nurses caring for clients at the end of life. These position statements serve as current practice standards for nursing care. The full text of the position statements can be found on the ANA website at http://www.ana.org. The six position statements are as follows:

   a. Promotion of Comfort and Relief of Pain in Dying Patients, 1997.
   b. Active Euthanasia and Assisted Suicide, 1997.
   c. Assisted Suicide, 1997.
   d. Nursing and the Patient Self-Determination Act, 1997.
   e. Nursing Care and Do-Not-Resuscitate Decisions, 1997.
   f. Foregoing Nutrition and Hydration, 1997.

3. A physician, Timothy Quill, has defined which requests for assistance at the end of life by clients are ethical, legal, and current standards of medical practice. Quill's list (2001, p.176) is also helpful for oncology nurses.

   a. Legal acceptability; ethical consensus; standards of practice.
      (1) Intensive pain and symptom management.
      (2) Not starting or stopping potentially life-sustaining therapies.
   b. Legal acceptability; growing ethical consensus.
      (1) Voluntarily stopping eating and drinking (VSED).
      (2) Terminal sedation (TS).
   c. Ethical controversy; legal prohibition in most states.
      (1) Physician-assisted suicide (PAS).
      (2) Voluntary active euthanasia (VAE).

INTERNET RESOURCES

American Nurses Association (ANA) Code of Ethics
website: www.nursingworld.org
Oncology clinical trials website: www.cancer.gov/clinical trials
Anenine Press
www.cancerwatch.org

REFERENCES

Ahronheim, J.C., Moreno, J.D., & Zuckerhman, C. (2000). *Ethics in clinical practice* (2nd ed.). Gaithersburg, MD: Aspen Publishers, pp. 368-381.

Arras, J.D., & Steinbock, B. (1995). *Ethical issues in modern medicine.* Mountain View, CA: Mayfield Publishing Co., pp. 1-39.

Beauchamp, T.L., & Childress, J.F. (2001). *Principles of biomedical ethics* (5th ed.). New York: Oxford University Press.

Beltran, J.E., & Coluzzi, P.H. (1997). Medical ethics: A model for comprehensive palliative care. *The Talbert Journal of Health Care,* Spring/Summer 1997, 47-57.

Buckman, R. (1992). *How to break bad news: A guide for health care professionals.* Baltimore: The Johns Hopkins University Press.

Health Insurance Portability and Accountability Act (HIPAA). (1996). Public Law No. 104-191.

Moss, A.H. (2003). *Course book for health care ethics.* Morgantown, WV: West Virginia University Center for Health Ethics and Law; www.wvethics.org.

Nelson-Marten, P., & Braaten, J.S. (2001). Common ethical dilemmas. In R.A. Gates & R.M. Fink (Eds.). *Oncology nursing secrets* (2nd ed.). Philadelphia: Hanley & Belfus, pp. 565-573.

Patient Self-Determination Act (PSDA). (1994). Public Law No. 101-508, '4206, 4751 (hereinafter OBRA) 104 Stat. 1388-115 to 117, 1388-204 to 206 (codified at 42 U.S.C.A.'1395cc(f)(l) & id. '1396a(a) (West Supp. 1994).

Quill, T. (2001). Palliative options of last resort: A comparison of practices, justifications, and safeguards. In *Caring for patients at the end of life: Facing an uncertain future together.* New York: Oxford University Press, pp. 175-202.

Rosse, P.A., & Garcia, M.T. (2001). Clinical trials. In R.A. Gates & R.M. Fink (Eds.). *Oncology nursing secrets* (2nd ed.). Philadelphia: Hanley & Belfus, pp. 97-102.

Scanlon, C., & Glover, J.J. (1995). A professional code of ethics: Providing a moral compass in turbulent times. *Oncology Nursing Forum* 22(10), 1515-1521.

Works, C. (2000). Principles of treatment planning and clinical research. In C.H. Yarbro, M.H. Frogge, M. Goodman, & S.L. Groenwald. (Eds.): *Cancer nursing: Principles and practice* (5th ed.). Sudbury, MA: Jones and Bartlett Publishers, pp. 259-271.

48 Cancer Economics and Health Care Reform

MOLLY LONEY

I. The national health care crisis.
   A. Definition.
      1. The United States is facing a critical shortage of health care resources to meet the complex and changing health care needs of individuals, families, and communities (Heinrich & Thompson, 2002; Oncology Nursing Society [ONS], 2002b).
      2. Health care resources include nurses and other health care providers; hospital support services; financial reimbursement from insurance companies, managed care providers, Medicare, and/or Medicaid to pay for the continuum of care; funding for nursing and medical education; and funding for ongoing research into disease prevention, diagnosis, treatment, and palliation.
   B. Historical perspective.
      1. Significant reorganization of hospitals in the United States in the last decade with merging and downsizing (eliminating positions and services) to reduce rising health care costs (Mee & Robinson, 2003).
      2. Managed care has become a predominant model for cost containment of health care, with 76% of all covered employees enrolled in either an HMO (health maintenance organization) or PPO (preferred provider organization).
      3. Goal of providing access to quality health care services to all in need has become conditional in reducing costs in managed care environments (Heinrich & Thompson, 2002; National Coalition for Cancer Survivorship [NCCS], 2002).
      4. Lack of adequate nursing work pool: 86% to 94% of oncology nurses said there are too few registered nurses (RNs) who specialize in cancer care (Lamkin et al., 2001). The nursing shortage is predicted to worsen over the next 10 to 15 years, at a time when increasing technology and scientific discoveries require highly skilled nurses to administer complex therapies (ONS, 2002a).
      5. Changes in care and work environments, with time-limited hospitalization for immediate acute care. Rehabilitation, supportive care, and end-of-life care have been shifted to ambulatory and home care settings. Seventy-four percent of oncology nurses said clients are sicker, and 47% said delegation to nurses by physicians has increased (Lamkin et al., 2001).
      6. While health care resources are diminishing, cancer incidence is rising, with a 50% increase in the number of cancer clients projected by 2020 (American Cancer Society [ACS], 2003).
II. Influencing factors.
   A. Aging population.

1. The population in America is aging rapidly.
    a. Approximately 39 million individuals will be over the age of 65 years by 2010.
    b. Approximately 69 million individuals will be over the age of 65 years by 2050, representing 23% of the total population in the United States (U.S. Bureau of the Census, 1989).
    c. Increased life expectancy is associated with increased incidence of disease, injury, and disability, with increased demands for ongoing health care.
    d. Participation in health screening decreases with age (Jemal et al., 2003).
    e. Age is the most important determinant of cancer risk. More than 57% of all cancers occur in individuals over the age of 65 years (Boyle et al., 1992; Lyman & Kuderer, 1998).
B. Nature of cancer care.
    1. Cancer is a major public health problem in the United States.
        a. National Cancer Institute (NCI) estimates that approximately 8.9 million individuals with a cancer history were living in 1999.
        b. Estimated new cases of cancer in 2004 are 1,368,030 in both genders.
        c. Since 1990, more than 17 million new cancer cases have been diagnosed (ACS, 2003).
        d. Lifetime probability of developing cancer has increased to 38.5% in women and 43.5% in men.
        e. One in four adult deaths is caused by cancer. Cancer is the second leading cause of death in children from ages 1 to 14 years (Jemal et al., 2003) and for individuals over the age of 55 years (Boyle et al., 1992).
        f. Estimated cancer deaths in 2004 are 563,700 , or more than 1500 deaths each day.
        g. From 1992 to 1999, cancer-related death rates declined slightly from 0.6% (in females) and 1.5% (in males).
        h. Probability of surviving cancer has increased significantly. The 5-year relative survival rate for all cancers is 62%—represents people living 5 years after diagnosis, whether disease free, in remission, undergoing treatment, or living with advanced disease (ACS, 2003).
    2. Recent changes.
        a. An increased risk for developing cancer and cancer-related deaths has been linked to environmental and lifestyle factors.
            (1) Includes smoking, high-fat diet and obesity, physical inactivity, infectious disease, and exposure to chemicals or radiation.
            (2) Associated with 75% of all cancer deaths in the United States (ACS, 2003; Jemal et al., 2003).
        b. Cancer care has become increasingly more specialized, sophisticated, and multimodal with the use of precise imaging equipment as well as gene assay, biotherapy, stereotactic radiation therapy, antiangiogenesis agents, chemoprotective agents, growth factors, and gene therapy (Pearce et al., 2001).
        c. Inpatient hospitalizations have shortened significantly as care has shifted to outpatient and home care, with families facing an increased burden of care (Jemal et al., 2003).
        d. The population of cancer clients is increasing as the general population is aging.
        e. Cancer has become a chronic, multifaceted disease. Many clients and their families are living with long-term side effects and accompanying

lifestyle changes from cancer and/or its treatment (NCCS, 2002; ONS, 2002c).

    f. Cancer care has been broadened to include palliative and hospice care (Institute of Medicine [IOM], 2003a).

3. Cost of cancer care.

    a. Health care costs have been rising over the past decade. In 1999, total health care administration costs were at least $294.3 billion in the United States. Costs for 2003 are estimated at more than $1 trillion (Woolhandler et al., 2003).

    b. National Institutes of Health (NIH) estimated the overall cost of cancer care in 2002 was $171.6 billion.

        (1) Direct medical costs were $60.9 billion.

        (2) Indirect morbidity costs (cost of lost productivity from cancer-related illness) were $15.5 billion.

        (3) Indirect mortality costs (cost of lost productivity from premature cancer-related deaths) were $95.2 billion (ACS, 2003).

        (4) Intangible costs to quality of life from unrelieved and distressing symptoms of cancer or its treatment cannot be measured in dollars and cents (i.e., pain and suffering, loss of control, loss of social supports, loss of autonomy, loss of family function) (IOM, 2003a; ONS, 2002c).

        (5) Cost of health care has been described by many consumers as a barrier to seeking medical care (ACS, 2003).

    c. Lack of integration of palliative care standards into the cancer care continuum has led to increased cost of care at the end of life.

        (1) Unresolved cancer symptoms can pose a financial burden for clients and their families. Direct, pain-related medical costs have averaged $891 per month per cancer client (Fortner et al., 2003).

        (2) Use of aggressive treatment until death often results in unresolved symptom management with emergency room visits and intensive care unit care (Scanlon, 2001).

        (3) Coordinated, expert end-of-life care that prevents emergency room visits and hospitalizations with early use of advanced directives may reduce end-of-life costs by 40% to 70% (Payne et al., 2002).

        (4) Cancer research dollars have been spent on understanding how cancer develops and its most effective cure and treatment. Little has been allocated for resolving or managing distressing symptoms and improving quality of life (IOM, 2003b; NCCS, 2002).

    d. Lack of cancer research funding is a national priority (ONS, 2003b).

4. Only 3% of cancer health care costs are associated with cancer research.

5. Fewer than 3% of adults with cancer participate in clinical trials of cancer therapies, yet 12% to 44% may be eligible to participate (National Coalition for Cancer Research, 2001).

C. Managed care.

    1. Definition: a type of health care delivery that aims to control costs by regulating and coordinating clients' use of health care services. Organized by insurance companies, hospitals, and employers.

    2. Payment is usually based on a fee for service (FFS) plan, with payment for each service provided that corresponds to a payment to the provider (i.e., health care system, physician).

> **3.** Types of managed care plans.
>> **a.** HMOs—tightly controlled staff model with a prepaid health plan that provides and restricts health care choice for its members.
>> **b.** PPOs—model that provides payment for health care at preestablished rates. Consumers have more choice, but rates are lowest for preferred list of providers.
>> **c.** Point-of-service contracts (POSs)—more liberal model that allows choice of physicians not affiliated with the primary HMO, especially for specialist referrals (Heinrich & Thompson, 2002).
>> **d.** In 2000, 80.9 million people were enrolled in HMOs and 84.5 million people were enrolled in PPOs (MCOL, 2003).
>> **e.** Growing enrollment in PPOs as consumers search for more choice in physicians and access to full range of health care services.
> **4.** Comparison of nonmanaged and managed care (Table 48-1).

TABLE 48-1
Comparison of Nonmanaged and Managed Care in the United States

	Nonmanaged Care	Managed Care
HEALTH SERVICE DELIVERY		
Focus	Episodic treatment	Prevention and continuity of care
Provider autonomy	Liberal	Routinely uses standard practice guidelines, care maps, clinical pathways, other methods
Referrals	Unlimited	Strict control
Physician usage	Multiple physician groups	Selected group of physicians
MARKET FACTORS		
Type of competing providers	Independent	Networks
Ancillary service use	High numbers	Lower numbers
Inpatient hospitalization rates/days	Higher	Lower
INFORMATION SYSTEMS		
Characteristics	Fragmented, episodic, financially focused	Mature managed market has well-developed client-focused information systems May include computerized medical record; data are outcome driven from financial, utilization, and clinical perspectives
REIMBURSEMENT		
Effect on volume	Uses fee-for-service system that provides incentive to increase or maintain high volume of services provided	Uses provider risk-sharing strategies to create an incentive to control volume
Type of reimbursement	Open-ended reimbursement; emphasizes productivity	Limited reimbursement with focus on efficiency
Type of care	Emphasized specialty care	Uses primary care model
Market share	Defined by number of inpatient admissions and/or clinic visits	Defined by number of covered lives for which it is liable to provide services if needed

5. Managed care organizations use a variety of methods to control health care costs and service use, including negotiating discounted fees from providers; offering financial incentives to "gatekeepers" (usually primary care physicians) to reduce costs; and paying a fixed fee per client regardless of the services used.

6. Ethical issues with managed care—provides an incentive to potentially undertreat clients who may need laboratory and diagnostic work-ups, as well as specialist referrals or specialized care (Heinrich & Thompson, 2002).

D. Medicare reimbursement system.

1. Definition: a government-regulated program that provides health insurance for all individuals at age 65 years and older, regardless of socioeconomic status or income. It covers people with any sensory loss or progressive or end-stage disease. Coverage is targeted for acute care, but limited benefits also cover hospice care (Pulcini et al., 2002).

2. In 2002, Medicare provided health care coverage for 40 million individuals; enrollment is expected to reach 77 million by 2031.

3. More than 60% of all new cancer diagnoses occur in the Medicare population.

4. Program has not kept pace with health care improvements.

   a. Four out of five cancer care visits occur in ambulatory settings, yet Medicare was designed to cover inpatient expenses.

   b. Medicare does not cover the full range of outpatient cancer care services available, including prescription drug coverage, prevention and screening, high cost of advanced cancer therapies, and the continuum of care provided by oncology nurses (ONS, 2002a, 2003c).

      (1) Lack of coverage for nurse-driven triage, client and family education, ongoing symptom assessment and management, financial counseling, health team collaboration.

      (2) Lack of coverage for other support services—pharmacy, social work, clinical trials.

   c. Reimbursement is based on the following:

      (1) DRGs (diagnosis-related groups) for inpatients with preset coverage fees determined by a client's primary and secondary diagnoses, age, gender, and complications (Pulcini et al., 2002).

      (2) AWPs (average wholesale prices) for outpatients with average reimbursement for preestablished drugs. Prices are set by pharmaceutical companies' drug reference publications and are currently higher than the cost of the drugs.

         (a) Coverage of expert nursing care comes from surplus of fees paid for AWPs.

         (b) In 2002 and 2003, Congress and regulatory agencies worked on Medicare reform by reducing AWPs without adding compensation for full range of nursing care and support services (ONS, 2003a, 2003c).

         (c) In January 2003, the Centers for Medicare and Medicaid Services (CMS) released a new payment system, hospital outpatient prospective payment system (OPPS)—with significant payment cuts for drugs.

         (d) Medicare reimbursement for outpatient chemotherapy was cut by 27% in 2003 (Braud, 2003).

         (e) Unbalanced reform threatens the future financial stability of outpatient cancer centers and oncologists' offices.

      (f) If reimbursement to pay for services is lacking, service cuts are projected—limiting cancer clients' access to the full range of quality cancer care (NCCS, 2002; ONS, 2003a, 2003c).

E. Disparities in access to care.

  1. Higher cancer incidence, morbidity, and mortality in African Americans.

    a. Ten percent higher incidence rate than in Caucasians, 50% to 60% higher than in Hispanics and Asians, and more than twice as high as American Indians.

    b. Poor probability of survival in African Americans. At time of diagnosis, cancer is less likely to be localized and easily treated.

    c. Thirty percent higher death rate from cancer than Caucasians and more than twice as high as death rates in Asians, Hispanics, and American Indians (ACS, 2003; Jemal et al., 2003)

  2. Less participation in cancer screening and early detection by African Americans and Hispanics than Caucasians.

    a. Influencing factors include socioeconomic status, cultural practices and beliefs, lifestyle behaviors, education, work status, social environment, access to health care, and migration trends.

    b. If health care access and use became more widespread with underserved populations, a 3% to 10% gain is estimated for early detection and treatment of cervical and breast cancers (Breen et al., 2001).

  3. Lack of access.

    a. More than 41 million individuals in the United States are uninsured (IOM, 2003b).

    b. According to the 2000 National Health Interview Survey, 17% of Americans under the age of 65 years had no health insurance and 27% of individuals over the age of 65 years had only Medicare coverage (Breen et al., 2001).

    c. African Americans are two times and Hispanics are three times more likely to be uninsured than Caucasians.

    d. The changing economy, with businesses merging, downsizing, and restructuring, will continue to increase unemployment and the percentage of uninsured.

    e. Being uninsured can increase the cost of medical care, with individuals and families delaying preventive and medical care.

    f. Growing numbers of uninsured can affect a community's stability, with reduced services available, poorer community health, and a less prosperous local economy.

    g. In 2001, $34 to $38 billion was paid for care delivered to the uninsured. The public was estimated to have paid for 85% of this care (IOM, 2003b).

F. Nursing shortage.

  1. American Nurses Association (ANA) estimated a nursing shortage of 126,000 unfilled hospital RN positions in 2001 (ANA, 2001).

  2. By 2020, the shortage is projected to total 808,400 nurses. The number of RNs not employed in nursing increased by 28% from 1992 to 2000 (U.S. Department of Health & Human Services, Health Resources & Services Administration [HRSA], 2000).

  3. A 50% increase in cancer clients is projected by 2020 (ACS, 2003), as the number of nurses to care for them decreases.

  4. Hospital cost cutting eliminated many RN positions. Remaining nurses have felt "overburdened" by short staffing, which has accelerated the "flight" of nurses from their profession (Mee & Robinson, 2003).

5. Almost 60% of the current RN workforce is over 40 years of age, with an average age of 45 years. Fifty percent of nurses working in 2003 will reach retirement age within 15 years.
6. Fewer people are going into nursing.
    a. Other professions are attracting young workers with diverse career options. The average age of a new graduate nurse is 31 years (Buerhaus et al., 2000).
    b. Nursing's public image is still not conveying the many ways nurses make a real difference. A recent ANA poll reflects public misunderstanding about what nurses do (ANA, 2001; Kimball & O'Neil, 2002).
    c. Since 1995, enrollment in all types of nursing schools has declined, resulting in 26% fewer RN graduates in 2000 than 1995 (U.S. Department of Health & Human Services, HRSA, 2000).
    d. Faculty shortages in schools of nursing have increased. The American Association of Colleges of Nursing (AACN) survey reported 379 faculty vacancies in 2000, with schools of nursing turning away almost 6000 qualified applicants (AACN, 2002; U.S. Department of Health & Human Services, HRSA, 2000).
    e. In 2000, the average age for doctoral-prepared nursing faculty was 53.5 years (AACN, 2002).
7. Fewer nurses are specializing in oncology nursing, as hospitals have merged oncology-designated units into general medical-surgical care (Lamkin et al., 2001).
    a. Many experienced oncology RNs, including expert advanced practice nurses, have lost their jobs with budget cuts.
    b. RNs are encouraged to generalize instead of specialize (ONS, 2002c).
8. Nurses are increasingly dissatisfied with health care's work environment and conditions.
    a. Nurses are working longer hours, with a reported average of 48 hours each week plus at least 7 hours of overtime (Bauer, 2001).
    b. More than 40% of hospital nurses in a multinational study reported dissatisfaction with their jobs (Aiken et al., 2002).
    c. Oncology nurses reported a 79% increase in client acuity and a 73% increase in paperwork (Lamkin et al., 2001).
    d. Reported sources of dissatisfaction include high nurse/client staffing ratios, lack of adequate support services, lack of administrative support, increased nonnursing work, lack of a collaborative professional practice environment, mandatory overtime, lack of tools to do one's job, inadequate compensation, and poor standards of care (Aiken et al., 2002; Mee & Robinson, 2003).
    e. In a 2001 earnings survey, 16% reported belonging to a nursing union (Bauer, 2001).
9. Significant impact on quality client care.
    a. Chemotherapy drugs are often administered by nurses lacking oncology knowledge (ONS, 2002c).
    b. A study of adult hospitals demonstrated a 7% higher death rate for each additional client assignment above four clients.
    c. Each additional client assigned per nurse was associated with a 23% increased risk of burnout and a 15% increased risk of job dissatisfaction (Aiken et al., 2002).
    d. A higher number of hours of RN-provided care has been associated with better care for hospitalized clients, including shorter length of

stay; lower rates of urinary tract infections, gastrointestinal bleeding, pneumonia, thrombosis, sepsis, shock, and cardiac arrest; and lower rates of "failure to rescue" (Needham et al., 2002).

  G. Competing economic demands.
    1. Factors such as the aging population, urbanization, competition for energy sources, terrorism, and war have reduced available governmental funds for addressing cancer care and nursing shortage issues (Pfoultz et al., 2002).

III. Health care reform: a call to action.
  A. ONS initiatives.
    1. Advocacy.
      a. Proactive health policy agenda with annual revisions—nursing shortage as number one priority.
      b. Health policy activities, such as the following:
        (1) Lobbying on Capitol Hill.
        (2) Representing ONS—seats at key legislative, regulatory, and advocacy group meetings.
        (3) Coordination of ONS advocacy groups.
          (a) State Health Policy Liaisons—regional advocacy.
          (b) Capitol Gang—national advocacy.
      c. Capitol Hill visits with legislators.
        (1) Congressional briefings.
        (2) Written and oral testimonies on key issues from expert ONS members.
      d. Grassroots support for passage of major health policy legislation.
        (1) 2002 Nurse Reinvestment Act (NRA) with funding allocated in 2003 to address growing nursing shortage.
          (a) National Cancer Act to double NCI funding.
          (b) Elimination of "zero work pool" terminology in 2002 as description of nursing care—proposals for Medicare reform.
      e. Honor awards to key legislators for support of nursing shortage and quality cancer care legislation.
    2. Education.
      a. Position statements and issue briefs published on issues affecting access, delivery, and cost of quality cancer care (see www.ons.org for current publications).
      b. Legislative website at www.onslac.org.
      c. Legislative alerts through ONStat.
      d. Nurse in Washington Internship and Association of Community Cancer Centers (ACCC) training conferences for State Health Policy Liaisons and ONS leadership.
      e. Regional legislative workshops
      f. ONS Health Policy Toolkit with practical advocacy tips.
      g. Leadership workshops in Washington, D.C. with visits to Capitol Hill.
      h. ONS publications addressing nursing shortage issues.
    3. Professional collaboration.
      a. Member of ANA's Nursing's Agenda for the Future with 60 other organizations.
      b. Member of Americans for Nursing Shortage Relief (ANSR) coalition with 37 other organizations.
      c. Joint testimony to Congress and CMS with ACCC and US Oncology.
      d. Hosted first congressional briefing in Washington, D.C. in 2002.

      e. Hosted summit on health care reform with members of the cancer care community in 2002.

      f. Joint advocacy activities with advocacy groups and health care organizations.

      g. 2002 ONS Workforce Study.

      h. Joint position statements with other health care organizations (e.g., ONS and Association of Oncology Social Work [AOSW] joint position on end-of-life care).

      i. Endorsement of positions and standards set by other health care groups and organizations (i.e., IOM report on palliative care).

  4. Community outreach.

      a. Public image promotion campaign.

          (1) Promoting Positive Professional Cultures—2002 steering council project.

          (2) ONS and Oncology Nursing Certification Corporation (ONCC) 2002 consumer awareness campaign—publication of consumer awareness brochure advocating for oncology and oncology certified nurse (OCN)–specialty nursing care.

          (3) Professional Image: Understanding Newer and Younger Nurses—2002 steering council project.

      b. Outreach to National Student Nurses Association (NSNA)—website link, dual ONS/NSNA membership.

      c. Job Shadowing Kit for chapters (Lamkin, 2003; www.ons.org).

B. Hospital initiatives.

  1. Major attention to recruitment and retention incentives.

  2. Changes in work conditions and work environment.

      a. Shared governance and nurse/physician partnerships—to give nurses more input and control over their practice.

      b. Growing success of magnet hospital accreditation and designation—to recognize hospitals with work environments that advocate for quality client care as well as supportive working environments (McClure & Hinshaw, 2002).

C. Nurses taking action.

  1. Education.

      a. Use ONS resources to become and/or stay informed on major issues affecting health care, both nationally and locally.

      b. Learn about managed care and Medicare reimbursement.

      c. Take advantage of opportunities to share stories about how oncology nurses make a difference for cancer clients, their families, the multidisciplinary team, health care organization, and/or the community.

      d. Explore opportunities to mentor and educate others in the oncology nursing specialty (i.e., job shadowing).

      e. Suggest chapter programs on health care reform as everyone's business—for oncology nurses and the public.

      f. Offer program on quality cancer care for local cancer support group.

  2. Advocacy.

      a. Contact State Health Policy Liaison for advocacy tips.

      b. Get involved—advocate for unrestricted access to full range of quality cancer care services with balanced reimbursement (ONS, 2002c, 2003b).

          (1) Vote in elections.

          (2) Call and/or visit local legislators in their home districts to discuss health care issues and needs.

        (3) Share stories of how local cancer clients are affected by the current health care reimbursement system.

        (4) E-mail legislators and/or their health policy contacts to encourage legislation support.

        (5) Schedule visit to local legislators when traveling to state capital or Capitol Hill (ONS, 2002c; Ruetter & Duncan, 2002).

        (6) Help clients access reimbursement information and resources through pharmaceutical companies.

    c. Find ways to meet personal and professional needs despite the changing health care system.

3. Changing the work environment.

    a. Share success stories.

    b. Find ways to improve oncology nursing practice. Identify evidence-based standards through ONS and other nursing organizations.

    c. Encourage brainstorming and constructive problem solving with coworkers and management.

    d. Volunteer for project work group.

    e. Help support orientation of new nurses and unlicensed assistive personnel.

    f. Recognize coworkers when they make a difference even in little ways (Mee & Robinson, 2003).

    g. Build multidisciplinary collaboration.

4. Community outreach.

    a. Explore opportunities to work with advocacy groups (i.e., Coalition for Cancer Survivors, ACS).

    b. Encourage local chapter to network with local student nurses association.

    c. Consider getting involved by recruiting voter turnout in local and national elections.

REFERENCES

Aiken, L., Clarke, S., Sloane, D., et al. (2002). Hospital nurse staffing and patient mortality, nurse burnout and job dissatisfaction. *Journal of the American Medical Association 288*(16), 1987-1993.

American Association of Colleges of Nursing (AACN). (2002). *2001-2002 Enrollments and graduations in baccalaureate and graduate programs in nursing*. Washington, DC: Author.

American Cancer Society (ACS). (2004). *Cancer facts and figures 2004*. Atlanta: Author.

American Nurses Association (ANA). (2001). *Analysis of American Nurses Association staffing survey*. Washington, DC: Author.

Bauer, J. (2001). Earnings survey—higher earnings, longer hours. *RN*, October, 36-47.

Boyle, D.M., Engelking, C., Blesch, K., et al. (1992). *Oncology Nursing Society position paper on cancer and aging: The mandate for oncology nursing*. Pittsburgh: Oncology Nursing Society.

Braud, E. (2003). Getting beyond the numbers—how Medicare reimbursement affects our patients. *Oncology Issues*, May/June, 23-24.

Breen, N., Wagener, D.K., Brown, M.L., et al. (2001). Progress in cancer screening over a decade: Results of cancer screening from the 1987, 1992, and 1998 National Health Interview Surveys. *Journal of the National Cancer Institute 93*, 1704-1713.

Buerhaus, P., Staiger, D., & Auerbach, D. (2000). Implications of a rapidly aging registered nurse workforce. *Journal of the American Medical Association 283*(22), 2948-2954.

Fortner, B., Pemarco, G., Irving, G., et al. (2003). Prescription and descriptors of direct and indirect costs of pain reported by cancer patients. *Journal of Pain and Symptom Management 25*(1), 9-18.

Heinrich, J., & Thompson, T. (2002). Organization and delivery of health care in the United States: A patchwork system. In D. Mason, J. Leavitt, & M. Chafee (Eds.). *Policy and politics in nursing and health care*. Philadelphia: W.B. Saunders, pp. 201-213.

Institute of Medicine (IOM). (2003a). *Improving palliative care: We can take better care of people with cancer*. Washington, DC: National Cancer Advisory Board Publication, National Academies Press.

Institute of Medicine (IOM). (2003b). *A shared destiny: Community effects on uninsurance*. Washington, DC: National Academies Press.

Jemal, A., Murray, T., Samuels, A., et al. (2003). Cancer statistics, 2003. *CA: A Cancer Journal for Clinicians 53*(1), 5-43.

Kimball, B., & O'Neil, E. (2002). *Health care's human crisis: The American nursing shortage*. Princeton, NJ: The Robert Wood Johnson Foundation.

Lamkin, L. (2003). *The nursing shortage and what ONS is doing about it*. Ohio Health presentation on March 28, Columbus.

Lamkin, L., Rosiak, J., Buerhaus, P., et al. (2001). Oncology Nursing Society workforce survey part I: Perception of the nursing workforce environment and adequacy of nurse staffing in outpatient and inpatient oncology settings. *Oncology Nursing Forum 28*(10), 1545-1552.

Lyman, G., & Kuderer, N. (1998). The diagnosis of cancer in the elderly: Cost-effectiveness considerations. In L. Balducci & W. Ersler (Eds.). *Comprehensive geriatric oncology*. Netherlands: Harwood Academic, pp. 533-543.

McClure, M., & Hinshaw, A. (Eds.). (2002). *Magnet hospitals revisited: Attraction and retention of professional nurses*. Washington, DC: American Nurses Publishing.

MCOL. (2003). Managed care fact sheet. Retrieved September 30, 2003 from the World Wide Web, Medicare HMO website: http://www.mcareol.com.

Mee, C., & Robinson, E. (2003). What's different about this nursing shortage? *Nursing 2003 33*(1), 51-55.

National Coalition for Cancer Research. (2001). *The NCCRF fact sheet: Cancer research makes sense*. Washington, DC: Author. National Coalition for Cancer Survivorship (NCCS). (2002). Imperatives for quality cancer care: Access, advocacy, action, and accountability. www.cansearch.org/policy/imperativesprin.html.

Needham, J., Buerhaus, P., Mattke, S., et al. (2002). Nurse staffing and quality of care in hospitals in the United States. *Policy, Politics, & Nursing Practice 3*(4), 306-308.

Oncology Nursing Society (ONS). (2002a). *The impact of the national nursing shortage on quality cancer care*. Pittsburgh: Author.

Oncology Nursing Society (ONS). (2002b). *Patients' bill of rights for quality cancer care*. Pittsburgh: Author.

Oncology Nursing Society (ONS). (2002c). *Quality cancer care*. Pittsburgh: Author.

Oncology Nursing Society (ONS). (2003a). *Average wholesale price (AWP) & oncology nursing practice expenses issue brief*. Pittsburgh: Author.

Oncology Nursing Society (ONS). (2003b). *Cancer research and cancer clinical trials*. Pittsburgh: Author.

Oncology Nursing Society (ONS). (2003c). *Ensuring high-quality cancer care in the Medicare program*. Pittsburgh: Author.

Payne, S., Coyne, P., & Smith, T. (2002). The health economics of palliative care. *Oncology 16*(6), 801-808, 811-812.

Pearce, S., Kelly, D., & Stevens, W. (2001). "More than just money"—widening the understanding of the costs involved in cancer care. *Journal of Advanced Nursing 33*(3), 371-379.

Pfoultz, S.K. , Price, S.A. , & Chang, C.F. (2002). Health economics. In D. Mason, J. Leavitt, & M. Chafee (Eds.). *Policy & politics in nursing and health care*. St. Louis: W.B. Saunders, pp. 229-240.

Pulcini, J.A., Neary, S.R., & Maloney, D.F. (2002). Health care financing. In D. Mason, J. Leavitt, & M. Chafee (Eds.). *Policy & politics in nursing and health care*. St. Louis: W.B. Saunders, pp. 241-264.

Ruetter, L., & Duncan, S. (2002). Preparing nurses to promote health-enhancing public policies. *Policy, Politics, & Nursing Practice 3*(4), 294-305.

Scanlon, C. (2001). Public policy and end-of-life care. In B. Ferrell & N. Coyle (Eds.). *Textbook of palliative nursing*. New York: Oxford University, pp. 682-689.

U.S. Bureau of the Census. (1989). *Projections of the population of the United States by age, sex, and race: 1988-2080*. Washington, DC: U.S. Bureau of the Census, Current Population Reports, Series P-25, #1018.

U.S. Department of Health & Human Services, Health Resources & Services Administration (HRSA). (2000). *The registered nurse report: Findings from the national sample survey of registered nurses*. Washington, DC: U.S. Department of Health & Human Services, Health Resources & Services Administration (HRSA), Bureau of Health Professions, Division of Nursing.

Woolhandler, S., Campbell, T., & Himmelstein, D. (2003). Costs of health care administration in the United States and Canada. *New England Journal of Medicine 349*(8), 768-775.

49 Professional Issues in Cancer Care

DIANNE N. ISHIDA

PROFESSIONAL DEVELOPMENT

I. Related professional standards.
   A. *Statement on the Scope and Standards of Oncology Nursing Practice* of the Oncology Nursing Society (ONS) (Brant & Wickham, 2004).
      1. Education—the oncology nurse acquires and maintains current knowledge in oncology nursing practice.
      2. Collegiality—the oncology nurse contributes to the professional development of peers, colleagues, and others.
   B. ONS's *Standards of Oncology Nursing Education: Generalist and Advanced Practice Levels* (Jacobs, 2002).
      1. Oncology nurse generalist.
         a. Assumes responsibility for personal professional development.
         b. Contributes to the professional growth of others.
      2. Advanced practice oncology nurse.
         a. Assumes responsibility for personal professional development.
         b. Contributes to the development of nursing theory, research, and practice.
         c. Disseminates nursing knowledge.
   C. Joint Commission on Accreditation of Healthcare Organizations (JCAHO) (JCAHO, 2004a, p. CX-29).
      1. All members of the nursing staff are competent to fulfill their assigned responsibilities.
      2. Each member of the nursing staff is assigned clinical and/or managerial responsibilities based on educational preparation, applicable licensing laws and regulations, and assessment of current competence.
      3. Nursing staff members participate in orientation and ongoing education to improve competence.
II. Professional development strategies (Dadich & Yoder-Wise, 2003).
   A. Identification of professional development needs and maintaining competence and versatility by continued learning.
      1. Conducts self-assessment of own learning needs and how and when to change behavior or position.
      2. Determines priorities, establishes goals, and determines a career development plan.
      3. Assesses personal resources while maintaining awareness of own beliefs, values, and biases.
      4. Learns from own experiences by self-reflection and seeks out resources to fill in the gaps.
      5. Discusses with colleagues critical incidents to enhance clinical decision making and level of performance.

6. Initiates independent learning activities (e.g., reading professional literature, participating in professional organizations, identifying resource staff, participating in professional support groups, joining clubs and study groups, using self-directed learning modules).
7. Participates in continuing education activities.
8. Seeks experiences to maintain and develop new clinical skills, including through formal education.
9. Selects an employment setting or position in which one can make the greatest contribution.

B. Professional certification—oncology certified nurse at the basic level (OCN), advanced oncology certified nurse (advanced practice level) (AOCN, AOCNP, AOCNS), and certified pediatric oncology nurse (CPON) (Oncology Nursing Certification Corporation [ONCC], 2004).
   1. Recognizes and promotes oncology nursing as an important specialty and gives certification to those with specialized knowledge in the field who have met minimum competency standards.
   2. Enables a profession to define and articulate for its members the new knowledge required for practice.
   3. Recertification enables a profession to validate the competency changes over time as knowledge and technology change.

C. Graduate education.
   1. Formalized university/college education to increase professional skills and depth of knowledge and skills.
   2. Formalized university/college education to redirect career path or fulfill career development plan.

III. Outcomes of professional development.
   A. Enhances the profession.
   B. Enhances the individual's professional growth, career development, and career enjoyment.
   C. Benefits the recipients of care.

MULTIDISCIPLINARY COLLABORATION

I. Related professional standards.
   A. *ONS Statement on the Scope and Standards of Oncology Nursing Practice* (Brant & Wickham, 2004). Collaboration involves the following:
      1. The oncology nurse partners with the client, significant others, interdisciplinary cancer care team, and community resources in providing client care.
         a. Rationale: the complexity of oncology care requires coordinated, ongoing interaction among the client, significant others, the interdisciplinary cancer care team, and community. Through the collaborative process, health care providers use their diverse abilities to assess, plan, implement, and evaluate oncology care.
      2. The oncology nurse collaborates with the client, significant others, and interdisciplinary cancer care team to formulate desired outcomes of care, the treatment plan, an evaluation of quality of care, and other decisions related to client care.
      3. The oncology nurse consults with other health care providers and makes appropriate referrals, including provisions for continuity of care, such as homecare, hospice, rehabilitation, palliative care, and community-based support groups to enhance the client's cancer experience.

       4. The oncology nurse collaborates with other health care providers in educational programs, consultation, management, and research endeavors as opportunities arise.

  B. ONS's *Standards of Oncology Nursing Education: Generalist and Advanced Practice Levels* (Jacobs, 2002).

    1. Oncology nurse generalist.

      a. Collaborates with the multidisciplinary team to assess, plan, implement, and evaluate across all levels of health care need.

    2. Advanced practice oncology nurse.

      a. Initiates collaboration with individuals and groups to minimize cancer risks and to promote health.

  C. JCAHO (JCAHO, 2004a, p. PC-4).

    1. Care, treatment, and services are provided in an interdisciplinary, collaborative manner.

  D. *Nursing, a Social Policy Statement* (ANA, 2003).

    1. Collaboration among health care professionals involves recognition of the expertise of others within and outside of one's (nursing) profession and referral to those providers when appropriate.

    2. Collaboration also involves some shared functions and a common focus on the same overall mission.

  E. *Code of Ethics for Nurses with Interpretive Statements* (ANA, 2001).

    1. The nurse collaborates with other health professionals and the public in promoting community, national, and international efforts to meet health needs.

II. Barriers to the development of collaborative relationships.

  A. Lack of identification with one's own profession.

  B. Tendency to regard professional expertise as bias.

  C. Discomfort with responsibility.

  D. Felt discrimination in relationships.

  E. Failure of others to value one's profession.

  F. Competency inconsistencies within one's profession with lack of uniform preparation.

  G. Lack of clearly defined, distinct domain of influence.

  H. Lack of understanding for another's perception.

  I. Overlapping and changing domains of practice that produce competition.

  J. Perceived threats to autonomy.

  K. Lack of administrative support for collaborative relationships.

  L. Lack of recognition for knowledge and expertise.

  M. Role confusion (role extension versus role expansion) within or among professions.

III. Opportunities for collaboration.

  A. Potential for collaboration among health care providers/agencies exists wherever and with whomever the client and family have contact.

    1. Although emphasis is often placed on physician-nurse collaboration, nurses have the potential for collaborative relationships with any member of the multidisciplinary health care team.

  B. Nurse-to-nurse collaboration may be influenced by the following:

    1. Role—clinician, educator, researcher, administrator. Examples include the following:

      a. Clinician-researcher collaboration in the identification of a clinical problem and evaluation of applicable research findings to address the problem.

       b. Educator-administrator-clinician collaboration in the development, implementation, and evaluation of staff graduate orientation.

       c. Clinician-administrator-researcher collaboration in the development and testing of a client acuity classification system.

  2. Domain of responsibility, such as shift and performance standards. Examples include the following:

       a. Day, evening, and night shift nurses collaborate on developing change-of-shift report guidelines.

       b. Primary nurse and associate nurse collaborate on the nursing process.

  3. Specialization, such as collaboration among nurses with different specialties.

  4. Subspecialization, such as collaboration among nurses with a subspecialty (e.g., medical oncology, surgical oncology, radiation oncology, biotherapy) in the development of educational cancer care materials for clients and families.

  5. Practice settings including acute care, outpatient, home care and hospice, ambulatory cancer treatment center, community hospital, rural community.

       a. For example, collaboration among nurses from a variety of practice settings to develop a chronic pain protocol.

C. Collaborative relationships may extend beyond direct care health care providers to members of voluntary agencies and organizations, including collaborating with clients in the development and implementation of client and family support groups.

D. Future of oncology nursing depends on critical collaborative partnerships being formed within clinical practice arenas as well as partnerships with other organizations.

IV. Benefits of collaborative relationships.

  A. Maximize and utilize the unique skills of each professional.

  B. Shared responsibility.

  C. Delineate shared and individual responsibilities and accountability.

  D. Expedite planned action.

  E. Enhance communication.

  F. Create and modify norms.

  G. Facilitate role clarification by revealing the uniqueness of each professional domain.

  H. Benefit recipients of service.

QUALITY IMPROVEMENT

I. Related professional standards.

  A. ONS's *Statement on the Scope and Standards of Oncology Nursing Practice,* (Brant & Wickham, 2004). Quality of care involves the following:

  1. The oncology nurse systematically evaluates the quality of care and effectiveness of oncology nursing practice (Brant & Wickham, 2004).

       a. Rationale: the complex and dynamic nature of the health care environment and the increasing body of oncology nursing knowledge and research provide both the impetus and the means for the oncology nurse to be competent in clinical practice, to continue professional development, to maintain competency in clinical practice, and to improve the quality of client care.

       b. Continuing peer review, interdisciplinary program evaluation, management, nursing quality assurance programs, and nursing research are used in this endeavor.

  B. *Nursing, a Social Policy Statement* (ANA, 1995).

     1. Each nurse remains accountable for the quality of her/his practice within the full scope of nursing practice.

     2. Nursing practice demands professional intention and commitment carried out in accordance with the ANA's *Standards of Nursing Practice* and its ethical code.

     3. All nurses are ethically and legally accountable for actions taken in the course of nursing practice as well as for actions delegated by the nurse to others assisting in the delivery of nursing care. Such accountability may be accomplished through the regulatory mechanisms of licensure, through criminal and civil laws, through the code of ethics of the profession, and through peer evaluation.

  C. ANA's *Code of Ethics for Nurses with Interpretive Statements* (ANA, 2001), addressing quality, states the following:

     1. The nurse's primary commitment is to the client, whether an individual, family, group, or community.

     2. The nurse promotes, advocates for, and strives to protect the health, safety, and rights of the client.

     3. The nurse is responsible and accountable for individual nursing practice and determines the appropriate delegation of tasks consistent with the nurse's obligation to provide optimum client care.

     4. The nurse owes the same duties to self as to others, including the responsibility to preserve integrity and safety, to maintain competence, and to continue personal and professional growth.

     5. The nurse participates in establishing, maintaining, and improving health care environments and conditions of employment conducive to the provision of quality health care and consistent with the values of the profession through individual and collective action.

  D. JCAHO.

     1. Requires hospitals to implement an effective, ongoing program to measure, assess, and improve the quality of nursing care, treatment, and services delivered to clients (JCAHO, 2004a, p. CX-51).

     2. Requires, as of January 1, 2004, all health care organizations surveyed to implement the 2004 National Patient Safety Goals in six areas, including the following that especially relate to oncology nursing (JCAHO, 2004b):

       a. Improve the effectiveness of communication among caregivers—standardized abbreviations, acronyms, and symbols used throughout organization (caution with use of abbreviation of drugs and protocols).

       b. Improve the safety of using high-alert medications—standardize and limit the number of drug concentrations available in the organization.

       c. Improve the safety of using infusion pumps—to ensure free flow protection on intravenous infusion pumps (e.g., chemotherapeutic drugs on infusion pumps).

       d. Reduce the risk of health care–acquired infections—oncology nurses care for immunosuppressed clients.

II. General statements about quality improvement.

  A. Society gives professional bodies the privilege to govern their concerns, empowering professions to manage their own functions; in return, professionals are accountable to society for their actions.

B. Self-regulation to ensure quality in performance and products is a hallmark of a profession.

C. Nurses have a professional responsibility to ensure quality control and improvement.

D. Nursing has the right and professional responsibility to define and control its own practice.

E. Professional and practice standards may be found in the following:
1. State nurse practice acts.
2. Published standards of professional organizations, such as the following:
   a. ANA's *Standards of Nursing Practice.*
   b. ONS's *Statement on the Scope and Standards of Oncology Nursing Practice.*
   c. ONS's *Standards of Oncology Nursing Education: Generalist and Advanced Practice Levels.*
   d. ONS's *Standards of Oncology Education: Patient/Significant Other and Public.*
   e. ONS's *Standards of Advanced Practice in Oncology Nursing.*
3. Agency guidelines and regulations (e.g., JCAHO, Social Security Administration).
4. Hospital or agency policy and procedure manuals.
5. Job description and performance evaluation criteria.
6. Professional organizations' publications (ANA's *Nursing: A Social Policy Statement;* ANA's *A Code of Ethics for Nurses with Interpretive Statements*).
7. Professional literature.

F. Professional continuous quality improvement strategies include the following:
1. Mandatory licensure.
2. Peer review—professional nurses evaluate the quality of care provided by other professional nurses in accordance with established standards.
3. Development and implementation of quality improvement programs.
4. Professional certification and educational credentialing.
5. Certification of education programs and continuing education programs.
6. Risk management.
7. Investigate what benchmark institutions are doing.

G. Concepts in continuous quality improvement process (Katz & Green, 1997).
1. Everyone in the organization needs to be committed to improving himself/herself and being quality conscious.
2. Quality standards or indicators should be data driven—for example, evidence-based practice.
   a. National Guideline Clearing House—developed by the Agency for Health Care Policy and Research (AHCPR) in partnership with the American Medical Association and the American Association of Health Plans has an Internet repository for evidence-based clinical practice guidelines (http://www.ahrq.gov).
3. Quality can be measured and defined.
4. Quality improvement is attaining a new higher level of performance than previously.
5. Quality should be achieved with the least cost while maintaining standards.
6. Quality increases the desired outcomes while minimizing the undesired outcomes.
7. Know your customers (internal as well as external customers).

8. Measure critical processes of the agency or unit, which can be based on the following criteria:
   a. High volume—50% or more with the same diagnosis, problem, concern.
   b. High cost—for example, uncovered services.
   c. Problem prone—for example, immunosuppressed clients.
   d. High risk—if performed or omitted leads to trauma, death, complications, litigation.
III. Institute of Medicine (IOM) of the National Academies has a concerted, ongoing effort to assess and improve the nation's quality of health care.
   A. IOM's definition of quality is the degree to which health services for individuals and populations increase the likelihood of desired outcomes and are consistent with current professional knowledge (IOM, 2003).
   B. IOM's committee on the quality of health care in America calls for fundamental changes to redesign the American health care system in order to close the quality gap.
   C. Included are the following 10 new rules to guide client relationships as performance expectations (Institute of Medicine, 2001, p. 3):
      1. Care is based on continuous healing relationships.
      2. Care is customized according to client's needs and values.
      3. Client is the source of control.
      4. Knowledge is shared, and information flows freely.
      5. Decision making is evidence based.
      6. Safety is a system property.
      7. Transparency is necessary, and information is available to clients and families to make informed decisions.
      8. Needs are anticipated.
      9. Waste is continuously decreased.
      10. Cooperation among clinicians is a priority.
IV. Nurse practice acts.
   A. The state law that governs the practice of nursing.
   B. Board of nursing (BON) is the administrative agency that implements the statutes, with power granted by the state legislature.
   C. Basic components of nurse practice acts include the following:
      1. Scope of practice of professional nursing.
      2. Requirements for licensure.
      3. Provision for endorsements or sanctioning of persons licensed in another state.
      4. Specifications of exemptions from licensure.
      5. Grounds for disciplinary actions, which may include the following:
         a. Improper procurement of a license.
         b. Conviction for a felony.
         c. Physical or mental incapacity.
         d. Unprofessional conduct.
         e. Incompetence, negligence, and malpractice.
         f. Substance abuse.
      6. Penalties for practicing without a license or substance abuse.
      7. Provisions for the board of nursing with an outline of their responsibilities.
V. Certification.
   A. Process by which a nongovernmental agency or association certifies that an individual licensed to practice in a profession has met certain predetermined standards specified by that profession for specialty practice.

    B. Its application to nursing means that a nurse has achieved competence in a field of specialty within the profession.

    C. Enables a profession to define and articulate for its members the new knowledge required to practice.

    D. Purposes include protection of the public and recognition of an expert practitioner.

CLIENT ADVOCACY

  I. Related professional standards/values.

    A. *Code of Ethics for Nurses with Interpretive Statements* (ANA, 2001).

      1. The nurse promotes, advocates for, and strives to protect the health, safety, and rights of the client.

    B. ONS's Core Values, (ONS).

      1. Advocate on behalf of people with cancer to ensure quality of life and their access to exemplary care throughout the continuum of care.

      2. Advocate for the nursing profession and oncology specialty to ensure respect and recognition, access to education, safe working environments, and fair reimbursement.

      3. Advocate for public policy, particularly in matters of health.

  II. Advocacy.

    A. The term *advocacy* denotes a variety of nursing roles, each derived from a specific set of beliefs and values.

    B. *Advocate* used to represent several related and occasionally opposing ethical perspectives.

      1. Beneficence—the principle of doing good.

      2. Nonmaleficence—the principle of doing no harm.

      3. Utilitarianism—an ethical doctrine in which actions are focused on accomplishing the greatest good for the greatest number of people.

    C. Types of advocacy.

      1. Simplistic advocacy—one who pleads the cause of another.

      2. Paternalistic advocacy—doing something for or to another without that person's consent and on the premise that it serves the person's own good.

      3. Consumer advocacy—nurse is required to provide the client with information to make a decision

      4. Consumer-centric advocacy—nurse provides information and then supports clients in their decision.

      5. Existential advocacy and human advocacy—the nurse's active participation with the client in determining the unique meaning that the experience of health, illness, suffering, or dying is for that individual.

      6. Human advocacy—when the whole nurse nurses, the whole person can be nursed; nurse discloses own views to the client (Hewitt, 2002).

    D. Advocacy is not without risk as issues of power and accountability need to be considered (Hewitt, 2002). Areas oncology nurses frequently deal with, including pain management, end-of-life care, and ethical decision making, have risks.

      1. Nurses may lack autonomy to take moral actions.

      2. Conflicting demands of different clients may create ethical conflicts.

      3. Independent action may be restricted by conflicting accountability to public, employer, and clients.

III. Avenues to be advocates.
- **A.** Within one's own work setting.
  1. By listening and speaking out for the needs expressed by clients and their families, thereby empowering clients and their families.
  2. By keeping abreast of current knowledge and sources of information on clinical trials, newly available evidence-based treatments, health legislation that affects practice and health care delivery, hospice and other resources that can benefit clients and families under their care.
- **B.** Within one's own community.
  1. By volunteering or practicing in minority, underserved, medically disadvantaged, or vulnerable populations to decrease health disparities in cancer and other areas that affect health and well-being (Centers for Disease Control and Prevention [CDC], 2003).
  2. By becoming active politically to ensure legislation protects the health of his/her community.
- **C.** Within professional organizations.
  1. By becoming actively involved in organizational legislative committees advocating for nurses, cancer care, and clients.
  2. By utilizing avenues available to ONS, ANA, and other professional organizations to provide testimony or letters to state legislators and/or congressional representatives to support health care and health care initiatives and reform.

IV. Important and useful Internet resources include the following:
- **A.** Oncology Nursing Society: http://www.ons.org.
- **B.** American Nurses Association: http://www.ana.org.
- **C.** Institute of Medicine: http://www.iom.edu.
- **D.** Joint Commission on Accreditation of Healthcare Organizations: http://www.jcaho.org.

REFERENCES

American Nurses Association (ANA). (2001). *Code of ethics for nurses with interpretive statements.* Washington, DC: ANA Publications.

American Nurses Association (ANA). (2003). *Nursing, a social policy statement,* ed 2, Washington DC, ANA Publications.

Brant, J.M., & Wickham, R.S. (Eds.). (2004). *Statement on the scope and standards of oncology nursing practice.* Pittsburgh: Oncology Nursing Society.

Centers for Disease Control and Prevention (CDC). Office of Minority Health. (2003). Retrieved October 29, 2003 from the World Wide Web: http://www.cdc.gov/omh/AMH.factsheets/cancer.htm.

Dadich, K.A., & Yoder-Wise, P.S. (2003). Career management: Putting yourself in charge. In P.S. Yoder-Wise (Ed.). *Leading and managing in nursing* (3rd ed.). St. Louis: Mosby, pp. 449-467.

Hewitt, J. (2002). A critical review of the arguments debating the role of the nurse advocate. *Journal of Advanced Nursing 38*(5), 439-445.

Institute of Medicine (IOM). (2003). Crossing the quality chasm: The IOM health care quality initiative. Retrieved December 4, 2003 from the World Wide Web: http://www.iom.edu/report.asp?id=5432.

Institute of Medicine (IOM). (2001). *Crossing the quality chasm: A new health system for the 21st century.* Washington, DC: National Academy Press.

Jacobs, L.A. (Ed.). (2002). *Statement on the scope and standards of advanced practice nursing in oncology* (3rd ed.). Pittsburgh: Oncology Nursing Society.

Joint Commission on Accreditation of Healthcare Organizations (JCAHO). (2004a). *Comprehensive accreditation manual for hospitals: The official handbook.* Oakbrook Terrace, IL: Joint Commission Resources.

Joint Commission on Accreditation of Healthcare Organizations (JCAHO). (2004b). 2004 National patient safety goals. Retrieved March 23, 2004 from the World Wide Web: http://www.jcaho.org/accredited+organization/patient+safety/04=npsg/index.htm.

Katz, J.M., & Green, E. (1997). *Managing quality: A guide to system-wide performance management in health care* (2nd ed.). St. Louis: Mosby.

Oncology Nursing Society Certification Corporation (ONCC). Retrieved March 23, 2004 from the World Wide Web: http://www.oncc.org/?v2_group=08g=13408p=11433.

Oncology Nursing Society. ONS vision, mission, and core values. Retrieved November 26, 2004 from http://www.ons.org/about/corevalues.shtml.

Index

Page numbers with "t" denote tables; those with "f" denote figures; and those with "b" denote boxes